Psychotherapy for the Advanced Practice Psychiatric Nurse

Kathleen Wheeler, PhD, PMHNP-BC, APRN, FAAN, is an advanced practice psychiatric nurse and a professor and director of the Psychiatric-Mental Health Nurse Practitioner (PMHNP) program at Fairfield University Egan School of Nursing and Health Studies in Fairfield, Connecticut. She developed this program in 1994 and it was one of the first PMHNP programs in the United States. Dr. Wheeler has been a leader in projects that are highly significant for psychiatric nursing. These include cochair of the National Panel that developed the first PMHNP Competencies and the first chair of National Organization of Nurse Practitioner Faculties' (NONPF) PMHNP special interest group. Both editions of her book, *Psychotherapy for the Advanced Practice Psychiatric Nurse: A How-To Guide for Evidence-Based Practice,* have been awarded AJN Book of the Year Awards. This book has been widely adopted by graduate PMHNP programs in the United States. Her leadership extends beyond psychiatric nursing as past president and advisory director of the Eye Movement Desensitization and Reprocessing International Association (EMDRIA) and in the development of an Integrative Trauma Psychotherapy Certificate Program for licensed mental health professionals at her university. Her awards include induction as a Fellow in the American Academy of Nursing (FAAN); the American Psychiatric Nurses Association (APNA) Media Award; the APNA Excellence in Practice Award; the APNA Excellence in Education Award; the EMDRIA Award for Outstanding Contributions and Service; and Distinguished Alumni of Cornell University-New York Hospital School of Nursing. Dr. Wheeler is a psychoanalyst and an EMDR Trainer and Consultant with expertise in treating trauma. Recently she chaired the Expert Panel that developed Trauma and Resilience Competencies for Nursing Education, which are now copyrighted and available online (https://www.acesconnection.com/blog/trauma-and-resilience-competencies-for-nursing-education). The Delphi survey supporting this work is published in the *Journal of the American Psychiatric Nurses Association.* Dr. Wheeler is on the Editorial Board of that journal as well as on the Editorial Board of *EMDR Journal of Practice and Research.*

Psychotherapy for the Advanced Practice Psychiatric Nurse

A How-To Guide for Evidence-Based Practice

Third Edition

Kathleen Wheeler, PhD, PMHNP-BC, APRN, FAAN

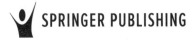
SPRINGER PUBLISHING

Springer Publishing Company, LLC
11 West 42nd Street, New York, NY 10036
www.springerpub.com
connect.springerpub.com/

Acquisitions Editor: Adrianne Brigido
Compositor: diacriTech

ISBN: 978-0-8261-9379-7
ebook ISBN: 978-0-8261-9389-6

Qualified instructors may request supplements by emailing textbook@springerpub.com
An Editable Appendices supplement is available at connect.springerpub.com/content/book/978-0-8261-9389-6

Instructor's Manual ISBN: 978-0-8261-9482-4
Instructor's PowerPoints ISBN: 978-0-8261-9481-7
DOI: 10.1891/9780826193896

20 21 22 23 24 / 5 4 3 2 1

Library of Congress Control Number: 2020910057

Contact us to receive discount rates on bulk purchases.
We can also customize our books to meet your needs.
For more information please contact: sales@springerpub.com

Kathleen Wheeler: https://orcid.org/0000-0003-0971-3763
Publisher's Note: New and used products purchased from third-party sellers are not guaranteed for quality, authenticity, or access to any included digital components.

Printed in the United States of America.

In memory of my parents, Sidney and Elizabeth Wheeler,
and my sister Betsy Wheeler

Contents

Contributors   ix
Foreword Michael J. Rice, PhD, APRN, FAAN, WAN   xi
Preface   xiii
Acknowledgments   xvii

PART I. GETTING STARTED

1. The Nurse Psychotherapist and a Framework for Practice   *3*
   Kathleen Wheeler

2. The Neurophysiology of Trauma and Psychotherapy   *57*
   Kathleen Wheeler

3. Assessment and Diagnosis   *105*
   Pamela Bjorklund

4. The Initial Contact and Maintaining the Frame   *185*
   Kathleen Wheeler with Michael J. Rice

PART II. PSYCHOTHERAPY APPROACHES

5. Supportive and Psychodynamic Psychotherapy   *249*
   Kathleen Wheeler

6. Humanistic–Existential and Solution-Focused Approaches
   to Psychotherapy   *289*
   Candice Knight

7. Eye Movement Desensitization and Reprocessing Therapy   *329*
   Kathleen Wheeler

8. Cognitive Behavior Therapy   *359*
   Sharon M. Freeman Clevenger

9. Motivational Interviewing   *401*
   Susie Adams and Edna Hamera

10. Interpersonal Psychotherapy   *419*
    Kathleen Wheeler and Marie Crowe

11. Trauma Resiliency Model® Therapy   *441*
    Linda Grabbe

12. Group Therapy   *469*
    Richard Pessagno

13. Family Therapy   *495*
    Candice Knight

PART III. INTEGRATING MEDICATION AND COMPLEMENTARY MODALITIES INTO PSYCHOTHERAPY

14. Psychotherapeutics: Reuniting Psychotherapy and Pharmacotherapy   *541*
    Barbara J. Limandri and Mary D. Moller

15. Trauma-Informed Medication Management   *569*
    Kathryn Kieran

16. Integrative Medicine and Psychotherapy   *601*
    Sharon M. Freeman Clevenger

PART IV. PSYCHOTHERAPY WITH SPECIAL POPULATIONS

17. Stabilization for Trauma and Dissociation   *643*
    Kathleen Wheeler

18. Dialectical Behavior Therapy for Complex Trauma   *689*
    Barbara J. Limandri

19. Psychotherapeutic Approaches for Addictions and Related Disorders   *711*
    Susie Adams

20. Psychotherapy With Children   *749*
    Kathleen R. Delaney, Janiece DeSocio, and Julie A. Carbray

21. Psychotherapeutic Approaches With Children and Adolescents   *779*
    Pamela Lusk and Anka Roberto

22. Psychotherapy With Older Adults   *823*
    Georgia L. Stevens, Merrie J. Kaas, and Kristin Linda Hjartardottir

PART V. TERMINATION AND REIMBURSEMENT

23. Reimbursement and Documentation   *869*
    Mary D. Moller

24. Termination and Outcome Evaluation   *907*
    Kathleen Wheeler and Danielle M. Conklin

Afterword   *933*
Index   *935*

Contributors

Susie Adams, PhD, RN, PMHNP, FAANP, FAAN Professor of Nursing and Faculty Scholar for Community Engaged Behavioral Health, Vanderbilt University School of Nursing, Nashville, Tennessee

Pamela Bjorklund, PhD, CS, PMHNP-BC, RN Professor, Department of Graduate Nursing, The College of St. Scholastica, Duluth, Minnesota

Julie A. Carbray, PhD, PMHNP-BC, PMHCNS-BC, APN Clinical Professor of Psychiatry and Nursing, Department of Psychiatry, University of Illinois at Chicago, Administrative Director, Pediatric Mood Disorder Clinic at University of Illinois Health, Chicago, Illinois

Sharon M. Freeman Clevenger, MSN, MA, CARN-AP, PMHCNS-BC Psychiatric Mental Health Clinical Nurse Specialist Nurse Practitioner, CEO, Indiana Center for Cognitive Behavior Therapy, P.C., Cognitive Psychotherapy and Integrative Medicine Psychiatric Practitioner, Adjunct Professor, Indiana/Purdue Universities, Fort Wayne, Indiana

Danielle M. Conklin, DNP, NP-P, PMHNP-BC Clinical Assistant Professor, Psychiatric-Mental Health Nurse Practitioner Program, Nurse Practitioner of Psychiatry, New York University Rory Meyers College of Nursing, New York, New York University

Marie Crowe, RN PhD Department of Psychological Medicine, University of Otago, Christchurch, New Zealand

Kathleen R. Delaney, PhD, PMHNP-BC, APRN, FAAN Rush College of Nursing, Chicago, Illinois

Janiece DeSocio, PhD, RN, PMHNP-BC, FAAN Professor, Sauvage Endowed Professor of Nursing, Psychiatric Mental Health Nurse Practitioner Track Lead, Psych Projects, Seattle University, Seattle, Washington

Linda Grabbe, PhD, FNP-BC, PMHNP-BC Clinical Assistant Professor, Nell Hodgson Woodruff School of Nursing, Emory University, Atlanta, Georgia

Edna Hamera, PhD, PMHCNS-BC, APRN Associate Professor (retired), University of Kansas School of Nursing, Kansas City, Kansas

Kristin Linda Hjartardottir, DNP, APRN   Allina Health, Abbott Northwestern Hospital, Minneapolis, Minnesota

Merrie J. Kaas, PhD, APRN, PMHCNS-BC, FAAN   Professor, Specialty Coordinator, Psychiatric Mental Health Nurse Practitioner Program, University of Minnesota School of Nursing, Minneapolis, Minnesota

Kathryn Kieran, MSN, PMHNP   Director of Nursing Operations at Hill Center, Hill Center for Women at McLean, Medford, Massachusetts

Candice Knight, PhD, EdD, APN, PMHCNS-BC, PMHNP-BC   Clinical Associate Professor, Program Director, Psychiatric-Mental Health Nurse Practitioner Program, Licensed Clinical Psychologist and Psychiatric Nurse Practitioner, New York, New York

Barbara J. Limandri, PhD, APRN, BC   Professor Emerita, Linfield College School of Nursing, Portland, Oregon

Pamela Lusk, DNP, RN, PMHNP-BC, FAANP   Clinical Associate Professor, University of Arizona College of Nursing, Tucson, Arizona

Mary D. Moller, DNP, ARNP, PMHCNS-BC, CPRP, FAAN   Associate Professor, Coordinator, PMH-DNP Program, Pacific Lutheran University School of Nursing, Tacoma, Washington

Richard Pessagno, DNP, PMHNP-BC, CGP, FAANP   Private Practice, Wimington, Delaware, Associate Professor, Psychiatric-Mental Health Program Coordinator, Catherine McAuley School of Nursing, Maryville University, St. Louis, Missouri

Michael J. Rice, PhD, APRN, FAAN, WAN   Endowed Chair of Psychiatric Nursing and Professor, College of Nursing, Anschutz Medical Center, University of Colorado

Anka Roberto, MPH, DNP, PMHNP-BC, APRN   Assistant Professor, School of Nursing, University of North Carolina Wilmington, Wilmington, North Carolina

Georgia L. Stevens, PhD, APRN, PMHCNS-BC   P.A.L. Associates: Partners in Aging and Long-Term Caregiving, Medication Management, Therapy and Consultation, Washington, DC

Kathleen Wheeler, PhD, PMHNP-BC, APRN, FAAN   Director of Psychiatric Mental Health Nurse Practitioner Program, Professor, Egan School of Nursing and Health Studies, Fairfield University, Fairfield, Connecticut

Foreword

Knowledge-driven evidence-based treatment models take time and effort but also must be provided by someone who is knowledgeable about the range of psychiatric mental health problems to be addressed. Dr. Wheeler is among a handful of people in the profession who offer an up-to-date evidence-based text of the knowledge and skills required by advanced practice psychiatric nurses. I am humbled to be asked to write this foreword for Dr. Wheeler's latest edition of *Psychotherapy for the Advanced Practice Psychiatric Nurse*.

Dr. Wheeler and I began our relationship as colleagues almost a quarter of a century ago. We first met during a 1994–1995 conference in Baltimore focused on the knowledge base and skills needed by the emerging advanced practice psychiatric nurse role. While many of us left the conference on a vociferous mission to define and shape the profession, Dr. Wheeler quietly designed, refined, and discussed the knowledge and skills needed and continues to influence us all today. The foundation for Dr. Wheeler's vision of advanced practice psychiatric nursing is reflected in the initial National Organization of Nurse Practitioner Faculties (NONPF) Psychiatric-Mental Health Nurse Practitioner (PMHNP) Competencies. Many do not realize that Dr. Wheeler and Dr. Judith Haber of New York University, penned the initial drafts of those competencies.

Dr. Wheeler continues to advocate for knowledge and skills, including "evidence-based" models for advanced practice psychiatric nurses. Then, as now, Dr. Wheeler's message, as in this book, is one of applying the best-known evidence and not DELIMITING skills of advanced practice psychiatric nurses in order to provide the best care for those with the greatest need. The knowledge and skills in this book serve as a foundation for all advanced practice psychiatric nurses. I also believe that faculty and current practitioners can improve the care they provide by using the content outlined in this book.

The foundation for defining the knowledge presented in the book is one of the tenants of the founder of psychiatric nursing, Dr. Hildegard Peplau. Every practicing psychiatric nurse realizes that the most effective outcomes result from developing a relationship with a patient that encourages treatment pathways relative to a patient's life. The content in this book applies Shapiro's adaptive information processing and Porges's polyvagal neurophysiological theories and research to practice. Understanding these theories based on brain-imaging studies, psychotherapy outcomes, and practice guidelines determines which treatment should be selected for a specific clinical problem.

Although the scope of the book may seem a bit overwhelming, the issues faced in clinical practice are consistent with the knowledge and skills addressed in this book. I agree with Dr. Peplau and Dr. Wheeler that relationships are the pathway to health. The road map to identifying and using which elements provide the best evidence-based outcomes are outlined in this book. To become skillful in selecting the right treatment approach requires knowledge, evidence, and skills. A serious practitioner will find those elements within the pages compiled by Dr. Wheeler in this impressive book. I highly recommend this book as the knowledge and skills foundation for the next generation of advanced practice psychiatric nurses.

Michael J. Rice, PhD, APRN, FAAN, WAN
Endowed Chair of Psychiatric Nursing
and Professor
College of Nursing
Anschutz Medical Center
University of Colorado

Preface

As I finish the 3rd edition of this book, we are living through a most extraordinary moment. COVID19 has emerged as a global crisis unlike anything we have seen in our lifetime. This is most certainly a time of anxiety for everyone, but especially for nurses and other healthcare personnel who are on the frontlines caring for those infected with this deadly virus. There are shortages of personal protective equipment (PPE), medicine, and supplies; psychiatric units converted to COVID units; hospital systems managing existing resources by rationing and triaging care; patients dying and losing loved ones; practice and academic changes. Providers are risking their own lives to care for others, all while worrying about infecting family and friends, facing financial hardship, caring for and educating children at home, and reckoning with social upheaval. Compounding the disturbance are conflicting messages from our government and the politicizing of common sense and health guidelines. Protecting ourselves requires isolation, distancing, and infringement of our freedom to live our lives in ways we previously took for granted. We are bracing ourselves for the tsunami of mental health problems coming our way as a result of the pandemic. It is essential that advanced practice psychiatric nurses (APPNs) care for themselves in order to be of assistance to others. I am hopeful that in some small way this book will be helpful during and after the chaos and crisis we are living through.

The framework for this book is trauma-informed and serves as a compass for building resilience for oneself and for our patients. This framework is based on three basic concepts for practice: resilience, relationship and patient-centered care. When I hear the term "patient-centered," it always seems obvious to me because who else would you be centered on? However, if you think about how the office visit is usually structured these days with data needing to be documented in short sessions…it is very hard to be patient-centered, as the concept implies that you will follow the patient through each visit, rather than setting an agenda and accomplishing predetermined tasks. Letting the session unfold according to the patient's needs is not encouraged or practiced in most settings. Yet this is one of three key principles of trauma-informed treatment, which includes #1: tailoring the therapy to the patient; #2: providing and ensuring safety; and #3: maintaining a positive and consistent therapeutic relationship (Briere & Scott, 2015).

Since the publication of the first edition in 2008 of *Psychotherapy for the Advanced Practice Psychiatric Nurse* significant developments for APPNs include: the Institute of Medicine (IOM) 2010 report on the Future of Nursing advocating removal of scope-of-practice barriers for advanced practice nurses; masters graduate programs transitioning to Doctoral Nursing Practice (DNP) programs; the Consensus Model for APRN Regulation (Licensure, Accreditation, Certification and Education, also known as LACE); revised Psychiatric-Mental Health Nurse Practitioner (PMHNP) Competencies; endorsement of the PMHNP as the one APPN role by American Psychiatric Nurses Association (APNA) and the International Society of Psychiatric Nursing (ISPN); a new

Diagnostic and Statistical Manual (DSM); new Current Procedural Terminology (CPT) codes for reimbursement; the Patient Protection Affordable Care Act; integrated behavioral care; parity of mental health with medical illness; explosion of telemental health; American Nurses Credentialing Center (ANCC) discontinuation of all APPN exams except PMHNP (across the lifespan); an exponential increase in the number of graduate psychiatric nursing programs; and an increasing need and shortage of APPNs, which is reflected in the PMHNP becoming one of the highest paid NP specialties. What do these major developments in healthcare, nursing, and mental health portend for PMHNPs and the practice of psychotherapy?

The PMHNP Competencies developed in 2003 and the adoption of these standards for evaluation by Commission on Collegiate Nursing Education (CCNE) for accreditation mandate that psychotherapy is an essential competency that all PMHNPs must achieve. This has been reaffirmed with the revision of the PMHNP Competencies in 2013. Nurse educators are now challenged to teach these competencies in addition to the essentials that are also required for graduate nursing curricula without increasing the total credit load. Psychotherapy skills must be acquired expeditiously in a short amount of time. Many of the jobs available to APPN graduates are in community mental health centers where 15- to 30-minute medication checks are the norm. APPN graduates are encouraged to negotiate for longer sessions as needed and for a broader role that includes psychiatric evaluations and psychotherapy if they wish, as well as prescribing medication. The marginalization of psychiatrists to the prescriber role should serve as a warning to APPNs who embrace a prescriber-only role without such negotiation. Often, more seasoned APPNs develop their own preferred private practice once confidence is gained.

Changes in this third edition of *Psychotherapy for the Advanced Practice Psychiatric Nurse* include a revised framework for practice based on new theory and research on attachment and neurophysiology. The confluence of new findings provides the science to support what nurses have known all along: the importance of relationship. It has been more than 75 years since Peplau proposed that it is the relationship between the nurse and the patient through which recovery and health are achieved. Relationship-centered care has always been the hallmark of psychiatric nursing. This book expands Peplau's interpersonal paradigm from a two-person model to a more contemporary holistic perspective. Interpersonal neuroscience and attachment research validate the scientific basis of the centrality of this relationship for healing. The overall framework for practice proposed in this book is built upon relationship science, with Shapiro's adaptive information processing and Porges's polyvagal theories providing the neurophysiological explanatory mechanism of action. APPNs who understand these theories can decide what treatment to use for which problem based on research from brain-imaging studies, psychotherapy outcome studies, and practice guidelines.

The nurse psychotherapist needs a context for practice: an overarching framework for when and how to use techniques germane to various evidence-based psychotherapy approaches for the specific client problems encountered in clinical practice. Given the complexity of people, no one-size-fits-all approach is espoused in this book. It is rare for a therapist to adhere to only one model in its pure form; most often the clinically-skilled therapist bases treatment choices on a formulation of the person's problem that takes into account such factors as the developmental history, pattern of relating, behavioral analysis, coping skills, support system, patient preference and learning style. Ethical psychotherapy practice demands no less. If the APPN has a solid theoretical understanding to guide interventions and training in several evidence-based approaches, it is possible to adapt the therapy to the needs of the patient, rather than requiring that the patient adapt to the demands of the therapist's orientation.

The skillful therapist knows how to respond, engage, and accurately assess the problem in order to formulate a treatment plan. A comprehensive and accurate assessment at the beginning of treatment, as well as throughout psychotherapy, serves as a compass to guide treatment. This book strives to assist the beginning therapist in accurate assessment through a comprehensive understanding of development and the application of neuroscience in order to make sense of what is happening for the patient in treatment. The aim is to provide helpful strategies, starting with the first contact through termination. The authors of these chapters have integrated the best evidence-based approaches into a relationship-based framework for APPN psychotherapy practice. This how-to compendium of evidence-based approaches honors our heritage, reaffirms the centrality of relationship for psychiatric advanced practice, and celebrates the excellence, vitality, depth, and breadth of knowledge of our specialty. We are fortunate to have the expertise of the esteemed colleagues who authored the chapters and I am honored and pleased to be able to share and disseminate their clinical wisdom.

In addition to the revised framework for practice in this edition, new chapters include Chapter 11, Chapter 14, Chapter 15, Chapter 16, and Chapter 21, so that there are now two chapters for psychotherapy with children, two chapters for medication management, and two new chapters with a focus on integrative and somatic therapies. These additions reflect the recognition of the job market and the need for mental health providers for children, as well as the burgeoning literature and interest in somatic processes for effective complex trauma therapy.

The contributing authors to this book are all expert APPNs. Throughout, liberal use of examples and case studies provide pragmatic examples for the novice as well as the expert nurse psychotherapist to use as a guide for practice. To aid the readers, Springer Publishing Company offers the appendices as an editable supplement, as well as faculty resources. The authors of the chapters in this edition have generously contributed PowerPoints, assignments, links to videos, and other resources designed to help faculty teach the content in their chapter.

This book, however, will only be as useful as the depth of the APPNs' own acceptance and knowledge of self. Compassion and wisdom cannot be taught in a book. Nurses who are healers understand that they can only accompany the patient on his or her journey if they have begun their own self-healing and that self-healing is a continuous process whereby one continues to develop clarity about one's own strengths and weaknesses. As an early supervisor of mine told our class at the beginning of graduate studies: "Don't walk around in someone's head with muddy boots." Openness and curiosity to self-discovery are essential in order to cultivate self-knowledge. Much of the work of psychotherapy takes place in the shared consciousness of two people and it is in those healing moments of connection that both participants grow. Indeed, the opportunity for personal growth in the transition from nurse to nurse psychotherapist is an exciting, rewarding journey leading toward a lifetime of professional satisfaction.

Kathleen Wheeler

REFERENCE

Briere, J.N., & Scott, C. (2015). *Principles of trauma therapy: A guide to symptoms, evaluation, and treatment* (2nd ed., DSM-5 update). Thousand Oaks, CA: Sage.

Qualified instructors may obtain access to an Instructor's Manual and PowerPoints by emailing textbook@springerpub.com.

An editable appendices supplement is available at http://connect.springerpub.com/content/book/978-0-8261-9389-6

Acknowledgments

I am deeply grateful to the expert clinicians and scholars who contributed chapters to this book. Their expertise is a gift to our current and future graduate students, advanced practice psychiatric nurses, and to our patients. I would like to especially thank Francine Shapiro for the gift of EMDR. Her Adaptive Information Processing model informed the theoretical and practice framework for this book. I continue to be inspired by all that she contributed to our understanding of the treatment of adverse life experiences and trauma. Thank you to my friend and colleague, Elaine Miller-Karas, for her elegant resiliency model that shows us how to clinically apply Porges's theory included in the revised framework for practice in this edition.

Thank you to my colleagues Uri Bergmann, for his careful review of the neurophysiology in Chapter 2; and to Michael Rice, who contributed the Foreword and the section on telepsychiatry in Chapter 4. Others who reviewed and edited selected chapters who I am indebted to include Robbie Adler-Tapia, Lee Combrinct-Graham, Joan Fleitas, Anne Harris, and Jessica Mack. I thank my supervisors, students, and patients who have taught me so much over the years. I am so grateful to those who allowed me to include some of our work together in this book. The assistance, professionalism, guidance, and attention to detail of the entire team at Springer Publishing Company, especially Adrianne Brigido, Publisher, Joanne Jay, Vice President of Production, Kris Parrish, Production Manager, and Cindy Yoo, Managing Editor, are greatly appreciated.

I am also deeply grateful to my family: my mother and father whose enduring presence is always with me; my connections to my brothers and sisters and their families, which sustain me; my husband, Robert Broad, who read every chapter and contributed case examples for Chapters 5 and 7; and my daughter, Elizabeth and her family, and Michael, my son, who are a source of joy and pride.

Getting Started

The Nurse Psychotherapist and a Framework for Practice

Kathleen Wheeler

This chapter begins with the historical context of the nurse's role as psychotherapist and the resources and challenges inherent in nursing for the development of requisite psychotherapy skills. Using a holistic paradigm, the framework for practice presented here is patient-centered and based on resilience and relationship. Mental health and illness are viewed through a cultural lens. The significant role of adverse life experiences in the development, contribution, and maintenance of mental health problems and psychiatric disorders is highlighted. A hierarchy of treatment aims is introduced on which to base interventions using a phase model for psychotherapy. This framework is based on the neurophysiology of adaptive information processing which posits that most mental health problems and symptoms of psychiatric disorders are due to a disturbance or dysregulation in the integration and connection of neural networks that occur in response to adverse life experiences. A case example is presented to illustrate the how to apply the framework proposed for psychotherapy practice.

WHO DOES PSYCHOTHERAPY?

The various disciplines licensed to conduct psychotherapy, depending on their respective state licensing boards, include psychiatrists, psychologists, social workers, marriage and family therapists, counselors, and advanced practice psychiatric nurses (APPNs) (Table 1.1). APPN is used throughout this book to include psychiatric-mental health clinical nurse specialists (PMHCNS) and psychiatric-mental health nurse practitioners (PMHNP). Educational preparation, orientation, and practice settings vary greatly among and within each discipline of practicing psychotherapists. In addition to basic educational requirements unique for that discipline, there are many postgraduate psychotherapy training programs that licensed mental health practitioners may pursue, such as psychoanalytic, family, eye movement desensitization and reprocessing (EMDR) therapy, cognitive behavioral, hypnosis, and others. Each of these training programs offer certification and require a specified amount of training for licensed mental health professionals: approximately 1 year for EMDR therapy (i.e., 40 academic didactic and 10 consultation hours for basic Parts 1 and 2 training; plus, in order to obtain certification an additional 20 consultation hours, 12 continuing educational units, 2 years' experience with a license in mental health practice, and a minimum of 50 sessions with 25 patients); and for psychoanalytic training 4 to 5 years (i.e., 4 years of coursework and supervision, ongoing practice, and one's own experience in psychoanalysis).

Postgraduate training and ongoing supervision are encouraged for APPNs who wish to gain proficiency and deepen their knowledge in a particular modality of psychotherapy.

TABLE 1.1 BASIC EDUCATION, ORIENTATION, AND SETTING OF PSYCHOTHERAPY PRACTITIONERS

Discipline	Education	Orientation/Setting
Psychiatrist	MD (medical doctor) or DO (Doctor of Osteopathy); 3-year psychiatric residency after medical school	Biological treatment, acute care, psychopharmacology and specific psychotherapy competencies for psychiatric MD residents; often inpatient orientation
Psychologist	PhD (research doctorate in psychology) or PsyD (clinical doctorate in psychology); both usually 1-year internship after doctorate	Psychotherapy and psychological testing
Master's level psychologist	MA (Master of Arts) or MS (Master of Science) or MEd (Master of Education)	Psychotherapy: some modalities, psychological testing
Social worker	MSW (Master of Social Work)	Psychotherapy: interpersonal, family, group; community orientation
Marriage and family therapists	MA (Master of Arts)	Systems and family therapy, marriage counseling; community outpatient orientation
Counselor	MA (Master of Arts in counseling) or MEd (Master of Education in counseling)	Counseling, vocational, and educational testing; outpatient orientation
Advanced practice psychiatric nurse (APPN; clinical specialist in psychiatric nursing or psychiatric-mental health nurse practitioner)	MSN (Master of Science in Nursing) or DNP (Doctor of Nursing Practice)	Psychopharmacology and psychotherapy; group and individual, sometimes family

Because it is highly unlikely that any one method will work for all problems for all people, the APPN who has additional skills such as hypnosis, EMDR therapy, family therapy, imagery, or ego state therapy will be more likely to help those who seek help. There are many ways to help the diverse number of patient problems and patients who seek our help, and beware of therapists who believe that "one size fits all"; in other words, if the only tool you have is a hammer, you are likely to treat every problem you encounter as a nail.

In 2002, the American Psychiatric Review Committee mandated that all psychiatric residency programs require competency training in psychodynamic therapy (PDT), cognitive behavioral therapy (CBT), supportive and brief psychotherapies, and psychotherapy combined with psychopharmacology in order to meet accreditation standards (Plakun, Sudak, & Goldberg, 2009). This list was further refined to what is termed the Y Model, with the stem of the Y being the shared elements or common factors in psychotherapy while the arms are PDT and CBT with supportive therapy at the base of the Y (Plakun et al., 2009). Delineation of these competencies is important in that this mandate was a direct response to the increasing emphasis on medication as *the* treatment for psychiatric disorders and reaffirmed the importance of psychotherapy in psychiatric treatment. These core competencies in psychiatrists' education indicate a significant cultural shift that may also herald academic changes for advanced practice psychiatric nursing education.

Many factors in graduate psychiatric nursing education challenge APPNs in attaining competency in psychotherapy. One challenge for nursing education is how to teach the requisite competencies and essentials that are required in graduate nursing curricula without increasing the total credit load. To remain competitive, programs need to offer coursework that can be completed in a reasonable amount of time and with a reasonable number of credits. It is not possible in a short period—usually 2 years for most full-time graduate master's degree nursing programs and 3 years or more for the Doctorate of Nursing Practice (DNP) degree, to attain *proficiency* in psychotherapy, but *competency* must be achieved. Psychotherapy competency was identified as necessary for all psychiatric-mental health nurse practitioner (PMHNP) programs as of 2003 (National Panel for Psychiatric Mental Health NP Competencies, 2003) and reaffirmed with the 2013 revised PMHNP Competencies (2013). With these competencies delineated and endorsed by the Commission on Collegiate Nursing Education (CCNE) for accreditation, all graduate APPN programs seeking CCNE accreditation must teach psychotherapy skills. In addition, to sit for the American Nurses Credentialing Center (ANCC) certification exam as a PMHNP, applicants are required to have clinical training in a minimum of two modalities of psychotherapy (ANCC, 2020).

Another change in nursing education that significantly impacts APPNs is the endorsement of the DNP by leaders in nursing, the NONPF, and the American Association of Colleges of Nursing (AACN). The DNP degree is envisioned as a terminal practice degree and is proposed to supplant the Master of Science in Nursing (MSN) degree for nurse practitioners by 2025 and will include a clinical research focus. Impetus for this shift came from the lack of parity with other healthcare disciplines, the high amount of credits required in current master's curricula, current and projected shortage of faculty, and the increasing complexity of the healthcare system (Dracup, Conenwett, Meleis, & Benner, 2005). Debate continues about whether this terminal practice doctorate will enhance or dilute advanced practice. It is not clear how curricula and program requirements will evolve to provide the needed practice expertise for APPN students. Faculty need current expertise in psychiatric advanced practice to effectively teach, and concerns have been expressed about whether graduate faculty have greater academic experience than practice experience because academia traditionally rewards faculty who publish and do research. Clinical practice and teaching are often overlooked in promotion decisions, and faculty members tend to emphasize research over practice, which may not bode well for APPN faculty expertise in psychotherapy skills.

A survey of APPNs in 2009 revealed that most APPN practice time is spent prescribing, conducting diagnostic assessments, and psychotherapy with medication management but rarely solely conducting individual psychotherapy (Drew & Delaney, 2009). A more recent national survey of 1,624 APPNs reveals that 82% provide education and 71% provide diagnostics, management, and prescribing, while 65% provide some type of psychotherapy, with 15% practicing psychotherapy alone. 65% is a significant increase from the 2009 data (Delaney, Drew, & Rushton, 2019). Perhaps given the current and projected shortage of psychiatrists, the need for APPNs who can provide the full spectrum of mental health services will continue (Burke et al., 2013).

A significant challenge for graduate nursing education is the difficulty of finding preceptors and clinical sites for psychiatric graduate nursing students to practice psychotherapy. Most settings have social workers who conduct psychotherapy while the APPNs most often prescribe. This is a cost-effective approach for the agency or clinic because APPNs usually earn more per hour than social workers, but it does not provide the student nurse psychotherapist with adequate experience to practice psychotherapy. APPN students can sometimes work out an arrangement in which the student can see the preceptor's patients for psychotherapy while the psychiatric APPN preceptor manages the medication, or preceptors from other licensed mental health disciplines who are conducting psychotherapy may be asked to serve as preceptors for a limited number of hours for APPN students. In addition to the liability issues with this arrangement, space constraints, agency policy, or lack of adequate psychotherapy supervision may prohibit the student from seeing an adequate caseload of patients for psychotherapy.

A national survey of 120 academic psychiatric-mental health nursing graduate programs confirmed the scarcity of sites and found a wide range of individual psychotherapy practice hours required for students, ranging from a minimum of 50 to a maximum 440 hours in the programs for which a certain number of requisite hours are required for psychotherapy (Wheeler & Delaney, 2005). For approximately 50% of programs, however, no designated number of psychotherapy practice hours was required, and medication management hours were integrated along with psychotherapy. A more recent survey reveals significant differences in how APPN programs teach psychotherapy (Vanderhoef & Delaney, 2017). The lack of consistency points to the need for more specific competencies and guidelines for what and how psychotherapy content should be taught.

Consequently, most graduate psychiatric nurses leave their graduate studies with a less than adequate knowledge base in this area, and often do not feel competent to practice psychotherapy. Faculty teaching students in graduate programs, when asked whether their students had achieved competency on graduation, felt decidedly mixed, with some stating that they did not envision a future role as psychotherapist and others suggested further training and supervision for competency to be achieved.

Working with people in the intimacy of psychotherapy is an honor, and much good can be done, as well as a great deal of harm. At vulnerable times in their lives, people see the psychotherapist as an expert, and this role often is imbued with a great deal of power and credibility. This privilege also comes with an ethical responsibility for the nurse psychotherapist to get as much training, supervision, and experience as possible in graduate studies and throughout her or his professional life. Expertise is a lifelong pursuit, and continuing education is imperative for those who wish to practice competently. Most licensed mental health professionals in other disciplines, which have considerably more psychotherapy practice in their programs than graduate psychiatric nursing programs, agree that it takes at least 10 years to become a skilled psychotherapist.

Stages of Learning

How then does one begin to learn psychotherapy? Psychotherapy is a learned skill like any other. The learning process begins with studying each component and practicing the technique and then blending it back together again with what you already know as each separate skill is acquired. Remember how you learned to take blood pressure or any other nursing skill? This can only be accomplished through learning discrete steps and practicing competencies in a skill set until that skill becomes automatic. If it seems like hard work at first, it probably means you are doing it well.

TABLE 1.2 COMPARISON OF BENNER'S MODEL AND THE STAGES OF LEARNING	
Stages of Learning	**Benner's Model**
Unconscious incompetency	Novice no experience, governed by rules and regulations
Conscious incompetency	Advanced beginner recognizes aspects of situations and makes judgments
Conscious competency	Competency/proficiency 2–5 years experience, coordinates complex care and sees situations as wholes, and long-term solutions
Unconscious competency	Expert flexible, efficient, and uses intuition

Benner (1984) offers a model of role acquisition from novice to expert that examines the levels of competency that can be applied for the novice nurse psychotherapist. It is likely that the graduate student who is pursuing a master's degree or postmaster's certificate as an APPN has practiced as an expert in an area of specialization before graduate studies. To transition from expert back to novice is often a painful and anxiety-provoking process. The beginning nurse psychotherapist has most likely interacted professionally with many different types of patients, but there is usually much anxiety about the first session in the role as psychotherapist. There is usually no one right thing to say. In psychotherapy, there is much ambiguity and often no right answers.

Juxtaposed to Benner's model is the four stages of learning model, which may help to allay anxiety for those who are beginning to learn psychotherapy (Table 1.2). Although there is some controversy regarding who developed this model, it is thought that learning takes place in four stages:

1. Unconscious incompetence (i.e., we do not know what we do not know).
2. Conscious incompetence (i.e., we feel uncomfortable about what we do not know).
3. Conscious competence (i.e., we begin to acquire the skill and concentrate on what we are doing).
4. Unconscious competence (i.e., we blend the skills together, and they become habits, allowing use without struggling with the components).

The challenge initially for novices is that they are becoming increasingly aware of being incompetent as progress is made. This is likely to generate anxiety.

Unique Qualities of Nurse Psychotherapists

The history of the one-to-one nurse–patient relationship and nurses conducting psychotherapy is detailed by Lego (1999) and Beeber (1995). Table 1.3 highlights the important events. The late 1940s were marked by the development of eight programs for the advanced preparation of nurses who cared for psychiatric patients. An extremely important debate took place over the next few decades about the nurse's role as psychotherapist. This culminated in the 1967 American Nurses Association (ANA) Position Paper on Psychiatric Nursing, which clarified the role of the clinical specialist in psychiatric nursing as psychotherapist, and certification for the specialty began in 1979. In the 1990s PMHNP programs were developed, and this culminated in the PMHNP competencies that included psychotherapy as an essential competency required for all PMHNPs (Wheeler & Haber, 2004).

TABLE 1.3	TIMELINE OF THE HISTORY OF THE NURSE PSYCHOTHERAPIST
1947	Eight programs established for advanced preparation of nurses to care for psychiatric patients
1952	Hildegard Peplau establishes the first master's in clinical nursing and a "Sullivanian" framework for practice for psychotherapy with inpatients and outpatients
1963	Perspectives in Psychiatric Care first published as a forum for interprofessional psychiatric articles
1967	American Nurses Association (ANA) Position Paper on Psychiatric Nursing—PCS (psychiatric clinical specialist) assumes role of individual, group, family, and milieu therapist
1979	ANA certification of psychiatric and mental health clinical nurse specialist (PMHCNS)
2000	American Nurses Credentialing Center (ANCC) certification of psychiatric-mental health nurse practitioner (PMHNP)
2001	Family PMHNP ANCC Exam
2003	PMHNP Competencies developed and delineate "conducts individual, group, and/or family psychotherapy" for PMHNP practice
2011	American Psychiatric Nurses Association (APNA) and International Society of Psychiatric-Mental Health Nurses (ISPN) endorse PMHNP as the entry role for all advanced practice psychiatric nurses
2013	PMHNP Competencies revised
2014	Only PMHNP Across the Life Span ANCC certification

The APPN role of psychotherapist has solid historical roots from the inception of advanced practice psychiatric-mental health nursing, whereas the prescribing role is a much more recent step in the evolution of the specialty. The current role of APPNs is focused on prescribing psychotropics which is more aligned with the medical model (Delaney, Drew, & Rushton, 2019).

After the issue of whether nurses should do psychotherapy was resolved, the literature examined the unique qualities that nurses might possess as psychotherapists compared with those in other disciplines who practice psychotherapy. Several strengths were cited: nurses have the ability to be patient because they have worked with the chronically ill and have respect for others' limitations; nurses are realistic and possess excellent observational skills, resourcefulness, innovation, and creativity (Smoyak, 1990); nurses are able to view the patient in a holistic way, understand crisis orientation, and have a knowledge of general health concerns (Lego, 1992); and nurses are familiar with the daily life and experience of the hospitalized patients (Balsam & Balsam, 1974). Nurses usually have had a breadth of life experience and exposure to many different ages, ethnicities, occupations, socioeconomic status, cultures, and personalities. The novice nurse psychotherapist is well served through experience with communicating and connecting with those from diverse backgrounds. Nurses being close to the patient's everyday experience is crucial for connection and collaboration. This connection is reflected in the public perception of nurses as positive and trustworthy. In 2019 for the 18th year in a row, the Gallup poll found that nurses top the list of most ethical professions, with Americans rating nurses among the most trusted professionals.

Eighty-five percent of respondents rated nurses' honesty and ethics as "very high" or "high" with medical doctors rated third at 65% (Gallup, 2020).

An additional quality that nurses bring to the role of psychotherapist is a pragmatic, problem-solving approach using the nursing process as an overall framework for practice. Usually, the patient has tried many things to feel better, and therapy is often a last resort. The patient's problems have brought the person into treatment, and if these problems could be solved outside of therapy with friends or family, he or she would have already done so. The problem-solving approach needed in the psychotherapeutic process is the same as in the nursing process. Both involve an assessment, diagnosis, plan, intervention, and evaluation. Nurses are used to collaborating with patients and thinking about what will solve the problem, what the patient's perspective is, what the person wants, and what the patient's strengths are. These approaches are derived from a problem-solving, health-oriented, holistic model fundamental to nursing practice and the nurse–patient relationship.

In my experience working with graduate psychiatric nursing students, this problem-solving approach is useful but one that novice nurse psychotherapists often struggle with. Because nurses are used to taking care of people and are action oriented, beginning students often want to rescue the patient and help the patient to feel better. Helping the patient feel better is not the main goal of psychotherapy, and a focus on amelioration of symptoms may even be counterproductive to the process, although feeling better overall most likely will be a by-product of successful therapy. In a well-intended effort to help the person feel better, the nurse may be too directive and offer fix it suggestions, and this is antithetical to promoting empowerment. Letting the psychotherapeutic process unfold takes time, and that has typically not been a part of nursing practice, especially within the current healthcare system.

Requisites for Nurse Psychotherapists

Nurse psychotherapists have the honor of participating in the healing process, and as nurse theorists Dossey and Keegan (2013) point out, in the nurse–patient relationship, the nurse enters into a shared experience or field of consciousness that promotes the healing potential of others. Through consciousness, intent, and presence, the nurse psychotherapist's therapeutic use of self facilitates others in their healing. To counter the learned patterns of nursing practice (i.e., busyness, task focused, and control), the nurse psychotherapist needs to cultivate reflection, mindfulness, and patience. According to Dossey and Keegan (2013), qualities essential for nurse healers include expansion of consciousness and continuing one's own journey toward wholeness and resilience. This can be accomplished through many different venues: nature, relationships, your own therapy, ongoing supervision, meditation, mindfulness, self-awareness exercises, spiritual practices, chanting, prayer, journaling, openness to receiving one's own healing treatments, and reflective activities such as hiking, walking, and yoga. Research has shown that the regular practice of mindfulness improves empathy, insight, immune function, attention, and emotional regulation (Dahlgaard et al., 2019). These changes correspond to changes in the brain that include increased activity and growth of regulatory and integrative regions which foster resilience.

Mindfulness is a skill that can be learned through practice and discipline and used as a tool in the psychotherapeutic process. The vast literature on the development of mindfulness crosses many disciplines and orientations, from Buddhism to psychoanalysis. Mindfulness is discussed more fully in Chapters 17 and 18. Safran and Muran (2000) state that mindfulness in psychotherapy has three characteristics:

(a) The direction of attention, (b) remembering, and (c) nonjudgmental awareness. The initial direction of attention involves intentionally paying attention to and observing

one's inner experience or actions. This involves cultivating an attitude of intense curiosity about one's experience. In mindful meditation, the individual can initially cultivate the ability to attend by focusing the attention on an object (e.g., the breath) and then noting whenever his or her attention has wandered and returning it to the intended focus of attention. By noting whatever one's attention has wandered toward (e.g., a particular thought or feeling) before redirecting one's attention, the individual develops the ability to observe and investigate his or her experience from a detached perspective rather from being fully immersed in or identified with it. (p. 59)

Peplau (1991) stressed the need for self-awareness in the nurse–patient relationship and stated: "The extent to which each nurse understands her own functioning will determine the extent to which she can come to understand the situation confronting the patient and the way he sees it" (p. x). However, with the rise of psychopharmacology and biological psychiatry, self-awareness has not been a priority. Self-awareness is key to understanding others, and it reduces the likelihood that therapists will act out their own agendas and use patients for gratification or self-esteem needs. For example, one novice nurse psychotherapist was so rewarded emotionally by his work with a particular patient that he went out of his way to meet with her when she needed him and to schedule additional office hours when he would not normally be in the office. The patient responded with gratitude, which enhanced the self-esteem of the nurse who was conscientious and overly responsible for this patient. It was only through supervision that he began to understand how his need for recognition fueled the overly accommodating stance; how his objectivity about the psychotherapeutic process had been compromised; and how this cultivated an unhealthy dependency in the patient.

Peplau (1991) says that there is a tendency for all those doing therapeutic work to generate inferences from limited data and to assume that these data are complete. It is only natural that we would try to fit the problem into our own limited schemata of experiences, but the richness of clinical data belies this belief. Attributing motivation to one simple reason, such as "she's borderline and manipulative," is simplistic and may assuage our anxiety but does not account for complex, multifaceted interactions and contributions that are more often the norm than the exception. Symptoms are usually multidetermined and have many different contributing factors.

Overdeterminism refers to the idea that a problem most often has many different causes. The patient may not be able to provide a full description of these contributions and most likely is unaware of the multiple reasons for the current symptom. For example, a young woman with bulimia may have factors that contributed to the development of her problem: a history of sexual abuse, feelings of deprivation and neglect in her family, a recent loss in her family, a genetic predisposition, a fear of weight gain, cultural pressures about weight, an overemphasis on weight in her family, an inability to self-soothe, a hormonal imbalance, the stress of a new job, and a best friend who is also bulimic. The friend with the same problem may have a few of these contributing factors and others, such as conflict in her home with an abusive, alcoholic father; a depressed, unavailable mother; and financial difficulties that contribute to the instability of her home environment and compromise her ability to manage her emotions. There are no simple answers, and two people with the same problem may have developed and maintained their symptoms for different reasons. Many factors, such as genetics, prenatal insults, parent–child interactions, abuse, neglect, school and social environments, family dynamics, and physical illness, have been studied, and all have been found to play a role in the cause of psychiatric disorders and mental health problems.

We all have preconceptions that are brought to every situation. It is not as important to eliminate these as to be aware of what they are and how they may influence our work. The extent of a nurse's self-knowledge determines the extent to which he or she can understand another person. Neuroimaging studies have confirmed that being aware of another's mind is related to a person's ability to monitor his or her own mental state (Siegel, 2012). A person does not have to be a paragon of mental health to help another. Some feel that to be truly empathic, a person should have experienced psychological suffering, which can serve to deepen the work in psychotherapy. Most expert therapists consider personal therapy and supervision essential for the novice psychotherapist to cultivate emotional genuineness, authenticity, and objectivity. Supervision is not therapy, but it does assist the therapist in discussing difficult cases and understanding his or her own blind spots and how personal issues may impact the therapeutic relationship. Ongoing group or individual supervision after graduation is necessary for continued growth and an ethical practice. Expert psychotherapists usually seek supervision and consultation throughout their professional lives. A sample of suggestions for presenting a case that may be covered in supervision is included in Appendix 1.1.

Irvin Yalom cogently makes a case for therapy for the therapist:

> *Therapists must be familiar with their own dark side and be able to empathize with all human wishes and impulses. A personal therapy experience permits the student therapist to experience many aspects of the therapeutic process from the patient's seat: the tendency to idealize the therapist, the yearning for dependency, the gratitude toward a caring and attentive listener, and the power granted to the therapist. Young therapists must work through their own neurotic issues, they must learn to accept feedback, discover their own blind spots, and see themselves as others see them; they must appreciate their impact upon others and learn how to provide accurate feedback.* (Yalom & Ferguson, 2002, pp. 40–41)

The student of psychotherapy who undergoes his or her own psychotherapy has a model for what the psychotherapeutic process is and understands the power and the process of psychotherapy in an immediate, experiential way that no amount of reading or didactic study can convey. Many expert psychotherapists report that they have experienced various modes of psychotherapy and this has enhanced their own technique as the skills others use are incorporated into their own practice.

In addition to self-awareness, enhancing one's own resilience through promoting self-care is fundamental in caring for others. Self-care strategies start with exercising regularly, eating healthily, spending time with friends, getting enough sleep, and limiting work hours to avoid exhaustion. When a flight takes off, the airline attendant announces that all adults must put the oxygen mask over their faces first before securing the mask on a child. This is an appropriate metaphor for all caregivers. Much has been written about the trauma inherent in nursing. Various terms have been used to describe this phenomenon, such as burnout, compassion fatigue, and vicarious or secondary traumatization. A 2017 survey of employed RNs in hospitals reported that 63% experience burnout (Kronos, 2017). Burnout may occur for many reasons: our collective history as a profession of women, the patriarchal medical system and nurses' subservient role, stressful healthcare environments, and caring for and witnessing trauma and pain in others. Most often, personal and professional trauma is unrecognized and therefore unaddressed. Sequelae of exposure to other's trauma may include fatigue, depression, anger, apathy, detachment, headaches, insomnia, and gastrointestinal distress (Foli & Thompson, 2019), all of which mitigate against the ability to adopt the psychotherapeutic stance necessary for conducting psychotherapy. It is only in the recognition and processing of one's own trauma that one can transcend it and be of help to others. A resource for understanding and overcoming compassion fatigue can be found at www.edumed.org/resources/compassion-fatigue-online-guide.

Competencies for Trauma and Resilience for Nursing Education have been developed and include self-resilience competencies for APPNs (Wheeler & Phillips, 2019).

These competencies build on those for undergraduate and graduate level education and are copyrighted. The full document with subcompetencies are included
online in the faculty resource website and at www.acesconnection.com/blog/
trauma-and-resilience-competencies-for-nursing-education.

HOLISTIC PARADIGM OF HEALING

In contrast to the biomedical model's goal to cure with symptom relief treatment, the
goal in a holistic paradigm is healing (see Figure 1.1). This is an important distinction,
because curing is not always possible but healing is (Dossey & Keegan, 2013). The word
heal comes from an old Anglo-Saxon word *haelen*, which means "to become whole,
body, mind, and spirit within oneself"; but it can also be defined in a broader context
as being in "right relationship" with oneself, others, and our world. Mariano defines
healing as "an emergent process . . . bringing together aspects of one's self and the body,
mind, emotion, spirit, and environment at deeper levels of inner knowing, leading to
an integration and balance" (2013, p. 60). Each component is interdependent and interrelated, based on the premise that when there is a change in one part of the system, the
change reverberates in all dimensions. For example, minor changes in one's emotions
may potentiate a change in all other spheres as well as in the person's relationship with
others and his or her world. Conversely, a change in the context or relationships with
others may create changes in other dimensions (e.g., body, mind, emotion, spirit) of the
person. The context or background is the person's culture as mediated by the person's
family and relationships.

Some of the goals of psychotherapy include the reduction of symptoms, improvement of functioning, relapse prevention, increased empowerment, and achievement of
the specific collaborative goals set with the patient. Within the biomedical model, symptoms are often thought to be the cause of the patient's problem and psychotropic medications are prescribed to target specific symptoms in an effort to eliminate or reduce
the symptoms. For example, prescribing a selective serotonin reuptake inhibitor (SSRI)
to increase serotonin levels is thought to treat the underlying cause of the depressive
disorder. However, whether this chemical imbalance causes depression or coexists with
some depressive disorders is a matter of speculation.

In contrast, in a holistic model, symptoms are seen as a form of communication and
are useful for understanding the meaning of the dysregulation and disharmony that are

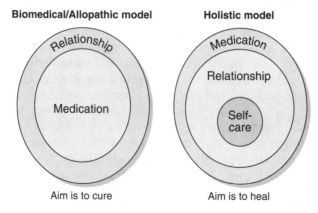

FIGURE 1.1 Paradigms of care.

occurring for this person at a given time. By eliminating the symptoms with medication, we are essentially "shooting the messenger." Often therapists find that therapy works best with full access to emotion; that is, if the person's emotions are damped down by benzodiazepines or other psychotropic medication, psychotherapeutic work may be compromised. For example, CBT seeks to allow the patient to become more comfortable with sensations and concomitant emotions related to panic attacks so that automatic thoughts about how dangerous these feelings seem can be confronted. If the patient reaches for medication for quick relief, the person may lose motivation to continue the treatment (Cloos & Ferreira, 2009). Of course when the patient's functioning is impaired, psychotropic medications do have their place in treatment. However, reframing symptoms as communication changes the way we view the relation of the problem to the person and enhances our ability to hear the meaning of the symptoms as we listen to our patient as well as access the person's emotion in order to facilitate the treatment of the patient.

The holistic paradigm is consistent with the mandate for recovery-oriented behavioral care. The Substance Abuse and Mental Health Services Administration (SAMHSA, 2020) provides a definition of recovery: "A process of change through which individuals improve their health and wellness, live a self-directed life and strive to reach their full potential." In addition to holistic care, elements of care aimed toward recovery include hope, respect, multidimensional care through many pathways, person-driven, supported by peers, culturally based, addresses trauma, supported through relationships and social networks, involving individual, family, and community strengths and responsibilities. Research has identified five gold standards of recovery for patients: hope, self-esteem, empowerment, self-responsibility, and a meaningful role in life (Livingston & Boyd, 2010; Siu et al., 2012). Practitioners who are recovery-oriented recognize the strengths and power of each person within the context of his or her life. The vehicle for recovery is through partnership and relationship with the practitioner and others so that the person is the driver of his or her own healing process (SAMHSA, 2020).

These elements and gold standards for recovery may feel familiar to APPNs because nurses have been educated to look at the context of the patient's life as they work in the reductionistic, symptom-oriented environment of the psychiatric biomedical paradigm. Biomedical psychiatry is based on a descriptive/biological approach of specialized knowledge that treats individuals as members of a diagnostic group. The diagnosis is based on observable clusters of symptoms or behaviors and there is no assumption about causation except for the *Diagnostic and Statistical Manual of Mental Disorders* (5th ed.; *DSM-5; American Psychiatric Association [APA], 2013*) category of trauma-related disorders. What is considered pathological is determined by societal values and behaviors that are considered acceptable at the time by a panel of, until most recently, exclusively psychiatrists. For example, the *DSM-III* considered homosexuality a psychiatric disorder while the *DSM-5* includes new diagnoses such as Binge Eating and Hoarding Disorders (APA, 2013).

The diagnosis may not tell us very much about the person sitting in front of us. The nurse is often the only person caring for the patient who sees the whole picture. The nurse knows the patient as "a grandmother who lives alone in a walk-up, estranged from her daughter and often terrorized by her own internal demons" while those practicing from a medical model might describe the same person as "an 88-year-old elderly woman with bipolar disorder." The former is relevant about who the person is while the latter tells us nothing about the uniqueness of that individual. Indeed the nurse practicing from a holistic paradigm respects the complexity of the person, and historically, this has been the foundation for nursing practice.

Relationship

Relationship has been considered foundational for psychiatric nursing since Peplau's seminal work in 1952 (D'Antonio, Beeber, Sills, & Naegle, 2014). The healing that takes place in psychotherapy occurs through the relationship between the therapist and the patient. Lego (1992) maintained that psychiatric nurses develop "a relationship designed to change the patient's interpersonal situation, changing the intrapsychic situation, thus changing the brain chemistry" (p. 148). Forchuk and associates (1998) observed that the nurse–patient relationship is the "active ingredient" in therapeutic change. Raingruber (2003) concurs and says that relationship and nurturing are hallmarks of psychiatric nursing. Dossey and Keegan (2013) say that the healing relationship occurs through the expansion of consciousness, during which a sacred space is created.

Emotional connection promotes interpersonal attunement, attachment, and coregulation of physiological states (Schore, 2019). Emotional connection with the patient through relationship has been found to be important for successful psychotherapy outcomes with 50% of positive outcomes due to therapist, relationship, and expectancy while the specific technique or theory used by the therapist accounts for only 17% of improvement; 33% of the variance is due to extratherapeutic factors such as spontaneous remission, patient, and community factors (Norcross & Lambert, 2019). The ability of the patient to connect through collaboration depends on the therapist's skills and on the patient's emotional developmental level, with some patients much better able to join in collaboration than others. Tryon and Winograd (2002) found that the more troubled, resistant, less-motivated patients are those most likely to need help and the least likely to engage and collaborate with therapists. Chronically disempowered patients, especially those who have been severely traumatized in childhood, often are unable to connect with others and use support to reach new solutions. The challenge for the APPN is how to facilitate connection, particularly with patients who have difficulty with relationships. Inherent in this connection is the APPN's curiosity and openness to learning about another's experience. The receptivity and openness of the therapist to what is presented offers the patient a model for developing curiosity about him- or herself and for an *observing ego*. It is thought that this capacity to develop the ability to observe one's own behavior with nonjudgmental curiosity is a hallmark of emotional health.

Caring in the nurse-patient relationship has been identified as essential for practice (Dossey & Keegan, 2013; Morse, Solberg, Neander, Bottorff, & Johnson, 1990; Schoenhofer, 2002; Watson, 2012). Caring encompasses and expands Carl Rogers's idea of unconditional positive regard that has been adopted by most mental health disciplines as essential to helping relationships (Rogers, 1951). A phenomenological study delineated the characteristics of the APRN–patient relationship that are foundational to caring (Thomas, Finch, Schoenhofer, & Green, 2004). They include the mutuality of nonromantic love based on a genuine knowing of the person, trust, and respect reflected in an acceptance of and authentic appreciation for the other. Every person is approached with acceptance with the nurse and patient as coparticipants in the process of healing. Inherent in caring is respect for the autonomy and agency of the other person. Fundamental to caring is the understanding of another person's unique configuration of attitudes, feelings, and values from that person's perspective.

The nurse psychotherapist creates a healing presence of acceptance, patience, lovingness, nonjudgmental attitude, understanding, good listening skills, honesty, and empathy. These qualities are the essence of presence (McKivergin, 1997) and allow the nurse psychotherapist to "be with" rather than "doing to" the patient. Bunkers (2009) says,

"True presence involves listening to what is important to the other and listening to what the meaning of a situation is in the moment for that person" (p. 22). Scaer (2005), a neurologist specializing in trauma, says that presence involves a personal interaction that contributes to physiological changes in the person. He states, "This healing, empathic presence affects and alters the parts of the brain that process pain, fear, anxiety, and distress" (p. 167). Presence may facilitate healing through mediation of neurotransmitters and hormones that promote optimal autonomic functioning.

The antithesis to empowerment is authority; in this situation, the therapist knows what is best for the person. The process of psychotherapy cultivates dependency because there is unavoidable inequality in the relationship with the patient, who naturally feels disempowered by needing help at a vulnerable time. This reality and the inevitable transference–countertransference responses create dependent feelings in the patient. The psychotherapist's competence lies in understanding that the patient's autonomy is always in the foreground of the process. The overall goal for patients is to deepen their understanding of themselves in order for them to make their own decisions. Caring is fundamental to creating an atmosphere conducive to the cultivation of relationship and empowerment.

Resilience

Both relationship and resilience are overarching pantheoretical concepts that apply to all approaches of psychotherapy and practice settings. The term *resilience* refers to the ability of an individual, family, or community to cope with adversity and trauma, and adapt to challenges through individual physical, emotional, and spiritual attributes and access to cultural and social resources (adapted from SAMHSA, 2014). In fact, there is speculation that surviving a crisis can actually be a growth-promoting experience for some people. However, other research supports that resilience and posttraumatic growth are inversely related; that is, those who cope well and are resilient after a traumatic event retain equilibrium and do not need to find positive meaning to the event while those who emerge with posttraumatic growth feel the need to reframe the event as positive (Levine, Lalufer, Stein, Hamama-Raz, & Solomon, 2009). A more recent study supports that moderate resilience and emotional intelligence is associated with the most growth (Li, Cao, Cao, & Liu, 2015). That is, there is a curvilinear relationship between posttraumatic growth and resilience.

An elegant yet simple resilience model based on neurophysiology is proposed by Elaine Miller-Karas and deepens our understanding how to help patients access their resources (2015). Miller-Karas says that one's resilient zone (RZ) is an internal state of adaptabiliy and flexibility that is regulated by our nervous system. We feel at our best and can think clearly and deal effectively with life when we are in our RZ. She states that there is a natural biological rhythm of the autonomic nervous system between the sympathetic nervous system and the parasympathetic nervous system and this corresponds to the RZ. The RZ is also referred to as the window of tolerance (Ogden, Minton, & Pain, 2006), or the therapeutic window of arousal (Siegel, 2012). Porges's polyvagal theory refers to the state of our nervous system as the myelinated ventral vagus social engagement response (Porges, 2011). The brain and the body communicate with each other unconsciously through the vagus nerve. Chapter 2 discusses the polyvagal theory and the neurophysiology of the RZ and its role in well-being and healing trauma. The skilled psychotherapist helps the person through various techniques that assist the person to mediate the autonomic nervous system and stay in their RZ, that is, not too hyperaroused (sympathetic system) and not too hypoaroused (parasympathetic system; see Figure 1.2). This is the optimal physiological state for the work of therapy and reflects the person's natural rhythm and flow of energy and vitality. Although the person may feel sad, happy, angry, and other emotions when in their RZ, the person is able to both feel and think at the same time.

If the person becomes too anxious and hyperaroused, resistances or defenses may increase, and the work of therapy will be thwarted, perhaps not consciously, but nevertheless, the person's brain will not be able to integrate memories or gain insight. Immediate strategies in a session to decrease arousal levels might include deep breathing exercises or imagery. There are also many patients who have suffered significant trauma and are in a chronic state of either hyperarousal or hypoarousal or swing from one physiological state to the other (see Figure 1.3). If the person is chronically hypoaroused, he or she may be unable to access emotions. Strategies for hypoarousal to increase arousal might include focusing on sensations in the body, mindfulness exercises, and self-regulation strategies. Self-regulation refers to one's ability to manage emotions and behavior and is further discussed in Chapter 2. Psychotherapy helps those with emotional dysregulation to widen and strengthen their RZ.

Severe trauma has been found to override constitutional, environmental, genetic, or psychological resilience factors (De Bellis, 2001). Studies have shown that factors that enhance resilience include the presence of supportive relationships and attachments as well as the avoidance of frequent and prolonged stress (Herrman et al., 2011). These factors are not inborn but can be fostered through psychotherapeutic interventions that focus on the strengths of the person, reducing risks, and improving relationships. Chapter 11 further discusses the RZ specific strategies to enhance resilience. Relationships form the foundation of resilience and serve to create new experiences that promote neuronal and synaptic connections that allow for learning new meaning for prior adverse experiences.

Figures 1.2 and 1.3 illustrate a user-friendly model that the APPN can teach patients at the beginning of therapy when making a treatment plan. Illustrating the RZ on paper and then drawing Figure 1.3 helps patients to understand their symptoms without judgment as something physiological that is happening to them. Many patients have no understanding why they feel so out of control, anxious, depressed, or numb and providing a simple explanation based on neurophysiology with visuals such as Figures 1.2 and 1.3 can be very helpful and destigmatizing. The message conveyed is, "It is not what is wrong with you but what has happened to you,"

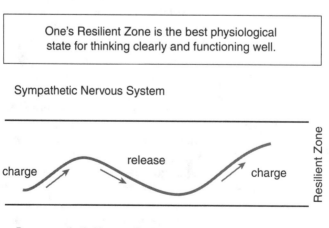

FIGURE 1.2 Therapeutic window of arousal/tolerance, or resilient zone.

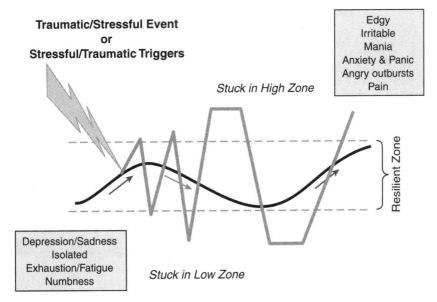

FIGURE 1.3 Out of the resilient zone.

Source: Adapted by Elaine Miller-Karas from an original graphic by Levine/Heller. Reprinted with permission from the Trauma Resource Institute, Claremont, CA.

which lays the foundation for a trauma-informed approach to your work together. Techniques and resources to widen or strengthen the patient's RZ will be further discussed within the context of the various psychotherapy approaches presented in this book. See Chapters 2 and 11, for a fuller discussion of the underlying neurophysiology of the RZ.

ANXIETY

Understanding, assessing, and managing anxiety is a cornerstone of Peplau's Interpersonal Relations Model for Nursing (1991). Anxiety is ubiquitous in the psychotherapeutic process, and the skilled APPN understands how to assist the patient in managing anxiety. Anxiety creates feelings of helplessness, which disempower the patient and prevent healing. Wachtel (2011) says:

> One of the chief aims of the psychotherapist is to help the patient overcome the fears and inhibitions that have led him to react to his normal and healthy feelings as if they were a threat; to help him reappropriate parts of himself that have been dissociated from full awareness, that have motivated avoidances, and that are likely to generate still further areas of vulnerability, deficits in crucial skills in living, and impediments to the very relationships that could in principle be correctives to the debilitating anxiety. (p. 87)

For the most part, people seek psychotherapy because anxiety or the effects of anxiety have in one way or another interfered with functioning. Sometimes, a person is seeking help for the anxiety itself, such as in cases of panic attacks or phobias, but often the presenting issue is related to the results of the person's efforts to avoid anxiety. For example, a person with borderline personality traits may present with depression as

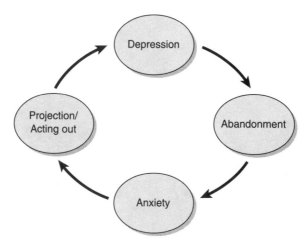

FIGURE 1.4 Cyclical psychodynamics of a person with borderline personality disorder.

a result of a lost relationship, but the central issue is a vulnerability to abandonment anxiety. It is likely that in the person's zeal to avoid the feared abandonments, that person inadvertently creates the very situation that he or she is trying so hard to avoid (Figure 1.4). Wachtel (2011) calls this *cyclical psychodynamics*, which is explained further in Chapter 5.

Inherent in all the theoretical approaches and basic principles discussed in this textbook is the centrality of anxiety as key to the patient's problems and the management of anxiety as key to solving these problems. In the safety of the therapeutic relationship, patients are encouraged to tolerate the feared experiences, memories, and thoughts. Cozolino (2017) says that a major role for the therapist is to assist the patient in using anxiety as a compass to explore unconscious fears. In deepening his or her understanding of anxiety as a trigger for avoidance or acting out, the person can then approach with curiosity what is feared. Strategies for working with anxiety are central to all therapy approaches. For example, behavioral techniques such as desensitization or flooding may be taught and increase anxiety initially, with the hope of decreasing anxiety later, so the person can face what was fearfully avoided. Cognitive techniques may involve "restructuring" thinking so that the threat that is anxiety-provoking is not considered as dire as originally believed. Psychodynamic techniques use interpretations to deepen the person's understanding of anxiously avoided thoughts, wishes, and feelings by making the unconscious conscious in order to understand the cause of anxiety.

For those patients with chronic hyperarousal and anxiety disorders, their RZ may be too narrow, and strategies and resources that help to widen their RZ may be needed. These can include basic stress management activities, such as exercise, decreasing caffeine intake, relaxation exercises, and imagery. A useful weekly plan for increasing resources and a weekly goal sheet is included in Appendices 1.2 and 1.3. Asking the person what he or she does to relieve anxiety or stress is part of good history taking, and developing a plan together that is not overwhelming is essential. Books such as Bourne's *The Anxiety and Phobia Workbook* (2015) can be very helpful and an important adjunct to therapy. The patient can be asked to read a chapter and complete the exercises in selected relevant chapters, and the next session is begun with a discussion about the person's experience with the material. Additional strategies to manage anxiety are especially important for those with dissociation and trauma-related disorders, and these are discussed further in Chapter 17.

However, a caveat is in order. Workbook exercises are only an adjunct to treatment and do not take the place of the real work in therapy, which is co-constructing a narrative and connecting through a therapeutic relationship. A consistent finding is that treatment manuals do not correlate positively with treatment outcome (Moncher & Printz, 1991; Strupp & Anderson, 1997; Truijens, Zühlke van Hulzen, & Vanheule, 2019). This may in part result from the constraints on creativity and flexibility with such a "cookbook" approach that is not context driven. Often, novice psychotherapists feel more comfortable with these structured approaches and with "doing" things; thus, it may help to manage the therapist's anxiety more than it does the patient's. In addition to monitoring the patient's anxiety, the beginning APPN must be aware of and manage his or her own anxiety.

It is easy to see why therapy in and of itself is highly anxiety provoking. Change, even a positive change such as we hope occurs in psychotherapy, is anxiety provoking. A seminal study by the Menninger Foundation found that patients who had positive outcomes from psychotherapy often reported an increase in anxiety, but they had learned to use anxiety as a signal rather than as a reality that danger was present (Siegel & Rosen, 1962). In the safety of the therapeutic relationship, the person is exposed to what has been avoided; and as the person begins to change toward healthier ways of functioning, increased anxiety is inevitable. It is important for the therapist to keep this in mind and monitor the patient's anxiety level as the therapeutic process unfolds. If anxiety becomes too unbearable in psychotherapy, there may be acting-out behaviors and increased resistance to change, or the person may leave treatment prematurely.

Anxiety is inherent in any new enterprise, and learning psychotherapy can be particularly anxiety provoking. In psychotherapy, we are trying to make sense of what is going on, and new information is emerging in every minute in our interaction with patients. One way the brain deals with ambiguous situations is to categorize information. This is largely what diagnosing is about—categorizing and labeling patients through a list of behavioral characteristics. The brain tries to fit the person into what is familiar, and this limits our ability to approach the patient with openness and without preconceptions. As anxiety increases, our focus becomes more limited, and it is harder to maintain the openness required to achieve a nonjudgmental, observational stance. Developing self-awareness about one's own anxiety is essential in empowering the therapist to allow the space needed for the relationship to develop.

MENTAL HEALTH AND CULTURE

To practice psychotherapy, the therapist must have a model on which to base interventions and some idea of what constitutes a mentally healthy person. Freud's simple idea that the goal of therapy is to be able to work and love remains relevant, because it can be applied generally to all cultures and people. In contrast, Sullivan (1947) thought that self-awareness was key to mental health and said, "One achieves mental health to the extent that one becomes aware of one's interpersonal relations" (p. 207). A more contemporary idea is offered by Siegel (2012) and is based on a systems perspective. He says that mental health emerges from integration in the brain/body through relationships. Integration is the core of resilience and vitality and reflects coherence of one's own states of mind. "Internal integration allows for vital interpersonal connections that are themselves integrative." (p. 351) Integration is accomplished through information processing that links disparate parts into a functional whole. The neurophysiological underpinnings of integration are explained further in Chapter 2.

BOX 1.1 Qualities of Self-Actualization

Appropriate perception of reality
Spontaneity
Ability to concentrate and problem solve
Acceptance of oneself and others
Intense emotional experiences
Peak experiences
Nonconformance
Creativeness and ethics
Interpersonal relationships
Independence and autonomy
Identification with humankind

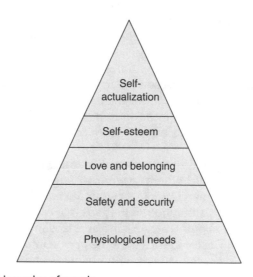

FIGURE 1.5 Maslow's hierarchy of needs.

Source: Adapted from Maslow, A. H. (1972). *The farther reaches of human nature.*
New York, NY: Viking.

Maslow delineated the ideal of a mentally healthy person as one who is self-actualized and who has the characteristics summarized in Box 1.1. Maslow's hierarchy of needs framework for problem solving is useful in conceptualizing the priority of patient needs (Maslow, 1972). Lower-level needs must be met before higher-level needs can be addressed. Meeting physiological needs is essential, with physical and emotional safety and security next (Figure 1.5). Safety in the world and the therapeutic relationship is essential to enable disclosure so that higher-level needs on the continuum, such as love, self-esteem, and self-actualization, can be achieved. This model is not fixed in that an individual may achieve self-actualization and then be faced with a trauma and have a need for physiological safety that would then take priority over self-actualization and needs higher in the hierarchy.

It is apparent from reviewing the characteristics of self-actualization in Box 1.1 that the meaning of mental health is culture bound; Maslow's self-actualized person, embodying independence, autonomy, individuation, and nonconformance, is largely a Western idea. For example, Eastern cultural values of interdependence, communal integration, and group harmony which does not fit with Western ideas of self-actualization. Some dimensions of this framework may apply to certain cultures but not to others. *Cultural relativity* is a term that Horowitz (1982) identified as important to consider in any discussion of mental health; behavior that is considered normal or abnormal depends on social and cultural norms.

Culture is an integral part of all relationships. Our cultural context shapes our perceptions, emotions, attributions, judgments, and ideas about ourselves and others (Barrett, 2017). The powerful influence of culture permeates all dimensions of our life in a way that is often unconscious. We are all multicultural in the sense that we belong to many different cultures simultaneously. For example, a young man who recently returned from combat belongs to the military culture, which values winning in battle and requires following orders and acting bravely. He may return to a society that does not value the war he fought and find a clash of values on his return. He may also belong to an Irish cultural heritage that does not sanction overt expression of emotion, and his male gender has another set of cultural expectations about behavior. He may be homosexual and belong to the gay culture, with the expectations and prejudices that accompany this orientation. His Roman Catholic upbringing adds another cultural layer that may contribute to his guilt, conflict, and confusion. It is easy to see how all of these multicultural influences provide the complex context that will impact his ability to resume his life in a healthy, productive way.

To diagnose and treat mental illness effectively, the APPN considers ethnicity, religion, race, class, cultural identity, cultural explanations of illness, and the cultural elements of the relationship between the individual and clinician. It is not possible to have extensive knowledge about many cultures, but a working knowledge of the backgrounds of those who most often seek treatment is essential. However, generalizations about another's culture do not tell us how to work with individuals. For example, knowing that those from a Hispanic culture often tend to somatize conflicts does not inform us about how to work with a Hispanic woman who hears the voice of her dead husband. It is highly likely that she may not be psychotic but is instead grieving according to acceptable cultural norms. Allowing time and support may be more appropriate than prescribing an antipsychotic drug.

The *DSM-5* includes cultural formulation with interview questions designed for assessing information about the impact of a person's social and cultural context and the person's perceptions of the problem. This is a very helpful resource for mental health clinicians for effective assessment and clinical management and helps to establish rapport and engage the patient. In addition, a glossary of cultural concepts of distress is included in the *DSM-5* Appendix, which illustrates syndromes in selected cultures. These syndromes illustrate the idiosyncratic nature of emotional concepts for various cultures; that is, it is how the culture perceives the emotional and bodily experiences that determines the characteristics and expressions of the disorder.

Recent cross-cultural research reveals that culture not only determines what is considered a psychiatric disorder but that neurobiological mechanisms linked to stress and trauma vary across cultures (Liddell & Jobson, 2016). For example, higher cortisol levels following a stressful event have been found in Chinese children compared with children from the United States (Doan et al., 2017) and in Brazilian older adults compared with Canadian older adults (Souza-Talarico, Plusquellec, Lupien, Fiocco, & Suchecki, 2014). This is important because relationships and culture shape not only our psychology but our biology. Research has also found that people from different cultural backgrounds vary in their interoceptive awareness (awareness of bodily states) (Ma-Kellams, 2014). Our bodily awareness, past experiences, and surroundings create emotions. Thus, emotions are constructed and predicted by the brain in the moment and learned in a relational context with the embedded values and norms of a particular culture (Barrett,

2017). One's perception about the world is shaped by predictions the brain is making about physical autonomic states; thus, we are deeply interacting with each other on a visceral level. Assisting the patient in labeling and identifying and exploring emotions without preconceived assumptions about what the person is feeling is essential in all psychotherapy.

If the APPN is unfamiliar with a particular person's culture, consultation may be in order. It is also important to research that culture and to ask the patient about his or her own experience. Asking the person of a culture different from yours how he or she feels about working with you is respectful and opens up a dialogue about the experience for the patient. It is okay to tell the patient that you may make mistakes about his or her culture and experience and to ask the person to let you know if you do. For people of color who come to a White therapist or vice versa, racial differences often are "the elephant in the living room" and should be addressed to enable the person to stay in treatment. Asking out of a genuine curiosity and admitting ignorance are collaborative and reduce the power imbalance in the relationship by allowing the patient to teach us. For example, one young Black woman who came to therapy for depression explained how she had experienced prejudice, and implicit in this communication was her concern that her White therapist might be prejudiced, too. Through acknowledging ignorance about the experience of prejudice and exploring her feelings and experiences, the therapist and patient deepened their understanding of her fears about therapy as a forum in which she might be judged. This strengthened the therapeutic alliance and connection, which allowed her to remain in treatment.

MENTAL ILLNESS

According to Luhrmann (2000), a cultural anthropologist, there are traditionally two frameworks for understanding mental illness. One framework is the psychodynamic approach, originally based on Freud's theoretical speculations, but that has evolved into many other frameworks. This model attributes mental illness more or less to environmental and psychosocial problems (i.e., nurture). In contrast, the biophysiological model attributes mental illness to chemical imbalance (i.e., nature). The latter framework attributes mental illness to an imbalance of neurotransmitters in the brain, and the answer lies in correcting these imbalances, largely through medication. This model has revolutionized psychiatry and has been dominant since the 1950s, when phenothiazines were discovered with great excitement for the treatment of those with chronic mental illness or psychosis.

How changes in neurotransmitters produce symptoms has been an intense focus of investigation, beginning in the 1990s with the "decade of the brain." These studies are based on the underlying premise that mental illness is a "brain disease" and should be treated as any other illness. This idea has been embraced by mental health providers and drug companies, as well as those diagnosed with a psychiatric disorder. However, a seminal research study found that this belief actually increases rather than decreases stigma and that people thought to have a brain disease are treated more harshly (Mehta & Farina, 1997). Perhaps diagnosing a person with a psychiatric disorder as "brain diseased" sets the person apart and further marginalizes the person as an "other." Stigma toward those with psychiatric disorders can be reduced through deepening our understanding of the effect of the environment on brain functioning. This knowledge may help to change the conversation from what is wrong with this person to what has happened to this person.

Both genetic vulnerability and environmental influences play significant roles in the development of mental illness. The term *epigenetics* has been coined to describe this interplay, that is, the environment selects, signals, modifies, and regulates gene activity. Heritable differences in gene expression are now thought to be not the result of DNA sequencing but the effects of the encryption of experience that can be transmitted and alter behavior over generations. Genetic, biological, traumatic, and social factors interact, and this complex interplay shapes thinking, feelings, and behavior.

The stress diathesis model of psychiatric disorders has evolved from the recognition that genetics (diathesis/nature) and environment (stress/nurture) both contribute to the development of psychiatric disorders (Hankin & Abela, 2005; Smoller, 2016). That is, for a person who has a genetic vulnerability and encounters significant early life stressors such as childhood trauma or neglect, loss, or viruses, the expression of the gene for the development of the psychiatric disorder most likely will be triggered. Evidence suggests that this is a result of changes in DNA through the process of methylation (Jiang, Postovit, Cattaneo, Binder, & Aitchison, 2019). Methyl groups affix genes that govern the production of stress hormone receptors in the brain and this prevents the brain from regulating the response to stress. Parental nurturing mediates this epigenetic response; however, in the absence of parental nurturing, regulatory and attention problems result.

Two psychiatric disorders that are thought to be strongly heritable, schizophrenia and bipolar disorder, are now thought to share epigenetic roots. Significant epigenetic chemicals were found in the genome of 22 pairs of identical twins diagnosed with either schizophrenia or bipolar disorder (National Institute of Mental Health [NIMH], 2009). That is, the twins had identical DNA but significant differences were noted in the gene activity caused by their environment. This is strong evidence that supports the hypothesis that epigenetic mechanisms may drive even those psychiatric disorders considered most heritable (Coghlan, 2011). In addition, genetically identical twins are 50% concordant for developing schizophrenia, which means that 50% of the variance is attributed to environmental or other nongenetic contributions (MacDonald & Schulz, 2009). Some psychiatric disorders such as PTSD, reactive attachment disorder, acute stress disorder, and adjustment disorders are identified in the *DSM-5* as trauma-related disorders and are triggered by exposure to extreme stress in people who otherwise may not be vulnerable (APA, 2013).

Animal and human studies strongly indicate that genetic factors of stress reactivity and greater physiological reactivity to stressful events may predispose one to a psychiatric disorder (Smoller, 2016). Those who have a stronger, more persistent response to stressors tend to withdraw from stressful situations and have internalizing traits. These people may be inhibited and more fearful, thus predisposing the person to anxiety and depressive disorders. Likewise, those whose temperament tends toward externalizing traits may be predisposed to develop psychopathology with symptoms of impulsivity, aggressiveness, and attentional difficulties. Caregivers who are not able to mediate arousal for their offspring with either of these traits are likely to exacerbate difficulties with affect and self-regulation that may lead to psychopathology (Schore, 2019).

Telomeres, DNA protein structures, have been found to be shortened in the presence of trauma. Telomere length is associated with the production of destructive radicals and molecules, chronic inflammation, co-occurring psychiatrc disorders, and a shorter life expectancy. A large meta-analysis found that PTSD was associated with shorter telomeres across gender (Li, Wang, Zhou, Huang, & Li, 2017). Research suggests that childhood adversity affects our genes (Papale, Seltzer, Madrid, Pollak, & Alisch, 2018). Gene expressions and salivary samples compared 22 girls who experienced high stress with those with normative stress. The high-stress group had more behavioral problems and 122 differentiated methylated genes. These genetic findings point to the transgenerational transfer of trauma from the first generation of trauma survivors to the second and further generations of offspring.

Adverse Life Experiences

It is now well established that adverse life experiences are associated with a wide range of psychiatric disorders and medical problems (Felitti & Anda, 2010; Hughes et al., 2017; Suglia et.al., 2018). Felitti's (1998) seminal study of the long-term sequelae of adverse childhood experiences (ACE) for 17,421 middle class adults found a graded, positive relationship between ACE and significant heart disease, fractures, diabetes, obesity, unintended pregnancy, sexually transmitted diseases, depression, anxiety, sleep disorder, dissociative disorders, eating disorders, and alcoholism.

Approximately 70% of adults world wide experience at least one traumatic event within their lifetime (Kessler, 2017). Exposure using *DSM-5* criteria is high (89.7%); exposure to multiple traumatic event types is the norm (Kilpatrick et al, 2013). Childhood adversity is common. Globally, the World Health Organization (WHO, 2018) estimates that 25% of all adults have been physically abused as children. In the United States, 59% of adults report at least one adverse childhood experience (Shonkoff & Gardner, 2012). One in ten children have experienced three or more ACEs and, in a number of states, the prevalence rate rises to one in seven (Sacks & Murphy, 2018). Notably, a significant dose response relationship has been established: the higher the ACE score, the greater the likelihood of physical and mental illness. With an ACE score of 4 or more, the likelihood of chronic pulmonary lung disease increases 390 percent; hepatitis, 240 percent; depression 460 percent; attempted suicide, 1,220 percent (Fellitti & Anda, 2010).

Children are particularly vulnerable to adverse events due to the plasticity of the developing brain; those who are brought up in a chaotic or non-nurturing environment suffer neurological consequences that are long-lasting and difficult to remediate (Shonkoff & Garner, 2012). Toxic stress and ACE have been found to result in lifelong consequences for both psychological and physical health that affect behavior, economics, education, and health outcomes (Shonkoff, 2010). A longitudinal study of 2,232 twins, which controlled for genetic effects, found that children who experienced maltreatment by an adult or bullying by peers were more likely to report psychotic symptoms at age 12 than those who did not experience traumatic events (Arseneault et al., 2011). Similarly, a large meta-analysis of prospective and cross-sectional cohort studies found that ACE are associated with psychosis and that psychosis would be reduced by 33% if that risk factor were removed (Varese et al., 2012). In one large study of 30,000 children, almost every diagnosis of depression, anxiety, substance abuse, or eating disorders was comorbid with PTSD (Seng et al., 2005). The effects of trauma on the developing brain are likely to be cumulative, profound, and long-lasting; they transcend the diagnosis of PTSD and contribute to a wide range of physical, emotional, and social problems (Afifi, Mota, Dasiewicz, MacMillan & Sareen, 2012; Nicholson et al, 2018; Porges, 2011; Schore, 2019; Teicher, 2012).

Toxic stress in early childhood also plays a role in the intergenerational transmission of disparities in health outcome (Braveman & Barclay, 2009). Research supports the long-term negative sequelae related to the neurobiological responses to childhood stress and trauma (Jiang et al., 2019; Heins et al., 2011; Nicholson et al, 2018; Perry, 2001; Schore, 2012; Stien & Kendall, 2006; Van Dam et al., 2012). These effects may then be inherited by subsequent generations: higher maternal ACE scores have been associated with measures of prenatal stress, autonomic nervous system reactivity, and psychopathology in her offspring (Esteves et al., 2020; Jones et al., 2019).

The link between trauma and mental illness is complex and interactive. Numerous studies have found that adults receiving treatment for severe and persistent mental illness, substance abuse, eating disorders, anxiety, and depressive disorders are highly likely to be survivors of trauma, such as childhood sexual abuse, domestic or community violence, combat-related violence, or poverty (Brown et al., 2009; Chu, 2011; Danese et al., 2009; Read, 2010; Stien & Kendall, 2006; Teicher, 2012). The majority of people served by public health mental health and substance abuse service systems have experienced repeated trauma since childhood and have been severely impacted by trauma (Grubaugh et al., 2011).

Racial trauma and the stress that results from danger related to real or perceived experiences of racial discrimination (Comas-Diaz, Hall, & Neville, 2019) – has been identified as a precipitant of PTSD symptoms and is distinguished by the ongoing nature of its threat to the affected individual, such as through racial microaggressions and vicarious experiences of bigotry (Helms, Nicolas, & Green, 2012). Higher PTSD prevalence and severity among African American and Latinx adults has been linked to a greater frequency of perceived experiences of racism and discrimination in these populations (Sibrava et al., 2019). In one large systematic review and meta-analysis, self-reported experiences with racism were correlated with negative mental health outcomes, including depression, anxiety, and PTSD (Paradies et al., 2015).

Judith Herman (1992), in her seminal book *Trauma and Recovery,* states: "Traumatic events are extraordinary, not because they occur rarely, but rather they overwhelm the ordinary human adaptation to life" (p. 33). Findings in the wake of the World Trade Center disaster indicate that many people experienced significant symptoms, such as insomnia, irritability, general anxiety, vigilance, and impaired concentration, but did not qualify for a diagnosis of PTSD as defined by the *DSM-IV-TR.* People sought help for a wide variety of disabling clinical responses, but their pathologies were not reflected in the available diagnostic categories (Amsel & Marshall, 2003). Similarly, in the absence of an identifiable Criterion A event (natural disasters, terrorist activities, war, incest, physical abuse, car accidents, or other major life-threatening events), those who experience PTSD symptoms as a result of racial trauma do not qualify for a DSM-5 PTSD diagnosis (Williams, Metzger, Leins, & DeLapp, 2018).

van der Kolk (2014) says that while single-incident traumas may sometimes account for those diagnosed with posttraumatic stress disorder (PTSD), most adults who seek psychotherapy have had numerous traumatic events and suffer from a variety of psychological problems, many of which do not fall within this diagnostic category. Broadly speaking, these are problems such as aggression, self-hatred, dissociation, somatization, depression, distrust, shame, relationship problems, and affect regulation. Studies of children have found similar results; two thirds of children with documented abuse do not suffer from PTSD but do suffer from a variety of other psychiatric disorders, such as dissociative identity disorder, borderline personality disorder, depression, substance abuse, and attention deficit hyperactivity disorder (Fellitti & Anda, 2010; Stien & Kendall, 2006; Teicher et al., 2003; Teicher, 2012).

Adults who encounter everyday hardships are also at risk. A survey of 832 people from a primary care practice found that there were more PTSD symptoms for those who had suffered stressful life events than for those who had PTSD Criterion A events (Mol et al., 2005). Relatively common life events, such as the loss of a relationship or job, result in more PTSD symptoms than an actual or threatened death (Mol et al., 2005; Robinson & Larson, 2010). Other studies confirm that even subthreshold PTSD results in significant functional impairments and a greater incidence of psychiatric disorders such as major depression, social anxiety, alcohol and drug use (McLaughlin et al., 2015; Mota et al, 2016).

Common sense dictates that suffering any emotional or physical illness is disruptive, disturbing, and stressful. Accordingly, those who experience acute or chronic illness have been found to develop post-traumatic stress symptoms, including those admitted to the ICU (Parker et al., 2015); cancer survivors (Cordova, Riba, & Spiegal, 2017); ischemic stroke patients (Stein et al., 2018); and people living with HIV (McLean & Fitzgerald, 2016). Edmondson and colleagues found that those who developed PTSD due to their acute coronary event doubled their risk of recurrent future cardiac events and mortality (2012). Negative childbirth experiences, cesarean sections, and perinatal depression are risk factors for postnatal PTSD (Ayers, Bond, Bertullies, & Wijma, 2016).

Pointedly, the experience of mental illness may in and of itself be regarded as a traumatic experience. For decades, studies have supported this possibility (McGorry et al., 1991; Meyer et al., 1999; Shaw et al., 1997). A diagnosis of PTSD plus depression and associated dissociative or borderline personality disorder appears to be a dose–response predictor for developing a chronic illness such as fibromyalgia, chronic fatigue syndrome, irritable bowel syndrome, chronic pelvic pain, and dysmenorrhea (Buskila & Cohen, 2007). Moreover, after an exhaustive review of the literature on psychosis and trauma, Morrison and colleagues (2003) state, "… it does seem that at least a significant proportion of psychotic disorders do arise as a response to trauma and that PTSD-like symptoms can be developed in response to people's experience of psychotic disorders" (p. 347). The literature suggests that trauma is both a cause and an effect of medical and psychiatric pathologies.

The above research supports Shapiro's (2001, 2012, 2018) expanded conceptualization of trauma from the Criterion A events for PTSD to include adverse life experiences that occur often and to most people, such as emotional neglect or indifference, humiliation, and family issues. For example, many childhood experiences, such as caregiver depression, chronic mother–infant misattunement, being bullied, chronic loneliness, significant loss, caregiver neglect, repeated separation from parents, betrayals, feeling stupid and humiliated in the classroom setting, abandonment, significant medical illness and procedures, relationship problems between parents, personality problems of parents, exposure to domestic violence, economic hardships, poverty, critical or negative comments from caretakers, social discrimination, prejudice, family instability, accidents, violence, frequent moves or changes of school, taking care of an alcoholic parent, and many other life events that impact the developing child, may contribute to mental health problems later in life. What is notable is that it is not just what has happened to the individual that is experienced as traumatic, but also what has not happened that should have happened, such as in situations of neglect and misattunement at critical periods of development.

The Substance Abuse and Mental Health Services Administration (SAMHSA) refers to trauma as:

> …. *experiences that cause intense physical and psychological stress reactions. It can refer to a single event, multiple events, or a set of circumstances that is experienced by an individual as physically and emotionally harmful or threatening and that has lasting adverse effects on the in-dividual's physical, social, emotional, or spiritual well-being (SAMHSA News, 2014).*

The word "trauma" is used in this book to denote this expanded conceptualization inclusive of all events and situations that are experienced by the person as overwhelming and affect brain functioning through the interruption of information processing. This disruption in brain circuitry, regulatory systems, and information processing, results in the disturbing event or situation being stored dysfunctionally, sometimes affecting the person even decades later (Shapiro, 2018). It is a basic tenet of this book that such experiences are the basis of most psychopathology. Trauma is a response – a disconnection from oneself,– not an event (Mate, 2003; Porges, 2019). It is not so much what has happened to the person, but what happens inside the person. Healing trauma involves the reconnection with self and is always possible.

An individual's response and the long-term sequelae of a disturbing event are highly individualistic and depend on a multitude of factors, such as the person's age, developmental stage, coping skills, support system, cognitive deficits, preexisting neural physiology, and the nature of the trauma. It is not just the event itself that determines the long- and short-term effects of trauma, but the individual differences that the person brings to the situation. Traumatic experiences disrupt brain functioning as mediated by genetics, social support, age, development, and many other factors. Healthy functioning of the brain is reflected in the optimal integration and coordination of neural networks. Chapter 2 discusses the neurophysiological theory and research that provide the underpinnings for the psychotherapeutic framework for this book.

A FRAMEWORK FOR PSYCHOTHERAPY PRACTICE

The adaptive information processing (AIP) model, developed by Shapiro as an explanatory theory for EMDR, is a metamodel for understanding mental health and psychopathology, and provides direction for planning therapeutic interventions (Shapiro, 2018). AIP is a metamodel because mechanisms of action for all psychotherapy approaches can be explained by the neurophysiological underpinnings of AIP about how the brain works. AIP posits that normally information is taken in through the senses and connected adaptively to other memory networks so that storing and learning occur. There is thought to be innate self-healing in the brain and just as the body strives for homeostasis, so too does the brain through the regulation and processing of information through neural transmission. However, if something is experienced as overwhelming emotionally, brain processing is interrupted owing to the massive influx of hormones and neurotransmitters. It is as if our brain is saying: "Don't forget this, this is important!" These unprocessed experiences are considered to be the basis of the symptoms of many mental health problems and psychiatric disorders (Bergmann, 2020; Cozolino, 2017; Shapiro, 2018).

Once information processing is interrupted, the memory of the event becomes fragmented. The emotion related to the experience may become disconnected from the words to describe the event and/or the sound and/or physical sensations. Thus, the fragmented memory is not integrated but stored in the brain with each component existing in discrete units that are disconnected or dissociated from each other. The memory is stored largely in implicit or unconscious memory and is experienced as being in the present once triggered. For example, a woman who was raped 40 years ago might be triggered by having sex with her partner and feel as though the rape was happening all over again, or she may be anxious and fearful around certain places or people that remind her of the event and be unaware of why she is anxious and does not connect her current anxiety to the original experience. These reactions are not in her control but come from neural associations deep within memory networks that are not connected with the conscious mind. Consciousness is defined as our subjective experience of being aware and having access to information about the experience (Siegel, 2012). It is understandable that a person who has experienced multiple traumas may not be very conscious or living in the present.

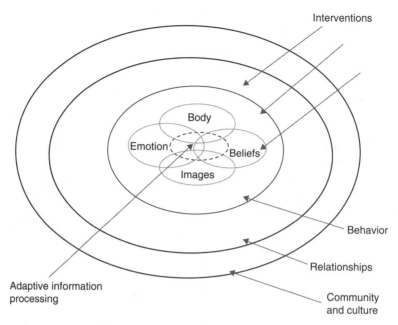

FIGURE 1.6 Where to target interventions.

Psychotherapy interventions can be designed to target any or all areas of the dis-sociated memory or experience—behavior, relationships, beliefs, the body, images, and/or emotions—to facilitate healing and promote neurophysiological harmony (see Figure 1.6). For example, the therapist using a CBT model would focus on the person's thoughts, beliefs, or behaviors; the therapist using a family therapy model would focus on the relationships and dynamics of the family; while the psychodynamic therapist would focus on emotions and thoughts assisting the person in deepening his or her understanding of how the past gets triggered and played out in the present. The EMDR therapist would target body, beliefs, images, and emotions in order to process trauma based on AIP. A change in any arena reverberates to all other dimensions for the overall purpose of facilitating healing and toward integration because all dimensions are inter-related and interconnected.

The treatment hierarchy framework for practice for this textbook based on AIP reflects a synthesis of research and theory developed by numerous clinicians and researchers (Briere & Scott, 2013; Cozolino, 2017; Davis & Weiss, 2004; Herman, 1992; Porges, 2011; Porges & Dana, 2018; Schore, 2019; Shapiro, 2018; Siegel, 2012; Wheeler, 2011). To begin the healing process, the APPN assesses where to target interventions, taking into con-sideration the patient's culture and building on the strengths and resources the person already has. In general, the lower the patient is on Maslow's hierarchy of needs, the more active the therapist must be. For example, the patient who is abusing substances, hungry, and homeless must first have physiological needs and safety met first, and the APPN attends to these needs largely through case management strategies.

The treatment hierarchy illustrates an overarching framework for therapeutic aims that must be ensured before the person can move up the levels in the triangle (see Figure 1.7). The patient's physiological needs, such as diet, sleep, and exercise, are essential to a healthy emotional life and the work of psychotherapy. Nurses are knowl-edgeable about what constitutes a healthy lifestyle and this knowledge is invaluable to integrate into psychoeducation with patients in psychotherapy. Overall, resources must be procured and stabilization guaranteed before trauma can be processed, and then a vision can be developed of a possible future. The aim is toward integration of neural

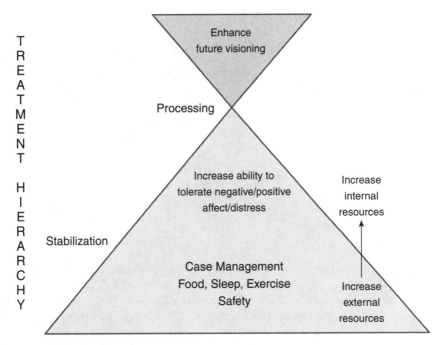

FIGURE 1.7 **Treatment** hierarchy framework for practice.

Source: Adapted from Davis, K., & Weiss, L. (2004). *Traumatology: A workshop on traumatic stress disorders.* Hamden, CT: EMDR Humanitarian Assistance Programs.

networks, of memories, of oneself and relationships, and of the person's connection in the world. The patient's ability to process information is variable, with some patients needing more stabilization so that adaptive memory and experiences are created or are reinforced if present, while other patients may be able to process information and quickly move toward integration. Stabilization strengthens and/or widens the person's RZ so that daily functioning is improved. Integration through the phases of stabilization and processing or memory reconsolidation can be accomplished through the various psychotherapeutic approaches and techniques discussed in this book.

Some psychotherapeutic approaches may have more utility than others, depending on the person's state of need, resources already present, emotional development, past traumas, and support system as well as the expertise of the therapist. The therapist's thorough and accurate assessment, as discussed in Chapter 3, helps to formulate a plan to assist the person to move upward on the treatment hierarchy to the next stage. Although treatment is discussed as a stage model, it is not static in that there is some fluidity of movement. Frequently, patients take two steps forward and then one backward; that is, often after therapeutic gain, a period of anxiety, confusion, and/or depression follows. This is because emotion is a powerful agent of change and creates disruption (Damasio, 1999). Even a positive change may have a disorganizing effect on the brain and behavior because of the proliferation of synapses that occurs with new learning (Stien & Kendall, 2006). This idea is supported by a developmental principle of all biological systems that "there can be no reorganization without disorganization" (Scott, 1979, p. 233). It is the therapist's responsibility to assist the person in understanding that the gains being made are often followed by increased sadness and anxiety. Explaining this to the person, keeping the overall plan and therapeutic aims in the foreground, and conveying hope is essential for the process and progress to continue.

BOX 1.2 Selected Stabilization Strategies

- Through therapeutic relationship
- Bibliotherapy/role play
- Case management
- Cognitive behavioral therapy
- Community resiliency model skills
- Dialectical behavioral therapy
- Education about RZ
- Managing physiological arousal
  - imagery

- Container
- Calm place
- Mindfulness/meditation
- Medication
- Stress management/education
- Provide safety
- Yoga/exercise

Stabilization

Essential to all approaches discussed in this book is providing for safety and increasing resources, if needed, to attain stabilization and a robust RZ. For positive psychotherapy outcomes, Norcross and Lambert state to "begin by leveraging the patient's resources and self-healing capacities" (2019, p. 13). Resources might include a person's positive memories of past experience, spiritual beliefs, the availability of nurturing and caring people, a sense of inner strength or a belief in oneself, and coping strategies. Techniques used during the stabilization stage are sometimes referred to as *case management* or *supportive psychotherapy* but may also include any of the strategies included in Box 1.2 and community resiliency model (CRM) skills, included in Chapter 11. Competency in case management includes the ability of the therapist to garner the necessary environmental resources on behalf of the patient and requires an active approach on the part of the therapist. Setting limits, educating, connecting the person to community resources, supporting the patient's ego functions, and assisting the patient in managing emotions are key to successful outcomes. A worksheet for treatment and case management strategies is included in Appendix 1.4 from *Seeking Safety: A Treatment Manual for PTSD and Substance Abuse*, by Najavits (2002); it is an excellent resource for case management.

Stabilization strategies assist the person to be better able to make state changes, that is, to change one's present physiology in order to function more effectively in the moment. Crucial in case management is the ability of the therapist to assess regressive and adaptive shifts in ego functioning and to recognize conflict to help the person to manage anxiety. Although the therapist may understand what is happening for the patient dynamically, this does not need to be interpreted to the person. Accurate assessment of where the person is in the change process is essential. A stage of change model is helpful in determining where the therapist needs to aim interventions. This is especially useful for interventions aimed at behavioral change. Stages of change are discussed in Chapter 9.

Along with behavioral change and shoring up external resources, if needed, internal resources often need to be increased before processing. Internal resources are less tangible than external resources, and include the person's ability to manage positive and negative emotions. Indicators that the person has sufficient internal resources include the person's ability to self-soothe, to demonstrate adequate impulse control, to identify stressful triggers, to regulate moods, and to communicate honestly. In general, the patient's resources and the traumas experienced need to be balanced. For the person who has a history of many adverse life experiences without positive memories

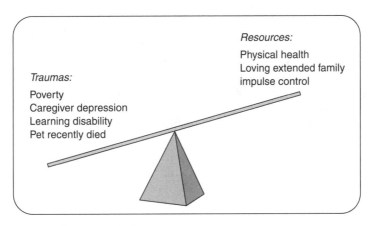

FIGURE 1.8 Trauma and resource balance.

or experiences, more resources may be needed to manage the deleterious effect of these experiences on functioning to enhance the RZ. For example, a 6-year-old, learning-disabled boy, whose dog recently died, started to wet his bed nightly and was brought to the clinic by his mother. He lived with his mother, who was single, chronically depressed, and had significant economic problems. Figure 1.8 illustrates that more resources may need to be developed for this child to counteract the imbalance between his traumas and resources or strengths. The assessment of adverse experience and resource balance is based on a comprehensive history and assessment as outlined in Chapter 3.

A stabilization checklist is included in Appendix 1.5 to help the clinician determine whether adequate stabilization has been achieved. The person does not need to meet all the criteria on this list before processing and the therapist's clinical judgment is essential in order to determine appropriate strategies. Sometimes the instability is driven by the trauma and once the traumatic memory has been processed, symptoms will dissipate. Specific strategies designed to widen or strengthen the RZ are delineated in the psychotherapy approaches included in this textbook.

Processing

After stabilization has been achieved, the person is ready to move to the next stage of processing. As represented toward the top of the treatment hierarchy in Figure 1.7, processing reflects access to all dimensions of memory: behaviors, affect, sensations, cognitions, and beliefs associated with the trauma (Shapiro, 2018). Processing usually involves assisting the person in constructing a narrative through the exploration of the meaning of significant adverse life experiences and traumas that impair functioning. Changes in physical and emotional responses occur as components of the dysfunctional memory are integrated with other, more adaptive networks. In contrast to state changes that occur in stabilization, processing creates trait changes, that is, enduring relationship and personality changes (Shapiro, 2018). The therapist assists the person in processing using the models and techniques discussed throughout this textbook. Some psychotherapy approaches involve components of stabilization as well as processing such as psychodynamic psychotherapy and EMDR therapy; others such as imaginal or in vivo exposure are designed primarily for processing a specific traumatic event. Processing strategies are included in Box 1.3.

BOX 1.3 Selected Processing Strategies

- Through therapeutic relationship
- Psychodynamic psychotherapy
- Imaginal or in vivo exposure
- Cognitive processing
- Somatic processing
- Eye movement desensitization and reprocessing

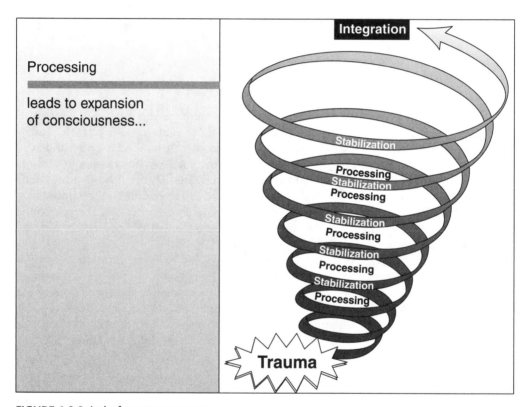

FIGURE 1.9 Spiral of treatment process.

Communication techniques can also facilitate stabilization or processing and are discussed in Chapter 4.

Processing is based on the idea that humans have an inherent information processing system that usually integrates experiences to a physiological adaptive state in which information can be taken in, and learning will occur (Shapiro, 2012, 2018). Memory is stored in neural networks that are linked together and organized around early events with associated emotions, thoughts, images, and sensations. Healthy functioning is reflected in the optimal integration and coordination of these neural networks, and this occurs through processing information. The neurophysiology underlying processing is discussed in Chapters 2 and 7.

Clinically, processing has been achieved once relationships are adaptive, work is productive, self-references are positive, there are no significant affect changes, affect is proportionate to events, and there is congruence among behavior, thoughts, and affect. A processing checklist is included in Appendix 1.6 to assist the therapist in determining whether processing has led to adaptive change. Periods of processing are usually followed by periods of destabilization, and the treatment process often looks more like a spiral alternating with interventions aimed at stabilization and then processing (Figure 1.9). Ongoing assessment and attunement to the person's therapeutic process are important in order to monitor progress and plan treatment strategies. The psychotherapeutic relationship is the vehicle for therapeutic change with the therapist's presence serving to stabilize the person and provides the foundation needed to assist the integration of dimensions of memory and all parts of the self at deeper levels of understanding. The therapeutic relationship may also facilitate processing as dimensions of earlier significant relationships through transference are triggered and reworked in the present. Empowerment and autonomy are fostered as the person moves toward envisioning and planning for the future.

CASE EXAMPLE

Ms. A is a 26-year-old married woman who works as a costume designer and seamstress for a theater company. She has been in psychotherapy numerous times since the age of 13 for past psychiatric diagnoses of major depressive disorder, bipolar II, panic disorder, and anorexia nervosa. She reports numerous psychosomatic complaints including frequent stomachaches, irritable bowel syndrome, acid reflux, headaches, restless legs syndrome, and generalized pain as well as cold chills all over her body. Her reason for seeking treatment was her anxiety and insomnia related to her loud, annoying neighbors at her condo. Ms. A's early history involved significant attachment problems with both her mother and father abusing drugs, and subsequently Ms. A was taken away from her parents and into custody by her aunt when she was 2,years,old. Ms. A said her aunt favored her own biological daughter and neglected her throughout her childhood. Her adult trauma history included two previous car accidents. On intake, she scored 63 on the Spielberger Trait Anxiety Scale; 22 on the Beck Depression Inventory; and 27 on

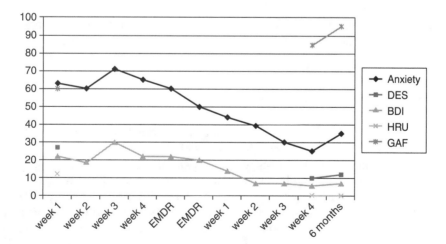

FIGURE 1.10 Ms. A's psychotherapy outcomes.

Anxiety, Spielberger trait anxiety scale; BDI, Beck depression inventory; DES, dissociative experiences scale; GAF, global assessment of functioning; HRU, health resource utilization

the Dissociative Experiences Scale. All scores were significant for anxiety, depression, and dissociation, respectively.

Because Ms. A had significant attachment problems by history, discomfort with her body and physical sensations, difficulty self-soothing, some dissociation, difficulty tolerating negative emotions, and inadequate trust of others, her RZ was quite narrow. Ms. A perceived her current problem with her neighbors as an unmanageable crisis. The RZ was explained to Ms. A: "There is a biological basis for the symptoms you are experiencing. When the nervous system is in balance we feel like our best self and are in our resilient zone. It sounds like you have been under a lot of stress lately and are being triggered by your neighbors' noise, which has knocked you out of your resilient zone so you are feeling anxious and depressed. It would be helpful to begin first with working on some strategies to help stabilize your nervous system. Would that be okay?" The beginning phase of therapy focused on developing a therapeutic alliance, teaching Ms. A stabilization strategies that were practiced in sessions such as imagery of safe/calm place (Appendix 1.7) and container exercises (included in Appendix 1.8); the Fraser Table Technique, which is an imagery exercise designed to facilitate knowledge of various parts of the self (Fraser, 1991); attachment imagery exercises (Steele, 2007); somatic awareness where she perceived feelings in her body (tracking in Chapter 11); and building resources outside therapy by increasing activities she liked such as regular exercise and yoga classes. Prozac 20 mg was also prescribed to help Ms. A manage her anxiety. Adequate resources must be present in order to ensure safe processing. EMDR therapy was integrated with these stabilization strategies to process her traumas. Ms. A was seen over a 6-month period.

At termination, Ms. A's scores on all measures showed significant improvement (see Figure 1.10). Ms. A's creativity, visual imaging skills, and humor were great assets to her in our work together. Less tangible outcomes than the reported quantitative data were qualitative outcomes, which included an integrative narrative about herself and her aunt that included a recognition of the impact of her past history; greater ability to express herself and advocate for her own needs; better emotional and physical self-regulation; a sense of security about herself and others; and greater access to full expression of emotion. Her somatic complaints greatly decreased and as illustrated in the graph in Figure 1.10, she did not need or seek medical care for her many illnesses during the course of her psychotherapy treatment in contrast to the 6 months prior to therapy when she had sought help from her primary care provider a total of 12 times. She appeared more robust and stronger at termination, stating that she had never felt this good before.

CONCLUDING COMMENTS

Psychotherapy has been identified as an important competency that all APPNs must achieve (ANA, 2013; National Panel for Psychiatric Mental Health NP Competencies, 2003; Wheeler & Haber, 2004). Nurses who are beginning graduate study in psychiatric nursing and expanding their roles to become psychotherapists have unique resources and challenges. The holistic paradigm inherent in nursing provides the context and a compass for psychotherapy practice, whereas the models of psychotherapy presented in this textbook provide the vehicle, anchored in the mooring of the healing nurse–patient relationship. Providing a context rich in resources enables further growth toward healing and wholeness. An appropriate metaphor is that of building a house with the foundation and frame necessary for support before furnishing and decorating. Providing for safety and stabilization by strengthening external and internal resources facilitates resilience so that healing can occur.

Adverse experiences have the potential to abort the wholeness of the brain, interfering with information processing, and this disruption and dysregulation, sometimes in tandem with neurobiologically encoded genetic vulnerabilities, are the basis for many mental health problems and psychiatric disorders. Psychotherapy assists in reintegration of neural networks that have become dysregulated or disconnected, enhancing the development of the brain so that continued growth and healing can occur. This framework is based on neurophysiology embedded in a holistic paradigm in that psychotherapy restores the harmony, balance, connection, and integration of neural networks on a cellular level, which is reflected in deeper connections with oneself and others. The neurophysiological basis for this model is discussed in Chapter 2.

DISCUSSION QUESTIONS

1. In light of Benner's model, where do you see yourself in relation to your past practice of nursing, and where are you now in your nurse psychotherapy practice?
2. How does your choice of intervention affect the outcome of treatment?
3. How can a person be healed and still have a diagnosed psychiatric disorder? How is curing different from healing? How do you know when healing has occurred?
4. Discuss a time when you and your patient had a different perception of health and illness and what this experience was like for you. How was this worked out then, and what would you do differently now?
5. Discuss how your self-understanding may affect your work with your patient. How has your own growth changed since you first began to work with others? Include your thoughts about how your prior practice as a nurse can be a help or hindrance to your practice as a psychotherapist.
6. What factors in your life led you to a nurse psychotherapist's role?
7. Discuss relationship and resilience and give a clinical example of each from your past nursing practice.
8. Describe a patient you have worked with, explain the person's traumas and resources, and discuss in general the priorities for treatment using the practice treatment hierarchy.

REFERENCES

Afifi, T. O., Mota, N. P., Dasiewicz, P., MacMillan, H. L., & Sareen, J. (2012). Physical punishment and mental disorders: Results from a nationally representative US sample. *Pediatrics, 130*, 184–192. doi:10.1542/peds.2011-2947

American Hospital Association. (2019). *For the 17th year in a row, nurses top Gallup's poll of most trusted profession*. Retrieved from https://www.aha.org/news/insights-and-analysis/2019-01-09-17th-year-row-nurses-top-gallups-poll-most-trusted-profession

American Nurses Association. (2013). *Psychiatric-mental health nursing: Scope and standards of practice*. Washington, DC: Author.

American Nurses Credentialing Center. (2020). *Psychiatric mental health nurse practitioner eligibility & instructions*. Silver Spring, MD: American Nurses Credentialing Center, American Nurses Association. Retrieved from https://www.nursingworld.org/our-certifications/psychiatric-mental-health-nurse-practitioner/

American Psychiatric Association. (2013). *Diagnostic and statistical manual of mental disorders* (5th ed.). Washington, DC: American Psychiatric Publishing.

Amsel, L., & Marshall, R. D. (2003). Clinical management of subsyndromal psychological sequelae of the 9/11 terror attacks. In S. Coates, J. Rosenthal, & D. Schechter (Eds.), *September 11: Trauma and human bonds* (pp. 75–97). Hillsdale, NJ: Analytic Press.

Arseneault, L., Cannon, M., Fisher, J., Polanczyk, G., Moffitt, T. E., & Caspi, A. (2011). Childhood trauma and children's emerging psychotic symptoms: A genetically sensitive longitudinal cohort study. *American Journal of Psychiatry, 168,* 65–72. doi:10.1176/appi.ajp.2010.10040567

Ayers, S., Bond, R., Bertullies, S., & Wijma, K. (2016). The aetiology of post-traumatic stress following childbirth: a meta-analysis and theoretical framework. *Psychological Medicine, 46*(6), 1121-1134.

Balsam, R., & Balsam, A. (1974). *Becoming a psychotherapist: A clinical primer.* Boston, MA: Little Brown.

Barrett, L. F. (2017). *How emotions are made: The secret life of the brain.* Boston, MA: Houghton Mifflin Harcourt.

Beeber, L. (1995). The one-to-one nurse patient relationship in psychiatric nursing: The next generation. In C. A. Anderson (Ed.), *Psychiatric nursing 1974–1994: A report on the state of the art* (pp. 9–36). St. Louis, MO: Mosby Year Book.

Benner, P. (1984). *From novice to expert.* Menlo Park, CA: Addison-Wesley.

Bergmann, U. (2020). *Neurobiological foundations for EMDR practice* (2nd ed.). New York, NY: Springer Publishing Company.

Bourne, E. J. (2015). *The anxiety and phobia workbook* (6th ed.). Oakland, CA: New Harbinger.

Braveman, P., & Barclay, C. (2009). Health disparities beginning in childhood: A life-course perspective. *Pediatrics, 124*(Suppl. 3), 163–175. doi:10.1542/peds.2009-1100d

Briere, J., & Scott, C. (2013). *Principles of trauma therapy: A guide to symptoms, evaluation, and treatment* (2nd ed.). Thousand Oaks, CA: Sage.

Brown, D. W., Anda, R. F., Tiemeier, H., Felitti, V. J., Edwards, V. J., Croft, J. B., & Giles, W. H. (2009). Adverse childhood experiences and the risk of premature mortality. *American Journal of Preventive Medicine, 37,* 389–396. doi:10.1016/j.amepre.2009.06.021

Bunkers, S. S. (2009). The power and possibility in listening. *Nursing Science Quarterly, 23*(1), 22–27. doi:10.1177/0894318409353805

Burke, B. T., Miller, B. F., Proser, M., Petterson, S. M., Bazemore, A. W., & Phillips, R. L. (2013). A needs-based method for estimating the behavioral health staff needs of community health centers. *BMC Health Services Research, 13,* 245. doi:10.1186/1472-6963-13-245

Buskila, D., & Cohen, H. (2007). Comorbidity of fibromyalgia and psychiatric disorders. *Current Science, 11*(5), 333–338. doi:10.1007/s11916-007-0214-4

Chu, J. A. (2011). *Rebuilding shattered lives: Treating complex PTSD and dissociative disorders* (2nd ed.). New York, NY: John Wiley & Sons.

Cloos, J.-M., & Ferreira, V. (2009). Current use of benzodiazepines in anxiety disorders. *Current Opinion in Psychiatry, 22*(1), 90–95. doi:10.1097/YCO.0b013e32831a473d

Coghlan, A. (2011). Epigenetic clue to schizophrenia and bipolar disorder. *New Scientist.* Retrieved from http://www.newscientist.com/article/mg21128323.400-epigenetic-clue-to-schizophrenia-and-bipolar-disorder.html

Comas-Diaz, L. Hall, G. N., & Neville, H. A. (2019). Racial trauma: Theory, research, and healing: Introduction to the special issue. *American Psychologist, 74*(1), 1-5.

Cordova, M. J., Riba, M. B., & Spiegel, D. (2017). Post-traumatic stress disorder and cancer. *The Lancet. Psychiatry, 4*(4), 330-338.

Cozolino, L. (2017). *The neuroscience of psychotherapy: Healing the social brain* (3rd ed.). New York, NY: W. W. Norton.

Dahlgaard, J., Jorgensen, M. M., van der Velden, A. M., Sumbundu, A., Gregersen, N., Olsen, R. K., . . . Mehlsen, M. Y. (2019). Mindfulness, health, and longevity. In S. I. S. Rattan & M. Kyriazis (Eds.), *The science of hormesis in health and longevity* (pp. 243–256). San Diego, CA: Academic Press.

Damasio, A. (1999). *The feeling of what happens: Body and emotion in the making of consciousness.* New York, NY: Harcourt Brace.

Danese, A., Moffit, T. E., Harrington, H., Milne, B. J., Polanczyk, G., Pariante, C. M., . . . Caspi, A. (2009). Adverse childhood experiences and adult risk factors for age-related disease: Depression, inflammation, and clustering of metabolic risk markers. *Archives of Pediatrics & Adolescent Medicine, 163*(12), 1135–1143. doi:10.1001/archpediatrics.2009.214

D'Antonio, P., Beeber, L., Sills, G., & Naegle, M. (2014). The future in the past: Hildegard Peplau and interpersonal relations in nursing. *Nursing Inquiry, 21,* 311–317. doi:10.1111/nin.12056

Davis, K., & Weiss, L. (2004). *Traumatology: A workshop on traumatic stress disorders.* Hamden, CT: EMDR Humanitarian Assistance Programs.

De Bellis, M. (2001). Developmental traumatology: The psychobiological development of maltreated children and its implications for research treatment, and policy. *Development and Psychopathology, 13*, 539–564. doi:10.1017/s0954579401003078

Delaney, K. R., Drew, B. L., & Rushton, A. (2019). Report on the APNA national psychiatric mental health advanced practice registered nurse survey. *Journal of the American Psychiatric Nurses Association, 25*(2), 146–155. doi:10.1177/1078390318777873

Doan, S. N., Tardif, T., Miller, A., Olson, S., Kessler, D., Felt, B., & Wang, L. (2017). Consequences of 'tiger' parenting: A cross–cultural study of maternal psychological control and children's cortisol stress response. *Developmental Science, 20*(3), e12404. doi:10.1111/desc.12404

Dossey, B., & Keegan, L. (2013). *Holistic nursing: A handbook for practice* (6th ed.). Burlington, MA: Jones & Bartlett.

Dracup, K., Conenwett, L., Meleis, A., & Benner, P. (2005). Reflections on the doctorate of nursing practice. *Nursing Outlook, 53*, 177–182. doi:10.1016/j.outlook.2005.06.003

Drew, B., & Delaney, K. R. (2009). National survey of psychiatric mental health advanced practice nursing: Development, process and findings. *Journal of the American Psychiatric Nurses Association, 15*, 101–110. doi:10.1177/1078390309333544

Edmondson, D., Richardson, S., Falzon, L., Davidson, K. W., Mills, M. A., & Neria, Y. (2012). Posttraumatic stress disorder prevalence and risk of recurrence in acute coronary syndrome patients: A meta-analytic review. *PLOS ONE, 7*(6), e38915. doi:10.1371/journal.pone.0038915

Elklit, A., & Blum, A. (2011). Psychological adjustment one year after the diagnosis of breast cancer: A prototype study of delayed post-traumatic stress disorder. *British Journal of Clinical Psychology, 50*, 350–363. doi:10.1348/014466510X527676

Esteves, K. C., Jones, C. W., Wade, M., Callerame, K., Smith, A. K., Theall, K. P., & Drury, S. S. (2020). Adverse childhood experiences: Implications for offspring telomere length and psychopathology. *The American Journal of Psychiatry, 177*(1), 47-57.

Felitti, V. J., & Anda, R. F. (2010). The relationship of adverse childhood experiences to adult medical disease, psychiatric disorders and sexual behavior: Implications for healthcare. In R. Lanius, E. Vermetten, & C. Pain (Eds.), *The impact of early life trauma on health and disease: The hidden epidemic* (pp. 77–87). Cambridge, UK: Cambridge University Press. doi:10.1017/CBO9780511777042.010

Felitti, V. J., Anda, R. F., Nordenberg, D., Williamson, D. F., Spitz, A. M., Edwards, V., . . . Marks, J. S. (1998). Relationship of childhood abuse and household dysfunction to many of the leading causes of death in adults: The adverse childhood experiences (ACE) study. *American Journal of Preventive Medicine, 14*(4), 245–258. doi:10.1016/S0749-3797(98)00017-8

Foli, K. J., & Thompson, J. R. (2019). *The influence of psychological trauma in nursing.* Indianapolis, IN: Sigma Theta Tau International.

Forchuk, C., Westwell, J., Martin, M. L., Azzapardi, W. B., Kosterewa-Tolman, D., & Hux, M. (1998). Factors influencing movement of chronic psychiatric patients from the orientation of the working phase of the nurse-patient relationship on an inpatient unit. *Perspectives in Psychiatric Care, 34*, 36–45. doi:10.1111/j.1744-6163.1998.tb00998.x

Fraser, G. (1991). The dissociative table technique: A strategy for working with ego states in dissociative disorders and ego state therapy. *Dissociation, 4*(8), 205–213.

Gallup. (2020). *Nurses continue to rate highest in honesty, ethics.* Retrieved from https://news.gallup.com/poll/274673/nurses-continue-rate-highest-honesty-ethics.aspx

Gilson, G., & Kaplan, S. (2000). *The therapeutic interweave in EMDR: Before and beyond: A manual for EMDR trained clinicians.* New Hope, PA: EMDR Humanitarian Assistance Programs.

Grubaugh, A. L., Zinzow, H. M., Paul, L., Egede, L. W., & Freuh, C. B. (2011). Trauma exposure and posttraumatic stress disorder in adults with severe mental illness: A critical review. *Clinical Psychology Review, 31*, 883–899. doi:10.1016/j.cpr.2011.04.003

Habibović, M., van den Broek, K., Alings, M., Van der Voort, P. H., & Denollet, J. (2011). Post-traumatic stress 18 months following cardioverter defibrillator implantation: Shocks, anxiety, and personality. *Health Psychology, 31*(2), 186–193. doi:10.1037/a0024701

Hankin, B. L., & Abela, J. (2005). *Development of psychopathology: A vulnerability-stress perspective.* Thousand Oaks, CA: Sage.

Heins, M., Simons, C., Lataster, T., Pfeifer, S., Vermissen, D., Lardinois, M., . . . Myin-Germeys, I. (2011). Childhood trauma and psychosis: A case-control and case-sibling comparison across different levels of genetic liability, psychopathology, and type of trauma. *American Journal of Psychiatry, 168*(12), 1286–1294. doi:10.1176/appi.ajp.2011.10101531

Helms, J. E., Nicolas, G., & Green, C. E. (2012) Racism and ethnoviolence as trauma: Enhancing profressional and research training. *Traumatology, 18*(1), 65-74.

Herman, J. (1992). *Trauma and recovery.* New York, NY: Basic Books.

Herrman, H., Stewart, D., Diaz-Grandos, N., Berger, E., Jackson, B., & Yuen, T. (2011). What is resilience? *The Canadian Journal of Psychiatry, 65*(5), 258–265. doi:10.1177/070674371105600504

Horowitz, A. V. (1982). *The social control of mental illness.* New York, NY: Academic Press.

Hughes, K., Bellis, M. A., Hardcastle, K. A., Sethi, D., Butchart, A., Mikton, C., Jones, L., & Dunne, M. P. (2017). The effect of multiple adverse childhood experiences on health: a systematic review and meta-analysis. *The Lancet. Public Health, 2*(8), e.356-e366.

Jennings, A. (2004). *Models for developing trauma-informed behavioral health systems and trauma-specific services.* Retrieved from http://theannainstitute.org/MDT.pdf

Jiang, S., Postovit, L, Cattaneo, A., Binder, E. & Aitchison K. (2019). Epigenetic modifications in stress response genes associated with childhood trauma. *Frontiers in Psychiatry*, 08, November. doi:10.3389/fpsyt.2019.00808

Jones, C. W., Esteves, K. C., Gray, S., Clarke, T. N., Callerame, K., Theall, K. P., & Drury, S. S. (2019). The transgenerational transmission of maternal adverse childhood experiences (ACEs): Insights from placental aging and infant autonomic nervous system reactivity. *Psychoneuroendocrinology, 106*, 20-27.

Kessler, R. C., Aguilar-Gaxiola, S., Alonso, J., Benjet, C., Bromet, E. J., Cardoso, G., . . . Koenen, K. C. (2017). Trauma and PTSD in the WHO world mental health surveys. *European Journal of Psychotraumatology, 8* (suppl. 5), 1353383.

Kilpatrick, D. G., Resnick, H. S., Milanak, M. E., Miller, M. W., Keyes, K. M., & Friedman, M. J. (2013). National estimates of exposure to traumatic events and PTSD prevalence using *DSM-IV* and *DSM-5* criteria. *Journal of Traumatic Stress, 26*(5), 537–547. doi:10.1002/jts.21848

Kronos. (2017). *Employment engagement in nursing.* Retrieved from https://www.kronos.com/about-us/newsroom/kronos-survey-finds-nurses-love-what-they-do-though-fatigue-pervasive-problem

Lego, S. (1992). Biological psychiatry and psychiatric nursing in America. *Archives of Psychiatric Nursing, 6*, 147–150. doi:10.1016/0883-9417(92)90025-E

Lego, S. (1999). The one-to-one nurse-patient relationship. *Perspectives in Psychiatric Care, 35*(4), 4–22. doi:10.1111/j.1744-6163.1999.tb00591.x

Levine, S., Lalufer, A., Stein, E., Hamama-Raz, Y., & Solomon, Z. (2009). Examining the relationship between resilience and posttraumatic growth. *Journal of Traumatic Stress, 22*(4), 282–286. doi:10.1002/jts.20409

Li, X., Wang, J., Zhou, J., Huang, P., & Li, J. (2017). The association between post-traumatic stress disorder and shorter telomere length: A systematic review and metaanalysis. *Journal of Affective Disorders, 218*, 322–326. doi:10.1016/j.jad.2017.03.048

Li, Y., Cao, F., Cao, D., & Liu, J. (2015). Nursing students' post-traumatic growth, emotional intelligence and psychological resilience. *Journal of Psychiatric and Mental Health Nursing, 22*, 326–332. doi:10.1111/jpm.12192

Liddell, B. J., & Jobson, L. (2016). The impact of cultural differences in self-representation on the neural substrates of posttraumatic stress disorder. *European Journal of Psychotraumatology, 7*(1), 30464. doi:10.3402/ejpt.v7.30464

Livingston, J. D., & Boyd, J. E. (2010). Correlates and consequences of internalized stigma for people living with mental illness: A systematic review and meta-analysis. *Social Science Medicine, 71*, 2150–2161. doi:10.1016/j.socscimed.2010.09.030

Luhrmann, T. M. (2000). *Of two minds: An anthropologist looks at American psychiatry.* New York, NY: Vintage Books.

MacDonald, A., & Schulz, S. C. (2009). What we know: Findings that every theory of schizophrenia should explain. *Schizophrenia Bulletin, 35*(3), 493–508. doi:10.1093/schbul/sbp017

Ma-Kellams, C. (2014). Cross-cultural differences in somatic awareness and interoceptive accuracy: A review of the literature and directions for future research. *Frontiers in Psychology, 5*, 1379. doi:10.3389/fpsyg.2014.01379

Mariano, C. (2013). Holistic nursing: Scope and standards of practice. In B. Dossey & L. Keegan (Eds.), *Holistic nursing: A handbook for practice* (6th ed., pp. 59–84). Burlington, MA: Jones & Bartlett.

Maslow, A. H. (1972). *The farther reaches of human nature*. New York, NY: Viking.

Mate, G. (2003). *When the body says NO*. New York, NY: John Wiley & Sons.

McGorry, P. D., Chanen, A., McCarthy, E., van Riel, R., McKenzie, D., & Singh, B. S. (1991). Posttraumatic stress disorder following recent-onset psychosis: An unrecognized postpsychotic syndrome. *The Journal of Nervous and Mental Disease, 179*, 253–258. doi:10.1097/00005053-199105000-00002

McKivergin, M. J. (1997). The nurse as an instrument of healing. In B. M. Dossey (Ed.), *Core curriculum for holistic nursing* (pp. 17–25). Gaithersburg, MD: Aspen.

McLaughlin, K. A., Koenen, K. C., Friedman, M. J., Ruscio, A. M., Karam, E. G., Shahly, V., . . . Kessler, R. C. (2015). Subthreshold posttraumatic stress disorder in the World Health Organization world mental health surveys. *Biological Psychiatry, 77*(4), 375–384. doi:10.1016/j.biopsych.2014.03.028

McLean, C. P., & Fitzgerald, H. (2016). Treating posttraumatic stress symptoms amoving people living with HIV: a criti cal review of intervention trials. *Current Psychiatry Reports, 18*(9), 83.

Mehta, S., & Farina, A. (1997). Is being "sick" really better? Effect of the disease view of mental disorder on stigma. *Journal of Social and Clinical Psychology, 16*, 405–419. doi:10.1521/jscp.1997.16.4.405

Meyer, H., Taiminen, T., Vuori, T., Aeijaelae, A., & Helenius, H. (1999). Posttraumatic stress disorder symptoms related to psychosis and acute involuntary hospitalization in schizophrenic and delusional patients. *Journal of Nervous and Mental Disease, 187*, 343–352. doi:10.1097/00005053-199906000-00003

Miller-Karas, E. (2015). *Building resilience to trauma*. New York, NY: Routledge.

Mintzer, L., Stuber, M., Seacord, D., Castaneda, B. A., Mesrkhani, V., & Glover, D. (2005). Traumatic stress symptoms in adolescent organ transplant recipients. *Pediatrics, 115*(6), 1640–1644. doi:10.1542/peds.2004-0118

Mol, S., Arntz, A., Metsemakers, J., Dinant, G.-J., Vilters-Van Montfort, P., & Knottnerus, A. (2005). Symptoms of post-traumatic stress disorder after non-traumatic events: Events from an open population study. *British Journal of Psychiatry, 186*, 494–499. doi:10.1192/bjp.186.6.494

Moncher, F. J., & Prinz, R. J. (1991). Treatment fidelity in outcome studies. *Clinical Psychology Review, 11*, 247–266. doi:10.1016/0272-7358(91)90103-2

Morrison, A., Frame, L., & Larkin, W. (2003). Relationship between trauma and psychosis: A review and integration. *British Journal of Clinical Psychology, 42*, 331–353. doi:10.1348/014466503322528892

Morse, J. M., Solberg, S. M., Neander, W. L., Bottorff, J. L., & Johnson, J. L. (1990). Concepts of caring and caring as a concept. *Advances in Nursing Science, 13*(1), 1–14. doi:10.1097/00012272-199009000-00002

Mota, N. P., Tsai, J., Sareen, J., Marx, B. P., Wisco, B. E., Harpaz-Rotem, L., . . . Pietrzak, R. H. (2016). High burden of subthreshold DSM5 post-traumatic stress disorder in U.S. military veterans. *World Psychiatry, 15* (2), 185–186. doi:10.1002/wps.20313

Najavits, L. M. (2002). *Seeking safety: A treatment manual for PTSD and substance abuse*. New York, NY: Guilford Press.

National Institute of Mental Health. (2009). *Schizophrenia and bipolar disorder share genetic roots: Chromosomal hotspot of immunity/gene expression regulation implicated*. Retrieved from https://www.nih.gov/news-events/news-releases/schizophrenia-bipolar-disorder-share-genetic-roots

National Organization of Nurse Practitioner Faculties. (2013). *Population-focused nurse practitioner competencies*. Retrieved from https://c.ymcdn.com/sites/nonpf.site-ym.com/resource/resmgr/competencies/populationfocusnpcomps2013.pdf

National Panel for Psychiatric Mental Health NP Competencies. (2003). *Psychiatric-mental health nurse practitioner competencies*. Washington, DC: National Organization of Nurse Practitioner Faculties. Retrieved from https://www.apna.org/files/public/NOPH_COMPETENCIES.pdf

Nicholson, W., Durand, S., Vance, D., McGuinness, T., & Carpenter, J. (2018). *Trauma-based disorders and the cardio-neural mechanisms involved in dysfunctional self-regulation*. Presented at the 2018 American Psychiatric Nurses Association Pre-Conference. Columbus, Ohio https://e-learning.apna.org/products/1035-18-trauma-based-disorders-and-the-cardio-neural-mechanisms-involved-in-dysfunctional-self-regulation

Norcross, J. C., & Lambert, M. J. (2019). *Psychotherapy relationships that work*. (3rd ed., Vol. 1). New York, NY: Oxford University Press.

Ogden, P., Minton, K., & Pain, C. (2006). *Trauma and the body: A sensorimotor approach to psychotherapy*. New York, NY: W. W. Norton.

Papale, L. A., Seltzer, L. J., Madrid, A., Pollak, S. D., & Alisch, R. S. (2018). Differentially methylated genes in saliva are linked to childhood stress. *Scientific Reports, 8*, 10785. doi:10.1038/s41598-018-29107-0

Paradies, Y., Ben, J., Denson, N., Elias, A., Priest, N., Pieterse, A., Gupta, A., Kelaher, M., & Gee, G. (2015). Racism as a determinant of health: A systematic review and meta-analysis. *PloS one, 10*(9), e0138511.

Parker, A. M., Sricharoenchai, T., Raparla, S., Schneck, K. W., Bienvenu, O. J., & Needham, D. M. (2015). Post traumatic stress disorder in critical illness survivors: a metaanalysis. *Critical Care Medicine, 43*(5), 1121-1129.

Peplau, H. (1991). *Interpersonal relations in nursing: A conceptual frame of reference for psychodynamic nursing*. New York, NY: Springer Publishing Company.

Perry, B. D. (2001). The neurodevelopmental impact of violence in childhood. In D. Schetky & E. P. Benedek (Eds.), *Textbook of child and adolescent forensic psychiatry* (pp. 221–238). Washington, DC: American Psychiatric Press.

Plakun, E., Sudak, D. M., & Goldberg, D. (2009). The Y model: An integrated, evidence-based approach to teaching psychotherapy competencies. *Journal of Psychiatric Practice, 15*, 5–11. doi:10.1037/a0022123

Porges, S. (2019, March 31). *The emergence of polyvagal informed therapies in the treatment of trauma*. Presented at The World Congress on Complex Trauma: Research | Intervention | Innovation.New York, NY.

Porges, S. W. (2011). *The polyvagal theory*. New York, NY: W. W. Norton.

Porges, S. W. & Dana, D. (Eds.). (2018). *Clinical applications of the polyvagal theory: The emergence of polyvagal informed therapies*. New York, NY: W. W. Norton.

Raingruber, B. (2003). Nurture: The fundamental significance of relationship as a paradigm for mental health nursing. *Perspectives in Psychiatric Care, 39*(3), 104–112, 132–135. doi:10.1111/j.1744-6163.2003.00104.x

Read, J. (2010). Can poverty drive you mad? 'Schizophrenia', socio-economic status and the case for primary prevention. *New Zealand Journal of Psychology, 39*(2), 7–19. Retrieved from https://www.psychology.org.nz/wp-content/uploads/NZJP-Vol392-2010-2-Read.pdf

Robinson, J. S., & Larson, C. (2010). Are traumatic events necessary to elicit symptoms of post-traumatic stress? *Psychological Trauma: Theory, Research, Practice & Policy, 2*(2), 71–76. doi:10.1037/a0018954(2010)

Rogers, C. R. (1951). *Client-centered therapy: Its current practice, implications, and theory*. Boston, MA: Houghton Mifflin.

Sacks, V., & Murphey, D. (2018, February 20). *The prevalence of adverse childhood experiences, nationally, by state, and by race/ethnicity*. Bethesda, MD: Child Trends. Retrieved from https://www.childtrends.org/publications/prevalence-adverse-childhood-experiences-nationally-state-race-ethnicity

Safran, J. D., & Muran, J. C. (2000). *Negotiating the therapeutic alliance*. New York, NY: Guilford Press.

SAMSHA (2020). Recovery and recovery support. Retrieved from https://www.samhsa.gov/find-help/recovery

Scaer, R. (2005). *The trauma spectrum: Hidden wounds and human resiliency*. New York, NY: W. W. Norton.

Schoenhofer, S. O. (2002). Philosophical underpinnings of an emergent methodology for nursing as caring inquiry. *Nursing Science Quarterly, 15*, 275–280. doi:10.1177/089431802320559173

Schore, A. (2019). *Right brain psychotherapy*. New York, NY: W. W. Norton.

Scott, J. (1979). Critical periods in organizational processes. In F. Falker & J. Tanner (Eds.), *Human growth neurobiology and nutrition* (Vol. 3, pp. 223–243). New York, NY: Plenum Press.

Seng, J. S., Graham-Bermann, S. A., Clark, M. K., McCarthy, A. M., & Ronis, D. L. (2005). Posttraumatic stress disorder and physical comorbidity among female children and adolescents: Results from service-use data. *Pediatrics, 116*(6), e767–e776. doi:10.1542/peds.2005-0608

Shapiro, F. (2012). *Getting past your past: Take control of your life with self-help techniques from EMDR therapy*. New York, NY: Rodale.

Shapiro, F. (2018). *Eye movement desensitization and reprocessing (EMDR)* (3rd ed.). New York, NY: Guilford Press.

Shaw, K., McFarlane, A., & Bookless, C. (1997). The phenomenology of traumatic reactions to psychotic illness. *The Journal of Nervous and Mental Disease, 185*, 434–441. doi:10.1097/00005053-199707000-00003

Shonkoff, J. P. (2010). Building a new bio-developmental framework to guide the future of early childhood policy. *Child Development, 81*(1), 357–367. doi:10.1111/j.1467-8624.2009.01399.x

Shonkoff, J. P., & Garner, A. S. (2012). The lifelong effects of early childhood adversity and toxic stress. *Pediatrics, 129*(1), 232–246. doi:10.1542/peds.2011-2663

Sibrava, N. J., Bjornsson, A. S., Perez Benitez, A. C. I., Moitra, E., Weisberg, R. B., & Keller, M. B. (2019). Posttraumatic stress disorder in African American and Latinx adults: Clinical course and the role of racial and ethnic discrimination. *American Psychologist, 74*(1), 101-116.

Siegel, D. (2012). *The developing mind, 2nd edition*. New York, NY: The Guilford Press.

Siegel, R. S., & Rosen, L. C. (1962). Character style and anxiety tolerance: A study of intrapsychic change. In H. Strupp & L. Luborsky (Eds.), *Research in psychotherapy* (Vol. 2, pp. 206–217). Washington, DC: American Psychological Association.

Siu, B. W., Ng, B. F., Li, V. C., Yeung, Y.-M., Lee, M. K., & Leung, A. Y. (2012). Mental health recovery for psychiatric inpatient services: Perceived importance of the elements of recovery. *East Asian Archive of Psychiatry, 22*, 39–48. Retrieved from https://www.easap.asia/index.php/find-issues/past-issue/item/151-1202-v22n2-39-oa

Smoller, J. W. (2016). The genetics of stress-related disorders: PTSD, depression, and anxiety disorders. *Neuropsychopharmacology, 14*(1), 297–319. doi:10.1038/npp.2015.266

Smoyak, S. (1990). The nurse psychotherapist as unique practitioner. In J. Durham & S. Hardin (Eds.), *The nurse psychotherapist in private practice* (pp. 15–24). New York, NY: Springer Publishing Company.

Souza-Talarico, J. N., Plusquellec, P., Lupien, S. J., Fiocco, A., & Suchecki, D. (2014). Cross-country differences in basal and stress-induced cortisol secretion in older adults. *PLOS ONE, 9*(8), e105968. doi:10.1371/journal.pone.0105968

Steele, A. (2007). *Developing a secure self: An attachment-based approach to adult psychotherapy*. Gabriola, BC, Canada: Author.

Stein, L. A., Goldmann, E., Zamzam, A., Luciano, J. M., Messe, S. R., Cucchiara, B. L., Kasner, S. E., & Mullen, M. T. (2018). Association between anxiety, depression, and post-traumatic stress disorder and outcomes after ischemic stroke. *Frontiers in Neurology, 9*, 890.

Stien, P., & Kendall, J. (2006). *Psychological trauma and the developing brain*. New York, NY: Hawthorne Press.

Strupp, H. H., & Anderson, T. (1997). On the limitations of treatment manual. *Clinical Psychology: Science and Practice, 4*, 76–82. doi:10.1111/j.1468-2850.1997.tb00101.x

Substance Abuse and Mental Health Services Administration [SAMHSA]. (2012) Trauma and justice strategic initiative. Retrieved from https://www.ncbi.nlm.nih.gov/books/NBK207192/

Substance Abuse and Mental Health Services Administration. (2012a). With peer support, recovery is possible. *SAMHSA Newsletter, 20*(3), 6–7. Retrieved from https://taadas.s3.amazonaws.com/files/0fd5cc121bdcc1b4089d24665849b552-Preventing%20Suicide%20Across%20the%20Nation%20Fall%202012.pdf

Substance Abuse and Mental Health Services Administration. (2020). *Recovery https://www.samhsa.gov/find-help/recovery*. Retrieved from http://www.apna.org/files/public/Recovery_to_Practice_Overview.pdf

Suglia, S. F., Koenen, K. C., Boynton-Jarrett, R., Chan, P. S., Clark, C. J., Danese, A., . . . Zachariah, J. P. (2018). Childhood and adolescent adversity and cardiometabolic outcomes: A scientific statement from the American Heart Association. Circulation, 137(5), e15–e28. doi:10.1161/CIR.0000000000000536

Substance Abuse and Mental Health Services Administration. (n.d) Resilience & Stress Management Retrieved from https://www.samhsa.gov/dbhis-collections/resilience-stress-management

Sullivan, H. S. (1947). *Conceptions of modern psychiatry*. Washington, DC: William Alanson White Institute.

Teicher, M., Polcari, A., Andersen, S., Anderson, C. M., & Navalta, C. (2003). Neurobiological effects of childhood stress and trauma. In S. Coates, J. Rosenthal, & D. Schechter (Eds.), *September 11: Trauma and human bonds* (pp. 211–238). Hillsdale, NJ: Analytic Press.

Thomas, J. D., Finch, L. P., Schoenhofer, S. O., & Green, A. (2004). The caring relationships created by nurse practitioners and the ones nursed: Implications for practice. *Topics in Advanced Practice Nursing eJournal*, 4(4). Retrieved from https://www.medscape.com/viewarticle/496420

Truijens, F., Zühlke van Hulzen, L., & Vanheule, S. (2019). To manualize, or not to manualize: Is that still the question? A systematic review of empirical evidence for manual superiority in psychological treatment. *Journal of Clinical Psychology*, 75(3), 329–343. doi:10.1002/jclp.22712

Tryon, G. S., & Winograd, G. (2002). Goal consensus and collaboration. In J. Norcross (Ed.), *Psychotherapy relationships that work* (pp. 109–125). New York, NY: Oxford University Press.

van Dam, D. S., van der Ven, E., Velthorst, E., Selten, J. P., Morgan, C., & de Haan L. (2012). Childhood bullying and the association with psychosis in non-clinical and clinical samples: A review and meta-analysis. *Psychological Medicine*, 42(12), 2463–2474. doi:10.1017/S0033291712000360

Vanderhoef, D. M., & Delaney, K. R. (2017). National organization of nurse practitioner faculties: Psychiatric mental health survey. *Journal of the American Psychiatric Nurses Association*, 23, 159–165. doi:10.1177/1078390316685154

van der Kolk, B. (2014). *The body keeps the score*. New York, NY: Penguin Books.

Varese, F., Smeets, F., Drukker, M., Lieverse, R., Lataster, T., Viechtbauer, W., . . . Bentall, R. P. (2012). Childhood adversities increase the risk of psychosis: A meta-analysis of patient-control, prospective and cross-sectional cohort studies. *Schizophrenia Bulletin*, 38(4), 661–671. doi:10.1093/schbul/sbs050

Wachtel, P. (2011). *Therapeutic communication: Knowing what to say when* (2nd ed.). New York, NY: Guilford Press.

Watson, J. (2012). *Jean Watson's theory of caring*. Retrieved from http://currentnursing.com/nursing_theory/Watson.html

Wheeler, K. (2011). A relationship-based model for psychiatric nursing practice. *Perspectives in Psychiatric Care*, 47(3), 151–159. doi:10.1111/j.1744-6163.2010.00285

Wheeler, K., & Delaney, K. (2005). Challenges and realities of teaching psychotherapy: A survey of psychiatric-mental health nursing graduate programs. *Perspectives in Psychiatric Care*, 44(2), 72–80. doi:10.1111/j.1744-6163.2008.00156.x

Wheeler, K., & Haber, J. (2004). Development of psychiatric nurse practitioner competencies: Opportunities for the 21st century. *Journal of the American Psychiatric Nursing Association*, 10(3), 129–138. doi:10.1177/1078390304266218

Wheeler, K. & Phillips, K. (2019). The development of trauma and resilience competencies for nursing education. *Journal of the American Psychiatric Nurses Association*. Advance online publication. doi:10.1177/1078390319878779

Williams, M. T., Metzger, I. W., Leins, C., & DeLapp, C. (2018). Assessing racial trauma within a DSM-5 frame work: The UCONN Racial/Ethnic Stress & Trauma Survey. *Practice Innovations*, 3(4), 242-260.

World Health Organization. (2016). *Child maltreatment: Key facts*. Retrieved from http://www.who.int/news-room/fact-sheets/detail/child-maltreatment

Yalom, I. D., & Ferguson, N. (2002). *The gift of therapy: An open letter to a new generation of therapists and their patients*. New York, NY: Harper Collins.

APPENDIX 1.1
Suggestions for Presenting a Case

Presenting a case can seem overwhelming, especially with complex patients. The following guidelines are intended to help you organize your thinking, summarize salient information about your patient in a coherent manner, identify areas where the therapy is stuck (resistance), and formulate questions that may offer insight into the process. Identifying information should be disguised.

BASIC INFORMATION

Demographics: age, race/ethnicity, gender, sexual orientation, education, and occupation.

Family: relationship status, living arrangement, members of immediate family, and extended relevant family members.

Working Diagnosis and Symptoms: dissociation, anxiety, depression, eating disorder, substance abuse, self-injury, and suicide attempts, destructive or violent behavior.

Relevant Medical Problems and Physical Disabilities: diabetes, asthma, chronic pain, birth defects, sensory impairment, impaired mobility, and so on.

Patient's Coping Mechanisms: both healthy and unhealthy, defenses, and ego functioning.

Treatment History: inpatient, outpatient, how long and intensive, treatment failures and responses.

Current Treatment: inpatient, outpatient, partial individual, group, and family.

Medication(s): current and past history.

CASE CONCEPTUALIZATION

1. What are the reasons the patient came for treatment now?
2. What are the patient's goals? How would the person know if the treatment was successful?
3. When did the current symptoms start?
4. What other situations may be contributing to the problem now?
5. Speculate on what experiential contributors from the past might be driving the current symptoms?
6. Is there a current crisis?
7. Resources and strengths.
8. Draw a timeline with the patient of the most disturbing and pleasant events in the person's life and rate disturbances on a 0 to 10 scale with 10 being the most disturbing. See Chapter 13 for example of timeline.

QUESTIONS TO PONDER

What's going well in the therapeutic process, and what is problematic? Have you established a therapeutic alliance? Is the patient's life stabilized? Is the patient avoiding or working on issues? Undermining the therapy? Flooding with memories or decompensating?

What makes you want to present this patient? What's unusual, special, difficult, confusing, arousing, frustrating, scary, overwhelming?

What do you experience with this patient that is unusual for you? Do you feel intense emotions, like or dislike, anger, admiration, humiliation, fear, revulsion, sleepy, dizzy, disoriented, a desire to nurture or rescue, and the urge to confront. Do you wish you could get rid of this patient, or are you afraid of losing him or her?

TREATMENT HIERARCHY

Based on this information and the hierarchy of treatment in your book, what do you think is the most appropriate interventions/treatment for this person now? What are treatment priorities?

APPENDIX 1.2
Weekly Plan for Increasing Resources

Check off, in the column to the left, all activities that you currently do and keep track of how often you do them for 1 week in the columns to the right. Then put a + in the column to the left of those activities you would like to try in the future. Select one with your therapist to try for the following week, and check off how often you do it. Some of these are learned skills that your therapist may teach you. The idea is to gradually build up and integrate more resources into your life.

		Mon	Tues	Wed	Thurs	Fri	Sat	Sun
	Practice deep breathing technique							
	Practice safe place							
	Practice yoga							
	Practice meditation/mindfulness							
	Practice progressive muscle relaxation							
	Exercise for 30 minutes							
	Keep a thought diary							
	Develop a list of positive attributes of self							
	Practice stopping negative self-talk							
	Use affirmations to counter mistaken beliefs							
	Practice imagery							

(continued)

	Mon	Tues	Wed	Thurs	Fri	Sat	Sun
Chant or pray or sing							
Engage in soothing activities (warm bath, nature walk, gardening, . . .)							
Practice real-life desensitization							
Keep a feelings journal							
Identify and rate feelings (0–10)							
Express feelings							
Practice assertive communication							
Develop a list of actual positive memories							
Practice grounding techniques (counting, holding object, stomping feet, . . .)							
Take a step toward achieving goal(s)							
Keep a dream journal							
Develop a healing ritual for a specific loss							
Implement a contingency contract							
Keep a food diary							
Eliminate caffeine/sugar/stimulants							

(continued)

	Mon	Tues	Wed	Thurs	Fri	Sat	Sun
Eat only whole unprocessed food (especially fruits & vegetables)							
Color, draw, or paint							
Keep a log about life's purpose and meaning							
Watch inspiring or funny movies							
Keep alcohol consumption to one or less drinks per day							
Use spiritual beliefs and practices							
Read self-help literature							
Listen to helpful audiotapes							
Reach out to others							
Listen to or play music							
Talk to a nurturing person							
Attend an appropriate group (AA, support group, . . .)							
Pet and/or play with dog or cat							
Sleep 6 to 8 hours at night							

APPENDIX 1.3
Weekly Plan

Please fill in two to three goals for the week and check off each day that you meet that goal.

Goal	Mon	Tues	Wed	Thurs	Fri	Sat	Sun

APPENDIX 1.4
Treatment and Case Management

Patient: _____

Address: _____

Date: _____

Phone: _____

Insurance: _____

Note: At the end of this form is the form for Patient Case Management Needs, which patients can fill out before the session to identify their key areas of need. However, it is still important for the therapist to assess each goal directly, because patients may not be aware of some needs.

1. **Housing Characteristics**
   Goal   Stable and safe living situation.
   Notes   Unhealthy living situations include short-term shelter, living with a person who abuses substances, an unsafe neighborhood, and a domestic violence situation.
   Status   If the goal is already met, check here _____ and describe.
           If the goal is not met, check here _____ and fill out the Case Management Goal Sheet.

2. **Individual Psychotherapy**
   Goal   Treatment that patient finds helpful.
   Notes   Try to get every patient into individual psychotherapy. Inquire whether the patient has any preferences (e.g., gender, theoretical orientation).
   Status   If the goal is already met, check here _____ and describe.
           If the goal is not met, check here _____ and fill out the Case Management Goal Sheet.

3. **Psychiatric Medication**
   Goal   Treatment that patient finds helpful for psychiatric symptoms (e.g., depression, sleep problems) or substance abuse (e.g., naltrexone for alcohol cravings).
   Notes   If the patient has never had a psychopharmacologic evaluation, one is strongly recommended, unless the patient has serious objections; even then, evaluation and information are helpful before making a decision.
   Status   If the goal is already met, check here _____ and describe.
           If the goal is not met, check here _____ and fill out the Case Management Goal Sheet.

4. **HIV Testing and Counseling**
   Goal   Test as soon as possible, unless one was completed in the past 6 months and there have been no high-risk behaviors since then. For a patient at risk for HIV infection who is unwilling to get testing and counseling, it is strongly suggested that the therapist hold an individual session with the patient to explore and encourage these goals.
   Notes   Assist patient with accessing community resources in your geographic area.
   Status   If the goal is already met, check here _____ and describe.

If the goal is not met, check here _____ and fill out the Case Management Goal Sheet.

5. **Job, Volunteer Work, and School**

   Goal   At least 10 hours per week of scheduled productive time.

   Notes   If the patient is unable to meet the goal of 10 hours/week, have the patient hand in a weekly schedule with constructive activities out of the house (e.g., library, gym).

   Status If the goal is already met, check here _____ and describe.

   If the goal is not met, check here _____ and fill out the Case Management Goal Sheet.

6. **Self-Help Groups and Group Therapy**

   Goal   As many groups as the patient is willing to attend.

   Notes   Elicit the patient's preferences, and consider a wide range of options (e.g., dual-diagnosis groups, women's groups, veterans' groups). For self-help groups (e.g., Alcoholics Anonymous), give the patient a list of local groups, strongly encourage attendance, and mention that the sessions are free. However, do not insist on self-help groups or convey negative judgment if the patient does not want to attend. If the patient participates in self-help groups, encourage seeking a sponsor.

   Status If the goal is already met, check here _____ and describe.

   If the goal is not met, check here _____ and fill out the Case Management Goal Sheet.

7. **Day Treatment**

   Goal   As needed and based on the patient's level of impairment, ability to attend a day program, and schedule.

   Notes   If possible, locate a specialty day program (e.g., substance abuse, PTSD). If the patient is able to attend (e.g., job, school, volunteer activity), do not refer to day treatment, because it is usually better to have the patient keep working; however, if the patient is working part-time, some programs allow partial attendance.

   Status If the goal is already met, check here _____ and describe.

   If the goal is not met, check here _____ and fill out the Case Management Goal Sheet.

8. **Detoxification and Inpatient Care**

   Goal   To obtain an appropriate level of care.

   Notes   Detox is necessary if the patient's use is so severe that it represents a serious danger (e.g., likelihood of suicide, causing severe health problems, withdrawal requires medical supervision, such as for painkillers or severe daily alcohol use). If the patient is not in acute danger but cannot get off substances, detox may or may not be helpful; many patients are able to stay off substances during the detox but return to their usual living environment and go back to substance use. For such patients, helping set up adequate outpatient supports is usually preferable. Inquiring about patient's history (e.g., number of past detox episodes and their impact) can be helpful in making a decision.

   Psychiatric inpatient care is typically recommended if the patient is a serious suicide or homicide risk* (i.e., not simply ideation, but immediate plan, intent, and inability to contract for safety) or the patient's psychiatric symptoms are so severe that functioning is impaired (e.g.,

(continued)

psychotic symptoms prevent a mother from caring for her child). In some circumstances, the patient may need to be involuntarily committed; seek supervision and legal advice on this topic.

Status   If the goal is already met, check here _____ and describe.
         If the goal is not met, check here _____ and fill out the Case Management Goal Sheet.

9. Parenting Skills and Resources for Children

Goal   If the patient has children, inquire about parenting skills training and about referrals to help the children obtain treatment, health insurance, and other needs.

Notes   You may need to gently inquire to assess whether the patient's children are being abused or neglected. If so, *you are required by law to report it to your local protective service agency.* The same rule applies for elder abuse or neglect.

Status   If the goal is already met, check here _____ and describe.
         If the goal is not met, check here _____ and fill out the Case Management Goal Sheet.

10. Medical Care

Goals   Annual examinations for (a) general health, (b) vision, (c) dentistry, and (d) gynecology (for women), including (e) instruction about adequate birth control and prevention of sexually transmitted diseases.

Notes   Other medical care may be needed if the patient has a particular illness.

Status   If all five goals are already met, check here _____ and describe.
         If any of the five goals is not met or other medical issues need attention, check here _____ and fill out the Case Management Goal Sheet for each.

11. Financial Assistance (e.g., food stamps, Medicaid)

Goal   Health insurance and adequate finances for daily needs.

Notes   It is crucial to help the patient obtain health insurance and entitlement benefits (e.g., food stamps, Medicaid), if needed. The patient may need help filling out the forms; the patient may be unable to manage the task alone, because the bureaucracy of these programs can be overwhelming. If much help is needed, you may want to refer the patient to a social worker or other professional skilled in this area. If the patient is a parent, be sure to check whether the children are eligible.

Status   If the goal is already met, check here _____ and describe.
         If the goal is not met, check here _____ and fill out the Case Management Goal Sheet.

12. Leisure Time

Goal   At least 2 hours per day in safe leisure activities.

Notes   Leisure includes socializing with safe people and activities such as hobbies, sports, outings, and movies. Some patients are so overwhelmed with responsibility that they do not find time for themselves. Adequate leisure is necessary for maintaining a healthy lifestyle.

Status   If the goal is already met, check here _____ and describe.
         If the goal is not met, check here _____ and fill out the Case Management Goal Sheet.

13. Domestic Violence and Abusive Relationships

Goal   Freedom from domestic violence and abusive relationships.

Notes   It may be extremely difficult to get the patient to leave a situation of domestic violence. Be sure to consult a supervisor and a domestic violence hotline representative.

Status   If the goal is already met, check here _____ and describe.

If the goal is not met, check here _____ and fill out the Case Management Goal Sheet.

14. Impulses to Harm Self or Others (e.g., suicide, homicide)

Goal   Absence of such impulses, or if such impulses are present, a clear and specific safety plan is in place.

Notes   Many patients have thoughts of harming self or others; however, to determine whether the patient is at serious risk for action and how to manage this risk, see the guidelines developed by the International Society of Study for Dissociative Disorders in Chapter 3.

Status   If the goal is already met, check here _____ and describe.

If the goal is not met, check here _____ and fill out the Case Management Goal Sheet.

15. Alternative Treatments (e.g., acupuncture, meditation)

Goal   The patient is informed about alternative treatments that may be beneficial.

Notes   Patients should be informed that some people in early recovery benefit from acupuncture, meditation, and other nonstandard treatments. Try to identify local referrals for such resources.

Status   If the goal is already met, check here _____ and describe.

If the goal is not met, check here _____ and fill out the Case Management Goal Sheet.

16. Self-Help Books and Materials

Goal   The patient is offered one or two suggestions for self-help books and other materials, such as audiotapes or Internet sites, that offer education and support.

Notes   All patients should be encouraged to use self-help materials outside of sessions as much as possible. For patients who do not like to read, alternative modes (e.g., audiotapes) are suggested. Self-help can address PTSD, substance abuse, or any other life problems (e.g., study skills, parenting skills, relationship skills, leisure activities, and medical problems).

Status   If the goal is already met, check here _____ and describe.

If the goal is not met, check here _____ and fill out the Case Management Goal Sheet.

17. Additional Goal

Goal

Notes

*For homicide risk or any other intent to physically harm another person, the therapist must follow "duty to warn" legal standards, which usually involve an immediate warning to the specific person the patient plans to assault. Always seek supervision and legal advice, and be knowledgeable in advance about how to manage such a situation.

CASE MANAGEMENT GOAL SHEET

Patient: _____

Date: _____

Goal: _____

Referrals given to patient, date given, and deadline (if any) for each:
Describe patient's motivation to work on this goal:
Emotional obstacles that may hinder completion (and strategies implemented to help patient overcome these):
Therapist to do:
Follow-up (date and update):

PATIENT CASE MANAGEMENT NEEDS

Do you need help with any of the following? (circle one)	
1. Housing characteristics	Yes/Maybe/No
2. Individual psychotherapy	Yes/Maybe/No
3. Psychiatric medication	Yes/Maybe/No
4. HIV testing and counseling	Yes/Maybe/No
5. Job, volunteer work, and school	Yes/Maybe/No
6. Self-help groups and group therapy	Yes/Maybe/No
7. Day treatment	Yes/Maybe/No
8. Detoxification and inpatient care	Yes/Maybe/No
9. Parenting skills and resources for children	Yes/Maybe/No
10. Medical care	Yes/Maybe/No
11. Financial assistance (e.g., food stamps, Medicaid)	Yes/Maybe/No
12. Leisure time	Yes/Maybe/No
13. Domestic violence and abusive relationships	Yes/Maybe/No
14. Impulses to harm self or others (e.g., suicide, homicide)	Yes/Maybe/No
15. Alternative treatments (e.g., acupuncture, meditation)	Yes/Maybe/No
16. Self-help books and materials	Yes/Maybe/No
17. Additional goal	Yes/Maybe/No

Source: Adapted from Najavits, L. M. (2002). Seeking safety: A treatment manual for PTSD and substance abuse. New York, NY: Guilford Press.

APPENDIX 1.5
Stage I

STABILIZATION CHECKLIST

Please check all indicators below to help assess whether patient is stabilized and ready to move to Stage II.

	Comfort with own body and physical experience
	Patient is able to establish a useful distance from the traumatic event
	No current life crisis such as impending litigation or medical problems
	Patient accepts diagnosis and has a working knowledge of trauma
	Patient's mood is stable, even if depressed
	Patient has at least two or more people to count on
	Patient knows and uses self-soothing techniques
	Patient gives honest self-reports
	Patient's living situation is stable
	Patient is able to communicate
	Patient has stable therapeutic relationship and adequate trust of others
	Patient has adequate impulse control, no injurious behavior to self or others
	Patient stays grounded and oriented x3 when distressed
	No major dissociation present
	Patient can identify triggers and reports significant symptoms
	Patient can set limits and is able to leave dangerous situations if necessary
	Patient can tolerate positive and negative affect, and shame
	If DID, is cooperative and has contractual agreement among parts
	Patient can establish "useful distance" from traumatic event

APPENDIX 1.6
Stage II

PROCESSING CHECKLIST

Please check all indicators below to help assess whether patient has adequately processed trauma and is moving to Stage III, future visioning. The stabilization checklist should already have been achieved.

	No significant affect changes
	Self-referencing cognitions are positive in relation to past event
	Can dismiss thoughts of trauma at will
	Relationships are adaptive
	Work is productive
	Good quality of decision-making
	Creativity begins to emerge
	Boundaries improve
	Complaints tend to deal with present-day events
	Affect is proportionate to current events
	Congruence between behavior, thoughts, and affect

APPENDIX 1.7
Safe-Place Exercise

The safe-place exercise described below helps the patient to enhance skills during stabilization as well as to decrease distress after processing. Through the ability to create one's own safe place, the person is empowered. As with all learning, the more it is practiced, the more readily available it is when needed. Thus, it should be used on a day-to-day basis. If a patient feels there is no place—real or imaginary—that is safe, have the patient focus on one time in his or her life when he or she felt safe or on a person he or she admires who exemplifies positive attributes, such as strength or control. If the person still cannot find a safe place, ask the person to think of a place where he or she feels relaxed or comfortable. Sometimes patients become more distressed when they relax and it may take some time before the person is able to identify a positive resource. Identifying a safe place resource may take several sessions. Ask the person to sit with his or her feet firmly planted on the floor. Sometimes this exercise is conducted with soothing music and/or background nature sounds. Some therapists tape the exercise with their voice to give to the patient to practice at home. The safe-place exercise follows.

Ask the person to identify an image of a safe place that he or she can easily evoke that creates a personal feeling of calm and safety. Use soothing tones to enhance the imagery, asking the person to "see what you see," "feel what you feel," "notice the sounds, smells, and colors in your special place." Once identified, ask the person to focus on the image, feel the emotions, and identify the location of the pleasing physical sensations and where he or she is in the body. "Concentrate on those pleasant sensations in your body and just enjoy as you breathe deeply, relaxing and feeling safe." After you have slowly deepened his or her experience of this, slowly ask the person to come back and tell you a description of the place. Ask for details so that you can assist the person in accessing this place in the future. Ask how he or she feels and if the experience has been difficult for the person and/or no positive emotions are experienced, explore other resources that might be helpful. If at any time the person indicates that he or she is not feeling safe, the exercise should be stopped immediately.

If successful in accessing a safe place, the person is asked for a single word that fits the picture (i.e., beach, forest . . .) and then asked to repeat the exercise using the person's words for the experience along with deep breathing. Then ask the person to repeat on his or her own, bringing up the image, emotions, and body sensations. Reinforce, after this exercise, that his or her safe place can be used as a resource and ask the patient to practice over the next week, once a day.

During the next session, practice again with the person. Then ask the patient to bring up a minor annoyance and notice the negative feelings while guiding the person through the safe place until the negative feelings have dissipated. Then ask the person to bring up a negative disturbing thought once again and to access the safe place but this time on his or her own without your assistance.

Occasionally the safe-place exercise triggers intense negative affect. Patients should be made aware about the possible activation of issues during the safe-place exercise. Reassure the person that even if temporary activation of issues does occur, this is not beyond the limits of expectation, and that it may identify issues that will be addressed in the course of therapy anyway.

APPENDIX 1.8
Container Exercise

This exercise is an important affect management strategy that can be taught to the patient and practiced so that the person can feel in control and develop mastery over his or her emotions. It also assists with self-soothing, decreasing arousal, and reinforcing a sense of safety. The person should already have a safe place. This exercise should be initiated toward the end of the session when the person has intense negative feelings of anxiety, anger, fear, and/or sadness.

The therapist introduces by saying something like: "Did you know that we can put those bad feelings into a container so you won't feel so overwhelmed when you leave?" The person's curiosity is usually piqued at this point even if he or she does not believe you. Continue with: "I can help you do this and then you can take out those feelings when you want and deal with them the next time we meet or when you decide it is okay." Usually the person agrees if for no other reason than he or she is curious and may think you are really strange to suggest such a thing. The therapist continues in a soothing tone: "So, just imagine you have a container; you can close your eyes or not as you wish. It can be made out of anything that you want and be any size you want but be sure it has a tight lid that you can cover or lock because we are going to put all those negative feelings in. Let me know once you have an image in your head." Once the person says he or she has the image, ask him or her for a few details regarding size and so on. Then ask the patient to "return to the image and imagine all those bad feelings going into the container. Once you have all the bad feelings in the container, lock it up. Let me know when they are in there." Once the person says they are in the container, ask the person whether there is any percentage that is still not in the container and usually the person will say something like 10% or 20%. At that point, ask the person: "Do you need a bigger container to accommodate all the bad feelings? You can make it as big as you want. See whether you can put the rest of those feelings in the container now. Let me know when the rest of the feelings are all in the container and locked." If more negative feelings come up, continue with either imaging another container or making the one he or she has bigger. Ask the person what this was like for him or her, checking to see whether he or she is okay.

It is important to do this exercise slowly and use pacing so that the person does not feel rushed. The session can then be ended with the safe-place exercise. Ask the person to practice the container exercise during the week when negative feelings come up. The patient can also practice allowing the feelings to come out if he or she thinks he or she can manage this and journal about these feelings between sessions. Asking the person at the next session: "What was different for you this past week?" and exploring how feelings were or were not manageable are important follow-up steps and help to assess how to increase the effectiveness of this exercise.

Source: Ginger Gilson, from Gilson, G., & Kaplan, S. (2000). *The therapeutic interweave in EMDR: Before and beyond: A manual for EMDR trained clinicians.* New Hope, PA: EMDR Humanitarian Assistance Programs.

The Neurophysiology of Trauma and Psychotherapy

Kathleen Wheeler

This chapter considers the neurophysiological basis for psychotherapy from the perspective of the polyvagal theory (PVT) and the adaptive information processing (AIP) model as theoretical underpinnings for practice. The confluence of neurobiology, attachment theory, and infant development research is transforming the way we think about and work in psychotherapy, deepening our understanding of what facilitates change and the role of trauma and its effects on the individual. A new age of psychotherapy is dawning with the ability to document differential responses to therapy and medication through positron emission tomography (PET), electroencephalography (EEG), and functional magnetic resonance imaging (fMRI). The ability to study brain activity enhances our potential to decide what treatments to use and how to use them based on neuroscience findings. Advanced practice psychiatric nurses (APPNs) who understand underlying neurophysiology can make informed decisions about what needs to change and how to benefit patients and family members in ways that we are only beginning to imagine. Neuroscience is a vast, complicated area of study, and this chapter highlights only selected relevant topics. It is not meant to be comprehensive, and some working knowledge of neurophysiology is assumed. Much exciting research is ongoing, and the references at the end of this chapter should be consulted for further information. Excellent reviews of neurophysiology for psychiatric nursing care can be found in the works of Boyd (2018) and Halter (2018).

Selected topics for discussion in this chapter begin with brain structures, the neurophysiological response to trauma, the PVT, AIP theory, brain development, memory, and the role of psychotherapy in restructuring neural networks. The word *trauma* is used throughout this chapter to reflect what happens inside a person when an adverse life experience or event is perceived as disturbing and overwhelms the person's ability to cope. The trauma response begins with the normal stress response but evolves into a failure to adapt or recover from extreme stress. It is thought that the more helpless and less in control of the situation a person feels, the more vulnerable he or she is to pathophysiological changes. Thus, stress can be conceptualized as existing on a continuum with mild stressors at one end and extreme helplessness/trauma at the other end. Trauma disconnects us from self, and thus, healing reflects a reconnection with oneself. Psychotherapy mediates the reintegration and connection of neural networks that have become maladaptively linked owing to overwhelming events. This is accomplished by changing implicit memory networks into more explicit adaptive connections and linking memory fragments through information processing. Neurophysiological research provides evidence that this memory reconsolidation or integration occurs primarily in the context of a healing relationship.

TRAUMA AND RELEVANT BRAIN STRUCTURES

Both significant traumatic events and adverse experiences affect brain development and structure. An overview of the brain structures that play the most significant role in memory is important to understand psychopathology. Brain structures are networks of neurons, and some, such as the thalamocortical circuitry or extensions of the locus coeruleus, project over wide areas of the brain. Through the neuromodulating chemistry of messenger molecules, these neural systems activate other neuronal networks. Figures 2.1 and 2.2 show the relevant structures of the brain.

The discussion that follows addresses some of the complex systems and brain structures affected by trauma. Further information on postraumatic stress disorder (PTSD) and dissociative disorders is included in Chapter 17. Although this chapter focuses on brain structure and function, brain structures are not isolated entities. Scaer (2005) says: "Sensory input from the body shapes and changes the structure of the brain, which concurrently shapes and alters the body in all its parts, particularly those that provided this sensory input to the brain" (p. 11). The brain and body are in constant reciprocal, dynamic interaction, adapting to and influencing each other.

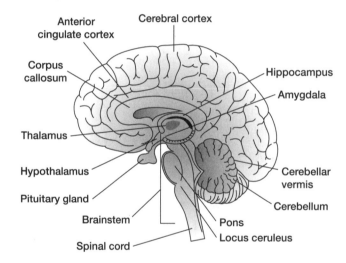

FIGURE 2.1 The structures of the brain.

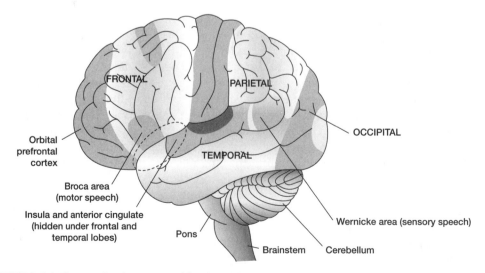

FIGURE 2.2 The cerebral cortex and brainstem.

Thalamus

The brainstem develops first in utero and is responsible for regulating bodily function such as heart rate, breathing, temperature, sleep, and states of alertness (Siegel, 2012). The thalamus, located deep in the brain, acts as a relay station for the top-down, bottom-up neural networks that connect the cortex to the limbic system. There is constant interaction between the thalamus and the cortex, and all sensory information, except for smell, which is routed through the thalamus to the cerebral cortex. The thalamus mediates the interaction between attention and arousal and is therefore relevant to the phenomenology of trauma. If neural networks in the thalamus are altered, neurological and psychiatric problems ensue. High levels of arousal during traumatic experiences are thought to lead to altered thalamic processing (Bergmann, 2012, 2020), and neuroimaging studies have found decreased thalamic activity in subjects with PTSD (Lanius, Paulson, & Corrigan, 2014). Thalamic dysregulation can result in significant memory problems, and the person may be unable to integrate memories into the present and personal memory into identity. These memories are isolated from consciousness and thought to underlie the experiences of flashbacks, nightmares, avoidances, and dissociation.

Cerebellum

The cerebellum is just above the brainstem and helps coordinate motor, social, emotional, and cognitive functioning. The cerebellum, known as the "little brain," has at birth around 90 billion neuronal connections and is fully developed by 2 years of age. This structure, along with the brainstem, is often referred to as the reptilian brain and is thought to process implicit memory. The brainstem regulates our level of arousal, some reflexes, and cardiovascular functions. The cerebellar vermis is a worm-shaped structure between both parts of the cerebellum. This structure helps regulate activity in the limbic system and is important for regulating emotional balance, attention, and posture. Reduced size of this structure has been found in traumatized children and has been linked to numerous disorders such as attention deficit hyperactivity disorder (ADHD), depression, bipolar disorder, schizophrenia, and autism (Teicher, 2000).

Locus Coeruleus

The locus coeruleus is a dense group of neurons found on both sides of the pons in the brainstem between the medulla oblongata and the midbrain, with projections to the amygdala, the prefrontal cortex, and the hippocampus. Stress activates this structure, which makes norepinephrine (NE; Charney, 2004). This contributes to sympathoadrenal medullary (SAM) axis and the hypothalamic–pituitary–adrenal (HPA) axis stimulation, which inhibits frontal cortex functions, allowing instinctual responses to override cognition. Complex feedback loops during acute stress, if unchecked, can result in chronic anxiety, fear, intrusive memories, and an increased risk for physical health problems, such as hypertension, tachycardia, bladder infections, asthma, migraines, fibromyalgia, irritable bowel syndrome, gastroesophageal reflux disease, ulcers, and sleep, thermoregulation, and eating disorders (Bergmann, 2012, 2020; Heitkemper et al., 2001; Scaer, 2005).

Hippocampus

The hippocampus is located deep within the brain's unconscious core, in the midbrain. It is important for explicit memory, reality testing, and inhibition of the amygdala. This area of the brain allows formation of a coherent narrative about personal history: what happened and where and when so that explicit memory can weave an autobiography. Normally, the hippocampus is not fully developed until the child is 16 to 18 months old (Siegel, 2003). The slow maturation and myelinization of the hippocampus is thought to be responsible for infantile amnesia. The hippocampus is necessary for forming new explicit memories while the amygdala organizes emotional experience and tells the hippocampus what is important to learn.

Research has found that the hippocampus in traumatized individuals is smaller for those who have suffered physical or sexual abuse (Bremner et al., 1997; Teicher et al., 2003; Zhang et al., 2011). Inability to integrate memories into a coherent narrative keeps images and bodily sensations distinct from other life experiences so that the person's experiences are fragmented and may feel ego-alien (not part of oneself) and timeless. For those who have been significantly traumatized, it is much harder to process any new experience if there are not enough cells in the hippocampus.

During high states of arousal, amygdala and hippocampal networks become dissociated so that learning is impaired. A lack of early attunement because of abuse or trauma can compromise the function of the amygdala and hippocampus (Kitchur, 2005). Decreased functioning of the hippocampus is caused by increased levels of cortisol combined with other substances, such as glutamate, which damages dendrites in the hippocampus and eventually causes cell death. Glucocorticoids secreted during a traumatic experience shut down the hippocampus and make it impossible for memory to be adaptively linked. These hormonal changes result in behavioral disinhibition and an inability to learn from experience. Arousing stimuli are then perceived as threatening, and the person may react through aggression or withdrawal. Research has found that both medication and psychotherapy ameliorate these problems and increase hippocampal size (Bossini, Fagiolini, & Castrogiovanni, 2007; Bossini et al., 2011). Earlier research found that recovery from dissociative identity disorder was associated with a 9% to 18% increase in hippocampal volume (Bremner et al., 1997). The hippocampus is an area of the brain where replication of new neurons is possible.

Amygdala

Nearby is another important structure, the amygdala, which is a bulbar structure at the end of the hippocampus. The amygdala, hippocampus, thalamus, hypothalamus, orbital medial prefrontal cortex (OMPFC), and anterior cingulate make up the limbic system, which is often referred to as the emotional brain. The amygdala mediates the crisis response and powerful emotions such as anger, fear, and rage. The amygdala makes connections with thalamic pain centers through a rich array of connections to visual and other sensory modalities. Neuroimaging studies show that people experiencing intense emotions, such as fear, sadness, anger, or happiness, have increased activation in these subcortical brain regions and significant reductions of blood flow in various areas of the frontal lobe (van der Kolk, 2006). Such research provides a neurophysiological understanding of why it is difficult to think straight when experiencing intense emotions. It is thought that a hyper-responsive amygdala causes the symptoms of irritability, anger, hypervigilance, and exaggerated startle responses in PTSD (Weiss, 2007).

The amygdala projects directly to cholinergic nuclei in the brainstem, geniculate nucleus of the thalamus, and the occipital nuclei and initiates REM sleep, triggering the eye movements that occur during REM sleep, and arbitrates REM-to-wake transitions (Bergmann, 2012, 2020; Woodward, 2004). Down-regulation of the amygdala results in better sleep because fear systems are inactivated. Sleep disturbances often occur in those with depression and PTSD, and it has been suggested that REM disturbances interrupt the emotional processing of traumatic memories that would normally occur in REM sleep (Bergmann, 2020). The REM dream state is thought to be a time when unprocessed memories are being integrated, and if the disturbance is too great, these memories cannot be assimilated and nightmares result (Stickgold, 2002, 2005, 2008).

Studies have found two types of reactions to traumatic events: in one there is emotional undermodulation with intrusive symptoms leading to hyperactivity of the medial prefrontal cortex and inhibition of the amygdala, and the other type indicates hypoarousal of the prefrontal cortex and activation of the amygdala (Felmingham et al., 2008; Lanius et al., 2014). These emotional memories are subcortical and indelible. When the amygdala is overactivated and irritable, kindling occurs. Kindling refers to lowering of the excitability threshold of neurons, rendering the person increasingly likely to develop certain symptoms (van der Kolk 2006). With repeated stress, kindling is thought to sensitize limbic neurons so that reactions are set off by stimuli that were previously subthreshold. The neuronal excitability of the amygdala may trigger panic attacks and even cause temporal lobe seizures (Teicher et al., 2003). Although panic attacks are triggered by stress and conflict in the person's life, seldom is this association made by the person, as the episodes are experienced as unrelated to any real threat. The person is left feeling as if he or she is going crazy or having a heart attack. Irritability of the amygdala has also been implicated in ADHD, PTSD, substance use disorders, and borderline personality disorder (Teicher et al., 2003). Research in animals has found that an intense, single stimulation of the amygdala produces lasting changes in neuronal excitability and behavior in stress responses (van der Kolk, 2003).

Hypothalamus

The amygdala can transmit signals directly to the hypothalamus through the orbitofrontal cortex and bypass other areas in the cerebral cortex so that we are in an immediate state of flight or fight without even thinking about it (Scaer, 2005). The hypothalamus is located deep in the middle and base of the brain and is the region of the brain where the nervous system intersects and communicates with the endocrine system. The hypothalamus regulates blood pressure, body temperature, sleep, appetite, glucose levels, and the autonomic nervous system (ANS). During stress, a cascade of physiological responses occurs, with the limbic–hypothalamic system modulating and coordinating the biochemical activity of the autonomic, endocrine, and immune systems (see Figure 2.1). Hormonal equilibrium is altered from severe stress in childhood so that genetic expression can be affected across generations. Thus, in early life, even in utero, brain growth is experience-dependent. What this means is that our ability to regulate stress is based on the stresses not only our parents but also our grandparents experienced (Bowers & Yehuda, 2016).

Cerebral Cortex

The cerebral cortex is considered to be the thinking part of our brain; it organizes experiences and determines how we interact with the world. Each of the four lobes that make up the cortex—frontal, temporal, parietal, and occipital—has specialized functions, with the prefrontal cortex the foremost portion of the frontal lobe (see Figure 2.2). The frontal lobe is responsible for motor behavior, expressive language, executive functioning, abstract reasoning, and directed attention, and the foremost area is referred to as the prefrontal cortex. The parietal lobe is responsible for linking the senses with motor abilities and for creation of the experience of a sense of our body in space. The occipital lobe is responsible for visual processing, and the temporal lobe is responsible for auditory processing, receptive language, and memory functions.

Axonal connections between the limbic system and the prefrontal cortex modulate arousal and emotional regulation and are developed between 10 and 18 months of age. The prefrontal cortex barely starts to myelinate in adolescence, and myelinization continues late into the 20s (Bergmann, 2012, 2020). This structure plays a role in the extinction of fear responses by exerting an inhibitory influence over the limbic system, modulating arousal by serving as a damper switch to the amygdala, thereby regulating emotions and the generalization of fearful behavior (van der Kolk, 2006). Sensations and impulses are compared with previous information for the integration of experience. Researchers have confirmed cortical neuronal loss and dysfunction in those who have suffered significant stress and trauma (Teicher et al., 2003; van der Kolk, 2003). Persons with an underdeveloped cortex are less able to modulate emotion, inhibit the emotional lower brain, and problem-solve. A decrease in cortical activation and an increase in anterior regions of the cingulate and insula occur in depression and anxiety symptoms (Kennedy et al., 2007).

Orbital Medial Prefrontal Cortex

A particularly relevant part of the prefrontal cortex for survival is the orbital medial prefrontal cortex (OMPFC); the first region of the frontal lobe to develop is located within the frontal lobes and just above the orbits of the eyes. This area of the brain serves an inhibitory function in response to stress in other regions of the brain, and it regulates planning behavior associated with reward and punishment and is considered part of the limbic system because of its role in emotional processing. The OMPFC assesses the reality of the danger and serves an inhibitory role when the amygdala is activated, modulating the timing of emotional response. The right OMPFC is thought to be the master regulator of the limbic system, modulating the person's response to threat and processing and regulating arousal-based information (Scaer, 2005). The reciprocal relationship between the amygdala and OMPFC determines how we handle emotional experience. These connections are shaped and rooted in early experiences and attachment experiences (Scaer, 2005; Schore, 2019).

Schore's work (2019) on attunement and self-regulation highlights the importance of the OMPFC in development. In a way, the mother serves as the OMPFC for the developing infant by regulating sensory input and emotions and inhibiting behavior. As this area of the brain matures, the child becomes better able to assume more and more of the reflective, regulatory, and inhibitory skills needed to function. Schore's research findings suggest that emotionally arousing interactions between the infant and caretaker lead to increases in dopamine concentrations, which trigger brain development, particularly in the OMPFC in the right hemisphere. This is accomplished through facial expressions of the caregiver that stimulate the production of opioids, which activate the dopamine neurons. In this way, positive attachments activate the dopaminergic and beta-endorphin systems, laying down implicit memory networks so that intimacy and connection continue to be rewarded throughout life. However, if attachment problems occur during early development, the OMPFC's ability to regulate cortical and autonomic processes is reduced, and long-standing regulatory and relationship difficulties may result (Schore, 2019; Siegel, 2012). Consequently, the child's development of a coherent sense of self is greatly impaired. A number of studies report that the OMPFC activity is inversely related to severity of PTSD symptoms (Shin, Rauch, & Pitman, 2006). That is, the activity of the OMFC decreases significantly during increased stress and consequently the problem-solving part of the brain is impaired.

Anterior Cingulate

Another important area in the cortex that is considered to be part of the limbic system and the OMPFC is the anterior cingulate, which is thought to be the last step before consciousness and serves as the gatekeeper of emotion (Stien & Kendall, 2004). This structure helps decide which emotional information to pay attention to and assists in processing emotion arising from the limbic system by recruiting other areas of the cortex to respond to emotions. Siegel (2003) calls this the chief operating officer of the brain because it plays a key role in orchestrating the autonomic, neuroendocrine, and behavioral expression of emotions. The volume of the anterior cingulate has been reported to be smaller in patients with PTSD (Shin et al., 2006).

Insula

The insula is another important area of the cortex and is buried beneath and within the folds of the cortex. The insula provides a means to connect body states to the expression and experience of emotions and behavior so that we are aware of what is happening inside our bodies and can reflect on emotional experiences. The insula, the OMPFC, and the anterior cingulate evaluate whether the information from the amygdala is threatening. These areas are especially sensitive to social interactions, are unconscious, and play a crucial role in coordinating perceptions with memory and behavior (Siegel, 2012). Imaging studies have found reduced activity in the anterior cingulate for those with PTSD symptoms (Bremner, 1999). Thus, it is thought that in PTSD the OMPFC is hyporesponsive, the amygdala is hyper-responsive, and the hippocampus and OMPFC fail to inhibit the amygdala (Shin et al., 2006). Early neglect, stress, and trauma affect the development of the anterior cingulate, and lifelong cognitive and emotional deficits may result (Cozolino, 2017).

Corpus Callosum and Hemispheres

An important brain structure relevant for discussion is the corpus callosum, which consists of long neural fibers connecting the right and left hemispheres of the cerebral cortex. Researchers have found that early stress results in decreased hemispheric integration and increased laterality (Teicher et al., 2003). A marked reduction in the size of this structure is associated with childhood history of neglect, especially for children who were sexually abused. This structural change results in diminished communication between the hemispheres. It is speculated that failure of left hemisphere functioning during states of extreme arousal is responsible for the de-realization and depersonalization experiences reported in PTSD. These left–right neural information loops need to communicate with each other and other processing neural information networks for optimal functioning in language, bodily awareness, emotional regulation, and many other processes (Cozolino, 2017).

The left hemisphere, which is usually dominant, is associated with problem-solving, analyzing, elaboration, processing of verbal communication, words, and numbers, and motor abilities (Feinberg & Keenan, 2005; McGilchrist, 2009). Research has shown that the left hemisphere is responsible for the tendency to seek solutions and take action (Stien & Kendall, 2004). The left hemisphere is also associated with positive emotions and prosocial behaviors, which help us to connect to others, while the right hemisphere has a proclivity toward negativity and keeps us vigilant to ward off danger (Harmon-Jones et al., 2010). This is sometimes referred to as a negativity bias in that we are built for survival. Explaining this is sometimes helpful to patients as a rationale for why reframing and practicing cognitive behavioral techniques are helpful in rerouting negative thinking.

Wernicke's area (i.e., comprehension of language) and Broca's area (i.e., expression of language) are located in the left hemisphere of the cerebral cortex. Left hemisphere deficits occur most frequently in those who have suffered trauma. There is speculation that interference of the myelinization of nerve fibers due to trauma may contribute to the underdevelopment of the left hemisphere (Teicher, 2000). If the left hemisphere is damaged, the right hemisphere may predominate.

Traumatic memories do not form a coherent narrative but persist as implicit, behavioral, and somatic memories (van der Kolk, 2003). Anything that is overwhelming to the individual results in information being linked dysfunctionally, that is, components of the traumatic memory are fragmented. Scaer (2005) posits that these fragmented memories are stored in procedural memory capsules dissociated for the most part from each other and from adaptive memory neural networks. Thus, you can see from Figure 2.3 that someone with many traumatic experiences may have difficulty staying in the present moment because experiences in the present may trigger these memory fragments. For example, a sound or image or feeling in the present can serve as a trigger for anxiety or depression without the person being aware of why this is happening. These memories are seemingly unattached to other experiences and are considered a right-brain phenomenon, stored as images, sensations, and emotions, not in a coherent narrative and context, which is a left-brain function. With entry into consciousness of previously warded off states through processing in therapy, the person can begin to develop self-regulatory capacities that were beyond their skill set previously.

The right hemisphere corresponds to Freud's idea of the unconscious and is mute in terms of responding verbally (Feinberg & Keenan, 2005). Neuroimaging studies have found that as trauma survivors reminisce about their terrifying experiences, activity in the right hemisphere of the brain increases. At the same time, there is a decrease in activity in the left hemisphere in Broca's area, which is our expressive speech area that allows us to put experiences into words. The idea of being speechless with terror is physiologically based. Perhaps this right or left hemisphere dysfunction also explains why those who have suffered trauma are unable to express feelings in words but instead somatize or act out feelings. Language is key for integration and putting words to our experiences forms new dendritic branches that activate and establish interhemispheric integration between the right and left brain. See Figure 2.4 for right- and left-brain functions.

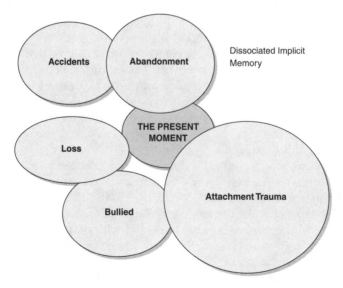

FIGURE 2.3 Dissociated implicit memory diagram.

Source: Adapted with permission from Scaer, R. (2005). *The trauma spectrum: Hidden wounds and human resiliency.* New York, NY:

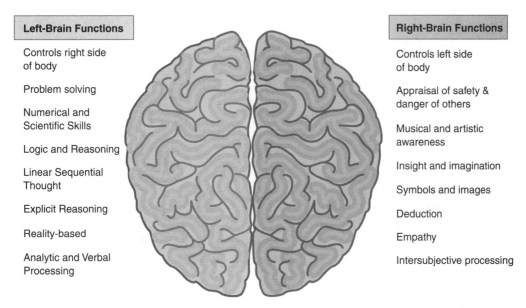

Left-Brain Functions	Right-Brain Functions
Controls right side of body	Controls left side of body
Problem solving	Appraisal of safety & danger of others
Numerical and Scientific Skills	Musical and artistic awareness
Logic and Reasoning	Insight and imagination
Linear Sequential Thought	Symbols and images
Explicit Reasoning	Deduction
Reality-based	Empathy
Analytic and Verbal Processing	Intersubjective processing

FIGURE 2.4 The right- and left-hemisphere functions of the brain.

The right hemisphere has been linked to implicit information processing, as opposed to the more explicit and more conscious processing of the left hemisphere (Bergmann, 2020; McGilchrist, 2009). The right hemisphere is dominant for the perception of nonverbal emotional expressions in facial expressions or voice patterns, nonverbal communication, processing bodily based visceral stimuli, implicit learning, and affect regulation. Right-brain to right-brain communication between mother and infant is thought to be responsible for affect regulation and interpersonal behavior. Schore (2019) says that the right hemisphere represents the unconscious and is the psychobiological core of the self. The right hemisphere mediates our somatic or emotional autobiographical memory, which is primarily unconscious (90%), and it is this area that drives emotion, cognition, and behavior. Our personalities are largely based on these accumulated memories mediated by the right hemisphere. Problems in connection and integration of the right and left hemispheres have been implicated in alexithymia, somatization, depression, dissociative disorders, borderline personality disorder, substance abuse, and mania (Cozolino, 2017; Teicher et al., 2003).

NEUROPHYSIOLOGICAL RESPONSES TO TRAUMA

Information from the body or the senses is matched or processed to previously stored patterns of activation, and a cascade of neuronal activity begins. Signaling pathways travel from the brainstem (i.e., locus coeruleus) through the thalamus to the amygdala (which evaluates emotional content) to the hippocampus (which evaluates the cognitive content) to the anterior cingulate and the orbitofrontal cortex, which activates the sympathoadrenal medullary (SAM) axis and the hypothalamic pituitary adrenal (HPA) axis to initiate the physiology of survival (Scaer, 2005). Often, the brain reacts even before the cerebral cortex has a chance to sort out and interpret what is happening (see Figure 2.5).

Once a significant threat occurs, information processing is disrupted. Neuronal pathways connect perceptual information with the amygdala and lower brain structures, bypassing the hippocampus, where conscious memory is mediated, and implicit memories of important emotional events may be triggered without knowing why.

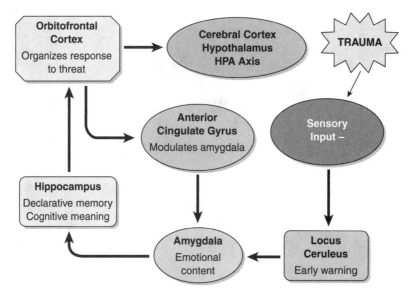

FIGURE 2.5 Trauma response pathway diagram. HPA, hypothalamic–pituitary–adrenal.

Source: Courtesy of Scaer, R. (2005). *The trauma spectrum: Hidden wounds and human resiliency.* New York, NY: W. W. Norton.

For example, characteristics of others such as tone of voice or appearance may be associated with a previous threat, or if unknown, an initial alarm response occurs, and a complex wave of physiological processes begins that are orchestrated to promote survival. This begins with the classic stress response involving the autonomic, endocrine, and immune systems and all the attending messenger molecules, such as vasopressin, oxytocin, norepinephrine (NE), dopamine, endorphins, serotonin, corticotropin (i.e., adrenocorticotropic hormone [ACTH]), corticotropin-releasing factor, glucocorticoids, and cytokines. The simultaneous activation of cortisol (HPA) and NE (SAM) stimulates active coping behaviors, whereas increased arousal in the presence of low glucocorticoid levels is thought to promote undifferentiated fight-or-flight reactions (Porges, 2011).

This response pattern continues after the initial alarm with an elevated heart rate, vigilance, increased startle response, behavioral irritability, and increased locomotion. Cortisol puts a brake on NE and modulates the arousal response so that if the person survives, cortisol manages ongoing stress through changes in circulation, metabolism, and immune response. Prolonged exposure to cortisol results in dysregulation through the release of glutamate, which inhibits its removal from the synaptic space, initiating long-term potentiation of synaptic connectivity, and as a consequence, fewer glucocorticoid receptors are available. The increased glutamate levels and chronic arousal cause atrophy of dendrites and neurons, especially in the prefrontal cortex and hippocampus, which results in impaired learning and memory. This in turn is thought to be the cause of avoidance, numbing, and memory loss (Weiss, 2007). See Box 2.1 for components of the stress response.

Research in the past decade has demonstrated that long-term physiological and structural changes in the brain and body often occur as a result of chronic stress. Victims of child abuse and neglect have been found to be at risk for high inflammation levels and clustering of metabolic risk biomarkers such as overweight, high blood pressure, high total cholesterol, low- or high-density lipoprotein cholesterol, high glycated hemoglobin, and low or maximum oxygen consumption levels (Heins et al., 2011). These physiological changes predispose the person to develop cardiovascular disease, and the risk for heart disease is doubled. Medical problems related to chronic stress and

BOX 2.1 Components of the Stress Response

1. The HPA axis regulates cortisol, a potent hormone that inhibits growth, immune responses, and inflammatory responses.
2. The amygdala, hippocampus, thalamus, hypothalamus, orbitofrontal cortex, and anterior cingulate make up the limbic system, which with the locus coeruleus, adrenal glands, and the sympathetic nervous system, mobilize a person for flight or fight.
3. Vasopressin and oxytocin peptide response causes the pituitary to release ACTH. The vasopressin–oxytocin response has been less researched than other aspects, but it is thought that early stress produces excessive levels of vasopressin and decreased levels of oxytocin throughout life and that this may result in enhanced sexual arousal but diminished capacity for sexual fulfillment.

ACTH, adrenocorticotropic hormone; HPA, hypothalamic–pituitary–adrenal.
Source: Teicher, M., Polcari, A., Andersen, S., & Navalta, C. (2003). Neurobiological effects of childhood stress and trauma. In S. Coates, J. Rosenthal, & D. Schechter (Eds.), *September 11: Trauma and human bonds.* Hillsdale, NJ: The Analytic Press.

increased cortisol levels are associated with suppression of the immune response and include infections and other immune system problems; increased levels of serum lipids, promoting atherosclerosis; storage of calories as fat in the abdominal region, promoting obesity; and increased blood volume, resulting in hypertension.

The adaptive physiological response to acute stress is called allostasis, and the burden borne by the brain and body adapting to physiological and psychological changes is called allostatic load (Charney, 2004). Allostasis and allostatic load illustrate how persistent stress is linked to adverse consequences in the body, and physiological markers have been identified that predict functional decline in the elderly. Allostatic load from chronic stress or trauma can cause neuronal death if prolonged because of the effect of hypercortisol and increased glutamate. Under normal stress, the hyperarousal in the sympathetic system is balanced by the parasympathetic system. In severe and prolonged stress, the HPA feedback to the pituitary gland is impaired and the hypothalamus does not decrease its activity, thus continuing to pump too much cortisol. Overwhelming chronic stress and trauma induce desensitization to the stress response through a negative feedback loop on the hypothalamus and the pituitary activity is increased, and this in turn decreases cortisol level production by the adrenal cortex (Briere & Scott, 2013). The dysregulation of cortisol during overwhelming stress and trauma results in suppression of cortisol and may be the brain's attempt to protect itself from hyperarousal.

A person with PTSD has chronically lower levels of cortisol and, when and if traumatized again, a blunted cortisol response occurs with a quicker return to baseline (Briere & Scott, 2013). Low levels of cortisol have been documented in combat veterans, in holocaust survivors and their offspring, and in pregnant women with PTSD after the 9/11 tragedy and their newborns (Yehuda et al., 2005). The offspring of holocaust and 9/11 mothers did not always develop PTSD but the hypocortisolemia puts them at risk for autoimmune diseases such as Crohn disease, Sjögren syndrome, Graves disease, fibromyalgia, rheumatoid arthritis, Hashimoto thyroiditis, type 1 diabetes, multiple sclerosis, chronic fatigue syndrome, lupus, and complex regional pain syndrome as adults (Bergmann, 2012, 2020).

For those with PTSD, it is hypothesized that the brain may become hypersensitive to the effects of cortisol. The person has a consequent loss of stimulus discrimination, and even minor triggers may cause the person to overreact. A variety of internal and external stimuli may result in extreme reactions as the amygdala is activated. Internal sensations include bodily sensations of anxiety, and external sensations include instances such as loud noises or specific reminders of the trauma. The person overreacts to minor events and underreacts to major problems and misinterprets stimuli that are not threatening as potentially dangerous. This person may function well in an emergency, but if something is spilled in the kitchen, he or she startles, overreacts, and exaggerates the significance of the event.

The capacity of triggers with diminishing strength to produce the same response over time is called kindling (van der Kolk, 2003, 2014). If a person has suffered multiple traumas, there is a stronger physiological response with triggers of diminishing strength. This tendency to overreact to cues can increase the potential for aggression and violence. Kindling explains why a bout of depression lowers the threshold for another bout of depression. The depressive state becomes linked with the state-dependent implicit memory with all the attending feelings, thoughts, and body memories. Consequently, the longer one stays in an untreated depression and the more frequent the episodes, the more resistant to treatment that person becomes because these neural networks become firmly established.

Hyperarousal of the sympathetic nervous system in times of significant stress is balanced by the parasympathetic nervous system like a brake on a car, which shuts down the sympathetic (accelerator) nervous system. Thus, following exposure to violence and trauma, the parasympathetic response triggers a hypoaroused state with dysregulation of the HPA axis resulting in dissociation. Dissociation is a disconnection of thoughts, emotions, sensations, and behaviors connected with a memory with some dissociation considered a normal experience for most people such as when we "space out" during a movie or when driving. However, severe dissociation or "mindflight" occurs for those who have suffered significant trauma (Steele, (2009)). This episodic failure of dissociation causes intrusive symptoms such as flashbacks, thus dysregulating cortisol, resulting in either too much or too little cortisol.

Neurotransmitters, particularly NE and vasopressin, produce long-term potentiation and help us to remember up to a point, whereas the opioids (i.e., endorphins) and oxytocin interfere with memory consolidation. Elevated levels of endogenous opioids are responsible for numbing, blunting of pain, and dissociation. Memories become disrupted or fragmented and may even be blocked from consciousness completely through dissociation that is mediated by the parasympathetic system. This has been called the immobilized freeze response, and it is posited that being repeatedly threatened in a state of helplessness can result in a parasympathetic-dominant response (Porges, 2011; Schore, 2019).

Trauma-induced neurohormonal changes mediate the reward systems in the brain. The arousal that occurs in stress states (i.e., sympathetic response) with the attending release of NE, serotonin, oxytocin, and endorphin is followed by decreases in the levels of these neurochemicals, which produces an opiate-like withdrawal with increased symptoms of restlessness and agitation that signal the need for physiological arousal again. The threat–arousal–endorphin cycle is activated, producing what van der Kolk, McFarlane, and Weisaeth (1996) call addiction to trauma. Massive secretion of neurohormones at the time of the traumatic event plays a role in the long-term potentiation and the overconsolidation of traumatic memories. These ANS changes become powerfully linked to implicit memory as templates of response for arousal. The physiological changes provide a compelling rationale for why trauma is reenacted as a conditioned response to related stimuli; that is, unconsciously and then triggered without the person's conscious awareness (Stavropoulos & Kezelman, 2018).

The release of endogenous opioids soothes the person temporarily so that abuse in the future triggers opioids and reflects the body's attempt to physiologically right itself. This is true for both individuals who have been significantly traumatized as adults as well as adults who have suffered early trauma as children (Waters, 2016). This mechanism explains why patients with early histories of childhood abuse often self-abuse by cutting or burning to relieve tension but do not experience such acts as painful because they are in a parasympathetic dissociated state. The brain is physiologically programmed or primed to recreate arousal or withdrawal states.

Dissociation can be useful, especially in childhood when no escape may be possible, except to temporarily leave the self in times of overwhelming danger. The dissociative processes of derealization and depersonalization allow the person to watch from a safe distance without experiencing the pain at that moment. However, dissociation at the time of the trauma is predictive for subsequent development of PTSD (Scaer, 2005). Development of dissociative memory networks of fear contributes to deficits in affect regulation, attachment, and executive functioning (van der Kolk, 2014). Particularly in patients with a history of early attachment trauma, rhythms of the body are severely dysregulated, and affective states of the self are not integrated. These unintegrated and dissociated self-states evolve from family environments that are chaotic, abusive, or neglectful (Howell, 2020; Schore, 2019).

Results of neuroimaging studies demonstrate different brain activation patterns for those with PTSD dominated by arousal symptoms from those with PTSD dominated by dissociative symptoms (Lanius et al., 2010). These differences point to different pathways of response for similar experiences. Scaer (2005) differentiates the diseases of stress from the diseases of trauma and he posits that the diseases of stress are related primarily to the sympathetic system, whereas the diseases of trauma result from the physiology of helplessness that occurs when the parasympathetic system is dominant, which is a physiological state of entrapment and disempowerment. The latter illnesses occur when a person enters into a state of physiological collapse and withdrawal that is characteristic of features of the parasympathetic freeze response, and can manifest when seemingly trivial life events represent a life threat based on the cumulative burden of negative life experiences and the similarity of the present event to any of the past experiences. This response occurs when autonomic regulatory functions are altered and there is a dramatic oscillation of autonomic activity, with manifestations of an exaggerated sympathetic and a parasympathetic response.

Dissociated neural networks are implicated in other psychiatric disorders, such as addictive disorders, eating disorders, obsessive–compulsive disorder, PTSD, borderline personality disorders, and dissociative disorders (Howell, 2020; Teicher et al., 2003). Other psychiatric disorders such as autism or schizophrenia are linked with impaired neuroception, the inability to detect whether the environment is safe (Porges & Dana, 2018). These individuals have difficulty with social engagement, with areas in the temporal cortex that inhibit ANS responses not activated. Compromised social behavior also occurs in those with anxiety disorders and depression with difficulties manifesting in the regulation of heart rate and reduced facial expressiveness. Children with reactive attachment disorder are either inhibited (emotionally withdrawn and unresponsive) or uninhibited (indiscriminate in their attachment), which also suggests faulty neuroception (Porges & Dana, 2018).

POLYVAGAL THEORY

Neuroception, a word coined by Porges, refers to the innate ability of the nervous system to detect safety, danger, and life-threat (Porges, 2004). Through evolution, the ANS has an information processing system that continually evaluates danger through neuroception, which modulates behavior and physiological states without our conscious awareness. Porges's (2011) research on the ANS has important implications for attachment and the brain's response to threat. His research led to the development of the PVT, which provides a more nuanced and fuller understanding of the stress/trauma response than described above. PVT posits that the ANS is composed of not just the sympathetic and parasympathetic systems but two parasympathetic branches, the myelinated ventral vagal, which originates in an area toward the front of the brainstem and develops around age 3 years, and the unmyelinated dorsal vagal, which originates in the back of the brainstem and is present early in fetal development. See http://www.debdanalcsw.com/resources/BG%20for%20ROR%20II.pdf for A Beginner's Guide to Polyvagal Theory.

The first response to the environment is that of social engagement through activation of the myelinated parasympathetic ventral vagus nervous system. The myelinated ventral vagus response corresponds to the resilient zone as described in Chapter 1. When in the "therapeutic window of arousal" or "resilient zone" (RZ), the person feels safe with others and is aware, curious, and responsive to the environment. The myelinated ventral vagal controls the face, neck, and head and develops rapidly after birth and supports attachment, inhibits the sympathetic system, and promotes a calm state that allows us to be interested in others and our surroundings. It is the vagal nerve that regulates heart rate; and heart rate variability provides an index of vagal tone so that your vagal tone helps to regulate cardiovascular, glucose, and immune responses. Ventral vagal tone is central to facial expressivity and the ability to tune into the human voice. The brain and the body communicate unconsciously with each other through the vagus nerve. By increasing ventral vagal tone, the capacity for empathy and interpersonal connection is increased so that one is more attuned to others. This explains why a lack of social contact diminishes people and why face-to-face contact is crucial for not only human development but to enhance the plasticity of the brain. It is through the predictability and familiarity of the caretaker that secure attachment and the ability to respond flexibly develops.

The second response or reaction of the nervous system if danger is sensed in the environment is through the sympathetic nervous system manifesting as fight or flight; finally, the third response, through the unmyelinated dorsal vagal, results in shutdown or immobilization if the sympathetic response does not prevent the attack. In the latter response, the parasympathetic system dominates and is responsible for states of hypoarousal manifested by symptoms of dissociation, pain blunting, depression, shame, loss of energy, and self-loathing (Corrigan Fisher, & Nutt, 2011). The dorsal vagal branch or third response to threat is activated and accompanied by a freeze immobility response once the sympathetic options of fight or flight are exhausted. See Figure 2.6 for the therapeutic window of arousal as conceptualized by Porges and Figures 1.2 and 1.3 in Chapter 1. These three systems are constantly adjusting our brains and bodies in response to our environments. If the person is in dorsal vagal shutdown or immobilization, Broca's area is likely offline and she or he may not be able to speak, that is, "speechless with terror." This is important for the APPN to know in order to reassure the rape victim who wanted to scream but couldn't that her brain did not allow the scream and that is a normal response to terror.

PVT provides a theoretical basis for the neuroscience of safety in relationship. Disconnection in relationship disrupts opportunities to co-regulate and thrusts the person into a state of "aloneness" (Porges, 2019). When we are not in our RZ, our perception changes and problem-solving is impaired. Safety in the therapeutic relationship is essential yet may be fraught with fear because a safe relationship may be a new experience for the patient. Through the APPN's compassion, presence, and empathy, the person may be able to experience what was previously a threatening relationship with new meaning, thus laying down new neural networks for relationship. Strategies on how to establish safety in a therapeutic relationship are discussed in Chapter 4.

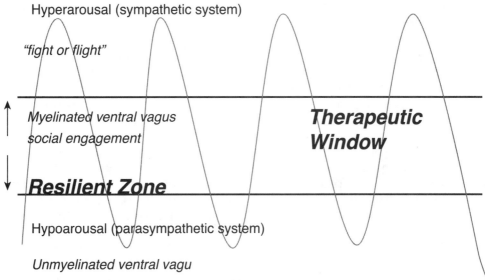

FIGURE 2.6 Therapeutic window of arousal or resilient zone.

Stabilization strategies discussed in Chapter 1 and throughout this book assist in widening one's window of arousal or RZ once the social engagement myelinated ventral vagus is activated. It is important to practice stabilization strategies when in the RZ so that those neural networks are reinforced; that is, "neurons that fire together, wire together." A robust RZ allows for a greater capacity for neurophysiological regulation. For those who have suffered errors of omission (neglect) or commission (physical, emotional, or sexual abuse) in childhood, their RZ is most likely narrow and a longer period of stabilization is needed. Porges's PVT provides the theoretical and neurophysiological basis for safety and the importance of the stabilization phase in psychotherapy as outlined in Chapter 1.

ADAPTIVE INFORMATION PROCESSING THEORY

AIP theory was developed by Shapiro through her development and observations of the effects of eye movement desensitization and reprocessing (EMDR) therapy (Shapiro, 2001, 2018). AIP hypothesizes that humans have an inherent information processing system that usually processes experiences to a physiological adaptive state in which information can be taken in and learning can occur. This model posits that there is an innate self-healing quality in the brain that strives to regulate its internal environment to survive and to maintain a stable, constant condition by means of dynamic regulation. Positive and negative experiences affect neurophysiological harmony. Optimally, memory is stored in a way that allows for connection with other adaptive memory networks (Shapiro, 2001, 2018).

Memory is stored in neural networks and learning is reflected as changes in synaptic strength among neural systems that are linked together and organized around early events with associated emotions, thoughts, images, and sensations (Bergmann, 2012, 2020). Interconnected neuronal and biochemical patterns are developed as templates for future experiences through interaction with others with specific profiles emerging that may be adaptive or nonadaptive. Information pathways exist throughout the brain and display synchronized oscillations so that neural networks entrain to each other's action potential. This synchronization allows for the creation of neural maps from the interactions of these neural networks. These pathways of neurons are forged by experience so that perception, memory, cognition, and emotion result and then are continually revised by new and ongoing experiences throughout life.

Learning changes the pattern of receptors in neural networks with integration and interconnections moving either top down (cortex to subcortical) or left right (across the two hemispheres of the brain). The top-down integration allows the processing of and organizing of impulses and emotions generated by the limbic and brainstem structures while the left-right integration allows for feelings to be put into words and for negative and positive emotions to be integrated. These systems are not necessarily independent of one another and involve multiple structures along the way (Cozolino, 2017). Adaptive processing means that neural connections are associated that allow the experiences to be integrated into positive emotional and cognitive schemas (Shapiro, 2001, 2018). Healthy functioning is reflected in the optimal integration and coordination of these neural networks with the brain existing in a balance of interconnectivity. "When the brain is operating efficiently, multiple assemblies of neurons are firing in unison, and information is flowing freely from one area to another" (Stien & Kendall, 2004, p. 19). Psychopathology is thought to result from a dysregulation that disrupts integrated neural processing of these networks. If an experience is perceived as emotionally intense or overwhelming, the event is registered as important as if your brain is saying: "This is important! Don't forget this!" We are hardwired for survival, so the experience is indelibly etched into our memory networks.

However, the memory is stored as it was at the time of the event and does not get linked to other networks in an adaptive way. The experience disrupts the biochemical balance of the information processing system and prevents the information from processing to an adaptive resolution by thwarting integration with other adaptive memory networks. Perceptions of the incident are etched into the information system as a result of the influx of messenger molecules, particularly NE for distressing experiences and dopamine for intensely positive experiences (Higgins & George, 2007). When a similar event occurs in the future, physiological information connected with the previous experience is matched against previous state-dependent memories that involve emotional, motor, and body memories. Reminders of these experiences by either internal or external factors trigger and continue to activate specific neurobiological responses that then drive behavior and the symptoms of most mental health problems and psychiatric disorders. To understand how experiences such as these affect brain function, it is helpful to review the stages of brain development and how the brain stores information.

BRAIN DEVELOPMENT

The brain allows us to accumulate and distill experiences through complex physiological processes. Elements of the collective experience of our species are reflected in the genome, and the experience of the individual is reflected in the expression of the genome. Life experience and environmental influences (epigenetics) determine the degree of expression of the genome through complex physiological processes (Champagne, 2010). Blood flow, energy use, and metabolism in various areas in the brain are determined by the person's environment and experience. The nuclei of various cells of the body modulate the expression of genes, and genes direct cells to produce various molecules that regulate the metabolism, growth, and activity level for every system of the body.

Genes are turned on and off by the messenger molecules that are chemical substances classified as hormones (i.e., endocrine system), neurotransmitters (i.e., ANS), immune cells (i.e., immune system), and neuropeptides. More than 300 messenger molecules have been identified. Some of these messenger molecules, such as hormones and neuropeptides, regulate the effects of the neurotransmitters and are specific for selected neural networks. Neurotransmitters have specific actions at receptor sites but are not considered the cause of mental illness (Melchitzky & Lewis, 2009). See Box 2.2 for the action of selected messenger molecules.

BOX 2.2

ACTION OF SELECTED MESSENGER MOLECULES

Acetylcholine: This neurotransmitter occurs in cholinergic tracts extending from the limbic structures to the cortex, and a decrease in concentration is associated with memory and cognitive impairments. Also it regulates mood, mania and sexual aggression. An increase is associated with depression.

Cortisol: This potent stress hormone mobilizes energy stores, stimulates the release of glucose, potentiates the release of adrenaline, increases cardiovascular tone, and inhibits growth, immune, and inflammatory responses.

Dopamine: This substance is produced in the substantia nigra and other areas in the brainstem; it is a key neurotransmitter for motor action, integration of emotions and thoughts, and decision-making; it stimulates the hypothalamic–pituitary–adrenal (HPA) axis to release hormones; and acts as the reward system. Elevated levels of dopamine may change mood, increase motor behavior, and disturb frontal lobe functioning, resulting in depression, memory impairment, and apathy. Parkinson disease and depression have been linked with decreased levels of dopamine and an increase is linked with schizophrenia and mania.

Endocrine messenger molecules: All are hormones composed of amino acids (in peptides, proteins, or glycoproteins) and are produced by one tissue and conveyed through the bloodstream to effect a change in growth or metabolism on another tissue. Moderate stress triggers the release of certain hormones that enhance cortical reorganization and new learning.

Endorphin: This endogenous opioid is found in a number of brain areas. It produces analgesia, reduces anxiety, and promotes calmness, and it is involved in self-harm and stress addiction.

Gamma-aminobutyric acid (GABA): This inhibitory neurotransmitter is found in most neurons in the central nervous system. It is involved in postsynaptic inhibition when benzodiazepines are given for anxiety, which further decreases the firing of the neurons. It plays a role in inhibition; reduces aggression, excitation, and anxiety; has anticonvulsant and muscle-relaxing properties; impairs cognition and psychomotor functioning. A decrease is associated with anxiety disorders, schizophrenia, and mania.

Glutamate: It is found in all cells, and its major receptor, N-methyl-D-aspartate (NMDA), helps to regulate brain development. Too much glutamate is toxic to neurons.

Immune messenger molecules: These substances are produced by the immune system and by nerve cells. Some produce neuropeptides and communicate directly and indirectly with the brain; others mediate behavioral responses, such as mild anxiety, avoidance, sleepiness, and lethargy. Selected substances include cytokines, interleukin-2, and immunocytes.

Norepinephrine (NE): Produced mainly in the locus coeruleus, NE is a key neurotransmitter in the flight, fight, or freeze stress response and affects mood, attention, and arousal. Too much can result in anxiety, vigilance, and aggressive behavior, but it can enhance memory and cognitive functioning up to a certain point. A decrease is associated with depression.

(continued)

On a cellular level, messenger molecules percolate across the synaptic space and bind to receptor sites found in cell walls, thereby changing receptor structure and cell wall permeability and causing ions to shift and second messenger molecules to direct the cell's activities. The receptors vibrate, and the messenger molecules are attracted to specific receptor sites. Receptors on each cell decrease or increase depending on the amount of their specific messenger molecule available at that moment (see Figure 2.7). A single neuron can get input from an average of 5,000 other neurons. With more than one-half million receptor sites per cell, 100 billion neurons in the brain, and 300 messenger molecules, it is easy to see that the number of possible interactions or communications is

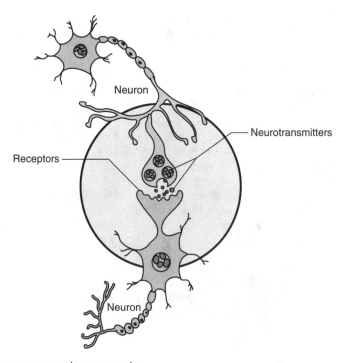

FIGURE 2.7 The neuron and receptor site.

enormous. Modulation of receptors regulates what information (i.e., memories, perceptions, and sensations) percolates across the synapse. The energy in the nerve impulse, the flow of ions down the axon, along with the information contained in the messenger molecules is fundamental to our subjective sense of self.

The brain stores experiences and creates templates, connections among neurons, against which everything is matched. These templates of neural networks begin to be laid down in utero and develop rapidly. The human brain develops many more neurons than it needs, and through apoptosis, or programmed cellular suicide, approximately 50% of them are eliminated before birth. The primary task of development is the sequential acquisition of various memories or networks of neurons. Sequential acquisition means that the brain develops from the bottom up, and templates of neurons are laid down to form these structures: from primitive regulation of body processes (e.g., respiration, sleep) to motor (i.e., simple to complex) to limbic (i.e., reaction to affiliation) to thought (i.e., concrete to complex). The brain develops from the lower brain structure of the brainstem to the midbrain through the limbic structures; the cortex is the last area and the most "plastic" area of the brain. Neuroplasticity refers to areas that are responsive to the environment and that can change. The lower brain structures such as the brainstem are more fixed than the higher brain functions of the cortex, which continue to develop throughout life. Figure 2.8 shows the stages of brain development, regulation, and memory.

Brain development consists of laying down neural networks during the various stages of development, and as synapses change, brain structures change on the basis of experience. The interplay of experience and developmental period is important in that there are certain critical periods, especially in the first 3 years of life, when specific neural networks are particularly malleable or plastic (Bergmann, 2020; Schore, 2019). The brain triples in size up to age 5 years, largely due to myelinization, and this increases the rate of information processing. Infancy and adolescence are two critical periods for the process of making new neurons, or neurogenesis.

A group of proteins called "neurotrophic growth factors" support neurogenesis. The most common is brain-derived neurotrophic factor (BDNF). (Higgins & George, 2013). BDNF binds to neurons and supports the growth, maturation, and survival of synaptic

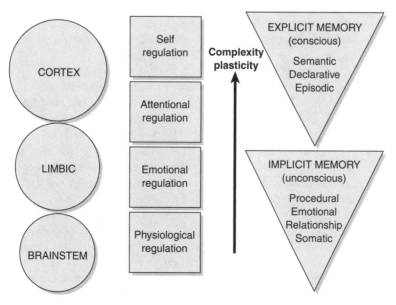

FIGURE 2.8 Stages of brain development, regulation, and memory diagram.

connections (Carasatorre & Ramirez-Amaya, 2013). The right hemisphere develops first, and a left hemisphere growth spurt occurs in the middle of the second year of life. The right hemisphere is more densely connected with subcortical areas and is associated with the sense of our bodies, images, perception of emotions, regulation of the ANS, and unconscious memories, whereas the left is primarily responsible for language, logic, and conscious problem-solving (Schore, 2019). See Figure 2.3.

Healthy brain development is contingent on early experience and sequential completion of critical windows of opportunity for establishing neural connections. All subsequent development is dependent on the basic circuitry of systems of neural networks. Given the timetable of the developing brain, it is easy to see that a frustrated 3-year-old child whose cortex is not fully developed will have a hard time modulating the arousal levels of the lower brain structures and may scream, kick, and bite, whereas the older child who has more cortex will be able to inhibit these urges when frustrated. This is consistent with theoretical speculations about the sequential development of ego and superego functions, which are cortically mediated functions that modulate impulse control. Loss of cortical functions can occur in many pathological processes, such as dementia or stroke, whereas loss of the cortical ability to modulate arousal and aggression in the brainstem and midbrain may result in hyperactivity and impulsivity and predispose the person to violence (Camchong & MacDonald, 2012).

The brain develops in a use-dependent fashion, which means that the more the neuronal network is activated, the more likely a template will be created and the connection and pattern formed between neurons and networks of neurons will be strengthened with the brain changing in response to this patterned neuronal activity. This process is called long-term potentiation (Siegel, 2012). According to Hebb's (1949) axiom, "any two cells or systems of cells that are repeatedly active, at the same time, will tend to become 'associated' so that activity in one facilitates activity in the other" (p. 70). This was summarized by Carla Schatz as "neurons that fire together wire together" (Schatz, 1992, p. 65). That is, the brain is more likely to activate this clustering of neurons in the future as a cohesive state of mind. Neural networks interconnect with multiple other neural networks so that if one network is activated, it can trigger another one and so forth. As the brain develops, there are increasingly synchronous patterns and activation of the neural networks of the cortex. As the cortex develops, top-down neural networks connect with the subcortical networks below. These synaptic connections or synaptogenesis continue throughout adult life supported by BDNF; however, aging and stress hormones can silence BDNF, suppressing synaptogenesis.

Unused neural connections are eliminated through a process called pruning. This occurs primarily during critical periods after a growth spurt: between 15 months and 4 years, between 6 and 10 years, during prepuberty, and during middle adolescence (Ornitz, 1996). Pruning results in decreases in cortical volume and decreases in gray matter and increases in white matter that are reflected in enhanced cortical connections and information processing (Bava & Tapert, 2010). A stimulating environment facilitates the development of dendritic branching in neurons, a process referred to as arborization. The proliferation of new connections among neurons increases the potential for learning. These changes develop as a result of experience through sensations from our external world or our internal world. Neural networks are shaped and continue to be developed by environmental experiences, which is reflected in increasingly complex behavioral patterns. Interconnected neuronal biochemical patterns are developed as templates for future experiences though interaction with others, and specific chemical and neuropeptide profiles emerge that may serve adaptive or nonadaptive functions. For example, sensations from a person's internal world arise from the brainstem, and the midbrain learns to respond to decreased temperature or increased glucose levels, and sensory input from the external world, such as light, sound, or pressure, comes in though our senses to our brain and tells our bodies how to respond.

MEMORY

Depending on when they are formed or the neural connections made, some memories are less plastic or harder to change than others (Siegel, 2012). Memory is determined by the stage of development when the neural connection was made, the area of the brain, and the nature of the memory itself. For example, structures in the brainstem, midbrain, and limbic areas are almost fully formed by the time the child is 3 years old. These memories are much harder to change than those in some areas of the cortex, which remain plastic throughout life.

The sequential acquisition of various memories is the primary task of development, and this is determined by genetics and interaction with the environment. Memory of a specific event is not stored in one particular place in the brain; it is distributed across neural networks in different brain areas. The brain takes associations from a single or specific event and generalizes to other events. For example, a scent memory can activate a chain of other associated memories connected with that odor based on that one sensation. Each memory has a particular biochemical profile depending on how it was perceived and stored in the brain. Each memory can be thought of as a particular state of consciousness that is triggered by a sensation unique to that physiological template. In this way, a somatic feeling such as an accelerated heart rate can trigger associated memories, thoughts, images, emotions, and sensations connected with it.

Memory is linked to the emotions surrounding the event from the moment it occurred and to the specific physiological state we are in when we have the experience. Emotions are the result of the physiological changes triggered by the experience (Damasio, 1999). Retrieval of this information depends on the chemical state of the brain at the time of storage and at the time of retrieval and also depends on where language is stored. Information can be stored verbally, emotionally, somatically, and in images, and what we learn depends on our physiological state at the time of the experience. The more intense the emotion, either positive or negative, the more likely the memory will be etched into an enduring neural template. This is what Rossi (1996) calls state-dependent learning. That is, state-dependent learning reflects the biochemical template for the specific emotions at the time of the experience, which reflects a specific physiological state we are in at the moment of the event. Research has found that retrieval of memory is best when the physiological state in which we learned the information matches the physiology of the current situation (Chu, 2011). For example, if we study for an exam while smoking cigarettes and drinking coffee, we will fare better in retrieving this information if we smoke cigarettes and drink coffee while taking the examination (Pert, 1999).

Pert (1999) observes that we are all like multiple personalities in that each emotional state has a specific template or profile that is linked to a specific physiological state along with its concomitant thoughts, images, sensations, and physiology. Different states of consciousness are triggered by stimuli throughout the day as we slip in and out of various physiological templates. We literally change our minds on a moment-to-moment basis, but unlike those with dissociative identity disorder, we are more or less aware of the interconnection of our experiences that define and unite our sense of self. Each experiential state is reflected in the specific activities of our external environment. For example, although we may "space out" when we are driving and cannot remember exactly how we got to where we were going, we do remember generally that we were driving. The numerous states of consciousness that occur throughout the day are part of the seamless whole we experience as ourselves and are fairly consistent through time. Other "normal" dissociative experiences include "spacing out" during a lecture or induced altered states of consciousness, such as those that occur while praying, chanting, drumming, or meditating. These specific dissociative periods are considered normal, and each has a specific physiological state and brain wave pattern that is triggered by the specific event (i.e., driving, listening to a lecture, or church attendance).

Memory research has expanded dramatically in the past few years, and our understanding about what happens in the brain when we learn and about the different types of memory has greatly increased. Usually, when we think of memory, we think of cognitive memory, such as learning phone numbers or names. This is referred to as explicit memory and includes declarative or semantic memory (Figure 2.8). This is the type of memory that Freud would have called conscious memory. Autobiographical memory is also explicit and sometimes called episodic memory or narrative memory and refers to knowing about oneself through recollection of the past, present, and possible future (Stavropoulos & Kezelman, 2018). In normal development, self-awareness and autobiographical narratives are interwoven, but in trauma, this type of memory may be greatly impaired. REM sleep is thought to be essential for consolidation of neocortical semantic memories (Bergmann, 2012, 2020).

The other type of memory, implicit memory, involves motor or procedural memories, emotional memories, and somatic memories that are most often formed earlier in development than explicit memories. Motor memories are procedural and include vestibular memories such as riding a bicycle, brushing your teeth, typing, or driving a car. These memories do not require conscious recall; after you know how to drive, you do not have to learn again. Other implicit memories include emotional and body memories. These experiences exist on a nonverbal, semiautomatic level and involve the here and now. These procedural, implicit memories ensure survival. It is thought that these implicit memory systems are essential for understanding development, psychopathology, and psychotherapy (Cozolino, 2017). This type of memory includes what Freud would have called the unconscious.

Emotional-state-dependent memories are implicit and include specific emotional experiences such as fear, grief, anxiety, and complex attachment feelings that form from interaction with caretakers based on the experiences of the developing child. When a mother and a child physically hold each other, their bodily autonomic states harmonize, connecting on a visceral level from distress to calm. There may not be words for somatic or emotional memories, only felt experiences. How we have a relationship is an implicit emotional memory. Implicit memories exist in our neural networks in a pattern of neural associations that are formed early in life from memories of attachment experiences. For example, a person may have a sense of sadness and agitation whenever alone, and it may be related to being left alone frequently as a child, with the subliminal connection patterned as a template in the brain. The person may not even be aware of why being alone triggers emotions of sadness and agitation. See Figure 2.9 for an example of one person's trigger of loneliness which is a specific physiological state activating various neurophysiological responses that are efforts to stay in the RZ yet which are largely unsuccessful and unconscious. The person needs resources and stabilization in order to widen the RZ or stay in a myelinated ventral vagal state.

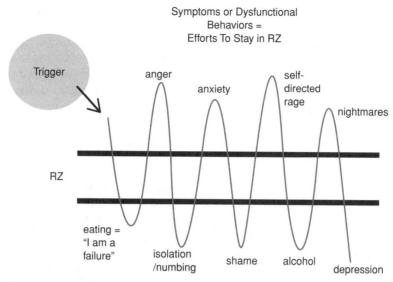

FIGURE 2.9 Triggers result in dysegulation of the nervous system

Defense Mechanisms

Defense mechanisms are implicit memory networks that develop through reciprocal interaction with caregivers and interpersonal experiences for the purpose of regulating anxiety, grief, anger, and self-esteem keeping from conscious awareness disturbing thoughts and feelings. Defense mechanisms are not categorical; they exist on a developmental continuum that evolves through parent, environment, and child interactions. Defenses serve the purpose of allaying anxiety and help the child survive painful emotional experiences and relational loss, but they may be dysfunctional in adulthood when no longer needed. For example, a child may need to deny that his mother's behavior is unloving in order to believe that he is safe; he can continue to survive "knowing" that he is cared about, thus preserving the attachment relationship. Later, as an adult, this denial may interfere with his ability to clearly see his mother as unloving, and as a result of cognitive immaturity, the person may conclude he is defective and that it is his fault because he is an unlovable person.

Early literature examined the development of specific defenses related to specific stages of psychosexual development, with the more immature defenses evolving earlier in development than those considered more mature (Brenner, 1982; Freud, 1966; Kernberg, 1975). It is thought that those with more primitive or immature defenses are "stuck" in an earlier, less neuroplastic way of reacting to the world that is more difficult to change. Primitive and immature defenses represent unintegrated neural networks that distort reality and result in functional impairment. Under stress, there is often regression to earlier, more immature defenses. Someone who is said to be defensive or well-defended seems impervious to change and may remain inflexible no matter what the situation.

Defenses are the good news and the bad news because they may enhance mental health or may contribute to mental illness if too reality distorting. Everyone needs defenses, and mature defenses allow a healthy, flexible, adaptive way of experiencing the world. Mature defenses are rooted in neural networks that allow the person to navigate reality with reactions that are reality-respecting with a minimum of defensiveness. We can speculate that a person with mature defenses has some facility and flexibility in using a variety of defenses and is not locked into a specific template of defense to be used no matter what the situation. Cozolino (2017) posits that mature defenses, such as humor and sublimation, allow us to lessen strong feelings, keep in contact with others, and remain attuned to a shared reality.

Sadock, Sadock, and Ruiz (2017) delineate defenses into three levels—immature, neurotic, and mature—to illustrate the continuum of defenses. Defenses are not static, and rarely does a person fall exclusively into one category. It is probable that there are clusters of defenses used more often in certain contexts and that differences are a matter of degree. Mature defenses are reality respecting and allow one to postpone immediate gratification and include sublimation and suppression. These defenses are often found in obsessive–compulsive and histrionic patients, whereas the primitive and immature defenses, such as projection and denial, are associated with adolescents and some non-psychotic patients. Those who use a preponderance of immature defenses often have greater problems in work and relationships. Those who have had a "nervous breakdown" are those whose defenses did not allow adaptation and the ability to ward off unpleasant affects. These individuals are flooded with anxiety and negative affect that render them incapacitated and unable to cope. Box 2.3 lists selected primitive or immature, neurotic, and mature defenses (Sadock et al., 2017).

BOX 2.3

DEFENSE MECHANISMS

Immature Defenses

Denial: avoiding the reality of painful reality by ignoring or refusing to acknowledge reality (e.g., a man with schizophrenia denies that he is ill and does not take his medication).

Projection: perceiving and reacting to unacceptable feelings and impulses as if they were outside the self (e.g., instead of the person feeling anger, anger is experienced as coming from others toward the person who is doing the projecting, as during paranoid delusions).

Acting out: avoiding conscious experience of the emotion through impulsive action (e.g., instead of feeling sad, a person gets drunk).

Regression: avoiding emotional pain through returning to an earlier level of development (e.g., a child begins wetting the bed after a sibling is born).

Hypochondria: exaggerating an illness arising from unacceptable feelings (e.g., anger and hostility are transformed into pain and somatic complaints).

Introjection: internalizing the qualities of the other (e.g., identification with the aggressor through which the person becomes aggressive to gain control).

Somatization: converting emotion into bodily symptoms (e.g., instead of getting angry, the person gets a headache).

Splitting: inability to integrate positive with negative aspects of oneself and then projecting this onto other people or situations (e.g., a woman tells her husband she loves him one day and hates him the next day, even though nothing has changed to warrant this).

(continued)

BOX 2.3

DEFENSE MECHANISMS (*continued*)

Neurotic Defenses

Displacement: shift of emotion from a person or object to one that is less distressing (e.g., instead of expressing anger at his boss, the man kicks his dog).

Dissociation: avoiding emotional distress through an altered state of consciousness, such as fugue states or conversion reactions (e.g., a person loses several hours of time and does not remember what happened).

Intellectualization: using intelligence to avoid intimacy and expression of disturbing feelings (e.g., a woman explains in great detail all the pluses of the new city where she is moving to assuage her anxiety about leaving a significant relationship).

Rationalization: offering explanations in an attempt to explain behaviors or feelings that are unacceptable (e.g., after doing poorly on a test, the student believes the test or teacher is stupid).

Reaction formation: transforming an unacceptable impulse into the opposite (e.g., a woman unexpectedly runs into someone she does not like on the street and is overly friendly).

Repression: thought to be the basis of all other defenses and involves withholding from consciousness an idea or feeling that is unacceptable (e.g., the child cannot remember her anger or hitting her mother).

Mature Defenses

Sublimation: channeling unacceptable impulses through pursuing socially acceptable goals (e.g., a young man who is aggressive and impulsive pursues a career as a boxing coach).

Suppression: consciously deciding to forget an unpleasant feeling (e.g., a woman is preoccupied with the illness of her father and decides to not worry about it because there is nothing she can do about it).

Altruism: using service to others and vicariously experiencing pleasure through doing good for others to avoid negative feelings about oneself (e.g., a young woman is a social activist).

Humor: using comedy to express feelings and thoughts without discomfort (e.g., a person uses self-deprecating humor to put others at ease).

Using a psychodynamic framework, the APPN assesses the level of the person's ego development through identification of the defenses that the person uses for the purpose of gauging ego strength (i.e., integration of neural networks). If someone primarily uses immature defenses, the person most likely has poor ego strength and early issues of trauma. This may indicate that a longer period of stabilization in psychotherapy is indicated. The therapist supports the defenses that are adaptive and helps the person to develop higher-level defenses, if needed. This can be accomplished through clarification and exploration so that the person's awareness of his or her defenses is enhanced. Conscious awareness of the defense often leads the person to experience the emotion against which the person is defending (Cozolino, 2017). For example, one man who was in rehabilitation for alcohol abuse told his therapist that he wanted his marriage to work but said he had to drink so that he could cope with his bad marriage. Pointing out the discrepancy between his actions and his stated wishes made the rationalization a less effective coping strategy. In subsequent psychotherapy sessions, he experienced much anxiety about the possibility of losing his wife and realized how angry he had been for a long time about not feeling cared about. The addiction assuaged his anxiety and the anxiety blocked his angry feelings. Through releasing emotion in the context of a supportive psychotherapeutic relationship, neural networks associated with state-dependent memories of not feeling loved were activated, and this enhanced growth because integration of more positive neural networks could then link to this experience.

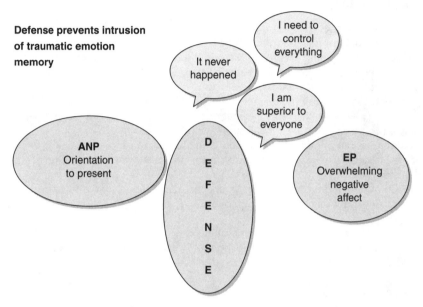

FIGURE 2.10 Defenses protect the ANP (apparently normal part). EP, emotional part.

Source: Adapted from Knipe, J. (2019). *EMDR toolbox: Theory and treatment of complex PTSD and dissociation* (2nd ed.). New York, NY: Springer Publishing Company.

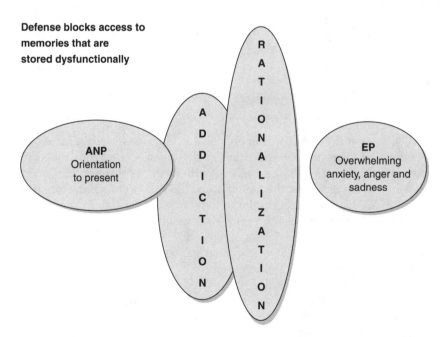

FIGURE 2.11 Addictive defense. ANP, apparently normal part; EP, emotional part.

Source: Adapted from Knipe, J. (2019). *EMDR toolbox: Theory and treatment of complex PTSD and dissociation* (2nd ed.). New York, NY: Springer Publishing Company.

Through the lens of more contemporary explanations of defense, PVT provides a neurophysiological explanation with the second (sympathetic arousal) and third response to threat (dorsal vagal shutdown) as defensive states while the first response mediated by the myelinated ventral vagus is reflected by openness to others and social engagement where defenses to threat are not activated. The second response (fight) may manifest as a resistant or angry patient or may manifest as acquiescence but the person does not adhere to the treatment.

Knipe (2019) provides an explanation of defense through the lens of AIP. He explains that the person who has suffered from a traumatic experience at any age often has memories that are fragmented and dissociated from consciousness. A trigger that is a fragment of the memory such as a feeling, image, thought, or sensation can occur and flood the person with unexpected emotion. Knipe states that a defense is any "mental action or behavior that has the function and purpose of blocking the full emergence into consciousness posttraumatic disturbance" (Knipe, 2019, p. 51). He expands the traditional idea about defenses to addictions and avoidance as well as the above-mentioned defense mechanisms. Thus, defenses serve to keep at bay disturbing feelings and memories.

This idea is consistent with structural dissociation theory that proposes that patients who have suffered trauma have not processed the traumatic experience and thus have different parts of their personality: the apparently normal part (ANP) or the adult perspective deals with daily life in the present; and the emotional part (EP) or trauma experience, which is not fully integrated with the ANP (Steele, Boon, & van der Hart, 2017; Steele, van der Hart, & Nijenhuis, 2005). The EP, or the part that holds the trauma, has split off from the ANP, or adult perspective, with the EP being that part of the personality that holds the emotions, somatic sensations, image, and cognition (memory fragments) of the traumatic experience while the ANP avoids the trauma. In order to function in daily life, the ANP blocks the EP with these dissociated parts not integrated. Memory fragments of the traumatic experience may occur as flashbacks and somatic sensations, which are triggers that can be quite startling to the ANP, who is phobic of any and all parts of the trauma.

The defense then blocks the trauma or EP out of the ANP or adult's consciousness (see Figure 2.10). In the clinical example described previously, the man's alcohol abuse was an acting out behavior that kept his sadness and anger dissociated from his awareness so he could avoid painful feelings of not being cared about. Thus, the man could continue to function in the present, seemingly oblivious to the disturbing feelings of anger and sadness that were numbed or kept at bay by his alcohol abuse. Figure 2.11 illustrates addiction and rationalization as defenses that keep the ANP from awareness of painful experiences and feelings (EP). See Chapter 17, for a further discussion of dissociation and structural dissociation theory and Chapter 19, for discussion of addictions.

Attachment

Attachment experiences are embedded in implicit somatic memory networks. Children are born biologically programmed to form attachments with others in order to survive. An internal working model of relationship is developed through the attachment to the caregiver (Bowlby, 1969). The brain develops only in the context of another brain (Schore, 2019). The human infant survives based on the caretaking abilities of those around them. Developmental and attachment research supports that the infant uses the parent to regulate inner states until psychoneurobiological functions are mature and autonomous. These shared states of affect, known as dyadic states of consciousness, shared attunement, or limbic resonance, are internalized and encoded as procedural memory, enabling stable and secure connections to others (Siegel, 2012). Moment-to-moment physiological attunement through neuroception is the capacity to read signals (often nonverbal) that indicate the need for engagement or disengagement (Schore, 2019). However, such attunement only needs to occur 30% of the time in order to build the scaffolding for a securely attached infant (Schore, 2019). The caregiver helps the infant to tolerate negative emotions as well as responds and enhances positive states of joy, exploration, and curiosity. These states of attunement begin the process of self-regulation through rhythmic autonomic cycling, which modulates the response to arousal, directing the flow of energy through the system. If there are problems in attachment, there are concomitant problems in the self-regulation of stress and core affects. Core affects refer to emotions hardwired from birth and include seeking/curiosity, fear, rage, and panic (Panksepp, 2004). As described in Chapter 1, these core affects evolve and are shaped by one's cultural milieu. Core affects are modulated by higher brain structures as we learn to express our feelings depending on the circumstance and culture.

Attachment research has classified attachment patterns or schemas that develop over the first few years of life in response to parental availability and attunement. Ainsworth developed the Infant Strange Situation, a test that categorized how infants reacted when their mother left them in a strange situation and how they reunited with their mother when she returned. She found four categories of response and labeled them: secure attachment, avoidant, ambivalent/preoccupied, and disorganized/disoriented patterns (Ainsworth, 1967). See Table 2.1 for attachment schemas. On maternal separation, the securely attached infant is easily comforted and resumes play and exploration when the mother returns. The avoidant infant remains aloof and disinterested when the mother returns, whereas the resistant/ambivalent infant is not easily soothed and remains preoccupied vigilantly scanning for mother's whereabouts. The disorganized or disoriented infant has not developed a consistent strategy for coping with the stress of separation (Meyer & Pilkonis, 2002). These neural pathways of infant attachment form blueprints of perceptions, feelings, and responses that manifest as personality characteristics that predict later adult attachment. A corresponding test for adults termed the Adult Attachment Interview has also been developed (Hesse, 1999). Attachment patterns have been found to be relatively stable and reflect how adults form attachment to others, including their partners and their therapist.

The newborn's brain development depends on interaction with others with relationships serving as regulators of physiological processes (Schore, 2019; Siegel, 2012). Schore describes the face-to-face and gaze-to-gaze connection of mother–infant bonding and posits that it facilitates development, especially of the right cerebral hemisphere which develops first. Biochemical reactions through these interactions with caregivers

TABLE 2.1   ATTACHMENT SCHEMAS

Infant Strange Situation	Adult Attachment Interview
Secure	Secure/Autonomous
Avoidant	Dismissing
Ambivalent/Resistant	Preoccupied
Disorganized/Disoriented	Unresolved/Disorganized

Sources: Data from Ainsworth, M. D. (1967). *Infancy in Uganda.* Baltimore, MD: Johns Hopkins Press; Hesse, E. (1999). The adult attachment interview: Historical and current perspectives. In J. Cassidy & P. R. Shaver (Eds.), *Handbook of attachment: Theory, research, and clinical applications* (pp. 395–433). New York, NY: Guilford Press.

enhance the development and connection of neural networks. The connection of neural networks allows discrete states of self to be integrated and linked. Siegel (1999) states, "The structure and function of the developing brain are determined by how experiences, especially within interpersonal relationships, shape the . . . maturation of the nervous system" (p. 149). These neural networks encoded in implicit procedural memories of sensory, motor, affective, and cognitive memories of caretaker experiences regulate physiological processes. Attuned caregivers share emotional states with the infant. This shared attunement, or limbic resonance, regulates emotions by modulating overstimulation or underarousal of the ANS for the cortically challenged infant. Through interaction, the mother creates a psychobiological state similar to her own (Schore, 2019; Stien & Kendall, 2004). Research has found that self-regulatory function is developed in a hierarchical fashion, as illustrated in Figure 2.8 (Feldman, 2009).

Schore (2019) says that higher levels of sympathetic activation increase production of endorphins, dopamine, and NE, which increase energy and pleasure in the child. BDNF is stimulated, modulating glutamate-sensitive N-methyl-D-aspartate (NMDA) receptors that regulate neuroplasticity and long-term potentiation, which appear to buffer the hippocampus from stress. Sympathetic dominance is associated with states of arousal, and parasympathetic dominance is associated with conservation withdrawal (Scaer, 2005; Schore, 2019). If misattunement is present, the infant may begin to frequently withdraw, and this is thought to be an early manifestation of dissociation. These are right-brain implicit memories and responses to early relational trauma. Secure attachment experiences are reflected in an optimal balance of the sympathetic and parasympathetic nervous systems, with synchronous connections among neural networks.

An important research finding about attachment and learning involves mirror neurons, which help us make sense of how we learn at critical periods by watching others (Ammaniti & Gallese, 2014; Dobbs, 2006). Mirror neurons are located in the lateral frontal cortex, the posterior parietal areas, and other regions that correspond to the ability to comprehend someone else's feelings and intention. Mirror neurons fire when we watch how someone else does something, and they fire as if we were doing the action ourselves. Neuroimaging studies have found that these neurons are present at birth. For example, if an infant watches an adult smile, the same neurons in the infant's brain will fire as if the infant were smiling. This occurs for visual stimuli and for sounds and other sensations. Our brain mirrors others' brains so that one does not have to experience something directly to feel what someone else is feeling. Mirror neurons are thought to play a key role in perceiving intentions, which is a first step in the development of empathy. The idea of shared minds and dyadic states of consciousness is a physiological reality that has implications for understanding the importance of attachment relationships for affect regulation and learning. It is thought that a dysfunction in mirror neurons may create significant problems in attachment, from autism to violence.

Attachment problems and unresolved trauma in the mother breed attachment problems and trauma in the child. Inability of the mother to connect and think about her own thoughts and feelings has been found to be a significant predictor of attachment problems. Results of one study illustrate the importance of affect attunement and regulation of affects in understanding the cycle of trauma and violence that persists across generations. This research on intergenerational maternal trauma found that the distressed child represents a possible posttraumatic trigger for the violence-exposed caretaker who has a history of violent trauma and insecurity of attachment that then adversely affects maternal perception (Schechter, 2003). The more negative and distorted the maternal perception of the child, the more the child is likely to be distressed and behaviorally disorganized. For children younger than 4 years, inability to regulate emotions is the norm, and this state in the child sometimes triggers in caregivers their own horror, helplessness, and outrage about violent perpetrators who had hostile aggression and difficulty with negative affect toward them. The caretaker with her own affect regulation problems due to trauma has great difficulty with soothing and connecting with her child and may attribute malevolent motivations to her child that are related to her earlier feelings about her perpetrators. This study points to the importance of the parents' role in the co-regulation of stressful states. In summary, attachment research has found that attachment neural networks impact learning, neural plasticity, the ability to cope with stress, and maternal behavior in adulthood.

Without the presence of a protective relationship with an adult, a child cannot develop the coping skills or sense of control to mediate stressors and regulate arousal. Early adversity and traumatic stress affect future stress reactivity through the development of neural circuits that control neuroendocrine responses (Roth, Lubin, Funk, & Sweatt, 2009; Szyf, 2009). Significant early trauma and lack of attachment have also been demonstrated to have effects on neurotransmitters, specifically irregular serotonin activity (Schlozman & Nonacs, 2008). Research has demonstrated that even in the absence of PTSD or a diagnosable psychiatric disorder, there may be abnormal cortisol activity so that through exposure to trauma, significant long-term physical changes in the body can occur (Scaer, 2005). Chefetz (2019) says that in disorganized attachment, the child has a parent who is frightening or unresponsive and inconsistent and the child can't figure out what to expect. Thus, the child ends up frozen, confused, and rejected/shamed. Long-term chronic shame is often present for those who have suffered impaired attachment.

Thus, interpersonal relationships play a significant role in either relieving or contributing to stress. These deeply etched attachment neural networks pattern limbic pathways from our earliest experiences and affect our susceptibility to disease. Those whose social engagement system or RZ is robust will have a map of relationships that sustains them through tough times and can be alone and still feel connected. The right brain continues to develop and be affected by close relationships throughout life (Schore, 2019). Without this map, hormonal and neurotransmitter responses predispose the person to physiological dysregulation and disease.

RESTRUCTURING NEURAL NETWORKS

While several decades of research have established the efficacy of psychotherapy in the treatment of various psychiatric disorders, experts are only beginning to understand exactly how psychotherapy works. Contemporary thinking about psychotherapy based on neurophysiological research about memory, trauma, and brain development led to the development of the AIP model (Shapiro, 2001, 2018). AIP provides a cogent explanation for a possible mechanism of psychotherapeutic action and serves as the underlying model for the treatment hierarchy framework discussed in Chapter 1. AIP posits that information is normally taken in and associated or connected to other memory networks to be used and stored constructively (Shapiro, 2001, 2018). For example, if we have an unpleasant interaction with a friend, we may talk about it or think about it until we feel better about the event, and then we know better in the future how to deal with this particular person; we have adaptively processed this information. Inherent in this model is the idea of self-healing, akin to the body's self-healing capacity. If there is a physical injury, natural mechanisms assist in healing the wound. Similarly, there is a natural healing mechanism in the brain for adaptively processing information. Scaer (2005) proposes that processing promotes limbic, autonomic, endocrine, and immune homeostasis.

A problem arises when an overwhelming traumatic event occurs and the brain is flooded with stress-related changes in messenger molecules, inhibiting the brain's ability to process or integrate this information in an adaptive way. The information is stored as it was experienced during the time of the event, with all the attending images, feelings, and sensations of that moment (Shapiro, 2001, 2018). This state-dependent information is then isolated and disconnected from more adaptive memory systems. Cozolino (2017) states that psychopathology is "a reflection of suboptimal development, integration, and coordination of neural networks" and that "unresolved trauma can cause ongoing information processing deficits that disrupt integrated neural processing" (p. 26). These unintegrated or underdeveloped neural networks create the problems for which people seek psychotherapy.

Dysfunctionally linked information that is isolated or disconnected must be linked or forged with adaptive neural networks to construct or return to full consciousness. If the person has had many traumas, there may be many areas of dissociated memories, with each containing its own somatosensory or autonomic and limbic or emotional cues (Scaer, 2005; see Figure 2.3). These cues, powerfully linked in neural networks, serve as triggers for the past and significantly limit the person's experience of the present. For example, a man who had suffered early emotional neglect and criticism from his perfectionist, distant parents experienced most interactions in his adult life as an evaluation of his worth. Consequently, he felt shamed and judged, and his moment-to-moment experience was filled with negative evaluations of himself and those around him. This left little room for the present reality because everything was filtered through a shame-based lens. Feeling like a disappointment and unlovable, he reacted to others with sarcasm or childlike passivity in an attempt to please, even though this created the experience he most feared: being rejected by others.

Because dysfunctional information needs to be linked to adaptive neural networks to enable synchronized integrated brain functioning to occur, the existence of positive memories or experiences is needed. For some patients who have suffered early neglect or trauma, positive experiences may need to be created first for adaptive networks to be present. For others, adaptive networks may exist, but need to be strengthened. Adaptive networks are created or strengthened through enhancing or creating internal resources and positive experiences. van der Kolk (2006) says that it is important to "explore previous experiences of safety and competency and to activate memories of what it feels like to experience pleasure, enjoyment, focus, power, and effectiveness before activating trauma-related sensations and emotions" (p. 289). Shapiro (2018) agrees and says that the person must be able to manage state changes before processing trauma. "State changes" refer to transient physiological states – such as anxiety – that can be assuaged through relaxation techniques or other strategies and resources that decrease sympathetic arousal. These therapeutic approaches contrast with treatment goals related to "trait changes," which Shapiro (2012, 2018) says can occur, but only after the person has fully processed the trauma. This speaks to the importance of an accurate assessment that includes not only deficits (i.e., what is wrong), but also the person's strengths (i.e., what is right) and available resources, so that an appropriate plan of care can be developed. This type of assessment is a hallmark of the holistic health-oriented model of nursing practice.

The person is stabilized after s/he can access external and internal resources and manage both positive and negative emotions. The development of adaptive memory networks then allows dysfunctional memory networks to be restructured. Clinical indices reflect whether the person is stabilized (see Appendix 1.5). According to Fuchs (2004), the focus of psychotherapy is to restructure "neural networks, particularly in the subcortical-limbic system, which is responsible for unconscious emotional motivations and dispositions" (p. 480). Schore (2012) agrees and says, "Both optimal development and effective psychotherapy promote an expansion of the biological substrate of the human unconscious, the right brain, which is considered the dynamic core of the implicit self." The unconscious serves as an emotion-processing regulatory system (Schore, 2019). Accessing dysfunctionally-linked material and connecting it to existing or newly created adaptive networks is the work of psychotherapy.

In processing, hyperarousal of the sympathetic nervous system must be modulated with anxiety-management strategies so that information can be brought to an adaptive resolution and further dissociation and dysregulation are prevented. High levels of emotional arousal decrease cerebral efficiency, which in turn inhibits emotional processing. The irritability of the amygdala must be decreased to enable effective integration to occur. Neuroplastic potential is maximized by moderate – but not excessive – arousal (Cozolino, 2017). When working with traumatized individuals, van der Kolk (2006) agrees and says, "Learning to modulate the arousal level is essential for overcoming the resulting passivity and dependency [that occurs in traumatized individuals]" (p. 284).

Imaging studies have found that for those with significant trauma, there is decreased activation in the prefrontal cortex, resulting in reduced cerebral efficiency and difficulty in modulating emotional arousal and in problem-solving. Increasing activation and functioning of the prefrontal cortex enhances the person's ability to manage emotions and to plan better for the future (van der Kolk, 2014). Mindful attention, such as occurs during meditation, has been found to increase the thickness of the prefrontal cortex and right anterior insula (Lazar et al., 2005). Exercises that incorporate dual awareness and mindfulness are helpful in increasing frontal lobe functioning so that the person learns to pay attention to his or her internal experience without being overwhelmed by the sensations. This attention is called interoceptive awareness. Traumatized individuals are afraid of themselves and their own physiological sensations because the situation is reminiscent of earlier states of helplessness and fear (van der Kolk, 2014). It is thought that through mindfulness, the person gradually becomes more aware of internal sensory stimuli, and this awareness increases the capacity to manage potentially stressful encounters. Mindfulness and dual awareness strategies may include somatic awareness, safe place, anchors, dual awareness exercises, progressive muscle relaxation, establishing boundaries, pacing the trauma narrative, and bridging the implicit with the explicit (Rothschild, 2017).

Through talking, a person is able to weave a coherent narrative with a past, present, and future. The narrative, primarily a language-based, left-brain activity, allows connections and expression of the images, feelings, and somatic/emotional autobiographical memories mediated by the right brain to connect with the language-based left brain. In addition, it is thought that this increases prefrontal activity, thus down-regulating negative emotional activation of the amygdala (Dolcos & McCarthy, 2006). Scaer (2005) says that this process also allows integration and reconsolidation of the implicit memory cues associated with a traumatic event. The narrative, in tandem with experiencing emotional components of the memory, allows processing and change to occur. Identifying emotions correlates with decreased amygdala response and an increase in prefrontal activity (Cozolino, 2017). Information in unconscious, implicit memory areas is brought to an adaptive resolution through connecting subcortical areas with cortically mediated higher brain functions for the purpose of changing dysfunctional symptoms.

Trait change, or meaningful shifts in personality, can occur through the processing of dysfunctional information (Shapiro, 2012, 2018). Processing de-traumatizes painful state-dependent memories by changing the pattern of receptors in existing synapses in the information network. Processing involves acquiring new learning, connecting adaptive neural networks with dysfunctionally linked information through activation of emotions associated with traumatic memories (Shapiro, 2001, 2018). Because trauma memories are stored in a state-specific form – frozen in time, and not connected to adaptive memory networks,– a similar state of consciousness must be re-created to access them. Thus, state-dependent memory has important implications for processing in psychotherapy: remembering events marked by sadness, anger, or fear activates areas where emotional memory is mediated, recreating dimensions of the experience. This provides the opportunity and a portal that allows for the restructuring of neural networks. Emotional arousal and novel sensory experiences are necessary to access these implicit memories and to change dysfunctional neural networks. Briere and Scott (2013) say that processing is primarily emotional, involving implicit, nonverbal, relational memories, and that cognitions do not necessarily need to be addressed. Chapter 5 provides a psychodynamic model for processing relational trauma; Chapter 7 discusses how to process with Eye Movement Desensitization and Reprocessing (EMDR) therapy; and Chapter 11 discusses somatic processing with the Trauma Resilience Model (TRM).

Different psychotherapies are thought to affect different areas in the brain. Research using brain imaging shows that mindfulness and EMDR operate primarily through bottom-up processing (limbic system to cortex) while cognitive behavioral therapy (CBT) seems to enhance top-down processing (cortex to limbic system; Wetherill & Tapert, 2012). Thus, CBT assists in inhibitory control and self-regulation through cortical changes, whereas mindfulness and EMDR therapy appear to improve attention and the tolerance of unpleasant feelings and thoughts through changes deeper in the brain in the limbic system. Neuroimaging studies have confirmed that changes in the cortical and limbic areas of the brain occur in response to psychotherapy for those with substance use (DeVito et al., 2012; Westbrook et al., 2011), obsessive–compulsive disorder (Apostolova et al., 2010; Baxter et al., 1992), panic disorder (Beutel, Stark, Pan, Silbersweig, & Dietrich, 2010), depression (Goldapple et al., 2004; Hirvonen et al., 2010; Karlsson et al., 2010; Kennedy et al., 2007; Martin, Martin, Rai, Richardson, & Royall, 2001), PTSD (Bossini et al., 2007, 2011; Felmingham et al., 2007), and social and specific phobias (Furmark et al., 2002; Paquette et al., 2003; Straube, Glauer, Dilger, Mentzel, & Miltner, 2006).

Most dysfunctional symptoms arise from the lower or limbic areas of the brain, which are more difficult to modify than the higher cortical areas. Highly emotionally arousing memories become powerfully linked in our brain and are mediated by amygdala functioning without connecting to the thinking part of our brain, the frontal cortex. Language and reason cannot change or access these memories. This is important for psychotherapists to understand, because intellectual understanding can take the patient only so far. Intellectual understanding, a prefrontal cortex activity, may not change the person's physiological reaction and responses. The subcortical areas involved with the emotional brain (i.e., brainstem and limbic areas) require us to utilize the language of the somatosensory (right hemisphere) rather than the symbolic and linear language of the left hemisphere. These types of procedural memories are much more difficult to learn than memorizing a phone number, for example, which is a cortically mediated memory. Relatedly, this explains why it is much harder for an adult to learn to play a musical instrument or a new sport because the lower areas of the brain are less plastic in adulthood than in childhood. The challenge for psychotherapists lies in changing implicit state-dependent memories that have formed through prolonged interaction, experience, and repeated activation of neurophysiological states of stress. These memory systems were adaptive and crucial for survival for people who have been threatened by an unsafe situation. A hungry infant who looks into the nonresponsive, lifeless eyes of a depressed mother may be just as threatened for survival as the caveman confronting a saber-tooth tiger (Cozolino, 2017). Maintaining vigilance and suspiciousness is a good idea in a potentially threatening environment because it enables a person to detect danger quickly and respond. The psychotherapy process has the potential to change state-dependent memories that are powerfully linked in the brain to more adaptive states of consciousness for the current circumstances, such as forming a loving, trusting relationship and remaining calm in situations when attachment is perceived as a threat.

In addition to changing implicit relational memories, psychotherapy can promote cognitive changes and resilience. Psychoeducation and learning skills assist in creating resources and provide a necessary foundation for the work, but they can take the person only so far because they are largely left-brain activities carried out in the cortex. Cozolino (2017) says that cortical processing from psychoeducation occurs through affective arousal and that this paired with relaxation allows cortical integration. Although the cortex rapidly learns new information, limbic information needs to be accessed for trait change to occur, and this requires repetition and a relational context. Education in the context of a supportive relationship allows implicit memory systems to be accessed. The process of psychotherapy is emotionally arousing because it is an attachment relationship. Changing implicit memory systems that are less accessible and amenable to change requires a safe attachment relationship.

Safety and stabilization are foundational to all psychotherapies for adaptive processing of traumatic memories. Strategies that enhance the therapeutic alliance and set appropriate boundaries provide a safe relationship. Stabilization strategies help the person to expand their RZ so that state changes are possible; that is, the person will be able to change their physiological state at the moment through strategies that decrease hyperarousal, such as deep breathing, self-soothing, and other approaches listed in Box 1.2 in Chapter 1. Adhering to the practice treatment hierarchy by increasing external and internal resources is essential and foundational for safe processing. Periods of stabilization alternate with periods of processing as therapy proceeds because processing can be destabilizing temporarily. For those who have had complex childhood-onset trauma, a long period of stabilization and resource development may be indicated. Specific resource strategies for stabilization are described throughout this book. See Appendix 1.6 for a checklist of outcomes for successful processing.

On Psychotherapy and Medication

Research continues to suggest that psychotherapy enhances the effects of psychotropic medications and may be a superior stand-alone treatment for some conditions. Better, longer-lasting, positive outcomes occur when psychotherapy is combined with medication compared with medication alone (Antonuccio, Burns, & Danton, 2002; Burnand, Andreoli, Kolatte, Venturini, & Rosset, 2002; DeRubeis, Gelfand, Tang, & Simons, 1999; Rothbaum et al., 2006). A recent meta-analysis found that the combination of CBT and antidepressant medication is superior to antidepressants alone (Cuijpers et al., 2014; Hollon et al., 2014). Meanwhile, the results of one study suggested that depressed patients with a history of child abuse responded better to psychotherapy than to medication, which only showed small benefits (Nemeroff et al., 2003), while another found that psychotherapy with EMDR was superior to medication for sustained reductions in symptoms for PTSD patients (van der Kolk et al., 2007). Shalev and associates (2012) found at 5-month follow-up that 20% of those who had received psychotherapy continued to meet criteria for PTSD compared to 60% of those on medication and 58% of those receiving placebo. Other meta-analyses of psychotherapy comparing psychopharmacology found a greater effect size for psychotherapy (0.73–0.85) compared to 0.17 for tricyclics and 0.24 to 0.31 for selective serotonin reuptake inhibitors (SSRIs; Shedler, 2010). An effect size of 0.8 is considered large, while an effect size of 0.2 is considered small. The greater change for those who receive psychotherapy makes sense because medications cannot change relationships, beliefs, and behavior; only emotional and interpersonal learning can do this. Medication can help the person ameliorate symptoms when taking the drug; however, the receptor sites compensate by increasing or decreasing depending on the amount of neurotransmitter available at the synaptic site.

Some studies have compared medication with psychotherapy and found that both produce physiological changes in the brain, but that the brain changes are different for medication than for psychotherapy (Goldapple et al., 2004; Karlsson et al., 2010; Kennedy et al., 2007; Martin et al., 2001). It is assumed that combining psychotherapy and psychopharmacology is more effective than either treatment alone; however, three large long-term studies suggest that medications may interfere with the learning that takes place during psychotherapy (Barlow, Gorman, Shear, & Woods, 2000; Haug et al., 2003; Marks et al., 1993). When medication was stopped, the groups in all the studies that received medication and psychotherapy did worse than the group that received psychotherapy alone. Thus, it is thought that the "therapeutic changes that occur in the brain with psychotherapy are impeded by the presence of the psychoactive medication" (Higgins & George, 2007, p. 248). This speaks to the importance of state-dependent learning, that is, if the person is in one physiological state with all the attending neurotransmitters, then whatever is learned in that state will be best remembered when the person is in that same physiological state (Chu, 2011). This means that the learning that takes place during psychotherapy when the person is on medication may need to be remediated once the medication is discontinued and the person is in a different physiological state.

There is evidence that antidepressants can enhance neural plasticity, which allows the person to be more receptive to the environment (Branchi et al., 2013). Some psychotropic medications, physical exercise, and mindfulness have been associated with increased hippocampal volume and BDNF (Cahn et al (2017); Gourgouvelis, Yielder, Clarke, Behbahani, & Murphy (2018) Warner-Schmidt & Duman, 2006). However, many studies of antidepressant outcomes have found only minimal benefits. Studies from 1990–2019 were reviewed and the authors conclude that the small effect sizes of these studies raise the question of efficacy and safety of antidepressants because there are potential harms such as sleep disturbances, suicide, and sexual dysfunction, as well as withdrawal symptoms with these medications (Jakobsen, Gluud, & Kirsch, 2019). Medication and lifestyle modifications are adjuncts to an overall treatment plan that includes psychotherapy as the primary treatment modality. APPNs should assess each individual in order to determine whether medication will help to stabilize the person. This is a decision that should be carefully decided in collaboration with the patient over several sessions. The holistic model of care outlined in Chapter 1, places relationship as central to care and medication as an adjunct to treatment.

Relationship and Emotion

The process of psychotherapy is not about uncovering the past so much as providing safety through a new attachment relationship and processing dysfunctional implicit memory so that new expectations can be formed through reintegration of neural networks. Schore (2019) says that the psychotherapeutic relationship is inherently physiological and that through limbic resonance, the limbic brain is restructured. Limbic resonance refers to communication between two mammals' limbic systems, and this connection is necessary for survival and growth. In seminal studies, Harlow's monkeys and Bowlby's attachment research provide early evidence of the parallels between bonding behavior and neurophysiology between animals and humans.

The psychobiological attachment relationship continues to be expressed throughout life (Schore, 2019). Relationships stabilize and regulate physiology, and in early relationships with others, when the brain is most plastic, long-lasting patterns are developed in the brain's neural networks. Repair and regulation of the patient's dysregulated states through psychotherapy is done in a supportive environment in which there is a sense of control and appropriate boundaries. A therapeutic alliance allows the person to stay safely within their RZ so that experiences can be verbalized instead of defenses mobilized. When a limbic connection has established a neural pattern, it takes a limbic connection to revise it (Lewis, Amini, & Lanon, 2000). As the patient becomes attached, relational templates are revealed within the context of the therapeutic relationship. Through attunement, developmental recapitulation is potentiated as opportunities are co-created for corrective emotional experiences that can generate a new relational template and neural integration (Cozolino, 2017). This is possible because the therapeutic relationship provides the optimal context neurophysiologically for neural plasticity. In psychotherapy, the patient encodes new information through numerous psychotherapeutic interactions that facilitate limbic connection. "Healing is a physical process within the brain that produces a physiological pattern of function that in turn promotes homeostasis and optimal autonomic arousal" (Scaer, 2005, p. 168). This is accomplished over time through connection and emotional responsiveness. Affect or emotional regulation is an essential element of the therapeutic alliance and thereby of the change process of psychotherapy (Schore, 2019; van der Kolk, 2014). The role of emotional regulation has been a significant focus of neurobiological studies and theoretical speculations. Emotional states are fundamentally physiological and involve basic bioregulation and homeostasis of all systems (Schore, 2019).

Affect development parallels affect regulation; that is, as a person develops emotional awareness, there is a greater capacity for increasing levels of affect regulation. Normal development in the context of an attuned caregiver facilitates the evolution of affects from their early form, in which they are experienced as bodily sensations, to subjective states that can gradually be verbally articulated (Stolorow & Atwood, 1996). This is consistent with Lane and Schwartz's (1987) theoretical speculations that there are various levels of emotional development, with the lowest level of emotions experienced as bodily sensations, such as occurs during infancy, and the highest level blending feelings and the capacity for fantasy, imagination, and empathy. Emotional development is derailed during trauma, whether through a specific traumatic event or the more chronic and insidious types of trauma, such as those that occur in attachment misattunements.

Emotions are physiological states, and reflect our conscious interpretation of visceral sensations (Damasio, 1999, 2018). Emotions are not caused by our thoughts but by our response to physiological changes in our body in response to external stimuli. The body tells us about our well-being. A simple exercise illustrates this. Think of an unpleasant event, situation, or person for a minute, and then tune into where that feeling registers in your body. Then think about a happy time or a person you like for a minute, and notice where you feel that in your body. Siegel (2002) says: "Emotion, body state, and a core consciousness of the self-emerge from the same brain circuitry" (p. 97). He further posits that emotion serves an integrative function and strengthens neural circuits through the release of neurotransmitters, which promotes self-regulation.

Healing is reflected in the capacity to experience a wider range and intensity of emotions. Experiencing all emotions fully is posited to be synonymous with being fully alive and salubrious to health (Maslow, 1972; Pert, Dreher, & Ruff, 1998). Contemporary theorists have further refined the idea that emotion serves to connect systems in the brain as well as connect people to each other, with emotional regulation being the key to integration. Too much emotional arousal creates chaos, while too little emotional arousal is manifested by rigidity and depletion of energy for life (Siegel, 2012). This balance or regulation of emotion is the outcome of orbital frontal prefrontal integration. The APPN psychotherapist assists the patient in clarifying and identifying nuances of emotion, facilitating neural connections and energy flow. However, emotions must be experienced and not just talked about; that is, the full range of emotions is expressed and communicated and received by an empathic person. In this way, psychotherapy assists in affect development and regulation.

The groundbreaking work of Pert and colleagues (1998) on neuropeptides theoretically supports the primacy of emotion and the importance of emotional expression in psychotherapy. Neuropeptides are the chemical substrates of emotion, and Pert says that emotional expression balances the flow of neuropeptides and that this generates a functional healing system throughout the body. Emotional regulation has a major impact on physical and psychological health. Pert says that emotional expression is salubrious to health and that some emotions are especially beneficial, such as the primary emotions of anger, joy, grief, sadness, and fear, whereas other emotions that produce long-term states of distress, such as helplessness, hopelessness, depression, and despair, create significant biochemical changes deleterious to psychological and physical health. Emotional regulation occurs through identification and expression of the primary emotions in an ambient emotional environment.

Emotional changes and affect regulation involve implicit memory systems and largely occur through right-brain communication between the therapist and patient in the therapeutic alliance (Schore, 2019). The therapeutic alliance forges a bond of emotional connection that is thought to be inherently psychobiological in that there is a mutual co-regulation of affects involving implicit right-brain communication with the right hemisphere dominant in psychotherapy (Schore, 2019). Siegel (2002) agrees and says that the therapist serves as an attachment figure and helps to assist the patient toward more autonomous self-regulation through co-regulation of internal states. Much of this communication is nonverbal, unconscious, implicit, and reflected in subtle shifts of positive and negative emotions. Nonverbal behavior, such as facial expression, respiration, body posture, gestures, eye contact, and the tone, rhythm, cadence, volume, and speed of verbal communication, determines the nature of the relationship and alliance (Scaer, 2005). These nonverbal aspects of the primary attachment relationship are functions of the right hemisphere, and they apply to the therapeutic alliance. Implicit communication precedes understanding words in development and in psychotherapy.

Psychotherapy offers the person the opportunity to transform and process implicit memories through relationship. Responses to early relational trauma are reenacted in the therapeutic relationship. Similar to one's original attachment relationship with a caretaker, the new attachment relationship with the therapist allows a secure base for the person to make changes. For those who already have a secure attachment schema, the capacity for reflection and mindfulness is present but may need to be supported through the unfolding narrative as they reflect on their experience. The securely attached patient can self-regulate, express feelings within the relationship, and generally function well in life; that is, he or she can both feel and deal.

In contrast, the person with an insecure/disorganized attachment style presents significant challenges because there often is intense anxiety and great difficulty in self-soothing and regulating emotion. This patient alternates between overwhelming emotion and dissociative states. Stabilization and resourcing are needed with the APPN teaching the person how to reflect on experiences and this in turn helps to regulate affects and to integrate experiences that have been dissociated. Through narrative and the "holding" (Winnicott, 1965/1976) of the therapeutic relationship, a more solid coherent sense of self can emerge. This parallels attachment research that demonstrates attachment security and self-reflective capacity can change over the life span and this change correlates with a coherent narrative (Siegel, 2012). This is because the OMPFC integrates social relationships, emotional regulation, and self-knowledge and remains plastic throughout life. For a more thorough discussion on working with those with attachment trauma, see *The Transformation of Affect: A Model for Accelerated Change* by Diana Fosha (2000).

BOX 2.4 Core Negative Beliefs of Defectiveness

- I am bad
- I am not good enough
- I am a failure
- I am worthless
- I am unlovable
- I am damaged
- I am invisible
- I am not important

Source: Shapiro, F. (2018). *Eye movement desensitization and reprocessing (EMDR)* (3rd ed.). New York, NY: Guilford Press.

Emotions serve as a portal to implicit memories and are considered the central agent of change. Accessing emotion engages relevant neurobiological processes for early trauma that may not be language based but reflect the right hemisphere language of emotions, images, sensations, and impressions. The emotional arousal inherent in psychotherapy provides an opportunity to access implicit memory to facilitate information processing. Even though implicit memory is unconscious, it is demonstrated through the person's feelings, attitudes, beliefs, behaviors, and symptoms. For example, faulty information processing may have led the person to core negative beliefs of defectiveness that are ingrained. These are false beliefs about oneself due to early developmental and/or attachment traumas and ingrained as part of the person's identity (see Box 2.4). Entrenched negative thoughts and beliefs of defectiveness coexist with chronic depression and arise from childhood neglect or abuse in an effort by the child to preserve the relationship with caretaker(s). For example, a child who is physically abused by her mother learns that those who love her hurt her, and owing to cognitive immaturity and in an effort to preserve the relationship, probably concludes, "There is something wrong with me." The negative emotion and sensations coupled with the thought are linked in memory networks and are triggered in future situations when similar feelings of powerlessness, despair, and worthlessness occur. The alternative that something is terribly wrong with those who have your life in their hands would lead to intolerable anxiety and utter hopelessness. Defenses evolve in the form of denial to protect the child from overwhelming anxiety and ultimately these false beliefs about oneself limit the person and are not linked to positive thoughts.

Otherwise the person may idealize her mother (reaction formation) or have no memories or feelings about her childhood (dissociation). Lack of memories before age 2 is normal because the hippocampus is not myelinated until 18 months. However, if there are no memories of childhood, this may suggest that dissociative defenses may be warding off a high level of anxiety. The child may have an ambivalent or dismissing attachment style and had to turn away from caretakers to self-regulate. Chapter 17, provides information on how to assess for early memories through use of a timeline that can be constructed with the patient on intake.

The plasticity and malleability of neural networks act as a double-edged sword in that the psychotherapist can play a significant role in the construction of beliefs for better or worse. In psychotherapy, therapeutic suggestions are powerful, and the therapist's beliefs, even if unspoken, influence the patient (Cozolino, 2017). The media attention to false memories as a basis for litigation highlights this issue. However, a recent examination of the study purporting that memories of childhood abuse can be implanted by psychotherapists found that there is no scientific research that supports this (Blizard & Shaw, 2019). In fact, studies on the suggestibility of children show that they cannot easily be persuaded to provide details of abuse if in fact, it did not happen. In addition, it is important to note that the reality is that there is no objective truth that the psychotherapist is seeking; there is only the pursuit of truth as the patient feels and remembers his or her experience. It is the person's perception that matters, not whether the memories are literal and true. This is important because a person's history is not destiny and what actually happened is not as relevant as how the people make sense of their lives. It is essential for the psychotherapist to remain impartial and listen with equal attention to all dimensions of the narrative without unwittingly encouraging elaboration in areas that the therapist feels are more interesting or valid. An important caveat is to not lead the patient toward the conclusion that she or he was abused, even if the therapist thinks it is true.

On the positive side, psychotherapists can use the malleability of memory for therapeutic change through creative use of the power of suggestion. Therapeutic communication, imagery, and the therapeutic alliance assist the person in enhancing internal resources to form new neural connections that enable patients to expand the possibilities for improved functioning. For example, one woman who was emotionally and physically abused severely as a child had great difficulty in enhancing internal resources because there was no memory of soothing interactions that she could draw on as a resource in stressful situations. Over time, as the therapeutic alliance deepened and with practice in sessions and then out of sessions, she was able to image her therapist with her, first in situations that were not stressful and then eventually during times of stress. The therapeutic alliance parallels the brain growth—promoting aspects of the mother–infant dyad—and it creates new dendritic connections in the brain that can serve as a resource for opening up possibilities for positive new experiences. Subsequently, the woman enrolled in yoga classes, which she previously found too stressful, and she extended her network of friends to include more supportive relationships. These changes can happen only when there is a strong therapeutic alliance providing a safe emotional relationship for the person.

Alexithymia

Alexithymia is an emotional regulation problem that has generated a considerable amount of research, and it is relevant for consideration in psychotherapy. Alexithymia is a specific communication style, which literally means no words for feelings. Individuals with alexithymia often express their emotions in bodily symptoms; for example, instead of feeling angry, the person may get a headache. Other patients may report a vague sense of dissatisfaction and may binge eat in an effort to alleviate this feeling. Somatizing may be the experiencing of emotion without the ability to translate the emotion into the feeling. Alexithymia is significantly associated with psychosomatic disorders (Taylor, Parker, Bagby, & Acklin, 1992), depression and childhood sexual abuse (Thomas, DiLillo, Walsh, & Polusny, 2011), substance use disorders (Aleman, 2007), eating disorders (Wheeler, Greiner, & Boulton, 2005), PTSD (Zahradnik, Stewart, Marshall, Shell, & Jaycox, 2009), and emotional neglect (Aust, Alkan Härtwig, Heuser, & Bajbouj, 2012).

Research supports a bidirectional interhemispheric transfer deficit for alexithymic and psychosomatic patients (Taylor, 2000). The emotional and somatic information systems of the right hemisphere are not connected optimally with the linguistic cognitive systems of the left. This is thought to be a problem in neural network connection and communication between the right and left hemispheres. A person may be born alexithymic (i.e., primary alexithymia), or alexithymia may be caused by trauma (i.e., secondary alexithymia; Freyberger, 1977). Whatever the cause, alexithymia can be thought of as a continuum because there are different degrees of this state or trait. Expression depends in part on the situation and the person. Under stress, an individual with primary or secondary alexithymia may have even more difficulty with affect regulation than during nonstressful times. Those with alexithymia have great difficulty in self-care, self-soothing, and self-regulating functions because they cannot identify their own sensations, emotions, and physical states, and there is an inability to gauge and modulate internal states. These individuals do not seem to have an inner sense of themselves and become easily overwhelmed if asked to attend to inner sensations. Other deficits include a marked absence of fantasy and lack of empathy.

This constellation of features has important implications clinically because traditional techniques used in talk therapy, such as role-playing, imaging, expressing feelings, and discussing dreams, are significantly compromised because the severely alexithymic patient may not have dreams or be able to image. For example, if the therapist asks the alexithymic patient to keep a feelings journal, the response is likely to be confusion or resistance because the person really does not know what feelings are and has no language with which to articulate emotions.

Assessment of alexithymia is indicated for all those whom the APPN suspects have been significantly traumatized, have chronic pain, have many somatic complaints with few identifiable causes, or have difficulty identifying their feelings beyond saying they are upset and appear confused when questioned further about their feelings. Assessment for alexithymia is described in Chapter 3. After confirmation through administration of tools that measure alexithymia, the therapist should explain to the person that she or he has a problem in identifying emotions and that this has created some of the problems he or she is experiencing. This is important, because people with alexithymia often do not know what is missing, especially if they have never experienced feelings. Alexithymia has been compared with color blindness in that a person with color blindness does not know what colors are, just as the alexithymic person does not know what feelings are (Krystal, 1979).

Overall treatment strategies for alexithymia include supportive psychotherapy, psychoeducation, and assisting the patient in labeling emotions by tracing antecedents to somatic complaints and symptoms so that the person can develop an understanding of trigger events and consequences (Wheeler, 2000). Tacon (2001) describes several staged approaches that are most helpful for the treatment of alexithymia. In one model, the first stage focuses on educating the person and observing; the second stage increases affect tolerance; and in the third stage, the person learns how to verbalize feelings and experiences. A similar staged model includes (1) ventilation of physical symptoms; (2) encouraging differentiation of somatic symptoms from feelings and using correct emotions to label feelings; and (3) guided reflections so that the person can understand past experiences. Dialectical behavior therapy (DBT), developed for working with borderline personality disorder, is also helpful in increasing affect tolerance and the ability to self-regulate, which helps those with alexithymia. Specific strategies are delineated in the *Skills Training Manual for Treating Borderline Personality Disorder* (Linehan, 1993). DBT is discussed in Chapter 18.

Overall, these strategies aid in increasing interhemispheric connection, strengthening right and left hemispheric integration, and the ability to regulate affect. Integration of the right and left hemispheres occurs through activation of conscious language (top left) with unconscious emotional (lower right) processes that have been dissociated by childhood stress or adult trauma (Cozolino, 2017). Siegel (2012) says that right and left hemispheric integration is achieved through coherent narratives. He believes that CBT, psychodynamic psychotherapy, and EMDR are successful in that they selectively activate processes in each hemisphere and promote integration through this activation.

Psychotherapy is about helping people to make sense of their inner lives, emotions, and interpersonal experiences. Siegel notes that integration of neurons may not just be about verbal recall but instead involve all images, emotions and sensations. "The sense of safety and the emotional 'holding environment' of a secure attachment within a therapeutic relationship . . . may be essential for these integrative processes to occur within the traumatized person's mind" (Siegel, 2003, p. 29). Using strategies that enhance the therapeutic alliance and setting appropriate boundaries provide a safe place for the work of healing. The evidence-based psychotherapeutic approaches included in this book—CBT, DBT, EMDR, motivational interviewing, humanistic existential therapy, psychodynamic therapy, family therapy, and group therapy—provide approaches that guide the APPN in working therapeutically and safely.

CONCLUDING COMMENTS

The neurophysiology discussed in this chapter lends support to the core concepts, resilience and relationship, identified in Chapter 1, as essential to psychotherapy. Resilience and relationship transcend all psychotherapy models and approaches and serve as the portal through which neural networks are integrated. Integration is accomplished through adaptive processing of dysfunctional information, which affects all dimensions of the person so that healing can occur. The neuroscience of psychotherapy is embedded in the paradigm of holism. Returning to the definition of healing from Chapter 1, "an emergent process . . . bringing together aspects of one's self and the body, mind, emotion, spirit, and environment at deeper levels of inner knowing, leading to an integration and balance" (Mariano, 2013, p. 60). This is the essence of healing and psychotherapeutic change. Information processing through psychotherapy restores regulation, connection, and integration of neural networks. This approach is key to wholeness and healing and is reflected in a deeper connection with oneself and others.

DISCUSSION QUESTIONS

1. Give a clinical example of each defense mechanism listed in this chapter from your practice or personal life. Identify which defense mechanism can be classified as primitive or narcissistic, immature, neurotic, or mature.
2. Discuss memory and how traumatic memories are stored differently than nontraumatic memories.
3. Discuss alexithymia, and present a case in which you thought the patient was alexithymic.
4. Define state-dependent learning and give an example from your own.
5. Identify five neurophysiological changes that can result from trauma.
6. Describe how psychotherapy works neurophysiologically.
7. Discuss the author's ideas about truth and false memories in psychotherapy.
8. What is meant by primacy of emotion in psychotherapy?
9. How does the neurophysiology discussed in this chapter lend support to the concepts of relationship and resilience as discussed in Chapter 1?

REFERENCES

Ainsworth, M. D. (1967). *Infancy in Uganda*. Baltimore, MD: Johns Hopkins.

Aleman, K. (2007). Four problems with psychodynamic assessment of drug abusers. *Nordic Psychology, 59*(4), 303–316. doi:10.1027/1901-2276.59.4.303

Ammaniti, M., & Gallese, V. (2014). *The birth of intersubjectivity: Psychodynamics, neurobiology, and the self*. New York, NY: W. W. Norton.

Antonuccio, D., Burns, D., & Danton, W. (2002). Antidepressants: A triumph of marketing over science? *Prevention & Treatment, 5*(1), 25. doi:10.1037/1522-3736.5.1.525c

Apostolova, I., Block, S., Buchert, R., Osen, B., Conradi, M., Tabrizian, S., . . . Obrocki, J. (2010). Effects of behavioral therapy or pharmacotherapy on brain glucose metabolism in subjects with obsessive-compulsive disorders as assessed by brain FDG-PET. *Psychiatry Resident, 184,* 101–116. doi:10.1016/j.pscychresns.2010.08.012

Aust, S., Alkan Härtwig, E., Heuser, I., & Bajbouj, M. (2012). The role of early emotional neglect in alexithymia. *Psychological Trauma: Theory, Research, Practice and Policy, 5*(3), 225–232. doi:10.1037/a0027314

Barlow, D. H., Gorman, J., Shear, M., & Woods, S. (2000). Cognitive behavioral therapy: Imipramine or their combination for panic disorder. *Journal of the American Medical Association, 283,* 2529–2536. doi:10.1001/jama.283.19.2529

Bava, S., & Tapert, S. (2010). Adolescent brain development and the risk for alcohol and other drug problems. *Neuropsychology Review, 29*(4), 398–413. doi:10.1007/s11065-010-9146-6

Baxter, L. R., Schwartz, J. M., Bergman, K. S., Szuba, M. P., Guze, B. H., Mazziotta, J. C., . . . Munford, P. (1992). Caudate glucose metabolic rate changes with both drug and behavior therapy for obsessive-compulsive disorder. *Archives of General Psychiatry, 49,* 681–689. doi:10.1001/archpsyc.1992.01820090009002

Bergmann, U. (2012). *Neurobiological foundations for EMDR practice*. New York, NY: Springer Publishing Company.

Bergmann, U. (2020). *Neurobiological foundations for EMDR practice* (2nd ed.). New York, NY: Springer Publishing Company.

Beutel, M. E., Stark, R., Pan, H., Silbersweig, D., & Dietrich, S. (2010). Changes of brain activation pre-post short-term psychodynamic inpatient psychotherapy: An fMRI study of panic disorder patients. *Psychiatry Research, 184*, 96–104. doi:10.1016/j.pscychresns.2010.06.005

Blizard, R., & Shaw, M. (2019). Lost-in-the-mall: False memory or false defense? *Journal of Child Custody, 16*(1), 1–22. doi:10.1080/15379418.2019.1590285

Boon, S., Steele, K., & van der Hart, O. (2011). *Coping with trauma-related dissociation: Skills training for patients and therapists*. New York, NY: W. W. Norton.

Bossini, L., Fagiolini, A., & Castrogiovanni, P. (2007). Neuroanatomical changes after eye movement desensitization and reprocessing (EMDR) treatment in posttraumatic stress disorder. *Journal of Neuropsychiatry and Clinical Neuroscience, 19*, 475–476. doi:10.1176/jnp.2007.19.4.475

Bossini, L., Tavanti, M., Calossi, S., Polizzotto, N. R., Vatti, G., Marino, D., & Castrogiovanni, P. (2011). EMDR treatment for PTSD, with focus on hippocampal volumes: A pilot study. *Journal of Neuropsychiatry and Clinical Neuroscience, 23*(2), E1–E2. doi:10.1176/jnp.23.2.jnpe1

Bowers, M. E., & Yehuda, R. (2016). Intergenerational transmission of stress in humans. *Neuropsychopharmacology, 41*, 232–244. doi:10.1038/npp.2015.247

Bowlby, J. (1969). *Attachment and loss: Attachment* (Vol. 1). New York, NY: Basic Books.

Boyd, M. A. (2018). *Psychiatric nursing: Contemporary practice* (6th ed.). Philadelphia, PA: Wolters Kluwer/Lippincott Williams & Wilkins.

Branchi, I., Santarelli, S., Capoccia, S., Poggini, S., D'Andrea, I., Cirulli, F., Alleva, E., (2013). Antidepressant treatment outcome depends on the quality of the living environment: A pre-clinical investigation in mice. *PLOS ONE, 8*, e62226. doi:10.1371/journal.pone.0062226.

Bremner, J. D. (1999). Alterations in brain structure and functioning associated with post-traumatic stress disorder. *Seminars in Clinical Neuropsychiatry, 4*, 249–255. doi:10.153/SCNP00400249

Bremner, J. D., Randall, P., Vermetten, E., Staib, L., Bronen, R. A., Mazure, C., . . . Charney, D. S. (1997). Magnetic resonance imaging-based measurement of hippocampal volume in post-traumatic stress disorder related to childhood physical and sexual abuse: A preliminary report. *Biological Psychiatry, 68*, 748–766. doi:10.1016/s0006-3223(96)00162-x

Brenner, C. (1982). *The mind in conflict*. New York, NY: International Universities Press.

Briere, J., & Scott, C. (2013). *Principles of trauma therapy: A guide to symptoms, evaluation, and treatment* (2nd ed.). Thousand Oaks, CA: Sage.

Burnand, Y., Andreoli, A., Kolatte, E., Venturini, A., & Rosset, N. (2002). Psychodynamic psychotherapy and clomipramine in the treatment of major depression. *Psychiatric Services, 53*, 585–590. doi:10.1176/appi.ps.53.5.585

Cahn, B. R., Goodman, M. S., Peterson, C. T., Maturi, R., & Mills, P. J. (2017). Yoga, medication and mind-body health: Increased BDNF, Cortisol aswakening response, and altered inflammatory marker expression after a 3-month yoga and medication retreat. *Frontiers in Human Neuroscience, 22*. doi:10.3389/fnhum.2017.00315

Camchong, J., & MacDonald, A. W. (2012). Imaging psychoses: Diagnosis and prediction of violence. In J. R. Simpson (Ed.), *Neuroimaging in forensic psychiatry: From the clinic to the courtroom* (pp. 114–129). Hoboken, NJ: John Wiley & Sons. doi:10.1002/9781119968900.ch7

Carasatorre, M., & Ramirez-Amaya, V. (2013). Network, cellular, and molecular mechanisms underlying long-term memory formation. In C. Belzung & P. Wigmore (Eds.), *Neurogenesis and neural plasticity* (pp. 73–115). New York, NY: Springer.

Champagne, F. A. (2010). Early adversity and developmental outcomes: Interaction between genetics, epigenetics, and social experiences across the life span. *Perspectives on Psychological Science, 5*, 564–574. doi:10.1177/1745691610383494

Charney, D. S. (2004). Psychobiological mechanisms of resilience and vulnerability: Implications for successful adaptation to extreme stress. *American Journal of Psychiatry, 161*(2), 195–216. doi:10.1176/appi.ajp.161.2.195

Chefetz, R. A. (2019). Psycho-neurobiology and its potential influence on psychotherapy: Being, doing, and the risk of scientism. *Psychodynamic Psychiatry, 47*(1), 53–80. doi:10.1521/pdps.2019.47.1.53

Chu, J. A. (2011). *Rebuilding shattered lives: The responsible treatment of complex post-traumatic and dissociative disorders* (2nd ed.). New York, NY: John Wiley & Sons.

Corrigan, F. M., Fisher, J., & Nutt, D. (2011). Autonomic dysregulation and the window of tolerance model of the effects of complex emotional trauma. *Journal of Psychopharmacology, 25*(1), 17–25. doi:10.177/0269881109354930

Cozolino, L. (2017). *The neuroscience of psychotherapy: Healing the social brain* (3rd ed.). New York, NY: W. W. Norton.

Cuijpers, P., Sijbrandij, M., Koole, S. L., Andersson, G., Beekman, A. T., Reynolds, C. F. (2014). Adding psychotherapy to antidepressant medication in depression and anxiety disorders: A meta-analysis. *World Psychiatry, 13*, 56–67. doi:10.1002/wps.20089

Damasio, A. (1999). *The feeling of what happens: Body and emotion in the making of consciousness.* New York, NY: Harcourt.

Damasio, A. R. (2018). *The strange order of things: Life, feeling, and the making of cultures.* New York, NY: Pantheon Books.

DeRubeis, R. J., Gelfand, L. A., Tang, T. Z., & Simons, A. D. (1999). Medications versus cognitive behavior therapy for severely depressed outpatients: Mega-analysis of four randomized comparisons. *American Journal of Psychiatry, 156*, 1007–1013. doi:10.1176/ajp.156.7.1007

DeVito, E. E., Worhunsky, P. D., Carroll, K. M., Rounsaville, B. J., Kober, H., & Potenza, M. N. (2012). A preliminary study of the neural effects of behavioral therapy for substance use disorders. *Drug and Alcohol Dependence, 122*, 228–235. doi:10.1016/j.drugalcdep.2011.10.002

Dobbs, D. (2006). A revealing reflection. *Scientific American Mind, 17*(2), 22–27. doi:10.1038/scientificamericanmind0406-22

Dolcos, F., & McCarthy, G. (2006). Brain systems mediating cognitive interference by emotional distractions. *Journal of Neuroscience, 26*, 2072–2079. doi:10.1523/JNEUROSCI.5042-05.2006

Dossey, B., Keegan, L., & Guzzetta, C. (2012). *Holistic nursing: A handbook for practice* (4th ed.). Burlington, MA: Jones & Bartlett..

Feinberg, T. D., & Keenan, J. P (2005). Where in the brain is the self? *Consciousness and Cognition, 14*, 647–790. doi:10.1016/j.concog.2005.01.002

Feldman, R. (2009). The development of regulatory functions from birth to 5 years: Insights from premature infants. *Child Development, 80*(2), 544–561. doi:10.1111/j.1467-8624.2009.01278.x

Felmingham, K., Kemp, A. H., Williams, L., Das, P., Hughes, G., Peduto, A., . . . Bryant, R. (2007). Changes in anterior cingulate and amygdala after cognitive behavior therapy of posttraumatic stress. *Psychological Science, 18*, 127–129. doi:10.1111/j.1467-9280.2007.01860.x

Felmingham, K., Kemp, A. H., Williams, L., Falconer, E., Olivieri, G., Peduto, A., . . . Bryant, R. (2008). Dissociative responses to conscious and non-conscious fear impact underlying brain function in posttraumatic stress disorder. *Psychology Medicine, 38*, 1771–1780. doi:10.1017/S0033291708002742

Fosha, D. (2000). *The transformation of affect: A model for accelerated change.* New York, NY: Basic Books.

Freud, A. (1966). *The writing of Anna Freud: (Vol. 2), 1936: The ego and the mechanism of defense.* New York, NY: International Universities Press.

Freyberger, G. (1977). Supportive psychotherapeutic techniques in primary and secondary alexithymia. *Psychotherapy Psychosomatics, 28*, 337–342. doi:10.1159/000287080

Fuchs, T. (2004). Neurobiology and psychotherapy: An emerging dialogue. *Current Opinion in Psychiatry, 17*, 479–485. doi:10.1097/00001504-200411000-00010

Furmark, T., Tilifors, M., Marieinsclatir, I., Fischer, H., Pissiota, A., Långström, B., . . . Fredrikson, M. (2002). Common changes in cerebral blood flow in patients with social phobia treated with citalopram or cognitive behavioral therapy. *Archives in General Psychiatry, 59*, 425–433. doi:10.1001/archpsyc.59.5.425

Goldapple, K., Segal, Z., Garson, C., Lau, M., Bieling, P., Kennedy, S., . . . Mayberg, H. (2004). Modulation of cortical-limbic pathways in major depression: Treatment specific effects of cognitive behavior therapy. *Archives of General Psychiatry, 61*, 34–41. doi:10.1001/archpsyc.61.1.34

Gourgouvelis, J., Yielder, P., Clarke, S., Behbahani, H., & Murphy, B.A. (2018, March 6). Exercise leads to better clinical outcomes in those receiving medication plus cognitive behavioral therapy for major depressive disorder. *Frontiers in Psychiatry.* doi:10.3389/fpsyt.2018.00037

Haller, M., Myers, U. S., McKnight, A., Angkaw, A. C., & Norman, S. B. (2016). Predicting Engagement in Psychotherapy, Pharmacotherapy, or Both Psychotherapy and Pharmacotherapy Among Returning Veterans Seeking PTSD Treatment. *Psychological Services, 13*(4), 341–348. doi:10.1037/ser0000093

Halter, M. J. (Ed.). (2018). *Varcarolis' foundations of psychiatric-mental health nursing: A clinical approach* (8th ed.). St. Louis, MO: Elsevier.

Harmon-Jones, E., Gable, P. A., & Peterson, C. K (2010). The role of asymmetric frontal cortical activity in emotion-related phenomena: A review and update. *Biological Psychology, 84*(3), 451–462. doi:10.1016/j.biopsycho.2009.08.010

Haug, T. T., Blomhoff, S., Hellstron, K., Holme, I., Humble, M., Madsbu, H. P., . . . Wold, J. E. (2003). Exposure therapy & sertraline in social phobia: 1 year follow-up of a randomized clinical trial. *British Journal of Psychiatry, 182*, 312–318. doi:10.1192/bjp.182.4.312

Hebb, D. O. (1949). *The organisation of behavior.* New York, NY: Wiley.

Heins, M., Simons, C., Lataster, T., Pfeifer, S., Vermissen, D., Lardinois, M., . . . Myin-Germeys, I. (2011). Childhood trauma and psychosis: A case-control and case-sibling comparison across different levels of genetic liability, psychopathology, and type of trauma. *American Journal of Psychiatry, 168*(12), 1286–1294. doi:10.1176/appi.ajp.2011.10101531

Heitkemper, M., Jarrett, M., Taylor, P. L., Walker, E., Landenberger, K., & Bond, E. I. (2001). Effect of sexual and physical abuse on symptom experiences in women with irritable bowel syndrome. *Nursing Research, 50*, 15–23. doi:10.1097/00006199-200101000-00004

Hesse, E. (1999). The adult attachment interview: Historical and current perspectives. In J. Cassidy & P. R. Shaver (Eds.), *Handbook of attachment: Theory, research, and clinical applications* (pp. 395–433). New York, NY: Guilford Press.

Higgins, E. S., & George, M. S (2007). *The neuroscience of clinical psychiatry: The pathophysiology of behavior and mental illness.* Philadelphia, PA: Wolters Kluwer/Lippincott Williams & Wilkins.

Higgins, E. S., & George, M. S (2013). *The neuroscience of clinical psychiatry: The pathophysiology of behavior and mental illness* (2nd ed.). Philadelphia, PA: Wolters Kluwer/Lippincott Williams & Wilkins.

Hirvonen, J., Hietala, J., Kajander, J., Markkula, J., Rasi-Hakala, H., Salminen, J. K., . . . Arlsson, H. (2010). Effects of antidepressant drug treatment and psychotherapy on striataland thalamic dopamine $D_{2/3}$ receptors in major depressive disorder studied with [^{11}C]raclopride PET. *Journal of Psychopharmacology, 25*(10), 1329–1336. doi:10.1177/0269881110376691

Hollon, S. D., DeRubeis, R. J., Fawcett, J., Amsterdam, J. D., Shelton, R. C., Zajecka, J., . . . Gallop, R. (2014). Effect of cognitive therapy with antidepressant medications vs antidepressants alone on the rate of recovery in major depressive disorder: A randomized clinical trial. *JAMA Psychiatry, 71*, 1157–1164. doi:10.1001/ jamapsychiatry.2014.1054

Howell, E. (2020). *Trauma and dissociation informed psychotherapy: Relational healing and the therapeutic connection.* New York, NY: W.W. Norton & Co.

Jakobsen, J. C., Gluud, C., & Kirsch, I. (2019, September 25). Should antidepressants be used for major depressive disorder? *BMJ Evidence-Based Medicine.* Advance online publication. doi:10.1136/bmjebm-2019-111238

Kamenov, K., Twomey, C., Cabello, M., Prina, A. M., & Ayuso-Mateos, J. L. (2017). The efficacy of psychotherapy, pharmacotherapy and their combination on functioning and quality of life in depression: A meta-analysis. *Psychological Medicine, 47*(7), 1337. Retrieved from https://www.ncbi.nlm.nih.gov/pubmed/28007047. doi:10.1017/S003329171600341X

Karlsson, H., Hirvonen, J., Kajander, J., Markkula, J., Rasi-Hakala, H., Salminen, J. K., . . . Hietala, J. (2010). Research letter: Psychotherapy increases brain serotonin 5-HT1A receptors in patients with major depressive disorder. *Psychological Medicine, 40*, 523–528. doi:10.1017/S0033291709991607

Karyotaki, E., Smit, Y., Holdt Henningsen, K., Huibers, M. J. H., Robays, J., de Beurs, D., & Cuijpers, P. (2016). Combining pharmacotherapy and psychotherapy or monotherapy for major depression? A meta-analysis on the long-term effects. *Journal of Affective Disorders, 194*, 144–152. doi: 10.1016/j.jad.2016.01.036

Kennedy, S. H, Konarski, J. Z., Segal, Z. V., Lau, M. A., Bieling, P. J., McIntyre, R. S., . . . Mayberg, H. S. (2007). Differences in brain glucose metabolism between responders to CBT and venlafaxine in a 16-week randomized controlled trial. *American Journal of Psychiatry, 164*(5), 778–788. doi:10.1176/ajp.2007.164.5.778

Kernberg, O. (1975). *Borderline conditions and pathological narcissism*. New York, NY: Jason Aronson.

Kitchur, M. (2005). The strategic developmental model for EMDR. In R. Shapiro (Ed.), *EMDR solution: Pathways to healing*. New York, NY: W. W. Norton.

Knipe, J. (2019). *EMDR toolbox: Theory and treatment of complex PTSD and dissociation* (2nd ed.). New York, NY: Springer Publishing Company.

Krystal, H. (1979). Alexithymia and psychotherapy. *American Journal of Psychotherapy, 33*, 17–31. doi:10.1176/appi.psychotherapy.1979.33.1.17

Lane, R. D., & Schwartz, G. E (1987). Levels of emotional awareness: A cognitive-development theory and its application to psychopathology. *American Journal of Psychiatry, 144*(2), 133–142. doi:10.1176/ajp.144.2.133

Lanius, R. A., Vermetten, E., Loewenstein, R. J., Brand, B., Schmahl, C., Bremner, J. D., . . . Spiegel, D. (2010). Emotion modulation in PTSD: Clinical and neurobiological evidence for a dissociative subtype. *American Journal of Psychiatry, 167*, 640–647. doi:10.1176/appi.ajp .2009.09081168

Lanius, U. F., Paulsen, S. L., & Corrigan, F. M. (Eds.). (2014). *Neurobiology and treatment of traumatic dissociation: Toward an embodied self*. New York, NY: Springer Publishing Company.

Lazar, S. W., Kerr, C. E., Wasserman, R. H., Gray, J. R., Greve, D. N., Treadway, M. T., . . . Fischl, B. (2005). Meditation experience is associated with increased cortical thickness. *Neuroreport, 16*, 1893–1897. doi:10.1097/01.wnr.0000186598.66243.19

Lewis, T., Amini, F., & Lanon, R. (2000). *A general theory of love*. New York, NY: Random House.

Linehan, M. M. (1993). *Skills training manual for borderline personality disorder*. New York, NY: Guilford Press.

Mariano, C. (2013). Holistic nursing: Scope and standards of practice. In B. Dossey & L. Keegan (Eds.), *Holistic nursing: A handbook for practice* (6th ed.). Burlington, MA: Jones & Bartlett.

Marks, I., Swinson, R., Basoglu, M., Kuch, K., Noshirvani, H., O'Sullivan, G., . . . Wickwire, K. (1993). Alprazolam and exposure alone and combined in panic disorder with agoraphobia. A controlled study in London and Toronto. *British Journal of Psychiatry, 162*, 776–787. *doi:10.1192/ bjp.162.6.776*

Maslow, A. H. (1972). *The farther reaches of human nature*. New York, NY: Viking.

Martin, S. D., Martin, E., Rai, S. S., Richardson, M. A., & Royall, R. (2001). Brain blood flow changes in depressed patients treated with interpersonal psychotherapy or venlafaxine hydrochloride. *Archives of General Psychiatry, 58*, 641–645. doi:10.1001/archpsyc.58.7.641

McGilchrist, I. (2009). *The master and his emissary: The divided brain and the making of the western world*. London, UK: Yale University Press.

Melchitzky, D., & Lewis, D. (2009). Chemical neuroanatomy of the primate brain. In A. E. Schatzberg & C. B. Nemeroff (Eds.), *The American publishing textbook of psychopharmacology* (4th ed., pp. 105–134). Washington, DC: American Psychiatric Publishing.

Meyer, B., & Pilkonis, P. (2002). Attachment style. In J. Norcross (Ed.), *Psychotherapy relationships that work* (pp. 367–382). New York, NY: Oxford University Press.

Nemeroff, C., Heim, C. M., Thase, M. E., Klein, D. N., Rush, A., Schatzberg, A., . . . Keller, M. B. (2003). Differential responses to psychotherapy versus pharmacotherapy in patients with chronic forms of major depression and childhood trauma. *Proceedings of the National Academy of Sciences of the United States of America, 100*(25), 14293–14296. doi:10.1073/pnas.2336126100

Ornitz, E. (1996). Developmental aspects of neurophysiology. In M. Lewis (Ed.), *Child and adolescent psychiatry: A comprehensive textbook* (pp. 39–49). Baltimore, MD: Williams & Wilkins.

Panksepp, J. (2004). *Affective neuroscience: The foundations of human and animal emotions*. New York, NY: Oxford University Press.

Paquette, V., Levesque, L., Mansour, B., Leroux, J. M., Beaudoin, G., Bourgouin, P., . . . Beauregard, M. (2003). Change the mind and you can change the brain: Effects of cognitive behavioral therapy on the neural correlates of spider phobia. *Neuroimage, 18*, 401–409. doi:10.1016/S1053-8119(02)00030-7

Pert, C. (1999). *Your body is your subconscious mind.* [CD]. Louisville, CO: Sounds True Recordings.

Pert, C., Dreher, H., & Ruff, M. (1998). The psychosomatic network: Foundations of mind-body medicine. *Alternative Therapies in Health and Medicine, 4*(4), 30–41.

Porges, S. (2004). Neuroception: A subconscious system for detecting threats and safety. *Zero to Three*, May, pp. 19–24

Porges, S. W. (2011). *The polyvagal theory.* New York, NY: W. W. Norton.

Porges, S. W. (2019, April 1). *The emergence of polyvagal-informed therapies in the treatment of trauma.* Presented at the World Congress on Complex Trauma: Research, Intervention, Innovation, New York, NY.

Porges, S., & Dana, D. (2018). *Clinical applications of the polyvagal theory: The emergence of polyvagal-informed therapies.* New York, NY: W. W. Norton.

Roth, T. L., Lubin, F. D., Funk, A. J., & Sweatt, J. D (2009). Lasting epigenetic influence of early-life adversity on the BDNF gene. *Biological Psychiatry, 65*(9), 760–776. doi:10.1016/j.biopsych.2008.11.028

Rothbaum, B. O., Cahill, S. P., Foa, E. B., Davidson, J. R., Compton, J., Connor, K. M., . . . Hahn, C. G. (2006). Augmentation of sertraline with prolonged exposure in the treatment of posttraumatic stress disorder. *Journal of Traumatic Stress, 19*, 625–638. doi:10.1002/jts.20170

Rothschild, B. (2017). *The body remembers: Revolutionizing trauma treatment* (Vol. 2). New York, NY: W. W. Norton.

Rossi, E. (1996). *The psychobiology of mind-body healing.* New York, NY: W. W. Norton.

Sadock, B. J., Sadock, V. A., & Ruiz, P. (2017). *Kaplan & Sadock's comprehensive textbook of psychiatry* (10th ed.). Philadelphia, PA: Wolters Kluwer/Lippincott Williams & Wilkins.

Scaer, R. (2005). *The trauma spectrum: Hidden wounds and human resiliency.* New York, NY: W. W. Norton.

Schatz, C. J. (1992). The developing brain. *Scientific American, 267*(3), 60–67. doi:10.1038/scientificamerican0992-60

Schechter, D. (2003). Intergenerational communication of maternal violent trauma. In S. Coates, J. Rosenthal, & D. Schechter (Eds.), *September 11: Trauma and human bonds* (pp. 115–142). Hillsdale, NJ: Analytic Press.

Schlozman, S. C., & Nonacs, R. M. (2008). Dissociative disorders. In T. A. Stern, J. F. Rosenbaum, M. Fava, J. Biederman, & S. L. Rauch (Eds.), *Massachusetts 02General Hospital comprehensive clinical psychiatry* (pp. 481–486). St. Louis, MO: Mosby.

Schore, A. (2012). *The science of the art of psychotherapy.* New York, NY: W. W. Norton.

Schore, A. (2019). *The development of the unconscious mind.* New York, NY: W. W. Norton.

Shalev, A. Y., Ankri, Y. L., Israeli-Shalev, Y., Peleg, T., Adessky, R. S., & Freedman, S. A. (2012). Prevention of posttraumatic stress disorder by early treatment: Results from the Jerusalem trauma outreach and prevention study. *Archives of General Psychiatry, 69*, 166–176. doi:10.1001/archgenpsychiatry.2011.127

Shapiro, F. (2001). *Eye movement desensitization and reprocessing (EMDR).* New York, NY: Basic Books.

Shapiro, F. (2012). *Getting past your past: Take control of your life with self-help techniques from EMDR therapy.* New York, NY: Rodale.

Shapiro, F. (2018). *Eye movement desensitization and reprocessing (EMDR)* (3rd ed.). New York, NY: Guilford Press.

Shedler, J. (2010). The efficacy of psychodynamic psychotherapy. *American Psychologist, 65*(2), 98–109. doi:10.1037/a0018378

Shin, L., Rauch, S., & Pitman, R. (2006). Amygdala, medial prefrontal cortex, and hippocampal function in PTSD. *Annals of the New York Academy of Sciences, 1071*, 67–79. doi:10.1196/annals.1364.007

Siegel, D. J. (1999). *The developing mind: How relationships and the brain interact to shape who we are.* New York, NY: Guilford Press.

Siegel, D. J. (2002). The developing mind and the resolution of trauma: Some ideas about information processing and an interpersonal neurobiology of psychotherapy. In F. Shapiro (Ed.), *EMDR as an integrative psychotherapy approach* (pp. 85–121). Washington, DC: American Psychological Association.

Siegel, D. J. (2003). An interpersonal neurobiology of psychotherapy. In M. Solomon & D. J. Siegel (Eds.), *Healing trauma: Attachment, mind, body, and brain* (pp. 1–56). New York, NY: W. W. Norton.

Siegel, D. (2012). *Pocket guide to interpersonal neurobiology: An integrative handbook of the mind.* New York, NY: W. W. Norton.

Spiegel, D., Loewenstein, R., Lewis-Fernandez, R., Sar, V., Simeon, D., Vermetten, E., . . . Dell, P. (2011). Dissociative disorders in DSM-5. *Depression and Anxiety, 28*, 824–852. doi:10.1002/da .20874

Stavropoulos, P., & Kezelman, C. *The truth of memory and the memory of truth: Different types of memory and the significance of trauma.* Milsons Point, NSW, Australia: Blue Knot Foundation National Centre of Excellence for Complex Trauma. Retrieved from https://www.blueknot. org.au/ABOUT-US/Blog/ID/189/The-Truth-of-Memory-and-the-Memory-of-Truth-Different-Types-of-Memory-and-the-Significance-for-Trauma

Steele, K. (2009). Reflections on integration, mentalization, and institutional realization. *Journal of Trauma and Dissociation, 4*(1), 1–8.

Steele, K., Boon, S., & van der Hart, O. (2017). *Treating trauma-related dissociation: A practical, integrative approach.* New York, NY: W. W. Norton.

Steele, K., van der Hart, O., Nijenhuis, E. R. S. (2005). Phase-oriented treatment of structural dissociation in complex traumatization: Overcoming trauma-related phobias. Journal of Trauma & Dissociation, 6(3), 11–53. doi:10.1300/J229v06n03_02

Stickgold, R. (2002). EMDR: A putative neurobiological mechanism of action. *Journal of Clinical Psychology, 58*(1), 61–75. doi:10.1002/jclp.1129

Stickgold, R. (2005). Sleep-dependent memory consolidation. *Nature, 437*, 1272–1278. doi:10.1038/nature04286

Stickgold, R, (2008). Sleep-dependent memory processing and EMDR action. *Journal of EMDR Practice and Research, 2*(4), 289–299, doi:10.1891/1933-3196.2.4.289

Stien, P. T., & Kendall, J. (2004). *Psychological trauma and the developing brain: Neurologically based interventions for troubled children.* New York, NY: Haworth Press.

Stolorow, R. D., & Atwood, G. E (1996). The intersubjective perspective. *Psychoanalytic Review, 83*(2), 181–194.

Straube, T., Glauer, M., Dilger, S., Mentzel, H. J., & Miltner, W. H (2006). Effects of cognitive-behavioral therapy on brain activation in specific phobia. *Neuroimage, 29*, 125–135. doi:10.1016/j.neuroimage.2005.07.007

Szyf, M. (2009). The early life environment and the epigenome. *Biochimica et Biophysica Acta, 1790*(9), 878–885. doi:10.1016/j.bbagen.2009.01.009

Tacon, A. (2001). Alexithymia: A challenge for mental health nursing practice. *Australian and New Zealand Journal of Mental Health Nursing, 10*, 229–235. doi:10.1046/j.1440-0979.2001.00215.x

Taylor, G. J. (2000). Recent developments in alexithymia theory and research. *Canadian Journal of Psychiatry, 45*, 134–142. doi:10.1177/070674370004500203

Taylor, G. J., Parker, J. D., Bagby, M., & Acklin, M. W. (1992). Alexithymia and somatic complaints in psychiatric outpatients. *Journal of Psychosomatic Research, 36*, 417–424. doi:10.1016/0022-3999(92)90002-J

Teicher, M. (2000). Wounds that time won't heal: The neurobiology of child abuse. *Cerebrum: The Dana Forum on Brain Sciences.* Retrieved from https://www.dana.org/article/wounds-that-time-wont-heal

Teicher, M., Polcari, A., Andersen, S., Anderson, C. M., & Navalta, C. (2003). Neurobiological effects of childhood stress and trauma. In S. Coates, J. Rosenthal, & D. Schechter (Eds.), *September 11: Trauma and human bonds* (pp. 211–238). Hillsdale, NJ: Analytic Press.

Thomas, R., DiLillo, D., Walsh, K., & Polusny, M. (2011). Pathways from child sexual abuse to adult depression: The role of parental socialization of emotions and alexithymia. *Psychology of Violence, 1*(2), 121–135. doi:10.1037/a0022469

van der Kolk, B. (2003). Posttraumatic stress disorder and the nature of trauma. In M. Solomon & D. Siegel (Eds.), *Healing trauma.* New York, NY: W. W. Norton.

van der Kolk, B. (2006). Clinical implications of neuroscience research in PTSD. *Annals of New York Academy of Sciences, 1071,* 277–293. doi:10.1196/annals.1364.022

van der Kolk, B. (2014). *The body keeps the score: Brain, mind, and body in the healing of trauma.* New York, NY: Penguin Books.

van der Kolk, B., McFarlane, A. D., & Weisaeth, L. (Eds.). (1996). *Traumatic stress: The effects of overwhelming experience on mind, body, and society.* New York, NY: Guilford Press.

van der Kolk, B., Spinazzola, J. Blaustein, M., Hopper, J. Hopper, E., Korn, D., . . . Simpson, W. (2007). A randomized clinical trial of EMDR, fluoxetine and pill placebo in the treatment of PTSD: Treatment effects and long-term maintenance. *Journal of Clinical Psychiatry, 68,* 37–46. doi:10.4088/JCP.v68n0105

Warner-Schmidt, J., & Duman, R. S. (2006). Hippocampal neurogenesis: Opposing effects of stress and antidepressant treatment. *Hippocampus, 16*(3), 239–249. doi:10.1002/hipo.20156

Waters, F. S. (2016). *Healing the fractured child: Diagnosis and treatment of youth with dissociation.* New York, NY: Springer Publishing Company.

Weiss, S. (2007). Neurobiological alterations associated with traumatic stress. *Perspectives in Psychiatric Care, 43*(3), 114–122. doi:10.1111/j.1744-6163.2007.00120.x

Westbrook, C., Creswell, J. D., Tabibnia, G., Julson, E., Kober, H., & Tindle, H. A. (2011). Mindful attention reduces neural and self-reported cue-induced craving in smokers. *Social Cognitive and Affective Neuroscience, 8*(1), 1–3. doi:10.1093/scan/nsr076

Wetherill, R., & Tapert, S. F. (2012). Adolescent brain development, substance use, and psychotherapeutic change. *Psychology of Addictive Behaviors, 27*(2), 393–402. doi:10.1037/a0029111

Wheeler, K. (2000). Emotional regulation and alexithymia: Treatment implications for nurse practitioners. *Clinical Excellence for Nurse Practitioners, 4*(3), 145–150.

Wheeler, K., Greiner, P., & Boulton, M. (2005). Exploring alexithymia, depression and binge eating in self-reported eating disorders in women. *Perspectives in Psychiatric Care, 41*(3), 112–121. doi:10.1111/j.1744-6163.2005.00022.x

Winnicott, D. W. (1976). *Maturational processes and the facilitating environment* (pp. 166–170). London, UK: Hogarth Press. (Originally work published in 1965)

Woodward, S. (2004). PTSD sleep research: An update. *PTSD Research Quarterly, 15*(4), 1–8. doi:10.1037/e400272008-001

Yehuda, R., Engel, S. M., Brand, S. R., Seckl, J., Marcus, S. M., & Berkowitz, G. S (2005). Transgenerational effects of posttraumatic stress disorder in babies of mothers exposed to the World Trade Center attacks during pregnancy. *Journal of Clinical Endocrinology and Metabolism, 90,* 4115–4118. doi:10.1210/jc.2005-0550

Zahradnik, M., Stewart, S. H., Marshall, G. N., Shell, T. L., & Jaycox, L. H (2009). Anxiety sensitivity and aspects of alexithymia are independently and uniquely associated with posttraumatic distress. *Journal of Traumatic Stress, 22,* 131–138. doi:10.1002/jts.20397

Zhang, J., Tan, Q., Yin, H., Zhang, H. X., Huan, Y., Tang, L., . . . Li, L. (2011). Decreased gray matter volume in the left hippocampus and bilateral cerebral cortex in coal mine flood disaster survivors with recent onset PTSD. *Psychiatry Research, 192,* 84–90. doi:10.1016/j.pscychresns.2010.09.0012

3

Assessment and Diagnosis

Pamela Bjorklund

A comprehensive assessment of the patient who presents for psychotherapy is necessary to develop an appropriate treatment plan. In some settings, a comprehensive assessment must be conducted during the initial session. This chapter presents the format and tools for such an assessment. The comprehensive psychiatric database and instruments included in this chapter can also be integrated in a setting that allows the therapist to conduct an assessment over several sessions. However, the therapist may bill for an initial, comprehensive assessment only once during the course of the assessment process. In reality, most assessments continue throughout the treatment, and therapists initially use only selected instruments in acquiring a database. The setting and population with whom a therapist works determine what is necessary and what is optional. Other screening tools not included in this chapter may be required by an agency or employer or are necessitated later by an evolving understanding of the patient.

INTRODUCTION

Even if the advanced practice psychiatric nurse (APPN) sees a patient only for the assessment, a sensitively crafted intake assessment can be a powerful therapeutic tool. It can establish rapport between patient and therapist, further the therapeutic alliance, alleviate anxiety, provide reassurance, and facilitate the flow of information necessary for an accurate diagnosis and appropriate treatment plan. For better or for worse, an assessment is a relational process. It represents a verbal and nonverbal dialogue between two therapeutic partners, whose behaviors reciprocally influence each other's style of communication and result in a specific pattern of interaction (Shea, 2017). To the degree this pattern of interaction transcends its question-and-answer format to constitute an authentic encounter between the patient and therapist; an assessment can play a significant role in the change process (Safran & Muran, 2000). At the very least, a sensitively crafted assessment can help ensure that a patient in distress returns for follow-up care.

Shea (2017) identified the broad goals of clinical assessment as follows:

1. To effectively engage the patient in the data-gathering process
2. To collect information and form a valid database
3. To develop an evolving and compassionate understanding of the patient
4. To develop an assessment from which a tentative diagnosis can be made
5. To collaboratively identify problems and therapeutic goals

6. To collaboratively develop a tentative treatment plan to achieve these goals
7. To effect some decrease in the patient's anxiety
8. To instill hope and ensure that the patient will return for the next appointment

The goals of engaging the patient in a therapeutic alliance, gathering data, uniquely understanding the patient as a person, and arriving at the most appropriate diagnosis and treatment plan are parallel assessment processes (Shea, 2017). Generally, the more powerfully engaged the patient and therapist are during the assessment process, the more valid are the data on which to base the diagnosis that will guide the choice of treatment plan.

In a clinical sense, *validity* refers to the accuracy of the database, that is, to whether the clinician actually elicited the information he or she tried to elicit (Shea, 2017). The more valid the database—and by implication, the more valid the diagnosis—the more confidence the therapist can have in the treatment plan and the more reassurance he or she can offer to patients about their probable course or expected outcomes. The successful engagement of patients in the assessment process is key to the validity of assessment data. It requires empathy, patience, a willingness to afford patients sufficient time to tell their stories in their own manner, the ability to structure patients when necessary, and careful attention to patients' needs for comfort, privacy, and security. Consequently, this chapter examines important areas for assessment and provides specific screening tools to aid in the assessment process while attending to the manner in which the therapist also fosters therapeutic engagement. It describes the process of taking a history and the comprehensive assessment of areas of patient functioning that are important to the practice of psychotherapy, including ego functioning, affective development, interpersonal relationships, and belief systems. The chapter ends with a discussion of diagnosis and case formulation, without which the treatment plan has no rationale.

TAKING A HISTORY

Fundamentally, the comprehensive psychiatric history is a form of life story told to the therapist by a patient in his or her own words and from his or her own point of view (Sadock, Sadock, & Ruiz, 2015). In some situations and with the patient's consent, excluding only emergency situations, the psychiatric history may include information from other sources, such as a parent, spouse, former therapist, other referral source, or medical record. The therapist must collaborate with a consenting patient in negotiating the details of how and when to obtain collateral information from other sources. A comprehensive history includes information about the current episode of illness with data related to the onset, chronology, and severity of current symptoms and stressors. It also includes past and present psychiatric and medical histories, a psychiatric review of systems, medication and substance use histories, a history of violence or self-destructive behavior, any history of trauma, and developmental, family, social, educational, occupational, and legal histories. Box 3.1 provides an outline of the major sections of the psychiatric history/initial psychiatric interview as adapted from *The American Psychiatric Association Practice Guidelines for the Psychiatric Evaluation of Adults* (3rd ed.; American Psychiatric Association [APA], 2016; Box 3.2) and *Kaplan & Sadock's Synopsis of Psychiatry* (11th ed.; Sadock et al., 2015). Appendix 3.1 outlines the content of a comprehensive psychiatric database developed from multiple sources, including professional experiences in various clinical assessment venues (APA, 2016; Gordon & Goroll, 2003; Marken, Schneiderhan, & Munro, 2005; Morrison, 2014; Sadock et al., 2015; Scully & Thornhill, 2012; Shea, 2017). Appendix 3.2 presents a sample intake assessment form adapted from Shea (2017) that includes all sections of the comprehensive psychiatric database.

BOX 3.1 Major Sections of the Psychiatric History

   I. Reason for the evaluation
      A. Identifying data
      B. Source and reliability of data
      C. Chief complaint
  II. History of the present illness (HPI)
      A. Symptoms
      B. Stressors
 III. Past psychiatric history
      A. Trauma history
 IV. Substance use/abuse history
  V. Past medical history
 VI. Family history
VII. Developmental and social history
      A. Strengths
      B. Support systems
      C. Values/belief systems
VIII. Review of systems
 IX. Mental status examination (MSE)
  X. Case formulation
 XI. *DSM-5* diagnoses
XII. Treatment plan

DSM-5, Diagnostic and Statistical Manual of Mental Disorders (5th ed.).

Source: American Psychiatric Association. (2016). *The American Psychiatric Association practice guidelines for the psychiatric evaluation of adults* (3rd ed.). Arlington, VA: Author; Sadock, B. J., Sadock, V. S., & Ruiz, P. (2015). *Kaplan & Sadock's synopsis of psychiatry: Behavioral sciences/clinical psychiatry* (11th ed.). Philadelphia, PA: Wolters Kluwer.

BOX 3.2 Websites for American Psychiatric Association (APA) Practice Guidelines

The American Psychiatric Association Practice Guidelines for the Psychiatric Evaluation of Adults (3rd ed):
psychiatryonline.org/doi/book/10.1176/appi.books.9780890426760
psychiatryonline.org/guidelines

Obtaining such a comprehensive history from the patient and, if necessary, from informed sources close to the patient is essential to making an accurate, culturally appropriate diagnosis and developing a specific, culturally sensitive, and effective treatment plan (Sadock et al., 2015). From this life story, the therapist can begin to paint a picture of the patient's personality characteristics, strengths and areas for growth, interpersonal style, cultural context, and development from his or her earliest years to the present moment. Taking a history, which also can be seen as a cocreative act of constructing a comprehensive life story, allows the therapist and ultimately the patient to more completely understand who the patient is, where the patient has come from, and how the patient may develop in the future (Sadock et al., 2015). It is an essential first step to reimagining the life story. That people in psychotherapy often come to change their life stories over the course of treatment is a positive development, because a patient's reflections on past circumstances in light of the changing present heralds the creation of a different future (Barker, 2001). The revision of life stories through narrative is the essential work of psychotherapy, which is a unique form of encapsulated experience that focuses on the life experiences of another such that those experiences can be reconsidered, more deeply understood, reframed, and thus reconstructed in healthier ways (Peplau, 1989). It all starts with taking a history.

CASE EXAMPLE

Opening Moves

In settings where a comprehensive history must be completed in one session, the therapist must accomplish a number of important alliance-building tasks in the first minutes of the initial assessment. These include an appropriate greeting, introductions (if not already made in an earlier contact), an indication of seating preference, a brief introduction to the assessment process, and an open-ended invitation to the patient to tell the therapist how he or she can be of assistance. In these moments, the therapist should indicate what the interview will be like, how much time it will take, what sort of questions will be asked, and what sort of information the patient is expected to share. The therapist needs to create a comfortable and secure environment that allows the patient as much control as possible (Morrison, 2014). Early in the assessment, a nondirective interview style with open-ended questions yields control to the patient, generally builds rapport, and garners facts that are more reliable (Morrison, 2014; Shea, 2017). Because studies have shown that patients give the most valid information when they are allowed to answer freely, in their own words, and as completely as they wish, it is generally desirable to initially employ open-ended questions that allow the widest possible scope of response (Morrison, 2014). To illustrate how a therapist may begin the data-gathering process, Box 3.3 summarizes the first moments of an initial clinical assessment with a fictive psychotherapy patient, who has indicated in an earlier phone contact her preference to be called by her first name, Beth.

In the medical model, the patient's response to the therapist's opening question is called the *chief complaint*, but it might better be called the *patient-identified problem* in a holistic nursing model. It is the patient's stated reason for seeking help and is

BOX 3.3 Beginning the Clinical Assessment

APPN:	Hello, Beth. It's nice to meet you in person. Please, sit down. You can make yourself comfortable here. [Points to a chair.]
Patient:	Okay, thanks.
APPN:	As I mentioned on the phone, I am an advanced practice psychiatric nurse, and in today's session, I hope to get a clearer sense of the difficulties you alluded to on the phone. I will be asking questions about important areas of your life, and with your permission, I would like to be able to take a few notes. I don't want to forget anything. [Smiles, waits for a response.]
Patient:	That's fine.
APPN:	I would like to get as much history as I can today, but if we aren't able to get to everything, we'll continue next week. I'll be asking lots of questions about your present circumstances and your past history, so if any of my questions make you uncomfortable, please let me know. I do not want to contribute to your distress, but I do want to hear as much about your thoughts and feelings as you are comfortable telling me.
Patient:	That's fair. I'll try.
APPN:	Could you tell me in whatever way you like what brings you in today?
Patient:	[Takes 5 to 10 minutes to tell her story, with open-ended prompts by the therapist only as needed, e.g., "What happened then?" "Could you tell me more about that?" "How were you feeling at that time?" "What else was going on?"]

recorded verbatim. It often reveals the problem uppermost in the patient's mind (Morrison, 2014) and can indicate the content region (Shea, 2017) or assessment area (APA, 2016) the therapist should explore first. When the patient's response to the therapist's opening question is a denial that anything is wrong, it is often helpful to rephrase the question in terms of why others may think the patient should seek help, such as "Can you tell me what went on that your (mother, spouse, friend, employer, primary care provider, court officer) thought you might benefit from coming in?" Another technique is to ally with the patient's resistance or sidestep it; for example, "Nothing may be wrong, but because you're already here, perhaps we can try to figure out if there is something else I can help with." Such denials are the first indication that the therapist may encounter significant resistance from the patient to engaging in psychotherapy, and they are cogent reminders that the first task of data gathering is alliance building.

During the minutes that follow the patient-identified problem, while the patient is freely telling his or her story, much is signaled that the therapist will need to explore in greater depth later in the interview. The therapist needs to mentally note or write down these areas of clinical interest, or content regions, so that specific questions can be asked at the appropriate time. Box 3.4 summarizes the content from Beth's response to the therapist's opening question.

BOX 3.4 Exploring the Patient-Identified Problem

APPN:	Can you tell me in whatever way you like what brings you in today?
Patient:	I don't know. [Long pause.] Donna N. [referral source] sent me. She and my mom and my advisor thought I had depression. Actually, I've been depressed on and off since the 10th grade. [Another long pause.] I have a lot of problems getting along with my parents, especially my mom. I've been thinking about dropping out of school until spring semester to get my head together, but my advisor talked me out of it. I am dropping only one class. I'm not really happy about deciding to stay in school. I cried for 3 hours about it. I'm overwhelmed with school. I can't catch up. I don't care about anything anymore. I'm happy just to stay in bed. The slightest things make me feel bad. I'm angry all the time. My mother thinks my personality has changed. I don't know. Maybe it has. I'm more irritable around my boyfriend. The slightest things he does put me on edge. My mother, too. She calls me every night in the middle of studying, and it gets on my nerves. If she didn't call me, I wouldn't even think about her.
APPN:	Beth, you mentioned you are quite irritable these days and have been crying a lot. Can you tell me more about the depressive symptoms you've been having?
Patient:	Well, I sleep okay, but I wake up tired, and I have no energy for anything. I'm not really sad, just angry and irritable and overwhelmed with everything.
APPN:	Anything else?
Patient:	A few days ago I thought about suicide. It just crossed my mind. I don't really want to die. I just want my problems to end.
APPN:	What did you think about? [Therapist takes this opportunity to thoroughly assess current suicide risk and to explore the past history of suicidal behavior. She then returns to the "depression" content region to more thoroughly assess the possibility of a diagnosable mood disorder, such as major depression or dysthymia.]

Expanding the Assessment

Although no rules dictate which content regions to explore first or in what order, it is generally advisable to thoroughly explore one before moving on to another (Shea, 2017). In this example, the therapist chooses to first explore the symptoms of a possible mood disorder and, when the patient (Beth) broaches the subject, to assess her current suicide risk. However, Beth makes a mental note to follow these content regions with the developmental, family, and social histories, focusing on Beth's strained relationships with her mother and boyfriend and on her academic decline. After a thorough assessment of the current suicide risk and any history of suicidal behavior, the therapist returns to the current mood symptoms and the history of the present illness (HPI) to get a more thorough sense of the onset, extent, severity, and chronology of mood symptoms and whether criteria are met for any particular mood disorder. In doing so, she learns more about Beth's hostile and enmeshed relationship with her mother. It seems the patient has been dysthymic since the 10th grade, when Beth's mother put her daughter's dog to sleep without her knowledge. This occurred on the day Beth got her braces removed from her teeth. A family celebration had been planned: "It was supposed to be a happy day for me. It wasn't." Apart from the fact that it is the humane thing to do, an engaged clinician should take this opportunity to further strengthen the therapeutic alliance— which facilitates continued data gathering—by empathizing with the patient's distress about what appears to have been a significant loss and a rather cruel act of sabotage by the patient's mother (e.g., "You must have been very hurt by this."). The therapist then needs to move to the developmental and family history to learn more about this incident and to more thoroughly assess the family dynamics, especially the patient's relationship with her mother (e.g., "Tell me more about that day, your relationship with your mother, and your family situation.").

In this way, the therapist proceeds to take a history, thoroughly exploring all the major sections of the comprehensive psychiatric database (see Box 3.1) by opening new content regions as opportunities arise. Open-ended questions invite exploration in new content regions, reveal what is uppermost in a patient's mind, and may yield important information about the patient's capacities, defenses, or degree of resistance to engaging in psychotherapy. Closed-ended questions elicit the specific details—such as symptom type, severity, frequency, duration, and the context in which a symptom occurs—that are necessary to thoroughly assess a content region or establish a diagnosis. Table 3.1 provides an outline of open-ended and closed-ended assessment questions along a continuum of openness. Opportunities to open new content regions do not always arise spontaneously; and in those cases, the therapist must guide the assessment into new clinical areas. Occasionally, time constraints may force a therapist to make an abrupt transition to unexplored content regions in order to complete the assessment within the allotted time. Nevertheless, the transition can be made skillfully, sensitively, and in a manner that continues to facilitate the therapeutic alliance. Box 3.5 illustrates the use of open-ended and closed-ended questions to facilitate skillful, even if abrupt, transitions to new content regions.

Organizing the History of the Present Illness

Of all the major content regions of the psychiatric history, the most important is the HPI. It represents the heart of the assessment interview. It is the most substantial part of the initial clinical assessment and includes a description of the patient's key symptoms, their timing and associated problems, and the stressors that account for their exacerbation. When well organized, the HPI develops much like a short story. It progresses chronologically through the onset and development of the patient's key symptoms to

TABLE 3.1 ASSESSMENT QUESTIONS: CONTINUUM OF OPENNESS	
Type	**Example**
Open-Ended Types	
Open-ended questions	What brings you in today?
	How can I help you?
	How would you describe your relationship with. . .?
Gentle commands	Tell me about your family situation.
	Try to describe how you felt when. . .
	Share with me what you think a good outcome would be.
Intermediate Types	
Swing questions (client can say "no" or client can elaborate)	Can you describe the depressive symptoms?
	Can you tell me anything more about that?
	Can you tell me what you're thinking right now?
Qualitative questions	How have you been sleeping?
	How is school going?
	How have you been getting along with your mom?
Statements of inquiry	So you have never before received any therapy?
	Your mother decided to go back to school when you did?
	You say you just want to stay in bed all the time?
Empathic statements	You must have been so hurt by that.
	That is very frustrating.
	It is hard to lose someone you love.
Facilitating statements	Go on.
	I see.
Closed-Ended Types	
Closed-ended questions	How many drinks did you have?
	How often do you feel that way?
Closed-ended statements	You can sit down here.
	We'll take about 50 minutes to. . .
	Medications can be very effective in these cases.

Source: Adapted from Shea, S. C. (2017). *Psychiatric interviewing: The art of understanding* (3rd ed.). New York, NY: Elsevier.

BOX 3.5 Transitioning to New Content Regions

APPN:	Beth, you've told me a great deal of very helpful information about your family situation. I'm beginning to understand the kinds of things you're dealing with. But I've noticed the clock, and we have only 15 minutes left. There are some other things I need to know before we can talk about where to go from here. Can you handle a few more questions? [closed-ended question] [Note: Using a patient's name judiciously can comfort, contain, invite closeness, and facilitate the therapeutic alliance. If used artificially or too often, it can seem ingratiating or insincere and can distance the patient and impede the therapeutic alliance.]
APPN:	You mentioned that you saw a school counselor when you were in the 10th grade and your dog was put to sleep. Can you tell me more about that treatment? [open-ended, swing question]
Patient:	Well, there's not much to tell. I saw her only once. It wasn't really a treatment. We talked for about 30 minutes. A teacher was concerned when she saw me crying at school. I didn't go back. She said I didn't have to if I didn't want to.
APPN:	Were there any other times that you saw a counselor, therapist, or psychiatrist? [closed-ended question]
Patient:	No.
APPN:	So you've never before received any therapy or any psychiatric treatment, either as an inpatient or outpatient? [closed-ended statement of inquiry]
Patient:	No.
APPN:	Okay. What about substance abuse? [open-ended question]
Patient:	Treatment? No, never. In fact, I don't use anything. I don't even drink coffee. I suppose . . .[long pause; therapist waits]
APPN:	Go on. [facilitating statement]
Patient:	Well, I have tried some things, but it was a long time ago.
APPN:	Tell me. [open-ended, gentle command]

the time of the patient's presentation for evaluation. By the end of a detailed HPI, an experienced clinician should be able to construct a near complete differential diagnosis. A thorough and well-constructed HPI contains the following components, roughly in the following order:

1. A statement of the patient's baseline functioning or last period of stability
2. Any previous diagnoses of psychiatric disorder and a brief synopsis of the course and treatment
3. The onset of the first symptom and its precipitant
4. A chronology of one to three key symptoms, including when they worsened and the precipitant events that caused them to worsen
5. Associated symptoms related to the one to three key symptoms
6. Documentation of the "why now," that is, why the patient presents for treatment now
7. Repetition of components 3, 4, and 5 if there is more than one diagnosable disorder
8. A list of pertinent negative symptoms, that is, symptoms that are not present
9. A list of additional stressors not mentioned

Box 3.6 documents the HPI in the case of Beth, inserting numbers 1 through 9 at appropriate points in the text to mark the essential HPI components as listed above.

BOX 3.6 Documenting the History of Present Illness

Beth is a 20-year-old college junior majoring in business administration who has felt chronically depressed since approximately the 10th grade, when her mother put her dog to sleep without her knowledge on a day the family planned to celebrate the removal of her braces (1).* She has no previous history of psychiatric treatment (2). In August, she moved away from home for the first time after having an argument with her parents about money and college expenses. The focus of the conflict was Beth's resentment about their refusal to help her more with college expenses when they had money for new recreational vehicles, house remodeling, and, most significantly, her mother's sudden enrollment in the Denton Business University, which coincided with Beth's change of majors from psychology to business administration. She moved in with her boyfriend of the past year and a half and found herself feeling increasingly irritated with him (3). Despite these stressors and her increasingly low mood, she functioned relatively well in school until approximately 3 weeks ago, when she began to feel more depressed, apathetic, and fatigued than usual. She wanted to drop out of school but was talked out of it by her academic advisor and ended up dropping only one course. She states she sleeps well but wakes up tired and has no energy. She "doesn't care about anything anymore" and is "happy to stay in bed." The "slightest things make me feel bad," and she has crying episodes three or four times per week. Beth has lost approximately 8 pounds in the past 3 weeks. She reports that she does not feel sad, hopeless, or helpless, just overwhelmed by school, work, changing majors, having to interact with her parents—her mother calls her every evening during her study time—and having to work harder to get along with her boyfriend in close quarters. All her symptoms have worsened over the past 1 to 2 weeks and are exacerbated by the seemingly daily conflict with her mother and boyfriend (4). Within the past week, she has begun scratching on her wrists with plastic, serrated knives—something she has not done since high school (5). Three days ago, a particularly loud and hostile phone conversation with her mother annoyed Beth's boyfriend, causing a bitter argument between the two of them. He stomped out of the apartment and did not return that night (6). She felt "abandoned" and "panicky"; thoughts of suicide (no plan or intent) crossed her mind, which scared her enough that she contacted her college vocational counselor, who referred her for psychiatric evaluation (7). She denies acute suicide ideation today, as well as any symptoms of mania or hypomania, psychosis, or severe anxiety (8). Additional stressors include 20 to 25 hours per week of work at McDonald's while carrying 12 semester credits, a substantial tuition bill that comes due very soon, and a growing sense that she needs to move again because she cannot tolerate the increased closeness with her boyfriend (9).

*Parenthetic numbers 1 through 9 mark the essential components of the history of present illness that are listed in the text.

Mental Status Examination

The mental status examination (MSE) has become a standard component of the initial clinical assessment. It is the clinician's description of the patient's current mental functioning. It is a direct examination of the patient's behavior and the examiner's inferences from what the patient says and does. In making these inferences, the clinician must carefully consider the patient's educational and cultural background. Illiteracy and differences in ethnic, cultural, and linguistic backgrounds can distort the results of the MSE (Jacob, 2012). The principles of symptom elicitation during the MSE are comparable to those employed in interpreting diagnostic laboratory tests, which require both sensitivity and specificity, and are employed to screen, exclude, or confirm abnormalities (Jacob, 2003, 2012). Although it is beyond the scope of this chapter to discuss in detail how to perform a formal MSE, Appendix 3.1 includes a comprehensive out-line of the content and possible organization of a formal MSE. Many of its sources (see Appendix 3.1) describe the performance of the MSE in great detail.

All APPNs must learn to perform a comprehensive, formal MSE, which has value even in the case of psychotherapy patients who present as cognitively intact. A formal MSE may elicit subtle abnormalities not readily apparent earlier in the assessment pro-cess. Although the volume of material to cover can seem daunting, much of the MSE is obtained during the general history-taking interview, requires no special questions or tests, and can be assessed through informal observation that begins the moment the therapist first encounters the patient. The key is to know what elements to look for and to be systematic in looking for them. When comfortable with a format for a complete MSE, the therapist can tactfully transition from informal observation to a direct, sys-tematic examination of the patient's cognitive status when a suitable opportunity pres-ents itself (Box 3.7). General introductory questions followed by specific confirmatory questions are standard. Open-ended formats and general probes are sensitive screening strategies (e.g., "Have you felt like odd things are happening that you cannot explain?"). More precise confirmatory questions provide specificity (e.g., "Are your thoughts read by other people?"; Jacob, 2003).

Sometimes, opportunities for a smooth transition to the formal MSE do not present themselves. Occasionally, a complete examination is impossible, such as with a very agi-tated or uncommunicative patient; and sometimes, it can seem insulting to ask appar-ently high-functioning people what today's date is or whether they can remember a "red ball" and "37 Elm Street" for a period of 5 minutes. Nevertheless, when a clini-cian inadvertently fails to perform a formal MSE or makes a deliberate decision not to perform one in a patient who seems unimpaired, the therapist risks missing impor-tant information that may emerge only through a direct, systematic examination of a patient's cognitive function. Until it becomes second nature, APPNs should choose a format, memorize it, and perform the MSE the same way each time (Morrison, 2014).

Box 3.8 presents one way of organizing data from the MSE. It summarizes the results of Beth's formal MSE as it might appear in a formal diagnostic report or on a clinical assessment summary. However, therapists must develop their own systematic method of obtaining, organizing, and recording the MSE so that the process becomes second nature. Although the results of Beth's MSE are essentially within normal limits, the doc-umentation of specific mental status abnormalities can help to substantiate a diagnosis and particular treatment needs.

Time Frames and Closing Moves

The patient's unique circumstances determine how much time the therapist spends on each major section of the psychiatric history. In Beth's case, the therapist will spend much of her time gathering data for the HPI and the family, developmental, and social histories.

BOX 3.7 Transitioning to the MSE

APPN:	You mentioned a short while ago that you're having trouble with your memory, so let's see exactly what that difficulty is. Can you tell me today's date?
APPN:	You say that you cannot concentrate. Let's take a closer look at that. I'm going to give you three things to remember and then ask you in a few minutes to recall them: a red ball, 37 Elm Street, and a clock radio. Can you repeat them now?

BOX 3.8 Documenting the Mental Status Examination (MSE)

Beth is an attractive, subdued, casually and appropriately dressed, 20-year-old single, White female who appears to be her stated age. She is quite distressed and is fighting back tears. However, she makes good eye contact and readily engages with the examiner. Her speech is fluent, soft, and quavering; her affect ranges from flat to sad and angry. Her mood is dysthymic and congruent with her affect. Her movements are graceful and without abnormality. She is alert and fully oriented. She evidences no problems with attention, concentration, or memory. She can recall 6/6 objects at 0 and 5 minutes, can subtract serial sevens without difficulty, repeats five digits forward and backward, can abstract proverbs, and has an adequate fund of general knowledge. Her thought processes are logical, linear, and goal directed with no evidence of a thought disorder. Prominent themes in her thought content include her smoldering resentment toward her parents, particularly her mother, and her feelings of being overwhelmed by her schoolwork. She denies current, active suicide or homicide ideation as well as all signs and symptoms of psychosis. Superficially, her judgment is intact. She appears to be of above-average intelligence; however, her problem-solving abilities are transiently overwhelmed. She is excessively worried about "not being ahead of the game," as she customarily would be.

15%:   Chief complaint and free speech

30%:   History of present illness; pursuit of information relevant to the differential diagnosis; histories of suicide, violence, or substance use

15%:   Medical history; review of systems; family history

25%:   Personal (developmental and social) history

10%:   MSE

5%:   Discussion of the diagnosis and treatment plan; plan for next visit

Very little time is needed for the psychiatric history, medical history, substance use history, and MSE because the patient is young, physically healthy, cognitively intact, and has no history of prior psychiatric treatment or significant substance use. Although the needs of the patient determine which content regions are most appropriate for deeper exploration, and taking into consideration time constraints (usually 60 minutes for an initial assessment), Morrison (2014) and Shea (2017) provide guidance on how to carve up the allotted time when the assessment data must be gathered in one session. Morrison (2014) suggests the following:

Shea (2017) suggests at least 5 to 7 minutes for the *scouting* period, which is what Morrison (2014) calls *free speech* and what is essentially the time it takes for the patient to narrate his or her story. By the end of the first 30 minutes of the initial assessment, the therapist should be nearing completion of the content regions that seem most pertinent for that patient. Often, during the third 15-minute period, the family history, medical history, social history, and the formal MSE are completed (Shea, 2017). In Beth's case, exploration of the family, developmental, and social issues would have been explored in depth earlier, because they are uniquely important content regions for her and might have extended into the third 15-minute assessment period.

In any case, Shea (2017) recommends that the therapist monitor, at least every 5 to 10 minutes, the progress of his or her data gathering and adjust the pace as necessary. It is probably a good idea to check with the patient by asking, "Is this okay for you?" During the last 15 minutes of the assessment period, regional content explorations of the major sections of the psychiatric history are completed; final points of clarification

BOX 3.9 Ending the Clinical Assessment

APPN:	[Summarizes diagnostic impression and treatment recommendations.] So that's what I'm thinking right now. What are your thoughts?
Patient:	What happens if the medication doesn't help?
APPN:	We have lots of options, including trying a different medication, but it is important to remember that medication is only one tool at our disposal. Even when it works, it doesn't solve relationship problems, although it can give you more energy to deal with them. That's why psychotherapy is so important. Do you have thoughts about that?
Patient:	Not really, except . . . [long pause; therapist waits] I don't really like talking about my family. It leaves me with a bad feeling.
APPN:	Yes, I have a pretty clear sense of how difficult that was for you. Is there anything I could have done differently to make that easier for you?
Patient:	No, I don't think so.
APPN:	Tell me more about what this [assessment] experience has been like for you?
Patient:	Actually, it wasn't as bad as I was thinking it would be. In a way, I feel relieved. I'm willing to try anything.
APPN:	I can hear how distressed you've been. On the other hand, that's a very positive attitude. I think there is every reason to believe you can feel significantly better very soon. And if not, we will work together to figure out why. How does that sound?
Patient:	Good. Sounds good.
APPN:	Will this time next week work for you? [details of follow-up are negotiated]

are pursued; and termination occurs. Time can get away from even experienced psychotherapists, especially when a patient is particularly distressed, verbose, vague, or disorganized. However, whenever possible, the last 5 to 10 minutes of the assessment period should be devoted to discussing the findings, treatment recommendations, and follow-up plan; answering whatever questions the patient may have about those findings; processing the patient's assessment experience; paving the way for the next visit; and in doing all that, continuing to build the strong therapeutic alliance on which a good psychotherapy outcome depends. Box 3.9 illustrates the closing minutes of Beth's initial clinical assessment.

Assessing Ego Functioning

The assessment of ego functioning from the perspective of ego strength, as opposed to ego deficit, is a valuable skill for nurse psychotherapists. The identification and assessment of ego strength help the therapist locate a patient on a developmental continuum, suggest a place to join with the patient to begin the therapeutic work, provide data to develop therapeutic goals, and create a valid construct for psychotherapy outcome measurement (Bjorklund, 2000; Burns, 1991). The person who gains ego strength as a result of his or her work with a therapist has made noteworthy therapeutic progress. Broadly defined, ego strength is the capacity for effective personal functioning (Burns, 1991). It encompasses specific capacities such as adaptability, resourcefulness, self-efficacy, self-esteem, interpersonal effectiveness, life satisfaction, and the many other mental health indicators succinctly encapsulated in Freud's (1923/1961) well-known phrase "to love and to work." Like the solid foundation of a well-built house, ego strength supports the individual in the pursuit of life goals, dreams, and ambitions, especially during times of trouble. It ensures coping abilities, provides an individual with a sense of identity, can be recognized during initial assessment and throughout therapy, and increases as patients grow in maturity (Bjorklund, 2000). To the degree each ego function can be identified and assessed in the clinical situation, ego strength can be acknowledged, rated, reinforced, supported, built upon, or "loaned" to some degree to lower-functioning patients by their relatively higher-functioning therapists in the process of identifying with the therapist's own ego strength (Bjorklund, 2000).

Identification occurs through the ongoing corrective emotional experience that constitutes therapy and the therapist's repetitive modeling of the kinds of coping behaviors indicative of ego strength. Table 3.2 identifies 12 ego functions and their definitions (Bellak, 1989). The list can be used as an assessment outline for the purpose of identifying patient strengths, or it can serve as the basis for self-reported or observer-rated

TABLE 3.2 EGO FUNCTIONS FOR ASSESSMENT	
Reality Testing	**Differentiating Inner From Outer Stimuli**
Judgment	Aware of appropriateness and likely consequences of intended behavior
Sense of reality of the world and of the self	Experiences external events as real; differentiates self from others
Affect and impulse control	Maintains self-control; can tolerate intense affect and delay of gratification
Interpersonal functioning	Sustains relationships over time despite separations or hostility
Thought processes	Attention, concentration, memory, language, and other cognitive processes are intact; thinking is realistic and logical
Adaptive regression in the service of the ego	Relaxation of ego controls, allowing creative perceptual or conceptual integrations to increase adaptive potential
Defensive functioning	Defenses satisfactorily prevent anxiety, depression, and other unpleasant affects
Stimulus barrier	Aware of sensory stimuli without stimulus overload
Autonomous functioning	Cognitive and motor functions (i.e., primary autonomy) and routine behavior (i.e., secondary autonomy) are free from disturbance
Synthetic-integrative functioning	Integrates contradictory attitudes, values, affects, behavior, and self-representations
Mastery competence	Performance consistent with existing capacity
Object constancy	Ability to provide for oneself, caretaking and soothing in the absence of the caretaker

Source: Adapted from Bellak, L. (1989). The broad role of ego function assessment. In S. Wetzler & M. Katz (Eds.), *Contemporary approaches to psychological assessment* (pp. 270–295). New York, NY: Brunner/Mazel.

ego strength assessment scales to measure more concretely a patient's emerging ego strength. Table 3.3 provides an example of an observer-rated ego strength assessment scale constructed in everyday language. The assessment items in Table 3.3 suggest specific questions the therapist may ask to elicit information about the ego functions outlined in Table 3.2 and Box 3.10.

TABLE 3.3 OBSERVER-RATED EGO FUNCTION ASSESSMENT TOOL*	
Assessment Item	**Ego Function**
Always (1) Almost Always (2) Usually (3) Sometimes (4) Hardly Ever (5) Never (6)	
1. When dealing with strong feelings, has trouble with getting too upset or losing control with words or actions	Regulation and control of affects and impulses
2. Explains problems as being caused almost entirely by others	Defensive functioning; interpersonal functioning
3. Has trouble sitting back and looking at own behavior in a realistic way	Defensive functioning; interpersonal functioning
4. Believes he or she is basically a good person, worth caring about, but with some problems	Synthetic-integrative functioning
5. Seems to feel good or bad about self, depending mostly on how others are feeling about him or her	Affect regulation and control of affect; synthetic-integrative functioning
6. Seems able to recognize how he or she is feeling	Regulation and control of affect; defensive functioning
7. Seems able to express his or her feelings in an appropriate manner	Regulation and control of affect and impulses
8. Seems really weird, bizarre, or out of touch with reality	Reality testing; sense of reality of the world and of the self; thought processes
9. Able to look at self fairly realistically in terms of good and bad qualities	Sense of reality of the world and of the self; synthetic-integrative functioning
10. Explains his or her problems by means of hallucinations, false beliefs, control by supernatural power	Reality testing; sense of reality of the world and of the self; thought processes
11. Seems as if he or she does not notice other people exist	Interpersonal functioning
12. Seems afraid of being close to others	Interpersonal functioning
13. Tends to see others as having both good and bad qualities	Synthetic-integrative functioning
14. Seems to need others to lean on	Interpersonal functioning

(continued)

TABLE 3.3 OBSERVER-RATED EGO FUNCTION ASSESSMENT TOOL* (*CONTINUED*)	
Assessment Item	**Ego Function**
Always (1) Almost Always (2) Usually (3) Sometimes (4) Hardly Ever (5) Never (6)	
15. Can structure his or her own time and enjoy it	Autonomous functioning
16. Tends to lump people together and see them as much the same	Interpersonal functioning
17. When left alone, has a hard time taking care of himself or herself	Autonomous functioning
18. Seems to perform up to his or her capabilities	Mastery competence
19. Seems basically to trust other people	Interpersonal functioning
20. Seems to use people to get things he or she needs	Interpersonal functioning
21. Sees his or her problems as resulting from being a bad person	Regulation of affect; synthetic-integrative functioning
22. Seems able to recognize and respond to the feelings of others in an appropriate manner	Regulation and control of affect and impulses
23. Is the type of person others want to be friends with	Interpersonal functioning
24. Recovers from significant emotional upset relatively quickly with previous capacities intact or improved	Adaptive regression in the service of the ego

*Not a validated tool.

Source: Adapted from Tulloch, J. D. (1984). Observer-rated ego function assessment tool. (Unpublished handout). Denver: University of Colorado Health Sciences Center.

BOX 3.10 Sample Questions to Assess Ego Functioning

- How do you deal with strong feelings? (1)*
- How would you describe yourself? (9)
- What kind of person is your mother? (13)
- Describe your most important relationships. (16)
- How do you think others view you? (23)
- What do you think is the cause of your problems? (2)
- What part do you play in these difficulties? (3)
- Tell me about your hobbies and interests. (18)
- How do you deal with downtime? (15)
- What is it like for you to be alone? (17)

---

*Parenthetic numbers refer to the assessment items in Table 3.3.

The assessment of ego functioning yields important information about a patient's sense of self and the degree to which he or she has consolidated a core identity. Where ego strength is lacking with respect to the ego functions identified in Table 3.2—particularly interpersonal functioning, defensive functioning, synthetic-integrative functioning, affect regulation, and a sense of the reality of the world and the self—identity diffusion can be discerned in the clinical interview, because a close connection exists between ego strength and identity (Bjorklund, 2000). The features of identity diffusion include markedly contradictory personality traits, temporal discontinuity in the self-experience, feelings of emptiness, gender dysphoria, and subtle body-image disturbances (Akhtar, 1995; Bjorklund, 2000). Even though not all these features can be elicited and explored to an equal degree through formal questioning, Akhtar (1995) believes it is almost always helpful to ask the individual to describe himself or herself. In the resulting description, "one should look for consistency versus contradiction, clarity versus confusion, solidity versus emptiness, well-developed and comfortably experienced masculinity or femininity versus gender confusion, and a sense of inner morality and ethnicity versus the lack of any historical or communal anchor" (p. 103). Box 3.11 provides an illustration in Beth's case, prompting the therapist to flag the possibility of identity diffusion.

Goldstein (1995) provides an alternative mode of assessing ego functioning. She discusses the nature of ego-oriented assessment as a process of data collection focused over several interviews on a patient's current and past functioning and on his or her inner capacities and external circumstances. The following five questions (Bjorklund, 2000, p. 126) are an important guide to the therapist in the overall assessment of ego strength:

1. To what extent is the patient's problem a function of stressors imposed by his or her current life roles or developmental tasks?
2. To what extent is the patient's problem a function of situational stress or of a traumatic event?
3. To what extent is the patient's problem a function of impairments in his or her ego capacities or of developmental difficulties or dynamics?
4. To what extent is the patient's problem a function of the lack of environmental resources or supports or of a lack of fit between his or her inner capacities and external circumstances?
5. What inner capacities and environmental resources does the patient have that can be mobilized to improve his or her functioning?

BOX 3.11 Assessing Identity Diffusion

APPN:	What sort of person are you?
Patient:	I don't know. [long pause] I don't feel like I know who I am.
APPN:	How would you describe yourself?
Patient:	It's funny . . . I hate being alone, but I'm not really very social. I keep to myself a lot. I want to be around people, but they really irritate me most of the time. I don't think I'm an irritable person. Not really. [long pause; therapist waits] Sometimes, I hate myself. I'm really bright, but I don't seem to accomplish much. I have friends, but I don't fit in anywhere. It seems like it doesn't take much for me to fall apart.
APPN:	You look troubled.
Patient:	[Silence]
APPN:	How would other people describe you?
Patient:	Some people think I'm really sweet. My mother thinks I'm very arrogant and conceited. I don't know. A lot of people tell me I look angry all the time, but I don't feel that way.

These questions are important, but questions 1 through 4 may be difficult to ascertain, especially if the person has had frequent or early trauma of which they may not even be aware. For question 5, collaboration with the patient about available resources may be helpful in the initial assessment. Although the assessment of ego functioning is not essential to all forms of giving help, it can assist a psychotherapist in determining whether initial interventions should be directed toward enhancing resources and stabilization, including nurturing, maintaining, enhancing, or modifying inner capacities; mobilizing, improving, or changing environmental conditions; or improving the fit between inner capacities and external circumstances (Bjorklund, 2000; Goldstein, 1995).

Those with impaired ego function most likely have significant early trauma and may not be able to answer some questions that assess ego function because experiences are dissociated from memory. Thus, all patients should be screened with the Dissociative Experiences Scale (DES). See Appendix 3.3 for a copy of this tool. This is a 28-item self-report screening tool that asks the respondent to circle the percent (0%–100%) of time that the experience happens to them. Sample questions include:

1. Some people find that they have no memory for some important events in their lives (for example, a wedding or graduation).
2. Some people have the experience of finding new things among their belongings that they do not remember buying.
3. Some people have the experience of looking in a mirror and not recognizing themselves.
4. Some people have the experience of feeling that other people, objects, and the world around them are not real.

A score of 28% or more indicates that a more thorough evaluation for a dissociative disorder is indicated. Further assessment measures for dissociation are included in Chapter 17. See Appendix 3.3 for the DES.

When a patient is overwhelmed by current stressors but shows good past ego functioning and has some environmental supports, the practitioner may use a brief, supportive, and cognitive approach aimed at stress reduction and more effective problem-solving. If the person is severely and persistently ill, a patient with limited ego strength and developmental deficits that interfere with his or her ability to cope with intimate relationships or current life roles may need interventions targeted toward improving ego function (Bjorklund, 2000; Goldstein, 1995), and a longer psychotherapy treatment with more frequent psychotherapy sessions may be indicated.

In Beth's case, given what turned out to be a significant lack of object constancy (see Table 3.2), dysregulation of affect and impulse control, an inability to tolerate the closeness of her most significant interpersonal relationships, and an inability to integrate contradictory feelings about those significant others—and about many other things, such as continuing her college career—she and her therapist will need to nurture, maintain, and modify some important inner capacities. Given the severity of current environmental stressors, such as the move away from home, withdrawal of her parents' financial support, her mother's hostility and intrusive neediness, significant debt, an unsatisfactory living situation, a stressful job, and a change in college majors, she will also need the therapist's support to mobilize, improve, or change environmental conditions.

Assessing Affective Development

When affective development has proceeded optimally, people have capacities for affect awareness, affect tolerance, and affect modulation (i.e., affect regulation and control). They are aware of their feelings and can identify and describe those feelings, express those feelings in socially appropriate ways, tolerate unpleasant feelings in themselves and others, and find ways to soothe themselves until unpleasant feelings pass. They can maintain their self-esteem and their generally positive outlook and feelings about others even when angry or hurt. They can contain the most intense feelings without losing control and can maintain their equilibrium and their boundaries in the midst of others' intense emotional expression. They can experience a full range of emotions and have developed an appropriate capacity for empathy, caring, and concern without falling prey to affect contagion (i.e., feeling exactly what another feels). They can orient to internal experience when necessary or desirable and have a capacity for fantasy and imagination.

Significantly, persons whose affective development has proceeded optimally can also realistically interpret the social meaning of emotional experience; it is an individual's interpretation of an unpleasant affect that leads to the experience of a specific negative emotion and to the intensity of the emotional arousal (Bradley, 2000). In other words, experience and cognition allow the individual to elaborate positive or negative affect throughout the gamut of emotional experience (Bradley, 2000). Compared with those whose affective development is impaired, persons whose affective development is optimal can tap into their inner worlds and use experience and cognition to interpret diffuse affective arousal as meaningful emotional experience—as both significant and less than catastrophic. They are simultaneously more affectively aware, less emotionally reactive, and able to achieve therapeutic distance from emotions if necessary. Their interpreted emotional experience is construed as manageable, and they have a repertoire of strategies to cope with it. These are the capacities the therapist examines when assessing a patient's affective development.

Much psychopathology ensues as a consequence of impaired affective development (Bradley, 2000). Conversely, much good therapeutic work has been done when a patient has grown in the capacity to identify, tolerate, regulate, and appropriately express affective experience. All types of psychotherapy promote affect regulation. Some therapies do this with the acquisition of specific behavioral skills to reduce the intensity of affect, such as breathing or distracting techniques to cope with anxiety. Others emphasize adaptive coping strategies, such as mindfulness, positive self-talk, or the correction of cognitive distortions to mitigate distress. Others involve reexperiencing and reprocessing of painful affects or repeated exposure to previously avoided situations so that desensitization and mastery can occur. Ultimately, they all work to modify the internal mental representations or cognitive–emotional schemas that produce automatic, maladaptive emotional responses (Bradley, 2000).

Affective regulation and control is an important ego strength (see Tables 3.2 and 3.3), and all effective therapy promotes it. However, some individuals described as *alexithymic* have such extreme difficulty experiencing, describing, and seeing connections between feelings and symptoms that they fare poorly in and frequently drop out of expressive psychotherapies, that is, those that discuss and examine affects (Bradley, 2000). These individuals are notably lacking in *psychological mindedness,* the awareness of internal experience and its relationship to external situations, events, or behaviors that are very important for successful psychotherapy outcomes (Bradley, 2000; Taylor, 1995). Defined as the inability to describe or be aware of emotions or mood (Sadock et al., 2015), alexithymia is a multifaceted construct that encompasses several different factors, including difficulty identifying subjective emotional feelings and distinguishing between feelings and the bodily sensations that constitute emotional arousal; difficulty describing feelings to other people; an impoverished fantasy life; and an externally oriented cognitive style (Taylor, Bagby, & Parker, 2003).

The most widely used measure of the alexithymia construct is the Toronto Alexithymia Scale (TAS-20; Bagby, Parker, & Taylor, 1994a, 1994b). The TAS-20 is a self-report scale

BOX 3.12 Sample Questions to Assess Affective Development

- Are you generally able to recognize how you feel at any given time? (6)*
- How would you describe your feelings right now? (6, 7)
- Can you describe how you felt when that happened? (6, 7)
- What is your internal experience like? (2)
- What do you suppose prompts/are the feelings that prompt your mother to call during your study time each evening? (22)
- What do you think your mother was feeling when you hung up on her? (22)
- How do you deal with especially strong feelings? (1)
- How do you think others feel about you? (23)
- What happens when you are upset? (1, 7)
- How do you calm yourself when you are upset? (1, 7)
- How long does it take to calm down? (24)
- How do you feel about yourself when you are angry/frustrated/upset? (4, 9)
- Are you still able to see yourself as a good person when she gets angry at you?

*Parenthetic numbers refer to the assessment items in Table 3.3.

with a three-factor structure that corresponds to the multifaceted construct described previously. Factor 1 assesses the ability to identify feelings and to distinguish them from the somatic sensations that accompany emotional arousal (i.e., "I am often confused about what emotion I am feeling," and "I have feelings that I can't quite identify"). Factor 2 assesses the ability to describe feelings to other people (i.e., "I am able to describe my feelings easily," and "It is difficult for me to reveal my innermost feelings, even to close friends"). Factor 3 assesses externally oriented thinking and, indirectly, reduced fantasy and imaginable activity (i.e., "I prefer to analyze problems rather than just describe them," and "Looking for hidden meanings in movies or plays distracts from their enjoyment;" Parker, Taylor, & Bagby, 2003; Taylor et al., 2003). A therapist can administer the TAS-20 at the outset of therapy as part of an overall diagnostic evaluation or to assess a patient's psychological mindedness, suitability for an expressive psychotherapy, or capacity for affect awareness and tolerance. Even if not administered directly, the TAS-20 and the observer-rated ego function assessment tool in Table 3.3 (Box 3.12) nevertheless suggest questions the therapist can ask in the context of an initial clinical assessment to assess affective development, that is, capacities for affect awareness, tolerance, modulation, regulation, and control.

Assessing Interpersonal Relationships

Identification of a patient's interpersonal strengths is a necessary first step in affirming and supporting them. It is also important in keeping a balanced view of the potential for adaptation, growth, and successful psychotherapeutic outcome in a patient with other areas of less optimal ego functioning. It is possible to assess the depth of a patient's interpersonal relationships—one indicator of ego strength—by reviewing the patient's past and present interpersonal environment to elicit detailed descriptions of significant others, including mothers, fathers, spouses, friends, and pets (Akhtar, 1995; Bjorklund, 2000; Horowitz, Rosenberg, & Bartholomew, 1993; Shea, 2017). The presence of the following three features in the patient's descriptions of significant others suggest some impairment in interpersonal functioning (Akhtar, 1995; Bjorklund, 2000):

1. An insistent emphasis on the patient's feelings and views about the person described rather than on that person's independent attributes (Box 3.13)

BOX 3.13 Insistent Emphasis on Own Feelings

APPN:	Can you tell me what sort of person your mother is?
Patient:	I hate her. I think she's a witch. It's always all about her, not me. I've tried and tried to get along with her, but it's impossible. If she didn't call me every night, I wouldn't even think about her. [As opposed to this: She's prickly. She's bright and beautiful, but she makes a lot of demands on people and likes to be the center of attention.]

BOX 3.14 Extreme Accounts of Others

APPN:	How would you describe your mother?
Patient:	She's a horrible mother. She is completely selfish. She has never done anything for anybody her entire life. She has never once told me she's proud of me or that she wants me to do well in school. [As opposed to this: She tries to be a decent mother. I imagine she loves me and my brother in her own way, but she competes with me. It's like she's jealous of me. When I changed my major to Business Administration, she enrolled in Denton (Business University). What does that tell you? I guess she's got some problems of her own to deal with.]

BOX 3.15 Inability to See Independent Motivations

APPN:	What do you suppose prompts your mother to call you and interrupt your studying every night?
Patient:	She wants me to fail. It makes her look good. Sometimes, I think she just likes upsetting me. She gets something out of it. I think she hates me as much as I hate her. [As opposed to this: I'm sure she has her reasons. I just can't figure out what they are. Like I said before, she's got problems of her own to deal with. Sometimes, I think she is having as hard a time with my moving away from home as I am. Other times, I think she really is jealous of my success. It's painful to realize, but I think she has mixed feelings about me, and I certainly have mixed feelings about her.]

2. An extreme and affectively charged verdict rather than a balanced account that permits mixed feelings toward the person described (Box 3.14)
3. An inability to see independent motivations in others (Box 3.15)

As conveyed in the alternative responses detailed earlier, descriptions of important relationships that evidence the ability to see significant others as separate individuals, with independent motivations and reasons of their own, suggest significant ego strength in the area of interpersonal relationships. The same is true for descriptions of significant others that show the patient has the capacity to experience others ambivalently—as whole people with good and bad qualities, who can simultaneously gratify and care for others as well as frustrate and disappoint them. More ominous are descriptions that indicate a patient functions in relationships at the level of need gratification (i.e., people have value only to the degree they can meet his or her needs); descriptions that indicate a patient cannot clearly differentiate people or differentiate self from others (i.e., people

BOX 3.16 Sample Questions to Assess Interpersonal Functioning

- **WHAT IS YOUR PART/THEIR PART IN THAT RELATIONSHIP PROBLEM? (2, 3, 21)***
- Can you trust people? (19)
- What is it like to have to trust or depend on someone else? (12, 19)
- What type of friend to others are you? (23)
- What makes a relationship a close one? (20)
- Do you have any close relationships? (12)
- How do you do with intimacy in relationships? (12)
- What do relationships mean to you? (20)
- What happens if there is no one around to lean on? (14, 17)
- How would you feel about the person if he or sher could no longer provide or could no longer meet your needs?

---

*Parenthetic numbers refer to the assessment items in Table 3.3.

are always "just like me" or "pretty much all the same"); or worse, descriptions that indicate a patient functions more or less autistically (i.e., other people seem not to exist or are experienced as aversive stimuli). Table 3.3 includes several assessment items that indirectly measure interpersonal functioning and suggest questions the therapist can ask to explore the quality of a patient's interpersonal relationships (Box 3.16).

One cannot overstate the importance of understanding the nature of a patient's interpersonal problems and the quality of his or her interpersonal functioning. Interpersonal problems are among the most common complaints reported in clinical interviews (Horowitz et al., 1993). Interpersonal relationships often are the focus of psychotherapy, and the work of psychotherapy occurs in an interpersonal environment through relational processes. The therapist can learn much about the patient's interpersonal functioning in the context of the therapeutic relationship, that is, through the manner of the patient's relating to the therapist and through the therapist's reactions to and feelings about the patient. From the way the patient relates to the therapist, particularly in the anxiety-provoking circumstance of crossing the boundary from everyday social discourse to interaction in the consulting room, the therapist can see firsthand the developmental phase that predominates in the patient's personality and interpersonal functioning (Scharff & Scharff, 2005). Ultimately, this firsthand experience may provide the best assessment data.

If, however, the therapist desires a more structured approach to assessing interpersonal functioning, perhaps for purposes of measuring psychotherapy outcomes, he or she can administer an instrument such as the Inventory of Interpersonal Problems (IIP; Horowitz, Rosenberg, Baer, Ureno, & Villasenor, 1988), which is a self-report inventory that has been used to identity dysfunctional patterns in interpersonal interactions. It describes different types of interpersonal problems and has been used to measure the level of distress associated with them before, during, and after psychotherapy (Horowitz et al., 1993). Each of its eight subscales describes a different interpersonal style (Box 3.17). This instrument can also be useful in clinic settings where the clinician completing the initial assessment is different from the eventual therapist. Although the IIP is not included in this chapter, Table 3.4 provides a fragment of it.

ASSESSING ADULT ATTACHMENT

The quality of the patient's earliest interpersonal relationships with caregivers may influence the adult personality. In particular, attachment insecurity in infancy and early childhood has been shown to predict various forms of psychopathology in adolescence

BOX 3.17 Interpersonal Styles

Domineering	I try to change other people too much.
Intrusive	It is hard for me to stay out of other people's business.
Overly nurturing	I put other people's needs before my own too much.
Exploitable	I let other people take advantage of me too much.
Nonassertive	It is hard for me to be assertive with another person.
Socially avoidant	It is hard for me to socialize with other people.
Cold	I keep other people at a distance too much.
Vindictive	I fight with other people too much.

TABLE 3.4   A FRAGMENT OF THE INVENTORY OF INTERPERSONAL PROBLEMS

It is hard for me to:	How much have you been distressed by this problem?				
Not At All (0) A Little Bit (1) Moderately (2) Quite a Bit (3) Extremely (4)					
Example					
1. Get along with my relatives	0	1	2	3	4
Part I. The following are things you find hard to do with other people:					
1. Trust other people	0	1	2	3	4
2. Say "no" to other people	0	1	2	3	4
3. Join in on groups	0	1	2	3	4
4. Keep things private from other people	0	1	2	3	4
5. Let other people know what I want	0	1	2	3	4
6. Tell a person to stop bothering me	0	1	2	3	4

Source: Adapted from Horowitz, L. M., Rosenberg, S. E., & Bartholomew, K. (1993). Interpersonal problems, attachment styles, and outcome in brief dynamic psychotherapy. *Journal of Consulting and Clinical Psychology, 61*(4), 549–560. doi:10.1037/0022-006X.61.4.549. Copyright 1993, with permission from the American Psychological Association.

and adulthood (Shmueli-Goetz, Target, Fonagy, & Datta, 2008). When the therapist suspects that attachment issues may be complicating the patient's interpersonal functioning, he or she may want to assess the patient's attachment system in a more structured way (Box 3.18). Provided that he or she has obtained training in administration procedure, the therapist may choose to utilize the Adult Attachment Interview (AAI) for the assessment. Numerous studies have established the reliability and validity of the AAI

BOX 3.18 Sample Questions to Assess Attachment

- How would you describe your relationship with your parents? As a child? Now?
- What words would you use to describe your mother/father? As a child? Now?
- With whom did you/do you now feel the closest?
- What did you/do you now do when you feel upset about something?
- Did your parents ever threaten or hurt you, even jokingly or to discipline you? Anyone else?
- What did you/do you now do with feelings of loss? Rejection? Threat?
- Were you ever separated from your parents as a child? Suffered a loss?
- How do you cope with losses/separations from significant others now?
- How do you think your overall experiences with your parents have affected your adult personality?
- What do you wish for your own children?

BOX 3.19 Screening/Assessment Tools

- Toronto Alexithymia Scale (TAS-20)*
- Beck Depression Inventory (BDI; copyright Psychological Corporation)
- Dissociative Experiences Scale (DES; see Appendix 3.3)
- Impact of Events Scale (IES; see Appendix 3.4); Zung Self-Rating Depression Scale (ZSRDS) (see Appendix 3.5)
- Geriatric Depression Scale (GDS; see Appendix 3.6)
- Patient Health Questionnaire (PHQ-9; see Appendix 3.7)
- Young Mania Rating Scale (YMRS; see Appendix 3.8); Hamilton Anxiety Rating Scale (HAM-A) (see Appendix 3.9)
- Generalized Anxiety Disorder Questionnaire (GAD-7; see Appendix 3.10)
- Yale-Brown Obsessive–Compulsive Scale (Y-BOCS; see Appendix 3.11)
- Mini-Mental State Examination (MMSE; www.dhs.state.or.us/spd/tools/cm/aps/assessment/mini_mental.pdf)
- Global Assessment of Functioning (GAF)
- Quality of Life Scale (QOL; see Appendix 3.12)
- CAGE Questionnaire (see Appendix 3.13)
- Alcohol Use Disorders Identification Test (AUDIT; see Appendix 3.14)
- Adult Attachment Interview (AAI; www.psychology.sunysb.edu/attachment/measures/content/aai_interview.pdf)
- Child Attachment Interview (CAI; see Appendix 3.15)
- Strange Situation Procedure (SSP; www.psychology.sunysb.edu/attachment/measures/content/ss_scoring.pdf)
- Adverse Childhood Experiences (ACE) Scale (see Appendix 3.16)

---

*The TAS-20 can be purchased directly from its developer, Dr. Graham J. Taylor, Department of Psychiatry, Mount Sinai Hospital, Toronto, Ontario, Canada.

(Shmueli-Goetz et al., 2008). Although the AAI protocol is readily available online (see Box 3.19), the scoring manual is available only in conjunction with training courses; and the published protocol, too lengthy to append in full, is not considered a substitute for AAI training (George, Kaplan, & Main, 1985; Main & Goldwyn, 1998). In general, the AAI focuses on the adult patient's childhood relationships with parents, thus facilitating an overall assessment of the quality of the attachment to parents, starting with childhood experiences that may have affected the patient's adult personality, and moving through adolescence to present-day, adult experiences.

More specifically, in a series of 20 assessment questions, with suggestions for follow-up probes, the AAI orients the interviewer to the patient's family constellation. It encourages the patient to remember and describe his or her earliest memories of relationships with parents and asks for descriptors of each parent that reflect the childhood relationships with them (George et al., 1985). The interview protocol covers areas with attachment implications, including the patient's childhood (and adult) experiences of separation, the person(s) to whom the patient as a child felt most close, what the patient did as a child when upset, how he or she coped with feelings of loss and/or rejection, whether or not the patient as a child ever felt threatened by parents, and how the patient understood and responded to such threats. The AAI protocol also explores other potentially traumatic experiences in both childhood and adulthood. It assesses the patient's experience of the impact of these events and explores the patient's wishes and hopes for his or her own children as well as the patient's present-day, adult relationships with living parents (George et al., 1985).

ASSESSING CHILD ATTACHMENT

The Child Attachment Interview (CAI; see Appendix 3.15) is similar in content to the AAI but focuses on the child-as-patient's current attachment relationships rather than the adult patient's memory of relationships in childhood (Shmueli-Goetz et al., 2008). Like the AAI, the CAI protocol elicits information about the family constellation but focuses on current and/or recent attachment-related events, including times of family conflict, distress, illness, hurt, separation, and loss (Shmueli-Goetz et al., 2008). It includes interview items that elicit self-descriptions and caretaker descriptions, which may illuminate the child's self-representations and representations of his or her primary caregivers as well as potentiate exploration of meaningful links between self-descriptions and attachment representations (Shmueli-Goetz et al., 2008). Because the CAI is a narrative-based assessment that relies on a level of linguistic competence (i.e., verbal ability), it requires a developmentally appropriate interviewer stance with age-specific cues, or follow-up probes to help children remember and express attachment experiences (Shmueli-Goetz et al., 2008). Throughout the CAI, such probes are used to assist the child to tell his or her story. Verbal and nonverbal behavior is coded and scored. Although the CAI is a systematic, valid, and reliable assessment of the school-age child's experience of parental availability (i.e., parent–child attachment), it cannot replace parental and teacher reports, nor is it appropriate for infants and toddlers for whom attachment is defined not by parental availability but rather by behavioral strategies to maintain proximity to attachment figures (Shmueli-Goetz et al., 2008).

For attachment assessment during very early childhood, a separation–reunion procedure such as the Strange Situation Procedure (SSP; Ainsworth, Blehar, Waters, & Wall, 1978) may be appropriate (Box 3.19). The SSP is conducted in an unfamiliar, or strange environment by an unfamiliar person (a "stranger") over a series of eight, brief, separation–reunion episodes that are designed to generate just enough stress to activate the infant's or toddler's behavioral attachment system. Separations are designed to be stressful but sufficiently manageable so that reunions become a reflection of the quality of the child–parent relationship (Ainsworth et al., 1978). Typically, the strange situation is videotaped and coded based on the child's observed behaviors. Categories of observed behavior include proximity- and contact-seeking behavior, contact-maintaining behavior, resistant behavior, and avoidant behavior. Based on SSP scoring, attachment security is classified as secure, insecure avoidant, insecure resistant, or insecure disorganized. Scoring methods for the SSP are detailed and include considerable commentary to facilitate valid and reliable scoring; thus, training in coding the SSP is advised (Ainsworth et al., 1978).

Assessing Belief Systems

The disorders for which patients seek out psychotherapists lie on the boundary between the natural world and the constructed social world (Wakefield, 1992). Whether a patient construes a particular symptom as harmful or a particular constellation of symptoms as a disorder or an illness for which help is required has a lot to do with his or her values and beliefs. A disorder exists when a person's internal psychological or physiological mechanisms fail to perform their functions as designed by nature *but only if* this impinges on the person's sense of well-being as defined by social values and meanings (Wakefield, 1992). Ultimately, the whole point of diagnosing a psychiatric disorder is to help a patient regain the ability to function effectively in social, occupational, and family roles. Most of the behaviors and feelings categorized as symptoms of mental illness in the *Diagnostic and Statistical Manual of Mental Disorders (DSM)* can be construed as what many people do or feel at various times *without* having a psychiatric disorder or suffering from a mental illness.

Belief systems, spiritual practices, religious affiliation, and other frameworks for meaning and purpose can have a profound impact on a person's well-being, resilience, or ability to adaptively cope with adversity. An inventory of the person's strengths is important to plan where to intervene in the treatment hierarchy see Chapter 1. At other times, a patient's symptoms may result from unrest in the person's belief systems or from conflict in his or her religious, spiritual, philosophical, ethical, or existential frameworks (Shea, 2017). It is therefore crucial that a therapist assess a patient's values, beliefs, and framework for meaning to identify problems and support important strengths. The information gleaned may suggest the utility of individual psychotherapy slanted toward existential concerns (Shea, 2017); or it may remind the therapist that patients sometimes find meaning and purpose in everyday, well-known activities, such as caring for their families, engaging in community service, or staying close to nature.

Although an understanding of the stages or processes of faith (Fowler, 1981) or spiritual development (Wink & Dillon, 2002) is not absolutely necessary to an understanding of how to assess belief systems (and is beyond the scope of this chapter), the therapist should consider that how people construct meaning in life is subject to developmental shifts (Fowler, 1981) and is the product of maturational processes that continue over the course of adult life (Wink & Dillon, 2002). Spiritual development is linked to other processes of development. It requires capacities for abstraction, ambiguity, and ambivalence (i.e., the ability to integrate paradox and disparate notions of self, other, and the world), which are some of the same capacities that constitute ego strength as earlier described. It involves going beyond the linear and strictly logical modes of apprehending reality described by Piaget's model of cognitive development to an integrated cognitive–emotional view of the world that embraces paradox and incorporates feelings and context as well as logic and reason in making judgments about the nature, meaning, and purpose of self, other, and the world (Wink & Dillon, 2002). Changes in or consolidation of belief systems, meaning frameworks, and other processes of making sense of life's meaning and purpose, occur more frequently during periods of adversity and crisis than during times of stability (Stokes, 1990). Such changes are more salient for women and older adults (Wink & Dillon, 2002), both of whom tend to experience more stress than other social groups (Mirowsky & Ross, 1992, 1995). The therapist assessing the quality, salience, and influence of his or her patients' belief systems should keep these findings in mind and use the energy existing in crisis to promote positive change.

Practically speaking, assessing the values and beliefs of patients is a standard part of taking a history (see Box 3.1). As a matter of course, the therapist should inquire about the patient's belief systems and values, both social and moral, including values about work, money, play, children, parents, friends, sex, community concerns, and cultural issues (Sadock et al., 2015). Much of this information is gleaned in the process of obtaining a patient's developmental, family, and social history. Specific assessment questions are illustrated in Box 3.20 and in Table 3.5, which is an adapted portion of the World Health Organization's (WHO) Quality of Life–Spirituality, Religiousness, and Personal Beliefs (WHOQOL–SRPB) field-test instrument. The WHOQOL–SRPB has been developed from an extensive pilot test of 105 questions in 18 centers around the world. The resulting 32-item instrument represents the finalized version currently in use in field trials (WHO, 2002).

BOX 3.20 Sample Questions to Assess Belief Systems

- What helps you cope with adversity?
- What gives you a sense of meaning and purpose in life?
- What matters most to you in life?
- What are your beliefs about health/illness/therapy/seeking help?
- To what extent do your spiritual/religious beliefs comfort you?
- What enables you to stay healthy/get better/find comfort/continue living?
- What do those spiritual/religious practices bring to your life?

TABLE 3.5   A PORTION OF THE WORLD HEALTH ORGANIZATION'S SPIRITUALITY, RELIGIOUSNESS, AND PERSONAL BELIEFS FIELD-TEST INSTRUMENT

1 = Not at all
2 = A little
3 = A moderate amount
4 = Very much
5 = An extreme amount

To what extent does any connection to a spiritual being help you to get through hard times?	1	2	3	4	5
To what extent does any connection to a spiritual being help you to understand others?	1	2	3	4	5
To what extent does any connection to a spiritual being provide you with comfort/reassurance?	1	2	3	4	5
To what extent do you find meaning in life?	1	2	3	4	5
To what extent do you feel your life has a purpose?	1	2	3	4	5
To what extent does faith contribute to your well-being?	1	2	3	4	5
To what extent does faith give you comfort in daily life?	1	2	3	4	5
To what extent does faith give you strength in daily life?	1	2	3	4	5
To what extent do you feel spiritually touched by beauty?	1	2	3	4	5
To what extent are you grateful for the things in nature that you can enjoy?	1	2	3	4	5

(continued)

TABLE 3.5 A PORTION OF THE WORLD HEALTH ORGANIZATION'S SPIRITUALITY, RELIGIOUSNESS, AND PERSONAL BELIEFS FIELD-TEST INSTRUMENT (*CONTINUED*)					
To what extent are you able to experience awe from your surroundings, for example, nature, art, music?	1	2	3	4	5
To what extent do you feel any connection between your mind, body, and soul?	1	2	3	4	5
To what extent do you feel the way you live is consistent with what you feel and think?	1	2	3	4	5
How much do your beliefs help you to create coherence between what you do, think, and feel?	1	2	3	4	5
How much does spiritual strength help you to live better?	1	2	3	4	5
To what extent does your spiritual strength help you to feel happy in life?	1	2	3	4	5
To what extent do you feel peaceful within yourself?	1	2	3	4	5
To what extent do you feel a sense of harmony in your life?	1	2	3	4	5
To what extent does faith help you enjoy life?	1	2	3	4	5
How satisfied are you that you have a balance between body, mind, and soul?	1	2	3	4	5
To what extent do you consider yourself to be a religious person?	1	2	3	4	5
To what extent do you consider yourself to be a part of a religious community?	1	2	3	4	5
To what extent do you have spiritual beliefs?	1	2	3	4	5

Source: Adapted from the World Health Organization. (2002). WHOQOL-SRPB field-test instrument. Retrieved from https://www.who.int/mental_health/media/en/622.pdf

ASSESSING FUNCTIONAL STATUS

For several important reasons, the APPN must be able to competently assess a patient's functional status and degree of functional impairment. First, for most psychiatric disorders to meet diagnostic criteria, the most commonly used diagnostic system (the *DSM*) requires that individuals meet a clinical significance criterion, which is that symptoms result in either clinically significant distress or impairment in social, occupational, or other important areas of functioning (McQuaid et al., 2012). Second, improved functioning in one or more domains is often a goal of psychotherapy. Thus, the means and methods by which the APPN assesses functional status are important to outcomes evaluation, that is, the process of determining the extent to which psychotherapy has been effective in targeting symptoms and improving the patient's health status and/or quality of life. Third, measures of functional status are important to patient for various reasons, including that degree of functional impairment has implications for compensation and pension procedures as well as decisions around the extent to which a psychiatric disorder is judged to have a military service connection (McQuaid et al., 2012). Fourth, functional status is often a better indicator of service needs and treatment outcomes than diagnosis alone (McQuaid et al., 2012). Thus, the APPN must be prepared to perform and document diagnostic evaluations that include competent functional assessments across the relevant domains of functioning.

Although this chapter addresses the assessment of mental health functioning broadly, its scope does not include detailed discussion of the many types, domains, and processes of assessing functional status. In some cases, the APPN may recommend a more comprehensive assessment of functional status from an occupational therapist or disability specialist. However, a number of screening instruments and rating scales are available to assess, measure, document, or monitor functioning in social, occupational, psychological, interpersonal, and other domains (Table 3.6). One of the most common and better known measures of functioning, included in Table 3.6 but no longer utilized in the *DSM-5* diagnostic system, is the Global Assessment of Functioning (GAF; APA, 2000), which is

TABLE 3.6 COMMONLY USED CLINICAL RATING SCALES

Scale	Reference*
Quality of Life Scales	
Quality of Life Enjoyment and Satisfaction Questionnaire Q-LES-Q	Endicott, Nee, Harrison, and Blumenthal (1993)
Quality of Well-Being Scale (QWB)	Kaplan and Anderson (1988)
Quality of Life in Depression Scale (QLDS)	Hunt and McKenna (1992)
Medical Outcome Survey (MOS)	Ware and Sherbourne (1992)
Mental Health Status and Functioning Scales	
Clinical Global Impression (CGI)	National Institute of Mental Health [NIMH] (1970)
Endicott Work Productivity Scale	Endicott and Nee (1997)
Global Assessment of Functioning (GAF)	American Psychiatric Association (APA), 2000: *DSM-IV-TR*
Sheehan Disability Scale	Leon, Shear, Portera, and Klerman (1992)
Social and Occupational Functioning Assessment Scale (SOFAS)	APA, 2000: *DSM-IV-TR*
Work and Social Adjustment Scale	Mundt, Marks, Shear, and Greist (2002)
Adverse Effects Scales	
Abnormal Involuntary Movement Scale (AIMS)	Guy (1976)
Simpson–Angus Extrapyramidal Symptom Rating Scale	Simpson and Angus (1970)
Cognitive Disorders Scales	

(continued)

TABLE 3.6 COMMONLY USED CLINICAL RATING SCALES (*CONTINUED*)	
Scale	**Reference***
Delirium Rating Scale Revised—98 (DRS—R98)	Trzepacz et al. (2001)
Mini-Mental State Examination (MMSE)	Folstein, Folstein, & McHugh (1975)
Alcohol Use Disorders Scales	
Alcohol Use Disorders Identification Test (AUDIT) CAGE Questionnaire	Saunders, Aasland, Babor, De La Fuente, and Grant (1993) Ewing (1984)
Michigan Alcoholism Screening Test (MAST)	Selzer (1971)
Mood Disorders Scales	
Beck Depression Inventory, 2nd Revision (BDI-II)	Beck, Ward, Mendelson, Mock, and Erbaugh (1961)
Hamilton Depression Rating Scale (HAM-D)	Hamilton (1960)
Inventory of Depressive Symptomatology (IDS)	Rush, Gullion, Basco, Jarrett, and Triveldi (1996)
Quick Inventory of Depressive Symptomatology (QIDS)	Rush et al. (2003)
Patient Health Questionnaire (PHQ-9)	www.pfizer.com
Geriatric Depression Scale (GDS)	Yesavage et al. (1983)
Montgomery–Asberg Depression Rating Scale (MADRS)	Montgomery and Asberg (1979)
Zung Self-Rating Depression Scale (ZSRDS)	Zung (1965)
Young Mania Rating Scale (YMRS)	Young, Biggs, Ziegler, and Meger (1978)
Anxiety Disorders Scales	
Hamilton Anxiety Rating Scale (HAM-A)	Hamilton (1959)
Yale-Brown Obsessive–Compulsive Scale (Y-BOCS)	Goodman et al. (1989)
Psychotic Disorders Scales	
Brief Psychiatric Rating Scale (BPRS)	Overall and Gorham (1962)
Positive and Negative Symptom Scale (PANSS)	Kay, Fiszbein, and Opler (1987)
Aggression and Agitation Scale	
Overt Aggression Scale—Modified (OAS-M)	Coccaro, Harvey, Kupsaw-Lawrence, Herbert, and Bernstein (1991)

*References in this table are listed at the end of the chapter.

DSM-IV-TR, Diagnostic and Statistical Manual of Mental Disorders (4th ed., text rev.).

Source: American Psychiatric Association. (2016). *The American Psychiatric Association practice guidelines for the psychiatric evaluation of adults* (3rd ed.). Arlington, VA: Author; Bresee, C., Gotto, J., & Rapaport, M. H. (2009). Treatment of depression. In A. F. Schatzberg & C. B. Nemeroff (Eds.), *The American Psychiatric Association Publishing textbook of psychopharmacology* (4th ed., chap. 53). Arlington, VA: American Psychiatric Publishing.

a clinician-rated, global measure of illness severity. Scores range from 0 to 100, with a higher score indicating better functioning. A GAF score is typically based on a patient's worst functioning within occupational, social, or psychological domains. It combines psychiatric symptomatology and social–occupational functioning into a single score even though they are distinct constructs, and even though research has found that GAF scores are most significantly associated with symptom ratings rather than social or occupational functioning (McQuaid et al., 2012). Table 3.6 lists several alternatives to the GAF. In addition, as an alternative to the GAF, McQuaid et al. (2012) offer a detailed description of the Inventory of Psychosocial Functioning (IPF), which is a newly developed, 80-item, self-report measure designed to assess functional impairment experienced by veterans and active-duty service personnel across multiple domains.

GENOGRAMS

The family genogram is a useful tool for the assessment of individuals, couples, and families; and it should be a routine part of any comprehensive patient or family assessment (Glick, Berman, Clarkin, & Rait, 2000). Encouraging or assigning a patient the task of drawing his or her family genogram is an effective assessment and intervention strategy at different points in the therapy. It can yield significant assessment data and lead to important, new patient understandings and insights as multigenerational patterns take shape and assume new meaning. In essence, the genogram is a graphic sketch of the patient and several generations of his or her family. Occupational and social roles, major life events, significant illnesses, and important dates—for example, births, deaths, marriages, and separations—are mapped. The quality and longevity of significant relationships are noted. The graphic presentation of family events and relationships facilitates the linkage of current issues, concerns, or circumstances to the multigenerational family's structure and evolving patterns of relationship (Glick et al., 2000). The family genogram has several purposes:

1. It provides the identified patient, family, and therapist with a graphic structure to explore past and present difficulties.
2. It provides the therapist with background information to put current patient difficulties in context.
3. It uses the assessment process as an opportunity for patient intervention, for example, as the patient begins to see patterns emerge (Glick et al., 2000).

In addition, based on genomics research findings, emerging standards of care for psychiatric assessment and treatment now include a more detailed family history or pedigree (genogram), assessment of environmental risk factors, genetic screening and testing if indicated, and application of individualized therapies based on assessment data (Pestka et al., 2010). While genetics is the examination of specific genes and their effects, genomics considers all the genes in a human genome and their interactions with each other, which has relevance for psychiatric practice along pathways of prevention, screening, diagnostics, prognostics, treatment selection, and monitoring of treatment effectiveness (Pestka et al., 2010). Nationally endorsed genomics competencies include the following nursing genomic assessments:

1. Gathering and/or clarifying family history information
2. Updating or constructing a family genogram
3. Assessing environmental factors
4. Assessing genomic physical findings

5. Assessing genetics/genomics learning needs (Consensus Panel on Genetic/
   Genomic Nursing Competencies, 2006, 2009; Greco, Tinley, & Seibert, 2012; Pestka,
   Meisheid, & O'Neil, 2008; Pestka et al., 2010)

Figure 3.1 shows a genogram with the inclusion of demographic, occupational, and
major life event information (Varcarolis, Carson, & Shoemaker, 2006). In Beth's case, a

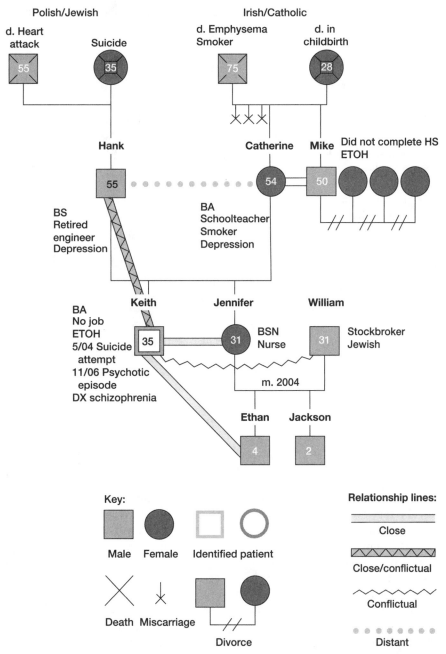

FIGURE 3.1 An elaborated genogram with demographic, occupational, and major
life event information.

d., died; DX, diagnosis; ETOH, alcohol; HS, high school; m., married.

Source: Adapted from Varcarolis, E. M., Carson, V. B., & Shoemaker, N. C. (Eds.). (2006).
Foundations of psychiatric mental health nursing (5th ed.). Philadelphia, PA: W. B. Saunders.

family genogram was not done because of her limited knowledge of family history and her refusal to participate in a family session. Had it been done, the family genogram would have revealed a multigenerational pattern of affective disorder, substance abuse, and early parent loss. Beth might have seen in graphic form some of the factors relevant to her strained relationship with her mother including her birth only 15 months after the birth of her older brother; a lengthy separation from her mother before age 3, precipitated by her mother's psychiatric hospitalization; and the death of Beth's maternal grandmother very early in Beth's mother's life, followed by a series of unstable living arrangements.

ASSESSING SPECIAL POPULATIONS

The initial psychiatric assessment follows an established, comprehensive format but also hones in on the specific content domains most relevant to the patient-identified problem and presentation. Some patient populations, if not most patients, will require ongoing assessment of missed or emerging symptoms as the patient becomes more comfortable disclosing them and/or the therapist better comprehends the clinical situation. For example, the patient who presented initially as depressed and anxious might later disclose the full extent of his or her bulimia, substance use, suicide ideation, violent fantasy, confusion, cognitive impairment, disability, personality disorder, or any of dozens of other symptoms, syndromes, or conditions. The literature is replete with specialized information, which is beyond the scope of this chapter, about focal assessments within given clinical domains; and the APPN should be comfortable turning to the scholarly literature whenever he or she experiences a knowledge gap. The literature includes, for example, information on psychiatric violence risk assessment (Buchanan, Binder, Norko, & Swartz, 2012); suicide risk assessment (Sadek, 2019); disability and occupational assessment (Williams, 2010); assessment of personality disorders (Widiger & Samuel, 2009); psychiatric evaluation of the agitated patient (Stowell, Florence, Harman, & Glick, 2012); specialized assessment of eating disorders (Berg, Peterson, & Frazier, 2012); and specialized assessment of cognitive function in older populations (Milisen, Braes, & Foreman, 2012).

SCREENING TOOLS

Screening tools can provide useful assessment data to supplement data obtained from the clinical interview. They can identify problem areas for psychotherapeutic focus and contribute to case formulation or to the determination of the differential diagnosis. For example, psychiatric rating scales can generate baseline measures of symptom severity, social and occupational functioning, or quality of life for purposes of monitoring changes over time or measuring psychotherapeutic outcomes. Although a single rating scale score at best provides only a snapshot of a complex clinical situation, repeated ratings can objectively describe longitudinal change over a defined treatment period and therefore provide some justification for the choice of treatment plan and some measure of its efficacy. Such ends are secondary to their overall purpose, which is to contribute to a deeper, more holistic, more empathic understanding of the person who presents for help and, in doing so, often risks so much.

Psychotherapists have long been challenged to quantify the impact on patients' lives of both psychiatric illness and the therapies employed to treat psychiatric illness (Bresee, Gotto, & Rapaport, 2009). Early on, Barrell and colleagues (Barrell, Merwin, & Poster,

1997) encouraged APPNs to use assessment tools to measure patient outcomes and to evaluate the efficacy of practice. Currently, with the arrival of "pay for performance" standards, a more rigorous approach to assessment and treatment is no longer optional (Bresee et al., 2009). The concept of *measurement-based* care, which refers to the use of rating scales to measure the outcome of psychiatric treatment, has arrived (Zimmerman, Young, Chelminski, Dalrymple, & Galione, 2012). The practice of assessing *psychiatric vital signs* also has arrived. Based on the prevalence of anxiety and depressive symptoms across diagnostic categories, Zimmerman et al. (2012) have recommended that anxiety and depression be regularly assessed and monitored as psychiatric vital signs in all patients regardless of diagnosis.

In addition, given the prevalence of childhood trauma and the long-term consequences, every adult should be screened with the Adverse Childhood Experiences (ACE) Scale. This is a 10-item scale that asks the person about disturbing events that occurred during childhood. A score of 4 or more indicates a highly significant increase in the development of chronic disease and mental illness (Felitti et al., 1998). See Appendix 3.16 for the ACE Scale. A more extensive instrument that evaluates specific traumatic experiences is the Traumatic Experience Checklist (TEC) which has 39 items (Nijenhuis, Van der Hart, & Kruger, 2002). This is a self-report measure that lists 29 traumatic events in the first column, the age when it happened in the second column, and how much impact the event had on the respondent on a 1 to 5 Likert-type scale in the third column. This tool is available in many languages and can be downloaded from www.enijenhuis.nl/tec.

The *American Psychiatric Association Practice Guidelines for the Psychiatric Evaluation of Adults* (3rd ed.; APA, 2016) and the *American Psychiatric Publishing Textbook of Psychopharmacology* (5th ed.; Schatzberg & Nemeroff, 2017) both emphasize the utility of structured instruments for patient assessment and outcomes evaluation; and both list commonly used clinical rating scales, screening tools, and structured instruments (Table 3.6). Fifteen screening tools commonly used by APPNs to assess psychotherapy patients and measure treatment outcomes are included in this chapter as appendices or are proprietary and can be purchased from their publishers (Box 3.19). They include several of the rating scales listed in Table 3.6.

DIAGNOSIS AND CASE FORMULATION

For any patient, the last steps in the assessment process are to formulate the case and determine the diagnosis. It is important to understand the relationship between a screening tool, along with the data it generates, and a diagnosis. Screening instruments are commonly used in many areas of healthcare and are well accepted by the general public and healthcare professionals. They are helpful in that they *suggest* the presence or absence of one or more diagnoses. In essence, screening tools identify the presence and severity of symptoms and therefore the *likelihood* of a diagnosis, but their results do not produce a diagnosis. The results of screening instruments have to be interpreted and put in the context of the broader assessment.

An important distinction exists between the presence of symptoms and the diagnosis of psychiatric disorder. Symptoms do not generate a diagnosis unless their nature, number, duration, and context (e.g., impaired social and occupational functioning) meet the established criteria of a diagnostic taxonomy such as the *DSM* for the suspected diagnosis. The distinction between symptoms and diagnoses underscores the importance of using systematic criteria to make a formal diagnosis. The data generated by screening tools can contribute to the systematic process of determining a diagnosis, but no one can assume that a score of 38 on a Beck Depression Inventory (BDI), for example, determines a diagnosis of major depression. What it indicates is the *likelihood* of a major depression. Further investigation, including the rest of the assessment process, which continues throughout treatment as the therapist observes how the patient responds to interventions, and the integration of findings across assessment areas are required to make that determination.

Diagnosis

Although a comprehensive assessment is essential to understanding a patient's concerns and capacities and to developing an appropriate treatment plan, a diagnosis is not central to psychotherapy. It is possible to help a person regain the ability to function effectively in social, occupational, and family roles without one. Nevertheless, skills in differential diagnosis are useful. They are among the specified competencies for APPNs, and a *DSM* diagnosis is required for purposes of insurance reimbursement. Some practice guidelines do specify the forms of psychotherapy to which research evidence points as most effective for certain diagnoses. Although it is beyond the scope of this chapter to address the development of skills in differential diagnosis, or to fully describe the historical development of the *DSM*, some discussion of the concept of *diagnosis* is warranted.

Psychiatric diagnosis is facilitated by psychiatric nosology, or classification. Attempts to classify mental illness began in ancient times and accelerated in the 19th century, first with the French physician, Philippe Pinel, who developed the first modern classification of psychiatric illness, and later in the 19th century with the German psychiatrists Wilhelm Griesinger, Richard von Krafft-Ebing, Karl Kahlbaum, and most important, Emil Kraepelin, whose classification system dominated European and (to a lesser degree) American psychiatry for the next 100 years (Brown, DePetro, & Whitaker, 2014; Shorter, 2015). Kraepelin's classification system was based upon close, systematic observation of psychopathology and data collected from large groups of patients, whose personal circumstances and individual characteristics were factored out. Kraepelin focused instead on the general characteristics patients held in common (Brown et al., 2014). His descriptive approach did not find expression in American psychiatry until *DSM-III* was published in 1980 with a new feature, that is, specific diagnostic criteria for clinically relevant categories of illness. Among other reasons for this change, by this time more effective psychotropic medications had emerged and explicit diagnostic criteria were needed to ensure homogeneity and validity of participant sampling for clinical trials of psychiatric drugs (Brown et al., 2014).

Influential as Kraepelin was in Europe, the immediate origins of the *DSM* lay in a psychiatric nosology developed in the United States by the psychoanalyst Karl Menninger, who had been a brigadier-general and head of psychiatry in the Office of the Surgeon General during World War II (Shorter, 2015). Thousands of war veterans were returning to civilian life with nonpsychotic, nonphysical disorders that seemed to have been environmentally triggered (e.g., by the war; Brown et al., 2014). Thus, Menninger published his psychiatric nosology in October 1945 as the *Technical Medical Bulletin* number 203 of the U.S. Army, which thereafter was known simply as *Medical 203*. Influenced by psychoanalysis, with its primary diagnosis of *psychoneurosis*, *Medical 203* became the basis of psychiatric classification in the postwar United States (Shorter, 2015). By 1948, however, the APA had become increasingly dissatisfied with the diagnostic system. It charged its Committee on Statistics to prepare an official taxonomy that was eventually published in 1952 as *DSM-I*, which was substantially a rehash of *Medical 203* (Shorter, 2015). Given the prestige of psychoanalysis, *DSM-I* went through 15 printings by 1962, with each successive edition less moored to psychoanalysis but only marginally more acceptable to the APA as a psychiatric taxonomy (Shorter, 2015).

By the late 1960s, the shift from psychoanalysis to biology was in full swing, and *DSM-II* was published to align American diagnosis with the 8th edition of the World Health Organization's *International Classification of Diseases* (Shorter, 2015). However, the structure of *DSM-II* was still very similar to *DSM-I* in terms of the main categories of disorder, including a Freudian section with what were called *psychoneurotic disorders* in *DSM-I* and *neuroses* in *DSM-II*. In 1973, the APA commissioned *DSM-III*, which was published in 1980 with a couple of major changes, including consensus-based diagnosis and the concept of *diagnostic criteria* (Shorter, 2015). *DSM-IV*, released in 1994, continued the multiaxial, empirically based, descriptive tradition of *DSM-III* but added a collection of culture-bound syndromes and a new criterion to roughly half of the disorders in the manual, namely, that symptoms must cause a clinically significant level of distress or impairment in the functioning of the patient (Brown et al., 2014).

The *DSM-IV-TR* described psychiatric disorders in terms of clusters of symptoms and relied heavily (and necessarily) on phenomenological description, that is, the subjective interpretation of experience as opposed to objective, physiological markers—of which there are very few in psychiatric illness. This edition attempted to reconcile multiple, competing theoretical notions about the cause of psychiatric illness in essence by avoiding the question of causality altogether, focusing only on symptom presentation. The *DSM* constitutes a consensus effort to achieve uniformity among mental health professionals with radically disparate theoretical orientations, ranging from the behavioral to the psychoanalytic (Mechanic, 2007). In sum, the *DSM* is a political document with clinical utility. It allows for greater precision in the use of psychiatric labels, which can facilitate clearer communication among mental health professionals with different disciplinary backgrounds; and it can define more clearly samples of patients for psychiatric research. Because the *DSM* is a tool for clustering symptoms and syndromes, a *DSM* diagnosis implies various therapeutic interventions. For clinicians, diagnosis serves one overriding purpose—to suggest an appropriate treatment plan that will further guide the discovery of information that will lead to the most effective methods of helping people regain optimal functioning in social and occupational roles (Shea, 2017).

In 2013, *DSM-5* was published with new categories of disorder, recognition of the dimensional nature of mental illness, a lifespan approach to the organization of contents, ever-increasing length (the *DSM* is now up to 947 pages), and some significant changes in the diagnostic understanding of selected categories of illness (e.g., eating disorders and autism spectrum disorders).

From its inception, the *DSM* has engendered controversy (Frances, 2013). A diagnosis is an extraordinarily complex concept. Few biological markers exist to substantiate a psychiatric diagnosis. The socially constructed aspects of diagnosis stem from the reality that the *DSM* is a sociopolitical document drafted by committee, that is, by consensus panels of experts who nevertheless are bound to their historical, cultural, social, political, moral, and professional contexts. Because most psychiatric disorders do not yet have known physiological correlates, a diagnosis is made by matching data from clinical interview, observations of behavior and mood, and patient self-report of symptoms to lists of diagnostic criteria. We cannot yet order imaging or laboratory studies to diagnose most psychiatric disorders. Moreover, what we see as constituting a psychiatric disorder shifts as cultural conditions change, knowledge grows, and time passes. Social conditions in particular historical eras create "niches" for psychiatric disorders such that new, sometimes gendered behavioral expressions of emotional distress and psychic suffering emerge, flourish for a time, and then disappear (Elliott, 2000). With each new version of the *DSM*, some diagnostic labels are discarded and new ones are added. In light of their complicated and controversial nature, perhaps diagnoses are best made, when they must be made at all, as a necessary evil and with an attitude of humility and profound respect for the complexity of human beings. Given the importance of *DSM* diagnoses for research purposes, their prominence within clinics and other medicalized practice sites, and their role in obtaining insurance reimbursement, diagnoses must also be made with a thorough understanding of the *DSM*, which is the most commonly used taxonomy of mental disorders in the United States and is now in its fifth edition.

The *DSM-5* significantly changes current processes of assessment and diagnosis with the addition of dimensional and cross-cutting assessments to the *DSM's* categorical diagnoses (Jones, 2012). A categorical diagnosis is either present or absent, and a categorical diagnostic system like the *DSM* assumes that psychiatric disorders are discrete entities with homogeneous populations that all display similar symptoms of a disorder (Jones, 2012). In reality, patient populations are widely heterogeneous and do not fall neatly into diagnostic categories, just as psychiatric disorders are neither homogeneous nor divided by distinct boundaries (Jones, 2012). This reality has highlighted some of the significant shortcomings of the current diagnostic system including excessive comorbidity (i.e., the need for multiple diagnoses); irresolvable boundary disputes with their corresponding conflicts among clinicians with differing diagnostic views; and excessive use of the *unspecified*, formerly known as *not otherwise specified* (NOS) diagnostic category (Jones, 2012).

To address these shortcomings, the *DSM-5* Task Force has proposed adding dimensional assessments to every diagnosis in the *DSM*. Dimensional assessments are rating scales with multiple (three or more) ordered values that measure the frequency, duration, severity, or other characteristics of a psychiatric disorder (Jones, 2012). A symptom cannot be either present or absent. Rather, it exists along a continuum of severity ranging from, for example, 0 = *not at all*, 1 = *for several days*, 2 = *more than half the days*, and 3 = *nearly every day* (Jones, 2012). In addition to including dimensional assessments for individual disorders, the *DSM* may also soon include cross-cutting assessments to measure symptoms such as depression and anxiety that commonly occur across patients regardless of the presenting problem or eventual diagnosis (Jones, 2012). Such symptoms have been conceptualized as *psychiatric vital signs,* given the evidence for their occurrence across diagnostic categories (Zimmerman et al., 2012).

In sum, a diagnosis is probably best understood as a descriptive tool, subject to change over time, which can assist in the identification of a current clinical syndrome for which a particular treatment is indicated. A diagnosis is a descriptive label that categorizes persons who evidence clusters of symptoms and behaviors considered clinically meaningful in terms of their course, outcome, and response to treatment—although no one fully agrees on the nature, significance, or utility of these designations (Mechanic, 2007). In some cases, a diagnostic label denotes an underlying condition with genetic and physiological antecedents (e.g., schizophrenia). In other cases, it refers to a pattern of response to various forms of stress not clearly connected to underlying physiological phenomena (e.g., adjustment disorder). The diagnosis is not itself the thing it connotes, that is, a disorder. However systematically or carefully it is crafted, a diagnosis represents a snapshot in time. Diagnostic error is common, and diagnoses tend to be fluid—that is, subject to the irresolvable boundary disputes identified by Jones (2012)—which is what accounts for the reality that, for example, what looks like attention deficit hyperactivity disorder at age 5 years might become oppositional defiant disorder at age 9 years, conduct disorder at age 12 years, antisocial personality disorder at age 18 years, and bipolar disorder at age 21 years. Here lies the need for diagnostic skill as well as humility and a lack of narcissistic investment in being "right" about the "correct" diagnosis.

Although *DSM-5* has eliminated multiaxial diagnoses, it has retained diagnostic categories and supplemented them with the addition of one or more dimensional assessments. In Beth's case, the diagnosis of major depression was determined from the fact she had the requisite number of designated *DSM* symptoms for the diagnostic category, including depressed mood and loss of interest or pleasure, in the 2-week period before her assessment. This represented a change from previous functioning, caused clinically significant distress and impairment in social and occupational functioning, and was not caused by the direct physiological effects of a substance or a general medical condition (APA, 2013). The dimensional assessment for the categorical diagnosis of major depression used the Patient Health Questionnaire-9 (PHQ-9; see Appendix 3.7), which assesses the severity of nine possible depressive symptoms over a 2-week period using a 4-point scale: 0 = *not at all*, 1 = *for several days*, 2 = *more than half the days*, 3 = *nearly every day*. Beth scored 16 out of a possible 27 points on the dimensional assessment, indicating a moderate level of major depression. Because she reported that some of these depressive symptoms had been present for longer than 2 years, a possibility emerged that this major depressive episode was superimposed on a dysthymic disorder, so dysthymia was provisionally included in the differential diagnosis. However, more information will be needed to make that diagnosis, including perhaps some collateral information from people who know Beth.

Beth's therapist also had concerns about a possible diagnosis of personality disorder given her history of intense and unstable relationships with her most significant others, the predominance of anger in her affective presentation, the apparent identity diffusion, her difficulty being alone, self-injurious behavior (wrist scratching), her inability to modulate interpersonal distance, and her apparent lack of object constancy (e.g., "If she [my mother] doesn't call me every night, I get extremely anxious."). Nevertheless, a diagnosis of personality disorder was deferred because it was not clear on the basis of a single interview, especially in the middle of a major depressive episode, that the impairments in personality functioning (self and interpersonal) were relatively stable across time and consistent across situations (APA, 2013; Good, 2012). In addition, it was not yet clear that Beth's individual personality trait expression, which seemed at first glance to include at least one pathological trait domain (negative affectivity), could not be better understood as normative for her developmental stage (APA, 2013; Good, 2012). Finally, it should be noted that Beth had no medical diagnoses to report and that the clinician's assessment of her overall level of functioning employed the GAF scale. Beth's GAF was scored at 41 due to suicide ideation, self-injurious behavior, and serious impairment in academic and social functioning.

A psychiatric assessment is not the completion of a symptom checklist; and a diagnosis cannot express the clinician's empathic understanding of the patient, even though accurate, empathic understanding of the patient may be essential to the diagnostic process (Silberman, 2010). Despite the comprehensiveness of the *DSM* diagnostic system, much is missing from this diagnostic picture. It has a flat, two-dimensional quality and does not really encapsulate the essence of Beth's case. It does not tell us enough. It does not clarify the boundaries between normality and illness in her case, establish an etiology for the diagnostic entities, or convey any understanding of the psychological or neurophysiological factors that might be contributing to her presentation (Silberman, 2010). It does not put Beth's case into a theoretical perspective, prioritize her problems, predict any sort of outcome, or most important, paint a rounded picture of her uniqueness and humanity. For that, we need a case formulation.

CASE FORMULATION

Case formulation lies "at the intersection of etiology and description, theory and practice, and science and art" (Sim, Gwee, & Bateman, 2005, p. 289). Case formulation fills the gap between the purely descriptive, atheoretical *DSM* criteria, which say nothing about the cause of a person's problems, and the practical art of prescribing a particular treatment approach for a given patient. Accurate diagnoses and effective treatment plans are essential to helping people; but in the gap that lies between, we need a process to link the patient's various complaints to one another, explain why these problems have emerged, and provide predictions about the person's probable course (Sim et al., 2005). We need a process to capture the essence of a case. Case formulation does so by succinctly describing the essential features of a case—by encapsulating the complaints, problems, diagnosis, etiology, treatment options, and prognosis with enough sensitivity and specificity so that the uniqueness of the individual appears and a more complete picture emerges of what is required in the way of help. Box 3.21 illustrates a formulation of Beth's case.

Sim and associates (2005) identify clear benefits to the therapist in having a case formulation. These are related to the following five aspects of any given case: integrative, explanatory, prescriptive, predictive, and therapist elements. Box 3.21 illustrates how a case formulation can attempt to integrate clinical data, including biological, psychological, and sociocultural data; summarize the salient features of a case; identify important issues quickly in the context of an explanatory framework that provides insight into the intraindividual and interindividual aspects of the case; prioritize the patient's problems and the interventions that will address them; and identify the target symptoms by which interventions will be evaluated (Sim et al., 2005). At the prescriptive level, it demonstrates how the case formulation guides the therapy in choice of goals, including the point at which intervention will begin. It demonstrates how a case formulation sheds light on the prognosis of the case and makes predictions about the probable course of treatment. It illustrates how a case formulation helps the therapist recognize and organize the complex issues that lie beyond the presenting problems such that greater empathy with the patient is possible (Sim et al., 2005).

In sum, a case formulation provides the context for an evolving therapeutic relationship. It allows the therapist to better understand the nature of the therapeutic relationship and to anticipate how to manage therapy-interfering events and resistance to change, including in Beth's case the possibility of self-injurious behavior or the impulse to flee from any further closeness with the therapist. Case formulation begins a process of actualizing in practice the holistic model of healing discussed in Chapter 1. More than integrating the physiological, emotional, spiritual, cognitive, and sociocultural *data* obtained through a comprehensive assessment process, it attempts to do so such that the *person* seeking help is more comprehensible as a complex, multidimensional being within specific cultural contexts. A particularly successful case formulation begins to actualize the practice treatment hierarchy discussed in Chapter 1, Figure 1.6. A good case formulation identifies, or begins a process of identifying in an ongoing way, a hierarchy of treatment interventions that can promote the patient's healing over time.

In Beth's case, a treatment hierarchy would move from a period of *stabilization*, through *processing* of past and present feelings and events, and on to *future visioning* and an integration of past, present, and future. It would move from a focus on increasing *external* resources to a focus on developing *internal* resources see Chapter 1, Figure 1.6. Beth's treatment may start with concrete, supportive, case-management interventions designed to promote safety and stabilization in physiological, emotional, and social spheres, such as medication to target her depressive symptoms, laboratory work to rule out complicating physiological conditions, a schedule of psychotherapy sessions and academic support services, a plan to seek financial and emotional support from her father, a new living situation, and a concrete plan to limit destabilizing phone calls with her mother. As therapy progresses, interventions would move up the treatment

BOX 3.21 Sample Case Formulation

Beth is a 20-year-old college junior with no previously diagnosed psychiatric problems. She presents with symptoms that meet criteria for a diagnosis of major depression, single episode, moderate severity, no psychosis, possibly superimposed on an underlying dysthymic disorder. Diagnostic criteria are met in the context of a 4- to 5-year history of family conflict, particularly with her mother, and a hostile-enmeshed family system that is not supportive of separation or individuation. The current episode is largely precipitated by Beth's moving away from home for the first time. Beth and her mother are both having a difficult time with the separation, but that is largely unacknowledged. Instead, they stay close with angry, conflict-ridden phone conversations initiated each evening by her mother and from which Beth does not or cannot separate herself.

Beth has considerable strengths: she has stayed in school despite her intense distress, has continued to work at a stressful fast-food job, and has not escalated her wrist-scratching behaviors. However, she might not be doing as well as she is but for the fact she has been living with a significant other since moving away from home. Of concern, that relationship is unstable, marked by some of the same intense conflict and abandonment anxiety that characterizes her relationship with her mother, and may not last much longer. In that case, I would expect to see an exacerbation of the self-injurious behaviors used previously to cope with stress. It is possible a low-level, chronic risk of passive suicide ideation may become transiently active and acute. An intense argument with her boyfriend, followed by his abandonment of her for an entire night, is the acute precipitant for the current therapy contact and evaluation. The vicissitudes of the therapeutic relationship are likely to precipitate similar responses.

To treat the major depression, I will start a selective serotonin reuptake inhibitor and order a thyroid-stimulating hormone test to rule out hypothyroidism. Because she gives a reliable history of birth control, I will not order a test for beta-human chorionic gonadotropin. Individual psychotherapy with a relational focus, starting at one session per week, begins next week. Ongoing assessment for a diagnosis of personality disorder will occur in the context of the therapeutic relationship. Given Beth's successful engagement in the assessment process, I expect she will be able to form a therapeutic alliance despite some difficulties modulating distance in close relationships. Family therapy with a colleague has been recommended and refused, but Beth may be more open to this option as individual gains are made. Beth will continue to receive academic support services at the college, and I will suggest that she investigate options for student housing on campus. She may be able to maintain her relationship with her boyfriend for a time if she gets a reprieve from the increased intimacy demanded by their close living quarters. I will also suggest she open a dialogue with her father about financial support, as she has an appropriately close and relatively conflict-free relationship with him. I will encourage her to continue to use her current support system and will work with her to expand and strengthen it as more pressing problems are addressed (e.g., as her depressed mood begins to lift, she is better able to modulate and tolerate contact with her mother, she achieves some stability in her living situation, and she is more able to negotiate the demands of work and school).

hierarchy to focus on building healthier relationships, improving communication and interpersonal effectiveness, processing thoughts and feelings, and developing internal resources, such as insightfulness; the ability to tolerate distress, unpleasant affect, and ambiguity; or the ability to integrate disparate feelings about her mother, herself, or other significant persons. Ultimately, integration is the goal, as defined by Beth within her own cultural context.

CONCLUDING COMMENTS

A comprehensive assessment of the patient who presents for psychotherapy is necessary to develop an appropriate treatment plan. In some practice settings, a comprehensive assessment is required in the initial session, and many tools are available to help the therapist. This assessment is a relational process that sets the tone for subsequent sessions. If sensitively crafted, an intake assessment can be a powerful therapeutic tool with the potential to further the therapeutic alliance, on which all good psychotherapy outcomes depend. Far from being a rote process with a simple question-and-answer format, a comprehensive intake assessment is a creative act (Havens, 1998). It begins the ongoing, essentially creative activity of two reciprocally influencing therapeutic partners in constructing the patient's life story. The more powerfully engaged the patient and therapist are in the assessment process, the more valid are the data on which to base the diagnosis that will guide the choice of treatment plan.

In addition to taking a comprehensive biopsychosocial history of the patient who presents for psychotherapy, the therapist must assess the patient's ego functioning, affective development, interpersonal relationships, and cultural belief systems. Genograms play an important role in the assessment process, as do the screening tools, diagnosis, and case formulation in the therapeutic process. Several rating scales, psychiatric databases, and other screening tools are commonly used to facilitate assessment and diagnosis or to measure psychotherapy outcomes. Although nothing substitutes for experience, the assessment format and rating scales presented in this chapter provide a foundation that equips the novice nurse psychotherapist for the creative collaboration that lies ahead.

DISCUSSION QUESTIONS

1. Discuss the ways in which a comprehensive clinical assessment presents a unique opportunity for intervention in the psychotherapeutic context.
2. How may an assessment interview in the psychotherapeutic context differ from conventional medical history taking?
3. Discuss the relationship between the therapeutic alliance and the validity of clinical assessment data.
4. Describe the major goals and tasks of assessment.
5. Describe the ways in which a psychotherapist facilitates and strengthens the therapeutic alliance in the process of completing an assessment.
6. How would you describe the connections among ego functioning, affective development, sense of self, and interpersonal functioning?
7. Think of a patient in your practice context with whom you have had a therapeutic relationship. What specific questions would you ask to assess that patient's ego functioning, affective development, and interpersonal functioning?
8. How does the therapeutic relationship with a psychotherapy patient serve as an assessment tool? Can you assess the areas of patient functioning mentioned in Question 7 without asking specific questions? If so, how?
9. What are the similarities and differences among screening, that is, employing a screening tool, diagnosing a disorder, and formulating a case?
10. Given what you have learned about Beth in this chapter, can you construct an alternative case formulation? Can there be multiple formulations of the same case? How so?

LIST OF VIDEOLINKS

1. Clinical interviewing: intake, assessment, and therapeutic alliance
   www.psychotherapy.net/video/clinical-interview-intake-assessment-training
2. The *DSM-5* and psychodiagnostic interviewing (4-video series)
   www.psychotherapy.net/video/dsm5-series
3. Conducting an MSE
   www.psychotherapy.net/video/mental-health-hospitals-mental-status-exam
4. Motivational interviewing step by step (4-video series)
   www.psychotherapy.net/video/motivational-interviewing-series
5. Advanced motivational interviewing: depression
   www.youtube.com/watch?v=3rSt4KIaN8I
6. Psychiatric interviews for teaching: depression
   www.youtube.com/watch?v=4YhpWZCdiZc
7. Psychiatric interviews for teaching: anxiety
   www.youtube.com/watch?v=Ii2FHbtVJzc
8. Psychiatric interviews for teaching: mania
   www.youtube.com/watch?v=zA-fqvC02oM
9. Psychiatric interviews for teaching: psychosis
   www.youtube.com/watch?v=ZB28gfSmz1Y
10. Psychiatric interviews for teaching: somatization
    www.youtube.com/watch?v=4-bH55MCa1U

REFERENCES

Ainsworth, M. D. S., Blehar, M. C., Waters, E., & Wall, S. (1978). *Patterns of attachment*. Hillsdale, NJ: Erlbaum.

Akhtar, S. (1995). Quest for answers: A primer of understanding and treating severe personality disorders. Northvale, NJ: Jason Aronson.

American Psychiatric Association. (2000). *Diagnostic and statistical manual of mental disorders* (4th ed., text revision). Washington, DC: Author.

American Psychiatric Association. (2013). *Diagnostic and statistical manual of mental disorders* (5th ed.). Washington, DC: Author.

American Psychiatric Association. (2016). *The American Psychiatric Association practice guidelines for the psychiatric evaluation of adults* (3rd ed.). Arlington, VA: American Psychiatric Association.

Bagby, R. M., Parker, J. D. A., & Taylor, G. J. (1994a). The twenty-item Toronto alexithymia scale. I. Item selection and cross-validation of the factor structure. *Journal of Psychosomatic Research*, *38*, 23–32. doi:10.1016/0022-3999(94)90005-1

Bagby, R. M., Taylor, G. J., & Parker, J. D. A. (1994b). The twenty-item Toronto alexithymia scale. II. Convergent, discriminant and concurrent validity. *Journal of Psychosomatic Research*, *38*, 33–40. doi:10.1016/0022-3999(94)90006-X

Barker, P. (2001). The tidal model: The lived-experience in person-centered mental health nursing care. *Nursing Philosophy*, *2*, 213–223. doi:10.1046/j.1466-769X.2000.00062.x

Barrell, L. M., Merwin, E. I., & Poster, E. C. (1997). Patient outcomes used by advanced practice psychiatric nurses to evaluate effectiveness of practice. *Archives of Psychiatric Nursing*, *11*(4), 184–197. doi:10.1016/S0883-9417(97)80026-X

Beck, A. T., Ward, C. H., Mendelson, M., Mock, J., & Erbaugh, J. (1961). An inventory for measuring depression. *Archives of General Psychiatry*, *4*, 561–571. doi:10.1001/archpsyc .1961.01710120031004

Bellak, L. (1989). The broad role of ego function assessment. In S. Wetzler & M. Katz (Eds.), *Contemporary approaches to psychological assessment* (pp. 270–295). New York, NY: Brunner/Mazel.

Berg, K. C., Peterson, C. B., & Frazier, P. (2012). Assessment and diagnosis of eating disorders: A guide for professional counselors. *Journal of Counseling & Development, 90*, 262–269. doi:10.1002/j.1556-6676.2012.00033.x

Bjorklund, P. (2000). Assessing ego strength: Spinning straw into gold. *Perspectives in Psychiatric Care, 36*(1), 14–23. doi:10.1111/j.1744-6163.2000.tb00685.x

Bradley, S. J. (2000). *Affect regulation and the development of psychopathology.* New York, NY: Guilford Press.

Bresee, C., Gotto, J., & Rapaport, M. H. (2009). Treatment of depression. In A. F. Schatzberg & C. B. Nemeroff (Eds.), *The American Psychiatric Association Publishing textbook of psychopharmacology* (4th ed., chap. 53). Arlington, VA: American Psychiatric Publishing.

Brown, C., DePetro, E., & Whitaker, H. (2014). The diagnostic and statistical manual: Historical observations. *Psicologia em Pesquisa, 8*(1), 85–96. doi:10.5327/Z1982-1247201400010009

Buchanan, A., Binder, R., Norko, M., & Swartz, M. (2012). Psychiatric violence risk assessment. *American Journal of Psychiatry, 169*(3), 340. doi:10.1176/appi.ajp.2012.169.3.340

Burckhardt, C. S., Woods, S. L., Schultz, A. A., & Ziebarth, D. M. (1989). Quality of life in adults with chronic illness: A psychometric study. *Research in Nursing and Health, 12*, 347–354. doi:10.1002/nur.4770120604

Burns, D. (1991). Focusing on ego strengths. *Archives of Psychiatric Nursing, 5*, 202–207. doi:10.1016/0883-9417(91)90047-9

Carlson, E. B., & Putnam, F. W. (1993). *Manual for the dissociative experiences scale.* Lutherville, MD: Sidran Foundation.

Coccaro, E., Harvey, P. D., Kupsaw-Lawrence, E., Herbert, J. L., & Bernstein, D. P. (1991). Development of neuropharmacologically based behavioral assessments of impulsive behavior. *Journal of Neuropsychiatry and Clinical Neurosciences, 3*(2), S44–S51.

Consensus Panel on Genetic/Genomic Nursing Competencies. (2006). *Essential nursing competencies and curricula guidelines for genetics and genomics.* Silver Spring, MD: American Nurses Association.

Consensus Panel on Genetic/Genomic Nursing Competencies. (2009). *Essentials of genetic and genomic nursing: Competencies, curricula guidelines, and outcome indicators* (2nd ed.). Silver Spring, MD: American Nurses Association. Retrieved from https://www.genome.gov/Pages/Careers/HealthProfessionalEducation/geneticscompetency.pdf

Elliott, C. (2000). A new way to be mad. *The Atlantic Monthly, 283*(6), 73–84. Retrieved from https://www.theatlantic.com/magazine/archive/2000/12/a-new-way-to-be-mad/304671

Endicott, J., & Nee, J. (1997). Endicott work productivity scale (EWPS): A new measure to assess treatment effects. *Psychopharmacological Bulletin, 33*, 13–16. doi:10.1037/t49981-000

Endicott, J., Nee, J., Harrison, W., & Blumenthal, R. (1993). Quality of life, enjoyment and satisfaction questionnaire: A new measure. *Psychopharmacology Bulletin, 29*, 321–326. doi:10.1037/t49981-000

Ewing, J. A. (1984). Detecting alcoholism: The CAGE questionnaire. *Journal of the American Medical Association, 252*(14), 1905–1907. doi:10.1001/jama.252.14.1905

Felitti, V. J., Anda, R. F., Nordenberg, D., Williamson, D. F., Spitz, A. M., Edwards, V., . . . Marks, J. (1998). Relationship of childhood abuse and household dysfunction to many of the leading causes of death in adults: The adverse childhood experiences (ACE) study. *American Journal of Preventive Medicine, 14*(4), 245–258. doi:10.1016/S0749-3797(98)00017-8

Folstein, M. D., Folstein, S. E., & McHugh, P. R. (1975). "Mini-mental state": A practical method for grading the cognitive state of patients for the clinician. *Journal of Psychiatric Research, 12*, 189–198. doi:10.1016/0022-3956(75)90026-6

Fowler, J. (1981). *Stages of faith.* New York, NY: Harper & Row.

Frances, A. (2013). *Saving normal.* New York, NY: Harper Collins.

Freud, S. (1961). The ego and the id. In J. Strachey (Ed. and Trans.), *The standard edition of the complete psychological works of Sigmund Freud* (Vol. 19, pp. 3–66). New York, NY: W. W. Norton. (Original work published 1923.)

George, C., Kaplan, N., & Main, M. (1985). *The adult attachment interview* [Unpublished manuscript]. University of California at Berkeley.

Glick, I. D., Berman, E. M., Clarkin, J. F., & Rait, D. S. (2000). *Marital and family therapy* (4th ed.). Washington, DC: American Psychiatric Press.

Goldstein, E. (1995). *Ego psychology and social work practice* (2nd ed., pp. 143–165). New York, NY: Free Press.

Good, E. M. (2012). Personality disorders in the DSM-5: Proposed revisions and critiques. *Journal of Mental Health Counseling, 34*(1), 1–13.

Goodman, W. K., Price, L. H., Rasmussen, S. A., Mazure, C., Fleischmann, R. I., Hill, C. L., . . . Charney, D. S. (1989). The Yale-Brown obsessive-compulsive scale I. Development, use, and reliability. *Archives of General Psychiatry, 46*, 1006–1011. doi:10.1001/archpsyc.1989 .01810110048007

Gordon, C., & Goroll, A. (2003). Effective psychiatric interviewing in primary care medicine. In T. A. Slavin, J. B. Herman, & P. L. Slavin (Eds.), *The MGH guide to psychiatry in primary care* (pp. 19–26). New York, NY: McGraw-Hill.

Greco, K. E., Tinley, S., & Seibert, D. (2012). *Essential genetic and genomic competencies for nurses with graduate degrees.* Silver Spring, MD: American Nurses Association and International Society of Nurses in Genetics. Retrieved from https://www.genome.gov/Pages/Health/ HealthCareProvidersInfo/Grad_Gen_Comp.pdf

Guy, W. (1976). *ECDEU assessment manual for psychopharmacology* (rev. ed.). DHEW Publication No. ADM 76–338. Washington, DC: U.S. Department of Health, Education, and Welfare.

Hamilton, M. (1959). The assessment of anxiety states by rating. *British Journal of Medical Psychology, 32*, 50–55. doi:10.1111/j.2044-8341.1959.tb00467.x

Hamilton, M. (1960). A rating scale for depression. *Journal of Neurology, Neurosurgery, and Psychiatry, 23*, 56–62. doi:10.1136/jnnp.23.1.56

Havens, L. (1998). Preface to the 1st edition. In S. C. Shea (Ed.), *Psychiatric interviewing: The art of understanding* (2nd ed.). Philadelphia, PA: W. B. Saunders.

Horowitz, L. M., Rosenberg, S. E., Baer, B. A., Ureno, G., & Villasenor, V. S. (1988). Inventory of interpersonal problems: Psychometric properties and clinical applications. *Journal of Consulting and Clinical Psychology, 56*(6), 885–892. doi:10.1037/0022-006X.56.6.885

Horowitz, L. M., Rosenberg, S. E., & Bartholomew, K. (1993). Interpersonal problems, attachment styles, and outcome in brief dynamic psychotherapy. *Journal of Consulting and Clinical Psychology, 61*(4), 549–560. doi:10.1037/0022-006X.61.4.549

Hunt, S. M., & McKenna, S. P. (1992). The QLDS: A scale for the measurement of quality of life in depression. *Health Policy, 22*, 307–319. doi:10.1016/0168-8510(92)90004-U

Jacob, K. S. (2003). The mental state examination: The elicitation of symptoms. *Psychopathology, 36*(1), 1–5. doi:10.1159/000069653

Jacob, K. S. (2012). Psychiatric assessment and the art and science of clinical medicine. *Indian Journal of Psychiatry, 54*(2), 184–187. doi:10.4103/0019-5545.99538

Jones, K. D. (2012). Dimensional and cross-cutting assessment in the *DSM-5. Journal of Counseling & Development, 90*, 481–487. doi:10.1002/j.1556-6676.2012.00059.x

Kaplan, R. M., & Anderson, J. P. (1988). A general health policy model: Updates and applications. *Health Services Research, 23*(2), 203–234.

Kay, S. R., Fiszbein, A., & Opler, L. A. (1987). The positive and negative syndrome scale (PANSS) for schizophrenia. *Schizophrenia Bulletin, 13*, 261–276. doi:10.1093/schbul/13.2.261

Leon, A. C., Shear, M. K., Portera L., & Klerman, G. L. (1992). Assessing impairment in patients with panic disorder: The Sheehan Disability Scale. *Social Psychiatry and Psychiatric Epidemiology, 27*, 78–82. doi:10.1007/BF00788510

Main, M., & Goldwyn, R. (1998). *Adult attachment scoring and classification system.* (Unpublished manual). Berkeley:University of California at Berkeley.

Marken, P. A., Schneiderhan, M. E., & Munro, S. (2005). Evaluation of psychiatric illness. In J. T. DiPrio, R. L. Talbert, G. C. Yee, G. R. Matzke, B. G. Wells, & L. M. Posey (Eds.), *Pharmacotherapy: A pathophysiologic approach* (6th ed., pp. 1123–1132). New York, NY: McGraw-Hill.

McQuaid, J. R., Marx, B. P., Rosen, M. I., Bufka, L. F., Tenhula, W., Cook, H., . . . Keane, T. M. (2012). Mental health assessment in rehabilitation research. *Journal of Rehabilitation Research & Development, 49*(1), 121–138. doi:10.1682/JRRD.2010.08.0143

Mechanic, D. (2007). *Mental health and social policy: Beyond managed care* (5th ed.). Cherry Hill, NJ: Pearson.

Milisen, K., Braes, T., & Foreman, M. D. (2012). Assessing cognitive function. In M. Boltz (Ed.), *Evidence-based geriatric nursing protocols for best practice* (pp. 122–134). New York, NY: Springer Publishing Company.

Mirowsky, J., & Ross, C. E. (1992). Age and depression. *Journal of Health and Social Behavior, 33*, 187–205. doi:10.2307/2137349

Mirowsky, J., & Ross, C. E. (1995). Sex differences in distress: Real or artifact? *American Sociological Review, 60*(3), 449–468. doi:10.2307/2096424

Montgomery, S. A., & Asberg, M. (1979). A new depression scale designed to be sensitive to change. *British Journal of Psychiatry, 134*, 382–389. doi:10.1192/bjp.134.4.382

Morrison, J. (2014). *The first interview* (4th ed.). New York, NY: Guilford Press.

Mundt, J. C., Marks, I. M., Shear, M. K., & Greist, J. H. (2002). The work and social adjustment scale: A simple measure of impairment in functioning. *British Journal of Psychiatry, 180*, 462–464. doi:10.1192/bjp.180.5.461

National Institute of Mental Health. (1970). CGI: Clinical global impression. In W. Guy & R. R. Bonato (Eds.), *Manual for the ECDEU assessment battery* (rev. 2nd ed., pp. 12.1–12.6). Chevy Chase, MD: National Institute of Mental Health.

Nijenhuis, E. R. S., Van der Hart, O., & Kruger, K. (2002). The psychometric characteristics of the traumatic experiences questionnaire (TEC): First findings among psychiatric outpatients. *Clinical Psychology and Psychotherapy, 9*(3), 200–210. doi:10.1002/cpp.332

Overall, J. E., & Gorham, D. R. (1962). The brief psychiatric rating scale. *Psychological Reports, 10*, 799–812. doi:10.2466/pr0.1962.10.3.799

Parker, J. D. A., Taylor, G. J., & Bagby, R. M. (2003). The 20-item toronto alexithymia scale. III. Reliability and factorial validity in a community sample. *Journal of Psychosomatic Research, 55*, 269–275. doi:10.1016/S0022-3999(02)00578-0

Peplau, H. E. (1989). General application of theory and techniques in psychotherapy in nursing situations. In A. W. O'Toole & S. R. Welt (Eds.), *Interpersonal theory in nursing practice: Selected works of Hildegard E. Peplau* (pp. 99–107). New York, NY: Springer Publishing Company.

Pestka, E. L., Derscheid, D. J., Ellenbecker, S. M., Schmid, P J., O'Neil, M. L., Ray-Mihm, R. J., & Cox, D. L. (2010). Use of genomic assessments and interventions in psychiatric nursing practice. *Issues in Mental Health Nursing, 31*, 623–630. doi:10.3109/01612840.2010.493266

Pestka, E. L., Meisheid, A., & O'Neil, M. (2008). Educating nurses on genomics. *American Journal of Nursing, 108*(2), 72A–72C. doi:10.1097/01.NAJ.0000310345.90872.0d

Rush, A. J., Gullion, C. M., Basco, M. R., Jarrett, R. B., & Triveldi, M. H. (1996). The inventory of depressive symptomatology (IDS): Psychometric properties. *Psychological Medicine, 26*, 477–486. doi:10.1017/S0033291700035558

Rush, A. J., Trivedi, M. H., Ibrahim, H. M., Carmody, T. J., Arnow, B., Klein, D. N., . . . Keller, M. B. (2003). The 16-item quick inventory of depressive symptomatology (QIDS), clinician rating (QIDS-C), and self-report (QIDS-SR): A psychometric evaluation in patients with chronic major depression. *Biological Psychiatry, 54*, 573–583. doi:10.1016/S0006-3223(02)01866-8

Sadek, J. (2019). *A clinician's guide to suicide risk assessment and management*. Cham, Switzerland: Springer Nature Switzerland.

Sadock, B. J., Sadock, V. S., & Ruiz, P. (2015). *Kaplan & Sadock's synopsis of psychiatry: Behavioral sciences/clinical psychiatry* (11th ed.). Philadelphia, PA: Wolters Kluwer.

Safran, J. D., & Muran, J. C. (2000). *Negotiating the therapeutic alliance: A relational treatment guide*. New York, NY: Guilford Press.

Saunders, J. B., Aasland, O. G., Babor, T. F., De La Fuente, J. R., & Grant, M. (1993). Development of the alcohol use disorders identification test (AUDIT): WHO collaborative project on early detection of persons with harmful alcohol consumption-II. *Addiction, 88*(6), 791–804. doi:10.1111/j.1360-0443.1993.tb02093.x

Scharff, J. S., & Scharff, D. E. (2005). *The primer of object relations* (2nd ed.). Lanham, MD: Jason Aronson.

Schatzberg, A. F., & Nemeroff, C. B. (2017). *The American Psychiatric Association Publishing textbook of psychopharmacology* (5th ed.). Arlington, VA: American Psychiatric Publishing.

Scully, J. H., & Thornhill, J. T., IV. (2012). The clinical examination. In J. T. Thornhill, IV (Ed.), *The national medical series for independent study: Psychiatry* (6th ed., pp. 1–16). Philadelphia, PA: Lippincott Williams & Wilkins.

Selzer, M. L. (1971). The Michigan alcoholism screening test: The quest for a new diagnostic instrument. *American Journal of Psychiatry, 127,* 1653–1658. doi:10.1176/ajp.127.12.1653

Shea, S. C. (2017). *Psychiatric interviewing: The art of understanding* (3rd ed.). Edinburgh, UK: Elsevier.

Shorter, E. (2015). The history of nosology and the rise of the *Diagnostic and Statistical Manual of Mental Disorders. Dialogues in Clinical Neuroscience, 17*(1), 59–68. Retrieved from https://www.ncbi.nlm.nih.gov/pmc/articles/PMC4421901

Shmueli-Goetz, Y., Target, M., Fonagy, P., & Datta, A. (2008). The child attachment interview: A psychometric study of reliability and discriminant validity. *Developmental Psychology, 44*(4), 939–956. doi:10.1037/0012-1649.44.4.939

Silberman, E. K. (2010). Patients' subjective experience as a component of psychiatric assessment: Where does it fit? *Psychiatry, 73*(4), 315–317. doi:10.1521/psyc.2010.73.4.315

Sim, K., Gwee, K. P., & Bateman, A. (2005). Case formulation in psychotherapy: Revitalizing its usefulness as a clinical tool. *Academic Psychiatry, 29*(3), 289–292. doi:10.1176/appi.ap.29.3.289

Simpson, G. M., & Angus, J. W. S. (1970). A rating scale for extrapyramidal side effects. *Acta Psychiatrica Scandinavica, 212*(S212), 11–19. doi:10.1111/j.1600-0447.1970.tb02066.x

Stokes, K. (1990). Faith development in the adult life cycle. *Journal of Religious Gerontology, 7,* 167–184. doi:10.1300/J078V07N01_13

Stowell, K. R., Florence, P., Harman, H. J., & Glick, R. L. (2012). Psychiatric evaluation of the agitated patient: Consensus statement of the American Association for Emergency Psychiatry project BETA psychiatric evaluation workgroup. *Western Journal of Emergency Medicine, 13*(1), 11–16. doi:10.5811/westjem.2011.9.6868

Taylor, G. J. (1995). Psychoanalysis and empirical research: The example of patients who lack psychological-mindedness. *Journal of the American Academy of Psychoanalysis, 23,* 263–281. doi:10.5811/westjem.2011.9.6868

Taylor, G. J., Bagby, R. M., & Parker, J. D. A. (2003). The 20-item Toronto alexithymia scale. IV. Reliability and factorial validity in different languages and cultures. *Journal of Psychosomatic Research, 55,* 277–283. doi:10.1016/S0022-3999(02)00601-3

Trzepacz, P. T., Mittal, D., Torres, R., Kanary, K., Norton, J., & Jimerson, N. (2001). Validation of the delirium rating scale-revised-98: Comparison with the delirium rating scale and the cognitive test for delirium. *Journal of Neuropsychiatry and Clinical Neurosciences, 13*(2), 229–242. doi:10.1176/jnp.13.2.229

Tulloch, J. D. (1984). Observer-rated ego function assessment tool. (Unpublished handout). Denver: University of Colorado Health Sciences Center.

Varcarolis, E. M., Carson, V. B., & Shoemaker, N. C. (Eds.). (2006). *Foundations of psychiatric mental health nursing* (5th ed.). Philadelphia, PA: W. B. Saunders.

Wakefield, J. C. (1992). The concept of mental disorder: On the boundary between biological facts and social values. *American Psychologist, 47*(3), 373–388. doi:10.1037/0003-066X.47.3.373

Ware, J. E., & Sherbourne, C. D. (1992). The MOS 26-item short-form health survey (SF-36), I: Conceptual framework and item selection. *Medical Care, 30,* 473–483. doi:10.1097/00005650-199206000-00002

Widiger, T. A., & Samuel, D. B. (2009). Evidence-based assessment of personality disorders. *Personality Disorders: Theory, Research, and Treatment, S*(1), 3–17. doi:10.1037/1949-2715.S.1.3

Williams, D. C. (2010). Disability and occupational assessment: Objective diagnosis and quantitative impairment rating. *Harvard Review of Psychiatry, 18*(6), 336–352. doi:10.3109/10673229.2010.527516

Wink, P., & Dillon, M. (2002). Spiritual development across the adult life course: Findings from a longitudinal study. *Journal of Adult Development, 9*(1), 79–94. doi:10.1023/A:1013833419122

World Health Organization. (2002). *WHOQOL-SRPB field-test instrument.* Retrieved from https://www.who.int/mental_health/media/en/622.pdf

Yesavage, J. A., Brink, T. L., Rose, T. L., Lum, O., Huang, V., & Adey, M. B. (1983). Development and validation of a geriatric depression screening scale: A preliminary report. *Journal of Psychiatric Research, 17,* 37–49. doi:10.1016/0022-3956(82)90033-4

Young, R. C., Biggs, J. T., Ziegler, V. E., & Meger, D. A. (1978). *The young mania rating scale.* Retrieved from www.formedic.com/Documents/PYRSLE.pdf

Zimmerman, M., Young, D., Chelminski, I., Dalrymple, K., & Galione, J. N. (2012). Overcoming the problem of diagnostic heterogeneity in applying measurement-based care in clinical practice: The concept of psychiatric vital signs. *Comprehensive Psychiatry, 53,* 117–124. doi:10.1016/j.comppsych.2011.03.004

Zung, W. W. (1965). A self-rating depression scale. *Archives of General Psychiatry, 12*(1):63–70. doi:10.1001/archpsyc.1965.01720310065008

APPENDIX 3.1
Outline of the Comprehensive Psychiatric Database

I. Reason for the evaluation
  A. Identifying data
    1. Age
    2. Sex/Gender preference
    3. Race/Ethnicity
    4. Marital status
    5. Children
    6. How arrived?
    7. Who referred? Why?
    8. Mental health providers?
    9. Sources of information
    10. Number of times seen in this setting
  B. Source and reliability of data
  C. Chief complaint
    1. What the patient states he or she wants help with
    2. Verbatim statement
      a. "I'm depressed."
      b. "My mother brought me. I don't need help."

II. History of present illness
  A. Onset, duration, or change in symptoms over time
    1. Organized chronologically
    2. Patient's perception of changes in himself or herself over time
    3. Others' perception of changes in the patient (e.g., spouse, employer, and friend)
  B. Stressors and precipitating factors
    1. Why now?
  C. Baseline functioning
  D. Last period of stability

III. Past psychiatric history
  A. Trauma history
    1. Ten most significant disturbing events in life

B. Inpatient
  1. Location, dates, and lengths of stay
  2. Diagnoses
  3. Previous episodes of current symptoms
  4. Previous episodes of other disorders not described in history of current illness
  5. Legal status
  6. Use of medications or other treatments, including doses, blood levels, clinical response
  7. Perception of helpfulness
C. Outpatient
  1. Dates, duration, and frequency of sessions
  2. Location, type, and focus of treatment or therapy
  3. Perception of helpfulness

IV. History of substance use and abuse
  A. Episodes of alcohol abuse
    1. What, how much, and consequences (e.g., charges for driving under the influence [DUI], other legal sequelae, and loss of relationships, jobs, and opportunities)
    2. Does the patient or others think he or she has a problem?
    3. Typical pattern of use
    4. History of blackouts, seizures, complicated withdrawal, or delirium tremens
    5. History of suicide ideation, gestures, or attempts while intoxicated or withdrawing
    6. Longest period of sobriety
    7. What facilitates sobriety?

(continued)

8. Previous treatments (e.g., detoxification, rehabilitation, counseling, and Alcoholics Anonymous)

B. Episodes of illicit or prescription drug abuse

1. What, amount, route of administration, and consequences (e.g., DUIs, other legal sequelae, and loss of relationships, jobs, and opportunities)
2. Does the patient or others think he or she has a problem?
3. Typical pattern of use
4. History of suicide ideation, gestures, or attempts while intoxicated or withdrawing
5. Longest period of sobriety
6. What facilitates sobriety?
7. Previous treatments (e.g., detoxification, rehabilitation, counseling, and Narcotics Anonymous)

C. Tobacco

1. Number of cigarettes or packs per day
2. Years patient has smoked
3. Cessation attempts

D. Caffeine

1. Form (coffee, cola, tea, and pills)
2. Amount consumed per day
3. Cessation attempts

E. Over-the-counter drugs or "herbal" medications

1. What, how much, purpose, frequency, side effects, and interactions with prescribed medications
2. Perceptions of helpfulness or efficacy

V. Medical history

A. Past and current medical problems

1. Illnesses, operations, and hospitalizations, especially history of open or closed head injury, birth trauma, seizure disorder, and encephalitis or meningitis

B. Past and current medications

1. Dosages, blood levels, and clinical response
2. Adherence

C. Primary care physician, specialists, and phone numbers

D. Allergies (and reactions)

VI. Family history

A. Psychiatric or substance use disorders

1. Have any family members undergone psychiatric or substance abuse treatment (inpatient or outpatient), attempted or completed a suicide, had problems with drugs or alcohol, and behaved strangely?
2. Have any family members successfully used any psychotropic medications for the same or similar symptoms?
3. Family attitudes toward mental illness

B. Pertinent medical disorders in blood relatives (e.g., seizure disorder or thyroid disease)

VII. Developmental history

A. Developmental milestones and family of origin

1. Information about mother's pregnancy and delivery
2. Were developmental milestones reached as expected?
3. Childhood temperament and important family events (e.g., death, separation, and divorce)

(continued)

4. Information about early experiences and relationships (e.g., school experiences, academic performance, delinquency, family of origin relationships, family stability, early sexual experiences, and history of abuse or neglect)
5. Important cultural or religious influences
6. Values, beliefs, or framework for meaning

B. Educational history

C. Occupational and military history
   1. Number and types of jobs; reasons for termination
   2. Highest rank attained; conditions of discharge
   3. History of disciplinary problems or combat

D. Legal history

VIII. Social history

A. Current social situation
   1. Living arrangements (e.g., where, with whom, for how long, how stable, and how satisfactory or desirable)
   2. Employment (e.g., where, for how long, how stable, and how satisfactory or desirable)
   3. Financial (e.g., current sources of income, how stable, and how adequate)
   4. Insurance coverage

B. Breadth of patient's social life
   1. Is he or she a loner or involved in an intimate relationship?
   2. How difficult is it to get into and out of relationships?
   3. Support system(s)

C. Past and present levels of functioning
   1. Marriage, parenting, and work
   2. Patient strengths and strategies used to manage stress, resources, or positive memories (draw a line and place important positive memories and events)
   3. Current functional deficits (e.g., activities of daily living, task performance, and relationships)

IX. Violence history

A. To self
   1. What, when, where, how, why; warning signs or symptoms, triggers, and consequences
   2. How intense, specific, and controllable is current ideation

B. To others or property
   1. What, when, where, how, why; warning signs or symptoms, triggers, and consequences
   2. How intense, specific, and controllable is current ideation

C. Current access to weapons
   1. What, where, why; plan for use; plan for disposition of weapon
   2. How will disposition of weapons be verified?

X. Psychiatric review of systems (ROS)

A. Includes all symptoms not part of the current episode or presentation

B. May have to ask specific questions about the presence or absence of these symptoms
   1. "Are you now or have you ever had any of the following . . ."

(continued)

C. Anxiety symptoms
  1. Shortness of breath, heart palpitations, panic attacks, sweating, flushing, hyperventilation, sense of doom, fear of death or collapse, cold or clammy skin, and tingling sensations in extremities
D. Mood symptoms
  1. Sadness, irritability, anergia, fatigue, lethargy, tearfulness, increased or decreased appetite or energy, changes in sleep or libido, suicide ideation, homicide ideation, hypomania (e.g., spending sprees, increased energy, and religious preoccupation beyond baseline), and feelings of hopelessness, helplessness, or worthlessness
E. Psychotic or cognitive symptoms
  1. Hallucinations, delusions, thought insertion, thought blocking, thought broadcasting, flight of ideas, hyperreligiosity, tangentiality, looseness of associations, and circumstantiality

XI. Mental status examination (MSE)
  A. Informal: begins immediately on contact with the patient and includes an informal assessment of the patient's characteristics
    1. Appearance
    2. Manner of relating
    3. Use of language
    4. Mood and affect
    5. Content of speech
    6. Perceptions
    7. Abstracting ability
    8. Judgment
    9. Insight
  B. Formal: focused, structured assessment of the patient's characteristics

1. Appearance: overall appearance, dress, grooming
2. Attitude: attitude toward examiner (e.g., hostile, cooperative, evasive)
3. Behavior and psychomotor activity: gait, carriage, posture, activity level
4. Speech
  a. Rate, amount, tone, impairment, aphasia
5. Mood and affect
  a. Mood (i.e., how the patient reports feeling) in relation to affect (i.e., emotional expression observed by the therapist)
  b. Depth and range of emotional expression
6. Perception
  a. Hallucinations
    i. Auditory
    ii. Visual
    iii. Gustatory: taste (temporal lobe dysfunction?)
    iv. Olfactory: smell (temporal lobe dysfunction?)
    v. Tactile: Skin sensations (alcohol withdrawal and intoxication?)
    vi. Kinesthetic: feeling movement when none occurs
    vii. Hypnagogic: occurs while falling asleep
    viii. Hypnopompic: occurs while waking up
  b. Illusions: misinterpretations of actual sensory stimuli
  c. Depersonalization: feels detached and views self as unreal
  d. Derealization: experiences objects and persons outside of self as unreal

(continued)

7. Thought process
   a. The pattern of a patient's speech allows the therapist to observe the quality of the thought process, including its flow, logic, and associations. Abnormalities include the following:
      i. Loose associations (LOAs)
      ii. Tangentiality
      iii. Circumstantiality
      iv. Thought blocking (TB)
      v. Thought insertion (TI)
      vi. Flight of ideas (FOAs)
      vii. Perseveration
      viii. Echolalia
8. Content of thought
   a. Delusions
      i. Paranoid or persecutory
      ii. Grandiose
      iii. Nihilistic
      iv. Somatic
      v. Bizarre
   b. Ideas of reference
   c. Obsessions
   d. Suicidal thoughts
   e. Homicidal thoughts
9. Judgment
   a. An assessment of social judgment involves determining whether a patient understands the consequences of his or her actions
   b. Must recognize differences in cultural values when assessing judgment
   c. "What would you do if you found a sealed, stamped, addressed envelope on the sidewalk?"

10. Insight
    a. Must assess whether a person is aware of a problem, the cause of the problem, and what type of help is needed to address the problem
11. Cognition
    a. A formal MSE measures the ability of the brain to function by assessing the following cognitive functions:
       i. Consciousness: alert, confused, drowsy, somnolent, obtunded, delirious, stuporous, and comatose
       ii. Orientation: knows who he or she is, where he or she is, and what day it is
       iii. Memory: can remember what was eaten for breakfast today; has remote memory for long-past events
       iv. Recall: can recall three objects after 5 minutes
       v. Registration: can name three objects immediately
       vi. Attention: can spell *world* forward and backward
       vii. Calculation: can do serial 7's or count backward from 20
       viii. Language: can name items, repeat a phrase, follow simple commands, read, write, and copy a design

(continued)

XII. *Diagnostic and Statistical Manual of Mental Disorders*, 5th ed. (*DSM-5*) differential diagnosis

  A. On a single axis, lists the principal psychiatric, neuro-developmental, neurocognitive, and other disorders requiring further assessment, along with the corresponding ICD code(s)

  B. Includes so-called "rule-out" and/or "provisional" diagnoses

  C. ICD-9 codes are listed before each disorder name, followed by ICD-10 codes in parentheses

  D. IDC-10 codes are used starting October 1, 2014.

XIII. Case formulation

  A. Presents a brief summary of the patient and rationalizes the diagnoses

    1. Minimal identifying data, including past diagnosis

    2. Abbreviated recapitulation of presenting symptoms, onset, and course

    3. Draws from all sections of the database as needed

  B. Outlines the contributing factors, precipitants, and stressors

  C. Summarizes the logic behind the differential diagnoses

  D. Identifies information still needed to confirm the diagnoses

XIV. Treatment plan

  A. Biological

    1. Medications (e.g., name, dose, route, for what purpose, and patient's level of understanding of medication education)

    2. Diagnostic tests (e.g., where, when, and who will administer)

    3. Referrals for primary care

  B. Psychological

    1. Therapeutic modalities to be used and with what focus

      a. Individual psychotherapy?

      b. Group psychotherapy?

      c. Family therapy?

      d. Case management?

  C. Social

    1. Support or self-help groups

    2. Mobilization of family resources

    3. Vocational rehabilitation

    4. Financial planning

  D. Strengths

    1. Overt identification of patient strengths, values, and beliefs to support or draw from in implementing the identified treatment plan

Source: Data from American Psychiatric Association. (2016). *The American Psychiatric Association practice guidelines for the psychiatric evaluation of adults* (3rd ed.). Arlington, VA: American Psychiatric Association; Gordon, C., & Goroll, A. (2003). Effective psychiatric interviewing in primary care medicine. In T. A. Slavin, J. B. Herman, & P. L. Slavin (Eds.), *The MGH guide to psychiatry in primary care* (pp. 19–26). New York, NY: McGraw-Hill; Marken, P. A., Schneiderhan, M. E., & Munro, S. (2005). Evaluation of psychiatric illness. In J. T. DiPrio, R. L. Talbert, G. C. Yee, G. R. Matzke, B. G. Wells, & L. M. Posey (Eds.), *Pharmacotherapy: A pathophysiologic approach* (6th ed., pp. 1123–1132). New York, NY: McGraw-Hill; Morrison, J. (2014). *The first interview* (4th ed.). New York, NY: Guilford Press; Sadock, B. J., Sadock, V. S., & Ruiz, P. (2015). *Kaplan & Sadock's synopsis of psychiatry: Behavioral sciences/clinical psychiatry* (11th ed.). Philadelphia, PA: Wolters Kluwer; Scully, J. H., & Thornhill, J. T., IV. (2012). The clinical examination. In J. T. Thornhill, IV (Ed.), *The national medical series for independent study: Psychiatry* (6th ed., pp. 1–16). Philadelphia, PA: Lippincott Williams & Wilkins; Shea, S. C. (2017). *Psychiatric interviewing: The art of understanding* (3rd ed.). New York, NY: Elsevier.

APPENDIX 3.2
Sample Assessment Form

INITIAL CLINICAL ASSESSMENT

Identifying Data

Name of Patient:_____

Date: _____

DOB: _____ Age: _____

Sex: _____ Sexual Preference: _____

Marital Status: _____ Children: _____

Race/Ethnicity:_____

Religious Preference:_____

Patient-Identified Problem (Patient's Own Words) and Referral Source

1. History of current illness
   A. Stressors and symptoms: include current stressors and detailed chronologic history of symptoms for each diagnosis on axes I and II. Detail current substance abuse and the amount and pattern of use.
   B. Recent suicide or homicide ideation or behavior: include all ideation, gestures, attempts, presence or absence of hopelessness, and extent of actions or plans in the past month.
2. Psychiatric history
   A. Episodes and treatment: describe previous episodes of current disorder and all other disorders, including treatment modalities such as hospitalization, psychotherapy, and medications and their dosages.
   B. History of trauma: list the 10 most significant traumas. Do a timeline, and rate the disturbance for each event on a scale of 0 to 10; you can also ask for significant positive and negative events in the person's life. Administer the Impact of Events Scale and Dissociative Experiences Scale if trauma is suspected or reported.
   C. History of violence
      To self:
      To others:
      To property:
3. Psychiatric review of systems: circle all relevant symptoms, and add any not listed
   A. Mood: sadness, tearfulness, depressed mood, irritability, fatigue, lethargy, anergia, anhedonia, sleep changes, appetite changes, decreased libido, hopelessness, helplessness, worthlessness, suicide ideation, homicide ideation, spending sprees, increased energy or activity, decreased need for sleep, increased libido, pressured speech, tangentiality, and flight of ideas.
   B. Anxiety: anxious mood, excessive worry, shortness of breath, heart palpitations, panic attacks, sweating, flushing, hyperventilation, sense of impending doom, fear of death or collapse, cold/clammy skin, and tingling sensations in extremities.

(continued)

    C. Thought disorder: auditory or visual hallucinations, other hallucinations, ideas of reference, paranoia, delusions, thought insertion, thought blocking, thought broadcasting, flight of ideas, hyper-religiosity, tangentiality, looseness of associations, and bizarre behavior.

4. Drug and alcohol history

    A. Episodes and treatment: describe previous episodes of current disorder and all other disorders, including treatment modalities such as hospitalization, psychotherapy, and medications and their dosages.

    B. Substance abuse profile:

Substance	Current Amount	Date Last Used
Alcohol (use CAGE if abuse suspected but denied)		
Tetrahydrocannabinol (THC)		
Cocaine, crack, speed		
LSD, mescaline, psilocybin		
Barbiturates, other sedatives		
Caffeine, tobacco		
Over-the-counter drugs, herbal medications		

5. Medical history: List significant past illnesses, surgeries, or hospitalizations

    A. Primary care physician: _____

    B. Allergies: _____

    C. Medications: use the table to document: _____

Current Medication	Dosage	Taken as Prescribed?	
		Yes	No

6. Psychosocial history

    A. Education:

    B. Family relationships, social relationships, and abuse history:

    C. Employment record and military history:

    D. Religious background, belief system, or meaning framework:

    E. Patient's strengths: include patient resources and how patient self-soothes and manages stress.

7. Family history

    A. Genogram:

(continued)

CASE FORMULATION

Assessment of suicide or violence risk: _____

Treatment recommendations: _____

Admit to: _____

One-time consultation: _____

Refer to: _____

Referred for:

_____ Physical examination

_____ Individual psychotherapy

_____ Psychological testing

_____ Group psychotherapy

_____ Hospitalization

_____ Medications

_____ Support group

_____ Community support program services

Diagnostic summary:

Axis	Diagnoses, Factors, or Status	Codes	Alternatives to Rule Out
I. Clinical psychiatric syndromes	1. 2. 3.		
II. Personality and specific development disorders	1. 2. 3.		
III. Medical problems	1. 2. 3.		
IV. Psychosocial stressors*	1. 2. 3.		
V. Global assessment of functioning (GAF)	Current GAF Highest GAF in past year		

*Prioritize and rank severity: 1, none; 2, mild; 3, moderate; 4, severe; 5, extreme; 6, catastrophic; 7, unspecified.

Clinician's signature: _____

Date: _____

Location of assessment: _____

Source: Adapted from Shea, S. C. (2017). *Psychiatric interviewing: The art of understanding* (3rd ed.). New York, NY: Elsevier.

APPENDIX 3.3
Dissociative Experiences Scale (DES)

Name _____ Date _____ Age _____ Sex _____

Directions: This questionnaire consists of 28 questions about experiences that you may have in your daily life. We are interested in how often you have these experiences. It is important, however, that your answers show how often these experiences happen to you when you are *not* under the influence of alcohol or drugs. To answer the questions, please determine to what degree the experience described in the question applies to you and circle the number to show what percentage of the time you have the experience.

Example:

0%	10	20	30	40	50	60	70	80	90	100%
(never)										(always)

1. Some people have the experience of driving a car and suddenly realizing that they don't remember what has happened during all or part of the trip. Circle a number to show what percentage of the time this happens to you.

   0%   10   20   30   40   50   60   70   80   90   100%

2. Some people find that sometimes they are listening to someone talk and they suddenly realize that they did not hear all or part of what was said. Circle a number to show what percentage of the time this happens to you.

   0%   10   20   30   40   50   60   70   80   90   100%

3. Some people have the experience of finding themselves in a place and having no idea how they got there. Circle a number to show what percentage of the time this happens to you.

   0%   10   20   30   40   50   60   70   80   90   100%

4. Some people have the experience of finding themselves dressed in clothes that they don't remember putting on. Circle a number to show what percentage of the time this happens to you.

   0%   10   20   30   40   50   60   70   80   90   100%

5. Some people have the experience of finding new things among their belongings that they do not remember buying. Circle a number to show what percentage of the time this happens to you.

   0%   10   20   30   40   50   60   70   80   90   100%

6. Some people sometimes find that they are approached by people that they do not know who call them by another name or insist that they have met them before. Circle a number to show what percentage of the time this happens to you.

   0%   10   20   30   40   50   60   70   80   90   100%

(continued)

7. Some people sometimes have the experience of feeling as though they are standing next to themselves or watching themselves do something as if they were looking at another person. Circle a number to show what percentage of the time this happens to you.

0%   10   20   30   40   50   60   70   80   90   100%

8. Some people are told that they sometimes do not recognize friends or family members. Circle a number to show what percentage of the time this happens to you.

0%   10   20   30   40   50   60   70   80   90   100%

9. Some people find that they have no memory for some important events in their lives (for example, a wedding or graduation). Circle a number to show what percentage of the time this happens to you.

0%   10   20   30   40   50   60   70   80   90   100%

10. Some people have the experience of being accused of lying when they do not think that they have lied. Circle a number to show what percentage of the time this happens to you.

0%   10   20   30   40   50   60   70   80   90   100%

11. Some people have the experience of looking in a mirror and not recognizing themselves. Circle a number to show what percentage of the time this happens to you.

0%   10   20   30   40   50   60   70   80   90   100%

12. Some people sometimes have the experience of feeling that other people, objects, and the world around them are not real. Circle a number to show what percentage of the time this happens to you.

0%   10   20   30   40   50   60   70   80   90   100%

13. Some people sometimes have the experience of feeling that their body does not belong to them. Circle a number to show what percentage of the time this happens to you.

0%   10   20   30   40   50   60   70   80   90   100%

14. Some people have the experience of sometimes remembering a past event so vividly that they feel as if they were reliving that event. Circle a number to show what percentage of the time this happens to you.

0%   10   20   30   40   50   60   70   80   90   100%

15. Some people have the experience of not being sure whether things that they remember happening really did happen or whether they just dreamed them. Circle a number to show what percentage of the time this happens to you.

0%   10   20   30   40   50   60   70   80   90   100%

(*continued*)

16. Some people have the experience of being in a familiar place but finding it strange and unfamiliar. Circle a number to show what percentage of the time this happens to you.

0%   10   20   30   40   50   60   70   80   90   100%

17. Some people find that when they are watching television or a movie they become so absorbed in the story that they are unaware of other events happening around them. Circle a number to show what percentage of the time this happens to you.

0%   10   20   30   40   50   60   70   80   90   100%

18. Some people sometimes find that they become so involved in a fantasy or daydream that it feels as though it were really happening to them. Circle a number to show what percentage of the time this happens to you.

0%   10   20   30   40   50   60   70   80   90   100%

19. Some people find that they are sometimes able to ignore pain. Circle a number to show what percentage of the time this happens to you.

0%   10   20   30   40   50   60   70   80   90   100%

20. Some people find that they sometimes sit staring off into space, thinking of nothing, and are not aware of the passage of time. Circle a number to show what percentage of the time this happens to you.

0%   10   20   30   40   50   60   70   80   90   100%

21. Some people sometimes find that when they are alone they talk out loud to themselves. Circle a number to show what percentage of the time this happens to you.

0%   10   20   30   40   50   60   70   80   90   100%

22. Some people find that in one situation they may act so differently compared with another situation that they feel almost as if they were different people. Circle a number to show what percentage of the time this happens to you.

0%   10   20   30   40   50   60   70   80   90   100%

23. Some people sometimes find that in certain situations they are able to do things with amazing ease and spontaneity that would usually be difficult for them (for example, sports, work, social situations, and so on). Circle a number to show what percentage of the time this happens to you.

0%   10   20   30   40   50   60   70   80   90   100%

24. Some people sometimes find that they cannot remember whether they have done something or have just thought about doing that thing (for example, not knowing whether they have just mailed a letter or have just thought about mailing it). Circle a number to show what percentage of the time this happens to you.

0%   10   20   30   40   50   60   70   80   90   100%

(continued)

25. Some people find evidence that they have done things that they do not remember doing. Circle a number to show what percentage of the time this happens to you.

0%   10   20   30   40   50   60   70   80   90   100%

26. Some people sometimes find writings, drawings, or notes among their belongings that they must have done but cannot remember doing. Circle a number to show what percentage of the time this happens to you.

0%   10   20   30   40   50   60   70   80   90   100%

27. Some people find that they sometimes hear voices inside their head that tell them to do things or comment on things that they are doing. Circle a number to show what percentage of the time this happens to you.

0%   10   20   30   40   50   60   70   80   90   100%

28. Some people sometimes feel as if they are looking at the world through a fog so that people or objects appear far away or unclear. Circle a number to show what percentage of the time this happens to you.

0%   10   20   30   40   50   60   70   80   90   100%

Source: Adapted from Carlson, E. B., & Putnam, F. W. (1993). *Manual for the dissociative experiences scale.* Lutherville, MD: Sidran Foundation.

APPENDIX 3.4
The Impact of Event Scale (IES)

The table contains comments made by people after stressful life events. Using the scale, please indicate how frequently each of these comments was true for you during the past 7 days.

Comment	0 Not at All	1 Rarely	3 Sometimes	4 Often
I thought about it when I did not mean to.				
I avoided letting myself get upset when I thought about it or was reminded of it.				
I tried to remove it from memory.				
I had trouble falling asleep or staying asleep because of pictures or thoughts about it that came into my mind.				
I had waves of strong feelings about it.				
I had dreams about it.				
I stayed away from reminders of it.				
I felt as if it had not happened or was not real.				
Pictures about it popped into my mind.				
Other things kept making me think about it.				

(continued)

Comment	0 Not at All	1 Rarely	3 Sometimes	4 Often
I was aware that I still had a lot of feelings about it, but I did not deal with them.				
I tried not to think about it.				
Any reminder brought back feelings about it.				
My feelings about it were kind of numb.				
Total Score _____ > 26 = moderate or severe impact				

Source: Adapted from Horowitz, M., Wilner, M., & Alvarez, W. (1979). Impact of event scale: A measure of subjective stress. *Psychosomatic Medicine, 41,* 209–218. doi:10.1097/00006842-197905000-00004; Weiss, D. S. (2004). The impact of event scale—Revised. In J. Wilson & T. Keane (Eds.), *Assessing psychological trauma and PTSD* (2nd ed., pp. 168–189). New York, NY: Guilford Press.

APPENDIX 3.5
Zung Self-Rating Depression Scale (ZSRDS)

Please read each sentence carefully. For each of the 20 statements, place a check mark in the column that best describes how often you have felt that way during the past two weeks.

Comment	None or Little of the Time	Some of the Time	Good Part of the Time	Most of the Time
1. I feel downhearted, blue, and sad.				
2. Morning is when I feel the best.				
3. I have crying spells or feel like it.				
4. I have trouble sleeping through the night.				
5. I eat as much as I used to.				
6. I still enjoy sex.				
7. I notice that I am losing weight.				
8. I have trouble with constipation.				
9. My heart beats faster than usual.				
10. I get tired for no reason.				
11. My mind is as clear as it used to be.				

(continued)

Comment	None or Little of the Time	Some of the Time	Good Part of the Time	Most of the Time
12. I find it easy to do the things I used to do.				
13. I am restless and can't keep still.				
14. I feel hopeful about the future.				
15. I am more irritable than usual.				
16. I find it easy to make decisions.				
17. I feel that I am useful and needed.				
18. My life is pretty full.				
19. I feel that others would be better off if I were dead.				
20. I still enjoy the things I used to do.				

Source: Adapted from Zung, W. W. (1965). A self-rating depression scale. *Archives of General Psychiatry, 12*(1):63–70. doi:10.1001/archpsyc.1965.01720310065008.

APPENDIX 3.6
Geriatric Depression Scale (GDS; Short Form)

Circle the appropriate answer.

1.	Are you basically satisfied with your life?	Yes	No
2.	Have you dropped many of your activities and interests?	Yes	No
3.	Do you feel that your life is empty?	Yes	No
4.	Do you often get bored?	Yes	No
5.	Are you in good spirits most of the time?	Yes	No
6.	Are you afraid that something bad is going to happen to you?	Yes	No
7.	Do you feel happy most of the time?	Yes	No
8.	Do you often feel helpless?	Yes	No
9.	Do you prefer to stay at home rather than go out and do new things?	Yes	No
10.	Do you feel you have more problems with memory than most?	Yes	No
11.	Do you think it is wonderful to be alive now?	Yes	No
12.	Do you feel pretty worthless the way you are now?	Yes	No
13.	Do you feel full of energy?	Yes	No
14.	Do you feel that your situation is hopeless?	Yes	No
15.	Do you think that most people are better off than you are?	Yes	No

Score: _____/15

Assign 1 point for "No" to questions 1, 5, 7, 11, and 13
Assign 1 point for "Yes" to other questions

Results:
0–4   normal, depending on age, education, and complaints
5–8   mild
8–11   moderate
12–15   severe

Source: Adapted from Yesavage, J. A., Brink, T. L., Rose, T. L., Lum, O., Huang, V., & Adey, M. B. (1983). Development and validation of a geriatric depression screening scale: A preliminary report. *Journal of Psychiatric Research, 17,* 37–49. doi:10.1016/0022-3956(82)90033-4

APPENDIX 3.7
Geriatric Depression Scale (GDS; Short Form)

Over the *past 2 weeks*, how often have you been bothered by any of the following problems?

	Not at All	Several Days	More Than Half the Days	Nearly Every Day
	0	1	2	3
1. Little interest or pleasure in doing things	☐	☐	☐	☐
2. Feeling down, depressed, or hopeless	☐	☐	☐	☐
3. Trouble falling/staying asleep, sleeping too much	☐	☐	☐	☐
4. Feeling tired or having little energy	☐	☐	☐	☐
5. Poor appetite or overeating	☐	☐	☐	☐
6. Feeling bad about yourself—or that you are a failure or have let yourself or your family down	☐	☐	☐	☐
7. Trouble concentrating on things, such as reading the newspaper or watching television	☐	☐	☐	☐
8. Moving or speaking so slowly that other people could have noticed. Or the opposite—being so fidgety or restless that you have been moving around a lot more than usual	☐	☐	☐	☐
9. Thoughts that you would be better off dead or of hurting yourself in some way	☐	☐	☐	☐

(continued)

If you checked off any problem on this questionnaire so far, how difficult have these problems made it for you to do your work, take care of things at home, or get along with other people?

Not Difficult at All	Somewhat Difficult	Very Difficult	Extremely Difficult
☐	☐	☐	☐

Total Score: _____

Source: Developed by Drs. Robert L. Spitzer, Janet B. W. Williams, Kurt Kroenke, and colleagues, with an educational grant from Pfizer Inc. No permission required to reproduce, translate, display, or distribute. Available at www.pfizer.com

APPENDIX 3.8
Young Mania Rating Scale (YMRS)

Elevated Mood:
0 Absent
1 Mildly, or possibly elevated on questioning
2 Definite subjective elevation: optimistic, cheerful, self-confident; appropriate to content
3 Elevated; inappropriate to content; humorous
4 Euphoric; inappropriate laughter; singing

Increased Motor Activity/Energy:
0 Absent
1 Subjectively increased
2 Animated; gestures increased
3 Excessive energy; hyperactive at times; can be calmed
4 Motor excitement; continuous hyperactivity; cannot be calmed

Sexual Interest:
0 Normal; not increased
1 Mildly, or possibly increased
2 Definitive subjective increase on questioning
3 Spontaneous sexual content; elaborates on sexual matters; hypersexual by self-report
4 Overt sexual acts (toward interviewer, staff, patients)

Sleep:
0 Reports no decrease in sleep
1 Sleeping less than normal by up to 1 hour
2 Sleeping less than normal by more than 1 hour
3 Reports decreased need for sleep
4 Denies need for sleep

Language/Thought Disorder:
0 Absent
1 Circumstantial; mild distractibility; quick thoughts
2 Distractible; loses goal of thought; changes topics frequently; racing thoughts
3 Flight of ideas; tangentiality; difficult to follow
4 Incoherent; communication impossible

Content:
0 Normal
2 Questionable plans; new interests
4 Special projects; hyper-religious
6 Grandiose or paranoid; ideas of reference
8 Delusions; hallucinations

Disruptive/Aggressive Behavior:
0 Absent; cooperative
2 Sarcastic; loud at times; guarded
4 Demanding; threats on ward
6 Threatens interviewer; shouting; interview difficult
8 Assaultive; destructive; interview impossible

Appearance:
0 Appropriate dress and grooming
1 Minimally unkempt
2 Poorly groomed; moderately disheveled; overdressed
3 Disheveled; partly clothed; garish makeup
4 Completely unkempt; decorated; bizarre garb

(continued)

Irritability:

0 Absent
1 Subjective increased
2 Irritable at times during interview; recent episodes of anger or annoyance on ward
3 Frequently irritable during interview; short and curt throughout interview
4 Hostile; uncooperative; interview impossible

Insight:

0 Present; admits illness; agrees with need for treatment
1 Possibly ill
2 Admits behavior change, but denies illness
3 Admits possible behavior change, but denies illness
4 Denies any behavior change

Speech (Rate and Amount):

0 No increase
2 Feels talkative
4 Increased rate or amount at times; verbose
6 Push; consistently increased rate or amount; difficult to interrupt
8 Pressured; uninterruptible; continuous speech

Guide for scoring items—the purpose of each item is to rate the severity of the abnormality in the patient. When several keys are given for a particular grade of severity, the presence of only one is required to qualify for that rating.

Source: Reproduced with permission from Young, R. C., Biggs, J. T., Ziegler, V. E., & Meyer, D. A. (1978). A rating scale for mania: Reliability, validity, and sensitivity. *British Journal of Psychiatry, 133*, 429–435.

APPENDIX 3.9
Hamilton Anxiety Rating Scale (HAM-A)

0 = None
1 = Mild
2 = Moderate
3 = Severe
4 = Grossly disabling

Anxious: worries, anticipates the worst, irritable	0	1	2	3	4
Tension: tense, fatigued, startles easily, trembling, restless, unable to relax	0	1	2	3	4
Fears: of the dark, strangers, animals, crowds, traffic, being alone	0	1	2	3	4
Insomnia: difficulty falling asleep or staying asleep, fatigue on waking, dreams, nightmares, night terrors	0	1	2	3	4
Intellectual: difficulty concentrating, poor memory	0	1	2	3	4
Depressed mood: loss of interest, lack of pleasure in activities, early waking, diurnal swing, depression	0	1	2	3	4
Somatic complaints (muscular): muscle aches and pains, bruxism, stiffness, myoclonus, unsteady voice	0	1	2	3	4
Somatic complaints (sensory): tinnitus, blurred vision, flushing, weakness, tingling sensations	0	1	2	3	4
Cardiovascular symptoms: tachycardia, chest pain, palpitations, throbbing vessels, feeling faint	0	1	2	3	4
Respiratory symptoms: shortness of breath, sighing, chest pressure or constriction, choking sensation	0	1	2	3	4
Gastrointestinal symptoms: difficulty swallowing, nausea, vomiting, constipation, bloating, weight loss	0	1	2	3	4
Autonomic symptoms: dry mouth, pallor, flushing, sweating, tension headache, goose bumps	0	1	2	3	4
Behavior at the interview: fidgeting, pacing, tremor, swallowing, sighing, belching, dilated pupils	0	1	2	3	4

Source: Adapted from Hamilton, M. (1959). The assessment of anxiety states by rating. *British Journal of Medical Psychology, 32,* 50–55. doi:10.1111/j.2044-8341.1959.tb00467.x

APPENDIX 3.10
Generalized Anxiety Disorder Questionnaire (GAD-7)

Over the past 2 weeks, how often have you been bothered by any of the following problems?

	Not at All	Several Days	More Than Half the Days	Nearly Every Day
	0	1	2	3
1. Feeling nervous, anxious, or on edge	☐	☐	☐	☐
2. Not being able to stop or control worrying	☐	☐	☐	☐
3. Worrying too much about different things	☐	☐	☐	☐
4. Trouble relaxing	☐	☐	☐	☐
5. Being so restless that it is hard to sit still	☐	☐	☐	☐
6. Becoming easily annoyed or irritable	☐	☐	☐	☐
7. Feeling afraid as if something awful might happen	☐	☐	☐	☐

If you checked off any problem on this questionnaire so far, how difficult have these problems made it for you to do your work, take care of things at home, or get along with other people?

Not Difficult at All	Somewhat Difficult	Very Difficult	Extremely Difficult
☐	☐	☐	☐

Total Score: _____

Source: Developed by Drs. Robert L. Spitzer, Janet B. W. Williams, Kurt Kroenke, and colleagues, with an educational grant from Pfizer Inc. No permission required to reproduce, translate, display, or distribute. Available at www.pfizer.com

APPENDIX 3.11
Yale-Brown Obsessive–Compulsive Scale (Y-BOCS)

Circle the average occurrence of each item during the prior week up to and including the time of interview.

Obsession Rating Scales

1. **Time spent on obsessions**
   0 = 0 hr/day
   1 = 0–1 hr/day
   2 = 1–3 hr/day
   3 = 3–8 hr/day
   4 = >8 hr/day
2. **Interference from obsessions**
   0 = None
   1 = Mild
   2 = Definite but manageable
   3 = Substantial impairment
   4 = Incapacitating
3. **Distress from obsessions**
   0 = None
   1 = Mild
   2 = Moderate but manageable
   3 = Severe
   4 = Near constant/disabling
4. **Resistance to obsessions**
   0 = Always resists
   1 = Much resistance
   2 = Some resistance
   3 = Often yields
   4 = Completely yields
5. **Control over obsessions**
   0 = Complete control
   1 = Much control
   2 = Some control
   3 = Little control
   4 = No control

Compulsion Rating Scale

6. **Time spent on compulsions**
   0 = 0 hr/day
   1 = 0–1 hr/day
   2 = 1–3 hr/day
   3 = 3–8 hr/day
   4 = >8 hr/day
7. **Interference from compulsions**
   0 = None
   1 = Mild
   2 = Definite but manageable
   3 = Substantial impairment
   4 = Incapacitating
8. **Distress from compulsions**
   0 = None
   1 = Mild
   2 = Moderate but manageable
   3 = Severe
   4 = Near constant/disabling
9. **Resistance to compulsions**
   0 = Always resists
   1 = Much resistance
   2 = Some resistance
   3 = Often yields
   4 = Completely yields
10. **Control over compulsions**
    0 = Complete control
    1 = Much control
    2 = Some control
    3 = Little control
    4 = No control

Obsession subtotal (add items 1–5):

_____

Compulsion subtotal (add items 6–10):

_____

Y-BOCS total score (add items 1–10):

_____

Range of severity (scores for patients who have both obsessions and compulsions):

Subclinical: 0–7
Mild: 9–15
Moderate: 16–23
Severe: 24–31
Extreme: 32–40

Source: Adapted from Goodman, W. K., Price, L. H., Rasmussen, S. A., Mazure, C., Fleischmann, R. I., Hill, C. L., . . . Charney, D. S. (1989). The Yale-Brown obsessive-compulsive scale I. Development, use, and reliability. *Archives of General Psychiatry, 46,* 1006–1011. doi:10.1001/archpsyc.1989.01810110048007

APPENDIX 3.12
Quality-of-Life Scale (QOL)

Please read each item and circle the number that best describes how satisfied you are at this time. Answer each item even if you do not currently participate in an activity or have a relationship. You can be satisfied or dissatisfied with not doing the activity or having the relationship.

Scoring
7 = Delighted
6 = Pleased
5 = Mostly satisfied
4 = Mixed
3 = Mostly dissatisfied
2 = Unhappy
1 = Terrible

Material comforts (e.g., home, food, conveniences, financial security)	7	6	5	4	3	2	1
Health (i.e., being physically fit and vigorous)	7	6	5	4	3	2	1
Relationships with parents, siblings, other relatives (e.g., communicating, visiting, helping)	7	6	5	4	3	2	1
Having and rearing children	7	6	5	4	3	2	1
Close relationships with spouse or significant other	7	6	5	4	3	2	1
Close friends	7	6	5	4	3	2	1
Helping and encouraging others, volunteering, giving advice	7	6	5	4	3	2	1
Participating in organizations and public affairs	7	6	5	4	3	2	1
Learning (e.g., attending school, improving understanding, getting more knowledge)	7	6	5	4	3	2	1
Understanding yourself (e.g., knowing your assets and limitations, knowing what life is all about)	7	6	5	4	3	2	1
Work (job or in home)	7	6	5	4	3	2	1
Expressing yourself creatively	7	6	5	4	3	2	1
Socializing (e.g., meeting other people, doing things, parties)	7	6	5	4	3	2	1

(continued)

Reading, listening to music, or observing entertainment	7	6	5	4	3	2	1
Participating in active recreation	7	6	5	4	3	2	1
Independence (i.e., doing for yourself)	7	6	5	4	3	2	1

Source: Adapted from Flanagan, J. D. (1982). Measurement of quality of life: Current state of the art. *Archives of Physical Medicine and Rehabilitation, 63,* 56–59; Burckhardt, C. S., Woods, S. L., Schultz, A. A., & Ziebarth, D. M. (1989). Quality of life in adults with chronic illness: A psychometric study. *Research in Nursing and Health, 12,* 347–354. doi:10.1002/nur.4770120604

APPENDIX 3.13
CAGE Questionnaire

Name: _____

Date: _____

CAGE score: _____

1. Have you ever felt you should **C**ut down on your drinking?   Yes   No

2. Have people **A**nnoyed you by criticizing your drinking?   Yes   No

3. Have you ever felt bad or **G**uilty about your drinking?   Yes   No

4. Have you had an **E**ye-opener first thing in the morning to steady nerves or get rid of a hangover?   Yes   No

Scoring: Assign 1 point for each "Yes" answer. A score of 1 to 3 should alert the examiner and warrants further evaluation.

Score of 1: 80% are alcohol dependent
Score of 2: 89% are alcohol dependent
Score of 3: 99% are alcohol dependent
Score of 4: 100% are alcohol dependent

Source: Adapted from Ewing, J. A. (1984). Detecting alcoholism: The CAGE questionnaire. *Journal of the American Medical Association, 252*(14), 1905–1907. doi:10.1001/jama.252.14.1905

APPENDIX 3.14
The Alcohol Use Disorders Identification Test (AUDIT)

Check the response that is correct for you.

1. How often do you have a drink containing alcohol?
   ____never (0 points)
   ____less than monthly / monthly (1 point)
   ____2-4 times/month (2 points)
   ____2-3 times/week (3 points
   ____4 or more times/week (4 points)

2. How many standard drinks containing alcohol do you have on a typical day when drinking?
   ____1-2 (0 points)
   ____3-4 (1 point)
   ____5-6 (2 points)
   ____7-9 (3 points)
   ____10 or more (4 points)

3. How often do you have six or more drinks on one occasion?
   ____never (0 points)
   ____less than monthly (1 point)
   ____monthly (2 points)
   ____weekly (3 points)
   ____daily or almost daily (4 points)

4. During the past year, how often have you found that you were not able to stop drinking once you had started?
   ____never (0 points)
   ____less than monthly (1 point)
   ____monthly (2 points)
   ____weekly (3 points)
   ____daily or almost daily (4 points)

5. During the past year, how often have you failed to do what was normally expected of you because of drinking?
   ____never (0 points)
   ____less than monthly (1 point)
   ____monthly (2 points)
   ____weekly (3 points)
   ____daily or almost daily (4 points)

6. During the past year, how often have you needed a drink in the morning to get yourself going after a heavy drinking session?
   ____never (0 points)
   ____less than monthly (1 point)
   ____monthly (2 points)
   ____weekly (3 points)
   ____daily or almost daily (4 points)

7. During the past year, how often have you had a feeling of guilt or remorse after drinking?
   ____never (0 points)
   ____less than monthly (1 point)
   ____monthly (2 points)
   ____weekly (3 points)
   ____daily or almost daily (4 points)

8. During the past year, have you been unable to remember what happened the night before because you had been drinking?
   ____never (0 points)
   ____less than monthly (1 point)
   ____monthly (2 points)
   ____weekly (3 points)
   ____daily or almost daily (4 points)

9. Have you or someone else been injured as a result of your drinking?
   ____no (0 points)
   ____yes, but not in the last year (2 points)
   ____yes, during the last year (4 points)

10. Has a relative or friend, doctor or other health worker been concerned about your drinking or suggested you cut down?
    ____no (0 points)
    ____yes, but not in the last year (2 points)
    ____yes, during the last year (4 points)

(continued)

Scoring the AUDIT

A score of 8 or more is associated with harmful or hazardous drinking. A score of 13 or more in women and 15 or more in men is likely to indicate alcohol dependence.

Source: Adapted from Saunders, J. B., Aasland, O. G., Babor, T. F., De La Fuente, J. R., & Grant, M. (1993). Development of the alcohol use disorders identification test (AUDIT): WHO collaborative project on early detection of persons with harmful alcohol consumption—II. Addiction, 88(6), 791–804. doi:10.1111/j.1360-0443.1993.tb02093.x. Tool is available in the public domain, online, at auditscreen.org.

APPENDIX 3.15
Child Attachment Interview (CAI) Protocol

Introduction: This is an interview not a test; want to know what things are like in your family; want to understand your point of view.

1. Can you tell me about the people in your family?
   - The people living together in your house?
   - Extended family?
2. Tell me three words that describe you, that is, what sort of person you are.
   - Examples.
3. Can you tell me three words to describe your relationship with your Mom, that is, what it is like to be with your Mom?
   - Examples for each.
4. What happens when your Mom gets cross with you or tells you off?
   - Story.
   (Questions 3 and 4 repeated for Dad or other main caregivers)
5. Can you tell me about a time when you were really upset and wanted help?
   - Story.
6. Do you ever feel that your parents don't really love you?
   - When? Do they know you feel that?
7. What happens when you are ill?
   - Example.
8. What happens when you get hurt?
   - Example.
9. Have you ever been hit or hurt by an older child or a grown-up in your family?
   - Story.
   - Have you been badly hurt by someone outside your family?
10. (Elementary school-age children:) Have you ever been touched in the private parts of your body by someone much older than you? (For older children:) Have you ever been touched sexually by someone when you did not want him or her to do it?
    - Story.
11. Has anything (else) really big happened to you that upset, scared, or confused you?
    - Story.
12. Has anyone important to you ever died? Has a pet you cared about died?
    - Story. What did you feel? What did others feel?
13. Is there anyone whom you cared about who is not around anymore?
    - Story.
14. Have you been away from your parents for longer than a day? (If child is not living with parents [e.g., is in foster care], ask about a time when he or she left parents.)
    - Story. How did you and your parents feel? What was it like when you saw them again?
15. Do your parents sometimes argue?
    - Story. How do you feel?
16. In what ways would you like/not like to be like your Mom/Dad?
17. If you could make three wishes when you are older, what would they be?

Source: Shmueli-Goetz, Y., Target, M., Fonagy, P., & Datta, A. (2008). The child attachment interview: A psychometric study of reliability and discriminant validity. *Developmental Psychology,* 44(4), 939–956. doi:10.1037/0012-1649.44.4.939. Adapted with permission from the publisher: American Psychological Association.

APPENDIX 3.16
Adverse Childhood Experiences Scale

While you were growing up, during your first 18 years of life:

1. Did a parent or other adult in the household **often or very often** . . .
   Swear at you, insult you, put you down, or humiliate you?
   or
   Act in a way that made you afraid that you might be physically hurt?
   Yes   No   If yes enter 1_____

2. Did a parent or other adult in the household **often or very often** . . .
   Push, grab, slap, or throw something at you?
   or
   Ever hit you so hard that you had marks or were injured?
   Yes   No   If yes enter 1_____

3. Did an adult or person at least 5 years older than you **ever** . . .
   Touch or fondle you or have you touch their body in a sexual way?
   or
   Attempt or actually have oral, anal, or vaginal intercourse with you?
   Yes   No   If yes enter 1_____

4. Did you **often or very often** feel that . . .
   No one in your family loved you or thought you were important or special?
   or
   Your family didn't look out for each other, feel close to each other, or support each other?
   Yes   No   If yes enter 1_____

5. Did you **often** or **very often** feel that . . .
   You didn't have enough to eat, had to wear dirty clothes, and had no one to protect you?
   or
   Your parents were too drunk or high to take care of you or take you to the doctor if you needed it?
   Yes   No   If yes enter 1_____

6. Were your parents **ever** separated or divorced?
   Yes   No   If yes enter 1_____

7. Was your mother or stepmother:
   Often or very often pushed, grabbed, slapped, or had something thrown at her?
   or
   Sometimes, often, or very often kicked, bitten, hit with a fist, or hit with something hard?
   or

(continued)

Ever repeatedly hit at least a few minutes or threatened with a gun or knife?
Yes   No   If yes enter 1_____

8. Did you live with anyone who was a problem drinker or alcoholic or who used street drugs?
Yes   No   If yes enter 1_____

9. Was a household member depressed or mentally ill, or did a household member attempt suicide?
Yes   No   If yes enter 1_____

10. Did a household member go to prison?
Yes   No   If yes enter 1_____

Now add up your "Yes" answers: . This is your ACE Score.

4

The Initial Contact and Maintaining the Frame

Kathleen Wheeler
with Michael J. Rice

The two most important goals of the first session are to initiate a therapeutic alliance and to assess safety. Both are foundational to the treatment hierarchy described in Chapter 1, and they provide the basis for the psychotherapeutic process. The psychobiological underpinnings of the therapeutic alliance are discussed in Chapter 2, in light of Porges's research on neuroception. Neuroception takes place without our conscious awareness and tells us whether situations or people are safe, dangerous, or life threatening (Porges, 2004). This chapter discusses strategies that enhance and/or allow the person who comes for help to feel safe in relationship in order to do the work of psychotherapy. It is only in a safe environment that one is able to inhibit defense systems and engage with the therapist. The therapeutic alliance fosters the ventral vagal response or resilient zone so that the emotional safety of the healing environment allows the patient to continue psychotherapy and to benefit from treatment. Safety issues also include assessment of how safe the patient is from himself or herself and from others. The first contact with the patient is described in this chapter along with issues germane to the first session, such as making practical arrangements, setting goals, how to end a session, and what records to keep. Therapeutic communication techniques are reviewed.

The other important dimension to psychotherapy is maintaining the frame of the session. The *frame* refers to the parameters of the psychotherapeutic relationship and includes maintaining appropriate boundaries and safeguarding the rules of therapy. Maintaining the frame is relevant for all models of psychotherapy and ensures that the patient is in a safe environment for the emotional intensity that often accompanies the therapy process. Although the rules may seem strange and arbitrary to the novice psychotherapist, they are of paramount importance in safeguarding the integrity, structure, consistency, and objectivity of the relationship. Attention to the frame of traditional psychotherapy facilitates the best possibility of clinical improvement and personal growth. The therapist is responsible for keeping the frame of the sessions.

The frame provides guidelines for the parameters of therapy, such as adherence to a schedule, fees, confidentiality, therapeutic relationship boundaries, and for minor but important issues during sessions, such as whether eating or smoking or interruptions are allowed during sessions, phone calls between sessions, and starting or stopping on time. By being consistent and trustworthy, punctual, unconditionally accepting, keeping commitments, maintaining boundaries while at the same time being caring, warm, and available, the advanced practice psychiatric nurse (APPN) facilitates neural integration. This chapter begins with a discussion of boundaries and countertransference, self-disclosure, fees, and how to deal with patients who are late or who do not show up for sessions. Change is always fraught with anxiety, and understanding violations of the frame as manifestations of anxiety is key to developing communication strategies that meet this challenge.

DEVELOPING A THERAPEUTIC ALLIANCE

The therapeutic alliance is initiated in the first contact with the patient, and the first several sessions are crucial for laying the foundation for the therapist's connection with the patient. The therapeutic alliance enables the patient to continue and benefit from treatment. Meta-analytic research studies have found that the therapeutic alliance is itself therapeutic and essential for the successful outcome of treatment no matter what model of therapy is used (Norcross & Lambert, 2019). The percentage of improvement in psychotherapy patients is a function of various therapeutic factors and includes patient expectancy (i.e., the placebo effect), technique, extratherapeutic change (e.g., friends, family, self-help, group participation, and clergy), and common factors (e.g., therapist empathy, genuineness, warmth, acceptance, encouragement of risk taking, confidentiality of relationship, and the therapeutic alliance). In other words, what the therapist does is less important than how the therapist does it. Thus, process is more important than the technique, because the latter only accounts for 10% of change in psychotherapy outcome (Norcross & Lambert, 2019).

A challenge for the therapist is to engage the patient so that he or she will continue treatment. A meta-analysis of 669 studies shows that the dropout rate after the initial session is 20%, that is, one out of five patients terminated treatment before meeting the goals of the proposed treatment (Swift, Greenberg, Whipple, & Kominiak, 2012). Another meta-analysis of psychotherapy dropout and the therapeutic alliance indicates a moderately strong relationship between dropout and therapeutic alliance, that is, the weaker the alliance, the more likely the person will be to drop out of treatment (Sharf, Primavera, & Diener, 2010).

The ideal is to develop a basic level of trust and a shared agenda with the patient, which includes the collaborative goals of therapy. Three elements of the therapeutic alliance that most theorists agree with are the collaborative nature of the relationship, the warm, emotional bond between the patient and therapist, and the agreement between the therapist and patient on the goals of treatment (Flückiger, Del Re, Wampold, & Horvath, 2019). Competencies that reflect the therapist's ability to develop a therapeutic alliance include the ability to establish rapport, enable the patient to actively participate in the process, establish a treatment focus, provide a healing environment, and recognize and attempt to repair the alliance if needed. Cultivating the therapeutic alliance is an ongoing process throughout the therapy.

Horvath elaborates on the therapeutic alliance:

> *Developing the alliance takes precedence over technical interventions in the beginning of therapy. Therapists need to be sensitive to the risk that their own estimate of the status of the relationship, particularly in the opening phases of therapeutic work, can be at odds with the patients and such misjudgment may have costly consequences. Thus it seems prudent to actively solicit from patients their perspective on various aspects of the alliance and to negotiate flexibly the goals of treatment and even the content of therapy to secure their active collaboration and engagement. Particularly close attention is warranted in the early phases of work with the patient who is diagnosed with relational problems . . . these patients not only find it difficult to engage in an intimate relationship*

such as the one between therapist and patient, but they also are likely to solicit nega-
tive or rejecting therapist responses. The value of an open, flexible stance as opposed to
relational control or rigid expectations on the part of the therapist is a consistent theme
across much of the literature. The therapists who can complement the patient's relational
style and are able to demonstrate a capacity to collaborate (e.g., adopt the patient's ideas;
using the patient's ideas or expressions) seem to have a better chance of guiding good
alliances. On the other hand, therapists who were seen by patients as rigid or cold; were
rated as less effective and had poorer alliances. Negative or rejecting transactions seem
to have a particularly insidious impact on the alliance, and there are preliminary indica-
tions that such hostile therapist responses may be related to the therapist's own negative
introject. (Horvath, 2001, pp. 369–370)

Although numerous tools are available to measure the alliance, most therapists test the waters of the therapeutic alliance without the use of elaborate tools. One way is to ask the patient at the end of the first session: "How do you feel about working with me?" or "How did you feel about talking to me today?" or "How did you feel about coming here today?" Alternatively, the therapist can question the patient at the beginning of the next session: "How did you feel after the last session?" Patients may respond positively, or they may say something negative, such as: "My last therapist always was very involved, and I'm not sure you will be." It is important to explore all negative feelings that the person brings up. Often, novice psychotherapists are hesitant to open up any suggestion of negative feelings with the patient for fear that the person will be more likely to leave treatment. The exact opposite is true; exploring the person's negative feelings makes it much more likely that the person will stay in treatment (Cozolino, 2017).

Additionally, besides not exploring the patient's negative feelings or thoughts about the therapist or therapy, ineffective qualities of the therapeutic relationship have been identified and include the use of confrontation; therapist's comments that are critical, rejecting, or blaming; therapists who assume they know what their patient is feeling or thinking without asking; the therapist's rigidity to a treatment method without adapting it to the person; the therapist's perspective on the therapy relationship not the patient's perspective; and cultural ignorance (Norcross & Lambert, 2019). Thus, balancing fidelity to the treatment protocol with flexibility to the person is essential. The more knowledgeable the therapist about various treatment approaches, the better able the therapist will be in accommodating the approach to the patient rather than allegiance to a particular therapy.

What is most important for the beginning psychotherapist is learning how to develop the therapeutic alliance. Strategies for initiating and maintaining the therapeutic alliance include asking detailed questions about the patient's main concern, validating affect, explaining the therapy process as it unfolds, listening empathically without minimizing or offering "fix it" statements, and goal consensus and collaboration (Tryon & Winograd, 2011). Matching the therapist's style to the patient's needs (i.e., the therapist's ability to be an "authentic chameleon") facilitates the alliance (Lazarus, 1993). This requires the therapist to have facility in a range of techniques and a flexible repertoire of relationship styles to suit different patients' needs and expectations. Essential relationship building skills have been identified by Perraud and colleagues (2006) in order to assess APPN students' ability and are included in Box 4.1.

A search of the nursing literature on the therapeutic nurse relationship from 2000 to 2019 found almost 2,000 articles on the nurse-patient relationship, so clearly this is an important area for nursing. Core attributes of the therapeutic relationship in advanced psychiatric/mental health nursing have been deconstructed into nine main

BOX 4.1 Essential Relationship-Building Skills

Therapist Contributions to the Therapeutic Alliance

Make the development of the alliance the highest priority early in therapy.

Enter a collaborative partnership.

Listen to the patient's theory of illness and avoid reinterpreting it to match your own theory.

Allow the patient to direct therapeutic choices.

Attend to and address what the patient considers is important and relevant.

Agree on interventions—only use those that you feel confident will work.

Find out what the patient thinks would represent improvement.

Tailor interventions and homework to accomplish goals set by the patient.

Recognize attitudes and behaviors that cause the patients to react negatively and avoid them.

Explore patient hostility when it is directed toward you.

Engage in supervision to explore relational difficulties.

Be in touch with your own experience of the patient.

Respond honestly and sincerely.

Goal Consensus and Collaboration Skills

Use your clinical expertise to help patients clarify problems.

Address topics of importance to patients that fit with why they feel they have these problems.

Be an understanding and sympathetic listener.

Discuss and agree upon goals frequently.

Check on homework if given.

Source: Modified and adapted from Perraud, S., Delaney, K. R., Carlson-Sabelli, L., Johnson, M. E., Shephard, R., & Paun, O.(2006). Advanced practice psychiatric mental health nursing, finding our core: The therapeutic relationship in the 21st century. *Perspectives in Psychiatric Care*, *42*(4), 215–226. doi:10.1111/j.1744-6163.2006.00097.x

constructs: conveying understanding and empathy, accepting individuality, providing support, being there/being available, being genuine, promoting equality, demonstrating respect, maintaining clear boundaries, and having self-awareness (Dziopa & Ahern, 2009).

For some patients, physical safety is an issue, whether real or imagined. For the psychotic patient, fears of fragmentation and annihilation may be the norm (McWilliams, 2011). Even though psychotic patients may be compliant, it does not mean that they trust the therapist; they may adhere only out of fear of retribution if they do not. Clinicians who work with psychotic patients use various strategies to reduce the overwhelming anxiety experienced by these patients. Strategies include sitting farther away from the patient than usual, leaving the door open, taking as few notes as possible, giving information, communicating with emotional honesty and judicious self-disclosure, providing education, normalization of the patient's experience, asking the person what would make him or her feel safe, assuming a more authoritative role, using simple communications, and creating opportunities for the person to demonstrate personal competency.

ASSESSING SAFETY

Assessing safety is of paramount importance in the initial contact. Every patient should be asked about suicidal or homicidal thoughts in the initial session. Suicide is a leading cause of death in the United States with rates in every state increasing every year since 1999 (Center for Disease Control and Prevention [CDC], 2018). Although the patient with major depressive disorder usually is considered to be at particularly high risk, research has found those with schizophrenia, bipolar disorder, and substance use disorder are also at high risk (Olfson et al., 2016). However, more than half of those who committ suicide do not have a known mental health problem (CDC, 2018). Other significant risk factors include previous attempts, social alienation, a family history of suicide, interpersonal violence, relationship difficulties, and recent discharge from psychiatric hospital. Demographic risk factors include males, single, elderly, adolescent and young adults, and Caucasian (Fowler, 2012). The highest risk factor according to the CDC is a relationship problem (2018).

Suicidality can be screened with questionnaires such as the self-report Beck Depression Inventory (BDI), which has a question about suicidality, or a rating scale such as the Columbia-Suicide Severity Rating Scale available at cssrs.columbia.edu/docs/C-SSRS_1_14_09_Baseline.pdf, which has good normative data (Posner et al., 2011). In addition, an assessment tool, the Suicide Assessment Five-step Evaluation and Triage (SAFE-T) developed by Substance Abuse and Mental Health Services Administration (SAMHSA) and derived from the American Psychiatric Association Practice Guidelines, can be downloaded for free from store.samhsa.gov/product/SMA09-4432 and a free app is available that helps providers integrate suicide prevention strategies into their practice at store.samhsa.gov/apps/suicide-safe. The SAFE-T offers comprehensive guidelines that include an assessment of risk factors, protective factors that can be enhanced, and a scale to determine the level of risk and possible interventions. See Box 4.2 for the SAFE-T. If an assessment tool is used, open interview questions should follow up on all positive items.

BOX 4.2 SAFE-T

1. RISK FACTORS
   - **Suicidal behavior:** history of prior suicide attempts, aborted suicide attempts, or self-injurious behavior
   - **Current/past psychiatric disorders:** especially mood disorders, psychotic disorders, alcohol/substance abuse, ADHD, TBI, PTSD, cluster B personality disorders, conduct disorders (antisocial behavior, aggression, impulsivity)

   Comorbidity and recent onset of illness increase risk.
   - **Key symptoms:** anhedonia, impulsivity, hopelessness, anxiety/panic, global insomnia, command hallucinations
   - **Family history:** of suicide, attempts, or Axis I psychiatric disorders requiring hospitalization
   - **Precipitants/stressors/interpersonal:** triggering events leading to humiliation, shame, or despair (e.g. loss of relationship, financial or health status—real or anticipated). Ongoing medical illness (esp. CNS disorders, pain), intoxication. Family turmoil/chaos. History of physical or sexual abuse. Social isolation
   - **Change in treatment:** discharge from psychiatric hospital, provider or treatment change

(continued)

BOX 4.2 SAFE-T (*continued*)

2. **PROTECTIVE FACTORS** *Protective factors, even if present, may not counteract significant acute risk*
   - **Internal:** ability to cope with stress, religious beliefs, frustration, frustration tolerance
   - **External:** responsibility to children or beloved pets, positive therapeutic relationships, social supports
3. **SUICIDE INQUIRY** *Specific questioning about thoughts, plans, behaviors, intent*
   - **Ideation:** frequency, intensity, duration—in the past 48 hours, past month, and worst ever
   - **Plan:** timing, location, lethality, availability, preparatory acts
   - **Behaviors:** past attempts, aborted attempts, rehearsals (tying noose, loading gun) vs. nonsuicidal self-injurious actions
   - **Intent:** extent to which the patient (1) expects to carry out the plan and (2) believes the plan/act to be lethal vs. self-injurious. Explore ambivalence: reasons to die vs. reasons to live
4. **RISK LEVEL/INTERVENTION**
   - **Assessment of risk** level is based on clinical judgment, after completing steps 1 through 3
   - **Reassess** as patient or environmental circumstances change

Risk Level	Risk/Protective Factor	Suicidality	Possible Interventions
High	Psychiatric diagnoses with severe symptoms or acute precipitating event; protective factors not relevant	Potentially lethal suicide attempt or persistent ideation with strong intent or suicide rehearsal	Admission generally indicated unless a significant change reduces risk. Suicide precautions
Moderate	Multiple risk factors, few protective factors	Suicidal ideation with plan, but no intent or behavior	Admission may be necessary depending on risk factors. Develop crisis plan. Give emergency/crisis numbers
Low	Modifiable risk factors, strong protective factors	Thoughts of death, no plan, intent, or behavior	Outpatient referral, symptom reduction. Give emergency/crisis numbers

5. **DOCUMENT** Risk level and rationale; treatment plan to address/reduce current risk (e.g., medication, setting, psychotherapy, ECT, contact with significant others, consultation), firearms instructions, if relevant; follow-up plan. For youths treatment plan should include roles for parent/guardian.

For Youths: ask parent/guardian about evidence of suicidal thoughts, plans, or behaviors, and changes in mood, behaviors, or disposition.

Homicide Inquiry: when indicated, especially in character disordered or paranoid males dealing with loss or humiliation. Inquire in four areas listed above.

ADHD, attention deficit hyperactivity disorder; CNS, central nervous system; ECT, electroconvulsive therapy; PTSD, posttraumatic stress disorder; SAFE-T, Suicide Assessment Five-step Evaluation and Triage; TBI, traumatic brain injury.

Research indicates that using both self-report and interview methods may be the best way to ensure accuracy, because some patients are thought to prefer the anonymity of a self-report form and the interviewer may get a negative response even though the patient is suicidal. Several questions can be asked: "Do you ever experience hopelessness or suicidal thinking?" "Do you ever think of hurting yourself?" Asking about suicide ideation does not give the person the idea or increase suicide risk. Most people are relieved to be able to discuss openly the painful feelings they have been struggling with in private. If the patient answers in the affirmative, the therapist can ask follow-up questions: "Do you have a plan?" or "How would you carry out a suicide?" This information is pursued because the more specific the plan, the more likely the person is to hurt himself or herself. Asking for specificity helps to determine the seriousness of intent.

Even so-called parasuicidal behaviors, such as cutting and self-mutilation, should be taken seriously. Understanding the person's underlying motivation for self-harm is important. There is a distinction between those who self-mutilate in an attempt to stay alive and those who attempt suicide and consider death a solution. Parasuicidal behaviors may reflect a reenactment of abuse dynamics with a physiological basis associated with poor attachment and early abuse (van der Kolk, 2014). Chapter 2 describes the neurophysiology associated with reenactment of early trauma. These reenactments may be experienced as normal because they mirror early experiences. The person with borderline personality disorder may want attention in the context of an abandonment crisis and may escalate the threat and self-destruct in a desperate bid for attention. Because these individuals may be suicidal in the context of an abandonment crisis, talking about the loss sometimes may be enough to assuage the suicidal feelings.

The therapist must openly and honestly express concern and engage in problem-solving with the patient so that a written plan can be developed. This collaborative plan should explicitly address the friends and community resources that would be available in an emergency so that the patient can be safe. A safety plan should be developed for all patients who are thought to be at high risk for self-harm. Guidelines developed by the International Society of Study for Dissociative Disorders (ISSD) with respect to suicidal behaviors can be applied to all patients who are at risk for self-harm. These guidelines include developing a safety plan that consists of a hierarchy of alternative behaviors, such as contacting friends, grounding techniques, medications as needed, and calling the therapist and waiting for a return call and/or going to the ED if the patient feels unable to maintain safety (ISSD, 2011). Although a safety plan and attention to protecting the life of the patient are paramount, it is important that the APPN is careful to avoid chronic crisis management as the purpose of the treatment. For example, one well-intended recent graduate adopted the role of constant savior and asked her patient to call her every morning to ensure her safety. This backfired because the patient ultimately viewed this as a strategy to relieve the therapist's anxiety and many frantic moments were spent on the part of the APPN attempting to call the patient when she had "forgotten" to call.

From a clinical and legal perspective, a written safety plan or a no-suicide contract, even if signed by the patient, is not a substitute for clinical judgment. Accurate assessment is imperative because the typical no-suicide contract may not be effective in a crisis situation, whether the patient is in the hospital or the community (Garvey, Penn, Campbell, Esposito-Smythers, & Spirito, 2009). A safety contract is only as good as the therapeutic alliance. Safety may be especially compromised if the patient is inebriated or psychotic. Although nurses are used to dealing with life and death situations, they usually do not occur in private practice or without others around to help. The therapist is often in just that situation and must make decisions independently. It is safest to err on the side of caution and believe your intuition that tells you the person may hurt himself or herself. Suicidal patients should be hospitalized immediately if the family or significant others cannot guarantee safety and the safety plan cannot be adhered to. The clinician must ensure that the patient is safe and may need to personally escort the patient to the ED if needed.

Other safety issues may need consideration, including the anorexic patient who is severely underweight (20% below the expected weight for the patient's height; Sadock, Sadock, & Ruiz, 2017); substance abuse patients who may overdose or pose a threat to others if inebriated and driving; actively self-mutilating patients; sexually promiscuous patients; and angry patients who want to hurt others. Each of these situations must be the first order of business in any treatment setting. Any acute mood disorder or psychosis, out-of-control substance abuse, or eating disorder may need to be treated in an inpatient program before traditional psychotherapy begins. If the patient comes to the session inebriated or high, the session should not be held, and the patient may need to be escorted to a safe place by the therapist, sent home in a taxi, or have a friend or family member called to escort the person home.

The therapist's safety must also be assessed. Some patients may be threatening, and the best predictor of violence has been found to be previous violent episodes (McWilliams, 2004). Often, intuition can tell you whether the patient may be violent, and it is better to err on the side of safety than to dismiss your feelings. Leaving your office door open and making sure that you are near the door may be warranted when working with hostile, unpredictable people, or it may be prudent to interview patients with a security guard nearby or with a colleague if you are working in a dangerous setting. One patient came to his session with a gun, which he told the APPN about. He was asked to leave the gun at home for future sessions, which he agreed to, and psychotherapy proceeded as planned.

THE FIRST CONTACT

APPNs work in varied public and private settings, such as inpatient psychiatric units, inpatient medical settings, outpatient community mental health centers and mental health clinics, residential care facilities, integrated behavioral care settings, intermediate and skilled nursing facilities, juvenile and criminal justice settings, private practice, primary care and medical outpatient settings, home care, managed care, homeless shelters, substance abuse units and programs, emergency or crisis settings, partial hospital settings, medical homes, and in rural, suburban, and urban areas. A 2018 survey reports that APPN practice sites include hospitals, ambulatory sites, community clinics, schools, and criminal justice facilities, as well as federal facilities such as the Veterans Administration (Delaney, Drew, & Rushton, 2019). This survey found that the majority of APPNs deliver a wide variety of mental health services including diagnosis and management of both acute and chronic mental illness, prescribing medications and providing psychotherapy to individuals across the lifespan. The unique practice setting determines how the initial contact with the patient unfolds, and the specifics of each cannot all be covered in this chapter. Guidelines and policies for the particular practice setting should be followed. Aspects of the suggestions offered here may be incorporated into specific settings, if applicable. However, the following discussion is probably most relevant for therapists in outpatient settings where psychotherapy is practiced.

The initial phone call is most likely from the patient seeking help, but it occasionally may be from a friend, family member, or professional colleague. It is important to speak to the patient directly, even if someone else has made the first phone call. To avoid telephone tag, it is helpful to leave a message with several times of the day and a number where you can be reached, as well as requesting that the person leave a message with a telephone number and the times when he or she can be reached if he or she has trouble reaching you. It is better to leave your first and last name when returning a call because the person may not want others who live in the house to know that he or she is seeking help. Recording a "Dr. Wheeler called" message on the patient's answering machine may leave the person in the uncomfortable situation of explaining to others when she or he does not wish to.

During the initial phone call, the therapist is already gathering information and begins the therapeutic alliance. Keeping the initial phone call as brief as possible is advised unless there are special circumstances. Occasionally, someone may ask whether you specialize in a particular problem or have had experience in a certain area, such as eating disorders or trauma. Answer the question factually, and refer the person elsewhere if that is warranted. Although at first you may not know what your areas of expertise are and feel you have none, it is probably best for you and the patients to start with populations and approaches with which you feel most comfortable. Knowing your own limits is essential, as is not using modalities with which you have little expertise, such as hypnosis, guided imagery, eye movement desensitization and reprocessing (EMDR therapy), or expressive therapies, because in incompetent hands, patient regression may be triggered.

If the person launches into a detailed description of the problem over the phone, it is appropriate to say that it would benefit the prospective patient to come in and set a mutually agreeable time for the first session. Most therapists do not ask about insurance or other specifics on the phone unless the patient asks for information regarding insurance or asks about fees or unless the therapist's agency requires that specific information ahead of the appointment. Others feel that it is important to discuss financial issues before committing to see the patient, because clarification of how the therapy will be paid for saves time for the patient and the therapist. Patients may not understand the terms of their insurance and may need to call the insurance company before setting up an appointment. Issues regarding which providers are covered, the number of sessions, copays, parity diagnoses, and preauthorization, may need to be explained first to allow the person to ask appropriate questions. Some APPNs make the phone call to the patient's insurance to ensure that the terms of reimbursement are clear before agreeing to see the patient. Another decision that needs to be made is whether to charge for the initial consultation. Some therapists do not charge for consultations, and the patient should be told whether you do or do not charge for the first session. Tell the person the times you have available, and end the conversation by giving directions to your office after an agreeable time to meet has been decided.

The patient comes to the first session with expectations, even if the person has never been in psychotherapy before. Some of these expectations are conscious and some are not. Expectations can tell you about the person's developmental level and what may be going on in the person's relationships. For example, some patients with magical thinking fully expect to have their problems solved in a few sessions; those with dependency needs may expect to be taken care of or to be given advice; those who have been criticized expect to be disapproved of or judged; and those who eroticize relationships may expect the therapist to have sex with them. Sometimes, asking the person how he or she feels about coming to the session can help to elicit some idea of expectations. Asking if the patient has ever known anyone who was in therapy can also give valuable information about expectations. The patient may have known someone who was greatly helped by psychotherapy or may associate treatment with Woody Allen and endless, self-absorbed neurosis. Some therapists elicit this information by giving the patient an intake form, such as the Multimodal Life History Inventory (Lazarus & Lazarus, 1991). This questionnaire contains questions that address patients' expectations regarding therapy. What do you think therapy is all about? How long do you think therapy should last? What personal qualities do you think the ideal therapist should possess?

If your office shares a waiting room, and you have not met the patient before, it is best to ask those in the room "Are you waiting for Kate Wheeler?" Doing so ensures that you will not be divulging the person's name to all those sitting there. In that way, the person can say yes without a breach of identity disclosure. Even the simple gesture of shaking hands is important to think about. If it is the therapist's custom to shake hands, and she naturally extends her hand to the patient, the patient may feel uncomfortable. It is better to take the lead from the patient. For patients who extend a hand, by all means shake hands. For a patient who does not offer, following his or her lead may allow the person control and to feel more comfortable. After the patient enters your office, asking what he or she would like to be called is a courtesy that sets a collaborative tone at the very beginning.

The therapist's office and seating arrangements are considered with respect to keeping the patient's best interests in the foreground. Seating arrangements may be constrained if you are seeing patients in a clinic setting, but it is usually best not to sit behind a desk because this puts a barrier between you and the patient. However, sitting at the desk with the person on one side of the desk may be conducive to conversation. Ideally chairs are set at approximately 3 to 4 feet away from each other and arranged so that the person is not directly across from you but at a 45-degree angle. In this way, the patient does not feel scrutinized and compelled to make eye contact and can look away if he or she wishes.

It is not appropriate to have your family pictures visibly displayed in the office. They may be comforting to you, but they may be distracting to the person seeking help and do not serve a therapeutic purpose for the patient. A clock can be placed across from the therapist's chair, so it can be easily seen unobtrusively by the therapist, or it can be placed where both the patient and therapist can monitor how much time is left in the session. Phone calls are not taken during sessions, and all phones and beepers are turned off. This is the patient's time, and it is courteous to ensure that the patient is the center of attention for the entire session. On the rare occasion when you are working with a professional or personal emergency, it is advisable to tell the person at the beginning of the session that you may be interrupted and to apologize. In most instances, a quiet, confidential setting where you will not be interrupted is imperative.

There are several ways to begin the session. "What brings you here?" usually gets the ball rolling, although for a very concrete-thinking patient, the answer may be "the bus." "What is going on that you are seeking help now?" or "How would you like to start?" may also be an effective way to begin. "How can I help?" may feel patronizing to the patient and implies something less than a collaboration. Small talk for a moment, such as asking if the person had any trouble finding the office, can be appropriate to put the person at ease because the last contact most likely was on the phone when directions were given. When the person is in the office and the APPN is ready to begin, the type of setting will determine how best to proceed.

The intake or first session for the patient may last for the usual 45 to 50 minutes to 1.5 hours, depending on the clinical site. In some settings, a different therapist does the intake, and the patient then may be assigned to another therapist, or sometimes, the same therapist may do the intake and continue with the person in therapy. If you are serving as the intake therapist in a setting in which forms must be completed by the patient, it may expedite the process to leave the forms with the receptionist so that as much information as possible is obtained before your meeting. Much of the information needs to be gathered initially, and if you do not have a receptionist, perhaps some of the assessment and intake forms can be mailed to the person ahead of time before the first session. Some APPNs give the patient forms to take home at the end of the first session and ask the person to bring them back the next week. In that case, the first session is used to gather only preliminary information and assess safety. Many therapists in private practice leave the first session less structured because this allows the person to tell his or her story in an unstructured way, and it can be invaluable in accomplishing one of the most important tasks of the first session: initiating a therapeutic alliance.

For those who work in settings in which a comprehensive assessment is required in the initial session, Chapter 3 provides guidelines on how to accomplish this while effectively initiating a therapeutic alliance. For those who are in settings in which the assessment can be conducted over several sessions, Chapter 3 provides excellent resources and screening tools to incorporate to ensure a thorough and accurate assessment. If you are the prescribing advanced practice nurse only, guidelines for assessment on how to combine medication management with or without psychotherapy are discussed in Chapters 14 and 15. No matter what type of setting you are working in and how you proceed, practical arrangements for continuing the work, establishing goals, ending the session, and keeping records must be considered.

Making Practical Arrangements

Practical arrangements must be made regarding the frequency and length of the sessions. Weekly sessions of 45 to 50 minutes are usually scheduled unless there is a significant reason to deviate from this standard plan. The session begins and ends at predetermined times. Meeting less often usually is not as effective and interferes with the momentum of treatment, unless the goal of treatment is maintenance of the status quo or the APPN is prescribing only and another person is conducting the psychotherapy. It may be best to see the patient more often initially if you are concerned about safety or the person is in crisis. However, starting several times a week often is too intense for most people and may be threatening and counterproductive. The number of sessions per week may be increased after a solid therapeutic alliance is formed and the patient wishes to intensify the work for faster resolution.

Some brief and cognitive psychotherapists advocate setting a termination date at the beginning of treatment, because it is thought that if the ending time is known, the goals and work may proceed faster. Toward the end of the time set, there can be renegotiation if more time is needed. Guidelines and principles for short-term psychotherapy are further discussed in Chapters 5, and 6. Sometimes, therapists prefer to allow the process to unfold and leave the termination date open-ended unless there is a specified number of sessions that the person is allowed by the insurance company or there are agency constraints. Frequently, what the person initially came to therapy for evolves into something somewhat different as the process unfolds, and goals are revised periodically. For example, one man came into treatment because he felt depressed and unhappy with his work. As this was explored, he began to examine his long-standing dysthymia and how this related to a childhood traumatic experience that had violated his trust and impacted all dimensions of his life. The goals then focused on resolving his early trauma in light of his deepening awareness of its significance.

A Health Insurance Portability and Accountability Act (HIPAA)–type form explaining confidentiality and a Therapy Contract delineating the terms of the psychotherapy should be given to the patient (see Appendices 4.1 and 4.2). A solo practitioner is held to the same HIPAA standards as organizations with respect to HIPAA. Some therapists also have a policy statement, posted in the waiting room, which describes consumer rights, confidentiality, missed sessions, and fees. A sample is available at www.guidetopsychology.com/compol.htm. The Therapy Contract and HIPAA form along with the packet of screening and assessment tools should be signed by the patient and brought back to the next session.

Confidentiality is discussed, and whether you will be discussing information about the person to a supervisor or other healthcare providers is disclosed. Permission for these discussions is authorized with a written release of information form, and care is taken to use discretion and reveal only what is necessary for medical care. If a treatment report requesting more sessions is to be sent to an insurance company, the form may be shared with the patient before sending it. In discussing patients with colleagues or in a professional forum such as a conference or paper, use a pseudonym or initial, and disguise identifying information to protect the person's identity. Even though the person's identity is kept confidential, permission should be obtained from the patient unless the information shared is an amalgam of cases and is not specifically about the patient. Permissions can also be explicitly stated in the initial treatment contract so that additional permissions are not needed. A formal Informed Consent document is required in some states; however, keep in mind that a written document signed by the patient does not demonstrate that informed consent has been obtained because it does not demonstrate the patient's comprehension. General risks and benefits should be discussed with the person and documented in the patient's records that such a conversation took place. Informed Consent specifically for nurse psychotherapists has not been addressed by our professional organizations but Ken Pope's website provides guidelines from other organizations about requirements. See kspope.com/consent/index.php and the sample of a practice contract in Appendix 4.2.

Confidentiality should be respected in all situations. That is, the APPN should not discuss the patient to the person's family members or spouse. If a family member calls and is concerned and wishes to tell the APPN something about the patient, the APPN can listen but is obligated to explain that therapy is confidential. The patient should also be informed of the family's concerns and call so that transparency between the therapist and patient is preserved. Of course, if the patient is a minor, this may change depending on the circumstances and the state law. If the APPN sees the patient in a public setting, it is best to not acknowledge the person's presence unless the patient says hello first. When asked by anyone for information about the patient, it is best to consult with an attorney experienced in mental health law before complying. Confidentiality should never be broken unless the patient is a danger to himself or herself. If you are concerned that the patient is a threat to others, it is important to document your assessment of the patient and to follow through if the risk is high. Every state has statutes about the duty to report when a patient is a risk to others, and it is important to be aware of your state's laws about how to manage these patients safely. The APPN is legally bound to report patients she or he suspects are abusing children to child protective service agencies, those who abuse the elderly to adult protective service agencies, and those threatening violence to the police. Familiarity with state statutes and services is essential, and the novice APPN should seek legal advice and consultation from the state board and professional associations before releasing any confidential records or filing a report with any agency.

Practical arrangement and issues relating to ethics, confidentiality, and scope of practice have become more complex with the advent of telepsychiatry for APPNs who wish to use technology to conduct psychotherapy or prescribe medications. For an overview of the use of Skype in tele–mental health, see www.zurinstitute.com/skype_telehealth. html#top. Prescribing and conducting psychotherapy for those who live out of state must be in compliance with the state regulations in which the patient resides and it is prudent to check with the respective state board of nursing before teleconferencing, Skyping, or prescribing. In addition, other issues are important considerations and are included in Box 4.3.

BOX 4.3 TELEPSYCHIATRY by Michael Rice

The rapid advance of Internet-based digital relationships are sparking a revolution in new models of "digital health." Digital health involves the use of all forms of digital communication used to interact with healthcare patients. These include the use of all forms of emails, texts, instant message services pagers, file transfers, social media platforms, and video conferencing. The rapid growth of these forms of digital communication must adhere to regulatory, licensure, and clinical standards of care in order to effectively maintain the frame of treatment. In general, all electronic devices sending receiving or transmitting a patient's personal health information should meet the criteria listed in Table 4.1, Digital Care Security.

TABLE 4.1 DIGITAL CARE SECURITY REQUIREMENTS
1. Active security encryption
2. Allows for remote wiping and/or remote disabling
3. Contains disabled and\or do not install file sharing applications
4. Active firewall protecting from unauthorized access
5. Active enabled security software
6. Periodic updates to security software
7. Downloaded mobile applications (apps) meet HIPAA security and do not allow tracking or user data authorization
8. Is always under the assigned user's physical control
9. Contains security encryption software that allows sending and receiving health information over public Wi-Fi networks
10. Users must delete all stored health information before discarding or repurposing the mobile device

HIPAA, Health Insurance Portability and Accountability Act.

Source: Centers for Medicare and Medicaid Services. (2018). Medical privacy of protected health information. Retrieved from https://www.cms.gov/Outreach-and-Education/Medicare-Learning-Network-MLN/MLNProducts/downloads/SE0726FactSheet.pdf

These major security issues are often misunderstood but are mandatory when providing any form of digital care, including telehealth video conferencing. The major difference between the social\public media platforms and professional digital and video conferencing is the level of protection of the healthcare information afforded the patient. Public social media do not meet the minimum standards and, often acceptance of the terms and agreements state that the company stores information and shares it with business partners. This is an automatic breach of the privacy guidelines and eliminates the potential use of these public video conferencing platforms.

Compliant Videoconferencing

The use of video conferencing has increased dramatically during the COVID19 pandemic. Federal and state laws, define video conferencing as care provided by a practitioner at a remote location using a telecommunications system (Centers for Medicare & Medicaid Services [CMS], 2011). The Drug Enforcement Administration further modified

(continued)

BOX 4.3 TELEPSYCHIATRY by Michael Rice (*continued*)

the criteria addressing prescribing across state boundaries. The DEA currently requires the criteria listed in Table 4.2.

TABLE 4.2   DRUG ENFORCEMENT AGENCY (DEA) PRESCRIBING CRITERIA VIA REMOTE TELECOMMUNICATIONS
A. The patient is physically located at a DEA registered hospital or clinic with a practitioner in accordance with state law and registered with the DEA in the state the patient resides.
B. The patient is treated by, and in the physical presence of, a DEA-registered practitioner in accordance with state law and registered with the DEA in the state the patient resides.
C. Practitioners must be registered in the primary state where they are physically located and the state in which the patient resides.
D. All records for FDA approved treatment of narcotic and opioid treatment must be kept in accordance with DEA requirements.

Source: Records and Reports of Registrants, 21 C.F.R. §§ 1304.01–1304.55 (2011); Registration of Manufacturers, Distributors, and Dispensers of Controlled Substances, 21 C.F.R. § 1301.12 (2016).

All healthcare professionals using video conferencing must meet the HIPAA security and CMS security compliance regulations, as previously mentioned. Access to the video conferencing system and software requires a unique identifier (user name) and a unique password. While many video conferencing systems comply with this standard, noncompliant systems often do not meet the Federal Information Processing Standards 140-2, often referred to as CMS (Medicare Rule) 140-2 at www.hhs.gov/hipaa/for-professionals/faq/2001/is-the-use-of-encryption-mandatory-in-the-security-rule/index.html. This set of regulations that required that all professional healthcare use meets requirements of the HITECH Act regulations were revised in 2018 and can be found at csrc.nist.gov/csrc/media/publications/fips/140/2/final/documents/fips1402annexa.pdf.   Although at first glance, these regulations appear intimidating, they are really quite straightforward. There are four basic rules that are applied, as noted in Table 4.3.

TABLE 4.3   BASIC RULES FOR COMPLIANT VIDEO CONFERENCING
1. Is the device(s) used for the video conferencing compliant with HIPAA security rules?
2. Is the software used for the video conferencing HIPAA compliant?
3. Is the software FIP 140-2 or CMS compliant?
4. Does the software encrypt the transmission of all information?

CMS, Centers for Medicare & Medicaid Services; FIP, Federal Information Processing; HIPAA, Health Insurance Portability and Accountability Act.

Encryption

The 140-2 rules are an encryption standard beyond the commonly used "Advanced Encryption Standard"(AES) found on most devices. The 140-2 regulations require an internal software program that mathematically encrypts the transmission of all protected health information, including patient records, and patient information at one of four levels based on a system defined by the Pentagon. While somewhat daunting, a simple check can verify the video conferencing software uses the 140-2 standard which should run within the background of the video conferencing software. Most institutional information technology (IT) departments operate these programs in the background and users are seldom aware of the presence of the security features. The absence of this encryption is one of the major problems associated with noninstitutional social media based video conferencing for psychiatric mental health issues. Failure to adhere to these guidelines can result in federal fines ranging from $100 to $1.5 million (Healthcare Compliance, n.d.). See Table 4.4 for a list of resources for digital care standards.

These aforementioned rules are incorporated into all states' regulations on reimbursement for telecommunication services as CMS sets the standard for all Medicaid services. The baseline standards for CMS, DEA, and other rules are listed in Table 4.5. All practitioners are advised to check with the state regulations on telehealth and what can and cannot be reimbursed within a state as there are some interstate variations (CMS, 2020).

TABLE 4.4 HYPERLINKS FOR DIGITAL CARE STANDARDS

Topic	Federal Hyperlink
HIPAA: Emergencies	www.hhs.gov/hipaa/for-professionals/faq/disclosures-in-emergency-situations/index.html
HIPAA, FERPA and Student Health Records	www.hhs.gov/hipaa/for-professionals/faq/ferpa-and-hipaa/index.html
HHS: Final Guidance	www.hhs.gov/hipaa/for-professionals/security/guidance/final-guidance-risk-analysis/index.html
Health Information Privacy Rights	www.hhs.gov/ocr/privacy/index.html
HIPAA: HITECH Act	www.gpo.gov/fdsys/pkg/FR-2013-01-25/pdf/2013-01073.pdf
HIPAA Privacy Rule	www.hhs.gov/ocr/privacy/hipaa/administrative/privacyrule/index.html
HIPAA Security Guidance	www.hhs.gov/ocr/privacy/hipaa/administrative/securityrule/securityruleguidance.html
HIPAA Text Messaging	www.hipaajournal.com/does-your-organization-need-a-secure-text-messaging-service-324
Notice of Privacy Practices	www.hhs.gov/ocr/privacy/hipaa/model notices.html
PHI: De-identification	www.hhs.gov/ocr/privacy/hipaa/understanding/coveredentities/De-identification/deidentificationworkshop2010.html
Security Risk Assessments	www.healthit.gov/providers-professionals/security-risk-assessment

(continued)

BOX 4.3 TELEPSYCHIATRY by Michael Rice (*continued*)

Topic	Federal Hyperlink
Security Final Rule	www.hhs.gov/hipaa/for-professionals/security/laws-regulations/index.html
Security and Electronic Signature Standards	aspe.hhs.gov/report/nrpm-security-and-electronic-signature-standards/electronic-signature-standard

FERPA, Family Educational Rights and Privacy Act; HHS, Department of Health & Human Services; HIPAA, Health Insurance Portability and Accountability Act; PHI, protected health information.

Source: Healthcare Compliance. (n.d.). *HIPAA compliance guide.* Retrieved from https://www.hipaaguide.net/hipaa-compliance-guide/#HIPAA_Resources

A final issue is the use of clinical standards of care. These are outlined in the American Telehealth Association for Videoconferencing. A summary of the guiding principles are listed in Table 4.5 (Richmond et al., 2017).

TABLE 4.5 TELECOMMUNICATION STANDARDS GUIDELINES

1. Professionals are aware of and comply with laws and regulations integrating nationally recognized professional standards.

2. Professionals are aware of and comply with all professional state board regulations and any guiding scope of practice policies.

3. Professionals who use information communication technologies are trained in equipment and software operation and have IT (information technology) support available for technical difficulties.

4. Professionals are performing services within professional standards of care, and the principles of evidence-based practice.

5. Professionals are aware of federal and state regulations for clinical documentation, storage of health data.

6. Professionals ensure the presence of a facilitator (caregiver, family member, or provider) is available before, during, and after the telecommunication session.

7. Professionals are responsible for the patient's safety. If, during the virtual encounter, the professional observes the patient's health is compromised, the patient is referred to local healthcare resources.

8. Professionals are aware of administrative telehealth guidelines affecting telecommunication services.

Source: Richmond, T., Peterson, C., Cason, J., Billings, M., Terrell, E. A., Lee, A., . . . Brennan, D. (2017). American Telemedicine Association's principles for delivering telerehabilitation services. *International Journal of Telerehabilitation, 9*(2), 63–68. doi:10.5195/IJT.2017.6232

A leader in the development and use of telecommunications is the American Telehealth Association (ATA). The ATA has developed a wide range of practice guidelines and updates them on a periodic basis. The ATA developed these guidelines to establish the baseline for use of all forms of digital and telecommunications and will evolve as the field advances.

Fees

Fees should be discussed during the first session. Novice nurse psychotherapists often feel conflicted about charging a fee for their services when they do not feel knowledgeable about what they are doing. Fees should reflect the level of education, the degree of expertise, and the going rate in the community for such services. Sometimes, beginning therapists overlook the extensive education and training required to do psychotherapy and the fact that to take care of the patient's emotional needs, it is necessary to get paid for their professional services. You may decide to offer a certain percentage of your patients a reduced fee, but having a pro bono practice in which you are paid by most of your patients less than others in your area is a recipe for resentment. Each therapist should decide on the basis of her finances whether a certain number of patients can be offered a lower fee and then fill that number of hours with low-fee or sliding-scale patients and refer others who cannot afford the standard fee to a low-cost clinic.

In agency settings, collecting fees is often taken care of by others, and it is not until the therapist is in private practice that collecting fees becomes an issue. In either setting, being clear about the fee and when payment is expected is part of the frame and should be discussed in the initial session. If you are in private practice or a setting that requires that you discuss fees with the person during the initial visit, information about the patient's insurance may need to be obtained by you. Usually, a limited number of sessions are authorized, sometimes after the deductible is met, and an outpatient treatment report (OTR) is required after the allotted number of sessions. This should be discussed with the patient, because many therapists believe that the OTR violates patient confidentiality and that the person should know what information will be provided to the insurance company. Sometimes, a creative solution can be worked out if the person already has a high copay with a managed care company that you are not a provider for. For example, seeing the person 30 minutes instead of the usual 45 to 50 minutes and charging one half of your usual fee may allow the person to pay about the same fee as he or she would if using the managed care company. In that way, the person can be seen for a shorter session and reduced fee, and confidentiality is preserved.

If the therapist is on the provider panel for a managed care company, the provider is contracted to charge a particular fee, and the patient pays a specified copay. Most therapists require payment at the end of the month for that month or the first session of the next month for the previous month. Other therapists expect payment at the end of each session. The provider submits the balance to the insurance company on a Health Care Financing Administration (HCFA) form and then gets paid by the managed care company or insurance company usually a month or more later. Psychotherapy sessions are given Current Procedural Terminology (CPT) codes that designate the type of service given for billing and documentation for all insurers. These codes were revised as of 2013 in an effort to better reflect the complexity and level of care for patients. See Chapter 23 for how to use these codes for reimbursement.

For those patients who do not have insurance or when the therapist is not a provider on the panel for the insurance they have, the fee may need to be paid by the patient out-of-pocket. In these cases, usually the patient pays the provider directly. The patient then is responsible for submitting the bill to the insurance company so that he or she can get reimbursed. Most therapists prefer this method of payment as it helps to avoid tracking down claims, wasting time on the phone with managed care companies, and trying to get paid for services already rendered. Whatever method you decide to use for payment, it is best to keep when and how you get paid consistent for everyone to avoid confusion for yourself.

Whether you charge for missed sessions is important information to share during the first session. A cursory survey of colleagues reveals that most APPNs in private practice do charge for missed sessions; some charge only for those who do not call and do not show up, whereas others charge if they do not receive 24 or 48 hours' notice and cannot reschedule for later that week. The idea behind charging for missed sessions is that the session time is *rented* much as a person would pay money for classes even if the person does not attend. The therapist has saved this time for the patient and should not be penalized financially for the patient's absence. Paying for missed sessions also emphasizes the importance of psychotherapy. Just as a person should not arbitrarily decide to not take a medication that was prescribed, psychotherapy is a prescribed treatment modality and, as such, is valuable. Some therapists feel that charging for missed sessions conveys to the patient the importance and value of their work together.

If the person cancels or does not come because of weather problems or significant illness, many therapists do not charge for the missed session. Most insurance companies do not allow reimbursement for missed sessions. If you are charging, be sure to state the specifics in the contract with the patient, and do not charge the insurance company because this violates the policy of most provider agreements. Many agencies do not have a cancellation policy and do not charge for missed sessions, and this may explain the high number of absences in such settings. Policies about attendance, missed appointments, and fees in the form of a contract should be provided to the patient at intake and should be signed by the patient.

Establishing Goals and Ending the Session

About 10 minutes before the end of the first session, it is a good idea to ask the person whether he or she has any questions. Then give the patient a brief idea without psychiatric jargon about what you think may be going on and what may help. For example: "From what you have told me, you have suffered several significant losses in the past year, and this could account for the difficulty concentrating, your sadness, and trouble sleeping that you have been having. I think it would be helpful to come and talk about what has been going on for you. I would like you to take some forms home with you to fill out this week, and over the next few sessions, I will be asking you additional questions so I can get to know you better. This will help me to determine what is the best way to help you." Conveying hope is also important, for example: "As you talk about some of these losses and begin to feel better, I have a hunch your sleeping will improve too."

The therapist then discusses the goals of treatment by asking the person: "How will you know this therapy worked. What will be different for you?" or "How would you like your life to improve?" or "What would you like your life to be like?" These are all open-ended questions that assist the person in formulating goals. Patients passively receiving suggestions fare far worse than patients who are actively involved in goal setting. Arriving at some consensus on therapy goals at intake helps the therapeutic alliance and engagement, which increases the probability that the patient will return after the initial session and will continue treatment. If the patient wants behavioral exercises between therapy sessions and the therapist is psychodynamically oriented, it will be apparent that there is a disagreement about therapy tasks at the outset, and these differences need to be explicitly negotiated. The therapist and patient need to jointly decide goals and reevaluate them together throughout therapy. Reflecting on your understanding of what the patient said helps to strengthen the alliance, and the person knows that you are listening and that you are on the same wavelength.

Although establishing goals is important, Gabbard (2017) cautions against the therapist being too wedded to goals, because the patient may begin to feel that the emphasis on attaining goals is the therapist's agenda and comply to please the therapist. Alternatively, the therapist who is too eager to achieve goals may elicit a stubborn resistance by the patient, who wishes to defeat the therapist by not changing. As a wise supervisor once told me: "The therapist should not be the most motivated person in the room." The therapist should not be too eager and respect the patient's ambivalence. Safran and Muran (2000) concur and place change in a framework of mindfulness. They state, "change merges out of nonjudgmental awareness, rather than through trying to force things to be different" (p. 116). A basic tenet of psychotherapy is to emphasize awareness rather than change.

Keeping Records

Taking notes during a session is a matter of individual preference. Sometimes, novice therapists take verbatim session notes and go over everything with a supervisor so that nothing will be missed that may be important because everything seems potentially important. This can be very distracting and distancing from the person sitting across from you. It is better to listen attentively, perhaps writing occasionally a word or two to pique your memory for constructing process notes that are more elaborate after the session.

It is important to keep two sets of notes:

1. Process notes include what you think is going on in terms of transference and countertransference, topics discussed, questions about your own intuition, issues for discussion during supervision, or verbatim notes, particularly about a difficult or problematic interaction.
2. A more formal record of the treatment progress covers the diagnosis, level of care, history of present illness, review of symptoms, past, family, and social history, examination components, medication reactions, suicidal thoughts, treatment decisions, and a description of the session for that particular session. These notes should be brief and respectful of the person's confidentiality. See Chapter 23, for an explanation of these components based on the 2013 CPT codes.

The formal progress notes are kept for legal purposes or for review if mandated by a managed care or insurance company for quality auditing, while the process notes do not need to be delivered if there is a legal action or a medical record is requested. Examples of process and progress notes can be found in Appendices 4.3 and 4.4.

THERAPEUTIC COMMUNICATION

Psychotherapy is considered the talking cure, and therapeutic communication skills are the hallmark of good psychotherapy. Nurses have learned communication skills as undergraduates and most likely have been talking to patients for years. However, as with any new role, the novice APPN psychotherapist may be anxious and forget what she or he already knows, and a review of therapeutic communication may be helpful. Therapeutic communication is embedded in the holistic model of nursing, with the overall aim of promoting integration toward the goals of wholeness and healing. This is accomplished by assisting the person in experiencing and expanding thoughts, feelings, and actions that enhance resources and/or processing. Therapeutic communication can be accomplished through the use of open-ended therapeutic communication techniques with the specific aims of promoting self-understanding and self-acceptance and of enhancing strengths. There is a vast literature on humanistic therapies such as Gestalt, patient-centered, and existential approaches to helping people become more connected with their feelings and more comfortable with expressing themselves directly (see Chapter 6). Most therapies encourage the patient to talk nondefensively about his or her emotional experiences, and through the ambient environment of a supportive, nurturing relationship, a narrative of the person's life unfolds.

The elements of psychotherapy as described in Chapter 1—resilience and relationship—provide the parameters for communication. Good communication is all about context and relationship. Therapeutic communication competency is based on the ability to listen nonjudgmentally, facilitate the patient to talk openly, and respond appropriately to what the person says. The psychotherapist assists the person in clarifying feelings and meanings and guides the person into areas that may not be fully conscious to enhance coping skills, deepen self-understanding, and improve the ability to make decisions. The patient does most of the talking, and the focus is on the patient's concerns. One criterion of effective communication is whether what you say enables the patient to speak more freely. If you are talking more than 10% to 20% of the time, it becomes your session, not the patient's. When you begin to feel concerned about what you are going to say, remember that less is best. During sessions, the therapist typically uses short sentences rather than long-winded explanations. Lengthy explanations have the potential for increasing the anxiety level of patients, especially during the initial session.

Barriers to listening include an emphasis on gathering information or getting the facts, giving information, and the therapist's bias and judgmental attitudes. For example, suppose you are listening to someone talk about an abortion with a cavalier attitude and you are pro-life. How would you hear what the person said? Alternatively, suppose you are an atheist, and the patient talks about reading scriptures every day and the solace that this brings him or her. Would you judge the person as being too religious? Everyone has prejudices and attitudes, and it is important for therapists, through supervision or their own therapy, to be aware of their attitudes and how they may interfere with their work with the different people encountered in practice. A respectful, nonjudgmental stance is essential for the development of rapport and connection.

Gabbard (2017) says that therapeutic communication interventions exist on a continuum from expressive to supportive. Those communication techniques that are most expressive are used by psychodynamic therapists to provide understanding and insight for processing while supportive interventions are less emotionally laden. This conceptualization is useful and applicable to the treatment hierarchy triangle described in Chapter 1. Some interventions, such as focusing, observation, immediacy, and interpretation may be emotionally arousing and are more likely to be employed for patients who are higher on the treatment hierarchy triangle, whereas patients needing stabilization are more likely to require more supportive techniques, such as broad openings, information giving, giving recognition, restating, clarification, and reflection. However, techniques considered more supportive and needed for stabilization are also used for processing, but the expressive techniques higher on the treatment triangle are most often used for processing, not stabilization.

Communication techniques used for processing may trigger implicit neural networks and, without the proper resources, may be experienced as overwhelming, unmanageable feelings. The supportive techniques are more likely to be resource building and less anxiety provoking. Cozolino (2002) speculates that supportive communication optimizes cortical executive functioning as the patient is invited and supported to experience a wide range of emotions. He states, "This simultaneous activation of cognition, emotion, enhanced perspective, and the emotional regulation offered by the relationship may provide an optimal environment for neural change" (p. 53). Figure 4.1 shows the treatment hierarchy triangle as outlined in Chapter 1, with the continuum of therapeutic communication.

It is not important to know the names of these techniques or to memorize each one, but a review and discussion may help the beginning psychotherapist to identify which skills he or she uses now and how to expand this repertoire of communication skills to include others. Each of us must find words that feel genuine so that we do not sound stilted and mechanical. The examples listed in Table 4.6 assist in advancing the

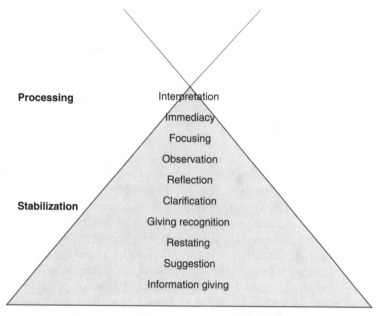

Processing

Interpretation

Immediacy

Focusing

Observation

Reflection

Stabilization

Clarification

Giving recognition

Restating

Suggestion

Information giving

FIGURE 4.1 Treatment hierarchy and continuum of therapeutic communication.

TABLE 4.6	SELECTED THERAPEUTIC COMMUNICATION TECHNIQUES
Technique	**Example**
Broad opening	Where shall we begin?
Information giving	I recommend that you take this medication at bedtime because it may make you feel tired.
Giving recognition	You were able to do well this week with the goals we set last week.
Restating	You cannot study and have trouble concentrating.
Suggestion	Some people find it helpful to keep a journal of their thoughts during the week.
Clarification	Would you tell me more about what you mean by "upset"?
Reflection	You are asking me what to do about your wife's drinking and are very frustrated by the situation.
Exploring	How did you feel when your friend said that to you?
Focusing	Yes, your relationship with your mother is important, and it may help you understand better what goes on for you in other relationships by discussing this further.
Observation	It seems that whenever you begin to talk about your mother, you change the subject.
Immediacy	Perhaps you are feeling that I am not giving you what you need here.
Interpretation	From what you have told me, it seems that when you get close in a relationship, you become anxious and then protect yourself by finding fault with the other person.

psychotherapeutic process and are embedded in the context of attending and listening, empathy, and exploration. Selected techniques are discussed as they relate to these processes of therapeutic communication. All techniques are included in the following discussion; however, those higher on the treatment triangle are most likely not used in the initial session.

Attending and Listening

The APPN psychotherapist attends and listens by paying close attention to what the patient is saying verbally and nonverbally. Therapists think of the manifest content as what patients are actually saying, whereas the latent content is what they mean by what they say, or the *process*. This dichotomy has also been referred to as *explicit versus implicit communication*. Often, a session or a series of sessions has a latent theme in the foreground, such as issues relating to trust, loneliness, abandonment, feelings of helplessness or inadequacy, or anger toward authority or about the carelessness of others. The therapist listens and hears the central issues and themes. Even though there may be manifest and latent content, the therapist most often does not directly address latent themes with the patient, but hearing and attempting to deepen understanding of the issues that the person is struggling with are relevant no matter what orientation or model of psychotherapy the therapist subscribes to. For example, a patient came to his session railing against authority figures he felt were controlling and unreasonable. This is the manifest content, whereas the latent content may relate to his feeling, perhaps unconsciously, that the therapist is authoritarian and controlling. It does not necessarily mean that the therapist is authoritarian and controlling, but for this person who is in a dependent position at this time, state-dependent neural networks of anger and resentment about helplessness or dependency from a past relationship are activated. The emotional arousal and novel sensory experience inherent in the psychotherapeutic process trigger implicit memory networks, or transference.

Transference refers to the patient's thoughts, feelings, and behaviors that are associated with early important relationships with caretakers and significant others and that are felt toward the therapist. Transference reflects state-dependent memories of specific physiological states of consciousness from the past. These neural networks are activated by the therapeutic relationship. Transference is ubiquitous and reflected in the way the patient acts, talks, and feels about the therapist. For example, a patient who is attending sessions regularly on time and is eager to share experiences and feelings most likely has a positive transference, and a person who is late, is reluctant to talk, and sits guardedly in sessions most likely has a negative transference. These are polarized extremes to illustrate vivid examples of transference, but most transference manifestations are much more subtle, nuanced, and complex.

There may be many different transference constellations and nuances over the course of treatment. The patient most likely is unaware of these feelings as transferential, especially at first, and it is often difficult for the novice therapist to identify them as well. Listening and responding empathically is usually the best strategy for any negative feelings that may arise. For example, one patient came to his initial session sullen and with arms crossed and informed the therapist that he did not trust her. Because the therapist had never seen this person before, the therapist first explored his feelings about coming. It is important to ascertain first whether the patient was forced to come, was responded to in a timely way when he called, or has any other reality-based reasons for the sullenness. If there seems to be no reality-based reason that needs to be addressed first, the therapist may understand his attitude as transferential. This can provide important information about the dynamics of this person. The therapist may empathically comment: "It may be hard to trust someone whom you do not know, and it makes sense to not trust me until you get to know me better."

If the transference is positive, it does not need to be addressed with the patient no matter what psychotherapy approach is used. Only if the therapeutic alliance is threatened or the transference is negative does the therapist explore with the person his or her feelings. Once the patient feels understood and validated, a negative transference is often dissipated. In some psychotherapy approaches such as psychodynamic, negative transference is addressed as an alliance rupture and that is the primary work in the treatment (Eubanks, Muran, & Safran, 2019) while in other types of psychotherapy such as cognitive behavioral, goals or tasks of treatment may be changed without addressing the transference. Listening for such themes and providing feedback in the form of a question, if appropriate, deepens the process and enhances self-understanding and empowerment. The therapist assists the patient in his or her healing journey with the humbling knowledge that the therapist's understanding may or may not be correct and that all observations require verification by the patient in terms of their probability. The therapist is not the authority on the patient's unconscious; the patient is. These observations are best delivered by emphasizing the therapist's subjectivity and nondefensive communication through the use of phrases such as "It seems to me . . ." or "I'm thinking that . . ." or "As I see it. . . ."

Body language speaks volumes about the patient, and the astute therapist is observant of how the patient sits, walks, speaks, and moves. The therapist listens to what the person is saying and considers the meaning of the body language. Where and how does the person sit, and what posture does the patient assume? Does the patient leave his or her coat on? The therapist needs to be aware of the patient's nonverbal behavior and its meaning. Following the patient's body language and mimicking the person's posture or breathing may signal the patient's unconscious that you are on the same wavelength and can deepen your understanding of the person. Students are sometimes hesitant to try this exercise because of concerns that the patient may notice, but informal reports from APPN students have not found this to be true, and *shadowing* the patient in this way often serves as an insightful exercise for both the novice and the experienced therapist.

The therapist assumes an open, receptive posture without fidgeting and with arms not crossed. Good eye contact without staring is important, although this is somewhat culturally determined; some people from Asian or aboriginal cultures prefer indirect eye contact. A neutral, expectant look is important, because smiling and friendliness may be experienced as a social interaction or as threatening, or it may imply that the therapist is not serious about the person's problems. Changes in the physiology of the therapist and the patient are important to observe to detect subtle or obvious dissociative shifts of consciousness in the patient (Schore, 2019). The therapist monitors his or her own body language and somatic experiences. These include changes in body position, shifts in facial expression or eye gaze, breathing, eye closing, yawning, swallowing, skin flushing, and tears that well up or flow.

In addition to following the patient's body language and your own, a rule of thumb for skillful communication is to use the patient's verbal language and to follow the affect. By following the affect, the therapist is attentive and listening to the emotions the person is expressing, whether verbal or nonverbal. Sometimes, there are discrepancies in what the person says, the manifest content, and how something is said. For example, if a person is recounting a tragic loss in a monotone that belies the seriousness of the situation, the therapist may point it out to the patient in the form of an *observation*: "You have had this horrible loss, but you do not look or sound sad about it." The person may laugh inappropriately when discussing an unloving marriage, and the therapist may offer this comment: "I am thinking that perhaps it is easier to laugh when feeling so unloved than to feel sad about your wife's neglect." Observations are made in a collaborative attempt at understanding and out of genuine uncertainty, not as objective truth.

Ralph Greenson (1967) discusses the use of language in his seminal text on technique:

> *My language is simple, clear, and direct. I use words that cannot be misunderstood, that are not vague or evasive. When I am trying to pin down the particular affect the patient might be struggling with, I try to be as specific and exact as possible. I select the word which seems to portray what is going on in the patient, the word which reflects the patient's situation of the moment. If the patient seems to be experiencing an affect as though she were a child, for example, if the patient seems anxious like a child, I would say, "You seem scared" because that is the childhood word. I would never say, "You seem apprehensive" because that would not fit, that is a grown-up word. Furthermore, "scared" is evocative, it stirs up pictures and associations, while "apprehensive" is drab. I will use words like bashful, shy, or ashamed, if the patient seems to be struggling with feelings of shame from the past. I would not say humiliation or abasement or meekness. In addition, I also try to gauge the intensity of the affect as accurately as possible. If the patient is very angry, I don't say: "You seem annoyed" but I would say: "You seem furious." I use the ordinary and vivid word to express the quantity and quality of the affect I think is going on. I will say things like: You seem irritable, or edgy, or grouchy, or sulky, or grim, or quarrelsome, or furious, to describe different kinds of hostility. How different are the associations to grouchy as compared with hostile? In trying to uncover and clarify the painful affect and the memories associated to that specific affect, the word one uses should be right in time, quality, quantity, and tone. (pp. 108–109)*

Following the person's affect and staying emotionally close to the patient's experience enhances connection and the therapeutic alliance while assisting the person in labeling his or her emotions. Expanding the patient's repertoire and emotional vocabulary and awareness is largely the work of psychotherapy. There are many nuances of feelings, and the therapist needs to know the language of emotions. For example, when hurt, a person may feel forsaken, crushed, devastated, destroyed, pained, wounded, disgraced, humiliated, anguished, or rejected. Unless the therapist is aware of his or her own nuances of emotion, it is not possible to convey this knowledge to others. Therapists must know themselves as much as the words for emotions, and even experienced therapists do not always have a rich vocabulary to describe feelings.

Giving information is customary for nurses and includes psychoeducation. Information giving normalizes the situation, provides hope, helps to set goals, identifies options, helps deal with obstacles, corrects misinformation, provides new perspectives, provides feedback, and helps to reframe the situation. However, therapists must be careful to not overload patients with information and should consider timing. Often, the person needs an empathic response and may not be ready to hear any information. Any information given should be clear, specific, and concise. Giving information is not giving advice or telling the person what to do. Giving advice is not compatible with promoting empowerment. If helpful comments and suggestions worked, the patient would not be sitting in your office. Moreover, advice that does not work may be blamed on the therapist, and even if the advice is successful, it is a reminder of the patient's inadequacy and can ultimately be demoralizing. A better strategy is to offer the person various options and explore each so that the patient can choose what to do. In my experience in teaching psychotherapy to nurses, being nondirective and not offering *fix it* statements are difficult for novice APPNs, because most nurses are used to telling patients what to do, particularly in inpatient settings.

Educating the person about the psychotherapy process is an important component of the initial contact and the ongoing sessions. Often, the psychotherapeutic process seems strange to patients, even if they have had previous treatment. For example, it is common practice and therapeutic for therapists to ask questions about how patients feel about them or about coming to see them, but patients may think therapists want reassurance rather than an honest answer. Patients should be told at the outset that they sometimes may not want to come to their sessions and that is okay to not want to come, but that it may mean that important issues are surfacing and that it is important to come anyway and to be honest about how they are feeling. This is important information, particularly for patients who are in treatment for the first time. It is also important to tell patients that psychotherapy is a relationship and that the feelings elicited sometimes are similar to those experienced in past relationships. For example, if a patient has generally felt vulnerable in relationships and distanced from these feelings by avoiding others in the past, this reaction is likely to occur in the relationship with the therapist. Instruct the patient to tell the therapist when she or he begins to feel this way, because the information is important to the continuing work of psychotherapy. As therapy progresses, there are many opportunities to educate patients about the process of psychotherapy, and they are discussed throughout this textbook.

Giving recognition is a form of attending. It means that the therapist notices what the person has done and validates dimensions that are successful, which helps to build on strengths already in place. This is different from praise, because indiscriminate praise can backfire. Although praise may make the therapist and patient feel better temporarily, it can also leave the patient wondering about the therapist's sincerity and the reality of the person's strengths. If everything is wonderful, perhaps nothing is wonderful. Being a cheerleader implies that the therapist has judged that certain actions are desirable, and this does not foster the patient's empowerment and decision making. A better reply to positive change would be: "How did you feel about being able to say no and set limits on your own behalf?" Another caveat about cheerleading is that the patient may try to please the therapist, often unconsciously; nonetheless, the therapy process is hijacked and turned into what the person senses the therapist wants without advancing the patient's self-direction and empowerment.

Empathy

Perhaps the most important element of therapeutic communication is empathy. Cozolino (2017) speculates that empathic connectedness stimulates the biochemical changes in the brain that increase brain plasticity and enhance learning. This makes sense in light of Schore's work (2019), which demonstrates that social interactions early in life result in the stimulation of neurotransmitters and neural growth hormones that shape brain development. Research in *mirror neurons* provides a scientific explanation for the development of empathy through attachment relationships. (See Chapter 2.) The attachment arousal of the therapeutic relationship provides the interpersonal context for integration and regulation of neural networks, with empathy serving as the vehicle for this connection. Empathic resonance is a physiological state of consciousness that helps the therapist connect, attune, and coregulate with the patient (Schore, 2019).

Historically, there has been a considerable amount of research on empathy in nursing (LaMonica, Wolf, Madea, & Oberst, 1987; Layton & Wykle, 1990; Määttä, 2006; Morse et al., 1992; Wheeler, Barrett, & Lahey, 1996). Empathy is a complex concept, and three phases have been delineated. In phase 1, empathy reflects the individual's empathic potential or ability; in phase 2, empathy is expressed; and in phase 3, empathy is received. Research does not support that a high degree of the nurse's empathy ability results in the patient receiving that empathy. The most accurate measure of empathy for patient outcome is phase 3, empathy received (Wheeler, 2003). This is important because therapists may *feel* very empathic toward patients, but it is conveying this understanding to patients and their hearing it as such that count. The most accurate definition for empathy is "a process of understanding whereby the nurse enters the patient's perceptual world, the patient perceives this understanding, and confirmation of self occurs as part of this process" (Wheeler, 2003, p. 207). Confirmation of self is reflected in the patient feeling more worthwhile, energetic, confident, hopeful, and comforted. This physiological state results from the attunement and empathic resonance that are cultivated through empathic communication techniques.

How does the therapist convey empathy and ensure that it is heard by the patient? The therapist's empathy is only as helpful as it is accurate. For example, one patient came to his session looking very stony faced. The therapist misunderstood the patient's silence as anger rather than fear and said: "Perhaps you are angry at me because I had to cancel our session last week." The reality was that the patient was afraid that he had made a big mistake with his girlfriend and that she was going to break up with him. This kind of breach of empathy can be harmful to the therapeutic alliance. A better response for the therapist would be to observe and ask for clarification: "You look unhappy. What is going on?" To deepen the perception of what others are feeling, it is sometimes useful to ask, "What would someone be feeling who experienced this? What is the implicit communication in this situation?" Empathy is about trying to understand the key elements of what the person's experiences, behaviors, decisions, values, and feelings are and about communicating these elements back to the person to see whether the perceptions were correct. It is responding to the context or implicit communication, not just to the words. Often, the person is unaware of what his or her feeling is, and it is the therapist's job to perceive the emotion and to convey the perception to help the person expand awareness (i.e., to make the implicit explicit).

A related concept to empathy but a barrier to effective listening is being overly sympathetic. Feeling sorry for the patient can reinforce self-pity, does not help problem-solving, and can weaken the patient because the therapist is not emphasizing strengths. One patient reported fleeing treatment from a therapist because she experienced the former therapist as "too kind." If the therapist feels too sympathetic toward the patient, it is most likely about the therapist's feelings, not the patient's. For example, one student nurse cared for a young woman about her own age who had just lost her father. The student's own father had died after a protracted illness several years earlier. Unable to hide her sadness, the student began to cry and was less than effective in being present and objective for her patient.

Empathy picks up on implied feelings and can be invaluable in deepening the process. For example, one patient complained about being charged for a session she had missed for which she had not given 24 hours' notice. The patient said: "All you care about is money. You don't care that I was sick and couldn't come!" The therapist answered empathically, *reflecting* "You feel angry because you believe that you are not cared about?" This response was less threatening than "You feel angry because you think that I do not care about you." Even though the latter response was not said and was undoubtedly the more empathic statement, this is an example of being empathic by not expressing empathy, because the therapist understood that the patient would have been humiliated and would have experienced the latter response as threatening and intrusive. The patient went on to discuss how unfair it was that the therapist could cancel sessions without repercussions, whereas she had to come or would be charged anyway. The power imbalance of the relationship revived how she felt in her relationship with her mother, who was cold and controlling. Being able to express her feelings in a supportive relationship allowed her to remain in therapy and feel understood, even though the framework of the therapy contract, which involved paying for missed sessions, remained the same.

Reflection is a form of empathic validation. It helps to provide direction, shows the patient that the therapist understands the person's perspective, helps to develop insight into problems, and encourages the patient to continue discussion. "You feel so hopeless . . ." encourages the patient to expand on his hopelessness. The therapist uses the same language as the patient but does so by paraphrasing and summarizing, not by restating what the person has said. Summarizing pulls together the main themes of the patient's conversation and can be done at the beginning of a conversation, when a conversation is disjointed, when the patient is "stuck," when the patient needs a new perspective, and at the end of a conversation. For example, the therapist may say, "You seem to feel very angry but feel that you are not supposed to be?"

Contributions from both the therapist and patient influence the degree of empathy the patient perceives from the therapist. In a review of the literature on the therapist-mediating factors, Elliott and associates found that similarity between the therapist and patient, a nonjudgmental attitude on the part of the therapist, attentiveness, openness to discussing any topic including countertransference, ability to regulate and awareness of one's own emotions, ability to encourage exploration using emotion words, ability to take others' perspective, abstract ability, in addition to the therapist's posture, and vocal quality influenced patient perception of therapist empathy (Elliott, Bohart, Watson, & Greenberg, 2011). Conversely, therapist behaviors seen as less empathic include talking too much, advice giving, interrupting, failing to maintain eye contact, and dismissing the patient's ideas. Patient contributions include the patient's self-esteem, less patient pathology, and the patient's intelligence that all predicted the patient's perception of the therapist's empathy. By enhancing self-awareness and continual work on improving communication skills using the therapeutic skill-building exercises described previously, empathy can be enhanced. Box 4.4 identifies skills and techniques that help to enhance empathy.

If the therapist's empathic statement is correct, the response of the patient is often one of endorsement and opening up further about what is being discussed, sometimes with an enthusiastic "That's exactly how I feel" or at least with a nod and further thoughtful comments about what is being discussed. Empathy advances the conversation. However, if the therapist is off base, the patient may pause, and the conversation may flounder, or the person may try to help the therapist get back on track. For example, one woman whose husband insisted she see a therapist because she criticized him

BOX 4.4 Skills and Techniques to Increase Positive Reception of Empathic Overtures

Accept and appreciate the patient's world but make sure that your understanding fits with the patient's ability to tolerate it.

If you suspect that the patient would rather not hear your empathic statements, do not share them.

Add to or carry forward the meaning in the patient's communication.

Listen beyond the words. Attempt to capture the nuances and implications and reflect back your understanding.

Focus on patients' feelings, perceptions, meanings, values, assumptions, and their views of the other people and situations.

Be nonjudgemental, attentive, and open to discussing any topic.

Avoid interrupting, talking too much, and advice giving.

Source: Modified and adapted from Perraud, S., Delaney, K. R., Carlson-Sabelli, L., Johnson, M. E., Shephard, R., & Paun, O. (2006). Advanced practice psychiatric mental health nursing, finding our core: The therapeutic relationship in the 21st century. *Perspectives in Psychiatric Care, 42*(4), 215–226. doi:10.1111/j.1744-6163.2006.00097.x

constantly complained, "This is such a waste of time! I wouldn't be here if my husband didn't want me to come. He has all the problems. I don't know what I am doing here!" The therapist responded with what was thought to be a reflective statement: "You are angry that he thinks you have mental health problems." The patient angrily responded, "No, that is not what I am angry about. I am being forced to come here and am resentful that he is unfairly blaming me for his problems!" The therapist obviously misunderstood, and after the patient explained further, the conversation focused on her feelings of being dominated in her marriage and how she criticized her husband as a response to her hurt about his disregard of her feelings.

Empathy is an important element of anxiety management in psychotherapy. Because anxiety often occurs when the patient changes, it is an important dimension for the therapist to be aware of, especially when the patient begins to feel anxious after a significant therapeutic gain. Any new behavior, feeling, or thought increases arousal in the brain and creates some anxiety, even if it is a change for the better. Change does not feel natural in the beginning, and it may take many tries or much time before it becomes integrated into the patient's brain and way of being. It is helpful for the therapist to educate the patient to expect anxiety when change occurs. For example, one patient who had been able to make significant changes in boundaries in her relationship with her boyfriend came to her session and commented about how anxious she had felt during the past week for no apparent reason. The therapist made this *interpretation*: "Perhaps the anxiety you are feeling now is not so much about being stuck as about being able to do things differently from before and your newfound ability to say no when it is not something you want to do." In psychotherapy, there are always two steps forward and one step back. Emotion is a powerful agent of change and causes disruption (Damasio, 1999). It is thought that this is due to a proliferation of synapses which disorganizes the brain (Stien & Kendall, 2004). In any case, an increase in anxiety or depression after a positive change follows the basic biological principle that "there can be no reorganization without disorganization" (Scott, 1979, p. 233). Knowing this and watching for therapeutic regressions as a normal part of the therapeutic process are essential to assist patients in healing. The therapist can then educate the patient that the setback is temporary and a temporary response to change. The APPN then helps the patient to manage by exploring anxiety management techniques that have been helpful for this person in the past, and assisting with learning new resources, if needed.

Exploration

Exploring or investigative questions encourage the person to clarify, expand, elaborate, and focus, moving the patient from the general to the specific. Listen carefully to the patient so that your questions follow from what the person is saying, have a therapeutic purpose, and are clear, concise, simple, and judicious. Asking a question to which you think you know the answer but which the person is busy denying most often alienates the person and increases defensiveness. For example, a therapist may suspect that a person is having anxiety because of angry feelings toward his mother who neglected him, but the person may not be ready to examine this idea and instead be aware only of feeling disturbed about a friend's negligence. A premature statement by the therapist ("Perhaps you are really angry at your mother, who was not there for you") may be met with silence or vehement denial, further strengthening defenses. A better *clarification* type of question may be "What is the worst part about feeling neglected?" Gently leading the person to examine his or her feelings helps the patient to engage and can be an appropriate therapeutic intervention because through the inquiry, the person's self-understanding is deepened.

A caveat is that asking questions centers the control in the therapist because the conversation is directed to an area the therapist wants to explore, and questions should therefore be used judiciously. Too many questions yield negative results and can be a barrier to listening. All questions should be patient centered, and only one question should be asked at a time. Sometimes, therapists ask multiple questions because they are uncomfortable, and this can leave the patient feeling overwhelmed or confused. Another problem is that asking many informational questions collects facts but often misses the point about the psychotherapy process and what is happening for the patient. *Restating* or paraphrasing may be less threatening and allows more space for the patient to pursue what he or she feels is relevant. For example, "What I hear you saying is that you have been having a great deal of trouble getting to sleep but, once asleep, you can sleep through the night."

Listen to the person contextually by focusing on key themes and messages. For example, a man who came into therapy recounted a number of unfortunate events in his life, explaining that "bad stuff always finds me. I will never be happy, and I never get a break." Rather than asking questions about each instance, it is beneficial for the therapist to identify the themes of hopelessness and helplessness and to explore other dimensions, such as genetic roots (when in the past did he feel this way?) or other more adaptive situations (has there been any time when he did not feel this way?) or future potential (what would he like to feel in the future?).

Exploring can be verbal or nonverbal; shaking the head yes or saying "I see" encourages the patient to continue with the story. It can be particularly helpful to use open questions that encourage the patient to be active in the conversation: "How did you feel when your friend told you that he did not want to see you?" Open questions begin with who, what, how, when, and where, and they invite the patient to elaborate and provide factual information. Open questions are preferable in therapy, but they should not be so broad that the person is confused. For example, rather than asking "What kind of person are you?" it may be more helpful to ask "How are you like your mother?" Hypothetical questions such as "What do you think would happen if you quit taking your medications?" or "What would being assertive in that situation be like for you?" help the person imagine future consequences or possibilities.

Avoid "why" questions because they tend to have a critical tone, are likely to make patients feel defensive, and may be associated with disapproval. For example, "Why did you say that to your son?" most likely will cause anxiety, leaving the person feeling put on the spot and explaining unnecessarily. Usually, why questions can be rephrased with "how" exploring-type questions that ask the person to give his or her perspective on the situation. For example, "How did you feel when you said that to your son?" or "What was going on with you when you said that to your son?" may lead to deepening the patient's understanding of her feelings.

Closed questions such as "Are you still feeling depressed?" usually elicit one syllable answers such as "No" without elaboration and may be used to clarify information, but if they are used too much, the therapist begins to feel as if she is conducting an interrogation and the patient is passive. However, it is sometimes appropriate to ask a closed question to obtain specific information and then follow with an open question that elicits more information from the patient. Closed questions tend to be less arousing than open questions and sometimes can be interspersed with open questions that may be more anxiety provoking to assist the person who is hyperaroused. The therapist should not ask leading questions that imply how the patient should answer, such as "Do you think that your depression affects your relationship with your family?" or "You do believe that abortion is acceptable, don't you?"

Observation, focusing, immediacy, and *interpretation* are higher on the treatment hierarchy continuum and are usually not used in the initial session, but they are employed later as therapy progresses. Making an *observation* is verbalizing what is perceived or observed, and this encourages the patient to recognize specific behaviors and compare his or her perception with those of others. Observation can be extremely helpful to the person. For example, a pattern of relating may contribute to the person's problem, and the therapist may point out the pattern by making an observation: "I've been noticing that you joke a lot whenever I mention how devoted you are to your husband" or "You seem tense today." The patient then can elaborate on the therapist's comments. *Observation can also* involve pointing out discrepancies and distortions between verbal and nonverbal behavior in a nonjudgmental, tentative way. These types of observations are best delivered using I statements such as "I wonder whether you are thinking that you are not really drinking if you only have two beers?"

Focusing is drawing attention to a potentially anxiety-provoking issue for further exploration. It can help the patient become more specific, move from vagueness to clarity, and further understanding about an issue. In addition to the example in Table 4.4, another form of focusing is to polarize the two parts of the patient that are in conflict by asking the person to examine each part. For example, "A part of you may feel like coming here to work on your problems while another part of you feels hesitant to share so many feelings with me." Alternatively, the therapist may say: "It seems that a part of you would really like to stop drinking but another part of you is afraid to consider this." The therapist can then explore each part with the patient in a way that assists in understanding relevant implicit issues through the matter-of-fact manner that the therapist accepts the two parts of the person: "Please tell me about the part that is afraid to stop." This type of comment can deepen the patient's understanding about implicit barriers to change, and it reframes resistance as anxiety. This type of communication points to the importance of the therapist's empathy in recognizing the emerging inclination of the patient to change.

Immediacy and *interpretation* are probably the most anxiety-provoking therapeutic communication skills for any therapist. *Immediacy* is a type of confrontation that is challenging and requires self-awareness by the therapist. Often, the patient is not aware of how he is affecting others and that the same pattern is occurring in the therapeutic relationship. Immediacy involves exploring what is occurring currently in the therapeutic relationship, and it can help with problem resolution. The therapist can address a change in the process. For example, if the patient is suddenly withdrawn or hostile, the therapist may say: "What are you feeling at this moment?" or "What do you want to say right now?"

Egan (2006) identifies three types of immediacy: exploring what is occurring in the relationship in general; assessing what is happening at the moment between the patient and therapist; and giving present tense feedback to the patient. Examples for each type include "It is hard for you when you feel so misunderstood." "What do you want to say right now?" and "It is hard for me when you cut me off while I am talking." Immediacy may be used in situations in which factors impact the relationship, such as when trust is a concern, when the patient is "stuck," when boundaries are violated, or when tension or dependency is an issue. The patient's acknowledgment of dependence can be invaluable. Assertiveness, self-awareness, and courage are prerequisites for using this skill.

Interpretations can take the form of pointing out to the patient what the therapist hears him or her saying regarding conflicts that he or she is struggling with (i.e., making the implicit explicit). An interpretation is a statement that explains how a feeling, thought, behavior, or symptom is related to its unconscious origin. Repeated attention to unconscious material results in gradually expanding awareness and the integration of top-down and right-left neural networks (Cozolino, 2017).

Interpretations are largely the work of psychodynamic psychotherapy, and they serve to defuse the potency of defenses as coping strategies. Cozolino (2002) says, "Conscious awareness of the defenses often leads to experiencing the feelings against which the patient has been defending. The networks containing the negative emotions become disinhibited and activated. For example, if intellectualization is being used to avoid the shame and depression related to early criticism, recognition of the defense will bring these feeling memories to awareness" (p. 51). For example, a patient who may be warding off feelings of abandonment is angry and critical of her boyfriend, and the therapist offered this interpretation: "It seems that you feel so angry when you feel dependent on Dan."

All communication techniques are only as good as the therapist's understanding of the patient and the therapist's sensitivity to nuances. How you understand your patient will inform what you say, and your understanding will deepen as you gently explore with your patient and expand your knowledge about human behavior and development. What is said is informed by the theoretical approach the therapist is using. For example, interpretations are largely used in psychodynamic or interpersonal psychotherapy, whereas suggestion is used most often in cognitive behavioral therapy (CBT) or supportive psychotherapy. Communication depends on your theoretical understanding of the patient, the approach used, the phase of therapy, the context, your relationship with the patient, and your own self-awareness.

Situations in which interpretations can be particularly helpful are when patients engage in negative statements about themselves, constant excuses, complacency, rationalization, procrastination, and passing the buck. Interpretations can increase the patient's awareness, but because interpretations can be threatening, the therapist should allow time for the comment to be heard and should offer support with empathic statements. Interpretations often are most effective if delivered in two parts, with empathy offered first and with the second part containing the interpretation with *but* or *however* linking the two parts (Wachtel, 2011). For example, Wachtel provides an example of such an interpretation for an adolescent who refused to clean her room and who kept her mother in a constant state of agitation. The therapist stated: "It is hard to keep your room clean and neat, and I could be wrong about this, but from what you say, it sounds as if your mom gives you a lot of attention when your room is a mess."

Therapeutic communication is a set of skills that can be improved for both experienced and novice APPNs. Expanding one's repertoire of skills can be accomplished through practice and by enhancing self-awareness. Therapists can gain understanding through their own psychotherapy and through reflection and mindfulness exercises. These include audio taping, clinical studies, assignments, clinical supervision, discussion, journaling, critical incident techniques, learning diaries, process recordings, literature or vignettes, montage, painting, poetry, role playing, videotaping, and reading books that help to develop self-awareness and reflective thinking. Although time consuming to write, process recordings provide an invaluable opportunity to scrutinize communication skills and require no special equipment. An example of a format and directions for a process recording are provided in Appendix 4.5. More information on selected exercises designed to enhance reflection can be found at www.nursingsociety.org/about/resource_reflective.doc. Mindfulness exercises are also helpful in deepening self-awareness and are included in Chapter 17.

MAINTAINING THE FRAME

Boundaries

The term *boundaries* in psychotherapy refers to the therapist's ability to establish and maintain a treatment frame, set a schedule, and honor times; maintain a professional relationship; and protect the patient from intrusions into privacy and confidentiality.

The frame of treatment is the APPN's responsibility, and it is important in creating a safe environment for both the patient and the therapist. For patients with dysfunctional, out-of-control behaviors, adherence to limits and boundaries may be a major focus of the treatment. Most therapists do not allow eating, drinking, or smoking during sessions or any type of interruption during the session. All phones and beepers should be turned off. This is the patient's time, and distractions from the business at hand are counterproductive to good psychotherapy.

Therapists' violations of the frame, such as extending sessions longer than usual, being late for sessions, forgetting the session, not following the standard protocol for all patients for any reason, making special allowances for a particular patient, feeling the patient is special having social contact with the patient, and violating confidentiality, are all breaches of boundaries and can alert the therapist to countertransference issues that he or she needs to address. The therapist is often not aware initially of feelings toward the patient and becomes aware only by taking note of his or her own behavior and the signs of countertransference (Box 4.5).

Countertransference reflects feelings that the therapist has toward the patient and is similar in some respects to transference. Countertransference involves past significant relationships and includes attitudes, feelings, and thoughts about another person. Contemporary theorists believe that countertransference is a response to the patient's transference, and as such, it can be used to understand the patient. Countertransference can serve as a barometer in the relationship with the patient for the self-aware therapist. Although countertransference is usually associated with breaches of boundaries or problems in relationship, such as those listed in Box 4.5, like transference, countertransference can also be positive, such as idealizing feelings or empathic resonance with the patient.

Countertransference involves activation of the therapist's state-dependent memories in the relationship with the patient. As occurs in transference, countertransference reflects a particular physiological state of consciousness triggered by the relationship, and therapists' bodies can inform them about what is occurring. For example, one therapist reported that narcissistic patients triggered her to become exceedingly tired in

BOX 4.5 Signs of Countertransference

- Extending sessions longer than usual
- Being late for sessions
- Forgetting the session
- Seeing the person socially
- Violating confidentiality
- Dreams about the patient
- Difficulty staying awake during sessions
- Anger at the patient's inability to change
- Arguing or irritability that occurs in sessions
- Sexual or aggressive fantasies about the patient
- Rescue fantasies and offering advice and "fix it" statements
- Anxiety or guilt about what you did or did not say
- Thinking a lot about or being preoccupied with the patient outside of sessions
- Dreading the session
- Postponing confrontations or questions about lateness or absence
- Unnecessary reassurances and oversolicitousness
- Denying the pathology, conflict, or resistance
- Allowing the person to run up a high unpaid bill
- Ignoring the therapist's errors and the subsequent effect on the patient's behaviors
- Therapist's body feelings, images, and thoughts during the session

sessions, so much so that she often struggled to stay awake. For another therapist, the same patient may elicit tension in the chest. This is because state-dependent memories are idiosyncratic biochemical profiles that depend on each therapist's experiences and development and on the interaction with the patient's contributions in the co-construction of the relationship.

Images and thoughts during the session can also alert the receptive therapist to what may be going on during the psychotherapeutic process. For example, one therapist had an image come to mind during a session with a patient from a movie scene he had seen that depicted a forbidden sexual encounter. This was a cue to the therapist about the erotic transference developing in the relationship, even though the manifest content of the session was seemingly about an unrelated topic. The astute therapist is aware of all emerging thoughts, images, and sensations, without judgment or censorship, as manifestations of countertransference. They are considered important data about the therapeutic relationship and deepen the therapist's understanding about the unfolding process.

A therapist using his or her feelings as a clue to what may be going on for a patient is referred to as *autognosis*, and this can be very helpful in understanding the patient. Autognosis is similar but different from the nursing concept of *therapeutic use of self*, originally described by Travelbee (1971). Therapeutic use of self is the ability to use oneself consciously and in full awareness in an attempt to establish relatedness and to structure nursing interventions (Travelbee, 1971). In contrast, autognosis is using one's feelings to deepen understanding of the patient and use of oneself to diagnose the nature of the patient's problems. Often, these feelings are implicit and not fully conscious.

Two types of countertransference identified are concordant and complementary (Racker, 1968). *Concordant identification* is a process in which the therapist takes on the experience of a patient's personality as if it were his or her own. For example, when interacting with a sad patient, the therapist begins to feel sad. *Complementary identification* occurs when the therapist is treated transferentially by the patient as if the feelings were true. For example, one patient who had a critical father began to feel criticized and judged by the therapist, and the therapist did feel induced to act punitively toward the patient. Often, these types of countertransferential responses are transitory and serve to deepen the therapist's understanding of the patient. The therapist who is able to monitor his or her own emotional reactions, thoughts, and fantasies throughout a session can deepen the process in a way that otherwise may not be possible.

Although we often think of countertransference feelings as strong sexual or hostile feelings or boredom, often the therapist's feelings toward the patient are more nuanced and may include judgments or unconscious stigmatizing beliefs. For example, one graduate nursing student working with a patient who decided he wanted to go back to school and become a nurse created an uneasy feeling in the student who told him that he needed to not take on too many stressors (Buck & Lysaker, 2010). Responses such as these that are not enthusiastic or perhaps overly enthusiastic may reveal deeply held stigmatizing beliefs about mentally ill adults and be barriers to treatment. All feelings—the good, the bad, and the ugly—occur and can be used in the service of the therapeutic process by self-aware therapists. Strategies to enhance self-awareness are included in Chapters 1 and 17.

The relational-psychodynamic therapist may address or interpret the cocreated countertransference, whereas the cognitive behavioral therapist more likely may notice but not address it directly. Chapter 5, on supportive and psychodynamic psychotherapy discusses countertransference further. Even if the therapist decides it is best not to address what is going on with the person, the work is enhanced. For example, one patient seemed so vulnerable and childlike that the therapist would often have fantasies of protecting and rescuing her. Even though this was not directly addressed with the patient in treatment, knowing this allowed the therapist to contain these feelings so that support could be provided without infantilizing the patient. Occasionally, feelings can be so intense about a patient that they may be difficult to contain and be therapeutic. "Strong countertransference feelings can be invoked when working closely with patients who are resistant to change" (Jones, 2004, p. 18).

Supervision and one's own therapy can help to process emotional reactions. Lifelong supervision is always a good idea, but extra consultation with an experienced therapist can help in managing countertransference. Supervision consists of meeting regularly, much like therapy sessions, and discussing issues germane to the work of psychotherapy that the therapist needs help with. Often, supervision is a mixture of the patient's issues and the therapist's issues, because the latter impacts the treatment process in significant, often unconscious ways. For example, one young woman who came for therapy was extremely demanding and devaluing to the point that the therapist was defensive and dreaded her appointment each week. Discussing this patient in supervision helped the therapist to be more objective and understand how her own issues were triggered by the patient's devaluation. The therapist then was able to be more empathic and understand how the patient must have felt in her relationship with her devaluing mother.

Empirical and clinical studies on countertransference have found five interrelated factors that are important for management of countertransference: (1) therapist qualities of self-insight (aware of one's own feelings), (2) self-integration (ability to set boundaries and manage internal reactions), (3) empathy, (4) therapist's ability to admit a mistake, and (5) conceptualizing ability (i.e., the therapist understands the patient's dynamics theoretically (Hayes, Gelso, & Kivlighan, 2019). Therapists who possess these characteristics are seen as excellent by peers and can control countertransference acting out, and it is thought that these qualities are positively related to treatment outcome. In contrast, the therapist may have personality characteristics that are called *chronic countertransference*, such as a tendency toward rescuing the patient, being overly supportive or solicitous, or being authoritarian or antiauthoritarian and frequently violating the rules or frame of treatment. These attitudes can create chaos in the therapeutic relationship, and the therapist may need psychotherapy in addition to a consultation to ameliorate such traits. It is essential to monitor countertransferential feelings throughout therapy because these feelings are implicit and state dependent, and they may come to awareness only through ongoing self-reflection. Countertransference can significantly enhance or inhibit the therapeutic process. Seeking consultation and keeping documentation in clinical notes are essential to protect the therapeutic relationship and patient from therapist boundary problems. Theory and personal awareness are key to managing countertransference. See Appendix 4.6 for an Inventory of Countertransference.

Relationship Boundary Violations

Dual or multiple relationships pose a transgression of boundaries because of the power differential between the psychotherapist and the patient and thus the potential for exploitation. This means that a psychotherapist who is a teacher should not see his or her students in psychotherapy; that a psychotherapist should not see his or her patient's immediate family members for individual psychotherapy; that the psychotherapist should not work with those with whom there is a business, family, or close personal relationship. All requests by the patient to see friends should be explored by the APPN to understand better the closeness of that relationship to the patient. If it is determined that the referral by the patient is more than an acquaintance, an appropriate referral should be made to another therapist. Explain to the patient that is it not ethical for therapists to see the patient's family members or close friends because there may be a conflict of interest. An excellent website with resources on dual relationships, multiple relationships, and boundary decision is available at kspope.com/dual/index.php.

It is customary if the therapist sees the patient at a party or somewhere outside the therapy office, that the therapist waits for the person to acknowledge him or her so the person does not feel embarrassed or have other conflicting feelings. This may be an extremely uncomfortable situation for the patient and it is important to ask the person at the beginning of the next session how they felt about seeing you outside treatment.

The most egregious violation of boundaries is that of a sexual relationship with the patient. Sexual misconduct ranks as one of the highest causes of malpractice actions against mental health providers (Norris, Gutheil, & Strasburger, 2003). Often, patients express wishes to be closer to the therapist, occasionally sexually or as a friend. It is the therapist's job to assist the person in understanding the wish for closeness and not to gratify it, no matter how well intended. Even a slight boundary violation sends the wrong signal and may lead to more serious violations. In discussing why the therapist should not hug the patient, even if requested, McWilliams (2004) says, "physical contact of this sort collapses the 'space' between the two parties—the area of symbolization, play, and 'as-if' relating—that has been so carefully constructed over the course of the therapeutic work. Such a collapse reduces to a concrete physical act the complex metaphorical meanings of the longing to be held, and it creates unconscious anxiety that other strivings—ones that are not so attractive (such as the wish to attack physically or exploit sexually)—may also be acted out" (pp. 190–191).

Nurses are used to touching their patients, and the emphasis in some psychiatric nurse practitioner roles as primary mental healthcare practitioner may leave the nurse psychotherapist on a slippery slope. The blurring of boundaries in advanced practice nursing was first addressed in the literature by McCabe & Burnett (2006). Relatively few studies on touching patients in psychiatric settings have been conducted, and none has addressed touching in the role of APPN psychotherapist. Gleeson and Timmins (2004) studied caring touch, in contrast to task touch, in a long-term setting for older patients who suffer from dementia. They conclude with the caution against the widespread adoption of caring touch as an intervention for ethical reasons. Another qualitative study of seven outpatients, who had previously been hospitalized for psychosis, found that some of the informants felt violated and oppressed when touched by someone with whom they did not have an established relationship (Salzmann-Erikson & Erikson, 2005). However, positive results were found for an inpatient adolescent population when therapeutic touch was utilized (Hughes, Meize-Grochowski, & Harris, 1996).

Although some forms of therapeutic touch do not involve actually touching the patient (i.e., the nurse may keep hands an inch or two away from the patient's body), use of this or any kind of touch significantly changes the parameters of the psychotherapy frame. The setting, situation, patient population, and other factors dictate boundaries for the APPN role. The blurring of boundaries mandates that each APPN set limits based on the patient's welfare. Because research on the APPN relationship with the patient and the integration of touch and psychotherapy has not been conducted, it is prudent to regard touch as a boundary violation. If the APPN conducts a physical assessment at intake or admission, it is not appropriate to continue with that person in ongoing psychotherapy. Erring on the side of caution ensures a judicious and ethical practice.

Chapter 19, further discusses maintaining the therapeutic frame and boundaries for those who have problems with addictions. However, the transference and therapeutic issues identified for this population are relevant in working with all patients, and the reader is referred to that chapter for a fuller discussion on how to work with those who have an idealized or erotic transference.

Self-Disclosure

Minimal self-disclosure is part of maintaining a professional relationship. Self-disclosure is defined as the therapist revealing something personal. However, the therapeutic technique of immediacy is a powerful type of self-disclosure, in which the therapist reveals feelings about himself or herself in relation to the patient or the therapeutic relationship. Therapists must be aware of their own motives and thoughts relating to self-disclosure. Gabbard (2010) says: "Because we cannot be sure what we are up to when we are disclosing our own feelings to the patient, self-disclosure should be thought about carefully before using it" (p. 159). Self-disclosure should not be used to meet the therapist's own narcissistic or intimacy needs in that the focus is shifted from the patient. This can interfere with the flow of the session and may confuse or burden the patient. It is essential for APPNs to be aware of patients with whom they would be more likely to confide, because this may herald a potential boundary issue.

Based on an extensive review of the research on self-disclosure, Hill, Knox & Pinto-Coelho (2019) suggest the following practice guidelines for therapists:

1. Be cautious, thoughtful, and strategic about self-disclosure.
2. Focus on the patient's needs rather than the therapist's.
3. Make sure the therapeutic alliance is strong before using self-disclosure.
4. Keep the disclosure brief with few details.
5. Monitor how patients respond by asking about their feelings about the self-disclosure.
6. Focus on similarities between therapist and patient.

In general, the less self-disclosure by the therapist, the more the transference is thought to be heightened. Less self-disclosure may be more helpful for some patients who are higher functioning so that through discussion of the transference, profound learning and change may occur.

However, for those who use more immature defenses, such as projection, it may be better if the therapist is judiciously self-disclosing and more real so that less implicit feelings, thoughts, and state-dependent memories from the past are transferred onto the therapist, resulting in less distortion. Patients who are paranoid especially may need the therapist to be candid because they may project so much that it is important to inform them what aspects of their observations are accurate and what is being misinterpreted. Answering nondefensively and without evasion is usually warranted. For example, one patient who was schizophrenic asked the therapist why she dressed like a hippie. The therapist responded good-naturedly, "I kind of like these 60s outfits; I think I look groovy." The inherent inequity in the therapeutic relationship creates a climate in which dependency and some distortion are inevitable, with one vulnerable person requesting caretaking from another. The dependency triggered by psychotherapy can be particularly problematic for those needing stabilization and for those who have been chronically disempowered.

Questions about one's credentials and qualifications should be answered. The patient has a right to know the APPN's general therapy orientation and the amount of experience with the type of problem the patient has. A thornier issue related to self-disclosure and maintaining boundaries is how to answer patients who ask personal questions. If the patient asks the therapist personal questions, the therapist can say, "I'll be glad to answer that, but first I'm wondering what your thoughts are about that and how is it that you are asking?" If the patient persists in asking personal questions that the therapist does not want to answer (e.g., "Are you divorced?" or "How many children do you have?") the therapist should listen for the latent content and explore what the patient is really asking for. For example, "Are you married?" may mean "Are you available?" or

"Are you gay?" Often, the question is really about the person wondering whether the therapist can be trusted and reflects concerns about whether the therapist likes him or her, can understand his or her culture, and can relate to the patient. The patient may be unsure about the intimacy of therapy versus the intimacy of a personal relationship. The therapist can say: "You are very curious about me. Can you tell me more about that?" or "This is your time to talk about you." If the person persists, and the therapist does not want to answer the question, it is best to say this honestly, "I am not comfortable answering personal questions about myself, but I am interested in how this information is important to you." It is possible to spend the whole session on the meaning of the person's question by reflecting: "It sounds as if you are feeling that if I am not married like you, I will not be able to understand how you feel." The therapist and patient then can explore the context for this belief. It is only through inviting the patient to express his or her reservations about therapy and about you that the process can proceed. Being curious, interested, and open to all communication are essential skills for all therapists.

Cancellations, Fees, and Lateness

Even though the patient has signed a contract about the cancellation policy and fees were discussed during the initial session, the policy may need to be revisited as therapy proceeds. Undoubtedly, the patient will cancel and forget that he will be charged for missed sessions as the policy proscribes. Understanding money issues in psychotherapy is essential. For example, paying late may be a signal that the patient unconsciously expects to be taken care of or forgetting to pay may be a passive aggressive act, and there may be any number of other unconscious reasons that the patient may deviate from the agreed fee structure and cancellation policy. Addressing and exploring the behavior to clarify the psychological meanings and to reiterate the frame for payment are imperative. Often, forgetting to pay reflects deeper meanings than at first glance.

It is not good practice for the patient or the therapist to allow a large outstanding bill to accumulate. A better alternative is to explore the meaning of not paying and help the person deepen his or her understanding while maintaining the frame of the contract. Higher-functioning patients usually honor the therapist's fee structure and are easier to work with when exploring money issues than those who are lower functioning. For example, one patient who was a therapist herself expected a reduced fee after her insurance company changed and she no longer had good coverage for outpatient psychotherapy. In exploring this subject with her, deep feelings of sadness and abandonment surfaced from her childhood related to the caretaking role she had played with her mother, who had significant emotional and financial problems. Implicit neural networks associated with dependency and entitlement were triggered in therapy when she was asked to take care of the therapist by paying more out-of-pocket fees for her sessions. As the therapist explored these issues and reworked them in the present, the patient was able to make new neural connections that allowed her to continue in treatment and pay the charged fee. This awareness reverberated to other areas of her life, and she benefited financially in her own practice as a consequence of her work on this issue. Often, money issues in treatment reflect similar difficulties for the person outside the therapy.

Essential to maintaining the frame is the therapist's reliability and consistency of sessions. The therapist must be on time for sessions. It is important to keep the time of the session the same each week because changing appointment times often creates chaos, and the patient may not honor the commitment if the therapist is a poor example. Informing the patient well ahead of time when you will be gone and trying to reschedule, if possible, are common courtesies and essential for integrity of the frame. The patient's lateness and not showing up for appointments are likely to be forms of resistance, but it is important to understand that tardiness and absence may be caused by an unforeseen circumstance. Emergencies, such as illness, lack of childcare, transportation problems, or weather problems do occur. It is important to determine whether this is an isolated event or whether a pattern is developing. If the lateness is a one-time event, you can open a discussion by observing: "I notice you were late today." However, if the person has been late two or three times in a row, the cause is most likely resistance, which should be addressed, or the person may leave treatment altogether. It may be better to wait until an opening in the session presents itself or the person's defenses may increase. If an opening does not present itself, the therapist can say: "You have been 10 minutes late for the past 2 weeks, and it seems hard for you to get here on time." The person may launch into the *real* reasons for the tardiness. The therapist can then ask, "Do you have any other feelings about coming here lately?" Approaching with curiosity and understanding conveys caring and allows the patient to explore what is going on. It is important for the therapist to adhere to the established time for the session and not extend the time another 10 minutes if the patient is 10 minutes late.

If the person does not show up for a scheduled session and does not call, most therapists assume that the patient will come to the next session and do not contact the person. However, if two sessions are missed, the person is usually called, and a message is left that states: "I had in my appointment book that you were coming yesterday at 3, and you did not come. I hope everything is okay. Please call if you would like to schedule an appointment. I look forward to hearing from you." Adding the last sentence is helpful, because the person may feel that the therapist is angry if he or she has missed several times. If the person calls, confirms, comes the following week, and has not missed before, the therapist must explore what is going on with the person, because the resistance must be addressed if the patient is to continue. If the person does not address the absence, the therapist can ask: "How did you feel about missing the past few weeks?" If this is the first time a session was missed, the therapist can reiterate the policy about paying for missed sessions once before instituting it the next time. If the patient calls and says she or he wants to end treatment, the therapist should suggest that the person come in to discuss the issue first.

Even when issues are discussed and the patient still wants to terminate against the therapist's best judgment, it can still be helpful to the patient to meet for a final session. The therapist can use this opportunity to explore what is going on and leave the door open for future work when the patient is ready. However, if the person does not call or come to the next confirmed appointment and has missed three sessions in a row, a termination of treatment letter (see Appendix 4.7) should be sent to the person. This official termination letter protects the therapist from legal liability if the person has difficulties later. Chapter 24, provides further discussion of termination.

Telephone Calls and Emails

Being responsible for patients 24 hours a day is often a new experience for most new APPNs, and it is essential that emergency coverage is in place. It is important to state explicitly whether you will be available for phone calls between sessions and adhere to clear limits. How the patient contacts you between sessions and in emergencies is included in the contract given to the patient during the initial session. Although you need not be available around the clock, suitable arrangements should be made. Reasonable examples include having a pager or cell phone and providing patients with a number so that they may contact you if needed, hiring an answering service that contacts you when contacted by a patient, and sharing coverage with colleagues who are each on call every few days, provides uninterrupted coverage throughout the week and weekend. Checking messages at least once each day and calling back within 24 hours are good practice habits that are relevant for legal and ethical professional responsibility. Some therapists leave a message on their answering machine that states that he or she will call back as soon as possible and that if this is an emergency, the patient should go to the ED or call a crisis hotline. In this way, you are not serving as the ED liaison and setting appropriate limits on your availability. Asking a colleague to cover is essential for vacations and time off, in addition to discussing fragile patients who may call while you are gone. It is helpful to write notes for the covering person with details about the patient's name, address, phone number, and narrative about issues that may arise. This is a courtesy to your colleague and your patient.

Occasionally a patient may call between sessions to hear the therapist's voice, and this can be quite soothing to those needing stabilization. Emails can also connect with patients and be helpful between sessions. However, this can create problems if the patient expects a timely response for lengthy journal entries. This puts an unnecessary burden on the therapist and complicates boundaries and the frame. Phone calls from patients between sessions should be discouraged by assessing quickly whether the call is truly an emergency and, if not, gently saying: "This sounds important, and we need to talk more about it when you come next week." However, sometimes a phone call from a patient who has been averse to seeking help or afraid to trust can signify that a positive shift has occurred in the therapeutic relationship. In other cases, a phone call may mean increasing desperation and loneliness. It may be necessary to strengthen affect management strategies for those who have difficulties in this area.

No matter what the reason, it is important to limit conversations, because giving away free sessions over the phone violates the frame and cultivates an unhealthy dependency. If the APPN is receiving several urgent phone calls each week, the possibility exists that such calls are inadvertently being encouraged, and consultation with an experienced therapist is indicated. Conducting phone sessions in lieu of office sessions is not routinely advised, but it may be necessary on occasion or in addition to a regularly scheduled weekly appointment. Fees for phone sessions are the same as for regular sessions. Phone sessions also may serve as a way to wean the patient from psychotherapy during termination. This topic is covered in Chapter 24.

WORKING WITH RESISTANCE

Resistance has traditionally been viewed as an inevitable and unfortunate occurrence in the psychotherapeutic process. Historically, resistance was thought to reflect the unconscious forces of the patient that inhibit change but more recently resistance is thought of as an opportunity to increase understanding of the patient (Gabbard, 2017). Resistance is seen primarily as a defense that shows the therapist that the patient's anxiety has increased and that defenses are near the surface, indicating an opportunity for insight. Despite this idea about resistance, research suggests that psychotherapy works best if the therapist induces as little resistance as possible while moving the patient toward his or her goals (Tryon, Birch, & Verkuilen, 2019). This is easier said than done, because change is always fraught with anxiety and resistance is a manifestation of anxiety. Resistance can be thought of as implicit memory networks created through earlier dysfunctional situations and relationships that serve a self-protective function. Resistances manifest in psychotherapy as aspects or issues in treatment that challenge the person's ability to change. It is often these implicit neural patterns and ways of being that have brought the person into therapy in the first place. These defenses or resistances have been helpful and were functional for the person in the past, and for this reason, understanding resistances can be valuable to the work of therapy. Chapter 5, discusses further how to work with resistance.

Often, a parallel process occurs, and the therapist's defenses are also triggered when the patient manifests resistance. Resistance is not always easy to recognize, and if the issue is not addressed, the patient may not return. Traditionally, resistances are thought to be caused by anxieties about the unknown, loss of control, rejection, loss of meaning, physical pain, isolation, and self-loathing (Gabbard, 2017). These manifest as agitation, demanding behaviors, silence, noncompliance, chronic lateness, not coming to sessions, anger, eagerness to leave treatment, superficial chit chat, paranoia, irritability, lack of progress, requests for special favors, eating or drinking during sessions, homework not done, nonpayment or late payment of bills, sexual interest in the therapist, frequent requests for personal information from the therapist, and doorknob disclosures (i.e., bringing up important material or intense emotion at the end of the session). When patients introduce new information as they are on the way out, this ensures that there will not be enough time to deal with the issues. This represents resistance in the form of ambivalence. If this occurs, it may be helpful to bring up the issue at the beginning of the next session to open up exploration.

A more contemporary view of resistance through the lens of adaptive information processing (AIP) theory is that resistance may reflect blocked processing. The blocked processing is due to reactance, that is, a failure of the therapist to fit the treatment to the receptivity of the patient. Expert therapists tailor interventions to meet the person's needs. For example, for those patients who are highly resistant, less directive models of therapy are used that allow more control for the patient. For example, directive therapies such as CBT may be better for patients who are less resistant, and nondirective forms such as psychodynamic therapy and interpersonal therapy may be better for highly resistant patients. A meta-analysis of 12 studies supports that nondirective techniques predict better treatment outcomes for highly resistant patients (Beutler, Harwood, Michelson, Song, & Holman, 2011). Clinically, it is important to identify those who are the low- or high-resistant patients. Several groups of those who are likely to be high resisters include adolescents, paranoid or distrustful patients, and those who are forced to come to treatment by the court, a spouse, a job, or a family member.

The therapist's competency in dealing with resistance includes identifying problems in collaboration, recognizing defenses and obstacles to change, and understanding ways to address resistance. Responses by the therapist to the patient have been identified as helpful: acknowledging and reflecting the patient's concern, discussing the therapeutic relationship, renegotiating the contract and goals, listening versus talking should shift more toward the patient, and using fewer instructions (Beutler & Harwood, 2000; Beutler et al., 2011). The therapist first observes and points out the behavior: "I notice that you have been pretty quiet the past couple of weeks during our sessions" or "You seem angry today" or "It is so hard for you to be here when you don't want to be here." Interventions that discuss the therapeutic relationship are called *process comments* and include questions such as "How did you feel when you left the last session?" or "How do you think things are going here?" These questions invite the patient's response. Sometimes, questions engender a limited or no response, but often such inquiries open up the process in a way that allows the patient to share feelings. The ensuing conversation may be surprising, because the person often responds quite honestly with feelings that are enlightening. If the person says that something is a problem or that things are not going so well, the therapist can explore further what would help to make it better. This can be very helpful for collaboration. On the other hand, the person may not know how he or she is feeling and may deny any negative feelings. The therapist can then explore with another question: "How did you feel when I asked you that?" These types of process questions encourage self-exploration and may enable the person to deepen self-awareness so that acting out can be minimized.

Renegotiating the contract and goals may not be feasible, but discussion and flexibility may be indicated if content and process comments are not working. Maintaining firm limits may be the focus of therapy for some patients, such as those who have borderline personality traits and who desperately need structure and consistency. Others may be better served by flexibility and the APPN moving with the resistance. Box 4.6 provides an example of moving with the resistance and renegotiating the contract for a patient who suffered an alliance rupture. Two things are important to remember about resistance. If resistance is increasing and not addressed, the patient may never return; however, once articulated by the patient and heard by a curious, nonjudgmental therapist, the resistance can be defused, often allowing the patient to continue with the work of therapy. Perhaps it is the empathic connectedness of the therapeutic relationship that allows new expectations and learning to occur.

During the session in Box 4.6, Ms. A's anger and hurt are acknowledged and validated empathically, and the therapist apologizes. This session illustrates an example of moving with resistance based on a real issue that the therapist acknowledges, not

---

BOX 4.6 Moving With Resistance and Renegotiating the Contract

Ms. A is a 28-year-old woman, who initially sought help for panic attacks. A major theme in her treatment was her intense neediness and struggle for love and safety. Asking for help was fraught with anxiety because she was ridiculed in her family for asking for anything, and this was compounded by the fact that on some level she felt that others should know what she wanted without telling them. The following process was from a session that addressed her leaving her last session seemingly angry (i.e., her face appeared angry, and she slammed the door as she left). The therapist had a cold during the session and had to struggle to stay awake.

APPN: How did you feel when you left the last session?

Ms. A: Angry; I wanted to shake you apart.

APPN: Tell me more about how you felt.

Ms. A: I felt lost; you don't talk to me enough. You weren't really with me.

APPN: Thank you for telling me how you felt. I'm sorry. I was not feeling well and really was not there for you. I understand how angry you must feel about being here and not being heard.

Ms. A: Yes, this is a waste of time, and I don't want to come here anymore.

APPN: You have been feeling that you are not getting better and that this is a waste of time?

Ms. A: I'm not that much better. I haven't had any more panic attacks, but maybe they are just going away on their own.

APPN: When you first came here, that was what you wanted to work on, and it seems that the panic attacks have lessened and are not such a problem for you anymore. Perhaps it would be helpful to discuss whether there are any other areas of your life in which you would like things to be different.

Ms. A: Well, can you find me a boyfriend? Jim [her boyfriend] is AWOL.

APPN: What do you mean by AWOL?

Ms. A: Jim wants his space and just wants to be by himself. [She then recounted numerous instances of his inattention to her needs and rude behavior toward her.]

APPN: How hurtful it is to feel so rejected and devalued. From what you have told me, you are feeling so vulnerable with Jim right now that it might be helpful to talk about some resources to help you feel stronger in situations in which you feel dependent and needy. Would it be okay to continue for a few more sessions and see if we can come up with a plan that will help you and then reevaluate whether this is the best time for you to stop?

Ms. A: Okay, I suppose, but only for a few more sessions.

on the patient's distortions, which is what we frequently think of as resistance. This is important in that the therapist needs to be prepared to take responsibility for mistakes. The therapist moves with the resistance by inviting Ms. A to talk about how she felt, even though she suspected that the patient would criticize her, and the therapist then thanks Ms. A for telling her how she felt. This patient risked criticizing the therapist, and the therapist was glad that Ms. A was able to trust the relationship enough to be honest about her feelings. Ms. A's feelings toward the therapist and Jim, her boyfriend, are similar and reflect current feelings and thoughts that are associated with implicit memories of being ignored and not responded to. Although not explicitly linked by the therapist, this issue is addressed by the renegotiating of goals. Setting new goals is another example of moving with the resistance, and although the therapist does think that the therapy has been helpful in decreasing Ms. A's panic attacks, she does not disagree with her about that because it will not serve to advance the process at this point. This also illustrates how the therapist moved with the resistance. This was a much different experience for Ms. A from what she remembers in her family when she asked for help. After a few more sessions, the therapist again asked Ms. A how she was feeling, how things were going, and whether they were on track with her goal of enhancing resources.

This example illustrates what is called an alliance rupture, that is, tension or breakdown in the collaborative relationship between the patient and the therapist (Eubanks et al., 2019). Such a rupture can occur at the beginning of treatment or anytime over the course of treatment. Unlike this example, sometimes patients may be only vaguely aware of their dissatisfaction and it is up to the APPN to help the person express negative feelings. These ruptures often leave the therapist feeling confused, incompetent, and guilty. An extensive review of the literature and research found a number of therapeutic strategies helpful to repair alliance ruptures (Eubanks et al., 2019). Please see Box 4.7.

Paradoxical Interventions

Paradoxical interventions are used for patients who are said to be highly resistant and experiencing much conflict about change. These communication strategies assist in looking at the problem in a new way and are paradoxical because they ask the person to embrace the behavior that the therapy is aiming to diminish (Wachtel, 2011). This approach often helps the person to become unstuck through bypassing the resistance and overloading the conscious mind with confusion. The problem that was thought to be uncontrollable becomes volitional and purposeful. Neurophysiologically, this may be arousing, particularly in the frontal and parietal lobes, which become activated during novel stimuli, and this allows a window of opportunity for new learning to occur. This parallels brain development in that repeated exposure to new stimuli in a supportive

---

BOX 4.7 Therapeutic Strategies for Alliance Repair

- Be aware of subtle indications of ruptures in the relationship and explore the patient's negative feelings.
- Respond nondefensively and accept responsibility for your contribution to the interaction.
- Emphasize with patient's experience and validate the patient for bringing it up.
- Consider changing the goals of treatment.
- Consider linking ruptures in session to interpersonal patterns in the person's life.
- Empathically explore your own negative feelings so you can do the same for your patient.

interpersonal context results in the brain's increased ability to tolerate increasing levels of arousal and permit ongoing neural integration (Cozolino, 2017). Paradoxical interventions challenge the established neural networks in the context of guidance and support that underlies all forms of successful therapy.

Paradoxical interventions are most appropriately used for patients who cannot see any other possibilities and are consistently self-defeating. The therapist connects with the person through understanding and empathy, agrees with the person, and then prescribes the problem behavior or may ask the patient to observe the behavior. One strategy is to ask the patient to not try to change the behavior but instead to observe it and keep track of it throughout the week. This changes the relation of the person to the behavior so that the behavior is no longer the enemy and becomes a curiosity because an antagonistic attitude often accompanies what should be changed. This also increases the therapeutic distance of the problem, and the person develops the capacity for an observing ego whereby the person is not the problem. For example, the insomniac who is battling to go to sleep dreads going to bed and may benefit from being told to try to stay awake and resist going to sleep. An analysis of two studies of treatment for chronic insomnia confirmed that paradoxical intention reported greater benefit compared to placebo (Morin et al., 1999). Another example of a paradoxical intervention is the therapist telling the person who is paranoid and highly distrustful, "It is probably a good idea not to trust me and wait until later to make sure that it is safe." For patients who are locked into being helpless, hopeless, and self-defeating, a useful paradoxical communication may be "I can understand believing that nothing will ever be better would make everything seem pretty impossible. Please continue this week to notice all the negative thoughts that come up for you without trying to make anything better."

These interventions have been used and are embedded in various psychotherapy approaches such as family, behavioral, solution focused, and psychodynamic therapies (Wachtel, 2011). Erickson, the master of paradox and metaphor, developed elaborate interventions designed to intentionally confuse the patient through contradictory commands during trance (Lankton & Lankton, 1991). Westerman and colleagues found that brief paradoxical treatment was more effective for resistant patients than brief behavioral treatment (Westerman, Frankel, Tanaka, & Kahn, 1987). A meta-analysis of 15 studies supports the idea that paradoxical treatments are more effective than nonparadoxical treatments for various behavioral problems (Hill, 1987).

Paradoxical interventions may be inappropriate for the beginning therapist because if not used sparingly and sensitively, the therapist may be experienced as sarcastic. For example, a patient who is plagued by distressing, negative thoughts may be advised to take 5 minutes of every hour to worry. Suggesting this without proper empathy may serve to humiliate and further alienate the person from his or her therapist. Prefacing such a suggestion with "I can see how having such negative thoughts would make things look pretty impossible" conveys an appreciation of the person's experience. There are a wide range of applications for paradoxical interventions such as smoking cessation, binge eating, anxiety disorders, behavioral problems, depressive thinking, or any problem where the person is entrenched in a self-defeating pattern of behavior that creates pain for the person.

Secondary gain means that the person develops an illness or perpetuates a behavior that results in favorable environmental, interpersonal, monetary, or situational benefits. Sometimes, these gains are explicit (i.e., in the person's awareness), and other times they are implicit and can be brought to consciousness through exploration. For example, for a depressed patient who was asked to list the pros and cons of being depressed, the person identified and clarified the secondary gains received from being depressed, which the person may only have been dimly aware of before. The areas identified included avoiding confrontation and possible abandonment by his partner, sex with his partner, and work in an area he did not like. Once identified, these underlying issues could then be explored. Open-ended exploration of what would happen if the person changed and asking how this change would affect his or her life and important relationships are relevant questions to ask at the beginning of any treatment to examine whether there are secondary gain issues. Often, secondary gains are more apparent to others than to the person. Skillfully leading the person to his or her own discovery can potentiate significant, long-lasting change.

CONCLUDING COMMENTS

In the initial session, assessing safety, developing an alliance, and goal consensus begin the psychotherapeutic process through the use of open-ended therapeutic communication. This applies to all models of psychotherapy and practice settings. Engagement of the patient is essential to ensure that the person returns after the intake process is complete. A review of early research on attrition reports that roughly 50% of patients drop out by the third session (Barrett et al., 2008). Despite managed care and the emphasis on brief treatment, keeping people in treatment until their goals are met is a hallmark of successful therapy. As you increase your skills in engagement and assessment, you will be able to achieve competency in assessment in a shorter period.

Both patients and therapists need to have the security of boundaries and a frame for practice to be comfortable with the anxiety-provoking work of psychotherapy. Early in the therapy process, it is thought that most patients consciously or unconsciously test the frame of the treatment. A person may *forget* to come or to pay, may be late, or continue to talk beyond the scheduled session time even when reminded that it is time to stop. It is always best to err on the side of consistency when setting boundaries. Both patients and therapists may have problems adhering to the frame. For example, ending the session and adhering to the time frame may be difficult for a variety of reasons for the therapist. The therapist may feel inadequate and extend the session, thinking perhaps that listening longer will make the person feel better or that it is okay to make up the time the person missed if he or she is late. It is important for the APPN to maintain the frame and start the session on time and end on time so that if the person has an appointment at 12 and comes at 12:30, the session that is scheduled for 45 minutes will still stop at 12:45 as previously planned. Patients may have separation issues and not want to leave. The person may linger while writing a check, talk about a scheduling problem, ask for a referral for a friend, or bring up an issue that seems important to address sooner rather than later (i.e., doorknob disclosure). Other patients may get intensely emotional during the last 5 minutes of the session. Offering the person a few extra minutes may be appropriate but difficult, particularly when other patients are waiting. The therapist can gently say something such as: "I'm sorry, but we do have to stop now. You have touched on some very sad feelings that would be important to talk more about. Would you like to wait in the waiting room until you feel better?" Ending the session on time is an area that well-intended therapists often struggle with in maintaining the frame.

For the novice APPN psychotherapist, the frame of treatment, payments, session times, phone calls, emergencies, and other factors are usually decided by the setting in which the therapist accepts employment, and have little to do with the therapist's preferences. Although the rules of the employing agency may not be what the therapist would choose, it is best for the patient if the therapist adheres to the policies. In opening a practice, the therapist is faced with a multitude of issues about the frame, such as setting fees, collecting money, availability, session times, cancellations, and records, that must be decided. The process of psychotherapy encourages powerful attachments for both participants, and these feelings may undermine the APPN's confidence about limits and sometimes obscure the importance of maintaining the frame. Boundaries, working with resistance, and setting limits are areas that challenge even experienced therapists. Errors will be made at times, but it is important to be able to recognize situations when boundary or resistance issues arise, to regain balance, and to follow the frame for treatment as closely as possible. This is what the work of psychotherapy is about, no matter what approach or model is used.

DISCUSSION QUESTIONS

1. Discuss transference, and give a clinical example from your practice. Describe how your understanding of transference affects your response as a therapist.
2. Develop specific goals for how and what therapeutic communication skills you would like to integrate and further develop in your practice.
3. Generate a list of words for the various nuances that can be used to describe the feeling of anger, and generate another list for the feeling of sadness.
4. Discuss the goals of the first session.
5. Discuss why the therapeutic alliance is important, and identify psychotherapeutic strategies that can help in developing this alliance.
6. Is empathy always a good thing? Give some examples of when it may be a problem.
7. Using the example of a practice contract from Appendix 4.2 or from the website cited in the chapter, develop a one-page contract or office policy that you could give to patients.
8. Identify from your clinical practice an example of complementary or concordant countertransference, and explain how your feelings might have helped you in understanding your patient.
9. Describe a clinical situation in which paradoxical interventions may be useful, and develop a plan to use this strategy.
10. Discuss communication techniques for dealing with three specific instances of resistance, and give examples for each.
11. Examine your own areas of chronic countertransference and what may be helpful to you in your future APPN practice.
12. What is meant by the *slippery slope* and what problems may arise as a result of integrating therapeutic touch and Reiki in your APPN practice? Discuss strategies for how you could address these issues.
13. A patient who has been depressed most of her life comes to therapy complaining that she is hopeless, helpless, and will never have a good life. Discuss your gut reaction with someone with this characterological issue and how this could impact frame issues such as money, time, and therapist availability.

REFERENCES

Barrett, M. S., Chua, W. J., Crits-Christoph, P., Gibbons, M. B., Casian, D., & Thompson, D. (2008). Early withdrawal from mental health treatment: Implications for psychotherapy practice. *Psychotherapy*, 45(2), 247–267. doi:10.1037/0033-3204.45.2.247

Beutler, L. E., & Harwood, M. T. (2000). *Prescriptive therapy: A practical guide to systematic treatment selection*. New York, NY: Oxford University Press.

Beutler, L. E., Harwood, T. M., Michelson, A., Song, X., & Holman, J. (2011). Resistance/reactance level. *Journal of Clinical Psychology: In Session*, 67(2), 133–144. doi:10.1002/jclp.20753

Buck, K., & Lysaker, P. H. (2010). Clinical supervision for the treatment of adults with severe mental illness: Pertinent issues when assisting graduate nursing students. *Perspectives in Psychiatric Care, 46*(3), 234. doi:10.1111/j.1744-6163.2010.00258.x

Center for Disease Control and Prevention. (2018). *CDC vital signs: Suicide.* Retrieved from https://www.cdc.gov/vitalsigns/pdf/vs-0618-suicide-H.pdf

Centers for Medicare & Medical Services. (2011). CMS manual system(*Pub. 100-02 Medicare benefit policy*). Retrieved from https://www.cms.gov/Regulations-and-Guidance/Guidance/Transmittals/downloads/R140BP.pdf

Centers for Medicare & Medicaid Services. (2020, March). *Telehealth services fact sheet.* Retrieved from https://www.cms.gov/Outreach-and-Education/Medicare-Learning-Network-MLN/MLNProducts/downloads/TelehealthSrvcsfctsht.pdf

Centers for Medicare & Medicaid Services. (2018). *Medical privacy of protected health information.* Retrieved from https://www.cms.gov/Outreach-and-Education/Medicare-Learning-Network-MLN/MLNProducts/downloads/SE0726FactSheet.pdf

Cozolino, L. (2002). *The neuroscience of psychotherapy: Building and rebuilding the human brain* (2nd ed.). New York, NY: W. W. Norton.

Cozolino, L. (2017). *The neuroscience of psychotherapy: Healing the social brain* (3rd ed.). New York, NY: W. W. Norton.

Damasio, A. (1999). *The feeling of what happens: Body and emotion in the making of consciousness.* New York, NY: Harcourt.

Delaney, K. R., Drew, B. L., & Rushton, A. (2019). Report on the APNA national psychiatric mental health advanced practice registered nurse survey. *Journal of the American Psychiatric Nurses Association, 25*(2), 146–155. doi:10.1177/1078390318777873

Dziopa, F., & Ahern, K. (2009). What makes a quality therapeutic relationship in psychiatric mental health nursing: A review of the research literature. *Internet Journal of Advanced Nursing Practice, 10*(1). Retrieved from http://ispub.com/IJANP/10/1/7218

Egan, G. (2006). *Essentials of skilled helping: Managing problems, developing opportunities.* Belmont, CA: Thomson.

Elliott, R., Bohart, A. C., Watson, J. C., & Greenberg, L. S. (2011). Empathy. *Psychotherapy, 48*(1), 43–49. doi:10.1037/a0022187

Eubanks, C. F., Muran, J. C., & Safran, J. D. (2019). Repairing alliance ruptures. In J. C. Norcross & M. Lambert (Eds.), *Psychotherapy relationships that work: Evidence-based responsiveness* (3rd ed., Vol. 1, pp. 549–579). New York, NY: Oxford University Press.

Flückiger, C., Del Re, A. C., Wampold, B. E., & Horvath, A. O. (2019). Alliance in adult psychotherapy. In J. C. Norcross & M. Lambert (Eds.), *Psychotherapy relationships that work: Evidence-based responsiveness* (3rd ed., Vol. 1, pp. 24–78). New York, NY: Oxford University Press.

Fowler, J. S. (2012). Suicide risk assessment in clinical practice: Pragmatic guidelines for imperfect assessments. *Psychotherapy, 49*(1), 81–90. doi:10.1037/a0026148

Gabbard, G. O. (2010). *Long-term psychodynamic psychotherapy: A basic text.* Washington, DC: American Psychiatric Publishing.

Gabbard, G. O. (2017). *Long-term psychodynamic psychotherapy: A basic text* (3rd ed.). Washington, DC: American Psychiatric Publishing.

Garvey, K., Penn, J., Campbell, A., Esposito-Smythers, C., & Spirito, A. (2009). Contracting for safety with patients: Clinical practice and forensic implications. *Journal of the American Academy of Psychiatry Law, 37*, 363–370. Retrieved from http://jaapl.org/content/37/3/363

Gleeson, M., & Timmins, F. (2004). The use of touch to enhance nursing care of older person in long-term mental health care facilities. *Journal of Psychiatric Mental Health Nursing, 11*, 541–545. doi:10.1111/j.1365-2850.2004.00757.x

Greenson, R. (1967). *The technique and practice of psychoanalysis.* New York, NY: International Universities Press.

Hayes, J. A., Gelso, C. J., Kivlighan, D. M. (2019). Managing countertransference. In J. C. Norcross & M. Lambert (Eds.), *Psychotherapy relationships that work: Evidence-based responsiveness* (3rd ed., Vol. 1, pp. 522–548). New York, NY: Oxford University Press.

Healthcare Compliance. (n.d.). *HIPAA compliance guide.* Retrieved from https://www.hipaaguide.net/hipaa-compliance-guide/#HIPAA_Resources

Hill, K. A. (1987). Meta-analysis of paradoxical interventions. *Psychotherapy, 24*, 266–270. doi:10.1037/h0085714

Hill, C. E., Knox, S., & Pinto-Coelho, K. G. (2019). Self-disclosure and immediacy. In J. C. Norcross & M. Lambert (Eds.), *Psychotherapy relationships that work: Evidence-based responsiveness* (3rd ed., Vol. 1, pp. 379–420). New York, NY: Oxford University Press.

Horvath, A. O. (2001). The alliance. *Psychotherapy, Theory, Research, Practice, Training, 38*(4), 365–372. doi:10.1037/0033-3204.38.4.365

Hughes, P., Meize-Grochowski, R., & Harris, C. N. (1996). Therapeutic touch with adolescent psychiatric patients. *Journal of Holistic Nursing, 14*, 6–23. doi:10.1177/089801019601400102

International Society of Study for Dissociative Disorders. (2011). Guidelines for treating dissociative identity disorders in adults, 3rd revision. *Journal of Trauma & Dissociation, 12*(2), 115–187. doi:10.1080/15299732.2011.537247

Jones, A. C. (2004). Transference and counter transference. *Perspectives in Psychiatric Care, 40*(1), 13–19. doi:10.1111/j.1744-6163.2004.00013.x

LaMonica, E. L., Wolf, R. M., Madea, A. R., & Oberst, M. T. (1987). Empathy and nursing care outcomes. *Scholarly Inquiry for Nursing Practice: An International Journal, 1*, 197–213.

Lankton, S., & Lankton, C. H. (1991). Ericksonian styles of paradoxical treatment. In G. R. Weeks (Ed.), *Promoting change through paradoxical therapy* (pp. 1434–1486). New York, NY: Brunner Mazel.

Layton, J., & Wykle, M. H. (1990). A validity study of four empathy instruments. *Research in Nursing & Health, 13*, 319–325. doi:10.1002/nur.4770130508

Lazarus, A. (1993). Tailoring the therapeutic relationship, or being an authentic chameleon. *Psychotherapy, 30*(3), 404–407. doi:10.1037/0033-3204.30.3.404

Lazarus, A., & Lazarus, C. (1991). *Multimodal life inventory*. Champaign, IL: Research Press.

Määttä, S. M. (2006). Closeness and distance in the nurse-patient relation. The relevance of Edith Stein's concept of empathy. *Nursing Philosophy, 7*(1), 3–10. doi:10.1111/j.1466-769X.2006.00232.x

McCabe, S., & Burnett, M. E. (2006). A tale of two APNs: Addressing blurred practice 7 boundaries in APN practice. *Perspectives in Psychiatric Care, 42*(1), 3–12. doi:10.1111/j.1744-6163.2006.00044.x

McWilliams, N. (2004). *Psychoanalytic psychotherapy*. New York, NY: Guilford Press.

McWilliams, N. (2011). *Psychoanalytic diagnosis*. New York, NY: Guilford Press.

Morin, C. M., Hauri, P. J., Espie, C. A., Spielman, A. J., Buysse, D. J., & Bootzin, R. R. (1999). Nonpharmacologic treatment of chronic insomnia. *Database of Abstracts of Reviews of Effects, 22*(8), 1134–1156. doi:10.1093/sleep/22.8.1134

Morse, J. M., Anderson, H., Bottoroff, G., O'Brien, O., Solberg, Y, B., Hunter, S. M., . . . Mellveen, K. H. (1992). Exploring empathy: A conceptual fit for nursing practice? *Image: The Journal of Nursing Scholarship, 24*(4), 273–280. doi:10.1111/j.1547-5069.1992.tb00733.x

Norcross, J., & Lambert, M. (Eds.). (2019). *Psychotherapy relationships that work: Evidence-based responsiveness* (3rd ed, Vol. 1). New York, NY: Oxford University Press.

Norris, D. M., Gutheil, T. G., & Strasburger, L. H. (2003). This couldn't happen to me: Boundary problems and sexual misconduct in the psychotherapy relationship. *Psychiatric Services, 54*(4), 517–522. doi:10.1176/appi.ps.54.4.517

Olfson, M., Wall, M., Wang, S., Crystal, S, Liu, S.M., Gerhard, T, Bianco, C. (2016). Short-term suicide risk after psychiatric hospital discharge. *JAMA, 73*(11), 1119–1126.

Perraud, S., Delaney, K. R., Carlson-Sabelli, L., Johnson, M. E., Shephard, R., & Paun, O. (2006). Advanced practice psychiatric mental health nursing, finding our core: The therapeutic relationship in the 21st century. *Perspectives in Psychiatric Care, 42*(4), 215–226. doi:10.1111/j.1744-6163.2006.00097.x

Porges, S. W. (2004). Neuroceiption: A subconscious system for detecting threats and safety. *Zero to Three, 24*(5),19–24.

Posner, K., Brown, G. K., Stanley, B., Brent, D. A., Yershova, K. V., Oquendo, M. A., . . . Mann, J. J. (2011). The Columbia-suicide severity rating scale (C-SSRS): Initial validity and internal consistency findings from three multi-site studies with adolescents and adults. *American Journal of Psychiatry, 168*, 1266–1277. doi:10.1176/appi.ajp.2011.10111704

Racker, H. (1968). *Transference and countertransference*. New York, NY: International University Press.

Records and Reports of Registrants, 21 C.F.R. §§ 1304.01–1304.55 (2011).

Registration of Manufacturers, Distributors, and Dispensers of Controlled Substances, 21 C.F.R. § 1301.12 (2016).

Richmond, T., Peterson, C., Cason, J., Billings, M., Terrell, E. A., Lee, A., . . . Brennan, D. (2017). American Telemedicine Association's principles for delivering telerehabilitation services. *International Journal of Telerehabilitation, 9*(2), 63–68. doi:10.5195/IJT.2017.6232

Sadock, B. J., Sadock, V. A., & Ruiz, P. (2017). *Kaplan & Sadock's comprehensive textbook of psychiatry* (10th ed.). Philadelphia, PA: Wolters Kluwer/Lippincott Williams & Wilkins.

Safran, J.D., & Muran, J.D. (2000). *Negotiating the therapeutic alliance.* New York: NY: Guilford Press

Salzmann-Erikson, M., & Erikson, N. (2005). Encountering touch: A path to affinity in psychiatric care. *Issues in Mental Health Nursing, 26*, 843–852. doi:10.1080/01612840500184376

Schore, A. (2019). *The development of the unconscious mind*. New York, NY: W. W. Norton.

Scott, J. (1979). Critical periods in organizational processes. In F. Falker & J. Tanner (Eds.), *Human growth neurobiology and nutrition* (Vol. 3, pp. 223–243). New York, NY: Plenum Press.

Sharf, J., Primavera, L. H., & Diener, M. J. (2010). Dropout and therapeutic alliance: A meta-analysis of adult individual psychotherapy. *Psychotherapy, 47*, 637–645. doi:10.1037/a0021175

Stien, P. T., & Kendall, J. (2004). *Psychological trauma and the developing brain: Neurologically based interventions for troubled children.* New York, NY: Haworth Press.

Swift, J., Greenberg, R. P., Whipple, J. L., & Kominiak, N. (2012). Practice recommendations for reducing premature termination in therapy. *Professional Psychology: Research & Practice, 43*(4), 379–387. doi:10.1037/a0028291

Travelbee, J. (1971). *Interpersonal aspects of nursing* (2nd ed.). Philadelphia, PA: F. A. Davis.

Tryon, G. S., Birch, S. E., & Verkuilen, J. (2019). Goal consensus and collaboration. In J. Norcross & B. E. Wampold. *Psychotherapy relationships that work: Evidence-based responsiveness* (3rd ed., Vol. 1, pp. 167–204). New York, NY: Oxford University Press.

Tryon, G. S., & Winograd, G. (2011). Goal consensus and collaboration. *Psychotherapy, 48*(1), 50–57. doi:10.1037/a0022061

van der Kolk, B. (2014). *The body keeps the score: Brain, mind, and body in the healing of trauma.* New York, NY: Penguin Books.

Wachtel, P. (2011). *Therapeutic communication: Knowing what to say when* (2nd ed.). New York, NY: Guilford Press.

Westerman, M. A., Frankel, A. S., Tanaka, J. S., & Kahn, J. (1987). Patient cooperative interview and outcome in paradoxical interview and behavioral brief treatment approaches. *Journal of Counseling Psychology, 34*, 99–102. doi:10.1037/0022-0167.34.1.99

Wheeler, K. (2003). Further development of the perception of empathy inventory. In O. Strickland & C. DiIorio (Eds.), *Measurement of nursing outcomes, Patient outcomes and quality of care* (2nd ed., Vol. 2, pp. 207–213). New York, NY: Springer Publishing Company.

Wheeler, K., Barrett, E., & Lahey, E. (1996). A study of empathy as a nursing outcome variable. *The International Journal of Psychiatric Nursing Research, 3*(1), 281–289.

APPENDIX 4.1
Notice of Privacy Practices

This notice describes how psychological and medical information about you may be used and disclosed and how you can get access to this information. Please review it carefully.

I. **Uses and Disclosures for Treatment, Payment, and Health Care Operations**
   I may use or disclose your protected health information (PHI), for treatment, payment, and health care operation purposes with your consent. To help clarify these terms, here are some definitions:
   - "PHI" refers to information in your health record that could identify you.
   - *"Treatment, payment, and health care operations"*
     - Treatment is when I provide, coordinate, or manage your healthcare and other services related to your healthcare. An example of treatment would be when I consult with another healthcare provider, such as your family physician or another psychologist.
     - Payment is when I obtain reimbursement for your healthcare. Examples of payment are when I disclose your PHI to your health insurer to obtain reimbursement for your healthcare or to determine eligibility or coverage.
     - Healthcare operations are activities that relate to the performance and operation of my practice. Examples of healthcare

operations are quality assessment and improvement activities, business-related matters such as audits and administrative services, and case management and care coordination.
   - "Use" applies only to activities within my (office, clinic, practice group, and so on) such as sharing, employing, applying, utilizing, examining, and analyzing information that identifies you.
   - "Disclosure" applies to activities outside my (office, clinic, practice group, and so on), such as releasing, transferring, or providing access to information about you to other parties.

II. **Uses and Disclosures Requiring Authorization**
   I may use or disclose PHI for purposes outside of treatment, payment, and healthcare operations when your appropriate authorization is obtained. An "authorization" is written permission above and beyond the general consent that permits only specific disclosures. In those instances when I am asked for information for purposes outside of treatment, payment, and healthcare operations, I will obtain an authorization from you before releasing this information. I will also need to obtain an authorization before releasing your psychotherapy notes. "Psychotherapy notes" are notes I have made about our conversation during a private, group, joint, or family counseling session, which I have kept separate from the

(continued)

rest of your medical record. These notes are given a greater degree of protection than PHI.

You may revoke all such authorizations (of PHI or psychotherapy notes) at any time, provided each revocation is in writing. You may not revoke an authorization to the extent that (1) I have relied on that authorization; or (2) if the authorization was obtained as a condition of obtaining insurance coverage, and the law provides the insurer the right to contest the claim under the policy.

III. Uses and Disclosures With Neither Consent nor Authorization

I may use or disclose PHI without your consent or authorization in the following circumstances:

- **Child abuse:** When in my professional capacity, I have received information that gives me reason to believe that a child's physical or mental health or welfare has been or may be adversely affected by abuse or neglect, I must report such to the county Department of Social Services, or to a law enforcement agency in the county where the child resides or is found. If I have received information in my professional capacity which gives me reason to believe that a child's physical or mental health or welfare has been or may be adversely affected by acts or omissions that would be child abuse or neglect if committed by a parent, guardian, or other persons responsible for the child's welfare, but I believe that the act or omission was committed by a person other than the parent, guardian,

or other persons responsible for the child's welfare, I must make a report to the appropriate law enforcement agency.

- **Adult and domestic abuse:** If I have reason to believe that a vulnerable adult has been or is likely to be abused, neglected, or exploited, I must report the incident within 24 hours or the next business day to the Adult Protective Services Program. I may also report directly to law enforcement personnel.

- **Health oversight:** The State Board of Examiners has the power, if necessary, to subpoena my records. I am then required to submit to them those records relevant to their inquiry.

- **Judicial or administrative proceedings:** If you are involved in a court proceeding and a request is made about the professional services I provided you or the records thereof, such information is privileged under state law, and I will not release information without your written consent or a court order. The privilege does not apply when you are being evaluated for a third party or where the evaluation is court ordered. You will be informed in advance if this is the case.

- **Serious threat to health or safety:** If you communicate to me the intention to commit a crime or harm yourself, I may disclose confidential information when I judge that disclosure is necessary to protect against a clear and substantial risk of imminent serious harm being inflicted by you on yourself or another person. In this situation, I must

(continued)

limit disclosure of the otherwise confidential information to only those persons and only that content which would be consistent with the standards of the profession in addressing such problems.

- **Workers' compensation:** If you file a workers' compensation claim, I am required by law to provide all existing information compiled by me pertaining to the claim to your employer, the insurance carrier, their attorneys, the South Carolina Workers' Compensation Commission, or you.

IV. Patient's Rights and Psychologist's Duties

PATIENT'S RIGHTS

- **Right to request restrictions:** You have the right to request restrictions on certain uses and disclosures of PHI about you. However, I am not required to agree to a restriction you request.
- **Right to receive confidential communications by alternative means and at alternative locations:** You have the right to request and receive confidential communications of PHI by alternative means and at alternative locations. (For example, you may not want a family member to know that you are seeing me. On your request, I will send your bills to another address.)
- **Right to inspect and copy:** You have the right to inspect or obtain a copy (or both) of PHI in my mental health and billing records used to make decisions about you for as

long as the PHI is maintained in the record. I may deny your access to PHI under certain circumstances, but in some cases you may have this decision reviewed. On your request, I will discuss with you the details of the request and denial process.

- **Right to amend:** You have the right to request an amendment of PHI for as long as the PHI is maintained in the record. I may deny your request. On your request, I will discuss with you the details of the amendment process.
- **Right to an accounting:** You generally have the right to receive an accounting of disclosures of PHI regarding you. On your request, I will discuss with you the details of the accounting process.
- **Right to a paper copy:** You have the right to obtain a paper copy of the notice from me on request, even if you have agreed to receive the notice electronically.

NURSE PSYCHOTHERAPIST'S DUTIES

- I am required by law to maintain the privacy of PHI and to provide you with a notice of my legal duties and privacy practices with respect to PHI.
- I reserve the right to change the privacy policies and practices described in this notice. Unless I notify you of such changes, however, I am required to abide by the terms currently in effect.
- If I revise my policies and procedures, I will mail you a copy of the new notice.

(continued)

V. Questions and Complaints

If you have questions about this notice, disagree with a decision I make about access to your records, or have other concerns about your privacy rights, you may _____. If you believe that your privacy rights have been violated and wish to file a complaint with our office, you may send your written complaint _____. You may also send a written complaint to the secretary of the U.S. Department of Health and Human Services.

You have specific rights under the Privacy Rule. I will not retaliate against you for exercising your right to file a complaint.

VI. Effective Date, Restrictions, and Changes to Privacy Policy

This notice will go into effect on April 14, 2004.

I reserve the right to change the terms of this notice and to make the new notice for all PHI that I maintain. I will provide you with a revised notice by mail.

APPENDIX 4.2
Contract

Welcome to my practice. The following includes some essential information regarding psychotherapy. Please read and sign at the bottom to indicate that you have reviewed this information.

LENGTH AND FREQUENCY OF TREATMENT

Psychotherapy typically involves regular sessions, usually 45 minutes in length. Duration and frequency vary depending on the nature of your problem and your individual needs.

Confidentiality

Information you share with me will be kept strictly confidential and will not be disclosed without your written consent. By law, however, confidentiality is not guaranteed in life-threatening situations involving yourself or others, or in situation in which children are put at risk (such as by sexual or physical abuse or neglect). If I need to discuss your treatment with a colleague, I will take pains to disguise identifying information, including using a pseudonym.

Fee Policies

My fee for an individual therapy session is _____ per session. If you need to cancel an appointment, please tell me at least 24 hours ahead of time; otherwise, you will be charged for the missed session. Please be aware that insurance carriers will not cover cancellation charges.

If you carry Anthem Blue Cross insurance coverage where I am a provider, I will bill your carrier and assist with insurance reimbursement. In this circumstance, the insurance carrier limits the fee charged for the session and you will not be charged for the difference between my ordinary fee and the cap placed by insurance. Any copayment necessary should be made at the time of the office visit. Unless we make another explicit arrangement, you are responsible for filing insurance claims for all other carriers where I am not a provider. I will give you a bill at the beginning of the month for the previous month and would like to receive payment at that time or at the next session.

Phone and Emergency Contact

If you need to contact me by phone, do not hesitate. When I am not available, my answering machine will take a message. I am usually able to return calls the same day. You will not be charged for phone calls unless we have a scheduled conversation of an information-exchanging or problem-solving nature that lasts more than 10 minutes. If you cannot reach me in an emergency, you can find help at the Emergency Services number of the local hospital at 203-852-2000.

Physician Contact

Physical and psychological symptoms often interact. I encourage you to seek medical consultation if warranted. It may benefit your treatment for me to speak to your primary care provider, in which case, I will ask your permission first.

(continued)

Freedom to Withdraw

You have the right to end therapy at any time. If you wish, I will give you the names of other qualified psychotherapists.

Informed Consent

I have read and understood the preceding statements. I have had an opportunity to ask questions about them, and I agree to enter a professional psychotherapy relationship with _____ _____.

Notice of Privacy Practices

I have read the NOTICE OF PRIVACY PRACTICES given to me by _____ _____. I have been given a copy to keep. I understand my rights and responsibilities and know that I may ask questions about my personal health information and its safekeeping at any time.

Signed: _____ Date: _____

APPENDIX 4.3
Process Note

This page is a psychotherapy process note under the Health Insurance Portability and Accountability Act (HIPAA) regulations. It must not be included in or attached to any other part of the patient's healthcare records except with other psychotherapy notes. Patients may request access to these notes only under exceptional circumstances and access may be denied if it is deemed harmful to the patient. Releasing these notes requires a special authorization.

Patient name:

(for each entry, date code, time, and signature)

APPENDIX 4.4
Progress Note

Kathleen Wheeler, PhD, PMHNP-BC, APRN, FAAN
69 Seabright Avenue
Bridgeport, CT 06605

Patient name: _____
Diagnoses *(DSM-5)*: _____
Date: _____
S:
O:
A:
P:
CPT code: _____
Prognosis: _____
Signature: _____
Visit time: _____

APPENDIX 4.5
Process Recording

Purpose

The process recording is a written account of a session between a patient and therapist. Through the reconstruction of the interaction, the student is provided with an opportunity to retrospectively examine and analyze your facilitative communication skills and therapeutic use of self and the patient's contribution to the interaction. Through an analysis of what is said (the content of the interaction) and the flow of the interaction (the process of the interaction), awareness is increased of your own feelings, values, attitudes, expectations, assumptions, and verbal responses and how all influence the interaction with the patient. The analysis also helps you to distinguish between your own thoughts and feelings and gain insight into how this influences the perception of the patient, the patient's situation, and how the patient is coping.

The therapist analyzes what is said (the content) and the flow of the interaction (the process of the interaction). This analysis is then used to increase self-awareness of your own feelings, values, attitudes, and beliefs and how they influenced the interaction with the patient. This analysis also helps to distinguish between your own thoughts and feelings, and gain insight about how each influences your perception of the patient. The process recording also provides you with an opportunity to retrospectively examine and analyze a patient's behavior. Through this analysis, inconsistencies or consistencies between what the patient says and does can be identified and used to help patient gain insight about their problems and function more effectively.

Directions

There should be four columns, the first designated as *Therapist Said*, the second, *Patient Said*, the third, *Therapist Thought/ Feeling* column, and the fourth, the *Analysis* column plus a *Summary* page. See criteria on the next page regarding what should be in each column and form for how to set up. At the end of the session, write down everything you can remember that the person said in the *Patient Said column*, then go back and fill in what you think you said in the *Therapist Said* column, then fill out the *Therapist Thought/Feeling* column, and the *Analysis* column last. After reading over, write a summary of the interaction on a separate page.

If you have gaps in your memory or cannot recall the exact flow of the interaction, indicate this in the *Analysis* column and examine why you think you might have "forgotten" (e.g., "I wonder whether the topic was anxiety provoking to me?"). Don't write while talking with the person. The process recording is an efficient way to provide students with help with their communication skills; therefore, choose an interaction that was difficult or problematic (e.g., you were stuck, speechless, and overwhelmed). You will probably think of alternative ways of dealing with the situation after reading it over. Openness about problems encountered during the interaction will facilitate helpful feedback that will enhance both your communication skills and therapeutic use of self.

Some of the patients that you will encounter come from very different cultural and socioeconomic backgrounds, and have very different values,

(*continued*)

expectations, perceptions, and behavior. An important part of the learning experience is to identify those differences and how they influence your ability to be sensitive, empathic, nonjudgmental, accepting, and therapeutic.

CRITERIA FOR EVALUATION OF PROCESS RECORDING

Therapist _____
Patient's initials_____
Date _____

In Therapist Said Column

Reconstruct an interaction with a patient using the assigned format.

Document, in the "therapist said" column, verbatim statements (what you said as closely as you can remember) during the interaction.

In Patient Said Column

Document, in the "patient said" column, verbatim statements (what the patient said as closely as you can recall) during the interaction.

In Therapist Thought/Feeling Column

Separate out your thoughts and feelings and indicate by a T for Thought or F for Feeling at the end of each sentence.

Document the cognitive responses (what you thought) during the interaction. (T)

Document your affective response (your feelings and emotions such as anxiety and sadness) in response to what occurred during the interaction. (F)

In Analysis Column

- Identify how thoughts and feelings influence own behavior.
- Identify own values, beliefs, attitudes, expectations, and assumptions, and how they influence perceptions and responses to the patient.
- Identify own expectations and how they influence perceptions and responses to the client. Identify inconsistencies between what the client is saying and doing, or between the patient's situation and efforts to function effectively.
- Identify discrepancies between verbal and nonverbal behavior.
- Identify discrepancies between the patient's perception of potential or existing problems and the reality of these problems.

On Summary Page

- Identify patient resistances to disclosing and examining potential or existing problems.
- Identify nonverbal behavior that indicates resistance to dealing with existing or potential problems.
- Identify verbal behavior that indicates resistance to dealing with existing or potential problems.
- Identify any defenses that you thought the patient manifested.
- Identify responses to the patient that were ineffective or nontherapeutic.
- Identify the verbal input that was a barrier to facilitating the relationship with patient.
- Label the barrier to facilitating the relationship with the patient.
- Identify alternative effective responses that would have facilitated the interaction with the patient.
- Identify examples of latent communication.

(continued)

Use the attached format to document the interaction

When documenting the interaction, set up the columns so that the reader can see the flow by staggering what is documented in the "therapist" and "patient" columns.

Therapist Said	Patient Said	Therapist Thought/ Feeling	Analysis

APPENDIX 4.6
Inventory of Countertransference

1. What are your reasons for becoming a nurse psychotherapist? How might these reasons hinder your effectiveness as a therapist?
2. Are you aware of reacting to certain types of people in overprotective ways or wanting to rescue people? If yes, what does this say about you?
3. Are you able to allow others to experience their emotional pain, or do you want to take the pain away and react quickly to alleviate the discomfort of others?
4. How do you feel when you are not appreciated by others who you have cared for?
5. How do you react when anger is expressed toward you?
6. How do you feel when your patients are not motivated to change or do not follow your instructions and suggestions?
7. What types of patients do you find yourself wanting to distance from?
8. What can you learn about yourself by looking at those who you are likely to reject?
9. Do you need approval of your patients? How willing are you to confront a patient even at the risk of being disliked?
10. Do you offer patients a lot of "fix it" statement and advice?
11. Do you have a lot invested in staying positive and find yourself reassuring patients that they will be all right?
12. Do you frequently extend the time of the sessions or feel in general that you are not enough?

APPENDIX 4.7
Sample Termination Letter

Date _____

Dear _____,

The last session we had was on _____ (date) and you have missed two scheduled appointments since then. I did leave you two telephone messages but you have not responded. I hope you are okay and will contact me in the near future to resume treatment. As the contract you signed stated when you initially came to therapy, regular appointments are important in order to continue to make progress. I believe it is not in your best interests to terminate now. I would like to continue to work with you but if you would like a referral elsewhere, please call me and I can make some suggestions for ongoing treatment. If I do not hear from you by _____ (date 2 weeks away), I will consider your treatment under my care to be terminated. If you have any difficulties, please go to your nearest emergency room. I hope to hear from you soon.

Best Regards,
Kathleen Wheeler, PhD, PMHNP-BC, APRN, FAAN

Psychotherapy Approaches

II

Supportive and Psychodynamic Psychotherapy

Kathleen Wheeler

This chapter begins with an overview of the underlying assumptions of psychodynamic psychotherapy, the history, and evidence-based research. Psychodynamic psychotherapy is discussed as on a continuum, with supportive, expressive, and psychoanalytic approaches considered. Rationale is provided for choice of approach based on developmental considerations for clinical decision-making. How to develop a case formulation and the working through phase of treatment is examined, as is working with alliance ruptures and dreams. Guidelines for brief psychodynamic psychotherapy are provided with case studies illustrating concepts and techniques throughout the chapter. Those skilled in psychodynamic psychotherapy recognize the difficulties in suggesting specific, standardized techniques because technique is driven by the context of the interaction.

In the current environment of managed care, in which a course of psychotherapy is often three to six sessions, practicing any meaningful relationship-based work is difficult, if not impossible. With these limitations in mind, an overview of relevant concepts and technical considerations is presented. The chapter ends with information about post-master's training and certification requirements for psychodynamic psychotherapy. Chapter 4 reviews the basic concepts of transference, countertransference, and resistance, which are foundational to understanding psychodynamic psychotherapy.

With the American Psychiatric Association's mandate that all psychiatric residency training programs teach long-term psychodynamic psychotherapy to meet standards of accreditation, the relevance and importance of this type of therapy were affirmed by the psychiatric establishment (Gabbard, 2010). Knowledge about psychodynamic psychotherapy is essential for all advanced practice psychiatric nurses (APPNs) to deepen understanding about development and how the patient's history is reenacted in the nurse–patient relationship in therapy and in life. Even if the APPN is using another approach, it is still important to understand the person's dynamics to inform decisions about treatment. The patient does not necessarily need to achieve dynamic insights to experience symptom reduction and personal growth, but developmental considerations, anxiety, transference, countertransference, implicit memory (unconscious), defenses, motivation, and resistance are relevant in any therapeutic encounter. Knowledge about psychodynamic theory is also important for APPNs when communicating with other mental health disciplines. The literature in nursing reiterates the importance of psychodynamic theory for understanding the psychodynamics in the nurse–patient relationship and the inner world of both the nurse and the patient (Gallop & O'Brien, 2003).

These authors stress that without knowledge of psychodynamic psychotherapy, nurses are at a tremendous disadvantage and at risk for acting inappropriately and not in the patient's best interests.

Psychodynamic psychotherapy requires intensive teaching and experience to attain competency. This chapter lays the foundation for the APPN who wishes to understand the basics of this approach. Competencies in psychodynamic psychotherapy include using developmental models to understand personality and psychopathology, formulating a psychodynamic explanation and plan treatment, tracking the issue that is the focus of treatment, implementing the process of therapy, and managing the relationship (Binder, 2004).

UNDERLYING ASSUMPTIONS OF PSYCHODYNAMIC PSYCHOTHERAPY

Psychodynamic psychotherapy is derived from psychoanalytic psychotherapy, which was developed by Sigmund Freud at the end of the 19th century. This type of therapy is also referred to as insight-oriented, intensive, exploratory, expressive, and depth psychotherapy. Underpinnings of psychodynamics are rooted in developmental theory, with the basic premise that what has happened in the past determines what we are doing today. It is thought that through understanding these factors, the person is empowered and then free to make more conscious decisions and consequently live a more satisfying and useful life.

Blagys and Hilsenroth (2000), in an extensive review of the literature, identify factors that distinguish psychodynamic from cognitive behavioral therapy (CBT). These factors include emphasis on the past; focus on the expression of emotion; identification of patterns in actions, thoughts, feelings, experiences, and relationships; emphasis on past relationships; exploration of and working with resistances that impede treatment; exploration of intrapsychic issues through asking about wishes, dreams, and fantasies; and emphasis on transference and the working alliance. Gabbard (2017) identifies seven key concepts of psychodynamic psychotherapy: the unconscious, a developmental perspective, transference, countertransference, resistance, psychic determinism, and unique subjectivity. Gabbard explains the concept of unique subjectivity as the therapist's challenge to pursue the patient's subjective truth and true self, which has most likely been thwarted by parents who cannot recognize, validate, and appreciate this self. This pursuit is informed by the underlying premise that we do not really know ourselves and that much of what determines our behavior is governed by unconscious memories.

Most psychodynamic schools emphasize the centrality of conflict among powerful desires, wishes, and fears. Psychodynamic clinicians believe that to help the person, it is essential to understand how these conflicts are enacted in the present. Psychodynamic theorists agree that understanding unconscious psychological structures and patterns in daily life, as well as how they interact and maintain each other, is essential to understanding the person (McWilliams, 2011; Wachtel, 2011). Wachtel points out that a key characteristic of this pattern is irony; the person ends up in the very position that he or she was trying hard to avoid. For example, the person who is fearful of feelings of anger may act overly nice, unassertive, and maintain a passive stance toward others. This allows others to ignore his or her needs and, consequently, he or she begins to feel frustrated and devalued, which leads to more anger and more anxiety, and the pattern is repeated. Another example is a person who fears hostility from others and interprets every interaction as potentially hostile, then preemptively enacts self-protective hostility toward others, which evokes hostility from them, which leads to more anxiety, and so on (Figure 5.1).

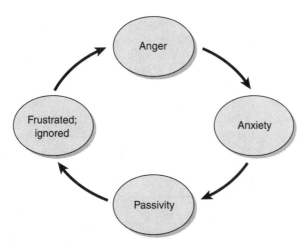

FIGURE 5.1 Cyclical psychodynamics diagram.

Anxiety is central to understanding these difficulties, and even if the person does not *feel* particularly anxious, defenses and characterological personality traits embedded in implicit memory systems bind the person to a life that is restrictive as compromises are made to keep anxiety at bay. Specific anxieties arise at every level of development, and various theorists posit that different tasks need to be accomplished in order to quell the anxiety for each stage of development (Tables 5.1 through 5.3). That is, for each developmental stage, anxiety revolving around a specific issue is negotiated, and if successful, the fear surrounding that phase is assuaged so that the person is then able to proceed to the next stage without being preoccupied by that threat (McWilliams, 1999). For example, in early infancy, a major preoccupation is security, with annihilation experienced as the threat if the attachment to the mother is endangered or absent; for early childhood, the issue is autonomy, with the concomitant anxiety revolving around separation (i.e., how to be an independent agent and still maintain a relationship with the caregiver); in later childhood, issues of identity must be resolved, particularly fears of punishment, injury, and loss of control. To regulate the anxiety and other painful affects associated with each stage, defense mechanisms develop in implicit memory networks through interaction with caregivers and interpersonal experiences.

The job of the psychodynamic therapist is to help the person understand both how fears and inhibitions in early life have led him or her to react to healthy feelings as if they were a threat and how the resulting anxiety plays an active role in generating his or her difficulties in the present. The person inadvertently and consistently brings about consequences that are not consciously intended. The psychodynamic therapist uses interpretations to expose the person to previously avoided experiences while offering empathy in a safe, therapeutic environment. Chapter 4 discusses interpretation, the focus of which depends on the school of psychodynamic thought the therapist subscribes to. Therapeutic exposure is not just aimed toward intellectual understanding, but it also emphasizes the facilitation of emotional experiencing at a gradual pace. Reexperiencing painful affects allows adaptive processing so that dissociated or disconnected memory networks can be integrated with other, more adaptive neural networks (Cozolino, 2017).

HISTORY

The history and theory of psychodynamic psychotherapy since Freud's time are complex, and his ideas have undergone numerous permutations and iterations. This evolution has paralleled paradigm shifts in science in the 20th century, which emphasize interconnections, mutual interactions, and subjectivity of phenomenon (Curtis & Hirsch, 2003). Each psychodynamic model evolved from previous approaches while establishing a new perspective that placed different emphases on human development and motivation for behavior. Successive interpretations addressed what was seen as the failure of Freud's theory (Mitchell, 1988). These competing schools of thought—Freudian, ego, self, existential, Lacanian, analytic, object relations, interpersonal, relational, and intersubjective—are somewhat insular and fragmented in that each seems to take little notice of the others. Each approach developed its own theoretical constructs and techniques. The following overview highlights selected theorists, but does not do justice to the complexity, richness, and nuances of psychoanalytic theory.

Sigmund Freud's classic model of psychoanalytic psychotherapy is based on drive theory; that is, that all behavior is determined by unconscious forces or instincts, either sexual or aggressive. Freud's structural model of the id, ego, and superego explains the idea of psychic conflict. Symptoms are thought to develop through a conflict between an instinctual wish (id) and the person's defense against the wish (ego). The superego is part of the unconscious that is formed through internalization of moral standards of parents and society and acts to censor and restrain the ego. The concept of *psychic determinism* is embedded within this model and refers to the idea that nothing happens by chance; everything on a person's mind and all behavior, pathological and nonpathological, has a cause, and is multiply determined. Freud delineated the psychosexual stages of development based on the idea that libidinal energy shifts between various erogenous zones in each stage. Freud posited that if a person had not successfully negotiated the previous stage, specific, problematic character traits or psychopathology would continue throughout life (see Table 5.1).

In the 1960s, the scope of psychoanalysis was widened by interpersonal theorists such as Harry Stack Sullivan, Karen Horney, and Eric Fromm, who stressed the importance of relationship. Sullivan believed that the details of the patient's interactions with others provided insight into what would help resolve intrapsychic difficulties. Sullivan's perspective of the therapist as participant–observer expanded the prevailing paradigm. He believed that the therapist was not just a passive observer of what was going on in the patient, but was a participant in the process of psychotherapy. Using Sullivan's framework, Hildegard Peplau developed the psychodynamic interpersonal model for psychiatric nursing.

Ego psychology and object relation theorists such as Margaret Mahler followed with increased emphasis on relationship as a vehicle for change. Mahler's object relation theory evolved from her observations of infants and children and the subsequent analysis of this qualitative data (Mahler, Pine, & Bergman, 1975). Stages of development based on separation–individuation were described and explanations were offered about how children develop a sense of identity separate from their mothers (see Table 5.2). The infant is described as being totally dependent, with relatively little self–other differentiation, and the child develops through relationship into a separate person with a high degree of differentiation.

Klein and Fairburn combined intrapsychic theory and drive theory with the idea that the primary motivation of the child is to seek objects (Curtis & Hirsch, 2003). Here, *object* refers to the internalization of experiences with other people. Object relation theorists posit that people are primarily motivated to seek other people and that this is the central motivating force in development, rather than drive gratification (Winnicott, 1965/1976). Winnicott (1965/1976) speculated that for a child to develop a healthy, genuine self, as opposed to a false self, the mother must be a *good enough mother* who relates to the child with *primary maternal preoccupation*. The child can then grow and explore without overwhelming anxiety, feeling that the world is safe. The child develops a sense of *me* and those aspects that are not part of him or her create a potential space between himself or

TABLE 5.1 FREUD'S PSYCHOSEXUAL STAGES

Stage	Age	Task	Problematic Traits
Oral	Birth to 18 months	To establish trust; comfortable expression and gratification of oral needs	Excessive dependency; envy and jealousy; narcissism; pessimism; excessive optimism
Anal	18 months to 3 years	Learning independence and control	Orderliness; obstinacy; frugality; heightened ambivalence; messiness; defiance; rage; obsessive compulsive; sadomasochism
Phallic/ Oedipal	3 to 6 years	Identification with same sex parent; development of sexual identity	Sexual identity issues; castration in males; penis envy in females; excessive guilt
Latency	6 to 12 years	Sexuality sublimated; emphasis on same sex peers	Inability to sublimate energies to learn; excessive inner control; obsessive traits
Genital	13 to 20 years	Establishment of separation from parents and mature nonincestuous relationships with others	Reworking all the previous developmental issues; establishing a life not dependent on parents

Source: Adapted from Sadock, B. J., Sadock, V. A., & Ruiz, P. (2017). *Kaplan & Sadock's comprehensive textbook of psychiatry* (10th ed.). Philadelphia, PA: Wolters Kluwer/Lippincott Williams & Wilkins.

TABLE 5.2 MAHLER'S STAGES OF SEPARATION–INDIVIDUATION

Phase	Age	Task
Normal autism	Birth to 1 month	Fulfillment of basic need for survival and comfort
Symbiosis	1 to 5 months	Awareness of external source for need fulfillment
Separation–Individuation		
Differentiation	5 to 10 months	Recognizes separateness from caretaker
Practicing	10 to 16 months	Increased independence and separateness of self
Rapprochement	16 to 24 months	Seeks emotional refueling from caretaker in order to maintain feeling of security; borderline pathology is thought to evolve from problems in this phase.
Consolidation	24 to 36 months	Sense of separateness established; on the way to object constancy; resolution of separation anxiety

Source: Adapted from Mahler, M., Pine, F., & Bergman, A. (1975). *The psychological birth of the human infant.* New York, NY: Basic Books.

herself and the mother. This space is the area of play and is an important dimension of the developing self. Winnicott (1965/1976) said that the therapist's chief task is to provide a *holding environment* for the patient so that the patient can have the opportunity to meet neglected ego needs and allow the true self to emerge. In contrast to the *good enough mother*, the not good enough mother is thought to create a dynamic in subsequent relationships in adult life in which the person feels never good enough. Alice Miller (1981) in her widely recognized book, *The Drama of the Gifted Child*, describes eloquently the adverse effects of certain types of parenting on the development of the child's true self.

Building on Freud's ideas about intrapsychic conflict, Erik Erikson, a lay psychoanalyst, expanded the theory of development to encompass the entire life cycle. He conceptualized life as a struggle of conflicting needs in the quest toward self-actualization (Erikson, 1964). These conflicting needs revolved around the need for stability versus the need for growth at each stage of development. Table 5.3 shows Erikson's stages of development. As we move from infancy to old age, Erikson posited that we face a stage-specific conflict that involves themes of inhibition versus desire. Although similar symptoms may be experienced in each stage, each of the eight stage-specific conflicts may have a different meaning, depending on the unique issues and emotions that arise within that period, and success at resolution depends on how successfully the person has negotiated the previous stages.

For example, a 21-year-old woman came to therapy after being raped in college. She had become significantly depressed and attempted suicide shortly after the rape. Her depression reflected a loss of identity that was shattered beyond repair. She had previously functioned as her parents expected her to and was generally motivated to meet

TABLE 5.3   ERIKSON'S PSYCHOSOCIAL STAGES

Age	Stage	Pathological Outcome
Infancy (birth to 18 months)	Trust vs. mistrust	Psychosis, addictions, depression
Early childhood (18 months to 3 years)	Autonomy vs. self-doubt	Paranoia, obsessions, compulsions, impulsivity
Late childhood (3 to 6 years)	Initiative vs. guilt	Conversion disorder, phobias, psychosomatic disorder
School age (6 to 12 years)	Industry vs. inferiority	Inertia, creative inhibition
Adolescence (12 to 20 years)	Identity vs. role confusion	Delinquency, gender-related identity disorders, borderline psychotic episodes
Young adulthood (20 to 30 years)	Intimacy vs. isolation	Schizoid personality
Adulthood (30 to 65 years)	Generativity vs. stagnation	Midlife crisis, premature invalidism
Old age (65 years to death)	Ego integrity vs. despair	Extreme alienation, despair

Source: Adapted from Erikson, E. (1964). *Insight and responsibility*. New York, NY: W. W. Norton; Erikson, E. (1968). *Identity, youth and crisis*. New York, NY: W. W. Norton.

others' expectations. Her depression precipitated an exploration of her own values and who she really was, a process that gradually allowed her to rebel against the need to conform. Finding her own voice was integral to the treatment, and she eventually was able to articulate the differences between her opinions and those of her parents. Her depressive symptoms represented the conflicting need for stability and conformity versus the need for self-awareness and growth.

Significantly departing from the idea of intrapsychic conflict, Heinz Kohut developed self psychology based on a deficit model of development. Kohut posited that the self was the central organizing frame of reference and that the self seeks out responses from others to maintain self-cohesion (Kohut & Wolf, 1978). Contrary to Freud's conception of the individual as primarily being driven by the quest for pleasure, Kohut's self strives for competence, self-esteem, and order, and these are the sine qua non motivators of behavior. Others serve self-object functions for the individual, and these include mirroring, idealizing, and alter ego experiences. Individuals never lose the need for self-object experiences throughout life. However, if self-object experiences are less than adequate in early life, the person may later have difficulty with self-soothing, self-regulation, and maintenance of self-cohesion. Kohut based this idea on the clinical observation that a certain subgroup of patients developed an idiosyncratic transference in therapy, which he called the *narcissistic transference*. These patients, unlike the typical analytic patient, needed mirroring and idealized the analyst. Those with this type of self-pathology formed attachments based on these needs. Kohut posited that empathy played a central role in the psychotherapy of those with narcissistic psychopathology.

The relational model evolved in the 1980s from object relations, self, interpersonal, existential, and feminist models. A basic tenet of the contemporary relational model is that the therapist and patient are always participating in a relational configuration and that understanding this process is how change occurs. Before relational theory, much discussion ensued about the differences between the transference relationship and the *real* relationship between the therapist and patient. The transference and the patient's feelings toward the therapist were artifacts of the past, whereas the *real* relationship was what was going on in the present. In the relational model, however, this is irrelevant because there are multiple truths and there is no real relationship, only a co-constructed interaction that is at best subjective (Gabbard, 2017). This interaction coupled with mindfulness is the agent of change, and developing and repairing problems in the therapeutic alliance are considered the work of relational psychodynamic psychotherapy.

Embedded in this idea of multiple truths is the concept of *multiple selves;* there is no unitary true self, but each person is constructed with many self-states. Different self-states are based on the various states of consciousness that we flicker in and out of throughout the day. Chapter 2, discusses the neurophysiology supporting this idea. These shifting, multiple self-states elicit complementary self-states in others through relationship. Dissociated self-states that are experienced as potentially dangerous are kept from the person's awareness. By *potentially dangerous,* Safran and Muran (2000) explain that these states are associated with actual traumatic experiences or disruptions of relatedness to significant others. Assisting the patient to experience and accept the various dimensions of the self through enhanced awareness of these traumatic states is considered crucial to the relational psychodynamic therapy process.

A synthesis of the literature on the relational model reveals significant differences between Freudian psychodynamic psychotherapy and relational psychodynamic therapy. Table 5.4 compares and contrasts these models.

The intersubjective movement evolved in 1984 with Stolorow and Atwood. An early formulation of this viewpoint was that psychoanalysis seeks to illuminate phenomena that emerge within a specific psychological field constituted by the interaction of two subjectivities, that of the patient and that of the analyst. This significant shift in the psychoanalytic paradigm changed what was called a one-person psychology to a *two-person*

TABLE 5.4   COMPARISON OF CLASSICAL PSYCHODYNAMIC THERAPY WITH RELATIONAL PSYCHODYNAMIC THERAPY

	Classical Psychodynamic	Relational Psychodynamic
Therapist role	Objective	Participant–observer
Perspective	One-person psychology	Two-person psychology
Motivation	Drives; sex and/or aggression	Emotional communication and affect regulation
Focus of exploration	Then and there; genetic roots of the problem (how a person's transference reaction is linked to feelings belonging to a person from the past)	Here and now; both patient and therapist contributions to the interaction; and patient's experience
Aim	Make the unconscious conscious	Resolve ruptures in the therapeutic alliance
Change agent	Insight	Mindfulness
Symptom	Psychopathology	A communication
Transference	Interprets in light of the past	Cautious about generalizing to past
Countertransference	Caused by the patient; less disclosure by therapist	Co-constructed; use of countertransference disclosure
Resistance	Intrapsychic event that involves a defense working against change	Co-constructed unconscious rupture of the therapeutic alliance; interpersonal ruptures outside therapy
Interpretation	Of wish/defense conflicts	Of alliance ruptures outside as well as inside therapy

psychology (Gabbard, 2017). This awareness of two separate minds interacting with one another is also referred to as *intersubjectivity*. The therapist is considered a coparticipant in the co-construction of the relationship, not an outside observer. It is only in the present moment as the process is unfolding that both participants' understanding is deepened. The need for relationship derives from the physical closeness to the mother and is thought to be the prime motivator for behavior. Self-regulation results from mutually regulatory interactions with caretakers and evolves within the mother–infant dyad. The presence of the other is necessary and inescapable, both in human development and in the therapeutic relationship. Relational psychodynamic theory heightens our understanding about the need for attachments for psychophysiological stability.

Schore's (2019) neurobiological research and theory on attachment provides a scientific basis for the importance of relationship to therapeutic action in psychotherapy. The growing capacity to self-regulate is contingent on transformations of underdeveloped functions that exist in the infant through early attachment experiences that assist the developing psychobiological, homeostatic regulatory processes. Cumulative early attachment problems are thought to produce chronic dysregulation in central and autonomic arousal, with deficits in mind and body. Chapter 2, discusses the neurophysiology underlying this dysregulation. Problems in self-regulation include difficulties in tension regulation, such as in addictive disorders, eating disorders, personality disorders, anxiety disorders, attention deficit hyperactivity disorder, and mood disorders.

EVIDENCE-BASED RESEARCH

Studies of the efficacy of psychodynamic psychotherapy began in earnest only within the past 20 years because this type of therapy developed outside universities and the academic world (Shedler, 2010, 2011). Education and training in psychoanalysis took place in institutes that were open only to medical doctors and excluded psychologists who are trained in research methodology. However, several compendiums of psychoanalytic research published within this period have attempted to address this deficiency by presenting reviews of psychodynamic research (Fonagy, 2002, 2015; Leichsenring et al., 2015; R. A. Levy & Ablon, 2009). These volumes report positive results for psychoanalytic psychotherapy.

The late start for research on psychodynamic therapy does not demonstrate that this approach is not effective, rather it may more accurately reflect inherent difficulties in experimental controlled design for this approach. Numerous methodological problems for research on psychodynamic psychotherapy have been identified, because psychodynamic techniques do not lend themselves to the precision required for a clinical trial (Curtis & Hirsch, 2003; Gabbard, 2017). The problems cited in the literature include the following:

1. Manualized, structured protocols, such as CBT and interpersonal psychotherapy (IPT), are easier to systematically evaluate.
2. There is great difficulty in randomizing subjects, which is the gold standard of experimental design. Patients who want to engage in psychodynamic psychotherapy must be motivated to engage in the self-reflected exploration needed and are self-selected.
3. If the treatment is long term, which some psychodynamic therapies are, the costs would be too great to follow patients over time.
4. Funding is lacking for studies in psychodynamic psychotherapy.
5. The complexity and variety of psychodynamic approaches and technique make adherence to a specific model for intervention in an experimental design difficult.
6. Because subjectivity and context are embedded in the psychodynamic process, it is not possible to study by traditional objective scientific inquiry.
7. Most psychodynamic research consists of case studies, which limits the ability to generalize to other situations and populations.
8. Outcomes involve internal change for psychodynamic psychotherapy, which is difficult to quantify.
9. Randomized clinical trials (RCTs) focus on patients with one specific diagnosis and symptom measurement. Patients treated with psychodynamic therapy present with complex problems that usually are not limited to one disorder.

Despite the preceding limitations, many RCTs in the literature report positive results. Several RCTs, for example, compared short-term psychodynamic therapy to cognitive behavioral therapy and demonstrated the effectiveness of this approach in the treatment of depression (Connolly Gibbons et al., 2016; Driessen et al., 2015, 2017). The most compelling evidence includes meta-analytic studies of randomized clinical trials, which are considered the most effective statistical method for synthesizing the findings of many studies through using effect size as a comparison. Effect size is the difference between the control and experimental groups, with 0.8 indicating a large effect size, 0.5 a moderate effect size, and 0.2 a small effect size. A review of meta-analytic studies of psychodynamic RCTs reveals overall large effect sizes for pretreatment to post-treatment outcomes. See Table 5.5 for selected meta-analytic studies. The large effect sizes for psychodynamic psychotherapy (0.69 to 1.46) are impressive, but even more so when compared with studies of the U.S. Food and Drug Administration (FDA) research, which found effect sizes for fluoxetine (Prozac) of 0.26, for sertraline (Zoloft) 0.26, citalopram (Celexa) 0.24, and escitalopram (Lexapro) 0.31 (Turner, Matthews, Linardatos, Tell, & Rosenthal, 2008). Meta-analyses that tested for equivalence of outcomes among various treatments have established that psychodynamic therapy is equally effective compared to other empirically supported interventions (Kivlighan et al., 2015; Steinert et al., 2017). Meanwhile, those meta-analyses that compared long-term psychodynamic psychotherapy (LTPP) to shorter forms of psychotherapy suggest LTPP may be superior treatment for complex mental disorders (Leichsenring, Abbass, Luyten, Hisenroth, & Rabung, 2013; Leichsenring & Rabung, 2011).

In addition, larger effect sizes have been reported for follow-up outcomes compared to immediate post-tests after treatment for those studies that included this measure (Shedler, 2010). More recently, the results of an RCT by Fonagy et al. (2015) suggested that the efficacy of long-term psychodynamic psychotherapy for treatment-resistant

TABLE 5.5 SELECTED META-ANALYTIC STUDIES OF PSYCHODYNAMIC PSYCHOTHERAPY

Study	Description	Effect Size	Number of Studies Analyzed
Anderson and Lambert (1995)	Short-term PDT for various disorders and outcomes	0.85	9 studies
Leichsenring and Leibing (2003)	Meta-analysis of PDT and CBT to treat personality disorders	Pretreatment to post-treatment 1.46 after 1.5 years follow-up	14 studies
Leichsenring, Rabung, and Leibing (2004)	Short-term PDT for various disorders	1.17 = change in target problems 1.57 after 13 months post-treatment	7 studies
Diener, Hilsenroth, and Weinberger (2007)	Therapist facilitation of affective experience and outcomes	0.30	10 studies
Leichsenring and Rabung (2008)	Long-term PDT treatment of personality disorders, pretreatment to post-treatment	1.8	7 studies

(continued)

TABLE 5.5   SELECTED META-ANALYTIC STUDIES OF PSYCHODYNAMIC PSYCHOTHERAPY *(continued)*

Study	Description	Effect Size	Number of Studies Analyzed
Abbass, Kisely, and Kroenke (2009)	PDT treatment for somatic disorders, and change in general psychiatric sx	0.69	8 studies
de Maat, de Jonghe, Schoevers, and Dekker (2009)	Systematic review of long-term psychoanalytic therapy, pretreatment to post-treatment	0.78 months 0.94 after 3.2 years post-treatment	10 studies
Messer and Abbass (2010)	Personality disorders, general sx improvement	0.91 after 18.9 months post-treatment	7 studies
Town et al. (2012)	The impact of audio/video recording, tx manuals, and checks on outcomes in PDT	1.01	46 studies
Abbass et al. (2014)	Short-term PDT compared to control conditions in RCTs	0.71 = general 1.39 = somatic 0.64 = anxiety	33 studies
Keefe et al. (2014)	PDT compared to control interventions for anxiety disorders	0.64	14 studies
Driessen et al. (2015)	Short-term PDT compared to control conditions	1.18 = general 1.15 = depression 0.79 = anxiety	54 studies
Christea et al. (2017)	PDT and other psychotherapies compared to control interventions for borderline-relevant outcomes (sx, self-harm, suicide) at post-test	0.41 = PDT 0.34 = DBT 0.24 = CBT	33 studies

BT, behavior therapy; CBT, cognitive behavioral therapy; DBT, dialectical behavior therapy; PDT, psychodynamic psychotherapy; RCT, randomized clinical trial; sx, symptoms; tx, treatment.

Source: Adapted from Shedler, J. (2010). The efficacy of psychodynamic psychotherapy. *American Psychologist, 65*(2), 98–109. doi:10.1037/a0018378

depression was equal to the control group at the time of termination, but superior to the control group at 24- and 42-month follow-up. What this suggests is that the patient continues to change for the better after leaving therapy, indicating that the changes are enduring and extend beyond symptom remission. As a result of this research, numerous practice guidelines include psychodynamic psychotherapy as a treatment for various psychiatric disorders (see Table 5.6).

TABLE 5.6 PRACTICE GUIDELINES FOR PSYCHIATRIC DISORDERS		
Practice Guideline	**Psychiatric Disorder**	**Special Considerations**
American Psychiatric Association (APA, 2009)	**Panic Disorder** Panic-focused psychodynamic psychotherapy recommended with moderate clinical confidence as an initial treatment	Special focus on transference as the agent promoting change and confront the emotional significance of the sx
APA (2010b)	**Borderline Personality Disorder** Two psychotherapeutic approaches have been shown in randomized clinical trials to have efficacy: psychoanalytic/ psychodynamic therapy and dialectical behavior therapy	The treatment provided has three key features: weekly meetings with an individual therapist, one or more weekly group sessions, and meetings of therapists for consultation/supervision
APA (2010c)	**Major Depressive Disorder** Psychodynamic therapy is named as psychotherapeutic treatment option	Manual-based model of psychodynamic therapy may be helpful in development of evidence for this approach
APA (2010d)	**Obsessive-Compulsive Disorder** No RCTs supporting use of psychodynamic therapy	Psychodynamic therapy may be useful in helping patients overcome their resistance to accepting a recommended treatment
APA (2010a)	**Post-Traumatic Stress Disorder** Use of psychodynamic therapy supported by descriptive studies, process-to-outcome analyses, and clinical experience	May be useful in addressing developmental, interpersonal, or intrapersonal issues that impact social, occupational, and interpersonal functioning
American Psychological Association (2019)	**Depression** Comparative effectiveness research finds similar effects between psychodynamic therapy and other treatments, including pharmacotherapy and CBT	When combining therapy with use of an antidepressant, APA recommends CBT or interpersonal psychotherapy

(continued)

Practice Guideline	Psychiatric Disorder	Special Considerations
TABLE 5.6 PRACTICE GUIDELINES FOR PSYCHIATRIC DISORDERS (*continued*)		
Department of Veterans Affairs, Department of Defense (2016)	**Major Depressive Disorder** Weak evidence supporting nondirective supportive therapy or short-term psychodynamic psychotherapy (STPP)	Recommended for patients who decline or cannot access first-line treatments
Medicus (2012)	**Children** Use of psychodynamic psychotherapy for a wide range of clinical problems in children aged 3 to 12 years	Provides specific recommendations for clinical standard and clinical guideline rating
National Collaborating Centre for Mental Health (2009)	**Schizophrenia** Not considered a first-line treatment for schizophrenia	Healthcare professionals may consider using psychoanalytic/ psychodynamic principles to help understand the experiences of people with schizophrenia and their interpersonal relationships in early postacute period
National Collaborating Centre for Mental Health (2011)	**Self-Harm** Refers to any act of self-poisoning or self-injury carried out by an individual irrespective of motivation (commonly involves self-poisoning with medication or self-injury by cutting)	Three to 12 sessions of a psychological intervention that is specifically structured for people who self-harm, with the aim of reducing self-harm

CBT, cognitive behavioral therapy; RCT, randomized clinical trial; sx, symptoms.

PSYCHODYNAMIC CONTINUUM

Psychodynamic psychotherapy can be seen as a continuum from supportive psychotherapy to expressive to psychoanalytic psychotherapies using the practice treatment hierarchy from Chapter 1, Figure 1.7, as an overall framework for practice. The goals and focus of each type of psychodynamic psychotherapy differ. The supportive end of the continuum is aimed toward stabilization through restoring functioning, reducing anxiety, strengthening defenses, and facilitating more effective problem-solving, whereas the psychoanalytic end is aimed toward processing through interpreting unconscious conflict and gaining insight (Gabbard, 2017).

Expressive and psychoanalytic therapies involve more emotional processing than supportive psychotherapy; periods of stabilization alternate with periods of processing, and therapy often shifts back and forth along this continuum. In Chapter 1, Figure 1.9 addresses the treatment process spiral that illustrates the process of psychotherapy. The degree to which the therapy is supportive versus psychoanalytic is based on the focus of transference issues and the frequency of sessions (Gabbard, 2017). In moving toward the psychoanalytic end of the continuum, the transference interpretations increase, as does the number of sessions per week. Through transference, unconscious conflicts are illuminated and then worked through. By increasing the number of sessions per week, it is thought that the transference intensifies, which is desired in psychoanalytic psychotherapy.

Along this continuum, some therapeutic communication techniques may be more appropriate for stabilization,while others aid in processing. See Figure 5.2 on treatment hierarchy, psychodynamic continuum, and communication. Briere and Scott (2013) describe the therapeutic window for emotional processing and say that trauma is processed when the activation of emotion accompanies its narrative. The APPN helps the patient to modulate experience through questions that increase or decrease activation. As described in Chapter 4, the communication techniques considered to be more supportive are less emotionally laden and appropriate for stabilization, whereas those higher on the treatment triangle may trigger implicit neural networks and facilitate processing. Without the proper resources, this may be experienced as overwhelming and accompanied by unmanageable feelings. The supportive techniques, which focus on resource-building, are considered to be less anxiety-provoking. Thus, for patients who primarily require stabilization through supportive psychodynamic psychotherapy, the communication techniques toward the lower level of the treatment hierarchy are most often used. Alternating supportive communication with those communication techniques higher on the hierarchy is appropriate for the emotional processing that occurs in expressive and psychoanalytic psychotherapies.

Expressive communication techniques may be implemented to increase arousal in avoidant patients. These techniques may include immediacy, interpretation, observation, and focusing, depending on the psychotherapy approach being used. Another strategy to increase activation is to ask the person to go over the memory slowly in detail using the present tense. The amygdala is thought to hold memory in the present tense because it has not yet been processed. The narrative naturally shifts from what is

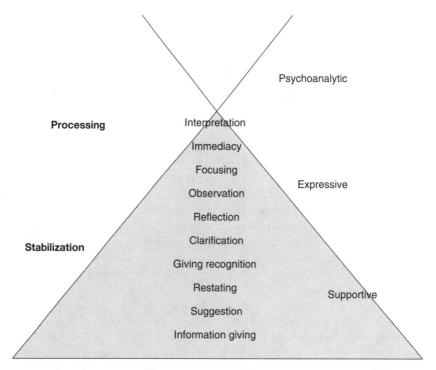

FIGURE 5.2 Psychodynamic case formulation diagram.

happening to what did happen after processing has occurred. The greater the detail of the event narrated in the present tense, the greater the activation and the processing of traumatic material (Briere & Scott, 2013).

Processing involves exposure to the trauma and assisting the person to construct a narrative through the exploration of the meaning of significant small and large traumas that impair functioning. The emotional dimension of the memory is essential for full processing to occur. Emotions are embedded in body sensations; both are experienced in tandem during processing. Talking about the event without addressing the attending emotions or body sensations may be a limited, intellectual exercise that precludes total processing. Briere and Scott (2013) emphasize that much of trauma activation and processing occurs at implicit, nonverbal, often relational levels.

Abreactions are intense emotional reactions to painful experiences that have been repressed. Chu (2011) delineates common phases that occur during abreactions: increased symptoms; intense internal conflict; acceptance and mourning; and mobilization and empowerment. Patients who do not have the capacity to withstand the intense feelings that occur during abreaction may instead use dissociation, substance abuse, distraction, and other avoidance responses (Knipe, 2019). Avoidance responses may take the form of missing sessions, lateness to sessions, increased distress, or self-injurious or impulsive behaviors after sessions. Therapists not skilled in working with abreactions should heed these signs as indicators that the therapeutic window for processing has been exceeded.

When overactivation or abreaction occurs, suggestions include shifting the focus away from the trauma with breathing exercises or relaxation techniques; directing the person's attention to less disturbing material; focusing on only one aspect or dimension of the experience such as the sounds or body sensations; distraction; using supportive communication techniques that are dearousing and supportive (see Figure 5.2); emphasizing intensity of emotion as doing good work; explaining activation before and after processing to normalize the person's reactions; problem-solving with the person to help mediate hyperarousal; using the safe place or container exercises (see Appendices 1.7 and 1.8); conveying optimism; and stabilizing with other affect management strategies (Steele, Boon, & van der Hart, 2017). If the person is abreacting, do not touch the person or make any sudden moves, and allow for personal space.

Periods of processing are often followed by periods of destabilization. The APPN paces and structures treatment so that work on traumatic material alternates with resources, such as grounding and containment. "Trauma should not be the focus of session after session. Instead, as material is retrieved, it is much more important to process that material in a manner that allows the patient to remain stable than it is to move on to find and/or deal with more material" (Kluft, 1999, p. 15). As Kluft points out, *slower is faster* because the overall therapy time is reduced if treatment is relatively stable. Periods after processing may include feelings of increased sadness, anxiety, loss of control, or confusion. Sometimes, normal functioning is impaired, and the person may become suicidal or unable to function, especially if there are memories of childhood abuse. More sessions per week sometimes offer more support, and the person then can have the opportunity to move beyond crisis intervention to address deeper underlying difficulties (Kluft, 1999).

The APPN emphasizes the importance of maintaining supportive relationships and regular activities because they provide a positive sense of self and allow the work to continue. If the crisis is not averted quickly, this is an indication that the patient is not ready to continue with emotional processing. Hospitalizing the person to process trauma only furthers regression and is counterproductive unless needed to ensure patient safety. As illustrated in Figure 1.9 in Chapter 1, the treatment process often looks more like a spiral, alternating interventions aimed at stabilization with processing that leads toward integration and future visioning. As life happens and job loss, serious illness, and other events may lead to destabilization, it may be necessary to stop processing and move to stabilizing again in the course of treatment.

Siegel (2012) posits that coherent narratives facilitate processing and interhemispheric integration. The left brain, which is language based, interprets the emotion-based autobiographical content of the right brain. Chapter 2, discusses right- and left-brain functions. The narrative in psychotherapy as told to an empathic other links self-states that have become dissociated due to trauma (Howell, 2005). This integration is considered the heart of mental health, with the successful resolution of trauma creating a deep sense of coherence (Siegel, 2012). The narrative helps the person to reconstruct a chronology to make sense of the experience by providing a context for time with a beginning, middle, and end. Research supports that through the reconstruction of the narrative, posttraumatic symptoms are reduced (Amir, Stafford, Freshman, & Foa, 1998). Because the disturbing experience is disconnected from other dimensions of the person's experience, it is important that the person integrate the event into his or her life and create meaning, allowing for closure. The literal recall of the event is not as important as how the person understands its meaning and how his or her sense of self or identity has been impacted.

As patients begin to accept their past, new perspectives about long-held assumptions begin to shatter. Those who have suffered abuse typically have conflicts in many areas of life. For example, one young woman who had been sexually abused by her father as a child felt intense shame about not having been *good enough* to stop the abuse. She had both love and hate for her father and, consequently, for herself. Her ambivalence was reflected in many areas: "I was loved/I was hated; I was powerless/it was my fault." These intense, ambivalent feelings were extremely painful, were repressed, and reflected entrenched neural networks of thought, emotion, and sensations. As she began to see her father more realistically, she was able to reformulate a more accurate view of herself. Over time, she began to see herself as a survivor instead of a victim. The reworking of traumatic material occurs over time in different ways. The person begins to understand the various elements of what happened and then interprets the same event and sense of self in a different way at a later date.

Another patient, a man who suffered horrific physical abuse from his sadistic father, examined various aspects of his traumatic experience. First, he understood and experienced the betrayal and pain he felt because of his father and, subsequently, he also understood the event as betrayal and humiliation by his neglectful mother, who did not intercede and passively witnessed his abuse. He then examined how this reverberated into all areas of his life, such as his feelings about himself in relationships, difficulty setting boundaries, inability to make decisions, lost job opportunities, self-esteem issues, somatic symptoms, difficulty managing feelings and self-soothing, and poor coping skills. Changes in physical and emotional responses occurred as the fragments of the traumatic memory were integrated with other more adaptive networks. The emotions elicited from the retelling are likely to be intense, and this expression is encouraged. Eventually, after they are fully processed, the events no longer increase emotional arousal. Over time, memories are woven into a narrative reflecting the integration of neural networks as new information is learned.

Educating the person about relapse prevention is important. The patient may always be vulnerable to symptoms when reexposed to stress because high states of arousal may trigger the retrieval of state-dependent memories, sensory information, or behaviors associated with prior disturbing experiences if the memories have not been fully processed. A plan for how to manage these times should be discussed, and this includes reviewing resource materials to enhance coping skills and booster sessions at vulnerable times. Explain to the patient that these high-risk periods may include developmental changes, periods of elevated stress, or reminders of partially processed traumas. Traumas that have not been previously identified may also be triggered at these vulnerable times. Resources should be increased prophylactically during these periods.

Supportive Psychotherapy

Frequently, supportive psychotherapy is recommended, and it is assumed that the therapist knows what this entails without training. Supportive psychotherapy is psychodynamic in that it is based on a knowledge of the patient's psychodynamics, which shapes the approach, but the goals of treatment differ considerably. Whereas psychoanalytic psychotherapy aims to restructure defenses and change personality organization through the interpretation of feelings, fantasies, and beliefs, supportive psychotherapy aims to strengthen defenses, promote problem-solving, restore adaptive functioning, and provide symptom relief. Left-brain frontal cortex problem-solving abilities are greatly impaired in some patients because of personality organization structure or current life stressors that have precipitated regression to an earlier stage of functioning. Supportive psychotherapy is indicated to assist the person in stabilization, as illustrated by the treatment hierarchy in Figure 1.7 in Chapter 1. This involves increasing external and internal resources.

In *A Primer of Supportive Psychotherapy*, Pinkster (1997) says that the supportive model is the preferred model for most patients and that it is only when the goals of treatment cannot be met through this model that more expressive therapies should be employed. Although Figure 5.3 indicates that supportive therapy is suggested for those who are on the psychotic end of the continuum, it is the treatment of choice for healthier patients, too. Most clinicians believe that the decision to use supportive psychodynamic psychotherapy should be based on the person's ego strength and weaknesses, present coping skills, highest level of functioning previously achieved, recent losses, and other life stresses and circumstances (Hollender & Ford, 2000). In a seminal article, 16 basic strategies are identified as supportive (see Table 5.7).

TABLE 5.7 BASIC STRATEGIES OF DYNAMIC SUPPORTIVE THERAPY	
Startegy	**Description**
Strategy #1: Formulate the case	Serves as a roadmap for future interventions; why does this person have this problem now; evolves as more information becomes available; involves a developmental assessment
Strategy #2: Be a good parent	"[T]o the extent that the patient is functioning at a childlike level in significant domains of life, the supportive therapist assumes a parental role" (p. 175)
Strategy #3: Foster and protect the therapeutic alliance	First and primary goal throughout the therapy; respect the patient with compassion, empathy, and commitment; align with the healthy parts of the person; collaboratively set goals and strategies to attain these; interpersonally active, treating the patient as the therapist would want to be treated
Strategy #4: Manage the transference	Do need to explore the childhood experiences that underlie negative transference feelings but they must be corrected or the person may leave treatment; therapist acknowledges openly, explicitly, and nondefensively and/or apologizes
Strategy #5: Hold and contain the patient	Provide empathy, understanding, soothing, helping the person to modulate affect, set limits when necessary, restrict acting out and impulsivity; may require medication and/or hospitalization, securing social services and so on while protecting the person's autonomy

(continued)

TABLE 5.7 BASIC STRATEGIES OF DYNAMIC SUPPORTIVE THERAPY (*continued*)	
Startegy	**Description**
Strategy #6: Lend psychic structure	Help as needed with reality testing, problem-solving, impulse control, affect modulation, interpersonal awareness, social skills, and empathy
Strategy #7: Maximize adaptive coping mechanisms	Support high level of defenses such as humor, altruism, sublimation, rationalization, and intellectualization and decrease use of denial, splitting, projection, and acting out; enhance coping skills such as mindfulness, dialectical behavior therapy and cognitive behavioral strategies to build distress tolerance skills and emotional regulation
Strategy #8: Provide a role model for identification	Use judicious self-disclosure; be present, available, and real
Strategy #9: Decrease alexithymia	Help the person to identify and name feelings; focus on somatic sensations associated with particular emotions; encourage use of metaphor to describe feelings
Strategy # 10: Make connections	Make associations between an event or situation and the person's feelings such as how false negative beliefs about himself or herself have undermined self-esteem and prevented the person from setting and/or achieving goals, seeking out healthy relationships, and so on
Strategy #11: Raise self-esteem	Foster competency in real skills; role-play skills; correct cognitive distortions; unravel unconscious guilt; normalize thoughts, feelings, and behaviors; explain why counterproductive behavior in the present may have been adaptive attempts to deal with earlier adverse life situations
Strategy #12: Ameliorate hopelessness	Use cognitive behavioral therapy, reframing, case management such as helping the person to obtain disability, housing, job, transportation, community resources
Strategy # 13: Focus on the here and now	Address primary issues: (1) safety, (2) therapy interfering behaviors, (3) future-foreclosing events or plans, (4) treatment noncompliance, (5) negative transference
Strategy #14: Encourage patient activity	Help the person to take action through setting concrete behavioral goals, devising a plan of action, behavioral rehearsal, role-playing, relaxation, visualization, imagery, graded exposure, and serving encouraging patient efforts
Strategy #15: Educate the patient and family	Teach about medication(s) side effects and so on, diagnosis/ illness, relapse symptoms, specific tasks or functions that the person cannot do on his or her own
Strategy #16: Manipulate the environment	Intervene as appropriate with agencies or persons in order to advocate for the person; do for the person what he or she cannot do for himself or herself, always with an aim toward maximum independence and growth

Source: Misch, D. (2000). Basic strategies of dynamic supportive therapy. *Journal of Psychotherapy Practice & Research, 9*(4), 173–189. Retrieved from https://www.ncbi.nlm.nih.gov/pmc/articles/PMC3330607

In assessing ego strength, it is important to identify the primary defenses the person uses to ward off anxiety. McWilliams (2011) lists the types of defenses most commonly associated with those in the psychotic level of personality organization and identifies these defenses as preverbal. They include denial, projection, splitting, primitive idealization and devaluation, withdrawal, omnipotent control, and dissociation. These defenses protect the person who is terrified of annihilation, who lacks a basic security in the world, and who is vulnerable to psychotic disorganization. Those on this end of the developmental continuum struggle with identity issues and confusion about who they are. Even if not overtly psychotic, the person is thought to be functioning at the symbiotic level of development, with little self–other differentiation. Some relational psychodynamic psychotherapists, such as Searles, Sullivan, and Fromm-Reichmann, advocate working with severe psychiatric disturbances such as schizophrenia using this model (Curtis & Hirsch, 2003).

Attachment research provides additional data for determining whether to use supportive or expressive interventions based on the person's attachment style (K. Levy, Ellison, Scott, & Bernecker, 2011). See Table 2.1 in Chapter 2. *Attachment style* describes the person's fear of rejection, yearning for intimacy, and preference of interpersonal distance in relationships. Determining the person's attachment style assists the APPN in understanding where to intervene on the psychodynamic continuum. The Adult Attachment Interview (AAI) is a semistructured interview that measures attachment style by analyzing how the patient describes childhood experiences (see Chapter 3). Those who are characterized as unresolved/disorganized are unable to form a coherent narrative about their life because of lapses in memory or reasoning; those with preoccupied attachment styles seem overwhelmed with early relationship experiences and are unable to elaborate a coherent narrative without being flooded with emotion; while securely attached individuals are able to communicate with coherence and emotional genuineness about difficult childhood experiences.

An unresolved/disorganized attachment style may need more active interventions that facilitate emotional expression and connection, whereas a preoccupied style may need more supportive interventions that help the person contain overwhelming emotions; those with a secure attachment are able to work productively anywhere on the continuum without customizing psychotherapy interventions. Preoccupied attachment has been strongly correlated with borderline personality disorder (BPD; Fonagy et al., 1996). Not surprisingly, the patient's attachment style predicts the nature of therapeutic alliance and the outcomes of treatment. The therapist's attachment style also influences treatment. One study found that therapists who measured as insecure on attachment tools tended to worry more about rejection and were less empathic with patients (Rubino, Barker, Roth, & Fearon, 2000).

In supportive psychodynamic psychotherapy, the content of sessions most often focuses on feelings, life stresses, and problem-solving, rather than on defenses. The therapeutic techniques most helpful in supportive psychotherapy are on the lower end of the continuum of therapeutic communication. These techniques include basic interpersonal skills such as reflection, empathic listening, encouragement, and helping people to explore and express their experiences and emotions (Cuijpers et al., 2012). Although giving advice is not on the continuum, it is sometimes prudent to offer a suggestion when the person cannot problem-solve. Suggesting that someone see an attorney in the context of an impending legal problem and suggesting that a patient see a medical specialist if those services are required are two examples of situations in which it is appropriate and necessary to offer a strong suggestion. It would be remiss in these situations to not offer this type of advice. In contrast, the therapist should not offer suggestions in other cases: suggesting that someone go to church, take a vacation, join a singles club, go back to school, or try online dating. These types of suggestions impose the APPN's values on the patient and shift the responsibility away from the patient to the therapist, which also encourages dependency and regression. Another way to help the person problem-solve without giving advice is to explore alternatives of action, expanding the possibility of choices with the person.

Often, supportive psychotherapy is most useful for people who need clarification and help in sorting out issues that they would be able to address under other circumstances. Patients may need to discuss situations, sort out the alternatives, and express feelings. Supportive psychotherapy focuses on safety, education, and assisting with enhancing coping skills. For example, Mrs. J came to therapy on the suggestion of a friend because of a crisis in her marriage. She recently found out her husband was having an affair and was quite despondent. She felt lonely, isolated, and useless. The therapist listened attentively as Mrs. J described her 30 years of marriage, the early years of their relationship, and her inability to forgive her husband. She felt stuck in her grief and anger and could not decide what course of action, if any, to take. The therapist suggested that it is sometimes better to wait to make decisions until feelings are clearer and that they would together explore the possible consequences of various courses of action. Through expressing her anger toward her husband in therapy, she felt somewhat better and was only then able to begin to examine other dimensions of disappointment that had been present in their relationship for a long time.

Sometimes, catharsis is all the person wants or needs from the therapy, without resolution of conflict. This is true especially in grief and the mourning process. Expression of feelings can be the first step in acknowledging other, more painful affects. For example, anger often masks underlying hurt, and anxiety often masks underlying anger. Through empathic exploring and open-ended questions, the person is gently guided to a full expression of the nuances of emotion. One caveat is warranted: With patients who are histrionic or overly emotional, emotion may need to be contained, rather than freely expressed, and affect regulation strategies may be needed before encouraging emotional expression. Chapters 17 and 18, discuss specific affect management strategies. The objective for supportive psychotherapy is to restore emotional equilibrium as quickly as possible.

Expressive Psychotherapy

The psychodynamic treatment of choice for those with borderline character structure is expressive psychotherapy (McWilliams, 2011). The American Psychiatric Association (APA) guidelines for BPD state that psychodynamic psychotherapy is the preferred psychotherapy, along with dialectical behavior therapy (APA, 2010b). Oldham (2005) reaffirms in a Guideline Watch that psychotherapy represents the core or primary treatment for BPD, with symptom-targeted psychopharmacology a secondary helpful adjunct. Those with borderline character structure as defined by McWilliams do not necessarily have a *DSM-5* diagnosis of BPD, but may encompass a wider diversity of diagnostic categories that rely on primitive and immature defenses. These individuals are not consistently operating in the mature spectrum of healthy defenses and, under stress, may even appear psychotic; hence, the term *borderline* is used. Defenses predominately include projection, acting out, and splitting when under stress, but higher-level defenses may also be used.

Some theorists speculate that the genesis of borderline traits occurs around 18 months of age in the rapprochement phase of separation–individuation (Masterson, 1976). It is thought that the child who still needs reassurance about his or her budding autonomy is thwarted developmentally by an unavailable caretaker or one who discourages separation. The child learns that independence equals loss of love (i.e., abandonment) and that closeness is associated with dependence and therefore fears of loss of control (i.e., engulfment). These early attachment issues can lead to a variety of adult relational problems and reflect unresolved attachment trauma. The ability to form and sustain reciprocal interpersonal relationships is notably disrupted in individuals who have experienced early traumatic attachment patterns (Schore, 2019). This essential dilemma gets played out in all subsequent relationships, including the psychotherapeutic relationship, creating chaos and unstable ego states.

Attachment trauma produces chronic problems in relationships, and processing relational trauma occurs largely through the therapeutic relationship. These individuals have difficulty in determining their own needs or sense of self and engaging in introspection. The relationally traumatized person has had to be hypervigilant, other-directed, and accommodating to survive. This focus on other precludes the inner work needed to develop a coherent sense of self (Briere & Scott, 2013). The child who has been emotionally or physically abused or neglected in early life learns that he or she is *not worth it* and, because of cognitive immaturity, arrives at the conclusion that he or she must deserve such treatment. Consequently, the person views himself or herself as weak, helpless, and inadequate, existing at the whims of an inherently rejecting, unavailable, and hurtful other. These implicit schemas of worthlessness and helplessness become powerful organizing determinants of personality. Sometimes, an exaggerated façade of independence, willfulness, and self-sufficiency develops to counter these vulnerable feelings.

Most often, those with borderline personality structure are anxious, depressed, self-harm in crisis, and are unable to tolerate ambivalence or defer gratification. These are individuals who are notoriously difficult to engage in treatment. Often, the precipitant for treatment is not because the person wants to change his or her personality, but because others have urged the person to seek help. These patients come to therapy with anxiety, depression, and dissatisfaction with their relationships. The challenge for the novice APPN is sorting out the focus of treatment and what to address first. Because the person with borderline personality structure can appear to be high-functioning and reality functioning seems intact, the nature of the underlying difficulties may not be readily apparent at intake.

As the transference evolves, it may take the form of idealizing or devaluing. The therapeutic relationship itself becomes a source of interpersonal triggers for implicit memories as the caring, empathic therapist often activates fears of abandonment. The growing feeling of emotional attachment to the therapist activates emotional responses from earlier childhood neglect or abuse experiences. These responses are often intense and may seem irrational and inappropriate. The therapist's first clue of a rupture in the therapeutic alliance may be the person reacting as if attacked to a comment that is intended to be helpful. For example, a man who is describing how angry he is that his boss is critical of him is asked by his therapist, "Does your boss remind you of anyone?" A higher functioning patient would most likely consider the question and answer, whereas the person with borderline personality structure may hear this as an accusation or criticism and feel angry at the therapist's perceived lack of attunement and "judgmental" comment.

However, it is important to note that processing may be on an implicit level and may not always occur in words (Blue Knot Foundation, 2019). Emotional processing can occur without the higher processing systems of the brain that involve explicit memory. For example, conditioned responses of shame or anger associated with abandonment and/or self-hatred that are present in implicit memory as a consequence of relationship or attachment trauma are triggered through relationship with the therapist, as well as with significant others. Within the safety of the therapeutic relationship, counterconditioning occurs as these schemas are not reinforced, and over time, the positive feelings in psychotherapy allow new learning to take place.

Expressive psychodynamic therapy provides a vehicle for the gradual processing of relational trauma through an ongoing therapeutic relationship. Briere and Scott (2013) identify healing components inherent in this approach:

1. The therapist offers consistent support for introspection through exploration, which allows the patient to develop an articulated and accessible sense of self.
2. The relationship itself provides a safe forum for activating and providing exposure to relational trauma.
3. The disparity between the therapeutic relationship and the expectation of abuse or neglect is demonstrated and experienced.
4. Counterconditioning occurs when the patient perceives safety, nurturance, and acceptance in the session, and consequently, fear is diminished.
5. Desensitization occurs as relationships are no longer perceived as dangerous, and triggers of fear, anger, distrust, and avoidant behaviors are changed so that relationships are seen as a source of support rather than pain.

As the therapeutic relationship deepens over time, the inevitable dependency of the patient provides an opportunity to rework these implicit memories so that new learning can occur. The therapist does not encourage dependency but does provide support and caring in a nurturing environment so that the patient can safely reexperience implicit, relational memories from childhood.

McWilliams (2011) says that the overall goal for expressive psychodynamic psychotherapy is the development of an integrated, complex, and positively valued self. This means that the person is able to tolerate ambivalent feelings and self-regulate emotions. Although there is no universal agreement about how to work with patients who have borderline character structure, several general principles of working in expressive psychodynamic psychotherapy with these individuals have been delineated: establishing consistent boundaries, using empathy before all interpretations, focusing on the here and now, asking the patient for help, rewarding assertiveness, discouraging regression and dependency, decreasing arousal levels so that communication can be heard, and understanding countertransference.

Countertransference is particularly challenging in working with those with borderline character organization and even experienced therapists seek supervision when working with these individuals. It is thought that powerful unconscious communication occurs with these patients, more so than with those who are psychotically or neurotically organized. The right-brain–to–right-brain communication often is more helpful in understanding the patient than what is actually said. Psychodynamic therapists identify *projective identification* as a specific type of countertransference that deepens the therapist's understanding of the patient.

Projective identification is considered a defense mechanism and a countertransference constellation. It essentially involves a patient behaving in such a way that subtle, interpersonal pressure is placed on the therapist to take on dimensions of the patient's experience or unconsciously identify with facets of him- or herself (Gabbard, 2017). Projective identification evokes a type of concordant countertransference, as described in Chapter 4 in which the therapist identifies with an aspect of the patient's self-experience (empathy). For example, a therapist may begin to feel afraid of the patient as the person is talking, which does not seem related to what the person is talking about. This out-of-the-blue feeling may reflect the patient's own fear being projected onto the therapist, which the therapist experiences in place of the patient.

Not only fear can be projected, but also anger, boredom, intrusiveness, passivity, and other feelings.

Alternatively, the therapist may identify with a patient's experience of an another that has been projected, which is known as complementary countertransference. For example, the therapist begins to behave, think, and feel as significant others felt when with the person. The therapist can identify whether or not this is occurring by noticing if she or he begins to feel or act unlike him- or herself. For example, the therapist may begin to feel angry or become verbally abusive toward the patient. The APPN is challenged to identify the powerful feelings that occur during a session.

Although projective identification has been touted as a useful tool to deepen therapists' understanding of patients, savvy therapists know that any feeling that may come up during a session may be from their own unconscious and not from a patient. Therapists should trust their own instincts, but only after taking emotional inventory and responsibility for their own dynamics. Sometimes, projective identification is so powerful that the therapist may feel confused, and, on reflection between sessions or with supervision, the therapist begins to sort out her or his own contributions from those of the patient. Contemporary psychoanalysts feel that countertransference and transference are co-constructed, and as such, the therapist uses her or his own feelings as a barometer to understand the patient's internal world only after considerable self-reflection. Relational psychodynamic psychotherapists believe that all transference–countertransference phenomena are forms of projective identification, in that the therapist always unwittingly lives out the reciprocal role of the significant other in the patient's early life.

Psychoanalytic Psychotherapy

Patients who are considered ideal candidates for psychoanalytic psychotherapy are those with neurotic-to-healthy personality organization and those who primarily rely on mature defenses. Some primitive defenses may be present, but along with these, mature defenses are also evident. These individuals have a sense of who they are, are in touch with reality, and have achieved object constancy. *Object constancy* refers to the capacity to be alone. When asked to describe others, they are able to give a fairly detailed account of the other person so that the APPN can get a clear picture of the person's characteristics. The patient with a neurotic-level personality most likely has had some satisfying relationships and is experienced by the therapist as capable of engaging in a therapeutic alliance. These persons may come to treatment because of obstacles in love or work that make them feel uncomfortable. Usually, they are the people who seek help without being forced. Problems for individuals with neurotic-level personality organization are often experienced as *ego dystonic* (i.e., alien to how they experience themselves). For example, patients may be troubled by disturbing thoughts about harm coming to them or loved ones. These experiences are felt as different from themselves, as *ego alien*. In contrast, persons with psychotically organized personality may be more likely to experience their problems as *ego syntonic*. This means that the problem is compatible with who they are. These individuals often feel that it is others who have the problem and want reassurance, for example, that they have good reason to be paranoid or acting out.

If the person wants to understand himself or herself deeply and significantly change, psychoanalysis may be indicated. Psychoanalysis is more intense than psychoanalytic psychotherapy in that session frequency is increased and the transference is intensified. Sometimes, the person comes to treatment and has some initial psychotherapy and then decides to deepen the work and undergo psychoanalysis. Psychoanalysis generally takes three to five sessions each week and requires the amount of time for natural or normal maturational change (3–7 years). Many of the candidates for psychoanalysis are those in training programs to become psychoanalysts. Therapists who want to work in a deeper way with patients and understand that knowing themselves is a prerequisite to this work sometimes seek their own psychoanalysis without the structure of a formal training program. Traditionally, the basic methods of psychoanalysis involve free association by the patient who is lying on the couch with the therapist sitting in back of him or her. The therapist listens and interprets resistance and transference as these elements are manifested in dreams and considers what the patient says or does in and outside sessions.

The development and facilitation of what is called the *transference neurosis* is integral to the process of Freudian psychoanalysis. The transference neurosis is a rerun of the developmental process through an intense relationship with the therapist. The patient experiences feelings toward the analyst that were similarly expressed toward significant others in early development. This enactment and resolution of the transference is the work of psychoanalysis. The deep analysis of the relationship with the therapist distinguishes psychoanalytic therapy from other types of therapies. The transference is intensified with the increased frequency of sessions and the neutrality of the analyst. The analyst listens with *evenly hovering attention*, which means without preconceptions, absorbing what the person says with an attitude of nonjudgmental, empathic neutrality designed to create a safe environment. As the transference unfolds, the patient and analyst work together in understanding unconscious processes that are triggered in the therapeutic relationship.

CASE FORMULATION

In order for the APPN to decide on a relevant therapeutic focus, realistic expectations of treatment, and the appropriate type of psychodynamic psychotherapy to use, a dynamic case formulation is essential. In general, the shorter the length of the psychotherapy, the more intense the pressure to determine a therapeutic focus, and this is done through a psychodynamic formulation. Safran and Muran (2000) state: "It is the establishment of a dynamic focus and the consistent interpretation of that focus over time, as it emerges in a variety of different contexts that facilitates the working through process and allows the patient to integrate treatment changes into his/her everyday life" (p. 178). As addressed in Chapter 1, The Nurse Psychotherapist and a Framework for Practice, Figure 1.7, the hierarchy of treatment aims is helpful in this regard, but a more sophisticated psychodynamic understanding of development and defenses further refines treatment choice and informs the work of psychodynamic psychotherapy. The case formulation identifies a central issue that underlies the person's presenting problem as it relates to the person's early developmental history. This involves conceptualizing presenting issues developmentally and understanding intrapsychic conflict. Three personality organization levels have been identified—neurotic to healthy, borderline, and psychotic—based on a synthesis of major developmental theories (McWilliams, 2011; Figure 5.3).

These organization levels may be thought of as a continuum that ranges from healthy to psychotic and cuts across all diagnostic categories, because virtually all diagnoses are represented at each level. Some diagnostic categories are more heavily represented on one end of the continuum or the other, depending on the primary category of the defense used: primitive, immature, neurotic, or mature. Chapter 2, The Neurophysiology of Trauma and Psychotherapy, lists defenses in each category. In general, the person who uses primarily primitive defenses is more likely in the psychotic range of the continuum, and the person who primarily relies more on mature, higher-level defenses more

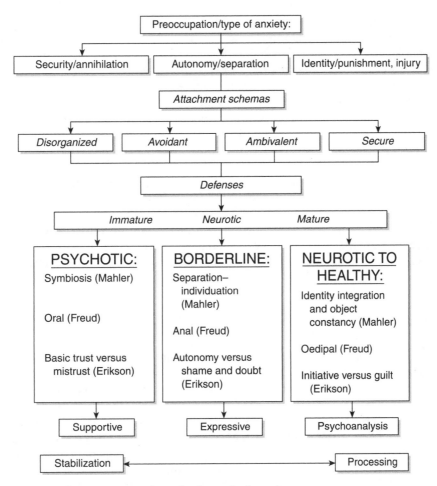

FIGURE 5.3 Case formulation and psychodynamic therapy.

likely is in the neurotic-to-healthy range. However, given enough stress, anyone can veer toward the psychotic end of the continuum. For example, the person with narcissistic traits can be primarily in the neurotic-to-healthy range, but with enough stress, can slip into the psychotic end of the spectrum. Under stress, we revert to methods of coping from earlier levels of development that feel similar to the current situation. Implicit memory networks of defenses are triggered by biochemical states reflecting state-dependent learning.

McWilliams (1994) says that dynamically oriented therapists make an assessment based on the following: "People with a vulnerability to psychosis may be understood as fixated on the issues of the early symbiotic phase; people with borderline personality organization are comprehensible in terms of their preoccupation with separation–individuation themes; and those with neurotic structure can be usefully construed in more oedipal terms" (p. 53). The importance of determining the primary defenses of the patient and assessing ego functions in light of these developmental levels is to determine a dynamic case formulation and what type of treatment can be most helpful for the person at this time. Chapter 3, Assessment and Diagnosis, explains how to assess ego development. The patient's core conflicts inform psychodynamic treatment more than a formal *Diagnostic and Statistical Manual of Mental Disorders* (*DSM*) diagnosis.

A tentative summary of the dynamic formulation should be shared with the patient and should include some idea about how the therapist sees the nature of the work to be accomplished. For example, Michele, a 27-year-old French woman, came to therapy because she felt "confused, depressed, and was losing control." She had several recent panic attacks accompanied by paranoid ideation, fearing that she might be attacked and possibly raped. At the end of the first session after taking her history, the therapist said: "The recent loss of your boyfriend has contributed to you feeling increasingly sad and panicky. We need to work on shoring up your resources so you can feel more in control when bad things happen. How does that sound to you?" The APPN felt that relational psychodynamic psychotherapy would be helpful, but was careful to not overwhelm Michele with too much information in the first session. Later in treatment, after an alliance was more firmly established, the APPN fleshed out the dynamic formulation to Michele by suggesting: "Most likely, the absence of your mother's presence in your early life and your father's anger made you feel unsafe and prevented you from learning and developing the coping skills you need to stay on an even keel. It would be helpful to deepen your understanding of how you seem to end up in relationships that are not good for you."

WORKING THROUGH

Working through is considered the heart of the therapeutic work. Freudian psychoanalysts see the working-through process as observing, clarifying, and interpreting defenses as manifested by the resistances and transferences again and again. In contrast, relational psychodynamic psychotherapists emphasize a restructuring of the person's relational schemas through working with therapeutic impasses or ruptures in the therapeutic alliance. This "involves a recognition of how the relationship with the therapist reflects relationships from childhood and current extratransference relationships" (Gabbard, 2017, p. 179). Working through is the consistent interpretation of this dynamic focus over time. Rarely is there one insightful comment or interpretation that changes things dramatically. Rather, the repeated, consistent interpretation of the same themes and patterns as they are manifested in myriad situations and relationships facilitates a person's transformation over time. Both Freudian and relational psychodynamic therapists conceive that change occurs gradually and includes changing internal and external representations. Patterns of interactions with other people are significantly changed, and this is accompanied by changes in the patient's internal representations, or how the person perceives himself or herself and others. This evolution reflects the adaptive information processing of memory networks that were previously dysregulated or dissociated in implicit memory systems.

Emphasis in relational psychodynamic psychotherapy in the working-through process is on facilitating the development of the capacity for mindfulness (Safran & Muran, 2000). *Mindfulness* is the ability to observe internal processes and actions in relation to other people. This goal is conveyed to the patient at the outset of therapy. The APPN explains to the patient that how he or she feels with the therapist can also occur outside therapy in other relationships. The patient is asked to monitor what dimensions of this situation are true or occur for him or her. The relational psychodynamic psychotherapist describes how, both with the therapist and with those outside therapy, patterns of relating are similarly fueled by the person's early experiences. The therapist observes characteristic patterns of implicit relatedness and shares these observations with the patient, providing a new perspective that is different from the person's own subjective impressions. Pointing out the person's tendency to be controlling, demanding, dependent, or passive increases his or her awareness of implicit modes of relatedness and the impact of these behaviors on others (Gabbard, 2017). This awareness often brings the patient a much greater sense of mastery, so that patterns of behavior can be reflected on before enacted in future relationships.

Meaningful change, however, involves more than interpretations about relationships. The psychotherapeutic relationship itself provides a different relationship experience for the person, so that new neural connections can be made. This inevitably leads to disillusionment as the person comes to accept his or her own separateness and that of the therapist, and it involves a mourning process in that the patient gives up an old way of being. Curtis and Hirsch (2003) state, "Salubrious new experience can only develop in a context in which old experience is first repeated, perhaps mourned, and let go of" (p. 81). Mourning the loss of possibilities and unhealthy relationships with significant others is considered curative because more energy is freed for current relationships. Unfulfilled desires are identified, tolerated, and then relinquished in a safe relationship.

The working-through process assists the person in recovering split-off and dissociated aspects of the self that developed to maintain a relationship with parents. The person who has not been attuned to or who suffered trauma in early life has had to comply to survive, and a false self is thought to have developed. This false self lacks spontaneity and may result in a pervasive sense of unreality, futility, and lack of vitality (Safran & Muran, 2000). Relational theorists posit that there is not one false self but multiple selves that need to be re-appropriated for the person to feel *real* and *alive*. These ways of being are embedded in important early relationships and templates of neural networks that at one time were adaptive. For example, the patient who was connected to her mother through chaos and unpredictability will experience sadness at giving up this state of consciousness, because this way of being is embedded in the fundamental attachment to the caretaker that ensured survival.

Various exploratory communication techniques assist in the working-through process. These include asking patients about their fantasies, daydreams, dreams, early memories, and ideas about what they perceive others are thinking, including what they imagine the therapist to be thinking. One way to help patients reflect on interactions outside therapy involves helping them to experience situations fully by comments such as: "Imagine being there right now" (Curtis & Hirsch, 2003). Another exploratory technique is to observe and reflect what seems to be happening for the patient. For example: "You sound very angry today. I wonder what this is about?" Gabbard (2017) says this increases mentalization (i.e., mindfulness), which is the person's ability to think about his or her own experiences and feelings, which invites further differentiation of emotions. In a similar vein, if the patient reports an impulsive act, the therapist may ask what was going on just before that happened. Using open-ended, exploring communication allows patients to deepen their capacity for reflection. As a patient integrates emotional information that has been dissociated, a more robust sense of self develops that is grounded in the person's own experience.

In contrast to cognitive therapy, in which there is a structured agenda for each session, psychodynamic psychotherapy is based on *psychic determinism* (Binder, 2004). This means that the patient's spontaneous verbalizations will reveal affectively charged themes; he or she does not need to have a specific topic in mind, but instead talks about whatever thoughts and feelings arise that are relevant to the agreed problem focus. Current, problematic relationships—or past ones—tend to be the most emotionally arousing. This free association is thought to allow space for the person's own experience and ways of interacting to emerge. The therapist listens with the idea of discerning latent patterns related to the person's underlying conflicts and issues. The therapist asks herself: "What is the central issue here? What is going on now?" It is the therapist's job to track salient themes and goals that were set at the outset of the treatment. Each session, then, is a continuation of the one before, meaning that themes reverberate, threading throughout sessions, and what is talked about in the current session reflects issues that felt important at the end of the previous session. Taking good process notes at the end of each session helps in tracking these themes.

Integral to the working-through process is identifying progress and supporting the person's strengths. The therapist points out positive changes to the patient and reframes experiences. For example, one patient who was struggling with rejection, neediness, and failed relationships was told by her therapist: "It is sad that things did not work out with Jim, but it seems that, unlike past situations, you were able to see much sooner that your needs were not being met and to say what you wanted, rather than just hanging in there, hoping that things would change." Encouraging risk-taking and tolerating anxiety-producing situations through such comments provides the support needed and points toward positive change. Tempered comments without cheerleading are most effective; making the therapist happy is not the point of therapeutic gains. The idea that the patient changes to please the therapist is known as *transference cure,* and the therapist needs to be vigilant to ensure that the patient's autonomy and self-actualization are the goal (Curtis & Hirsch, 2003).

Challenging situations in psychotherapy can be structured through the gradual tolerance of anxiety-provoking situations, as facilitated through psychoeducation, role-playing, imagery, rehearsal, and modeling. For example, a man who came to treatment for marital problems was extremely passive in his relationship with his wife and often expected her to know what he wanted without articulating his needs. He grew up the youngest of six children with an angry father and depressed mother, and he spent much time alone in his room, withdrawing passively from the chaos around him. This typical response to conflict, coupled with his fear of rejection and his wife's anger, paralyzed him in attempts to address anything with her that he was unhappy about. The therapist role-played a typical scenario, with the patient playing the role of his wife and the therapist playing his role. This exercise provided a new way of responding that he eventually was able to try at home. The role-playing helped to build his confidence, see new ways of relating, and enabled him to deepen his understanding about his anxiety in a safe context.

Because problems in relating to others are a core focus in relational psychodynamic psychotherapy, the therapist helps the person to understand his impact on others, deepening understanding of other people, too (Wachtel, 2011). Flexibility in relationships is considered a sign of health, with healing defined as the ability to assimilate new experiences and to transcend unhealthy identifications with others and the constraints of the past (Curtis & Hirsch, 2003). For example, in the previous situation, the therapist pointed out to the patient: "Given what you have told me about your wife, she seems to strike out and get angry when she is feeling neglected, and she likely feels neglected when you withdraw and do not communicate." This type of comment enables the patient to see the cyclical nature of the patterns of relating that perpetuate the difficulties she or he is experiencing. In this situation, the patient's passivity created the very situation that he was trying to avoid: his wife's rejection and anger.

REPAIRING ALLIANCE RUPTURES

Many relational psychodynamic theorists believe that alliance ruptures are inevitable in therapy and that resolving these ruptures creates positive change (Eubanks, Muran, & Safran, 2019). Any psychotherapy that goes too smoothly is thought to reflect the therapist's accommodation of the person's false self and is likely to remain superficial and preclude change. In general, the therapeutic alliance may be stable from session to session, but instances of strained interpersonal interactions between the therapist and patient will arise. If the therapy is particularly brief, alliance ruptures may not develop because of the limitations of the treatment. Research suggests that repairing the alliance results in positive outcomes. This is accomplished by the APPN first recognizing the rupture and then acknowledging the rupture openly and nondefensively; empathizing and validating the patient for sharing his or her dissatisfaction; and then accepting one's own responsibility for the patient's concerns.

Immediacy, a therapeutic communication technique described in Chapter 4, is useful in relational psychodynamic psychotherapy, especially in the throes of an alliance rupture. For example, one patient, a 46-year-old woman named Susan, came to therapy for depression because of a series of failed relationships. Her history revealed early deprivation with both parents, who were extremely self-involved and neglectful of their children. Her experience was one of chronically feeling devalued, which reinforced her schema that she was not lovable and not worth it. This theme played out in all her relationships in that no one could ever meet her needs or be there in the way she needed them to be. Chronic dissatisfaction and feelings of deprivation permeated every situation as she upped the ante, no matter what was offered to her. Whatever was given was not enough, providing proof of the person's neglect or ill intentions. She presented an *unpaid bill demanding to be paid* in every interpersonal encounter. This was repeated in therapy, with Susan wanting more time, continuing to talk at the end of sessions, making frequent demands for changes of appointment times, and offering relentless criticisms of others. The therapist began to feel demoralized and tense up before each session, almost as if to shore up in order to withstand the barrage of negativity. The therapist felt hopeless and helpless, caught in the throes of a negative transference–countertransference enactment. After discussing the situation in supervision, the therapist understood that she was feeling as Susan must have felt, devalued in her family and hopeless, and the therapist offered this interpretation in the next session: "Perhaps you are feeling that I am not giving you what you need here." This helped bring the process into the here and now, focusing on the therapeutic relationship, which allowed Susan to explore the reasonableness of her needs and her inevitable disappointment and hurt when she felt slighted. An interpretation is considered timely and relevant if it opens a productive avenue of therapeutic inquiry. The therapist encouraged and explored, listening empathically and nondefensively. She stated: "It is so hard to be here and feel so vulnerable and not get what you want or need."

Negative Therapeutic Reaction

A negative therapeutic reaction is a specific type of therapeutic impasse in which the patient gets worse and becomes entrenched in maintaining his or her problems despite the help of the therapist. Gabbard (2017) says that these reactions likely result from revenge fantasies, in that the therapist—serving as parent in the transference—is defeated by the patient not getting better. This reaction is usually unconscious. The patient is often not aware of ill intentions, only that he or she is stuck or unhappy in treatment. In relational psychotherapy, this situation is not one-sided. The therapist may have too much invested in helping the person and begins to feel demoralized because no effort seems to be beneficial. It is often necessary for the therapist engaged in the throes of a negative therapeutic reaction with a patient to seek supervision and consultation to sort out the situation. Evaluating the relational dynamics with a colleague can be helpful, but sometimes, even then, the only solution is to refer the patient to someone else. The patient sometimes makes significant improvements only after treatment is terminated.

WORKING WITH DREAMS

Research on dreams has confirmed their importance and relevance for understanding the unconscious and implicit memory (Solms & Turnbull, 2002). Dreams are the brain's attempt to process information and to integrate the *day's residue* into the existing memory networks. Dreams represent current conflicts, and work on dreams focuses on the here and now, rather than the past, although current conflicts usually have roots in the past. Many psychodynamic psychotherapists consider dream work a useful tool to assist patients in deepening their understanding about themselves. A basic tenet of dream work is that dreams represent wishes, fears, and conflicts, as well as the person's attempts to master unresolved issues and process traumatic experiences. Dreams are fertile ground for work in psychodynamic psychotherapy.

As in communication, dreams contain both manifest and latent content. The manifest content is what the dreamer says the dream is about, and the latent content is the meaning of the dream. The latent content is disguised by defenses so that the person will not awaken. Although dream symbol books are interesting, they are not particularly useful in interpreting dreams because the meaning and symbols in dreams are highly idiosyncratic, not universal. Dreams have multiple levels of meaning, and the symbols represented in the dream are unique for that person. Two people may have the same exact dream, and it may mean completely different things to each individual. However, dreaming about a house or type of house may symbolize the person and feelings about him- or herself. Another theme that seems to appear for many people is the act of going someplace in a car or train, which sometimes heralds movement or change, either in therapy or in a person's life. There are often transferential dimensions to the dream; its content may reflect feelings the dreamer has about the therapist, albeit in disguised form. Dreams can reveal feelings that have arisen in the therapeutic relationship that have not yet been addressed (Curtis & Hirsch, 2003).

Dream interpretation is a little like trying to understand a poem or a work of art. It is undoubtedly a right-brain endeavor, and it is helpful to use right-brain functions when working with dreams. This can sometimes be accomplished through a mindful state, whereby the APPN attends to the patient by suspending usual left-brain problem-solving thinking and listens with empathic receptivity and resonance. Dreams are not experienced as linear; the constraints of time and space are suspended. To understand the patient's dream, it is important to know the basic mechanisms associated with dreams, which include secondary revision, symbolic representation, condensation, and displacement (Gabbard, 2017). *Secondary revision* refers to a right-brain, implicit message being translated into a coherent story. *Symbolic representation* refers to an image that represents a complex set of emotions that may be highly charged. *Condensation* is a mechanism that combines more than one wish, feeling, or impulse into a single image. *Displacement* is similar to defense in that feelings for one person are displaced onto another person in the patient's life.

Dream work can be introduced to the patient in the assessment by asking about recurring dreams, memorable childhood dreams, and recent dreams. These dreams can be useful in gaining insight. It is helpful to suggest that the patient keep a dream log next to the bed, so that he or she can jot down significant dreams upon awakening. Even if patients do not usually remember their dreams, they can be trained to do so by beginning to keep track of their dreams in this way. After discussing the idea of working with dreams with patients, it is better to not bring up the subject again and to allow patients to report dreams when they are ready. Not all patients are able to recall dreams and alexithymic patients, in particular, have great difficulty in remembering their dreams because of their impoverished ability to symbolize (Hollender & Ford, 2000).

Bringing in the first dream often heralds a deepening of the therapeutic alliance and should be positively acknowledged by the APPN. This first dream often illustrates the dynamic focus for the work of treatment. For example, one woman, who came to treatment with significant long-term depression, but was fairly high-functioning, had suffered significant attachment trauma from her early relationship with her mother, who had BPD. The patient reported her first dream in the sixth session: "My daughter and I are taking care of a baby, a baby girl, about 2 years old. She is dead and in parts, and we can't seem to get her back together. I am trying to call the funeral home but can't get through, and for some reason, I have only 45 minutes. That is not enough time. I wake up thinking that I won't be able to put her together in such a short time." Her thoughts about the dream were that the baby represented herself and the 45 minutes corresponded with the length of our session time. This was a graphic illustration of how the patient felt about herself and the work that needed to be accomplished in therapy.

Although dreams can advance the work of therapy, they can also serve as a resistance. If the patient comes in with several dreams and floods the session with dream material, it may not be possible to examine any dimension of the dream in the detail needed to be helpful. As with all therapy, the process or context should be dealt with first. What is going on in the process of psychotherapy that causes the person to overwhelm the therapist with so much material now? If a dream is reported in a session, the whole session's latent content usually is about the dream, even if the dream content itself is not the topic of conversation. Asking the person: "What are your thoughts about the dream?" is often a good way to encourage the patient to share his or her associations about the dream. Another way to work is to ask the person what stands out the most about the dream, or to identify the worst part of the dream. If the dream is readily understood and the manifest content is obvious, it is considered *transparent*, which may sound like a derogatory term, but means that the content is not highly disguised or defended against. In contrast, the dream that is difficult to understand may reflect the strength of the defense against this implicit material coming to consciousness. Sometimes, novice therapists are hesitant to do dream work because they feel they must come up with a grand interpretation at the end. Often, however, the therapist merely receives the person's thoughts on the dream without much comment. It is thought that the act of relating the dream is therapeutic because right-brain material is translated into left-brain information, which is an integrative process in and of itself. It is not incumbent on the therapist to make sense of the dream; after all, it is the patient's dream, and it is his or her thoughts about it that count. The following example illustrates these concepts.

Sarah, a 22-year-old English woman from an orthodox Jewish family, was seen for depression and low self-esteem. She described her mother as depressed, sometimes staying in bed for weeks, and her father as hypersensitive, depressed, tense, and domineering. Sarah had moved to the United States to go to school the previous year. She began her 15th psychotherapy session by saying that she was too hard on herself and that she always feels she is going to be judged because she sees others as superior to her and wonders how they will perceive her. She wanted to be different, but was anxious about changing. Her parents always implied that they knew the real Sarah and that she was too introspective. Her older sister was always down on everything and saw Sarah as emotional, selfish, and a troublemaker, and Sarah tended to agree with her. She then reported the following dream: "I was at home in my parents' house in London. Dad died in the dream and was out in the front yard without his head. Blood was pouring out of his neck, but he was still talking. I was crying 'no, no, no.' I felt awful that he had died."

When the therapist asked what she thought about this dream, Sarah said she thought that she was trying to kill off parts of herself that were like her dad. She thought that the dream was telling her that she loved her father and did not really hate him and that she could love him after she was in control of herself and did not feel as if he controlled her. The therapist responded: "You care a great deal about your father, but you have issues to work out about yourself before you can improve your relationship with him." In understanding the session in light of the dream, Sarah had started the session being concerned about being judged and perhaps wondered what the therapist would think of such a murderous dream. This is the latent transferential part of the session. By listening nonjudgmentally and accepting her thoughts about the dream, the therapist provided a different experience for her from the one she had in her family. The therapist offered no new interpretation, but agreed and reflected what Sarah said about the dream. The following illustrates the basic mechanisms in Sarah's dream:

Secondary revision

Sarah recounts the dream in story form.

Symbolic representation

The house in London may represent her childhood experiences.

Condensation

She sees her anger at her father and her own murderous impulses toward him on the one hand; his death brings freedom from his tyranny. On the other hand, he is still talking, and this may reflect the embedded wish that she can still maintain a relationship with him despite her anger, or that his words would continue to influence her even though he is dead. Perhaps his talking head reflects her wish that her anger would not kill him and he would still be alive.

Displacement

Sarah is in part displacing her own anger about herself toward her father. She focuses on her father as the source of her unhappiness in the dream, but in her associations to the dream, she says that she wants to kill off parts of herself that are like her dad, which illustrates the utility of the dream in illuminating her displacement.

BRIEF PSYCHODYNAMIC PSYCHOTHERAPY

In contrast to psychoanalysis, brief psychodynamic psychotherapy takes place in fewer days per week and lasts for a shorter duration. Although techniques are similar, less regression is encouraged, and the patient is not encouraged to use the couch, but to sit facing the therapist. For those wishing to work on a particular issue or conflict, shorter-term psychodynamic psychotherapy may be indicated. This approach is sometimes called *focal psychodynamic psychotherapy*. Although psychodynamic psychotherapy is frequently thought of as long-term therapy, brief psychodynamic psychotherapy is probably most often practiced given the current climate of managed care.

How many sessions constitute brief therapy? It could be one session, although we might question what this one session would consist of and how helpful it would be. Most often, a course of 20 to 30 sessions is considered brief therapy. Here, psychodynamic assumptions and techniques are the same as if longer-term treatment was conducted; there is no qualitative difference between brief and long-term psychodynamic psychotherapy. "There are not specific techniques that hold the key to the practice of brief therapy. Instead, the most expeditious means to achieve efficient and effective therapeutic outcomes is to practice 'good' psychotherapy, regardless of the anticipated or planned length" (Binder, 2004, p. 22). Wolberg (1977) developed general guidelines for conducting brief psychodynamic psychotherapy. A slightly modified version is provided in Box 5.1.

Proponents of brief psychodynamic psychotherapy believe that setting a termination date at the beginning of treatment assists in the progress and resolution of the patient's problems. Setting the termination date is thought to provide a focus that can link or thread unrelated experiences together for the therapist and the patient. This deadline is thought to be integral to the treatment in that the patient is helped to work through the meaning of termination. This central issue in the therapy parallels the separation–individuation developmental issue of life. Loss is a central theme for everyone, along with the tension of connecting through relationship while remaining a self-agent. Termination in psychotherapy can be a forum for addressing and exploring these central dilemmas in life. Specific issues related to termination that frequently arise in therapy are abandonment fears, disappointments, and anger about not getting what a person hoped for. The therapist listens empathically, and this noncritical acceptance of the patient's needs and wants helps the patient to accept the limitations of others. This approach is thought to help the person access dissociated wishes and needs that have been split off due to early relationships. Through the process of acknowledging and relinquishing the pursuit of an idealized, unattainable goal, the limitations and realities of relationships are accepted. Because there may not be enough time for transference to develop sufficiently, the therapist can use the relationship to work through as just described. Here, the focus of therapy is on interpersonal relationships outside the therapeutic relationship.

BOX 5.1 General Principles for Conducting Brief Psychodynamic Psychotherapy

- Establish a therapeutic alliance
- Set a termination date (within 30 sessions)
- Deal with initial resistances
- Gather historical and other data
- What is the most important problem? Why now? What has been done so far?
- What does the patient think caused the problem? What does the patient want from therapy?
- Select the symptoms (focus) most amenable to treatment within the first three sessions
- Define the precipitating event
- Identify developmental issues and defenses to understand how to proceed
- Share the case formulation with the patient
- Enlist the patient as an active participant through a verbal contract
- Use the most effective techniques to help the patient
- Identify resistances or alliance ruptures, and address them with the patient
- Be sensitive to how the past is influencing the present
- Examine countertransference feelings
- Give homework (optional)
- Stress the need for continuing work

Source: Adapted from Wolberg, L. R. (1977). *The technique of psychotherapy* (3rd ed.). New York, NY: Grune & Stratton.

CASE EXAMPLE

Ms. S is a 32-year-old intelligent, attractive woman who is very successful in her career. Her reason for seeking treatment is related to her dissatisfaction with her chronic tendency to choose men who eventually abuse her emotionally. Ms. S stated that her father had abused her sexually, as well as other female relatives in the family. When Ms. S got older and objected to his advances, her father accused her of being *uptight* and compared her unfavorably to her younger and more compliant sister, who obviously had no problem because she willingly accepted his behavior. Ms. S had a good early relationship with her mother. The sexual abuse left Ms. S with a profound mistrust of men. She was active and controlling in relationships with men (e.g., she was always the one who initiated sex). When her partner expressed an interest in sex, it felt analogous to her father's sexually controlling, intrusive, and abusive behavior. In addition to initiating sex, she was giving in other ways (e.g., gifts, dinners, and arranging activities for her and her boyfriend to enjoy). The unfortunate side of this behavior was that it obscured the essentially narcissistic character structure of these men. In other words, they were fine as long as they were on the receiving end. Inevitably, the relationship would flounder when she risked expressing needs of her own.

Developmentally, her anxiety and conflict seemed to lie in the area of identity and loss of control in that she experienced much anxiety in relationships with men if she did not control what happened. Ms. S had good object constancy and could be alone without much separation anxiety, could self-soothe, was self-directed, and was fairly autonomous, even though controlling, in relationships. In Erikson's framework, issues of intimacy versus isolation were apparent in that the crux of her problems was in establishing an intimate relationship. Neurotic-level defenses of displacement and rationalization were evident, as well as denial, which is considered a primitive defense. Her displacement took the form of an inability to recognize her own deep feelings of worthlessness, and she became a compulsive giver and cared about the needs of others in order to avoid the fact that she was being exploited in her relationships with men. Whenever she was not treated well in a relationship, she rationalized that she was needed: only she could help her boyfriend feel better about himself. She *should* care for men and was plagued with guilt if she did not give more. The *should* often indicates oedipal issues in that a harsh superego predisposes the person to be overly hard on himself or herself. This, coupled with her denial about the selfish, exploitative characteristics in the men she chose to date, corresponded to her denial on some level of her father's motives. Her high level of functioning with use of the defenses of humor and sublimation led her male therapist to conclude that she was probably a good candidate for psychoanalytically oriented psychotherapy. Twice-weekly psychotherapy was conducted over a 2-year period.

Ms. S initially related to the therapist in a guarded, hypervigilant state, which sometimes made the therapist feel uneasy and constricted. At other times, she was quite seductive and incredulous that her male therapist would not have sex with her. The following excerpt from a session illustrates the exploration of the importance of her sexual quest. She arrived characteristically late for her session and alluded to the previous session, which involved her declaring her sexual feelings for the therapist.

Ms. S:	I finally understand why you won't have sex with me, and although it's frustrating, at least I understand why you are doing this.
APPN:	What is it that you understand?
Ms. S:	It's your goddamn ethics, your code.
APPN:	My code of ethics prevents me from having sex with you?

Ms. S:	Yes.
APPN:	Anything else about me that may contribute to my not having sex with you?
Ms. S:	[after a long pause] Well maybe, just maybe you feel it would hurt me.
APPN:	So, on the one hand, I want to have sex with you, but don't because of my ethical code, and on the other hand, I may care enough about you to not want to hurt you, as you have in the past been hurt.
Ms. S:	Perhaps I'm trying here to create a situation that is familiar to me.
APPN:	Perhaps, but you also consider that I may have different, more caring motives, and that is very new for you.

This session highlights the use of the relational model of psychodynamic psychotherapy. Relational psychodynamic psychotherapy is based on the idea that problems are caused by disturbances in relationships with early caretakers that pattern subsequent relationships. The therapist's understanding emerged over time as the relationship unfolded. The therapist initially explained to Ms. S the importance of mindfulness and the observation of her own thoughts and feelings in the therapy relationship as it is taking place in the present moment. Through this exploration in the here and now with the therapist, Ms. S was able to consider that the therapist cared about her, which introduced a new hypothesis about what ingredients constitute relationships. She spent numerous sessions struggling with a shift in her thinking that someone would care about her and not want to exploit her. As she mourned the loss of the illusion of a loving father and saw her father more realistically, she was able to see men in her life more realistically, too. Over time, she developed better object choices in that she looked for indicators that the men who she dated overtly cared about her, and she was able to make a better assessment of their intentions. Her defenses were modified, and she no longer had to compulsively control and give in intimate relationships. The patient learned new, more adaptive information in implicit memory networks through the processing that took place in her relationship with the therapist.

POST-MASTER'S PSYCHODYNAMIC PSYCHOTHERAPY TRAINING AND CERTIFICATION REQUIREMENTS

Although there is no one certifying body or national certification in psychodynamic psychotherapy, there are many psychodynamic training programs in most major cities in the United States. Psychodynamic training is most often offered at an analytic institute and requires the therapist's own analysis, coursework, and supervised psychoanalytic treatment of a requisite number of patients, culminating in a written case presentation and an oral defense, much like an oral dissertation defense. There are a number of 2-year programs with a focus on psychodynamic psychotherapy and 4-year programs in traditional psychoanalysis. In the past, programs affiliated with the American Psychoanalytic Association limited training to doctors of medicine (MDs), but most of these programs now allow APPNs, social workers, and psychologists to matriculate into their programs.

The American Psychoanalytic Association (2018) sets standards for candidates eligible for admission and includes doctors of osteopathic medicine, medical doctors, and mental health professionals with a doctorate, as well as those with a clinical master's degree. The many institutes of psychodynamic psychotherapy represent the various schools of psychodynamic thought, and their respective curricula reflect their orientation. These include ego psychology, self psychology, traditional Freudian psychoanalysis, intersubjectivity approaches, interpersonal therapy, and relational therapy. APPNs who wish to pursue this type of training are advised to obtain information about the institute's orientation before matriculation, because the theoretical foundation and practice approach may differ greatly.

CONCLUDING COMMENTS

As new knowledge about implicit unconscious processes continues to be generated, the field of psychodynamic psychotherapy is forging new connections with neurobiology to validate existing clinical practices. It is this meeting of psychology with physiology that Freud envisioned more than 100 years ago. The contemporary model of relational psychodynamic psychotherapy builds on the important contributions of interpersonal psychodynamic theory and is consistent with the centrality of relationship that nursing espouses. The interpersonal psychodynamic model of psychotherapy has been the dominant paradigm for psychiatric nursing for the past three decades, since Hildegard Peplau based her framework of psychiatric nursing on the work of Harry Stack Sullivan. The contemporary psychoanalytic theory discussed here for APPN psychotherapy practice is moored in the one-to-one relationship, which builds on that model. The evolving, expanding knowledge of psychodynamic psychotherapy is based on a developmental, neurophysiological model that deepens the understanding of others and offers the APPN relevant principles important for clinical practice.

DISCUSSION QUESTIONS

1. Diagram (as in Figure 5.1) and discuss the cyclical dynamics of a patient you are currently working with or have worked with in the past.
2. Identify at least five reasons why evidence-based research is difficult to conduct in psychodynamic psychotherapy.
3. Compare and contrast the developmental models (i.e., Freud, Mahler, and Erikson) presented in this chapter.
4. Discuss the evolution of psychoanalytic thought.
5. What is the relational psychodynamic model of psychotherapy, and how can you integrate the concepts and techniques described in this chapter in your work with patients?
6. Using the diagram in Figure 5.3, present a case formulation for a specific patient, covering all the dimensions (e.g., anxiety, developmental issue, attachment schema, defenses, and developmental level), and then discuss what type of psychodynamic therapy you think would be appropriate and why.
7. Describe supportive psychodynamic psychotherapy, and discuss the various techniques for this type of therapy.
8. Discuss the dynamics of borderline personality organization, and describe general principles for how to work with patients with this character structure.
9. A patient comes to you for brief psychotherapy, and you believe that psychodynamic psychotherapy would be helpful. Discuss the beginning steps of treatment, and elaborate on how you would go about establishing a therapeutic alliance.

REFERENCES

Abbass, A., Kisely, S., & Kroenke, K. (2009). Short-term psychodynamic psychotherapy for somatic disorders: Systematic review and meta-analysis of clinical trials. *Psychotherapy and Psychosomatics, 78*, 265–274. doi:10.1159/000228247

Abbass, A., Kisely, S., Town, J., Leichsenring, F., Driessen, E., De Maat, S., . . . Crowe, E. (2014). Short-term psychodynamic psychotherapies for common mental disorders. *Cochrane Database of Systematic Reviews,* (7), CD004687. doi:10.1002/14651858.CD004687.pub4

American Psychiatric Association. (2009). *Practice guideline for the treatment of patients with panic disorder* (2nd ed.). Washington, DC: American Psychiatric Publishing. Retrieved from https://psychiatryonline.org/pb/assets/raw/sitewide/practice_guidelines/guidelines/panicdisorder.pdf

American Psychiatric Association. (2010a). *Practice guideline for treatment of patients with acute stress disorder and posttraumatic stress disorder.* Retrieved from https://psychiatryonline.org/pb/assets/raw/sitewide/practice_guidelines/guidelines/acutestressdisorderptsd.pdf

American Psychiatric Association. (2010b). *Practice guideline for treatment of patients with borderline personality disorder.* Retrieved from https://psychiatryonline.org/pb/assets/raw/sitewide/practice_guidelines/guidelines/bpd.pdf

American Psychiatric Association. (2010c). *Practice guideline for treatment of patients with major depressive disorder* (3rd ed.). Retrieved from https://psychiatryonline.org/pb/assets/raw/sitewide/practice_guidelines/guidelines/mdd.pdf

American Psychiatric Association. (2010d). *Practice guideline for treatment of patients with obsessive-compulsive disorder.* Retrieved from https://psychiatryonline.org/pb/assets/raw/sitewide/practice_guidelines/guidelines/ocd.pdf

American Psychoanalytic Association. (2018). *Standards for psychoanalytic education.* Retrieved from https://apsa.org/sites/default/files/StandardsForPsaEducation.pdf

American Psychological Association. (2019). *Clinical practice guideline for the treatment of depression across three age cohorts.* Retrieved from https://www.apa.org/depression-guideline/guideline.pdf

Amir, N., Stafford, J., Freshman, M. S., & Foa, E. B. (1998). Relationship between trauma narratives and trauma pathology. *Journal of Traumatic Stress, 11*, 385–392. doi:10.1023/A:1024415523495

Anderson, E. M., & Lambert, M. J. (1995). Short-term dynamically oriented psychotherapy: A review and meta-analysis. *Clinical Psychology Review, 15*, 503–514. doi:10.1016/0272-7358(95)00027-M

Binder, J. L. (2004). *Key competencies in brief dynamic psychotherapy.* New York, NY: Guilford Press.

Blagys, M., D., & Hilsenroth, M. J. (2000). Distinctive of short-term psychodynamic-interpersonal psychotherapy: A review of the comparative psychotherapy process literature. *Clinical Psychology: Science and Practice, 7*, 167–188. doi:10.1093/clipsy.7.2.167

Briere, J., & Scott, C. (2013). *Principles of trauma therapy: A guide to symptoms, evaluation, and treatment* (2nd ed.). Thousand Oaks, CA: Sage.

Christea, I., Gentili, C., Cotet, C., Palomba, D., Barbui, C., & Cuijpers, P. (2017). Efficacy of psychotherapies for borderline personality disorder: A systematic review and meta-analysis. *JAMA Psychiatry, 74*(4), 319–328. doi:10.1001/jamapsychiatry.2016.4287

Chu, J. A. (2011). *Rebuilding shattered lives: Treating complex PTSD and dissociative disorders* (2nd ed.). Hoboken, NJ: Wiley.

Connolly Gibbons, M., Gallop, R., Thompson, D., Luther, D., Crits-Christoph, K., Jacobs, J., . . . Crits-Christoph, P. (2016). Comparative effectiveness of cognitive therapy and dynamic psychotherapy for major depressive disorder in a community mental health setting: A randomized clinical noninferiority trial. *JAMA Psychiatry, 73*, 904–911. doi:10.1001/jamapsychiatry.2016.1720

Cozolino, L. (2017). *The neuroscience of psychotherapy: Healing the social brain* (3rd ed.). New York, NY: W. W. Norton.

Cuijpers, P., Driessen, E., Hollon, S. D., van Oppen, P., Barth, J., & Andersson, G. (2012). The efficacy of non-directive supportive therapy for adult depression: A meta-analysis. *Clinical Psychology Review*, *32*(4), 280–291. doi:10.1016/j.cpr.2012.01.003

Curtis, R. C., & Hirsch, I. (2003). Relational approaches to psychoanalytic psychotherapy. In A. S. Gurman & S. B. Messer (Eds.), *Essential psychotherapies: Theory and practice* (pp. 69–106). New York, NY: Guilford Press.

de Maat, S., de Jonghe, F., Schoevers, R., & Dekker, J. (2009). The effectiveness of long-term psychoanalytic therapy: A systematic review of empirical studies. *Harvard Review of Psychiatry*, *17*, 1–23. doi:10.1080/16073220902742476

Department of Veterans Affairs, Department of Defense. (2016). *VA/DoD clinical practice guideline for the management of major depressive disorder (MDD)*. Retrieved from https://www.healthquality.va.gov/guidelines/MH/mdd

Diener, M. J., Hilsenroth, M. J., & Weinberger, J. (2007). Therapist affect focus and patient outcomes in psychodynamic psychotherapy: A meta-analysis. *American Journal of Psychiatry*, *164*, 936–941. doi:10.1176/appi.ajp.164.6.936

Driessen, E., Hegelmaier, L., Abbass, A., Barber, J., Dekker, J., Van, H., . . . Cuijpers, P. (2015). The efficacy of short-term psychodynamic psychotherapy for depression: A meta-analysis update. *Clinical Psychology Review*, *42*, 1–15. doi:10.1016/j.cpr.2015.07.004

Driessen, E., Van, H., Don, F., Peen, J., Kool, S., Westra, D., . . . Dekker, J. (2013). The efficacy of cognitive-behavioral therapy and psychodynamic therapy in the outpatient treatment of major depression: A randomized clinical trial. *American Journal of Psychiatry*, *170*(9), 1041–1050. doi:10.1176/appi.ajp.2013.12070899

Driessen, E., Van, H., Peen, J., Don, F., Twisk, J. W. R., Cuijpers, P., & Dekker, J. (2017). Cognitive-behavioral versus psychodynamic therapy for major depression: Secondary outcomes of a randomized clinical trial. *Journal of Consulting and Clinical Psychology*, *85*(7), 653–663. doi:10.1037/ccp0000207

Erikson, E. (1964). *Insight and responsibility*. New York, NY: W. W. Norton.

Erikson, E. (1968). *Identity, youth and crisis*. New York, NY: W. W. Norton.

Eubanks, C. F., Muran, J. C., & Safran, J. D. (2019). Repairing alliance ruptures. In J. C. Norcross & M. Lambert (Eds.), *Psychotherapy relationships that work: Evidence-based responsiveness* (3rd ed., Vol. 1, pp. 549–579). New York, NY: Oxford University Press.

Fonagy, P. (2002). *An open door review of outcome studies in psychoanalysis*. London, UK: International Psychoanalytical Association.

Fonagy, P. (2015). The effectiveness of psychodynamic therapies: An update. *World Psychiatry*, *14*(2), 137–150. doi:10.1002/wps.20235

Fonagy, P., Leigh, T., Steele, M., Steele, H., Kennedy, R., Mattoon, G., . . . Gerber, A. (1996). The relationship to attachment status, psychiatric classification, and response to psychotherapy. *Journal of Consulting and Clinical Psychology*, *64*, 22–31. doi:10.1037/0022-006X.64.1.22

Fonagy, P., Rost, F., Carlyle, J., McPherson, S., Thomas, R., Fearon, R., . . . Taylor, D. (2015). Pragmatic randomized controlled trial of long-term psychoanalytic psychotherapy for treatment-resistant depression: The Tavistock adult depression study (TADS). *World Psychiatry*, *14*(3), 312–321. doi:10.1002/wps.20267

Gabbard, G. O. (2010). *Long-term psychodynamic psychotherapy: A basic text* (2nd ed.). Washington, DC: American Psychiatric Publishing.

Gabbard, G. O. (2017). *Long-term psychodynamic psychotherapy: A basic text* (3rd ed.). Arlington, VA: American Psychiatric Publishing.

Gallop, R., & O'Brien, L. (2003). Re-establishing psychodynamic theory as foundational knowledge for psychiatric mental health nursing. *Issues in Mental Health Nursing*, *24*, 213–227. doi:10.1080/01612840305302

Hollender, M. H., & Ford, C. V. (2000). *Dynamic psychotherapy: An introductory approach*. Northvale, NJ: Jason Aronson.

Howell, E. (2005). *The dissociative mind*. Hillsdale, NJ: Analytic Press.

Keefe, J. R., McCarthy, K. S., Dinger, U., Zilcha-Mano, S., & Barber, J. P. (2014). A meta-analytic review of psychodynamic therapies for anxiety disorders. *Clinical Psychology Review*, *34*(4), 309–323.

Kivlighan, M., Goldberg, S., Abbas, M., Pace, B., Yulish, N., Thomas, J., . . . Wampold, B. (2015). The enduring effects of psychodynamic treatments vis-à-vis alternative treatments: A multilevel longitudinal meta-analysis. *Clinical Psychology Review, 40*, 1–14. doi:10.1016/j .cpr.2015.05.003

Kluft, R. P. (1999). Current issues in dissociative identity disorder. *Journal of Practical Psychiatry and Behavioral Health, 5*, 3–19. doi:10.1097/00131746-199901000-00001

Kohut, H., & Wolf, E. (1978). The disorders of the self and their treatment. *International Journal of Psychoanalysis, 59*, 413–425.

Knipe, J. (2019). *EMDR toolbox: Theory and treatment of complex PTSD and dissociation.* New York, NY: Springer Publishing Company.

Levy, K., Ellison, W., Scott, L. N., & Bernecker, S. L. (2011). Attachment style. In J. Norcross (Ed.), *Psychotherapy relationships that work: Evidence-based responsiveness* (2nd ed.). New York, NY: Oxford University Press.

Levy, R. A., & Ablon, J. S. (2009). *Handbook of evidence-based psychodynamic psychotherapy: Bridging the gap between science and practice.* New York, NY: Humana Press.

Leichsenring, F., Abbass, A., Luytn, P., Hilsenroth, M., & Rabung, S. (2013). The emerging evidence for long-term psychodynamic therapy. *Psychodynamic Psychiatry, 41*(3), 361–384.

Leichsenring, F., & Leibing, E. (2001). The effectiveness of psychodynamic therapy and cognitive behavior therapy in the treatment of personality disorders: A meta-analysis. *American Journal of Psychiatry, 160*, 1223–1232. doi:10.1176/appi.ajp.160.7.1223

Leichsenring, F., Luyten, P., Hilsenroth, M., Abbass, A., Barber, J., & Keefe, J. (2015). Psychodynamic therapy meets evidence-based medicine: A systematic review using updated criteria. *The Lancet Psychiatry, 2*(7), 648–660. doi:10.1016/S2215-0366(15)00155-8

Leichsenring, F., & Rabung, S. (2008). Effectiveness of long-term psychodynamic psychotherapy: A meta-analysis. *Journal of the American Medical Association, 300*, 1551–1565. doi:10.1001/jama .300.13.1551

Leichsenring, F., & Rabung, S. (2011). Long-term psychodynamic psychotherapy in complex mental disorders: Update of a meta-analysis. *The British Journal of Psychiatry: The Journal of Mental Science, 199*(1), 15–22. doi:10.1192/bjp.bp.110.082776

Leichsenring, F., Rabung, S., & Leibing, E. (2004). The efficacy of short-term psychodynamic psychotherapy in specific psychiatric disorders: A meta-analysis. *Archives of General Psychiatry, 61*, 1208–1216. doi:10.1001/archpsyc.61.12.1208

Mahler, M., Pine, F., & Bergman, A. (1975). *The psychological birth of the human infant.* New York, NY: Basic Books.

Masterson, J. F. (1976). *Psychotherapy of the borderline adult: A developmental approach.* New York, NY: Brunner/Mazel.

McWilliams, N. (1994). *Psychoanalytic diagnosis.* New York, NY: Guilford Press.

McWilliams, N. (1999). *Psychoanalytic case formulation.* New York, NY: Guilford Press.

McWilliams, N. (2011). *Psychoanalytic diagnosis* (2nd ed.). New York, NY: Guilford Press.

Medicus, J. (2012) Practice parameter for psychodynamic psychotherapy with children. *Journal of the American Academy of Child & Adolescent Psychiatry, 51*(5), 541–57. doi:10.1016/j.jaac.2012 .02.015

Messer, S., & Abbass, A. (2010). *Evidence-based psychodynamic therapy with personality disorders.* Washington, DC: American Psychological Association.

Miller, A. (1981). *The drama of the gifted child.* New York, NY: Basic Books.

Misch, D. (2000). Basic strategies of dynamic supportive therapy. *Journal of Psychotherapy Practice & Research, 9*(4), 173–189. Retrieved from https://www.ncbi.nlm.nih.gov/pmc/articles/ PMC3330607

Mitchell, S. A. (1988). *Relational concepts in psychoanalysis: An integration.* Cambridge, MA: Harvard University Press.

National Collaborating Centre for Mental Health. (2009). *Schizophrenia: Core interventions in the treatment and management of schizophrenia in adults in primary and secondary care.* Leicester, UK: British Psychological Society. Retrieved from https://www.ncbi.nlm.nih.gov/books/ NBK11681

National Collaborating Centre for Mental Health. (2011). *Self-harm: Longer-term management.* Leicester, UK: British Psychological Society. Retrieved from https://www.ncbi.nlm.nih.gov/books/NBK126777

Oldham, J. M. (2005). *Guideline watch: Practice guidelines for the treatment of patients with border-line personality disorder.* Retrieved from https://psychiatryonline.org/pb/assets/raw/sitewide/practice_guidelines/guidelines/bpd-watch.pdf

Pinkster, H. (1997). *A primer of supportive psychotherapy.* Hillsdale, NJ: Analytic Press.

Rubino, G., Barker, C., Roth, T., & Fearon, P. (2000). Therapist empathy and depth of interpretation in response to potential alliance ruptures: The role of therapist and patient attachment styles. *Psychotherapy Research, 10,* 408–420. doi:10.1093/ptr/10.4.408

Sadock, B. J., Sadock, V. A., & Ruiz, P. (2017). *Kaplan & Sadock's comprehensive textbook of psychiatry* (10th ed.). Philadelphia, PA: Wolters Kluwer/Lippincott Williams & Wilkins.

Safran, J. D., & Muran, J. C. (2000). *Negotiating the therapeutic alliance.* New York, NY: Guilford Press.

Schore, A. (2019). *The development of the unconscious mind.* New York, NY: W. W. Norton.

Shedler, J. (2010). The efficacy of psychodynamic psychotherapy. *American Psychologist, 65*(2), 98–109. doi:10.1037/a0018378

Shedler, J. (2011). Science or ideology? *American Psychologist, 62(2),* 152–154. doi:10.1037/a0022654

Siegel, D. (2012). Pocket guide to interpersonal neurobiology: An integrative handbook of the mind. New York, NY: W. W. Norton.

Solms, M., & Turnbull, O. (2002). *Dreams and the inner world.* New York, NY: Other Press.

Steele, K., Boon, S., & van der Hart, O. (2017). *Treating trauma-related dissociation: A practical integrative approach.* New York, NY: W. W. Norton.

Steinert, C., Munder, T., Rabung, S., Hoyer, J., & Leichsenring, F. (2017). Psychodynamic therapy: As efficacious as other empirically supported treatments? A meta-analysis testing equivalence of outcomes. *The American Journal of Psychiatry, 174*(10), 943–953. doi:10.1176/appi.ajp.2017.17010057

Town J. M., Abbass, A., Driessen, E., Diener, M., Leichsenring, F., & Rabung, S. (2012). A meta-analysis of psychodynamic psychotherapy outcomes: Evaluating the effects of research-specific procedures. *Psychotherapy, 69*(3), 276–290. doi:10.1037/a0029564

Turner, E. H., Matthews, A. M., Linardatos, E., Tell, R. A., & Rosenthal, R. (2008). Selective publication of antidepressant trials and its influence on apparent efficacy. *New England Journal of Medicine, 358,* 252–260. doi:10.1056/NEJMsa065779

Wachtel, P. (2011). *Therapeutic communication: Knowing what to say when* (2nd ed.). New York, NY: Guilford Press.

Winnicott, D. W. (1976). The aims of psychoanalytic treatment. In *The maturational processes and the facilitating environment* (pp. 166–170). London: Hogwarth Press.

Wolberg, L. R. (1977). *The technique of psychotherapy* (3rd ed.). New York, NY: Grune and Stratton.

Humanistic–Existential and Solution-Focused Approaches to Psychotherapy

Candice Knight

This chapter provides an overview of humanistic–existential therapy and solution-focused therapy (SFT) for the advanced practice psychiatric nurse (APPN). It addresses the influence of the humanistic–existential approach in nursing and traces its historical evolution. Four major humanistic–existential approaches are described, explicating their key concepts, goals, and therapeutic interventions: person-centered therapy, existential therapy, Gestalt therapy, and emotion-focused therapy (EFT). Motivational interviewing, an important humanistic–existential approach, is covered in Chapter 9, and is not addressed in this chapter. SFT, a postmodern, social constructivist psychotherapy with humanistic–existential elements, is also included. Attention is focused on the practical aspects of conducting psychotherapy and delivering therapeutic interventions that a beginning level APPN would be able to use. Evidence-based research in humanistic–existential therapy and SFT is presented. Case examples are provided to illustrate therapeutic interventions. The chapter concludes with a description of post-master's training and certification programs for humanistic–existential therapy and SFT.

NURSING AND THE HUMANISTIC–EXISTENTIAL APPROACH

The humanistic–existential approach has long served as a foundation for psychiatric nursing with its emphasis on holism, self-actualization, facilitative communication, and the therapeutic relationship. In undergraduate programs, psychiatric nursing students are commonly taught Abraham Maslow's theory of human needs and Carl Rogers's facilitative communication techniques.

Important humanistic–existential nursing theorists include Joyce Travelbee, Josephine Paterson, Loretta Zderad, and Jean Watson. Their work is commonly found in nursing theory courses. Travelbee's Human-to-Human Relationship Model of Nursing is an application of the existential work of Søren Kierkegaard and Victor Frankl and emphasizes free will and the search for meaning in experiences of pain, illness, and distress (Travelbee, 1971). Paterson and Zderad's humanistic nursing approach views nursing as a lived dialogue between patient and nurse and places the phenomenological method of inquiry at the center of importance (Paterson & Zderad, 1988). Watson's Theory of Human Caring emphasizes a caring relationship with patients that includes

Carl Rogers's unconditional acceptance and positive regard as well as creating caring moments of healing (Watson, 2011).

In advanced practice psychiatric nursing as well as in all mental health disciplines, the humanistic–existential concepts of empathic attunement and the therapeutic relationship are emphasized in psychotherapy courses. The major theoretical orientations of person-centered psychotherapy, Gestalt psychotherapy, and existential psychotherapy have stood the test of time and are commonly taught as the three foundational psychotherapies of the humanistic–existential approach. Other important humanistic–existential therapies include transactional analysis, focusing, actualizing therapy, and redecision therapy. More recently, EFT and motivational interviewing have received much attention. These two empirically validated therapies have placed the humanistic–existential school in a position of importance.

HISTORICAL ROOTS

The historical roots of humanistic–existential psychotherapy extend back in time to the birth of the philosophies of humanism, existentialism, and phenomenology. Humanism, a reform movement of the 14th-century European renaissance, developed in response to medieval religious ideologies and focused on human values rather than the divine. Humanism's dominant themes were happiness, spontaneity, creativity, actualization, holism, and the goodness of the human spirit (Kendler, 1986).

Existentialism emerged as a reaction to the dominant philosophy of rationalism and the objectivity of science during the mid-19th century. Beginning with the writings of Kierkegaard (1813–1855), existentialism focused on personal choice and commitment. Later existential leaders such as Friedrich Nietzsche (1844–1900) introduced existential themes of responsibility and courage. Jean-Paul Sartre (1905–1980) later recognized the importance of human freedom, emotions, and imagination (Kendler, 1986).

During the early 20th century, Edmund Husserl's (1859–1938) phenomenological philosophy broke with the dominant science of positivism and focused on a person's lived experience as the source of knowledge and truth (Husserl, 1925). Phenomenology is dedicated to the descriptive study of consciousness and subjective experience, completely free of preconceptions, interpretation, explanation, and evaluation. Martin Heidegger (1889–1976), another phenomenological philosopher, later applied phenomenological methods to understanding the meaning of experience (Heidegger, 1962).

In the United States, the philosophies of humanism, existentialism, and phenomenology merged into the humanistic–existential movement soon after World War II. Although articles began to emerge in the late 1950s, scholars consider the birth of humanistic–existential philosophy to be in 1964, when a group of psychologists, including Carl Rogers, Abraham Maslow, Rollo May, Clark Moustakas, Gordon Allport, and others, met in Old Saybrook, Connecticut, and unmistakably defined and described humanistic–existential psychology. After that historic meeting, the movement gained widespread popularity.

Psychoanalysis and behaviorism, respectively known as the "first force" and "second force" of psychotherapy, were joined by humanistic–existential psychotherapy, which became known as the "third force," a term coined by Abraham Maslow in his text, *Toward a Psychology of Being* (Maslow, 1962). Humanistic–existential psychology's ideas and values became incorporated into and nourished the great social upheavals of the 1960s and 1970s including the feminist, civil rights, antiwar, and human potential movements. Humanistic–existential psychotherapy also spawned a plethora of pop psychology texts that are widespread today. Five decades of substantial advances in theory, practice, and research have accumulated, supporting the effectiveness of humanistic–existential psychotherapy (Cain & Seeman, 2002; Elliott, 2002; Kirschenbaum & Jourdan, 2005).

HUMANISTIC–EXISTENTIAL PSYCHOTHERAPY

The humanistic–existential psychotherapy approach includes a diverse group of psychotherapies. Each shares philosophical assumptions that rest on the philosophies of humanism, existentialism, and phenomenology.

Characteristics of Humanistic–Existential Psychotherapy

Seven distinctive characteristics of humanistic–existential psychotherapy distinguish it from the characteristics of other approaches. A list of these characteristics can be found in Box 6.1 and are described in more detail here.

COMMITMENT TO THE PHENOMENOLOGICAL PERSPECTIVE

A phenomenological perspective strives to understand the subjective experience of the patient in the context of his or her unique experience. The therapist brackets (sets aside) all presuppositions and preconceptions that interfere with the ability to attend to the immediate experience and enters into the patient's frame of reference without prejudgment about what content is real or false or which is significant or trivial. The patient, rather than the therapist, generates explanations and interpretations (Rogers, 1980). Commitment to the phenomenological approach is grounded in the belief that patients are uniquely capable of reflective consciousness and this capacity leads to self-determination and self-actualization (Greenberg & Rice, 1997). In most psychotherapeutic approaches, the therapist conceptualizes the patient's narrative using preconceptions removed from the direct, unfiltered experience of the patient. In a phenomenological perspective, the patient's lived experience is paramount. For example, a victim of a traumatic assault may experience fear years after the event, even when no apparent threat exists. What does this fear mean? Where does it come from? How is it experienced from the patient's perspective? The answers bring the therapist closer to the phenomenon that is lived by the patient.

CENTRALITY OF THE THERAPEUTIC RELATIONSHIP

The therapist–patient relationship is the primary source for constructive change in the humanistic–existential approach. The relationship, described by Martin Buber as a genuine "I–Thou" encounter, stresses a collaborative, authentic, dialogic encounter (Buber, 1937). The therapist focuses on empathic understanding of the patient and trusts that the patient has the capacity to make choices and strive toward meaningful life goals. The humanistic–existential literature has been foremost in publishing research on the centrality of the therapeutic relationship. In fact, Carl Rogers (1957) was the first to empirically discover that the therapist's characteristics of empathy, genuineness, and unconditional positive regard, along with the patient's ability to perceive these characteristics, are the

---

BOX 6.1 Characteristics of Humanistic–Existential Psychotherapy

- Commitment to the phenomenological perspective
- Centrality of the therapeutic relationship
- Belief in holism
- Focus on the here and now
- Emphasis on humanistic–existential themes
- Prominence of process
- Use of experiential techniques

necessary elements for therapeutic change. Contemporary research has consistently shown that the therapeutic relationship is the common factor responsible for positive therapy outcomes and that therapists who are empathic, caring, and congruent are more effective (Duncan, Miller, Wampold, & Hubble, 2010; Wampold, 2001).

BELIEF IN HOLISM

The etymological roots of the word *holism* stem from the Greek word *holos,* meaning the total or entirety. Holism was brought to the attention of psychology by the South African statesman and philosopher, Jan Smuts, who described the holistic nature of the personality in his text *Holism and Evolution* (1926). Smuts had a profound influence on Frederick Perls, the founder of Gestalt therapy, who integrated the concept of holism into Gestalt therapy (Perls, 1942). It soon became a major tenet in the humanistic–existential approach to psychotherapy. Holism recognizes that people are unique, whole individuals who cannot be reduced to separated parts, encapsulated in the expression, "the whole is greater than the sum of its parts." It posits that each person is a unified whole of mind, body, and spirit and that these aspects work together in a synergistic fashion, mutually and reciprocally influencing and modifying each other (Smuts, 1926). Holism understands dysfunction from an integrated perspective seeking to comprehend the entirety of the person and rejects a reductionist point of view, which understands dysfunction by identifying a specific part such as a thought or a chemical imbalance.

FOCUS ON THE HERE AND NOW

Humanistic–existential therapy believes that authentic contact and change can happen only in the present; thus, the here and now is the focus of therapy. The here and now, a frequently misunderstood concept, is not merely talking about what is currently happening in the patient's life, nor is it an exclusion of the past or the future. Instead, the past, present, and future are *experienced* in the here and now through various interventions introduced by the therapist. For example, if the patient begins to tell a story about something that happened in the past, the therapist might say, "Tell me the story as if it were happening now, in the present tense," so that the past comes alive in the moment. The patient who begins to tell a difficult situation that happened during the week may be asked, "What are you experiencing right now as you impart this information?" The humanistic–existential approach is also interested in what is emerging in the moment within the therapeutic relationship. For example, a person who believes that the world is bereft of support may at times feel unsupported within the therapeutic relationship. Addressing the issues that emerge during the session poignantly brings the here and now into focus.

EMPHASIS ON HUMANISTIC–EXISTENTIAL THEMES

Humanistic–existential themes are concerned with the universal human experiences of life (the givens of existence). Most prominent themes include awareness, authenticity, freedom, choice, responsibility, meaning, and self-actualization. Awareness allows one the freedom to choose and organize life in a meaningful way. Authenticity, rather than self-deception, allows a person to be fully responsible and live life with aliveness rather than with feelings of dread, guilt, and anxiety. The humanistic–existential approach believes that a person is faced at every moment with choice and is responsible for the choices that are made. There is also a belief in the self-actualizing tendency and the notion that if a person is provided with the appropriate conditions, he or she will automatically grow in positive ways and find meaning in existence (Cain & Seeman, 2002).

The approach holds that a person is endlessly remaking or discovering himself or herself and there is no essence of human nature to be discovered once and for all. The humanistic–existential approach is concerned with the significant experiences of being human.

PROMINENCE OF PROCESS

Humanistic–existential therapies focus more on the process rather than the content of therapy. The process of therapy describes the flow of action and reaction within the session. It includes pacing (the rate of movement in the session progression), timing (judgment at what point of time to initiate a response or intervention), and tracking (close observation and following of the process). The content of therapy, in contrast, refers to what is being discussed in therapy. The content is easier to observe than the process for it refers to the specific facts such as the patient's description of problems and perspectives about their causality. Humanistic–existential therapy does not ignore the content, for knowledge of content is necessary for empathy and connection. The emphasis, however, is on the process, for the process is what provides the essential information as to how the patient is experiencing and provides an avenue for real change to occur. For example, while listening to the content of the patient's narrative, the humanistic–existential therapist pays attention and notices the how of experiencing. The therapist may ask, "What just happened inside when you told me about this difficult situation?" An example of process versus content is as follows:

Patient: "I discovered that my son is using heroin again and I don't know what to do."

APPN: "I notice tears in your eyes when you said that." (process response)

APPN: "When did you discover he was using again?" (content response)

USE OF EXPERIENTIAL TECHNIQUES

Humanistic–existential therapists do not interpret or give advice, but use experiential techniques that are reflective and experimental in style. They work actively with patients, using interventions to heighten awareness, promote the expression of emotionally laden material, support contact, and guide attentional focus to stimulate novel experience (Greenberg & Goldman, 1988). Experiential techniques are carefully tailored to a patient's specific wants and needs at a given moment, and serve the purpose of enhancing a patient's experience in the here and now. Experiential techniques give the patient a chance to try out, in the safety of the therapeutic situation, variations of current behavior. The possibilities of experiential techniques are unlimited and may include attention to the body such as the breath and the voice, exaggeration to emphasize awareness, and reenactments of problematic scenes of the past in the here and now to create healing moments. They may include the use of creative arts, including drawing, music, and movement. They may include working with dreams or the empty chair (Greenberg, 1979). Experiential techniques vary and depend on the developmental readiness of the patient, the characteristics of the patient, the stage of the therapeutic relationship, and the style and creativity of the therapist in the moment.

Beliefs About Patients in the Humanistic–Existential Approach

The humanistic–existential approach has specific beliefs about patients. A list of these beliefs can be found in Box 6.2 (Cain & Seeman, 2002).

BOX 6.2 Humanistic–Existential Beliefs About Patients

Patients are:
- Endowed with an inherent tendency to develop their potential
- Resourceful and have the capacity to draw on inner and outer resources
- Free to choose how to live and are responsible for the choices made
- Resilient in manifesting their natural inclination to survive and grow
- Holistic and not reducible to the sum of their parts
- Contextual and best understood in relationship to others and their environment
- Meaning making and find meaning by creating and constructing realities from experience
- Social beings and have a powerful need to feel valued and belong
- Diverse in worldviews and viable lifestyles that result in satisfying lives

Humanistic–existential therapists attempt to receive patients with curiosity and openness, endeavoring to grasp their subjective world, and believing that patients are the experts on their own experience. They use the phenomenological approach of suspending preconceptions and bracketing anything that may interfere with their ability to attend to immediate experience. They view patients as unique beings who are understood only in the context of their experiences. They appreciate multiple perspectives on reality and believe that the same experience can be interpreted in diverse ways. Humanistic–existential therapists have an implicit optimism in patient's capacity for growth and change, while not denying the existence of dark, destructive aspects of self and the extremes of emotional pain. They have a commitment to democratic principles in negotiating differences and are inclined to engage in relationships that are collaborative, are authentic, and provide optimal freedom (Cain & Seeman, 2002).

PERSON-CENTERED THERAPY

Overview

Person-centered psychotherapy, also known as patient-centered psychotherapy, was founded by Carl Rogers (1902–1987), the most influential psychotherapist of the 20th century (Cook, Biyanova, & Coyne, 2009). He developed a nondirective, patient-centered approach to psychotherapy that recognized the importance of facilitative counseling techniques such as reflection, exploring, and clarification (Rogers, 1942) as well as the three facilitative conditions necessary for positive therapeutic outcomes: unconditional positive regard, empathic understanding, and congruence (Rogers, 1961). Rogers popularized the term *patient* rather than *patient,* emphasizing the egalitarian relationship between the therapist and the patient. Initially, he named his approach patient-centered psychotherapy as a way to highlight the prominence of the patient's knowledge in determining the focus and direction of therapy. He rigorously trained students as well as conducted extensive research by recording, transcribing, and studying transcripts of audio-recorded therapy sessions in an attempt to understand therapy processes (Kirschenbaum & Jourdan, 2005). His book *Counseling and Psychotherapy: Newer Concepts in Practice* (Rogers, 1942) contained the first complete transcript of an actual therapy session, the case of Herbert Bryan, which was the first phonographically recorded verbatim transcript of an entire course of psychotherapy ever published. Rogers's approach to psychotherapy training was later used by graduate psychiatric nursing programs in the form of audio and written process recordings.

Later in his career, Rogers became increasingly interested in working with groups and systems including education, industry, and politics and renamed his approach person-centered psychotherapy, reflecting its application to diverse populations. His last years were devoted to international relations, applying his theories to situations of political conflict in his pursuit of world peace, and he was nominated for a Nobel Peace Prize. The influence of Rogers's work has continued today, with over 200 training institutes worldwide (Kirschenbaum & Jourdan, 2005). Natalie Rogers (1993) has integrated person-centered therapy with the creative arts and developed expressive arts psychotherapy. Virginia Axline (1947/1992) has applied the person-centered approach to children and play therapy. Eugene Gendlin (1981) developed experiential techniques such as focusing as a way to enhance patient experiencing. Person-centered therapy also serves as an integral component of motivational interviewing (Miller & Rollnick, 2002) and EFT (Greenberg, 2011), two contemporary, humanistic–existential psychotherapy approaches.

The central belief of person-centered therapy is that people are basically good and have a vast potential for self-growth if their potential is tapped within a special type of therapeutic relationship that provides the necessary, facilitative conditions of empathic understanding, unconditional positive regard, and congruence (Rogers, 1957, 1961). Over the last decade, research has repeatedly demonstrated that successful psychotherapy depends on these common factors (Duncan et al., 2010; Wampold, 2001).

Key Concepts

BELIEF OF HUMAN NATURE

A central belief in the person-centered approach is that there is a positive center at the core of all individuals. People are thought to be trustworthy, creative, and resourceful. They are capable of self-understanding and self-direction and able to live effective and productive lives. People become destructive only when a poor self-concept or external constraints override the core sense of goodness (Rogers, 1961).

SELF-CONCEPT

An organized, consistent set of perceptions about the self, continually influenced by experience and its interpretation, self-concept includes self-worth (what a person thinks about self), self-image (how a person sees self), and ideal self (how a person would like to be). People are in a state of congruence with a higher sense of self-worth when their self-image and ideal self are similar to each other, a necessary state for self-actualization (Rogers, 1951).

ACTUALIZING TENDENCY

The actualizing tendency is the innate drive, basic motivational force, and directional process in humans to grow, develop, and strive toward self-realization and fulfillment (Rogers, 1951). Rogers stated, "The organism has one basic tendency and striving—to actualize, maintain, and enhance the experiencing organism" (Rogers, 1951, p. 487). A belief in the actualizing tendency places trust in the patient's capacity to know what needs to be worked on and what choices to make.

FULLY FUNCTIONING PERSON

An individual who is fully engaged in the process of self-actualization is a fully functioning person. A fully functioning person demonstrates the following: (a) knowledge of subjective experience, (b) existential living emphasizing choice, freedom, and responsibility, (c) awareness of emotions, (d) ability to take risks and seek new experiences, and (e) engagement in a continual process of change (Rogers, 1961).

Goals of Therapy

The goal of person-centered therapy is for the patient to become a fully functioning person engaged in the process of self-actualization. When achieving this level of development, the patient is able to live life more authentically and cope well with current and future problems. The therapist provides a climate conducive to helping the person achieve these goals (Rogers, 1961).

Psychotherapeutic Interventions: Assessment

The therapist begins the assessment by asking the patient where to begin and what issues to work on. The patient's phenomenological experience, rather than the presenting problem, is the focus. The therapist is genuine, empathic, and caring and sets aside preconceptions in an attempt to understand the inner world of the patient. The therapist creates an understanding atmosphere that encourages clarification and reflection of present feelings. For example, to the patient's comment, "I'm depressed most of the time," the therapist might respond with, "You constantly feel unhappy?" The patient is then able to pursue his or her own line of thought, resulting in a fuller exposure of the patient's subjective experience.

Traditional assessment procedures such as taking a psychiatric history or using psychometric tests are not used because these approaches encourage an external focus and give the patient the message that the therapist is the expert who provides the solutions. The patient is not considered a sick patient in need of treatment, but a person who is prevented from realizing his or her potential. Diagnosing is not highly regarded in this approach. Rogers believed that diagnostic constructs are inadequate, prejudicial, and often misconstrued (Rogers, 1942). If providing a diagnosis is necessary, a collaborative approach is used in which the patient and therapist together formulate the diagnosis (Bohart & Watson, 2011).

Psychotherapeutic Interventions: Psychotherapy Techniques

In the person-centered approach, each session is considered fresh and unpredictable. Structured techniques and process interventions beyond facilitative listening are avoided. The therapist honors the wisdom of the patient and the ability of the patient to determine the direction of therapy. This encourages greater self-exploration and improves self-understanding (Rogers, 1961).

NONDIRECTIVE–FACILITATIVE COUNSELING

The person-centered approach emphasizes a nondirective–facilitative counseling approach with the aim of helping patients become aware of their inner experiences and processes. This approach is quite different from the directive and interpretive approaches that were practiced during the time when the person-centered approach was developed. In Rogers's early text, *Counseling and Psychotherapy: Newer Concepts in Practice* (1942), the practice of nondirective counseling and facilitative counseling techniques were explicated. The therapist attempts to understand the inner world of the patient and the patient's lived experiences through a discovery-oriented approach. While techniques such as giving advice, persuasion, and interpretation are discouraged, techniques such as reflecting, clarifying, and exploring are encouraged: "So, when you initiate cuddling, he pushes for more intimacy, and that frustrates you." "Is this what you are experiencing?" "Say more about that." Other techniques include presence and immediacy, which are being completely attentive to and immersed in the patient's expressed concerns and addressing what is specifically going on between the patient and therapist, respectively (Cain, 2010).

It is important to note that the person-centered approach is not just a repertoire of techniques or merely reflecting the last part of the patient's statement, which some critics of the approach often state. The attitude of the therapist and the therapeutic relationship are the heart of person-centered psychotherapy rather than the technique. The relationship provides a supportive structure within which patients' self-healing capacities are activated and where change occurs. A psychotherapist who is too directive or too busy guiding the patient toward goals will find it difficult to establish the essence of a therapeutic relationship (Rogers, 1961).

PSYCHOLOGICAL CONDITIONS NECESSARY FOR PERSONALITY GROWTH

In the person-centered approach, the therapist embodies and implements the three core conditions, which are both necessary and sufficient for successful therapy. Rogers believed that the therapist needs to be evolved as a person in order to provide these conditions (Rogers, 1961). They are fully explicated in Rogers's seminal text, *On Becoming a Person* (Rogers, 1961) and include:

- **Congruence.** The therapist who is genuine and authentic during the therapy session embodies the core condition of congruence and serves as a model to the patient. Congruence involves having inner and outer experiences that match. The therapist openly expresses feelings, thoughts, and reactions with the patient, which may include the expression of a range of feelings including annoyance, but in a well-timed, constructive fashion that is attuned to the emerging needs of the patient. As the patient experiences the genuineness of the therapist, pretenses drop and authenticity prevails.
- **Unconditional positive regard.** The therapist has a deep caring for the patient best achieved through empathic identification. The therapist is nonjudgmental of the patient and warmly accepts him or her without placing stipulations on the acceptance. The greater the degree of caring and accepting, the greater the chance the therapy will be successful (Rogers, 1957). It is uncommon to feel acceptance and unconditional caring at all times, but if there is little caring or an active dislike for the patient, therapy is not likely to be fruitful. If the therapist's caring stems from his or her own need to be liked and appreciated, change is also inhibited. The greater the degree of caring, prizing, accepting, and valuing of the patient, the greater chance the patient will begin to see worth and value in himself or herself.
- **Accurate empathic understanding.** Accurate empathic understanding is the cornerstone of the person-centered approach. Empathy is a very deep understanding of the patient and requires attunement to the patient's experience as it is revealed moment to moment during the session. To sense the subjective experience in this way encourages the patient to feel more deeply and to recognize and resolve the incongruity that exists within himself or herself. It goes beyond recognition of the obvious feelings to a sense of the less clearly experienced feelings. The therapist attempts to understand the meanings expressed by the patient that often lie at the edge of awareness. Showing empathy requires understanding the patient's feelings and reflecting them back to the patient to help him or her understand these feelings (Elliott, Bohart, Watson, & Greenberg, 2011). The therapist can share the subjective world of the patient by drawing from his or her similar experiences, which helps the patient process his or her own experience. Sixty years of research has consistently demonstrated that empathy is the most powerful determinant of patient progress in therapy (Cain, 2010).

GESTALT PSYCHOTHERAPY

Overview

Gestalt therapy, founded by Fritz Perls (1893–1970) and Laura Perls (1905–1990), is a theoretically and clinically complex approach to psychotherapy. Gestalt, a German word meaning organized whole, recognizes the unity of humans as integrated wholes, not divided into parts, taken out of context, or generalized. Fritz Perls, a German physician, was influenced by Jan Smuts's views of holism, Kurt Goldstein's ideas of organismic self-regulation, Kurt Lewin's field theory, Martin Buber and Paul Tillich's views on relationships and existentialism, and his own analysts: Wilhelm Reich, a body-oriented psychoanalyst who stimulated his interest in how unexpressed energy is held within the body, and Karen Horney, an interpersonal psychoanalyst, who inspired his interest in neurotic structures and layers of the personality. His training in theater and Zen Buddhist practices were also an important influence for therapeutic interventions. Laura Perls, a German psychologist, studied Gestalt psychology with Kurt Goldstein and Max Wertheimer, phenomenological and existential philosophy with Paul Tillich and Martin Buber, and field theory with Kurt Lewin. As a psychoanalyst she trained with Otto Fenichel, an analyst interested in sociological explanations, and had her personal analysis with Frieda Fromm-Reichmann and Karl Landauer. Laura Perls's early training as a classical pianist and modern dancer influenced her therapeutic interventions as well.

Soon after Nazism descended on Germany, the Perls left Germany and settled in South Africa, where they became directors of the South African Psychoanalytic Institute and collaborated on the book, *Ego, Hunger and Aggression: A Revision of Freud's Theory and Method* (Perls, 1942). This book broke with the traditional psychoanalytic approach to include concepts of holism, existentialism, and phenomenology. After immigrating to the United States, they broke away from the psychoanalytic community and officially launched Gestalt therapy in 1951, with the publication of *Gestalt Therapy: Excitement and Growth in the Human Personality* (Perls, Hefferline, & Goodman, 1951). Within a short time, the New York Institute for Gestalt Therapy was formed and workshops and study groups began throughout the country. Fritz Perls eventually settled at the Esalen Institute in California, where he trained numerous clinicians in his well-known Gestalt therapy workshops. Gestalt therapy has continued to develop and thrive, further expanding its concepts and methodologies (Wheeler, 1991; Yontef, 1993; Zinker, 1977), and establishing training institutes worldwide (Knight, 1996).

Gestalt therapy can be described as a humanistic–existential psychotherapy with theoretical roots firmly grounded in holism, phenomenology, existentialism, humanism, Gestalt psychology, organismic theory, interpersonal psychoanalysis, and Eastern philosophy. It integrated aspects of these theories to create a unified, unique approach to psychotherapy.

Key Concepts

FIGURE AND GROUND

Figure and ground are concepts in Gestalt therapy that refer to the theoretical explanation for how the self develops and organizes experiences as it interacts within the environmental field. The field is differentiated into figure (foreground) and ground (background). People organize aspects of the field into meaningful patterns in which one element stands out as the figure of interest, while the others recede into the ground. The figure is the dominant need at a given moment. As soon as the need is met or interest is lost, it recedes into the ground and a new figure emerges. All behavior is organized around emerging needs and their satisfaction. With healthy individuals, there is a natural flow of Gestalt formation and completion (Perls, 1973). In contrast, people with more dysfunctional patterns have incomplete Gestalts that clamor for attention. These incomplete Gestalts usurp the full attending powers for meeting new situations and dampen aliveness (Perls, 1969).

ORGANISMIC SELF-REGULATION

Organismic self-regulation is a natural process whereby the organism is continually disturbed by the emergence of a need and strives to restore equilibrium by constantly reorganizing and adapting to changing circumstances. It is a growth process by which a person moves toward wholeness and integration and has been operationalized into a cycle of experience: (a) awareness of sensation, (b) figure and ground formation, (c) mobilization, (d) action, (e) contact, and (f) withdrawal. This cycle provides a way to understand health and dysfunction as well as guide therapeutic process interventions.

Awareness of sensation (e.g., feelings, drives, or perceptions) commences the cycle as an experience from within or in response to an environmental stimulation. Figure formation organizes sensation into a meaningful want or need in relationship to the environment. Mobilization is the surge of energy that impels the figure formation into action. Action is the movement that brings the person into contact with self or an environmental object. Contact is the meeting of self and other at the boundary to either assimilate or reject the object. Withdrawal is the fading of the figure into the background, disengagement, and the closure of the Gestalt. When people are functioning well, they move through the cycle of experience in a rhythmic, sequential fashion with awareness, excitement, and aliveness. When functioning poorly, they are unaware and interrupt the organismic process, reducing vitality and creating dysfunction (Perls, 1973).

LAYERS OF THE PERSONALITY

When natural self-regulatory processes are disrupted, interruptions to awareness occur with frequency, parts of the self are disowned, and incomplete Gestalts become abundant. Each incomplete Gestalt represents an unfinished situation, which interferes with the formation of any novel Gestalt. Instead of growth, a person lives life within inauthentic layers of the personality (cliché, role, impasse, and implosion) rather than by organismic self-regulation. Cliché is the ordinary social chitchat and the most superficial, top layer of the personality; role is the part played in an interpersonal context such as the "good person" or the "invulnerable person"; impasse is a layer of confusion and stuckness, representing the conflict of moving to a deeper layer versus returning to role or cliché; implosion is the death or paralyzed layer where a part of self has been cut off or interrupted. Explosion is the last, authentic layer where contact with the genuine self occurs and feelings of joy, grief, anger, or orgasm explode into awareness. During therapy, specific interventions by the therapist help the patient move through the layers to contact the authentic self (Perls, 1973).

INTERRUPTIONS

Interruptions to awareness and contact, also known as boundary disturbances, refer to dysfunctional processes, developed early in life, that people employ in an attempt to meet their needs. Gestalt therapists bring awareness to these interruptions and create experiments to reduce them and restore organismic self-regulation. Some examples follow:

- **Introjection.** To uncritically accept others' beliefs and standards without discriminating and assimilating what belongs to self and eliminating what does not. Examples are, "be a good girl," "don't be angry," and "boys don't cry."

- **Projection.** To disown certain unacceptable aspects of self by ascribing them to other people or the environment. Examples are blaming others for problems within the self or believing others do not like you when you actually have strong negative feelings toward them.
- **Retroflection.** Turning back onto self what is meant for someone else. Instead of engaging with the environment and directing energy outward, energy is redirected inward. Examples of retroflection include biting one's lip, self-harm behaviors, and symptoms of depression and psychophysiological disorders.
- **Confluence.** Blurring the differentiation between self and the environment where there is no clear demarcation between internal experience and outer reality. Confluence allows a person to blend in and get along with everyone. Examples include extreme agreeability or the belief that people experience similar thoughts and feelings to self.
- **Deflection.** Distractions that diminish the intensity and sustained sense of awareness and contact. Examples include avoiding direct eye contact, overuse of humor, generalizations, asking questions rather than making statements, and being overly polite (Polster & Polster, 1973).

Goals of Therapy

The goal of Gestalt therapy is to assist the patient in restoring his or her natural state of organismic self-regulation. Disowned parts of self are reintegrated, inauthentic layers of existence are worked through, and unfinished Gestalts are completed (Perls, 1973). New Gestalts can then emerge and complete with fluidity. The patient returns to a natural state of excitement, aliveness, and growth and is able to live a more vital, integrated, authentic, and meaningful life.

Psychotherapeutic Interventions: Assessment

Assessment in Gestalt therapy is a discovery process that allows for understanding the patient's experience and recognizing factors that hinder organismic self-regulation. Assessment occurs during the initial session and is ongoing throughout the course of therapy. It is both individualized and collaborative and addresses process and content factors. Process factors are figural and include such things as how the patient relates to the therapist, the manner in which the narrative is related, the level of awareness and contact, interruptions to awareness, and nonverbal behavior such as body language, voice tone, mannerisms, posture, and energy level. Content factors are background and include information such as the precipitating problem, symptoms, stressors, developmental and family history, and mental status.

A goal of assessment is for the therapist to develop an empathic understanding of the patient's experience and unfolding story. To a major extent, this occurs by the use of facilitative communication and empathic responses. The therapist approaches assessment with a respect for the patient's figure and ground movement, allowing the patient to bring to the foreground what is deemed important. The therapist has a notion of areas of the patient's life that are important to explore, yet these notions are bracketed to allow for the natural unfolding of the session; thus, assessment is not viewed as a linear questioning procedure.

Collaboratively, the patient and therapist come to a shared understanding of what is poignant, salient, and relevant for exploration. An agreed-on case formulation and goals are determined, which are tentative and always take second place to the patient's flow of experiencing (Watson, Goldman, & Greenberg, 2007). Process diagnoses such as retroflected anger or deflected sadness during a session take precedence and serve as a guide for interventions.

Psychotherapeutic Interventions: Psychotherapy Techniques

Change occurs in the here and now; thus, Gestalt therapists are interested in what is emerging in the moment and in making the past, present, and future come alive in the here and now. They pay close attention to the patient's organismic self-regulation and interruptions to awareness and contact. Gestalt therapists closely track the patient's process and content with moment-to-moment awareness in order to understand what is immediate and to guide and tailor appropriate interventions. Two critical therapeutic skills for the Gestalt therapist are the ability to establish an authentic I–Thou relationship and to craft creative experiments (Perls, 1973).

I–THOU RELATIONSHIP

An authentic, nonjudgmental, dialogic relationship is carefully nurtured between the patient and the therapist. This relationship, first discussed by the existential philosopher Martin Buber (1937), is a major component of Gestalt therapy and is necessary for change to occur. It is an encounter between the patient and therapist in which both persons are subjects, rather than one being subject and the other object. The patient is not "talking to" an aloof expert, but rather "communicating with" a therapist who is aware, authentic, vulnerable, and fully human. The therapist strives to understand the patient's phenomenological field by experiencing his or her own reactions to the patient and the therapeutic process, while also attending to the patient's thoughts, feelings, and behavior.

A Gestalt I–Thou relationship involves suspending preconceptions and bracketing anything that may interfere with an ability to attend to immediate experience. It also requires an attitude of openness and humility and to approach the patient with genuine interest, curiosity, and profound respect. In this relationship the therapist creates a safe environment where the patient feels understood rather than concerned with being judged or criticized (Yontef, 1993).

CREATIVE EXPERIMENTATION

Designing and implementing creative experiments is the cornerstone of Gestalt therapy interventions. Experiments heighten awareness, promote the expression of emotionally laden material, support contact, and guide attentional focus to stimulate novel experience. Creating experiments requires the therapist to be very aware and attend to the nonverbal as well as the verbal content of the patient's narratives in order to understand and focus on what is alive and immediate for the patient. The specific experiment is not merely a technique imitated from an experienced Gestalt trainer or a technique to apply at whim, but a spontaneous, one-of-a-kind, tailored experiment, emerging from the dialogic interaction (Zinker, 1977). Experiments are creative and unlimited. Gestalt therapists bring their unique life experiences and skills to the creation of the experiment; thus, each Gestalt therapist's work is different. For example, one Gestalt therapist may pay close attention to the body such as the rate and depth of breath or the volume, timbre, or tone of the voice, while another may pay close attention to the syntax, fluidity, and meaning of language. Another Gestalt therapist may use metaphor and imagery to deal with a problematic situation, while another may use movement or the creative arts to deal with the same situation. Some well-known Gestalt experiments follow:

- **Body awareness.** Patients frequently have blocked body energies manifested by shallow breathing, speaking in a restricted voice, shaking legs, or fidgeting fingers. Gestalt therapists pay close attention to the patient's body and create experiments to heighten body awareness. A therapist may ask, "What are you experiencing right now in your body?" or "Go inside and see what is emerging in your body now." An example of this in-session process is as follows:

Patient:	Last night, I was so angry at my partner. After I finished telling him something important that happened to me during the day, I saw he was not paying attention to a word I said.
APPN:	As you tell me this story, what are you experiencing?
Patient:	I am feeling angry and want to yell at him, but I can't.
APPN:	Where are you experiencing the anger in your body?
Patient:	In my throat, my voice.
APPN:	Can you support that part of your body and tell him how angry you are?

There are varied experiments that a Gestalt therapist may use to heighten body awareness to blocked energy. A patient may be asked to exaggerate a body movement where energy is blocked. For example, a patient who is moving the foot back and forth might be asked to do it more and exaggerate the movement. Or a patient may be asked to allow an image to emerge from a blocked body sensation. For example, a patient experiencing confusion was asked to create an image and came up with a slide carousel going round and round. When asked to stay with the image, the patient realized that the carousel could not stop because then a slide would pop up on the screen and she might not be able to deal with what she might see. This image was symbolic of the patient's fear of going deeper into her experience of traumatic memories that were beginning to move closer to the surface of her awareness (Knight, 1996).

- **Focusing.** Focusing is used to make contact with disowned or alienated aspects of self (Gendlin, 1981). For example, in the following dialogue, the APPN notices that a person who is speaking calmly about a recent loss starts blinking:

APPN:	I noticed when you told me the story of your recent loss, your eyes began blinking. Can you give a voice to your blinking eyes?
Patient:	I am my blinking eyes—I am sad—blinking keeps my tears from flowing.
APPN:	Just breathe deeply into your blinking eyes.
Patient:	After a few moments, the patient's tears begin to flow. …

There are numerous experiments that a Gestalt therapist may use to deepen contact through focusing. Especially useful are the creative arts, such as music and art (Rogers, 1993).

- **Empty-chair dialogues.** Empty-chair dialogues may be used to complete unfinished business with a significant other (Paivio & Greenberg, 1995) or with two conflicting aspects of self (Greenberg, 1979). The purpose is to evoke associated sensations and engage in dialogue with the significant other or with the conflicting parts of self. An example of the former is a person who is not able to express his or her feelings to another person, and he or she will be asked to put the person in an empty chair and tell him or her what needs to be expressed. An example of the latter is when two parts of self are in conflict. For example, a female patient who was told as a child (introject) not to express anger will be in conflict with her authentic self who wants to express healthy anger when experiencing a violation:

Patient:	I would like to express my anger at my partner but I stop myself.
APPN:	Would you agree to an experiment where you imagine each of these parts of yourself in an empty chair?
Patient:	Okay.
APPN:	The part of you that would like to express your anger sits in one chair and the part that cannot express anger sits in another.
Patient:	I would like to sit in the chair that can't express my anger first.
APPN:	Go ahead and start in the chair that cannot express your anger.
Patient:	I can't express my anger, but I want to. I am afraid something bad will happen if I express my anger.
APPN:	Now switch chairs.
Patient:	You'll never be able to express anger. You should not express anger. Something bad will happen. You will be destroyed.
APPN:	Now switch chairs.
Patient:	I have a right to my anger. You can't stop me any longer.

- **Language of responsibility.** This technique focuses specifically on deflected language that a patient may use to decrease the intensity of awareness and contact. For example, patients may use questions rather than statements to keep themselves safe or use pronouns such as "it" or "you" to deflect the intensity of feelings. When using the language of responsibility, the therapist asks the patient to put a question into a statement or use a first person pronoun to heighten awareness.

Patient:	It is so difficult to find a partner.
APPN:	Would you be willing to say, "I am finding it so difficult to find a partner"?

- **Dreamwork.** In Gestalt therapy, working with dreams is a common intervention. The characters and objects in the dreams are viewed as projections of disowned parts of self that need to be reintegrated. When working with dreams, the therapist has the patient assume all parts of the dream and tell the dream as if it were happening in the here and now, using present tense rather than past tense (Perls, 1969). For example:

Patient:	I'd like to recount a dream I had last night. I was climbing a precipitous mountain and felt exhausted. About halfway to the top, the mountain suddenly turned into meatloaf. I became immobilized, unsure if I should continue climbing or stop.
APPN:	Can you retell the dream using the present tense—as if the dream was happening right now.
Patient:	Sure. I am climbing a precipitous mountain and I feel exhausted. I am halfway to the top. The mountain has turned into meatloaf.

	I don't know what to do. I am immobilized. I don't know if I should continue climbing or stop.
APPN:	What are you experiencing now retelling the dream?
Patient:	I am confused.
APPN:	Would you be willing to speak as different parts of the dream—the steep mountain, the mountain made of meatloaf, yourself?
Patient:	(as the meatloaf mountain) I am alive, rich, tasty, vital, nourishing. (as the mountain) I am barren, rocky, lacking vegetation, without much life, and dying.

As the dreamwork continued, the parts of the dream were asked to speak to each other and eventually the patient became very tearful, realizing that the dream represented her struggle between her inauthentic desire to live a life of sheer ambition and her authentic desire to live a more balanced, nourishing, and fulfilling life. The patient was eventually able to create a new ending for the dream where she stopped climbing the mountain.

These are merely a few examples of the many types of experiments used in Gestalt therapy. Gestalt therapists pay close attention to the patient's process and create experiments based on the patient's needs that emerge moment to moment during the session (Knight, 1996).

EXISTENTIAL PSYCHOTHERAPY

Overview

The formal beginning of existential psychotherapy in the United States can be traced to 1958 with the publication of the text *Existence: A New Dimension in Psychiatry and Psychology* by May, Angel, and Ellenberger (1958). Although many people helped shape the existential psychotherapy movement, Rollo May (1909–1994), Victor Frankl (1905–1997), and Jim Bugental (1915–2008) were the leaders who played an early role in developing and promoting existential psychotherapy, while Irving Yalom (b. 1931) and Kirk Schneider (b. 1956) are the contemporary leaders involved in further developing this approach.

Rollo May, a psychologist often referred to as the father of American existential psychology, was concerned with the importance of anxiety for self-growth as well as themes of freedom and responsibility. May believed that psychotherapy should be concerned with the problem of *being* rather than problem-solving (Bugental, 1996). Victor Frankl, a physician and philosopher sent to a concentration camp when Hitler came to power, wrote *Man's Search for Meaning* (1963) based on his experiences. This compelling book introduced Frankl's logotherapy, an existential therapy that translates into *meaning therapy*, which supports the view that people have the freedom to choose their attitude in any given set of circumstances and discover meaning (Frankl, 1963). James Bugental, a psychologist, focused on living an authentic and responsible life (Bugental, 1965). He contributed a great deal to the practice of therapeutic presence rather than therapeutic techniques in conducting existential psychotherapy (Schneider & Greening, 2009). Irving Yalom, a psychiatrist, addressed the four *givens of existence*: freedom and responsibility, isolation, meaninglessness, and death (Yalom, 1980). Yalom's existential application to group therapy, seen in his widely used and respected text *Theory and Practice of Group*

Psychotherapy (Yalom, 2005), has solidified a continued place for existential therapy in the group therapy modality. Kirk Schneider, a psychologist and contemporary spokesperson for existential–humanistic psychotherapy, is well known for his development of the existential concept of *awe* and how to cultivate awe in existential psychotherapy (Schneider, 2009). Schneider, co-founder of the Existential–Humanistic Institute in San Francisco, has been integral in fostering global dialogue of existential themes in psychotherapy, a framework for psychotherapy integration, and a link between existential theory and postmodernism (Schneider & May, 1995).

Existential psychotherapy, a philosophical approach to psychotherapy, addresses the large, universal themes of life. These themes, considered to be the *givens of existence*, are frequently found not only in psychotherapy but are written about in great novels. For example, Albert Camus, in his well-known novel *L'Etranger*, has Meursault, the main character, accept his mortality, reject the constrictions of society he previously placed on himself, and become unencumbered to live his life as he chooses. These themes of death, choice, and freedom as well as others create a focus for existential psychotherapy.

Key Concepts

Existential psychotherapy is centered in resolving life's existential themes. Dysfunction occurs when existential themes are unresolved and people live a meaningless life. A list of common existential themes can be found in Box 6.3, with more detailed descriptions to follow:

CHOICE

A range of choices exists that is available to everyone. Although choices may be somewhat limited by external circumstances, the existential approach embraces the idea that people are free to choose and rejects the notion that choice is predetermined or restricted.

FREEDOM

Freedom is an openness, readiness, and flexibility to grow and change, which necessitates a capacity to choose among alternatives. People are free to shape their destiny and are the authors of creating their own world.

RESPONSIBILITY

With freedom comes accepting responsibility for the choices made and actions taken in determining a self-directed life. Existential therapy is rooted in the premise that people are responsible for their lives, their actions, or their failure to take action (Bugental, 1987).

BOX 6.3 Existential Themes

- Choice
- Freedom
- Responsibility
- Awareness
- Aloneness
- Meaning
- Anxiety
- Death
- Authenticity
- Awe

AWARENESS

Increasing self-awareness leads to an emphasis on choice and responsibility and the view that a worthwhile life is one that is authentic and genuine. Existential therapy believes that it takes courage to become aware of self and live from a place of authentic choice. Through self-awareness, people are able to choose their actions and create their own destiny.

ALONENESS

Part of the human condition is that people enter and depart the world alone. Strength and meaning are derived from the experience of looking to oneself and sensing this separation and aloneness. People nevertheless desire to be significant to others and thus need to create close relationships with others while accepting the existential aloneness (Yalom, 1980).

MEANING

A part of the human condition is the struggle for a sense of meaning and purpose in life. Meaninglessness leads to emptiness and an existential vacuum. Faced with the prospect of mortality, people may ask: "Is there any point to what I do now, because I will eventually die? Will what I do be forgotten once I am gone?" The existentialist position encourages people to search for meaning by living fully and responsibly, accepting the consequences of their choices, and engaging in a commitment to creating, loving, working, and building a meaningful life (Frankl, 1963).

EXISTENTIAL ANXIETY

An essential part of existence entails accepting existential anxiety as a condition of living. As awareness of the consequences of freedom, choice, responsibility, isolation, and death increases, anxiety is inevitable. Existential anxiety is a stimulus for growth and an appropriate response to having the courage to be. The aim of therapy is not to eliminate anxiety but to be aware of it and embrace it in order to live a fulfilling life.

DEATH

Awareness of death is the terrible truth and ultimate human concern that gives significance to life. The fear of death and the fear of life are related, for the fear of death looms over those who are afraid to participate fully in life. Existentialists believe that those who fear death also fear life; thus the fear of death must be faced before one can truly live (Schneider & May, 1995).

AWE

Awe is a state of being that incorporates wonder, dread, mystery, veneration, and paradox. Cultivating awe in existential therapy requires a movement away from many contemporary values of consumerism, conventionality, mindless entertainment, competitiveness, and the "quick fix," efficiency-oriented culture (Schneider, 2009).

Goals of Therapy

The goals of existential psychotherapy center on the given themes of existence and helping patients face the anxieties of life, freely choose their life direction, take responsibility for their choices, and create a meaningful existence. Patients are encouraged to face the anxieties generated by personal freedom, choice, aloneness, and death.

Existential therapy can be viewed as an invitation to help patients recognize how they are not living fully authentic lives and make choices that will lead to living life authentically (Corey, 2011).

Psychotherapeutic Interventions: Assessment

In existential psychotherapy, the emphasis of assessment is on a phenomenological understanding of the subjective world of the patient rather than employing traditional assessment procedures and diagnostic constructs. Preconceptions are bracketed in order to be present with the immediate experience. The existential psychotherapist is generally not concerned with the patient's past; instead, the emphasis is on the choices to be made in the present and future.

The first session is extremely important for building an authentic therapeutic relationship. Patient's values and assumptions about the world are examined during the assessment. The therapist attempts to understand the patient's current life situation, freedom of choice, potential for meaningful change, and expectations for therapy (Corey, 2011).

Psychotherapeutic Interventions: Psychotherapy Techniques

A fundamental characteristic of existential psychotherapy is that the approach does not identify with a set of specific techniques. Existential therapists have themselves examined and worked through the universal themes of life. Interventions are thus based on an understanding of what it means to be more fully human. The existential psychotherapist is free to draw on techniques from other orientations (Schneider, 2008). To follow are some notions related to interventions:

THERAPEUTIC RELATIONSHIP

Existential therapy places a high premium on the quality of the therapeutic relationship as a healing agent. It emphasizes an authentic I–Thou encounter between the patient and therapist. It supports equality in the therapeutic relationship and an encounter characterized by mutuality, authenticity, openness, immediacy, and dialogue. The use of the therapeutic self is the core of therapy; thus, the therapist needs to be mature and have a personal philosophy that is congruent with the theoretical underpinnings associated with the existential psychotherapy approach.

PRESENCE

The existential psychotherapist cultivates the quality of presence. Presence is a subjective experience of being here and now in a relationship and intending, at a very deep level, to participate as fully as one is able (Schneider, 2008). Bugental (1987) wrote that therapists need to maintain full presence to the patient's experience in the moment and to closely attend to patient's immediate inner flow of experience. "Be there!" and "Insist that the patient be there!" were well-known mantras of Bugental's existential approach (Schneider & Greening, 2009).

EXPERIENTIAL REFLECTION

The existential psychotherapist asks in-depth questions about universal themes in order for patients to experientially reflect on how their life is being lived in the present. The patient is challenged to grapple with complexities and paradoxes of the human condition and to face the givens of existence. Experiential reflection through in-depth questioning helps the patient recognize the range of life choices, remove obstacles to freedom, find meaning, and take responsibility (Yalom, 1980). For example, a question such as, "How is your freedom impaired?" seeks to bring awareness to the patient's obstacles to freedom. Prototypical questions include:

- What is the purpose of your life?
- Where is the source of meaning for you?
- You want to live an authentic life, yet you stay in a relationship and a job that give you little satisfaction. How are you keeping yourself stuck?
- What might be accomplished in treatment that would help you live a more authentic life?

A recent patient of mine was confronting the possibility of disability and an early death from Parkinson disease. As an existential therapist, I encouraged him to confront the probable disability and possible early death and, accordingly, face decisions that this disease has thrust upon him. Questions focused on helping him reflect on understanding that his life, akin to everyone else's life, is finite but that he is still capable of finding meaning and making different decisions about his illness and his life's path. The focus in therapy was on choosing a life he wanted to live and assuming responsibility for his choices. He was in a difficult and unsatisfying relationship with a partner who abused substances and who had an Internet addiction. He was very unhappy in his job as well. In therapy, he was encouraged to evaluate his choices and his accompanying anxieties regarding change. He was asked, "What prevents you from living an authentic life?" He was helped to understand that making difficult choices in the face of illness is actually a way to find wholeness and meaning. This patient eventually chose to live a less encumbered life and discard some of the constraints he previously placed on himself. He ended his relationship, quit his job, and moved to a city where there were more medical facilities and support and where he could avail himself of public transportation. He joined a support group for people with Parkinson disease. He found a new life direction that gave him purpose and meaning. Once he was able to face his own mortality, he truly developed the courage to be.

EMOTION-FOCUSED THERAPY

EFT is an evidence-based, short-term humanistic–existential psychotherapy approach. Developed in the 1980s, primarily by Canadian psychologist Leslie Greenberg (b. 1945), EFT has invigorated the central role of emotion in psychotherapy, which has been routinely eclipsed in importance by cognition and behavior in the last few decades. "You need to feel to heal" and "I feel, therefore I am" are mantras frequently touted in the EFT community.

EFT integrates person-centered therapy, Gestalt therapy, and the neuroscience research of emotions. When the approach was predominantly a blend of person-centered and Gestalt therapy, it was called process-experiential therapy; however, when the Neuroscience Theory of Emotions was integrated in the 1990s, the name was changed to EFT. Nevertheless, person-centered therapy and Gestalt therapy have retained their strong influence, especially in regard to therapeutic interventions. Extensive evidence-based research has been conducted using EFT with very positive results. It has also been manualized and many of its interventions operationalized. Nonetheless, learning this approach requires a great deal of training and psychotherapeutic sophistication (Greenberg, 2011).

Key Concepts

EMOTIONS

An affective state of information processing, emotion informs a person of important needs and creates an action readiness that prepares the self for action. For example, fear sets in motion a search for danger, sadness informs of loss, and anger signals a violation.

Emotions exert influence on cognition and behavior. They are signals that keep people energized, interested, and connected to others (Greenberg, 2011).

Emotion Schemes

Complex memory networks within the amygdala and neocortex pathways, formed in response to emotional life experiences, are the basis of adult emotional responses. They are activated rapidly, without thought or awareness, by learned situational cues (e.g., visual images and verbal triggers) of evoked emotion from prior life experiences. Schemes are oriented toward action and serve to satisfy needs and goals. If adaptive, they form positive, flexible emotional-processing systems with clear pathways. Maladaptive schemes, caused by unprocessed emotions from difficult situations (e.g., betrayal, abandonment, and trauma) may form negative, inflexible emotional-processing systems. Changing the negative emotion scheme is the target of therapeutic intervention and central to change (Greenberg, 2011).

MEMORY CONSOLIDATION

Memory consolidation is a process during a time period after an emotional life experience when memory of the experience is fragile and can be disrupted. The memory becomes permanent fairly soon after the event. The more highly aroused the emotion, the more the experience and evoking situation will form a memory (Greenberg, 2010).

MEMORY RECONSOLIDATION

Memory reconsolidation occurs during a time period after a memory is reactivated later in life when it is again fragile and can be disrupted. Changing an emotion scheme during EFT occurs during this memory reconsolidation period (Greenberg, 2010).

PRIMARY EMOTIONS

Genuine, authentic emotional reactions initially activated in response to a situation, primary emotions may be adaptive or maladaptive (Greenberg, 2011).

- **Primary adaptive emotions.** Direct reaction consistent with the situation and resulting in appropriate action. Primary adaptive emotions are accessed for their useful information and capacity to meaningfully organize action and include sadness, fear, anger, joy, love, and surprise. Sadness, for example, occurs in response to a loss, anger in response to a violation, and fear in response to danger (Greenberg, 2011).
- **Primary maladaptive emotions.** Also a direct reaction to a situation but an overlearned response based on prior traumatic experiences that does not result in appropriate action. They are maladaptive emotional states that are familiar, occur repeatedly, and neither change in response to different circumstances nor provide adaptive direction for problem-solving. Examples include a core sense of abandonment, worthlessness, or shame. A person who experienced extreme fear to early sexual abuse, for example, may as an adult experience fear in response to closeness rather than warmth and pleasure. Primary maladaptive emotions are accessed and transformed during EFT (Greenberg, 2010).

SECONDARY EMOTIONS

A secondary emotion is an emotional reaction to a primary emotion or thought that follows, replaces, or obscures a primary emotion. Examples include feeling guilty about feeling angry or feeling angry in response to feeling hurt. Therapeutic interventions in EFT attempt to reduce the secondary emotions in order to access primary emotions (Greenberg, 2011).

INSTRUMENTAL EMOTIONS

Instrumental emotions are used to control, manipulate, and elicit support. An example of an instrumental emotion is crying insincere "crocodile tears" to manipulate the environment and elicit support.

MARKERS

Markers are in-session, problematic emotional-processing states that patients enter during therapy that are indicative of underlying affective problems. They are identified by certain statements and behaviors and are used by the therapist to guide therapeutic interventions. Examples of markers include problematic reactions, conflict splits, unclear felt sense, and unfinished business. Currently, more than 15 process markers have been identified (Greenberg, 2011).

Goals of Therapy

The goal in EFT is to help patients move toward wholeness and self-actualization by helping them develop emotional awareness and adaptive emotional processing. Patients develop the ability to access important information that emotions provide and use that information to live a full, vital life. Patients are able to use emotions as signals to inform them of their needs and deal effectively with life experiences. Patients learn how to access their primary adaptive emotions and transform primary maladaptive emotions. Maladaptive emotion schemes are evoked for reprocessing, thereby enabling patients to create new emotional narratives. A goal is also to decrease the use of secondary and instrumental emotions so that patients are not encumbered by them (Greenberg & Goldman, 1988).

Psychotherapeutic Interventions: Assessment

Assessment in EFT occurs in the first phase of therapy called the bonding and awareness phase. In this phase, a strong therapeutic relationship is developed based on the person-centered work of Carl Rogers, emphasizing empathy, congruence, and unconditional positive regard. The therapist enters the patient's frame of reference, validates the patient's feelings, and empathically follows the patient's experience to deepen emotional experiencing and access core emotions. Emotional functioning is assessed including emotional awareness, emotional regulation skills, and emotion schemes. The therapist provides a rationale for working with emotion, establishes a collaborative focus, and promotes the patient's awareness of emotional experience (Greenberg, 2011). Assessment also occurs continuously throughout the therapeutic process.

Psychotherapeutic Interventions: Psychotherapy Techniques

The second phase of therapy called the evoking and exploring phase utilizes therapeutic interventions that access and evoke problematic feelings, primary maladaptive emotions, and maladaptive core schemes using process-directed Gestalt therapy style experiments. Therapeutic interventions are marker guided; thus, in-session states of underlying affective problems are identified and specific process interventions employed that flow from the in-session markers (Greenberg, 2011). The therapeutic process is construed as a sequence of events in which specified markers repeatedly present themselves in therapy as opportunities to employ effective process interventions. Thus, the psychotherapist is constantly engaged in assessing for the presentation of a marker and must be proficient both at making process diagnoses of markers as well as implementing appropriate interventions to help resolve the problem indicated by the marker. Perceptual skills are needed for recognizing markers and determining the appropriate intervention (Greenberg, Rice, & Elliott, 1993).

MARKER EXPERIMENTS

In-session markers (problematic emotional-processing states) are identified that guide experiments to help patients access and transform their maladaptive primary emotions and negative emotion schemes (Greenberg, 2011). Numerous markers have been identified in EFT. A list of the more common markers can be found in Box 6.4. Examples follow to illustrate these markers and their interventions (Greenberg, 2011).

- **Problematic reactions.** Emotional overreactions to particular stimulus situations perceived as problematic and expressed by puzzlement. An example is a comment a patient made during a recent session: "On my way to therapy, I saw a plume-tailed dog and became very fearful and I don't know why." The intervention is a systematic unfolding procedure that allows the patient to arrive at the implicit meaning of the situation, make sense of the reaction, and resolve the problematic reaction. The patient is asked to provide detailed and concrete descriptions of the situation and the emotional reaction through the use of evocative language. The therapist then amplifies the description with the use of vivid, imagistic language, which promotes reexperiencing the situation (Greenberg, 2011).
- **Unclear felt sense.** An inability to get a clear sense of an experience perceived as problematic. The patient may say, "I just have this inner tenseness, but don't know what it is." The intervention is a focusing technique whereby the therapist guides the patient to approach the unclear felt sense with attention and willingness to access and create a symbolic expression of it in the form of a metaphor or image. The therapist may say to the patient, "I'd like you to attend to your inner tension, breathe into the area in your body with curiosity, stay with it, and allow an image to emerge." Resolution involves a bodily felt shift to the creation of new meaning (Greenberg, 2011).
- **Conflict split.** When one aspect of self is critical toward another aspect. The patient may say, "A part of me feels so inadequate while the other feels very competent." The intervention is two-chair work where the two parts of self are put into contact by dialoguing with each other in two separate chairs. Thoughts, feelings, and needs within

BOX 6.4 Common Emotion-Focused Therapy (EFT) Markers

- Problematic reactions
- Unclear felt sense
- Conflict splits
- Self-interruptive splits
- Unfinished business
- Vulnerability
- Trauma narrative

each part of self are explored and communicated. Resolution involves a softening of the critical voice, integration of the two sides, and self-acceptance (Greenberg, 2011).

- **Self-interruptive split.** When a patient interrupts a part of self. For example, a patient states, "I can feel the tears coming up, but I just tighten and suck them back in; no way am I going to cry." A two-chair enactment is used to make the interrupting part of self explicit. The patient is guided to enact the way the tightening and sucking back the tears occur in order to experience the self as an agent in the process of shutting the part of self down. The patient is invited to challenge the interruptive part of self. Resolution involves expression of the previously blocked experience (Greenberg, 2011).

- **Unfinished business.** Unresolved feelings toward a significant other. For example, a man abandoned by his mother may be resentful when his wife is busy and pays little attention to him. An empty-chair intervention may be used whereby the patient activates his internal view of his mother and expresses unresolved feelings and needs. "You were never there for me. I have never forgiven you. I will never feel support. I needed you to be there and comfort me." The resolution involves holding the other accountable or understanding and forgiving the other with shifts in views of both self and other (Greenberg, 2011).

- **Vulnerability.** A state in which the self feels fragile, ashamed, or insecure. The patient states, "I feel like I've got nothing left. I just can't carry on." The intervention is affirming empathic validation and attunement from the therapist who must capture the feeling content; mirror the tempo, rhythm, and tone of experience; and validate and normalize the experience of vulnerability. Resolution involves a strengthened sense of self (Greenberg, 2011).

- **Trauma narrative.** When the patient experiences internal pressure to tell a difficult life story. The patient states, "I am remembering a very traumatic situation that happened when I was in college, but even though I want to, I am having difficulty speaking about it." The intervention is to assist the patient to retell the trauma narrative. Resolution brings relief, restoration of narrative gaps, and creation of a new narrative (Greenberg, 2011).

The unique aspect of working with markers in EFT is that specific interventions have been identified for each type of marker. This gives the beginning therapist clear guidelines as to how and when to use a specific intervention (Greenberg, 2011). The reader is referred to the work of Greenberg (2011) for a comprehensive list of markers and their interventions. At the end of an intervention, reflection of the experience occurs between the patient and therapist in order to make sense of the experience. This is the third phase of EFT called generating new emotions and creating new narrative meaning. In this phase, validation for new feelings and support for an emerging sense of self are given. There is a deep experiential self-knowledge that occurs as new meanings and coherent narratives are created to explain the experience (Greenberg, 2011).

SOLUTION-FOCUSED THERAPY

Overview

SFT is a brief psychotherapy embedded in the philosophy of postmodernism and the theory of social constructionism, a psychological application of the postmodern worldview. Postmodernism and social constructionism emerged in the 1960s as a reaction to the assumed certainty of scientific and objective efforts to explain reality and an awareness of an increasingly more diverse, complex, and uncertain world.

Both postmodernism and social constructionism are, in many respects, similar to humanistic–existential worldviews and share common beliefs about psychotherapy. Some of the early postmodern philosophers were existentialists (e.g., Kierkegaard and Nietzsche) and phenomenologists (e.g., Husserl and Heidegger; Schneider & May, 1995).

Postmodernism recognizes that there are no objective or absolute universal truths, and it is skeptical of explanations that claim to be valid for all cultures and groups. Instead, it believes that there are multiple ways of knowing, and reality is believed to exist only through the interpretation of each person. Postmodernism relies on individual experience, knowing that the outcome of a person's experience will necessarily be fallible and relative, rather than certain and universal. Postmodernism denies the existence of ultimate scientific or philosophical truth that will explain everything for everybody. It promotes the restructuring of theory and methodology to include more ethics, diversity of representation, and cultural relativism (Kvale, 1992).

Social constructionism places emphasis on truth, reality, and knowledge as socially embedded. Reality is based on the use of language and the situations in which people live. Language is viewed as the vehicle through which people attribute meaning to their experience (Gergen, 1985, 1999). For example, a person is bipolar when he or she accepts a definition of self as bipolar. Once this definition of self is assumed, it is difficult to recognize behaviors opposed to the definition, such as a period when the person had a stable mood. Some basic premises of postmodernism and social constructionism can be found in Box 6.5.

Postmodernist thought has influenced the development of a number of contemporary psychotherapies. The most well known are SFT, narrative therapy, and feminist therapy. SFT, a brief therapy that is easily understood and mastered, was codeveloped by husband and wife Steve de Shazer and Insoo Kim Berg in the early 1980s with their team at the Brief Family Therapy Center in Milwaukee, Wisconsin. It has been strongly influenced by the work of Milton Erikson, Gregory Bateson, and the Mental Research Institute in Palo Alto, California, as well as the philosophies of Buddhism and Taoism (Corey, 2011).

Insoo Kim Berg (1935–2007), a social worker and psychotherapist, applied the approach to working with couples and families as well as patients with addictions (Berg & Miller, 1992). Steve de Shazer (1940–2005), a social worker and psychotherapist, wrote several seminal texts on SFT (de Shazer, 1985, 1988, 1991, 1994). Both were popular workshop leaders and trained therapists in SFT throughout North America, Europe, Australia, and Asia. Other well-known leaders and trainers in this approach include

---

BOX 6.5 Basic Premises of Postmodernism and Social Constructionism

- The subjective experience of the patient is most important and valued
- Problems and solutions take shape and have meaning within a dialogic context.
- Patients are viewed as experts about their own lives.
- Patients are cocreators and cofacilitators of the therapy process.
- Hierarchy and power differential increase the potential for exploitation.
- Therapist and patient are collaborative in the psychotherapy structure and process.
- Knowledge and skill of the therapist are not as paramount as the relationship.
- Therapists disavow the role of expert.
- Manualized and empirically supportive treatments (EST) are flawed.
- Diagnosing and pathologizing patients should be avoided.
- Self-report ratings of dysfunction are inadequate interventions.

Source: Gergen, K. (1985). The social constructionist movement in modern psychology. *American Psychologist, 40,* 266–275. doi:10.1037/0003-066X.40.3.266; Gergen, K. (1999). *An invitation to social construction.* Newbury Park, CA: Sage.

Michele Wiener-Davis, Bill O'Hanlon, Yvonne Dolan, Eve Lipchik, Scott Miller, John Walter, and Jane Peller. They applied SFT to a number of different problems including alcoholism, domestic violence, and trauma and have added greatly to the SFT literature (Corey, 2011).

SFT believes that the therapy process does not necessitate processing problems in order to resolve them. Therapy is solution focused rather than problem focused and is present and future oriented rather than past oriented. Therapy seeks to empower the patient and is positive and nonpathologizing. The patient is viewed as competent, having resources needed to construct solutions. Therapy is expected to result in change. Even long-standing issues are resolved in a relatively short period of time. SFT believes that smaller changes lead to bigger changes, and the effects of change tend to multiply (De Jong & Berg, 2008; de Shazer, 1985, 1988, 1994).

Key Concept

SOLUTION TALK

From social constructionism, the belief that language creates reality was applied to SFT with the key concept of *solution talk*. SFT espouses the view that a problem-focused approach using "problem talk" actually helps maintain the problem, but that a solution-focused approach using "solution talk" helps the patient change in a positive direction. Solution talk highlights what the patient wants to achieve through therapy rather than the problem that made the patient seek help. By identifying what is desired, the therapist invites the patient to construct a concrete vision for a preferred future. Thus, to change a problem, the language must be shifted from problem talk to solution talk (de Shazer, 1991).

Goals of Therapy

The goal of SFT is to help the patient change by constructing solutions to problems rather than dwelling on them. The two key therapeutic goals are to determine (a) how the patient wants his or her life to be different, and (b) what it will take to make it happen. Creating a detailed picture of what it will be like in the future when things change creates a feeling of hope and makes the solution seem possible to the patient (de Shazer, 1991).

Psychotherapeutic Interventions: Assessment

During the assessment, the therapist creates a positive climate of hope, respect, dialogue, inquiry, and affirmation. The focus is on understanding the subjective experience of the patient as well as developing a collaborative therapeutic relationship. The patient is given the message that he or she is viewed as the expert and the therapist assumes a *not knowing* position in order for the patient to construct the solutions and develop well-formed goals. SFT focuses on the present and future rather than the past. The therapist pays little attention to history taking and traditional assessment data, for this type of knowledge is believed to be inconsequential and may actually hamper the development of solutions. The therapist also does not give the patient a diagnosis, for this is believed to be irrelevant to finding solutions (Berg & Miller, 1992).

During the assessment, a goal that is important and meaningful to the patient is established. The goal focuses on desirable behaviors (e.g., I will, rather than I will not) and is concrete, specific, and behavioral. It includes a detailed explanation as to how it will be accomplished, which increases the ability to achieve the goal (Berg & Miller, 1992).

Psychotherapeutic Interventions: Psychotherapy Techniques

SFT uses specific types of questions to help the patient access solutions. The following questions are examples of the most popular SFT questions.

PRESESSION CHANGE QUESTIONS

These questions ask the patient what improvements have been made during the time period of contracting for services and the first session. Scheduling an appointment starts the change process and asking this question encourages the patient to engage in solution-building conversations from the beginning (de Shazer, 1985, 1988). For example, the therapist might say:

- During the next few days, before we meet, I would like you to think about what I can do to be helpful to you.
- or
- Between now and when we meet, think about what the perfect therapist would do.

JOINING

Joining involves the therapist connecting and accommodating to the patient's world (de Shazer, 1985, 1988). Some examples of joining questions are:

- What improvement have you noticed since you made the call to come in?
- On the way here, what were you most worried I would or would not do?
- What needs to happen today so that when you leave you'll think this was a good session?

MIRACLE QUESTIONS

These questions ask the patient to imagine how things would be different if the problem were solved. This helps the patient identify goals and envision the future without the problem. The intent is to help the patient describe realistic steps toward the solution (de Shazer, 1991). The therapist uses a hypnotic voice quality to ask the miracle question:

Suppose that one night there is a miracle and while you were sleeping the problem that brought you to therapy is solved. How would you know? What will you notice different the next morning that will tell you that there has been a miracle?

Therapists may become very concrete with the miracle question, asking what they would notice first, what would happen next, and so forth (De Jong & Berg, 2008).

EXCEPTION QUESTIONS

These questions seek to determine times in the patient's life when the identified problems were not as problematic. SFT believes that there were *always* times when the problem was less severe or absent for the patient. The therapist seeks to encourage the patient to describe what different circumstances existed or what the patient did differently.

The goal is for the patient to repeat what has worked in the past, and to help him or her gain confidence in making improvements for the future (De Jong & Berg, 2008).

- When was a time that a problem could have occurred but didn't?
- Tell me about times when you don't get angry.
- Was there ever a time when you felt happy in your relationship?

SCALING QUESTIONS

These questions help the patient assess and track progress on different dimensions (e.g., motivation, hopefulness, and confidence). The poles of a scale range from the worst the problem has ever been (0) to the best things could ever possibly be (10; De Jong & Berg, 2008). On a scale from 1 to 10 with 0 being the lowest and 10 the highest:

- How bad is the problem?
- On a day when you are one point higher on the scale, what would tell you that?
- Where would you place your depression when you first came in and where would it be now?
- What would it take to move from a 3 to a 4?

FUTURE-ORIENTED QUESTIONS

These questions focus on guiding the conversation from problems to envisioning a better life in the future. When a problem is stated, the therapist asks questions to explore what could be better if the problem were resolved (De Jong & Berg, 2008).

- How will this make you happier?
- What will be better for you after this occurs?
- What do you see down the road after this is resolved?

COPING QUESTIONS

These questions are designed to elicit information about the patient's resources that may have gone unnoticed. Such questions work well when the patient is going through a difficult time, for even the most hopeless story has within it examples of coping that can be explicated (De Jong & Berg, 2008). With coping questions, the first part of the intervention is a validating statement and the second part gently challenges the patient:

- I can see that things have been really difficult for you. How have you managed to carry on and prevent things from becoming worse?
- I am struck by the fact that, even with all of your losses, you manage to get up each morning and do everything necessary to get the kids off to school. What keeps you going under such difficult circumstances?
- It is admirable how you have been able to keep on going under such difficult circumstances. How did you do that?

COMPLIMENTS

This type of question reinforces the patient's successes through validating the difficulty of the problem and acknowledging what the patient is doing well and what is working. It invites the patient to self-compliment by virtue of answering the question (De Jong & Berg, 2008).

- Wow! How did you manage to finish that task so quickly?
- What do your colleagues appreciate in how you work?

ENDING

Experiments or homework assignments are suggested by the therapist for the patient to try between sessions. For example, suppose the patient states that she wants to feel more competent (De Jong & Berg, 2008). An experiment and homework might be:

- Let yourself envisage that when you leave the office today, you feel more competent. What will you be doing differently? Try that during the week.
- During the week, record any time you feel competent and then notice what you were thinking and doing.

SUBSEQUENT SESSIONS

At the start of each new session, the therapist will ask about what learning has occurred since the last session (De Jong & Berg, 2008). The therapist reviews experiments and homework assignments:

- So what is better, if anything, since our last meeting?
- What would need to happen so you did not need to come back to therapy anymore?

EVIDENCE-BASED RESEARCH

Since 1964 in Old Saybrook, Connecticut, when humanistic–existential psychotherapy was launched, five decades of substantial advances in theory, practice, and evidence-based research have accumulated supporting the effectiveness of humanistic–existential psychotherapy for a wide range of patient problems. The research demonstrates that the humanistic–existential psychotherapies are as effective or more effective than other major psychotherapy approaches. Person-centered therapy, Gestalt therapy, existential therapy, and EFT have effect sizes comparable with therapies such as cognitive behavioral therapy (CBT; Cain & Seeman, 2002; Elliott, 2002; Elliott, Greenberg, & Lietaer, 2004; Kirschenbaum & Jourdan, 2005) and therapy gains are maintained over time (Elliott, Greenberg, Goldman, & Angus, 2009). Much of the research that has been done in humanistic–existential therapies is process research, which looks at what occurs during the session to bring about positive results. Theories of change processes have been tested empirically by using a task-analytic approach to the study of therapeutic change processes (Greenberg, 1986, 1991; Greenberg & Rice, 1997). Readers are referred to Cain and Seeman's *Humanistic Psychotherapies: Handbook of Research and Practice* (2002) for an extensive review of the research in humanistic–existential psychotherapies.

A great deal of research has been done in person-centered therapy by Carl Rogers and his colleagues on the importance of the therapeutic relationship. Much of the current research on psychotherapy outcomes, which calls Rogers's core conditions the common factors or the therapeutic working alliance, has validated Rogers's original work (Duncan et al., 2010; Wampold, 2001). Rogers's work, far ahead of his time, is experiencing a major revival. Increasingly, most schools of psychotherapy recognize the importance of the core conditions (Kirschenbaum & Jourdan, 2005). A compilation of the extensive research in the person-centered approach can be found in Kirschenbaum and Jourdan's article, "The Current Status of Carl Rogers and Person-Centered Approach" (2005) and Cain's text, *Person-Centered Psychotherapies* (2010). See Table 6.1 for Selected Humanistic–Existential Therapy Research.

TABLE 6.1 SELECTED HUMANISTIC–EXISTENTIAL THERAPY RESEARCH

Overview of research in humanistic and experiential therapies	Elliott, Greenberg, and Lietaer (2004); Schneider, Bugental, and Pierson (2001)
Person-centered therapy with LGBT youth helped in accepting sexual identity	Lemoire and Chen (2005)
Person-centered therapy with lesbian and gay patients experiencing violence and trauma	Brice (2011)
Person-centered therapy more effective than medication for patients with personality disorders	Teusch, Bohme, Fink, and Gastpar (2001)
Person-centered therapy more effective than antidepressant medication in the assimilation of problematic experiences	Teusch, Bohme, Fink, Gastpar, and Skerra (2003)
Person-centered therapy effective in the treatment of borderline personality disorder	Quinn (2011)
Person-centered therapy effective in the treatment of social anxiety disorder	Stephen, Elliott, and Macleod (2011)
Person-centered therapy effective in the treatment of bulimia nervosa	Schutzmann, Schutzmann, and Eckert (2010)
Person-centered play therapy effective with children experiencing disasters and catastrophic events	Jordan, Perryman, and Anderson (2013)
Person-centered therapy effective with patients with Alzheimer disease	Reisberg et al. (2017)
The challenge of person-centered therapy facilitates emotional growth and a sense of personhood and agency inolder adults	Von Humboldt and Leal (2015)
Person-centered therapy promotes coherence with older adults	Von Humboldt and Leal (2013)
Existential therapy effective with patients facing chronic and terminal illness	Schneider et al. (2001); Travelbee (1971)
Existential therapy effective with patients experiencing HIV	Farber (2009)
Existential therapy effective with patients having sexual dysfunctions	Barker (2011)
Existential therapy effective with adolescents with anxiety and depression	Shumaker (2012)
Existential therapy on spiritual health in women with infertility	Taghvaeinia, Dehghani, Jobaneh, and Nikoo (2017)
An update of existential therapy institutions worldwide	Correia, Cooper, and Berdondini (2016)

(continued)

TABLE 6.1 SELECTED HUMANISTIC–EXISTENTIAL THERAPY RESEARCH (*continued*)	
Gestalt therapy with children	Oaklander (1978)
Gestalt therapy with families	Resnikoff (1995)
Gestalt therapy with groups	Feder and Ronall (1980)
Gestalt therapy with organizational systems	Nevis (1987)
Effects of Gestalt therapy on body image	Clance, Thompson, Simerly, and Weiss (1994)
Gestalt therapy cycle effective with patients with attentional problems	Root (1996)
Overview of research in Gestalt therapy	Barber (2006); Brownell (2008)
Gestalt therapy effective with veterans with PTSD	Nazari, Mohammadi, and Nazeri (2014)
Gestalt therapy treatment effective with patients with schizophrenia	Greenberg (2015)
Gestalt sand-tray processing work with adult patients	Timm and Garza (2017)
Effectiveness of EFT versus CBT with patients with depression	Watson, Gordon, Stermac, Kalogerakos, and Steckley (2003)
EFT in resolving childhood trauma with patients diagnosed with autism spectrum disorder	Robinson (2018)
EFT in changing trauma narratives and complex childhood trauma	Mundorf and Paivio (2011); Paivio and Pascual-Leone (2010)
Solution-focused therapy success stories	Berg and Dolan (2001)
Solution-focused therapy for the problem drinker	Berg and Miller (1992)
Solution-focused therapy in improving university student's well-being	Pakrosnis and Cepukiene (2015)
Solution-focused therapy group therapy for common mental health problems	Carrera et al. (2016)
Solution-focused therapy for adults recovering from child sexual abuse	Gonzalez (2017)

Note: References cited in this table are listed at the end of the chapter.

CBT cognitive behavioral therapy; EFT, emotion-focused therapy; PTSD, posttraumatic stress disorder.

CASE EXAMPLE

Assessment

Joy, a 40-year-old nurse practitioner, has been married for 16 years and has three children, aged 6, 8, and 10. She entered therapy with symptoms of anxiety that began when she realized her husband was viewing excessive amounts of Internet pornography on a daily basis. She has not revealed to him that she knows about his Internet addiction. Joy has been dissatisfied with her marriage for a number of years and states she has fallen out of love with him. She has frequently thought of leaving her husband in the past but concluded that the prospect was too frightening. Recently, she has experienced her relationship with her husband as particularly emotionally void and empty. From her perspective, he is very emotionally restricted so that she dreads being alone with him and is embarrassed to be in his company with friends. The discovery of his pornography addiction has increased her desire to leave. She met her husband on graduation from college at the age of 22, a time when she was insecure and unstable. He had a stable, corporate job and seemed to be supportive of her. She married him 4 years later. She feels that there is a part of herself that is still unstable, and fears without the safety of the marriage, she might be unable to cope with the vicissitudes of life. During most of their married life, Joy worked part-time as a nurse, and when not working, immersed herself in the tasks of childcare. Her husband pursued his professional corporate business career and sports activities. They tried marriage counseling on two occasions without success and she believes that strategy is fruitless. She desires individual therapy to help end the marriage. She realizes that what prevents her from leaving the marriage resides within her.

Conceptualization

Joy is a woman who has difficulty accessing and expressing her primary emotions. Underneath the secondary emotion of anxiety, which emerged with the discovery of her husband's Internet addiction, is a significant amount of unaware anger and sadness that cannot be contacted, used as a signal to heal from her losses, or used to help propel her out of the marriage. She feels betrayed and violated by his Internet addiction as well as sad over the inevitable loss of her marriage and breakup of her family. Responsibility is an important issue thwarting her decision to leave, both a moral responsibility of not depriving her children of their father and the responsibility she feels for her children's future. She fears he would be an inadequate parent and realizes he will have the children half of the time. Further, she has never faced her existential aloneness and has difficulty with authenticity, freedom, choice, and responsibility. In addition, she has a number of introjects including:

- It is not okay to get divorced.
- I will fall apart if I am alone.
- He will be a derelict single parent.

Facilitating Change and Working on Problems

Joy's therapy was an integrated humanistic–existential approach with a few solution-focused techniques. Several existential themes emerged during the course of therapy including her fear of aloneness and taking responsibility for her life. During therapy, she reconnected with a former boyfriend on social media and "fell in love" with him. Although the state of being "in love" is one of the great experiences in life, it usually prevents therapy from moving forward in a deep fashion, for the pull of love is so great that it engulfs even the most well-directed therapeutic endeavors. Joy found her new love to be the "ideal man" and no other man existed for her. What finally made it possible for Joy to work in therapy was that her new male friend, hoping for a long-term commitment, became somewhat frightened by the prospect of having a relationship with a woman who was not yet out of her marriage and told her that he would not see her until she was divorced. Only then was she willing to look at her fear of being alone, her anxiety regarding her children, her desire to merge with a man to eliminate her anxiety, and her fear of freedom, choice, and responsibility.

After 6 months of intensive therapy, she gradually became comfortable with the thought of her aloneness. She realized that she could give up some control of her children, and although she knew she was the better parent, she realized that the children would be parented "well enough." She gradually learned that only she was the architect of her life and learned to take responsibility for her choices. She gained awareness and was able to access her primary emotions and use these emotions to move forward with her life. Some excerpts from the work with Joy that represent the humanistic–existential and postmodern–social constructionist approaches follow:

APPN: Where would you like to begin?

Joy: Well, I've been having a great deal of anxiety.

APPN: Say more about that.

Joy: I want to get out of my marriage. I am clear about that. I discovered he is watching Internet pornography on a daily basis.

APPN: Suppose that one night there is a miracle and while you were sleeping the problem is solved. How would you know? What would be different?

Joy: I would be calm without anxiety. I would be divorced. I would have my own house. I wouldn't worry about the children being taken care of by my ex-husband, for I would be okay with his parenting.

APPN: What would you need to do for this to happen?

Joy: Well, I would need to be less anxious. I would need to confront him about the pornography, for I don't want my children to follow in his footsteps. I would need to visit an attorney and know my choices. And I would need to look at real estate and see what I can afford. And I would need to work full time to get some savings.

The miracle question gave the APPN and the patient an understanding of the necessary solutions. A combination of person-centered, Gestalt, existential, and EFT was initiated with Joy. She remained in therapy for 6 months, at which time she was able to leave her husband and move into the world with less anxiety and more authenticity and awareness of her emotions.

APPN: If you divorce, what might that look like?

Joy: If we divorce, I do not think he will take care of the children when he has them. He doesn't even have them brush their teeth or help them with their homework. He is oblivious to what goes on around him.

APPN: So it's scary to imagine the children in his care without you there to monitor him.

Joy: Yes, I am also fearful of making the change. We have a nice house and a good life from the outside. I feel sad that everything we have worked for will end.

APPN: As you speak, where do you experience that sadness in your body?

Joy: I feel a tightness in my abdomen, like a bunched up fist. [Joy places her hand palm down on her abdomen.]

APPN: I notice your hand on your abdomen. Can you give the sadness some support?

Joy:	[Joy begins to gently rub her abdomen in small circles and tears form at the corners of her eyes.]
APPN:	Can you give the sadness a voice, first person, present tense? I am the sadness …
Joy:	I am your sadness. You push me down all the time. You are so afraid to feel me. If you cry, you will need to leave sooner, and you don't feel ready. I am feeling another emotion now trying to take over.
APPN:	Give that emotion a voice.
Joy:	I am your anxiety. I have an overwhelming sense of fear to move forward. It's so safe here, even though I am so unhappy. I will have to start all over. I will lose the house, for his parents will give him money to buy me out. He will have the kids three or four nights a week and won't help them or supervise their homework. He will let them play video games all night.
APPN:	Umm, and you're helpless to change what happens?
Joy:	[Joy still speaking as her anxiety with her voice rising.] Yes, here I have all the control, especially with the children. I can make sure the kids are well cared for. If I leave, I have absolutely no control over what happens.
APPN:	Umm, so scary … yet, in some ways you have not taken charge of your life and have surrendered control in not deciding and in living a life that is very unhappy and inauthentic.
Joy:	Yes, I am dying in this relationship and I have given up control of my life in an attempt to protect the children—control how the children are taken care of. [Joy becomes tearful and cries.]
APPN:	If you had a wise fairy godmother right now, what would she say to you?
Joy:	[Joy speaks in the pert, matter-of-fact voice of a spunky, intelligent old woman.] Now dearie, just dry those lovely tears. Let them wash away your fear. It can't be half as bad to go as staying. Besides your children's well-being is best served by an emotionally whole mother.
APPN:	How does that feel to hear?
Joy:	[Sighs heavily] I feel supported, like I have the answers right inside me.

These brief session dialogues from the work with Joy illustrate some of the ways the APPN would work with a patient in individual therapy. An integration of several humanistic–existential and SFT therapeutic interventions were used throughout the dialogue.

POST-MASTER'S HUMANISTIC–EXISTENTIAL PSYCHOTHERAPY TRAINING AND CERTIFICATION REQUIREMENTS

Considerable training is necessary in order to conduct humanistic–existential psycho-therapy effectively (Greenberg & Goldman, 1988). Experiential learning in a group setting, where theory and practice are interwoven throughout the training experience, is at the heart of humanistic–existential psychotherapy training and serves to differentiate it from other major schools of psychotherapy training (Feder & Ronall, 1980; Knight, 1996). Trainers may sometimes bring their own patients to training sessions for trainees to observe, but typically, trainees observe experienced trainers conducting live therapy sessions with patients culled from the training group. Trainees also conduct live therapeutic sessions in the training group where they work as therapists, patients, and supervisors. Although reading lists, watching master psychotherapists on videotapes, and supervision with trainees' own patients are typically part of organized training programs, theoretical concepts are taught primarily through informal lectures and processing experiential work in the here and now, rather than talking about therapy sessions that occur outside the group. Individual therapy is usually included as part of the training as well (Bohart, 1995; Gladfelter, 1997; Greenberg & Goldman, 1988; Greenberg, Rice, & Elliott, 1993; Kerfoot, 1998; Wiseman, 1998).

Organized training programs are found in private, postgraduate training institutes, approximately 2 to 4 years in length. Intensive weekend and summer programs are also available at most institutes. There are no national certifying exams in humanistic–existential therapy. Institutes generally provide a certificate of completion and place their graduate's name on their website for referral purposes. Leading humanistic–existential and SFT institutes are listed in Box 6.6.

There are many associations throughout the world for the humanistic–existential therapies. The following two are highly recommended:

- Association for Humanistic Psychology, Alameda, CA, www.ahpweb.org
- Division of Humanistic Psychology (Division 32), American Psychological Association, Washington, DC, www.apa.org

BOX 6.6 Leading Humanistic–Existential and Solution-Focused Therapy Institutes

- Association for the Development of the Person Centered Approach, Chicago, IL, www.adpca.org
- Center for the Studies of the Person (CSP), La Jolla, CA, www.centerfortheperson.org
- World Association for Person Centered & Experiential Psychotherapy & Counseling, Monmouth, UK, www.pce-world.org
- Focusing Institute, Spring Valley, NY, www.focusing.org
- Carl Rogers Institute for Patient-Centered Therapy, Chicago, IL, www.thenewcenterchicago.com
- Gestalt Institute of Cleveland, Cleveland, OH, www.gestaltcleveland.org
- Gestalt Center for Psychotherapy and Training, New York, NY, www.gestaltnyc.org
- Gestalt Therapy Institute of Philadelphia, Philadelphia, PA, www.gestaltphila.org
- Gestalt Therapy Institute of Los Angeles, Los Angeles, CA, www.gatla.org
- New York Institute for Gestalt Therapy, New York, NY, www.newyorkgestalt.org
- Existential-Humanistic Institute, San Francisco, CA, ehinstitute.org
- International Institute for Humanistic Studies, Petaluma, CA, www.human-studies.com
- International Collaborative of Existential Counsellors and Psychotherapists, London, UK, www.icecap.org.uk
- Emotion-Focused Therapy Clinic, Toronto, Ont., Canada, www.emotionfocusedclinic.org
- Institute for Psychotherapy Training & Supervision, Flemington, NJ, www.parkplacepractice.com
- Institute for Solution Focused Therapy, Chicago, IL, and Sturgeon Bay, WI, www.solutionfocusedinstitute.com
- Solution-Focused Brief Therapy Association, www.sfbta.org

CONCLUDING COMMENTS

This chapter provides an overview of humanistic–existential therapy and SFT, highlighting the importance of these approaches for the APPN. It explicates five major psychotherapeutic approaches (person centered, Gestalt, existential, emotion focused, and solution focused), describing their key concepts, goals, interventions, and evidence-based research. It includes a case study with patient–therapist dialogue as well as information on how to obtain postgraduate training. It is hoped that the chapter gives the reader a solid introduction to the rich field of humanistic–existential psychotherapy and that the reader will want to learn more and continue training in these powerful approaches. There are other approaches to humanistic–existential therapy not mentioned in this chapter such as redecision therapy, actualizing therapy, transactional analysis, and focusing. It is suggested that the APPN explore these other types of humanistic–existential approaches as well. For a comprehensive compilation of humanistic–existential approaches, two texts are recommended for the APPN new to these approaches: (a) Cain and Seeman's *Humanistic Psychotherapies: Handbook of Research and Practice* (2002) and (b) Schneider, Bugental, and Pierson's *The Handbook of Humanistic Psychology: Leading Edges in Theory, Research, and Practice* (2001). Original texts are highly recommended for the advanced practitioners and can be found in the reference list.

DISCUSSION QUESTIONS

1. What are the similarities and differences among the four major humanistic–existential approaches (e.g., person centered, Gestalt, existential, and EFT) discussed in this chapter?
2. Why is it important for the APPN to have theoretical knowledge and clinical competency in the three facilitative conditions: unconditional positive regard, congruence, and empathic understanding?
3. Identify one existential theme that you commonly find in your work with patients and explain how the theme would be addressed in an existential approach.
4. Gestalt therapy is based on a natural theory of organismic self-regulation. Explain how this flow can be interrupted.
5. EFT uses in-session markers to determine interventions. Select a marker and explain how you would intervene.
6. SFT is based on the philosophy of postmodernism and social constructionism. How are these philosophies similar to humanism and existentialism?
7. SFT has specific solution-oriented questions that are used as therapeutic interventions. Select one question and prepare a patient–therapist dialogue reflecting a positive outcome.
8. Which humanistic–existential therapy approach do you find the most interesting and hope to further explore? Why?

REFERENCES

Axline, V. M. (1947/1992). *Play therapy.* New York, NY: Churchill Livingstone.

Barber, P. (2006). *Becoming a practitioner researcher: A gestalt approach to holistic inquiry.* London, UK: Middlesex University Press.

Barker, M. (2011). Existential sex therapy. *Sexual and Relationship Therapy, 26*(1), 33–47. doi:10 .1080/14681991003685879

Berg, I. K., & Dolan, Y. (2001). *Tales of solutions: A collection of hope-inspiring stories*. New York, NY: W. W. Norton.

Berg, I. K., & Miller, S. D. (1992). *Working with the problem drinker: A solution-focused approach*. New York, NY: W. W. Norton.

Bohart, A. C. (1995). The person-centered psychotherapies. In A. S. Gurman & S. B. Messer (Eds.), *Essential psychotherapies* (pp. 85–127). New York, NY: Guilford Press.

Bohart, A. C., & Watson, J. C. (2011). Person-centered psychotherapy and related experiential approaches. In S. B. Messer & A. S. Gurman (Eds.), *Essential psychotherapies: Theory and practice* (3rd ed., pp. 223–260). New York, NY: Guilford Press.

Brice, A. (2011). "If I go back, they'll kill me…" Person-centered therapy with lesbian and gay clients. *Person-Centered & Experiential Psychotherapies*, 10(4), 248–259. doi:10.1080/14779757.2011.626624

Brownell, P. (2008). *Handbook for theory, research and practice in gestalt therapy*. Newcastle, UK: Cambridge Scholar Publishing.

Buber, M. (1937). *I and thou*. New York, NY: Scribner & Sons.

Bugental, J. F. T. (1965). *The search for authenticity: An existential-analytic approach to psychotherapy*. New York, NY: Holt, Rinehart, & Winston.

Bugental, J. F. T. (1987). *The art of the psychotherapist*. New York, NY: W. W. Norton.

Bugental, J. F. T. (1996). Rollo May (1909–1994). *American Psychologist*, 51, 418–419. doi:10.1037/0003-066X.51.4.418

Cain, D. J. (2010). *Person-centered psychotherapies*. Washington, DC: American Psychological Association.

Cain, D. J., & Seeman, J. (Eds.). (2002). *Humanistic psychotherapies: Handbook of research and practice*. Washington, DC: American Psychological Association.

Carrera, M., Cabero, A., Gonzalez, S., Rodriguez, N., Garcia, C., Hernandez, L., & Manjon, J. (2016). Solution-focused group therapy for common mental health problems: Outcome assessment in routine clinical practice. *Psychology and Psychotherapy: Theory, Research and Practice*, 89, 294–307. doi:10.1111/papt.12085

Clance, P. R., Thompson, M. B., Simerly, D. E., & Weiss, A. (1994). The effects of the gestalt approach on body image. *The Gestalt Journal*, 17, 95–114.

Cook, J. M., Biyanova, T., & Coyne, J. C. (2009). Influential psychotherapy figures, authors, and books: An internet survey of over 2,000 psychotherapists. *Psychotherapy: Research, Practice, Training*, 46(1), 42–51. doi:10.1037/a0015152

Corey, G. (2011). *Theory and practice of counseling and psychotherapy* (9th ed.). Belmont, CA: Brooks/Cole.

Correia, E. A., Cooper, M., & Berdondini, L. (2016). Existential therapy institutions worldwide: An update of data and the extensive list. *Existential Analysis*, 27(1), 155–200.

De Jong, P., & Berg, I. K. (2008). *Interviewing for solutions* (3rd ed.). Belmont, CA: Brooks/Cole, Cengage Learning.

de Shazer, S. (1985). *Keys to solution in brief therapy*. New York, NY: W. W. Norton.

de Shazer, S. (1988). *Clues: Investigating solutions in brief therapy*. New York, NY: W. W. Norton.

de Shazer, S. (1991). *Putting difference to work*. New York, NY: W. W. Norton.

de Shazer, S. (1994). *Words were originally magic*. New York, NY: W. W. Norton.

Duncan, B. L., Miller, S. D., Wampold, B. E., & Hubble, M. A. (Eds.). (2010). *The heart and soul of change* (2nd ed.). Washington, DC: American Psychological Association.

Elliott, R. (2002). The effectiveness of humanistic therapies: A meta-analysis. In D. J. Cain & J. Seeman (Eds.), *Humanistic psychotherapies: Handbook of research and practice*. Washington, DC: American Psychological Association.

Elliott, R., Bohart, A. C., Watson, J. C., & Greenberg, L. S. (2011). Empathy. In J. C. Norcross (Ed.), *Psychotherapy relationships that work: Evidence-based responsiveness* (2nd ed., pp. 132–152). New York, NY: Oxford University Press.

Elliott, R., Greenberg, L. S., Goldman, R. N., & Angus, L. (2009). Maintenance of gains following experiential therapies for depression. *Journal of Consulting and Clinical Psychology*, 77, 103–112. doi:10.1037/a0014653

Elliott, R., Greenberg, L. S., & Lietaer, G. (2004). Research on experiential psychotherapies. In M. J. Lambert (Ed.), *Bergin & Garfield's handbook of psychotherapy and behavior change* (5th ed., pp. 493–539). New York, NY: Wiley.

Farber, E. W. (2009). Existentially informed HIV-related psychotherapy. *Psychotherapy, Theory, Research, Practice, Training, 46*(3), 336–349. doi:10.1037/a0016916

Feder, B., & Ronall, R. (Eds.). (1980). *Beyond the hot seat: Gestalt approaches to group* (pp. 167–175). New York, NY: Brunner/Mazel.

Frankl, V. (1963). *Man's search for meaning: An introduction to logotherapy.* New York, NY: Pocket Books.

Gendlin, E. (1981). *Focusing.* New York, NY: Random House.

Gergen, K. (1985). The social constructionist movement in modern psychology. *American Psychologist, 40*, 266–275. doi:10.1037/0003-066X.40.3.266

Gergen, K. (1999). *An invitation to social construction.* Newbury Park, CA: Sage.

Gladfelter, J. (1997). Training redecision therapists. In C. Lennox (Ed.), *Redecision therapy: A brief action-oriented approach* (pp. 289–298). Northvale, NJ: Jason Aronson.

Gonzalez, C. (2017). Recovering process from child sexual abuse during adulthood from an integrative approach to solution-focused therapy. *Journal of Child Sexual Abuse, 26*(7), 785–805. doi:10.1080/10538712.2017.1354954

Greenberg, E. (2015). A new look at the treatment of schizophrenia from a gestalt therapy perspective. *Gestalt Review, 19*(1), 2–7. doi:10.5325/gestaltreview.19.1.0002

Greenberg, L. S. (1979). Resolving splits: Use of the two-chair technique. *Psychotherapy: Theory, Research & Practice, 16*, 316–324. doi:10.1037/h0085895

Greenberg, L. S. (1986). Change process research. *Journal of Consulting and Clinical Psychology, 54*, 4–9. doi:10.1037/0022-006X.54.1.4

Greenberg, L. S. (1991). Research on the process of change. *Psychotherapy Research, 1*, 3–16. doi:10.1080/10503309112331334011

Greenberg, L. S. (2010). Emotion-focused therapy: A clinical synthesis. *Focus: The Journal of Lifelong Learning in Psychiatry, 8*, 32–42. doi:10.1176/foc.8.1.foc32

Greenberg, L. S. (2011). *Emotion-focused therapy.* Washington, DC: American Psychological Association.

Greenberg, L. S., & Goldman, R. L. (1988). Training in experiential therapy. *Journal of Consulting and Clinical Psychology, 56*, 696–702. doi:10.1037/0022-006X.56.5.696

Greenberg, L. S., & Rice, L. N. (1997). Humanistic approaches to psychotherapy. In P. L. Wachtel & S. B. Messer (Eds.), *Theories of psychotherapy* (pp. 97–128). Washington, DC: American Psychological Association.

Greenberg, L. S., Rice, L. N., & Elliott, R. (1993). *Facilitating emotional change: The moment-by-moment process.* New York, NY: Guilford Press.

Heidegger, M. (1962). *Being and time.* New York, NY: Harper & Row.

Husserl, E. (1925). *Phenomenological psychology* (J. Scanlon, Trans.). The Hague, Netherlands: Martinus Nijhoff.

Jordan, B., Perryman, K., & Anderson, L. (2013). A case for child-centered play therapy with natural disaster and catastrophic event survivors. *International Journal of Play Therapy, 22*(4), 219–230. doi:10.1037/a0034637

Kendler, H. (1986). *Historical foundations of modern psychology.* Belmont, CA: Brooks/Cole.

Kerfoot, E. M. (1998). TART: Redecision therapy training in academia. *Journal of Redecision Therapy, 1*, 80–93.

Kirschenbaum, H., & Jourdan, A. (2005). The current status of Carl Rogers and person-centered approach. *Psychotherapy: Theory, Research, Practice, Training, 42*(1), 37–51. doi:10.1037/0033-3204.42.1.37

Knight, C. (1996). *A Gestalt therapy training manual.* Flemington, NJ: Center for Gestalt Therapy.

Kvale, S. (1992). *Psychology and postmodernism.* London, UK: Sage.

Lemoire, S. J., & Chen, C. P. (2005). Applying person-centered counseling to sexual minority adolescents. *Journal of Counseling & Development, 83*, 146–154. doi:10.1002/j.1556-6678.2005.tb00591.x

Maslow, A. H. (1962). *Toward a psychology of being.* Princeton, NJ: Van Nostrand.

May, R., Angel, E., & Ellenberger, H. F. (Eds.). (1958). *Existence: A new dimension in psychiatry and psychology.* New York, NY: Basic Books.

Miller, W. R., & Rollnick, S. (2002). *Motivational interviewing: preparing people for change* (2nd ed.). New York, NY: Guilford Press.

Mundorf, E. S., & Paivio, S. C. (2011). Narrative quality and disturbance pre- and post-emotion-focused therapy for child abuse trauma. *Journal of Traumatic Stress, 24*(6), 643–650. doi:10.1002/jts.20707

Nazari, I., Mohammadi, M, & Nazeri, G. (2014). Effectiveness of Gestalt therapy on PTSD symptoms on veterans of Yasuj City. *Amaghane Danesh Journal, 19*(4), 295–304.

Nevis, E. (1987). *Organizational consulting: A Gestalt approach*. New York, NY: Gardner Press.

Oaklander, V. (1978). *Windows to our children: A gestalt therapy approach*. Gouldsboro, ME: Gestalt Journal Press.

Paivio, S. C., & Greenberg, L. S. (1995). Resolving "unfinished business": Efficacy of experiential therapy using empty-chair dialogue. *Journal of Consulting and Clinical Psychology, 63*, 419–425. doi:10.1037/0022-006X.63.3.419

Paivio, S. C., & Pascual-Leone, A. (2010). *Emotion-focused therapy for complex trauma: An integrative approach*. Washington, DC: American Psychological Association.

Pakrosnis, R., & Cepukiene, V. (2015). Solution-focused self-help for improving university students' well-being. *Innovations in Education and Teaching International, 52*(4), 437–447. doi: 10.1080/14703297.2014.930352

Paterson, J. G., & Zderad, L. T. (1988). *Humanistic nursing*. New York, NY: National League for Nursing.

Perls, F. S. (1942). *Ego, hunger and aggression: A revision of Freud's theory and method*. New York, NY: Gestalt Journal Press.

Perls, F. S. (1969). *Gestalt therapy verbatim*. Highland, NY: Gestalt Journal Press.

Perls, F. S. (1973). *The Gestalt approach and eyewitness to therapy*. New York, NY: Science and Behavior Books.

Perls, F. S., Hefferline, R., & Goodman, P. (1951). *Gestalt therapy: Excitement and growth in the human personality*. Highland, NY: Gestalt Journal Press.

Polster, E., & Polster, M. (1973). *Gestalt therapy integrated*. New York, NY: Vintage Books.

Quinn, A. (2011). A person-centered approach to the treatment of borderline personality disorder. *Journal of Humanistic Psychology, 51*(4), 465–491. doi:10.1177/0022167811399764

Reisberg, B., Shao, Y., Golomb, J., Monteiro, I., Torossian, C., Boksay, I., … Kenowsky, S. (2017). Comprehensive, individualized, person-centered management of community-residing persons with moderate-to-severe Alzheimer's disease: A randomized controlled trial. *Dementia Geriatrics Cognitive Disorders, 43*(1–2), 100–117. doi:10.1159/000455397

Resnikoff, R. (1995). Gestalt family therapy. *The Gestalt Journal, 18*(2), 55–76.

Robinson, A. (2018). Emotion-focused therapy for autism spectrum disorder: A case conceptualization model for trauma-related experiences. *Journal of Contemporary Psychotherapy, 48*, 133–143. doi:10.1007/s10879-018-9383-1

Rogers, C. R. (1942). *Counselling and psychotherapy: Newer concepts in practice*. Boston, MA: Houghton Mifflin.

Rogers, C. R. (1951). *Client-centered therapy: Its current practice, implications, and theory*. Boston, MA: Houghton Mifflin.

Rogers, C. R. (1957). The necessary and sufficient conditions of therapeutic personality change. *Journal of Consulting Psychology, 21*, 95–103. doi:10.1037/h0045357

Rogers, C. R. (1961). *On becoming a person*. Boston, MA: Houghton Mifflin.

Rogers, C. R. (1980). *A way of being*. Boston, MA: Houghton Mifflin.

Rogers, N. (1993). *The creative connection: Expressive arts as healing*. Palo Alto, CA: Science & Behavior Books.

Root, R. W. (1996). The Gestalt cycle of experience as a theoretical framework for conceptualizing the attention deficit disorder. *The Gestalt Journal, 19*, 9–50.

Schneider, K. J. (Ed.). (2008). *Existential-integrative psychotherapy: Guide posts to the core of practice*. New York, NY: Routledge.

Schneider, K. J. (2009). *Awakening to awe: Personal stories of profound transformation*. Lanham, MD: Jason Aronson.

Schneider, K. J., Bugental, J. F. T., & Pierson, J. F. (Eds.). (2001). *The handbook of humanistic psychology: Leading edges in theory, research, and practice*. Thousand Oaks, CA: Sage.

Schneider, K. J., & Greening, T. (2009). James F. T. Bugental (1915–2008). *American Psychologist, 64*, 151. doi:10.1037/a0014551

Schutzmann, K., Schutzmann, M., & Eckert, J. (2010). The efficacy of outpatient client-centered psychothereapy for bulimia nervosa: Results of a randomized controlled trial. *Psychotherapy, Psychosomatic Medicine Psychology, 60*(2), 52–63. doi:10.1055/s-0029-1234134

Shumaker, D. (2012). An existential-integrative treatment of anxious and depressed adolescents. *Journal of Humanistic Psychology, 52*(4), 375–400. doi:10.1177/0022167811422947

Smuts, J. (1926). *Holism and evolution*. New York, NY: Macmillan.

Stephen, S., Elliott, R., & Macleod, R. (2011). Person-centred therapy with a client experiencing social anxiety difficulties: A hermeneutic single case efficacy design. *Counselling and Psychotherapy Research, 11*(1), 55–66. doi:10.1080/14733145.2011.546203

Teusch, L., Bohme, H., Fink, J., & Gastpar, M. (2001). Effects of client-centered psychotherapy for personality disorders alone and in combination with psychopharmacological treatment. *Psychotherapy and Psychosomatics, 70,* 328–336. doi:10.1159/000056273

Teusch, L., Bohme, H., Fink, J., Gastpar, M., & Skerra, B. (2003). Antidepressant medication and the assimilation of problematic experiences in psychotherapy. *Psychotherapy Research, 13*(3), 307–322. doi:10.1093/ptr/kpg029

Taghvaeinia, A., Dehghani, F., Jobaneh, R. G., & Nikoo, S. J. (2017). Effectiveness of existential psychotherapy on spiritual health of infertile women. *Health, Spirituality and Medical Ethics, 4*(4), 13–17. Retrieved from http://jhsme.muq.ac.ir/article-1-140-en.html

Timm, N., & Garza, Y. (2017). Beyond the miniatures: Using gestalt theory in sandtray processing. *Gestalt Review, 21*(1), 44–55. doi:10.5325/gestaltreview.21.1.0044

Travelbee, J. (1971). *Interpersonal aspects of nursing*. Philadelphia, PA: F. A. Davis.

Von Humboldt, S., & Leal, I. (2013). The promotion of older adults' sense of coherence through person-centered therapy: A randomized controlled pilot study. *Interdisciplinaria, 30*(2), 235–251. doi:10.16888/interd.2013.30.2.4

Von Humboldt, S., & Leal, I. (2015). Disclosing the challenges of older clients in person-centered therapy: The client's perspective. *Person-Centered & Experiential Psychotherapies, 14*(3), 248–261. doi:10.1080/14779757.2015.1058290

Wampold, B. E. (2001). *The great psychotherapy debate: Models, methods, and findings*. Mahwah, NJ: Lawrence Erlbaum Associates.

Watson, J. (2011). *Human caring science: A theory of nursing* (2nd ed.). Sudbury, MA: Jones & Bartlett.

Watson, J. C., Goldman, N., & Greenberg, L. S. (2007). *Case studies in emotion-focused treatment of depression*. Washington, DC: American Psychological Association.

Watson, J. C., Gordon, L. B., Stermac, L., Kalogerakos, F., & Steckley, P. (2003). Comparing the effectiveness of process-experiential with cognitive-behavioral psychotherapy in the treatment of depression. *Journal of Consulting and Clinical Psychology, 71,* 773–781. doi:10.1037/0022-006X.71.4.773

Wheeler, G. (1991). *Gestalt reconsidered: A new approach to contact and resistance*. New York, NY: Gardner Press.

Wiseman, H. (1998). Training counselors in the process-experiential approach. *British Journal of Guidance & Counselling, 26,* 105–118. doi:10.1080/03069889808253842

Yalom, I. D. (1980). *Existential psychotherapy*. New York, NY: Basic Books.

Yalom, I. (2005). *The theory and practice of group psychotherapy* (5th ed.). New York, NY: Basic Books.

Yontef, G. M. (1993). *Awareness, process and dialogue: Essays on gestalt therapy*. Highland, NY: Gestalt Journal Press.

Zinker, J. (1977). *Creative process in gestalt therapy*. New York, NY: Vintage Books.

Eye Movement Desensitization and Reprocessing Therapy

Kathleen Wheeler

This chapter discusses eye movement desensitization and reprocessing (EMDR) therapy, the only major evidence-based psychotherapy that has emerged with the explicit goal of neural network integration. Although other therapies, such as psychodynamic or humanistic–existential therapy, can involve processing because implicit memories are accessed and new information is learned, EMDR has been developed specifically for the purpose of processing adverse life experiences and traumatic events with the goal of neural network integration. EMDR is both a psychotherapy approach on its own as well as a psychotherapy that can be integrated into other psychotherapy models such as cognitive behavioral, transpersonal, family, psychodynamic, experiential, feminist, hypnosis, schema-focused, and behavioral therapies (Shapiro, 2018) as an adjunct to treatment. This chapter begins with an introduction to EMDR and presents evidence-based research. Stabilization and processing are discussed along with general guidelines for processing. The eight-phase protocol for EMDR is described and a case example illustrates the use of EMDR. The chapter ends with information about post-master's EMDR certification.

WHAT IS EMDR THERAPY?

EMDR therapy has emerged in the past two decades as one of the most innovative and effective approaches to treat symptoms of adverse life experiences and trauma. Dr. Francine Shapiro, a brilliant visionary, humanitarian, and psychologist, developed eye movement desensitization (EMD) in the late 1980s as a behavioral technique to treat posttraumatic stress disorder (PTSD). Subsequently EMDR evolved, as it became apparent that more than desensitization occurred and that dysfunctional memories were actually being reprocessed (Shapiro, 1991). EMDR therapy is now viewed as an integrative eight-phase psychotherapy based on a comprehensive three-pronged approach that includes earlier life experience, present-day stressor (i.e., triggers), and desired thoughts and actions for the future. The therapist guides the patient in processing affective, cognitive, and somatic material with procedures and protocols that include some form of bilateral stimulation (BLS) during a session. The BLS may take the form of eyes moving horizontally back and forth, sounds alternating in each ear, or alternate tapping on each hand or knee. The goal is to bring the trauma to an adaptive resolution.

Research indicates that trauma involves right-brain processing and most psychotherapy is a left-brain endeavor, so there may be areas that talk therapy does not reach.

Processing in EMDR therapy seems to rapidly connect left-brain ways of processing information with emotional right-brain information. Both limbic and prefrontal changes have been found in brain scans after EMDR treatment; that is, the prefrontal cortex shows increased activation with increased inhibition of the amygdala so that patients with PTSD are less hyperaroused and have fewer symptoms of flashbacks and hallucinations (Pagani, Högberg, Fernandez, & Siracusano, 2013). In addition, functional MRI studies have found an increase in hippocampal volume after PTSD patients are treated with EMDR (Bossini et al., 2012). These neurobiological changes correspond with significant clinical improvement in PTSD symptoms. EMDR therapy is the only evidence-based trauma psychotherapy that includes a somatic component that provides therapists the ability to access all dimensions of memory.

Evidence-Based Research

EMDR therapy has a solid research base demonstrating effectiveness in treating PTSD with over 44 randomized clinical trials (RCTs) and 28 RCTs supporting EMDR therapy's use in other disorders including major depression, bipolar disorder, substance use, anxiety disorders, psychosis, and pain (Maxfield, 2019). See Table 7.1 for selected meta-analysis. EMDR therapy is included in many practice guidelines for the treatment and processing of trauma (see Box 7.1). Researchers and clinicians have developed and researched EMDR protocols for a wide variety of clinical problems and diagnoses such as combat trauma, anxiety disorders, depression, unresolved grief, medical trauma, dissociative disorders, chemical dependency, eating disorders, and somatic problems. Please see Table 7.2 for some populations that have been successfully treated with EMDR therapy. EMDR therapy protocols for many different clinical problems are published in Luber's manuals (2010a, 2010b, 2014, 2016a, 2016b, 2019a, 2019b).

Studies of single trauma, in contrast to complex multiple trauma, indicate a 77% to 100% remission of PTSD after three to six EMDR sessions (Lee, Gavriel, Drummond, Richards, & Greenwald, 2002). When comparing trauma-focused cognitive behavioral therapy (TF-CBT), the other Level A treatment for PSTD, with EMDR therapy, both are considered effective. "Like CBT with a trauma focus, EMDR therapy aims to reduce subjective distress and strengthen adaptive beliefs related to the traumatic event. Unlike CBT with a trauma focus, EMDR therapy does not involve (a) detailed descriptions of the event, (b) direct challenging of beliefs, (c) extended exposure, or (d) homework" (World Health Organization, 2013, p. 1). EMDR is less time intensive (Ironson, Freund, Strauss, & Williams 2002, Lee et al., 2002; Power et al., 2002; Rothbaum, Astin, & Marsteller, 2005; Taylor et al., 2003), treatment effects are long lasting (J. G. Carlson, Chemtob, Rusnak, Hedlund, & Muraoka, 1998; van der Kolk et al., 2007; Wilson, Becker, & Tinker, 1997), and dropout rates are significantly lower for EMDR therapy than for TF-CBT (J. G. Carlson et al., 1998; Congressional Budget Office, 2012).

Mechanism of Action

The exact mechanism of action is unclear just as any other psychotherapy's action is unclear. However, because EMDR therapy is such an unusual and powerful therapy, there has been much speculation about how it works. EMDR therapy was the first psychotherapy to demonstrate a neurophysiological effect, that of altered brain wave activity in response to treatment (Pagani et al., 2013). There are five hypotheses about how and why EMDR therapy works. (a) It is thought that the dual attention stimulation that is required during EMDR facilitates interhemispheric connection and jumpstarts the natural information processing system. Cozolino (2017) agrees and says that the activation in both temporal lobes with the BLS enhances neural network connectivity and the

TABLE 7.1 EMDR RESEARCH: META-ANALYSES

Author	Study	Results
Bisson and Andrew (2007)	Psychological treatment for PTSD	Trauma-focused CBT and EMDR have the best evidence for efficacy at present and should be made available to PTSD sufferers.
Bradley, Greene, Russ, Dutra, and Westen (2005)	A multidimensional meta-analysis of psychotherapy for PTSD	EMDR is equivalent to exposure and other cognitive behavioral treatments. It should be noted that exposure therapy uses 1 to 2 hours of daily homework and EMDR uses none.
Y.-R. Chen et al. (2014)	Efficacy of EMDR for patients with PTSD	EMDR therapy significantly reduces the symptoms of PTSD, depression, anxiety, and subjective distress in PTSD patients.
R. Chen et al. (2018)	Efficacy of EMDR in complex trauma	EMDR significantly reduced PTSD symptoms, depression, and/or anxiety compared to CBT and other therapies.
Davidson and Parker (2001)	A meta-analysis of EMDR	EMDR is equivalent to exposure and other CBT treatments. Exposure uses 1 to 2 hours of daily homework and EMDR uses none.
Ho and Lee (2012)	CBT vs. EMDR for PTSD	No difference between EMDR and TF-CBT on PTSD; EMDR better at reducing depression plus no homework for EMDR.
Khan et al. (2018)	CBT vs. EMDR with PTSD	EMDR better than CBT in reducing PTSD and in reducing anxiety but not depression.
Lee and Cuijpers (2013)	Meta-analysis of the contribution of eye movements	Effect size for eye movements was moderate and significant for one group and large and significant for second group
Maxfield and Hyer (2002)	Relationship between efficacy and methodology in studies investigating EMDR for PTSD	Meta-analysis reported that the more rigorous the study, the larger the effect.
Rodenburg, Benjamin, de Roos, Meijer, and Stams (2009)	Efficacy of EMDR in children: a meta-analysis	Results indicate efficacy of EMDR when effect sizes are based on comparisons between EMDR and nonestablished trauma treatment or no-treatment control groups, and incremental efficacy when effect sizes are based on comparisons between EMDR and established (CBT) trauma treatment.

(continued)

TABLE 7.1 EMDR RESEARCH: META-ANALYSES (*CONTINUED*)

Author	Study	Results
Seidler and Wagner (2006)	Comparing the efficacy of EMDR and trauma-focused CBT in the treatment of PTSD: a meta-analytic study	Supports use of EMDR and Narrative Exposure Therapy for PTSD.
Thompson, Vidgen, and Roberts, (2018)	Efficacy of interventions for refugee and asylum seekers	CBT and EMDR are both effective.
Watts et al. (2013)	Meta-analysis of efficacy of treatments for PTSD	Results suggest that in the treatment of PTSD, both therapy methods tend to be equally efficacious.

CBT, cognitive behavioral therapy; EMDR, eye movement desensitization and reprocessing; PTSD, posttraumatic stress disorder; TF-CBT, trauma-focused cognitive behavioral therapy.

integration of traumatic memories into normal information processing. (b) Accessing adaptive information and integration of memory networks has been linked to the processes of rapid eye movement (REM) sleep, and there is some empirical support for this explanation for EMDR therapy (Shapiro, 2018; Stickgold, 2008). (c) The BLS that is part of the EMDR protocol promotes the dual attention to internal and external stimulation. Thus, this is thought to disarm arousal by coupling attention to the disturbing dimensions of the memory (internal stimulation) with attendant relaxation that occurs with BLS (external stimulation) allowing the linkage of dysfunctional material with more adaptive memory networks. (d) The working memory hypothesis explains that the dual attention in EMDR therapy requires people to divide their attention between the BLS and an aversive memory so that the aversive memory becomes reconsolidated and less emotionally salient and vivid than previously. (e) A more recent explanation based on the earlier models and research on eye movements and neurophysiological studies of PTSD involves activation of the default mode network and cerebellum. Thus, this model emphasizes the cerebellum's role in associative learning, memory reconsolidation, and event-timing (Calancie, Khalid-Khan, Booij, & Munoz, 2018).

BOX 7.1 International Practice Guidelines

American Psychiatric Association. (2004). *Practice guideline for the treatment of patients with acute stress disorder and posttraumatic stress disorder*. Arlington, VA: American Psychiatric Publishing. Retrieved from https://psychiatryonline.org/pb/assets/raw/site-wide/practice_guidelines/guidelines/acutestressdisorderptsd.pdf

Bleich, A., Kotler, M., Kutz, I., & Shalev, A. (2002). *A position paper of the (Israeli) National Council for Mental Health: Guidelines for the assessment and professional intervention with terror victims in the hospital and in the community*. Jerusalem, Israel : Israeli National Council for Mental Health.

Bisson, J. I., Roberts, N. P., Andrew, M., Cooper, R., & Lewis, C. (2013). Psychological therapies for chronic post-traumatic stress disorder (PTSD) in adults. *Cochrane Database of Systematic Reviews*, (12), CD003388. doi:10.1002/14651858.CD003388.pub4

(continued)

BOX 7.1 International Practice Guidelines (*continued*)

Clinical Resource Efficiency Support Team. (2003). *The management of post-traumatic stress disorder in adults*. Belfast, Northern Ireland: Author. Retrieved from http://www. spitjudms.ro/_files/protocoale_terapeutice/psihiatrie/managementul%20stresului%20 posttraumatic.pdf

Department of Veterans Affairs & Department of Defense. (2017). *VA/DoD clinical practice guideline for the management of post traumatic stress* disorder and acute stress disorder. Washington, DC: Author. Retrieved from https://www.healthquality.va.gov/ guidelines/MH/ptsd/VADoDPTSDCPGClinicianSummaryFinal.pdf

Dutch National Steering Committee Guidelines Mental Health Care (2003). *Multidisciplinary guideline: Anxiety disorders*. Utrecht, the Netherlands: Quality Institute Heath Care CBO/Trimbos Institute.

Foa, E. B., Keane, T. M., Friedman, M. J., & Cohen, J. A. (Eds.). (2009). *Effective treatments for PTSD: Practice Guidelines from the International Society for Traumatic Stress Studies*. (2nd ed.) New York, NY: Guilford Press.

INSERM Collective Expertise Centre. (2004). *Psychotherapy: Three approaches evaluated*. Paris, France: French National Institute of Health and Medical Research. Retrieved from https://www.ncbi.nlm.nih.gov/books/NBK7123.

International Society of Traumatic Stress Studies Guidelines Committee. (2019). *Posttraumatic stress disorder prevention and treatment guidelines: Methodology and recommendations*. Retrieved from https://istss.org/getattachment/Treating-Trauma/New-ISTSS-Prevention-and-Treatment-Guidelines/ISTSS_Prevention TreatmentGuidelines_FNL-March-19-2019.pdf.aspx

National Institute for Health and Care Excellence. (2018). *Post-traumatic stress disorder*. Retrieved from https://www.nice.org.uk/guidance/ng116

World Health Organization. (2013). *Guidelines for the management of conditions that are specifically related to stress*. Geneva, Switzerland: Author. Retrieved from https://apps.who.int/iris/bitstream/handle/10665/85119/9789241505406_eng.pdf? sequence=1

TABLE 7.2 EMDR CLINICAL APPLICATIONS

Population	Selected Research Studies
Acute trauma/PTSD	Y.-R. Chen et al. (2014); van der Kolk et al. (2007); Tofani and Wheeler (2011); van den Berg and van der Gaag (2012); Rousseau et al. (2019); Van Woudenberg et al. (2018)
Addictions	Abel and O'Brien (2010); Little, van den Hout, and Engelhard (2016); Brown, Gilman, Goodman, Adler-Tapia, and Feng (2015); Knipe, (2019); Bae and Kim (2015); Tapia, (2019)
Anxiety disorders	Faretta and Farra (2019); Rudiger Bohm (2019)
Attachment disorder	Zaccagnino and Cussino (2013); Sukumaran, (2015); Paulsen and O'Shea (2017); Shapiro, Wesselmann, and Mevissen (2017)
Bipolar	Valiente-Gómez et al. (2019)

(*continued*)

TABLE 7.2 EMDR CLINICAL APPLICATIONS (*CONTINUED*)	
Population	**Selected Research Studies**
Pain	Grant, (2016); Marcus, (2008); Tesrarz, Wicking, Bernardy, and Gunter (2019)
Complex trauma	Bongaerts, Van Minnen, and de Jongh (2017)
Depression	Grey, (2011); Ostacoli et al. (2018); Hase et al. (2018)
Dissociative disorders	van der Hart, Groenendijk, Gonzalez, Mosquera, and Solomon (2014); Wong (2019); Knipe (2019)
Eating disorders	Seubert (2018);
First responders, police, firefighters	Behnammoghdam, Kheramine, Zoladi, Cooper, and Shahini (2019); Jarero, Schnaider, and Givaudan (2019); emdrresearchfoundation.org/research-grants/toolkit/
Grief and mourning	Cotter, Meysner, and Lee, (2017); Murray, (2012)
Medical illness	Civilotti et al. (2014); Jarero, Artigas, Uribe, and García (2016); Nia, Afrasiabifar, Behnammoghadam, and Cooper (2019); Broad and Wheeler (2006)
Pedophilia	Ricci (2006), Ricci and Clayton (2016)
Performance anxiety	Barker and Barker (2007); Foster and Lendl (1995, 1996); Graham, (2004); Maxfield and Melnyk (2000); Silverman (2011)
Phantom limb pain	de Roos et al. (2010); Schneider, Hofmann, Rost, and Shapiro (2008); Rostaminejad, Behnammoghadam, Rostaminejad, Behnammoghadam, and Bashti (2017)
Phobias, panic disorder, obsessive-compulsive disorder, and generalized anxiety disorder	de Jongh (2012); Faretta and Leeds (2017); Doering, Ohlmeier, de Jongh, Hofmann, and Bisping (2013); Marsden, Lovell, Blore, Ali, and Delgadillo (2018)
Psychosis	de Bont, de Jongh, and van den Berg (2019); Abel and O'Brien (2010); van den Berg et al. (2015); de Bont, van der Vleugel, et al. (2019)
Sexual assault and victims	Allon (2015); Edmond, Lawrence, and Voth Schrag (2016); Rost, Hofmann, and Wheeler (2009)
Victims of natural and manmade disasters	Fernandez, Callerame, Maslovaric, & Wheeler (2014); Natha and Daiches (2014); E.Shapiro & Laub, (2015)
Victims of family, marital, and sexual dysfunction	Jebelli, Maaroufi, Maracy, and Molaeinezhad (2018); Wong (2018); Okawara and Paulsen (2018)

EMDR, eye movement desensitization and reprocessing; PTSD, posttraumatic stress disorder.

There may be both right and left hemisphere stimulation of attention that triggers the integration of affect with cognition, sensations, and emotion in the brain along with top-down cortical–hippocampal circuits and bottom-up amygdala–cortical activation with subsequent processing. The activation of emotion and the right hemisphere along with the simultaneous activation of the language-based left hemisphere may aid in integration of these functions, thus enhancing the person's ability to gain cognitive perspective and emotional regulation. This multilayered process produces a new information-processing matrix in the brain that is essential for the resolution of trauma and integration of the left hemisphere, which is language based, with the right hemisphere, which contains the somatic and autobiographic components of the self.

Although EMDR therapy contains aspects of numerous psychotherapy approaches, the BLS and the unique components of the EMDR protocol are crucial ingredients for the efficacy of this approach. A meta-analysis of 14 EMDR studies comparing eye movement with no eye movement evaluated the efficacy of eye movements in processing emotional memories with eye movements averaging a significant medium effect size with respect to outcomes over those studies with no eye movements (Lee & Cuijpers, 2013). Thus, contrary to some early classifications of EMDR therapy as a type of CBT, eye movements are essential for the efficacy of EMDR. The mechanism of action for TF-CBT and exposure is different than for EMDR therapy. EMDR strategies include frequent brief exposure to the disturbing memory, interrupted exposure, and free association, while CBT relies on habituation and prolonged exposure, which often creates high levels of anxiety. A meta-analysis of EMDR studies found larger effect sizes for studies that cited use of a treatment manual and that adhered to the EMDR protocol (Maxfield & Hyer, 2002). These studies support the use of eye movements and fidelity to the treatment protocol for best results.

STABILIZATION

Specific stabilization strategies are the focus of Chapter 11, and Chapter 17, as well as inherent in other approaches in this book including CBT, supportive therapy, solution-focused, group, family therapy, and motivational interviewing. Stabilization and resourcing the patient are integral to EMDR especially in Phase 2, the preparation phase. The therapeutic relationship and attunement serve as resources and help to stabilize the person. Patient collaboration and empowerment are integral to all phases of the EMDR protocol. It is crucial to explain to the patient that current symptoms may be driven by experiences from the past, how the present serves as a trigger for these past experiences, and how the therapy can help.

Three general types of resources used in stabilization are identified by Shapiro (2018) and include mastery resources such as patient's memories of past coping, relational resources such as memories of positive role models or supportive others, or symbolic resources from dreams, nature, religion, music, and future positive image(s). EMDR has specific protocols for stabilization and these usually combine imagery, safe place, therapeutic interweaves, and containment exercises with BLS. The person is taught the safe place in the preparation phase in addition to other resource strategies if needed. See Appendix 1.7 for the safe place exercise, Appendix 1.8 for the container exercise, Appendix 7.1 for the lightstream exercise, and Appendix 7.2 for the circle of strength exercise. See Chapter 17, for stabilization strategies, many of which can be combined with or without BLS.

Although EMDR has been most researched for processing trauma, extension of the EMDR protocol for resource development and installation (RDI) has been found to increase stabilization in a series of cases (Korn & Leeds, 2002). RDI is often used to prepare the patient so that positive resources increase affect regulation and coping skills prior to trauma processing. See Table 7.3 for the steps in RDI. If the person has had few positive experiences in his or her life, there may need to be a longer period for resourcing. In general, patients who have suffered complex early trauma need a longer period of stabilization because adaptive memory networks may need to be strengthened and created in order to tolerate processing. However, it should be noted that most patients presenting with PTSD do not need RDI (Leeds, 2006). RDI exercises can be used with or without BLS and should be practiced in the session with the patient as well as at home so that they can be used to assist the person in decreasing hyperarousal at the end of disturbing sessions, as well as other times outside of sessions when disturbing memories may be reexperienced.

Signs that the person is stabilized include no current life crisis, acceptance of the diagnosis, an ability to set and adhere to limits, the ability to identify triggers, ability to self-soothe and to reach out to supportive people, and the ability to communicate honestly with the clinician. In terms of mood stability, the person's mood may be depressed but not labile (Davis & Weiss, 2004). The Stabilization Checklist provided from Chapter 1, in Appendix 1.5 is a general guideline, and not all of these parameters must be met before processing. Clinical judgment is essential in assessing the patient's ability to tolerate processing. Because of the intensity of the experience, the patient must have the ability to maintain a dual awareness during processing and sustain increased arousal with little or no dissociating or avoidance of the content. The person needs to be in the here and now of the therapy session while also in the then and there of the traumatic event. After stabilization has been achieved, the person is ready to move to the next stage, processing.

TABLE 7.3	RESOURCE DEVELOPMENT AND INSTALLATION PROCEDURE	
Step #1	Identify needed resources	Ask the patient what personal positive qualities are needed (confidence, self-worth, patience, etc.)
Step #2	Explore types of resources	Ask for a memory of experiencing that quality or other resources related to that quality
Step #3	Access more information	Ask to access sensory information related to the memory or resource identified in Step #2
Step #4	Check the resource	Check to ensure that the memory/resource is a positive one
Step #5	Install the resource	Ask the patient to focus on memory/resource while experiencing several sets of six to 12 eye movements (or tapping or sounds), and ask the person after each set what they are experiencing

(continued)

TABLE 7.3	RESOURCE DEVELOPMENT AND INSTALLATION PROCEDURE (*CONTINUED*)	
Step #6	Strengthen the resource linking with verbal/sensory cues	Instruct the patient to use words, imagery, and affect to further strengthen the resource
Step #7	Establish a future template	Ask the patient, while experiencing short sets of eye movements, to focus on using the resource in a future situation

Source: Adapted from Shapiro, F. (2001). *Eye movement desensitization and reprocessing (EMDR): Basic principles, protocols, and procedures* (2nd ed.). New York, NY: Guilford Press.

PROCESSING

Processing involves acquiring new learning and connecting adaptive neural networks with dysfunctionally stored information by activating emotions associated with traumatic memories or adverse experiences in tandem with the relaxation induced through BLS. Processing, represented toward the top of the Treatment Hierarchy Triangle see Chapter 1, Figure 1.6, reflects accessing of all dimensions of memory: behaviors, affect, sensations, cognitions, and beliefs associated with the experience (Shapiro, 2018). Current situations activate or trigger unprocessed memories, and the person feels the attending emotions and sensations of the stored memory. The memory that informs the basis of the current problem is called the touchstone memory or event. This may be one event, a Criterion A event for PTSD, or a situation that represents or reflects the origin of the problem. For example, a patient who has an early attachment trauma history may repeatedly be triggered by her relationship with the therapist and expects to be emotionally abused and criticized. In this situation, there is not one specific event but most likely many implicit memories that get activated. Because the therapist is consistently caring and nonjudgmental, this expectation is eventually diminished through counterconditioning through the therapeutic relationship without the person being explicitly aware that this has happened. Chapter 5, describes how to work with and process this type of attachment trauma using psychodynamic psychotherapy, but when EMDR is used, often the results are much faster.

Processing promotes neural integration and association of dysregulated memory fragments, removing blocks to the flow of information and energy. This is a basic tenet of the adaptive information processing (AIP) model (Shapiro, 2018). AIP posits that dysfunctional information is blocked from adaptive resolution and connection to other memory networks. The other important tenet of AIP is that this integration can occur much faster than previously thought possible with appropriate accessing of information. Nonadaptive self-beliefs, negative emotions, bodily sensations, and intrusive images that contribute to psychopathology can be positively integrated as fast as these elements were disturbed in the first place.

Research and theory support that unprocessed, dimensions of memory improperly stored, fragmented, and dissociated from one another are the basis of most psychopathology (Bergmann, 2020; Cozolino, 2017; Shapiro, 2018; van der Kolk, 2014). As discussed in Chapter 2, high levels of emotion with the resulting physiological changes contribute to traumatic memories being stored in dysfunctional memory networks (Shapiro, 2018). The person may experience anxiety without the attending context for the anxiety or experience a body sensation, and these feelings and sensations may be disconnected from other, more adaptive memory networks. For example, one man came to psychotherapy for depression and subsequently had a panic attack after undergoing sinus surgery. On exploration in psychotherapy, he discovered that the panic attack was triggered by an earlier body memory of swallowing blood after a tonsillectomy in which he had almost died as a child. He had no memory of this incident as particularly disturbing prior to the EMDR processing of his panic attack (Broad & Wheeler, 2006).

Another patient heard only sounds without understanding the context but knew that these sounds were associated with disturbing memories that occurred when she was a child. These dissociated memory networks may also manifest as behaviors or personality traits that are compartmentalized and triggered in specific situations or contexts. For example, in intimate relationships at home, a woman is emotionally and physically abused by her husband; but at work, she is decisive and assertive. All these examples reflect state-dependent memories or states of consciousness that are physiologically based and triggered by stimuli in the present. The latter example illustrates that resources, like trauma, may be stored in one state of consciousness and may not be available in another state.

Transforming traumatic memories through processing opens up access to positive emotions and thoughts as the negative event is integrated into the larger networks where positive memories are stored (Shapiro, 2018). The traumatized person may be numb to both positive and negative emotions because we cannot numb emotions selectively; that is, we cannot numb negative emotions without numbing the positive emotions as well. As emotional awareness increases and the attending anger, sadness, and hurt are experienced, the person will also be able to access more positive feelings.

When processing in EMDR therapy, dysfunctionally stored implicit memories are accessed, and this occurs in the context of a safe therapeutic relationship with adequate resources in place. This is important so that the person's experience is safe, because activating the disturbing memory has the potential to further entrench the negative memory network. The more the dysfunctional memory network is activated, the more likely it is that this template is reinforced and the connection and pattern formed between neurons and networks of neurons are strengthened (i.e., long-term potentiation). Chapter 2, describes the neurophysiology supporting this phenomenon. This explains why the traumatized person is prone to reenact the experience. To counter this, adaptive memory networks need to be linked to the traumatic memory during the arousal generated by the event so that processing and new learning can occur. This speaks to the importance of preparing the person so that positive neural networks exist that can be accessed spontaneously during processing so that state changes are possible. The reparative process begins when catharsis and abreaction are possible in a supportive relationship.

Indicators that the person is processing during EMDR therapy include changes in facial expression, body movements, and sensations; sighing; changes in feelings; changes in cognitions; the memory becomes either more distant or more clear; and the incident or image of the event changes (Dodgson, 2009). The experience and memories are not held in isolation and are connected or linked to other memory networks so that during processing, there are emotional or body sensation associations to other related memories. Each person processes information differently and a unique dimension of EMDR processing is that the therapist allows and facilitates the process to unfold without being too directive.

The Therapeutic Window of Processing

In processing, the hypothalamic–pituitary–adrenal (HPA) axis needs to modulate sympathetic arousal so that the person can regulate affect while accessing arousing memories that must be activated for neural reintegration to occur. This activation must occur in the therapeutic window or resilient zone see Chapter 1, Figure 1.3; the person must not be too overwhelmed and hyperaroused (i.e., sympathetic dominant) but not be too numb and hypoaroused (i.e., parasympathetic dominant) to engage the emotional memory. Research has shown that high levels of arousal interfere with frontal lobe functioning. It is thought that trauma is relegated to the right posterior hemisphere and to its hormonal counterpart, the HPA axis. EMDR therapy works best if the person is in their resilient zone so that the skillful advanced practice psychiatric nurse (APPN) needs to assess whether the person is avoiding the material, is dissociating, and has too little activation; or is hyperaroused with too much activation. Some patients may need activation decreased, especially if they are hyperventilating, overwhelmed with emotion, and in a highly anxious state. Hyperarousal sometimes manifests as REMs, increased respirations, and increasing levels of anxiety.

During processing, an *abreaction*, which is the intensive discharge of emotions related to the trauma, may occur. During abreaction, the person experiences some or all of the same sensations, thoughts, and emotions that occurred during the time of the trauma and becomes immersed in the event. Abreactions indicate that the person has accessed the memory with all the attending emotions of the original event. The abreaction should be titrated and monitored so that the person does not reexperience the trauma with overwhelming negative affect, identity fragmentation, or feelings of loss of control (Briere & Scott, 2013). The key to reexperiencing the trauma with manageable affect is maintaining dual awareness so that the person knows he or she is in the present with one foot in the traumatic memory. Dual awareness is cultivated during EMDR processing through the use of BLS in tandem with explaining to the person prior to processing to just note what comes up as if the person is on a train and watching out the window as the memories and experiences come up, much as scenery passes while on a moving train (Shapiro, 2018).

Shapiro (2018) differentiates abreactions that occur with EMDR from those that occur with hypnosis or other therapies. In EMDR, abreactions occur more rapidly as processing is accelerated, and abreactions can be an indicator of movement toward healing. Helpful strategies during abreactions include a calm voice, detached compassion, changing the rate or direction of BLS, allowing the process to unfold without judgment, grounding techniques see Chapter 17, calling the person by name, and orienting the person: "It's okay, Jeanne. You are at my office and can hear my voice. It is old stuff; let it go. You are right here with me, and you are safe."

For a significant subgroup of patients, dissociation presents a barrier to processing trauma, especially for those who have suffered complex trauma. Dissociation is a right-brain phenomenon and therefore may not be linked to declarative memory networks see Chapter 17. For those who are victims of complex trauma, there may not be a felt sense of their whole body. Accessing procedural somatic memories through words and left-brain activities may not be possible. For those who are mildly dissociating (see Chapter 17, Boxes 17.1 and 17.2 for signs of dissociation), the therapist may be able to bring the person back by asking questions and observing that the person seems to be *away*. Grounding techniques as described in Chapter 17, may be needed to bring the person back to the present. For an avoidant patient, asking detailed information about the specifics can increase activation and encourage comments if the patient is processing: "Stay with that. You're doing well."

General Guidelines for Processing

Processing in EMDR involves accelerated learning as the targeted memory is accessed and brought to a successful resolution so that trait changes can occur (Shapiro, 2018). A *trait change* refers to a permanent personality change, whereas a *state change* is a temporary change of emotions. For example, a person who is anxious driving over a bridge may learn deep breathing, distraction, safe place, or container exercises so that he or she could manage to get across the bridge. Trait change, on the other hand, would be total removal of anxiety about driving over a bridge without the need to use any anxiety-relieving strategies to accomplish this. The person would just not feel anxious about that anymore. The therapist's role in EMDR is to facilitate the patient's own natural healing ability to deal with stored, unprocessed experiences, which manifest as dysfunctional symptoms.

In EMDR, processing occurs according to procedures that track the progress through memory networks. As part of the protocol all dimensions of the memory—the image, the thoughts, the emotion, and the body sensations—are accessed with the therapist administering the BLS in the form of eye movements, auditory tones, or tapping, while at the same time the patient pays attention to the disturbing memory. This dual attention to the here and now with the then and there is foundational to EMDR. During the bilateral sets of stimulation, the patient free-associates according to protocols to elicit information and associated memories. Through EMDR, patients follow their own associative memory networks to process painful memories and integrate new information. The goal of treatment is to link dysfunctional memory networks to other, more adaptive networks.

In processing, the trauma recounted is often connected to other dysfunctional memory networks and can trigger other traumas, so that there may not be a discrete, coherent account of one specific memory but a collage of traumatic memories. For example, one patient was focusing on a recollection of an abusive relationship with a boyfriend and then had another memory triggered that reminded her of being bullied by her brother. This led to a memory of an earlier abusive relationship with her father. Following the narrative with empathic attunement and allowing the person to go where he or she needs to go is a good principle for all therapies but of paramount importance for the significantly traumatized patient. It is especially important when working with a patient with significant trauma to honor feelings, go slowly, and give the person as much control as possible. The APPN empowers the patient by planning interventions collaboratively, allowing the process to unfold by staying out of the way so that the person's natural healing ability can be accessed. The person's ability to follow through with trauma processing depends on his or her affect regulation skills, support from others, and life stress at the time as well as on the safety of the therapeutic relationship.

Most people are not eager to reexperience upsetting material, and this is essentially what we are asking the traumatized person to do. Trauma survivors have spent considerable effort avoiding thinking about the traumatic event(s) and naturally question the wisdom of this idea. It is essential for the therapist to educate the person about how the flashbacks, symptoms, and intrusive memories are the brain's effort to heal and how the avoidance serves to keep the trauma alive. The memories need to be integrated with other memory networks to dissipate. Reassure patients that you will teach them methods of managing arousal so that they will not be overwhelmed and assure them that they can stop or take a time out anytime they wish. However, it is more than the therapist's reassurance that enables the patient to trust that processing trauma will be helpful. It is the psychoeducation in tandem with the safety and trust that has been cultivated in the therapeutic relationship that allows the person to process traumatic material.

Processing only in the middle of the session and helping the person to leave in a calm state are essential. Patients who have been processing need special closure at the end of the session so that they can leave in a comfortable state. Immediately after processing, sometimes patients report that they feel scattered or spacey. The APPN might suggest that the patient walk around first or sit quietly before driving home. It is important to inform the patient that processing may continue between sessions. Summing up the session at the end and telling the person the date of the next session helps to provide closure. Reframing the emotional distress with a statement such as, "You did some good processing today," or returning to the safe place (see Appendix 1.7) or using the container exercise (see Appendix 1.8) for negative feelings, visualizing a healing image, or using art to draw a new belief or feeling are ways to soothe and contain at the end of processing.

Suggestions for assisting patients in managing emotions between sessions include offering to be available by phone if needed, journaling, walks in nature, artwork, meditation, stress-reduction strategies, group work, exercise, eating well, and other resource-enhancing skills. These are all skills that have been learned before processing in the stabilization phase. Sometimes, patients report a deep sleep after an EMDR processing session, and perhaps this heralds the healing that is taking place. Ask the person to keep track between sessions of any increase in flashbacks, nightmares, and disturbing feelings or memories and to bring this information to the next session. It can also help patients if the APPN records CDs for relaxation and guided imagery in one's own voice so that the patient can play these in between sessions to reinforce stabilization outside of sessions. These strategies help the person to stay connected and feel supported between sessions by providing a link to the *holding environment* of the therapeutic relationship.

Clinically, processing has been achieved once the subjective unit of disturbance (SUD) is 0 on a 0 to 10 scale and there are no reported bodily disturbances when thinking about the event. Shapiro (2018) says that the clinician can tell that processing has occurred by positive somatic, behavioral, and cognitive trait changes that occur after treatment. These changes are not temporary state changes, but enduring trait changes with the person able to talk about the event without the attending hyperarousal that was present before processing (Shapiro, 2018). The patient will not feel the trauma in the body after it has been processed. Asking the patient near the end of processing to scan his or her body is useful to determine whether processing has occurred. Significant body changes will be noticed after trauma is processed and the dysfunctional memory is integrated. Appendix 1.6 provides a processing checklist to assist the therapist in determining whether processing has led to adaptive change. The traumatic memory should be reaccessed at the next session after processing and again before termination to determine whether the changes reflect trait changes (Shapiro, 2018). Asking the person to rate the SUD on a 0 to 10 scale of the memory assists the therapist and patient in determining the degree of processing that has been accomplished.

Overall, successful processing has occurred after relationships are adaptive, work is productive, self-references are positive, there are no significant affect changes on exposure to trauma triggers, affect is proportionate to events, and there is congruence among behavior, thoughts, and affect (Davis & Weiss, 2004). As the trauma loses its arousal capacity and losses are mourned, the person is able to be more future oriented and may decide to pursue life goals, such as relationships, education, or professional goals, that previously were not thought about. Remediation of life skills that were missed during crucial developmental periods because of trauma may be needed. For example, one patient who suffered incest as a child processed this trauma in psychotherapy, and only then began to envision a future for herself with a partner. The therapist taught her basic skills about dating and how to develop, pace, and deepen a relationship safely.

PROTOCOL FOR EMDR

EMDR therapy for most traumas involves three stages: targeting the original traumatic memory, targeting the present trigger, and incorporating a positive template for the future (Shapiro, 2018). The theoretical assumption is that the present dysfunctional emotions are related to past events that feed or keep alive the present problems. Current situations serve as triggers that activate implicit or episodic memories, and these unprocessed memories contain the emotions, thoughts, and sensations from the original event. Interventions for processing involve targeting the specific trauma with an eight-phase protocol that guides the person through a description of the disturbing event related to the presenting problem (Shapiro, 2018). The current triggers are also processed in order to address the possible effects of conditioning. Table 7.4 describes the eight phases of EMDR.

In the first phase, screening for dissociation and identification of targets begins the initial assessment. Assessing the person's readiness for EMDR includes the person's ability to manage intense emotions. The Dissociative Experiences Scale (DES; E. B. Carlson & Putnam, 1993) is usually given as a screening tool for a dissociative

TABLE 7.4	EIGHT-PHASE PROTOCOL FOR EMDR
One	Patient History and Treatment Planning—assessment of stability and current life constraints; evaluation of clinical symptoms (affect tolerance and dissociation); screening for use of EMDR; identification of targets including small traumas and big traumas; developing a treatment plan
Two	Preparation—establish therapeutic alliance; educate the person about AIP and EMDR; evaluate secondary gains; practice relaxation and safe place; resource development if needed
Three	Assessment—identify components of the target (see Figure 7.1); patient identifies: an image that represents the experience or worst part of it; an NC associated with the incident or image and a PC that represents what the person would like to feel about himself or herself now; the patient then rates the PC on a 1 to 7 VOC scale that represents how true the PC feels now; then the emotions associated with the event are identified with an SUD on a 0 to 10 rated scale; finally, the person is asked where he or she feels this in his or her body
Four	Desensitization—begin sets of bilateral stimulation with eye movements, sound, and/or tapping and continue until the SUD is 0 or 1
Five	Installation—install PC with bilateral stimulation
Six	Body Scan—note tension and sensations in body for any residual
Seven	Closure—instruct about keeping a log and educate about disturbances that may occur post session
Eight	Reevaluation—reassess and review targets that were processed at the beginning of the next session

AIP, adaptive information processing; EMDR, eye movement desensitization and reprocessing; NC, negative cognition; PC, positive cognition; SUD, subjective unit of disturbance; VOC, validity of cognition.

Source: Adapted from Shapiro, F. (2018). *Eye movement desensitization and reprocessing* (EMDR) (3rd ed.). New York, NY: Guilford Press.

disorder. If the total score is above 30, which indicates possible significant disso-ciation, the APPN should proceed with caution in that EMDR may be destabilizing because dissociative barriers and defenses are dissolved in EMDR processing. See Chapter 3, for the DES. A history of seizures or eye pain is a contraindication for using eye movements.

If a significant single incident trauma is apparent, the Impact of Events Scale is administered. Chapter 3 and Chapter 17 describe assessment tools and how to take a history for trauma. To further identify significant traumas, the patient is asked to identify his or her five to 10 most disturbing memories or events that are stressful or upsetting in his or her life. Some clinicians use this opportunity to construct a time-line of negative and positive memories or events so that the positive memories can be used later as resources and negative events are rated as to their level of disturbance. See Chapter 17, for how to construct a trauma history timeline.

Sometimes, patients minimize traumas and may not remember anything. This does not necessarily mean that this is the rare person who is trauma free; more likely, these memories may be dissociated and not in conscious awareness. If any disturbing memories or traumas are recounted, ask the person to rate each on the 0 to 10 SUD scale. This is a good indicator for current arousal levels for the trauma. This scale is used later in the assessment phase of EMDR, with 0 reflecting no disturbance at all and 10 indicating the worst disturbance imaginable. These levels may change after the incident is accessed in treatment. It is important to identify the memory of the event and any related flashbacks, nightmares, and triggers that are associated with the event (Shapiro, 2018). Nightmares may represent unprocessed trauma and can also be targeted with EMDR.

The memory or target that is chosen to process first is usually that which the per-son has identified as the first and worst with the idea that once this event is processed, there will be generalization to other disturbing similar memories. Components of the identified target are developed (Phase 3). The following is a summary as devel-oped by Shapiro (2018). Asking the patient what was the worst part helps to hone in on the specific image or incident. For example, a patient who suffered from injuries in an automobile accident reported that the worst part was being alone, not the injuries sustained. After an image or picture of the worst part is clearly identified, the person is asked to think about that and to identify the negative cognition (NC) associated with the event. This can sometimes be challenging for patients, and the person can be helped in focusing by asking: "What words best go with the picture that express your negative belief about yourself now?" The patient may then offer: "I am powerless" or "I am not lovable." Often, the NC is not readily apparent to the patient, and the APPN helps the person in exploring the most accurate words that capture the self-referencing thoughts. After the NC is identified, the patient is asked to develop a positive cognition (PC) by the therapist, who asks: "When you bring up that picture or incident, what would you like to believe about yourself now?" This is important to do at this point to plant the seed for future adaptive associations. Examples might include "I am competent" or "I am lovable." After the PC is identi-fied, the patient is asked to rate how true the PC feels on a 1 to 7 scale, with 1 being completely false and 7 being completely true. This is called the *validity of cognition* (VOC) scale.

The next components of the target, which are all parts of Phase 3, are identifying the emotion, the SUD, and the body sensations. After the emotion is identified, the patient is asked to rate the disturbance on the SUD scale of 0 to 10. This gives a baseline so that the patient and clinician can monitor the processing as it unfolds. This then leads to the last question in activating the target, which is to identify the body sensations: "Where do you feel it in your body?" Some patients who are particularly shut off from their bodies may have difficulty accessing this dimension of the memory, and the APPN may need to coach the person. "Becoming conscious of one's body is a prerequisite for naming emotion and experiencing affect. This can be taught through sensate focusing exercises, such as asking the person to feel a feather on his or her skin, an ice cube on the arm, or any touch sensation to heighten awareness of sensations. These exercises require time before true processing can be accomplished and may be included during stabilization if needed. Asking patients to close their eyes and think of a person or place they love and to notice where they feel this in their body may help to discriminate between the body sensations of the trauma memory and other bodily feelings. Asking patients where they feel blocked can help to focus their attention on their body.

After these components are identified, the person has accessed all dimensions of the memory and may already be processing. The patient focuses on all these aspects together and the clinician begins BLS. Sets of approximately 24 BLS are interspersed with the person noticing changes in thoughts, images, and sensations related to the targeted event. The clinician guides the patient to concentrate on various aspects of the associations, and at times asks the patient to return to the memory of the event in order to make sure that the entire memory network is accessed and processed. After the SUD reaches 0, the person is asked if their PC is still correct and, if yes, the person is asked to think about this while thinking of the event during BLS. The person is asked to scan his or her body to check for any residual body sensations, and if any disturbance is reported, the therapist continues with BLS until it dissipates. The session is closed with a safe place exercise and instructions to observe any distress between sessions. The SUD level is reevaluated at the beginning of the next session. See https://www.emdria.org/emdr-training-education/become-an-emdr-training-provider/emdr-international-association-definition-of-emdr/ for the official definition of EMDR and delineation of the protocol. The following case example illustrates the use of EMDR to process trauma.

CASE EXAMPLE

Mr. S, a 32-year-old, successful, single man was referred for treatment because he felt stuck in his grief and had obsessive thoughts, guilt, and difficulty concentrating. Five months earlier, he had found his roommate, J, dead from an apparent overdose. An initial assessment was completed, and his trauma history revealed that he had worked near the World Trade Center during the 9/11 attack. Mr. S said he felt guilty when he thought about others who had suffered so much. He also reported his childhood was "rocky" with many arguments occurring between his parents in front of him when he was quite young. These events were not disturbing at the time of assessment and reported only as facts. After several sessions, the therapist felt that Mr. S was adequately stabilized, and EMDR was offered in order to process the trauma of finding his roommate dead. Mr. S was given information about the EMDR procedure, the potentially intense nature of the treatment, and a safe place practice session. Mr. S reported that the worst part of the trauma at this point was his difficulty with calling J's father after the funeral. After this target for processing was accessed, relevant components were identified (Figure 7.1). Mr. S said that when he thought about calling J's father, he became grief stricken, and the image of his roommate's body flashed before his mind. The following is a verbatim session using EMDR to process this traumatic incident:

APPN: What words best go with that image that expresses your negative belief about yourself now?

Patient: I'm helpless. I should have known. (NC)

APPN: When you think of that image, what would you like to believe about yourself now?

Patient: I did okay. (PC)

APPN: When you think of that image, how true do those words *I did okay* feel to you now on a scale of 1 to 7 where 1 feels completely false and 7 feels totally true? (VOC)

Patient: 2.

APPN: When you bring up that image and those words *I'm helpless. I should have known* what emotion do you feel now?

Patient: Grief, sadness.

APPN: On a scale of 0 to 10, where 0 is no disturbance and 10 is the highest disturbance you can imagine, how disturbing does it feel now? (SUD)

Patient: 8 or 9.

APPN: Where do you feel it in your body?

Patient: All over my head and eyes.

APPN: Okay. Now bring up that image and your words *I'm helpless. I should have known* and notice where you feel it in your body. Follow my fingers with your eyes. [Therapist holds two fingers upright, about 12 to 14 inches from the patient's gaze, and slowly moves his fingers horizontally from the left to the right of the patient's visual field while the patient follows with his eyes for approximately 24 bidirectional movements.]

Patient: I feel the door whacking his head as I open the door. I get a picture of his dad and the brother a couple of days later.

APPN: Go with that (eye movement #2).

Patient: There are different angles on his body. I asked someone not to cover him. There is blood on the floor under his nose . . . shock and grief, crying, calling, telling J's friends. I talked to my other roommate, and I said we have to talk more.

APPN: Go with that (eye movement #3).

Patient: I had your fingers in mind. I feel more at peace. The funeral, the wake was sad but necessary . . . lot less trauma . . . feel more relaxed now.

APPN: Go with that (eye movement #4).

Patient: The first part was weird. J is alive, hanging out at a Christmas party . . . then 9/11 . . . an image of towers falling . . . moments when I was on the roof.

APPN: Go with that (eye movement #5).

Patient: 9/11 some more . . . saw the second plane hit . . . big ball of flame . . . fuel line fire . . . talking with people . . . people running and jumping . . . hear people hitting the ground . . . then walked uptown to a friend's place.

APPN: Go with that (eye movement #6).

Patient: Kind of moved past 9/11 . . . younger . . . childhood . . . seeing dead grandparents in the coffin . . . my parents . . . the big fight . . . now I am really mad. I was 6. My mom calls me in and asks how would you feel if we split up? Later, I wondered why are you asking me?

APPN: Go with that (eye movement #7).

Patient: Really angry . . . tense all over.

APPN: Go with that (eye movement #8).

Patient: There was a total shit storm when dad came home . . . he didn't know. She started yelling at him . . . words exchanged . . . I was in the living room . . . dad was in his robe . . . he had to explain his whereabouts . . . dad cried . . . weird . . . he was held up and got a ticket and produced the ticket. Clearly there were larger issues at play. Somebody said you are going to burn in hell for what you are doing. I couldn't believe it. They made up, and I said promise that you won't break up.

APPN: Go with that (eye movement #9).

Patient: Mixed emotions . . . anger . . . relaxing . . . feeling of understanding between mom and me . . . she knows . . . she is sorry.

The session ended with Mr. S down to a 3 or 4 SUD, which indicated incomplete processing because 0 means that there is no subjective disturbance and that processing is complete. In the next session, Mr. S said he felt much better and wanted to work on some disturbing memories he had over the week about his childhood. He said: "EMDR was amazing and 9/11 was done." This indicated that he had continued to process after the last session because his SUD level was now 0 when he thought about his roommate's death. He said: "I never felt that kind of rage before; my whole body felt it." The disturbing memory he wanted to work on in the session was the fight his parents had when he was younger that he had described in the previous session. When asked for the worst part about that situation, he reported that it was his parents crying and saying bad things to each other.

APPN: What words go best with that incident that express your negative belief about yourself now?

Patient: I'm a troublemaker (NC).

APPN: When you think of that image, what would you like to believe about yourself now? (PC)

Patient: I'm okay, a good person.

APPN: When you think of that image, how true do those words *I'm okay, a good person* feel to you now on a scale of 1 to 7 (SUD), where 1 feels completely false and 7 feels totally true? (VOC)

Patient: I guess a 3 or 4, sometimes.

APPN: When you bring up that incident and those words *I'm a troublemaker* what emotion do you feel now?

Patient: Anger for being exposed to it.

APPN: On a scale of 0 to 10, where 0 is no disturbance and 10 is the highest disturbance you can imagine, how disturbing does it feel now? (SUD)

Patient: Probably a 6.

APPN:	Where do you feel it in your body?
Patient:	My stomach.
APPN:	Now, bring up that incident and your words *I'm a troublemaker* and notice where you feel it in your body and follow my fingers (eye movement #1).
Patient:	Parents crying . . . saying bad things to each other . . . my family unit shattering. Is there anything to do to put it back together? I've moved onto episodes of getting hurt . . . mundane . . . getting hit for knocking some curlers over. Mom would hit me for trivial reasons . . . Spanked . . . pissed at my folks . . . the fight . . . the rage . . . anger subsided . . . witnessing how painful marriage can be. I don't want to be an instrument of pain.
APPN:	Go with that (eye movement #2).
Patient:	Mixed emotions . . . happy memories with parents . . . home in Boston . . . baby-sister . . . regret that it happened . . . tired of carrying this around.
APPN:	Go with that (eye movement #3).
Patient:	None of the same scenes . . . feeling crampy in my stomach . . . There's nothing you can do about it.
APPN:	Go with that (eye movement #4).
Patient:	Moving away from the pain . . . feeling of absolution.
APPN:	Go with that (eye movement #5).
Patient:	I was a kid . . . not doing anything abnormal . . . she washed my mouth out for just doing kid shit . . . came back to J's dad, and I'm feeling better about that whole situation . . . coping better.
APPN:	Go with that (eye movement #6).
Patient:	Stomach . . . always an acid stomach . . . started thinking about good things . . . hanging out with J . . . feels good to not feel guilty . . . absolving myself . . . a feeling of liberation.
APPN:	Go with that (eye movement #7).
Patient:	Thought back at age 14 about getting grounded . . . Parents going to my little league games . . . I'm happier . . . going about things the right way.
APPN:	Go with that (eye movement #8).

Mr. S ended the session with a SUD level down to 0. He was instructed to keep a log over the course of the next week and told that other feelings or disturbing thoughts might occur. At the beginning of the next session, Mr. S was asked to return to the disturbing memory he had discussed the week before, and when asked how he felt now on a 0 to 10 scale, he reported that the incident remained a 0. The PC *I'm okay, a good person* was installed with short sets of eye movements, and a body scan revealed no residual tension. After a total of five sessions, Mr. S terminated treatment successfully.

The trauma of the roommate's death had reactivated guilt and responsibility schemas from long ago, when Mr. S felt responsible for his family's difficulties. He reported after EMDR that he felt freer and not so guilt ridden and responsible. His belief that he had created the conflict in the family was processed, and he was able to normalize his childhood transgressions as normal kid stuff that his parents had

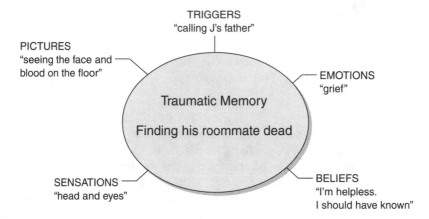

FIGURE 7.1 Components of the assessment phase of EMDR therapy.

reacted to with punishments that were inappropriately severe. He had always felt that he had to make up for something and was overly giving in relationships. With the processing of J's death, he was able to resolve other associated memory networks. Mr. S said that he was less giving in friendships after EMDR in that he was looking out for himself and his own needs more. He realized that he did not have to make up for anything. The resolution of his guilt allowed him to increase his sense of worth and self-esteem.

This case was included because it is a simple demonstration of the successful use of EMDR therapy, and it illustrates how memory networks are accessed and connected. Until Mr. S had processed his grief and early adverse childhood experiences, he did not have access to positive emotions of his childhood. This then resulted in significant trait changes in his personality because he was able to be in a relationship without the attending guilt feelings that he needed to make up for something. EMDR therapy is a powerful therapeutic approach and perhaps the best way to understand this type of therapy is to experience an EMDR session. A certified EMDR therapist can be found on the website EMDRIA.org. Often dramatic outcomes occur after only a few sessions of EMDR therapy, particularly with simple PTSD or symptom-focused EMDR.

POST-MASTER'S EMDR TRAINING AND CERTIFICATION REQUIREMENTS

Although EMDR therapy may seem at first glance to be a simple technique, it is a complex psychotherapy approach that requires a high degree of clinical skill. Certification is needed to practice EMDR effectively and safely. EMDR certification is available for licensed mental health clinicians who have 2 years of clinical experience in their field through EMDR International Association (EMDRIA). EMDR training is offered by private trainers, the EMDR Institute, or the EMDR Trauma Recovery Humanitarian Assistance Programs (HAP). The latter training is offered at half price for those who work 30 hours or more per week at a not-for-profit, are a student, or are university faculty. See the HAP website at www.emdrhap.org for schedule and location of future trainings. EMDR trainings must be approved by EMDRIA, which sets the standards for training programs. Approved EMDRIA training programs through the Institute or with private trainers are listed on the website www.emdria.org. The Basic Training usually consists of two weekend EMDR workshops (20 academic didactic and 20 supervised practice hours) plus 10 additional consultation hours. In order to receive EMDR certification, additionally a minimum of

50 sessions with a minimum of 25 patients, 12 continuing education units (CEUs), and 20 hours of consultation from an approved EMDRIA consultant are required. It usually takes at least a year to complete all the requirements for EMDR basic training and certification.

CONCLUDING COMMENTS

During the past 10 years, our understanding of trauma and effective psychotherapy for trauma has increased owing to the development of brain imaging techniques and biochemical research studies of the physiology and sequelae of trauma. We now understand that trauma causes short- and long-term effects on the body. This expanding knowledge has inspired new approaches to treatment and new ways to consider what happens in the brain when trauma occurs. The AIP model evolved as a result of this work. AIP posits that trauma is any information that cannot be processed to an adaptive conclusion, based on the idea that the brain has an inherent ability to process information and integrate with other memory networks (Shapiro, 2018). AIP provides the underpinnings for how to conduct psychotherapy with the person who has suffered adverse life experiences as well as significant trauma.

EMDR therapy is a comprehensive psychotherapy approach used to treat depression, anxiety, phobias, pain, addictions, behavioral and personality disorders, trauma-related disorders, relationship and sexual problems, and other mental health and somatic problems due to adverse life experiences. It is used for those with complex and attachment disorders with special considerations and advanced training. Complex trauma often involves more resource installation and longer treatment than a few sessions. It is important to keep in mind that the APPN must be skilled in working with the type of issue or problem that is presented. For example, in working with a patient with a dissociative disorder, skills and knowledge about this population are imperative prior to using EMDR. Because EMDR therapy breaks down dissociative barriers, the APPN should seek consultation and advanced training in treating those who are highly dissociative.

EMDR therapy is highly congruent with nursing's holistic model of care and recovery principles. The process and protocol is patient centered with the therapist facilitating and following the person's lead. The EMDR trained APPN will be richly rewarded as brain changes are literally witnessed during processing and profound changes occur in a short amount of time. Not only does the patient experience deep feelings of gratitude, the therapist too feels grateful and moved by the power and miracle of this remarkable healing therapy.

DISCUSSION QUESTIONS

1. Discuss your understanding of processing and how you would know whether a patient was ready for processing.
2. What is an abreaction, and how would you handle this if it occurred in an EMDR session?
3. Identify strategies to pace treatment and mediate arousal levels.
4. Discuss a patient you have cared for and describe how you would conceptualize the problem and treatment based on the AIP model.
5. Identify some strategies that may be helpful in closing a session when the person has processed some traumatic material.
6. How would you support the person who has processed trauma between sessions?
7. What are the components of the EMDR protocol?

8. Although EMDR training is required before using the protocol, Phases 1 and 2 can be integrated into your practice before training. Discuss specifically using a case example how you could include components of these phases in your work with your patient.

REFERENCES

Abel, N. J., & O'Brien, J. M. (2010). EMDR treatment of comorbid PTSD and alcohol dependence: A case example. *Journal of EMDR Practice and Research, 4*(2), 50–59. doi:10.1891/1933-3196.4.2.50

Allon, M. (2015). EMDR group therapy with women who were sexually assaulted in the Congo. *Journal of EMDR Practice and Research, 9*(1), 28–34. doi:10.1891/1933-3196.9.1.28

Bae, H., & Kim, D. (2015). Desensitization of triggers and urge reprocessing for pathological gambling: A case series. *Journal of Gambling Studies, 31*(1), 331–342. doi:10.1007/s10899-013-9422-5

Barker, R. T., & Barker, S. B. (2007). The use of EMDR in reducing presentation anxiety. *Journal of EMDR Practice and Research, 1*, 100–108. doi:10.1891/1933-3196.1.2.100

Behnammoghadam, M., Kheramine, S., Zoladi, M., Cooper, R. Z., & Shahini, S. (2019). Effect of EMDR on severity of stress in emergency medical technicians. *Psychology Research and Behavior Management, 12*, 289–296. doi:10.2147/PRBM.S190428

Bergmann, U. (2020). *Neurobiological foundations for EMDR practice* (2nd ed.). New York, NY: Springer Publishing Company.

Bisson, J., & Andrew, M. (2007). Psychological treatment of post-traumatic stress disorder (PTSD). *Cochrane Database of Systematic Reviews*, (3), CD003388. doi:10.1002/14651858. CD003388.pub3

Bongaerts, H., Van Minnen, A., & de Jongh, A. (2017). Intensive EMDR to treat patients with complex PTSD: A case series. *Journal of EMDR Practice and Research, 11*(2), 84–95. doi:10.1891/1933-3196.11.2.84

Bossini, L., Casolaro, I., Santarnecchi, E., Caterini, C., Koukouna, D., Fernandez, I., . . . Fagiolini, A. (2012). Evaluation study of clinical and neurobiological efficacy of EMDR in patients suffering from post-traumatic stress disorder. *Rivista di Psichiatria, 47*Suppl.(2), 12–15. doi:10.1708/1071.11733

Bradley, R., Greene, J., Russ,E., Dutra, L., & Westen, D. (2005). A multidimensional meta-analysis of psychotherapy for PTSD. *American Journal of Psychiatry, 162*(2), 214–227. doi:10.1176/appi.ajp.162.2.214

Briere, J., & Scott, C. (2013). *Principles of trauma therapy: A guide to symptoms, evaluation, and treatment* (2nd ed.). Thousand Oaks, CA: Sage.

Broad, R. D., & Wheeler, K. (2006). An adult with childhood medical trauma treated with psychoanalytic psychotherapy and EMDR: A case study. *Perspectives in Psychiatric Care, 42*, 95–105. doi:10.1111/j.1744-6163.2006.00058.x

Brown, S. H., Gilman, S. G., Goodman, E. G., Adler-Tapia, R., & Feng, S. (2015). Integrated trauma treatment in drug court: Combining EMDR and seeking safety. *Journal of EMDR Practice and Research, 9*(3), 123–136. doi:10.1891/1933-3196.9.3.123

Calancie, O. G., Khalid-Khan, S., Booij, L., & Munoz, D. P. (2018). Eye movement desensitization and reprocessing as a treatment for PTSD: Current neurobiological theories and a new hypothesis. *Annals of the New York Academy of Sciences, 1426*(1), 127–145. doi:10.1111/nyas.13882

Carlson, E. B., & Putnam, F. (1993). An update on the dissociative experiences scale. *Dissociation: Progress in the Dissociative Disorders, 6*(1), 16–27.

Carlson, J. G., Chemtob, C. M., Rusnak, K., Hedlund, N. L., & Muraoka, M. Y. (1998). Eye movement desensitization and reprocessing treatment for combat related posttraumatic stress disorder. *Journal of Traumatic Stress, 11*, 3–24. doi:10.1023/A:1024448814268

Chen, R., Gillespie, A., Zhao, Y., Xi, Y., Ren, Y., & McLean, L. (2018). The efficacy of eye movement desensitization and reprocessing in children and adults who have experienced complex childhood trauma: Systematic review of randomized controlled trails. *Frontiers in Psychology, 9*, 534. doi:10.3389/fpsyg.2018.00534

Chen, Y.-R., Hung, K.-W., Tsai, J.-C., Chu, H., Chung, M.-H., Chen, S.-R., . . . Chou, K.-R. (2014). Efficacy of eye-movement desensitization and reprocessing for patients with posttraumatic-stress disorder: A meta-analysis of randomized controlled trials. *PLOS ONE, 9*(8), e103676. doi:10.1371/journal.pone.0103676

Civilotti, C., Sacchezin, S., Agazzi, T., Modolo, G., Poli, E., Callerame, C., & Faretta, E. (2014). EMDR and cancer: A pilot study to evaluate the effectiveness of EMDR in a sample of cancer patients. *Psycho-Oncology, 23*(Suppl. 3), 226–227. doi:10.1111/j.1099-1611.2014.3695

Congressional Budget Office. (2012). *The Veterans Health Administration's treatment of PTSD and traumatic brain injury among recent combat veterans.* Washington, DC: Congress of the United States. Retrieved from https://www.cbo.gov/publication/42969

Cotter, P., Meysner, L., & Lee, C. W. (2017). Participant experiences of EMDR vs CBT for grief: Similarities and differences. *European Journal of Psychotraumatology, 8* (Suppl. 6) , 1375838. doi:10.1080/20008198.2017.1375838

Cozolino, L. (2017). *The neuroscience of psychotherapy: Healing the social brain* (3rd ed.). New York, NY: W. W. Norton.

Davidson, P. R., & Parker, K. C. H. (2001). Eye movement desensitization and reprocessing (EMDR): A meta-analysis. *Journal of Consulting and Clinical Psychology, 69*, 305–316. doi:10.1037/0022-006X.69.2.305

Davis, K., & Weiss, L. (2004). *Traumatology: A workshop on traumatic stress disorders.* Hamden, CT: Humanitarian Assistance Program.

de Bont, P. A. J. M., de Jongh, A., & van den Berg, D. (2019). Psychosis: An emerging field for EMDR research and therapy. *Journal of EMDR Practice and Research, 13*(4), 313–324. doi:10.1891/1933-3196.13.4.313

de Bont, P. A. J. M., van der Vleugel, B. M., van den Berg, D. P. G., de Roos, C., Lokkerbol, J., Smit, F., . . . van Minnen, A. (2019). Health–economic benefits of treating trauma in psychosis. *European Journal of Psychotraumatology, 10*(1), 1565032. doi:10.1080/20008198.2018.1565032

de Jongh, A. (2012). Treatment of a woman with emetophobia: A trauma focused approach. *Mental Illness, 4*(1), e3. doi:10.4081/mi.2012.e3

de Roos, C., Veenstra, A. C., de Jongh, A., den Hollander-Gijsman, M. E., van der Wee, N. J. A., Zitman, F. G., & van Rood, Y. R.(2010). Treatment of chronic phantom limb pain (PLP) using a trauma-focused psychological approach. *Pain Research and Management, 15*(2), 65–71. doi:10.1155/2010/981634

Dodgson, P. W. (2009). EMDR & PTSD. In A. Rubin & D. Springer (Eds.), *Treatment of traumatized adults and children: Clinician's guide to evidence-based practice* (pp. 257–348). Hoboken, NJ: Wiley.

Doering, S., Ohlmeier, M.-C., de Jongh, A., Hofmann, A., & Bisping, V. (2013). Efficacy of a trauma-focused treatment approach for dental phobia: A randomized clinical trial. *European Journal of Oral Sciences, 121*(6), 584–593. doi:10.1111/eos.12090

Edmond, T., Lawrence, K., & Voth Schrag, R. (2016). Perceptions and use of EMDR therapy in rape crisis centers *Journal of EMDR Practice and Research, 10*(1), 23–32. doi:10.1891/1933- 3196.10.1.23

Faretta, E., & Farra, M. D. (2019). Efficacy of EMDR therapy for anxiety disorders. *Journal of EMDR Practice and Research, 13*(4), 325–332. doi:10.1891/1933-3196.13.4.325

Faretta, E., & Leeds, A. (2017). EMDR therapy of panic disorder and agoraphobia: A review of the existing literature. *Clinical Neuropsychiatry, 14*(5), 330–340.

Fernandez, I., Callerame, C., Maslovaric, G., & Wheeler, K. (2014). EMDR Europe humanitarian programs: Development, current status, and future challenges. *Journal of EMDR Practice & Research, 8*(4), 215–224. doi:10.1891/1933-3196.8.4.215

Foster, S., & Lendl, J. (1995). Eye movement desensitization and reprocessing: Initial applications for enhancing performance in athletes. *Journal of Applied Sport Psychology, 7*, 63.

Foster, S., & Lendl, J. (1996). Eye movement desensitization and reprocessing: Four case studies of a new tool for executive coaching and restoring employee performance after setbacks. *Consulting Psychology Journal, 48*, 155–161. doi:10.1037/1061-4087.48.3.155

Graham, L. (2004). Traumatic swimming events reprocessed with EMDR. *The Sport Journal, 7*(1), 1–5. Retrieved from https://thesportjournal.org/article/traumatic-swimming-events-reprocessed-with-emdr

Grant, M. (2016). *The new change your brain, change your pain: Based on EMDR.* Melbourne, Australia: Author.

Grey, E. (2011). A pilot study of concentrated EMDR: A brief report. *Journal of EMDR Practice and Research, 5*, 14–24. doi:10.1891/1933-3196.5.1.14

Hase, M., Plagge, J., Hase, A., Braas, R., Ostacoli, L., Hofmann, A., & Huchzermeier, C. (2018). Eye movement desensitization and reprocessing versus treatment as usual in the treatment of depression: A randomized-controlled trial. *Frontiers in Psychology, 9*, 1384. doi:10.3389/fpsyg.2018.01384

Ho, M. S. K., & Lee, C. W. (2012). Cognitive behaviour therapy versus eye movement desensitization and reprocessing for post-traumatic disorder—Is it all in the homework then? *Revue Européenne de Psychologie Appliquée/European Review of Applied Psychology, 62*(4), 253–260. doi:10.1016/j.erap.2012.08.001

Ironson, G. I., Freund, B., Strauss, J. L., & Williams, J. (2002). A comparison of two treatments for traumatic stress: A pilot study of EMDR and prolonged exposure. *Journal of Clinical Psychology, 58*, 113–128. doi:10.1002/jclp.1132

Jarero, I.N., Artigas, L., & Hartung, J. (2006). EMDR integrative group treatment protocol: A postdisaster trauma intervention for children and adults. *Traumatology, 12*, 121–129. doi:10.1177/1534765606294561

Jarero, I. N., Artigas, L., Uribe, S., & García, E. L. (2016). The EMDR integrative group treatment protocol for patients with cancer. *Journal of EMDR Practice and Research, 10*(3), 199–207. doi:10.1891/1933-3196.10.3.199

Jarero, I. N, Schnaider, S. & Givaudan, M. (2019). Randomized controlled trail: Provision of EMDR protocol for recent critical incidents and ongoing traumatic stress to first responders. *Journal of EMDR Practice and Research, 13*(2), 100–110. doi:10.1891/1933-3196.13.2.100

Jebelli, F., Maaroufi, M., Maracy, M. R., & Molaeinezhad, M. (2018). Effectiveness of eye movement desensitization and reprocessing (EMDR) on the sexual function of Iranian women with lifelong vaginismus. *Sexual and Relationship Therapy, 33*(3), 325–338. doi:10.1080/14681994.2017.1323075

Kahn, A. M., Dar, S., Ahmed, R., Bachu, R., Adnan, M., & Kotapati, V. P. (2018). Cognitive behavioral therapy versus eye movement desensitization and reprocessing in patients with post-traumatic stress disorder: Systematic review and meta-analysis of randomized clinical trials. *Cureus, (9)*, e3250. doi:10.7759/cureus.3250

Knipe, J. (2019). *EMDR toolbox: Theory and treatment of complex PTSD and dissociation*. New York, NY: Springer Publishing Company.

Korn, D. L., & Leeds, A. M. (2002). Preliminary evidence of efficacy for EMDR resource development and installation in the stabilization phase of treatment of complex posttraumatic stress disorder. *Journal of Clinical Psychology, 58*, 1465–1487. doi:10.1002/jclp.10099

Lee, C. W., & Cuijpers, P. (2013). A meta-analysis of the contribution of eye movements in processing emotional memories. *Journal of Behavioral Therapy and Experimental Psychiatry, 44*(2), 231–239. doi:10.1016/j.jbtep.2012.11.001

Lee, C. W., Gavriel, H., Drummond, P., Richards, J., & Greenwald, R. (2002). Treatment of PTSD: Stress inoculation training with prolonged exposure compared to EMDR. *Journal of Clinical Psychology, 58*, 1071–1089. doi:10.1002/jclp.10039

Leeds, A. M. (2006, September 8). Criteria for assuring appropriate clinical use and avoiding misuse of resource development and installation when treating complex posttraumatic stress syndromes. Presented at EMDR International Association Annual Conference, Philadephia, PA.

Littel, M., van den Hout, M. A., & Engelhard, I. M. (2016). Desensitizing addiction: Using eye movements to reduce the intensity of substance-related mental imagery and craving. *Frontiers in Psychiatry, 7*, 14. doi:10.3389/fpsyt.2016.00014

Luber, M. (2010a). *Eye movement desensitization and reprocessing (EMDR) scripted protocols: Basics and special situations*. New York, NY: Springer Publishing Company.

Luber, M. (2010b). *Eye movement desensitization and reprocessing (EMDR) scripted protocols: Special populations*. New York, NY: Springer Publishing Company.

Luber, M. (2014). *Implementing EMDR early mental health interventions for man-made and natural disasters: Models, scripted protocols and summary sheets*. New York, NY: Springer Publishing Company.

Luber, M. (2016a). *EMDR with first responders: Models, scripted protocols, and summary sheets for mental health interventions*. New York, NY: Springer Publishing Company.

Luber, M. (2016b). *Eye movement desensitization and reprocessing (EMDR) therapy scripted protocols and summary sheets: Treating anxiety, obsessive-compulsive, and mood-related conditions.* New York, NY: Springer Publishing Company.

Luber, M. (2019a). *Eye movement desensitization and reprocessing (EMDR) scripted protocols and summary sheets: Treating eating disorders, chronic pain and maladaptive self-care behaviors.* New York, NY: Springer Publishing Company.

Luber, M. (2019b). *Eye movement desensitization and reprocessing (EMDR) therapy scripted protocols and summary sheets: Treating trauma in somatic and medical related conditions.* New York, NY: Springer Publishing Company.

Marcus, S. V. (2008). Phase 1 of integrated EMDR: An abortive treatment for migraine headaches. *Journal of EMDR Practice and Research, 2,* 15–25. doi:10.1891/1933-3196.2.1.15

Marsden, Z., Lovell, K., Blore, D., Ali, S., & Delgadillo, J. (2018). A randomized controlled trial comparing EMDR and CBT for obsessive–compulsive disorder. *Clinical Psychology & Psychotherapy, 25*(1), e10–e18. doi:10.1002/cpp.2120

Maxfield, L. (2019). A clinician's guide to the efficacy of EMDR therapy. *Journal of EMDR Practice and Research, 13*(4), 239–246. doi:10.1891/1933-3196.13.4.239

Maxfield, L., & Hyer, L. (2002). The relationship between efficacy and methodology in studies investigating EMDR treatment of PTSD. *Journal of Clinical Psychology, 58*(1), 23–41. doi:10.1002/jclp.1127

Maxfield, L., & Melnyk, W. T. (2000). Single session treatment of test anxiety with eye movement desensitization and reprocessing (EMDR). *International Journal of Stress Management, 7,* 87–101. doi:10.1023/A:1009580101287

Murray, K. (2012). EMDR with grief: Reflections on Ginny Sprang's 2001 study. *Journal of EMDR Practice and Research, 6*(4), 187–191. doi:10.1891/1933-3196.6.4.187

Natha, F., & Daiches, A. (2014). The effectiveness of EMDR in reducing psychological distress in survivors of natural disasters: A review. *Journal of EMDR Practice and Research, 8*(3), 157–170. doi:10.1891/1933-3196.8.3.157

Nia, N. G., Afrasiabifar, A., Behnammoghadam, M., & Cooper, R. Z. (2019). The effect of EMDR versus guided imagery on insomnia severity in patients with rheumatoid arthritis. *Journal of EMDR Practice and Research, 13*(1), 2–9. doi:10.1891/1933-3196.13.1.2

Okawara, M., & Paulsen, S. L. (2018). Intervening in the intergenerational transmission of trauma by targeting maternal emotional dysregulation with EMDR therapy. *Journal of EMDR Practice and Research, 12*(3), 142–157. doi:10.1891/1933-3196.12.3.142

Ostacoli, L., Carletto, S., Cavallo, M., Baldomir-Gago, P., Di Lorenzo, G., Fernandez, I., . . . Hofmann, A. (2018). Comparison of eye movement desensitization reprocessing and cognitive behavioral therapy as adjunctive treatments for recurrent depression: The European depression EMDR network (EDEN) randomized controlled trial. *Frontiers in Psychology, 9,* 74. doi:10.3389/fpsyg.2018.00074

Pagani, M., Högberg, G., Fernandez, I., & Siracusano, A. (2013). Correlates of EMDR therapy in functional and structural neuroimaging: A critical summary of recent findings. *Journal of EMDR Practice & Research, 7*(1), 29–38. doi:10.1891/1933-3196.7.1.29

Paulsen, S. L., & O'Shea, K. (2017). *When there are no words: Repairing early trauma and neglect from the attachment period with EMDR therapy.* Bainbridge Island, WA: Bainbridge Institute for Integrative Psychology.

Power, K. G., McGoldrick, T., Brown, K., Buchanan, R., Sharp, D., Swanson, V., . . . Karatzias, A. (2002). A controlled comparison of eye movement desensitization and reprocessing versus exposure plus cognitive restructuring, versus waiting list in the treatment of post-traumatic stress disorder. *Journal of Clinical Psychology and Psychotherapy, 9,* 299–318. doi:10.1002/cpp.341

Ricci, R. J. (2006). Trauma resolution using eye movement desensitization and reprocessing with an incestuous sex offender: An instrumental case study. *Clinical Case Studies, 5,* 248. doi:10.1177/1534650104265276

Ricci, R. J., & Clayton, C. (2016). EMDR with sex offenders: Using offense drivers to guide conceptualization and treatment. *Journal of EMDR Practice and Research, 10*(2), 104–118. *EMDR International Association.* doi:10.1891/1933-3196.10.2.104

Rodenburg, R., Benjamin, A., de Roos, C., Meijer, A. M., & Stams, G. J. (2009). Efficacy of EMDR in children: A meta-analysis. *Clinical Psychology Review, 29,* 599–606. doi:10.1016/j.cpr.2009.06.008

Rost, C., Hofmann, A., & Wheeler, K. (2009). EMDR treatment of workplace trauma: A case series. *Journal of EMDR Practice and Research, 3*(2), 80–90. doi:10.1891/1933-3196.3.2.80

Rostaminejad, A., Behnammoghadam, M., Rostaminejad, M., Behnammoghadam, Z., & Bashti, S. (2017). Efficacy of eye movement desensitization and reprocessing on the phantom limb pain of patients with amputations within a 24-month follow-up. *International Journal of Rehabilitation Research, 40*(3), 209–214. Retrieved from https://www.ncbi.nlm.nih.gov/pubmed/28368869

Rothbaum, B. O., Astin, M. C., & Marsteller, F. (2005). Prolonged exposure versus eye movement desensitization and reprocessing (EMDR) for PTSD rape victims. *Journal of Traumatic Stress, 18*, 607–616. doi:10.1002/jts.20069

Rousseau, P.-F., Khoury-Malhame, M. E., Reynaud, E., Boukezzi, S., Cancel, A., Zendjidjian, X., . . . Khalfa, S. (2019). Fear extinction learning improvement in PTSD after EMDR therapy: An fMRI study. *European Journal of Psychotraumatology, 10*(1), 1568132. doi:10.1080/20008198.2019.1568132

Rudiger Bohm, K. (2019). EMDR's efficacy for obsessive compulsive disorder. *Journal of EMDR Practice and Research, 13*(4), 333–336. doi:10.1891/1933-3196.13.4.333

Schneider, J., Hofmann, A., Rost, C., & Shapiro, F. (2008). EMDR in the treatment of chronic phantom limb pain. *Pain Medicine, 9*, 76–82. doi:10.1111/j.1526-4637.2007.00299.x

Seidler, G. H., & Wagner, F. E. (2006). Comparing the efficacy of EMDR and trauma-focused cognitive-behavioral therapy in the treatment of PTSD: A meta-analytic study. *Psychological Medicine, 36*, 1515–1522. doi:10.1017/S0033291706007963

Seubert, A. (2018). Becoming known: A relational model utilizing gestalt and ego state- assisted EMDR in treating eating disorders. *Journal of EMDR Practice and Research, 12*(2), 71–86. doi:10.1891/1933-3196.12.2.71

Shapiro, E., & Laub, B. (2015). Early EMDR intervention following a community critical incident: A randomized clinical trial. *Journal of EMDR Practice and Research, 9*(1), 17–27. doi:10.1891/1933-3196.9.1.17

Shapiro, F. (1991). Eye movement desensitization and reprocessing procedure: From EMD to EMDR: A new treatment model for anxiety and related traumata. *Behavior Therapist, 14*, 133–135.

Shapiro, F. (2001). *Eye movement desensitization and reprocessing (EMDR): Basic principles, protocols, and procedures* (2nd ed.). New York, NY: Guilford Press.

Shapiro, F. (2018). *Eye movement desensitization and reprocessing (EMDR)* (3rd ed.). New York, NY: Guilford Press.

Shapiro, F., Wesselmann, D., & Mevissen, L. (2017). Eye movement desensitization and reprocessing therapy (EMDR). In M. A. Landolt, M. Cloitre, & U. Schnyder (Eds.), *Evidence based treatments for trauma-related disorders in children and adolescents* (pp.273–298). New York, NY: Springer Publishing Company.

Silverman, S. (2011). Effecting peak athletic performance with neurofeedback, interactive metronome, and EMDR: A case study. *Biofeedback, 39*, 40–42. doi:10.5298/1081-5937-39.1.08

Stickgold, R. (2008). Sleep-dependent memory processing and EMDR action. *Journal of EMDR Practice and Research, 2*, 289–299. doi:10.1891/1933-3196.2.4.289

Sukumaran, B. (2015). Treating body dysmorphophobia with EMDR. *International Journal of Psychosocial Research*, Special Issue, 219–222.

Tapia, G. (2019). Review of EMDR interventions for individual with substance use disorder with/without comorbid PTSD. *Journal of EMDR Practice and Research, 13*(4), 345–353. doi:10.1891/1933-3196.13.4.345

Taylor, S., Thordarson, D. S., Maxfield, L., Fedoroff, I. C., Lovell, K., & Ogrodniczuk, J. (2003). Comparative efficacy, speed, and adverse effects of three PTSD treatments: Exposure therapy, EMDR, and relaxation training. *Journal of Consulting and Clinical Psychology, 71*, 330–338. doi:10.1037/0022-006X.71.2.330

Tesarz, J., Wicking, M., Bernardy, K., & Gunter, J. (2019). EMDR therapy's efficacy in the treatment of pain. *Journal of EMDR Practice and Research, 13*(4), 337–344. doi:10.1891/1933-3196.13.4.337

Thompson, C. T., Vidgen, A., & Roberts, N.P. (2018). Psychological interventions for post-traumatic stress disorder in refugees and asylum seekers: A systematic review and meta-analysis. *Clinical Psychology Review, 63*, 66–79. doi:10.1016/j.cpr.2018.06.006

Tofani, L. R., & Wheeler, K. (2011). The recent-traumatic episode protocol: Outcome evaluation and analysis of three case studies. *Journal of EMDR Practice and Research, 5*, 95–110. doi:10.1891/1933-3196.5.3.95

Valiente-Gómez, A., Moreno-Alcázar, A., Gardoki-Souto, I., Masferrer, C., Porta, S., Royuela, O., . . . Amann, B. L. (2019). Theoretical background and clinical aspects of the use of EMDR in patients with bipolar disorder. *Journal of EMDR Practice and Research, 13*(4), 307–312. doi:10.1891/1933-3196.13.4.307

van den Berg, D. P. G., de Bont, P. A. J. M., van der Vleugel, B. M., de Roos, C., de Jongh, A., Van Minnen, A., & van der Gaag, M. (2015). Prolonged exposure versus eye movement desensitization and reprocessing versus waiting list for posttraumatic stress disorder in patients with a psychotic disorder: A randomized clinical trial. *JAMA Psychiatry, 72*(3), 259–267. doi:10.1001/jamapsychiatry.2014.2637

van den Berg, D. P. G., & van der Gaag, M. (2012). Treating trauma in psychosis with EMDR: A pilot study. *Journal of Behavior Therapy & Experimental Psychiatry, 43*, 664–671. doi:10.1016/j.jbtep.2011.09.011

van der Hart, O., Groenendijk, M., Gonzalez, A., Mosquera, D., & Solomon, R. (2014). Dissociation of the personality and EMDR therapy in complex trauma-related disorders: Applications in phases 2 and 3 treatment. *Journal of EMDR Practice and Research, 8*(1), 33–48. doi:10.1891/1933-3196.8.1.33

van der Kolk, B. (2014). *The body keeps the score: Brain, mind, and body in the healing of trauma.* New York, NY: Penguin Books.

van der Kolk, B. A., Spinazzola, J., Blaustein, M. E., Hopper, J. W., Hopper, E. K., Korn, D. L., . . . Simpson, W. B. (2007). A randomized clinical trial of eye movement desensitization and reprocessing (EMDR), fluoxetine, and pill placebo in the treatment of posttraumatic stress disorder: Treatment effects and long-term maintenance. *Journal of Clinical Psychiatry, 68*, 37–46. doi:10.4088/JCP.v68n0105

Van Woudenberg, C., Voorendonk, E. M., Bongaerts, H., Zoet, H. A., Verhagen, M., Lee, C. W., . . . de Jongh, A. (2018). Effectiveness of an intensive treatment programme combining prolonged exposure and eye movement desensitization and reprocessing for severe post-traumatic stress disorder. *European Journal of Psychotraumatology, 9*(1), 1487225. doi:10.1080/20008198.2018.1487225

Watts, B. V., Schnurr, P. P., Mayo, L., Young-Xu, Y., Weeks, W. B., & Friedman, M. J. (2013). Meta-analysis of the efficacy of treatments for posttraumatic stress disorder. *Journal of Clinical Psychiatry, 74*, e541–e550. doi:10.4088/JCP.12r08225

Wilson, S. A., Becker, L. A., & Tinker, R. H. (1997). Fifteen-month follow-up of eye movement desensitization and reprocessing (EMDR) treatment for PTSD and psychological trauma. *Journal of Consulting and Clinical Psychology, 65*, 1047–1056. doi:10.1037/0022-006X.65.6.1047

Wong, S. -L. (2018). EMDR-based divorce recovery group: A case study. *Journal of EMDR Practice and Research, 12*(2), 58–70. doi:10.1891/1933-3196.12.2.58

Wong, S. -L. (2019). Flash technique group protocol for highly dissociative clients in a homeless shelter: A clinical report. *Journal of EMDR Practice and Research, 13*(1), 20–31. doi:10.1891/1933-3196.13.1.20

World Health Organization. (2013). *Guidelines for the management of conditions specifically related to stress.* Geneva, Switzerland: Author. Retrieved from https://apps.who.int/iris/bitstream/handle/10665/85119/9789241505406_eng.pdf

Zaccagnino, M., & Cussino, M. (2013). EMDR and parenting: A clinical case. *Journal of EMDR Practice and Research, 7*(3), 154–166. doi:10.1891/1933-3196.7.3.154

APPENDIX 7.1
Lightstream Exercise

This exercise can be used for any problem, such as obsessive-compulsive disorder, pain, and so on. The therapist can ask the patient to draw what the problem or pain would look like on a piece of paper with colors or else to use the following without the drawing and to visualize:

"Concentrate on the feeling in your body . . . if the feeling had a shape: what would it be? If it had a size . . . what would it be? If it had a color . . . what would it be? If it had a sound . . . would it be high pitched or low?

Which of your favorite colors might you associate with healing?

Imagine that this favorite colored light is coming in through the top of your head and directing itself at the shape in your body. Let's pretend that the source of the light is the cosmos; the more you use, the more you have available. . . . The light directs itself at the shape, and permeates and penetrates it . . . resonating and vibrating in and around it. As it does, what happens to the shape, size, or color?

As the light continues to direct itself to that area, you can allow the light to come in and gently and easily fill your entire head, easily and gently. . . . Now allow it to descend through your neck into your shoulders, and flow down your arms into your hands and out through your fingertips. Now allow it to come down your neck and into the trunk of your body easily and gently. Now allow it to descend down through your trunk and into your legs, streaming down your legs and flowing out your feet. . . ."

Give peaceful and calm suggestions until the next session.

An audiotape version is available from eye movement desensitization and reprocessing-humanitarian assistance program (EMDR-HAP).

Source: Adapted with permission from Shapiro, F. (2001). *Eye movement desensitization and reprocessing (EMDR): Basic principles, protocols, and procedures* (2nd ed.). New York, NY: Guilford Press.

APPENDIX 7.2
Circle of Strength

This exercise is designed to assist the person in developing an internal resource for support. This exercise is most helpful if used with those who have positive relationships and memories and may not be appropriate for attachment and relationship trauma. It may create distress for those whose relationships are not working so well.

"If it is okay, close your eyes, leaving them open is okay too. Take a nice deep breath and imagine yourself in the center of a wheel with people surrounding you like spokes in a wheel who are resources for you. Each person is a person who you like who has been there for you and who you feel comforted by and represents a source of strength for you. It could be someone you know from the past or a current person. As you think of each person, tell me who they are (say the name after each person is named to strengthen the image). Make the image of you surrounded by your resource people as vivid as you can with each person's image as clear as you can make it with faces, colors. Just notice as you are surrounded by (name the people again who they named) and how you feel in your body . . . taking a nice deep breath as you feel the strength and comfort of your resources surrounding you with caring and comfort, those who like you for you and have been there for you. Feel their love around you supporting you and notice where you feel this in your body . . . let me know where this is. Now, as you breathe in, notice your _____ (body part mentioned by patient) and memorize that feeling and notice how calm and strong you feel as you image your circle of strength with you in the middle. Continue for a few minutes enjoying your circle of special people. Take a nice deep breath knowing that you can return to this image anytime you need."

(Ask the person to practice the image during the week several times a day. The more this is practiced, the easier it is to bring to mind when needed.)

8

Cognitive Behavior Therapy

Sharon M. Freeman Clevenger

This chapter provides a brief overview of cognitive behavior therapy (CBT) beginning with defining concepts of CBT, an overview of the guiding principles, and examples of evidence-based research using CBT as the psychotherapeutic model. Basic cognitive and behavioral techniques are presented that Advanced Practice Psychiatric Nurses (APPNs) can integrate into practice. The chapter has been updated in this edition to include acceptance and commitment therapy (ACT) and mindfulness-based CBT, behavioral plans integrated with operant conditioning, and expanded information on schema focused and dialectical behavioral therapies as well as the application of different models of CBT treatments for specific populations. The chapter concludes with a case study illustrating the use of CBT and a brief discussion of competencies for the CBT practitioner.

CBT is based on the belief that psychological health depends on how well a person is able to positively adapt, both cognitively and functionally, to changing conditions and situations in the environment. Functional adaptation includes modification of behavioral skills to meet common, uncommon, and crisis-related challenges as they occur, within a reasonable period of time. Cognitive adaptation adds the component of learning from consequences and conditions in a manner that is rational and useful. People who are psychologically healthy tend to be more active socially, engage in enjoyable activities, and have a feeling of confidence, or mastery in their environments, and are more capable of finding hopeful, positive views when navigating life's responsibilities and challenges. The goal of the CBT therapist is to help the patient observe, evaluate, monitor, and adapt the patient's problematic views and behaviors toward a more hopeful, flexible, inclusive, rational, and confident skill set. Cognitive and behavioral skill training that includes the person's goals and abilities in a respectful, collaborative, structured manner is the hallmark of CBT-based psychotherapy.

CBT has undergone numerous modifications and adaptations over the past 50 to 60 years; however, the structural "bones" of CBT are apparent in each adaptation. The basic structure of CBT is based on the understanding that a person's views of a situation will influence his or her assumptions, behaviors, and reactions to that situation. Modification of unrealistic, or dysfunctional/distorted thinking patterns toward realistic present-time useful and positive observations and attributions will result in enduring patterns of emotional, cognitive, and behavioral changes. A wide range of emotional and behavioral problems has been researched using CBT as a psychotherapeutic model with demonstrated effectiveness around the world (DeRubeis, Hollon, Evans, & Bemis, 1982; Hollon, Stewart, & Strunk, 2006; Leichsenring & Leibing, 2003; McLean et al., 2001; Mohr, Boudewyn, Goodkin, Bostrom, & Epstein, 2001; Paunovic & Öst, 2001). Therapy begins with a conceptualization, or understanding of the individual's core beliefs, ways of reacting, and behaviors combined with available internal resources and coping skills. Once a clear, specific problem is identified, the therapist, in collaboration with the patient, develops a structured plan that includes measurable, reasonable, and specific goals so that both participants know when progress has been made. Goals might include problems to overcome, positive changes that need to be made, or clarification of troubling, but elusive, understanding of a situation or experience. Sessions are structured with a beginning (agenda), middle (work and practice), and end when homework is assigned. The homework is then reviewed at the beginning of the next session when the agenda is set for that session. The session structure becomes familiar and recognizable as the person moves through therapy. Each session has an expected flow and is based on plans that are clearly conceptualized and based on well-researched protocols and theories that guide the clinician through each action, session, and overall plan of care.

GUIDING PRINCIPLES

Cognitive therapy "is a collaborative process of empirical investigation, reality testing, and problem solving between the therapist and the patient" (Beck & Weishaar, 1986, p. 43.). For example, the basic premise regarding the development of depression is that it is a result of systematic bias in the way individuals interpreted experiences creating distorted thinking, skewed attributions, and eventually, maladaptive emotions and behaviors (Beck, Rush, Shaw, & Emery, 1979; Beck, 2011). Cognitive therapy evolved out of the work of Aaron T. Beck in the early 1960s at the University of Pennsylvania. Beck, who was originally trained in psychoanalysis, observed that individuals with depression had similar distortions in their thinking that created dysfunctional, inaccurate conclusions that fueled depressogenic emotions, thoughts, and behaviors. He decided to explore the dysfunctional cognitions with depressed patients and discovered that realistic modifications, even modest ones, resulted in improvement of mood and function. Beck explored further by departing from his psychoanalytic roots and began to study Adler, Horney, and Sullivan, expanding upon and testing thinking in here-and-now patient life problems. By concentrating on a person's distortions in self, the world, and others, in a series of studies focused on depression and suicidal thinking, Beck developed a more systematic cognitive-behavioral conceptualization of both psychiatric disorders and personality structure (Beck, 1976; Beck & Lester, 1976).

Behavior theories were integrated with cognitive theory during the 1970s as researchers observed that traditional behavior theory only focused on guided experiments to shape measurable behaviors such as avoidance and suicidal ideation. Very little attention was paid to the cognitive processes involved in the behavioral changes. Observations made by researchers who combined theories found that fearful cognitive reactions and thought patterns were extinguished with behavioral exposure protocols highlighting that modifications of thought and behavior occur together (Lewinsohn, Hoberman, & Teri 1985; Meichenbaum, 1977). The work of Meichenbaum and Lewinsohn incorporating behavioral interventions within cognitive theoretical structures added depth, context, and deeper understanding to therapeutic outcomes. Since that time, continued extensive research has repeatedly shown significant efficacy with the combined approach of cognitive techniques (i.e., cognitive restructuring) along with behavioral techniques (i.e., exposure therapy and relaxation training), a model called "CBT."

Cognitive-behavior therapy as it is known today is a "system of psychotherapy based on a theory which maintains that how an individual structures his or her experiences largely determines how he or she feels and behaves" (Beck & Weishaar, 1986, p. 43). The model posits that dysfunctional (or maladaptive) thoughts relating to self, world, and/or others (the "cognitive triad") is rooted in irrational or illogical assumptions. The individual's view of self and the world are central to the determination of emotions and behaviors and thus by changing one's thoughts, emotions and behaviors can also be changed. In addition, CBT is structured hierarchically with cognitive processes understood in terms of primary and secondary thinking. Secondary thinking views the social and cultural world in determinate, positive, rational terms while primary thinking recognizes the indeterminate, negative, and irrational as forever part of human action. Finally, CBT places significant importance on cognitive information processing and behavioral change (Beck, 1989; Beck & Weishaar, 1986). The resultant theoretical model combines features of traditional psychotherapy within a unique conceptual framework that focuses on the interplay between thoughts, feelings, and behaviors within one's environment. Psychotherapy must therefore target all three foci to affect sustainable changes, with cognition being the pivotal point.

EVIDENCE-BASED RESEARCH

The amount of research conducted evaluating the efficacy of CBT is massive, and therefore, almost impossible to summarize in a brief page or two. A short list of publications validating the efficacy of CBT for both medical and psychiatric disorders as well as many mental health problems is included in Table 8.1.

TABLE 8.1   EVIDENCE-BASED RESEARCH FOR CBT

Medical Disorder	Citation
Tinnitus	Kaldo, Cars, Rahnert, Larsen, and Andersson (2007); Robinson et al. (2008)
Chronic pain	Buhrman et al. (2015); Morasco et al. (2016)
PMDD	Hofmeister and Bodden (2016); Hunter et al. (2002)
Sexual dysfunction	G. Andersson, Cuijpers, Carlbring, Riper, and Hedman (2014); Brotto et al. (2012)
Chronic insomnia	Blom, Jernelöv, Rück, Lindefors, and Kaldo (2017); Morris et al. (2016); Ritterband et al. (2017); D. J. Taylor et al. (2017)
Chronic fatigue syndrome	Deale, Chalder, Marks, and Wessely (1997); Deale, Husain, Chalder, and Wessely (2001)
Myocardial infarction	Carney et al. (2004); Roest et al. (2013)
Depression	G. Andersson, Hesser, Hummerdal, Bergman-Nordgren, and Carlbring (2013); Fava et al. (2004); Freedland, Carney, Rich, Steinmeyer, and Rubin (2015); Johansson, Nyblom, Carlbring, Cuijpers, and Andersson (2013); Johansson et al. (2012); Nakagawa et al. (2014)

(continued)

TABLE 8.1   EVIDENCE-BASED RESEARCH FOR CBT (*CONTINUED*)

Medical Disorder	Citation
Anxiety, PTSD, and panic disorders	E. Andersson et al. (2011); Caudle et al. (2007); Forman et al. (2012); Hedman et al. (2014); Hedman, Hesser, Andersson, Axelsson, and Ljótsson (2017); Hendriks, Kampman, Keijsers, Hoogduin, and Voshaar (2014); Herbert et al. (2009); Lovato, Lack, Wright, and Kennaway (2014); Mansson et al. (2016); Nixon, Sterk, Pearce, and Weber (2017); Schienle, Schafer, Hermann, Rohrmann, and Vaitl (2007); M. A. Stanley et al. (2009); Steketee, Frost, Tolin, Rasmussen, and Brown (2010); L. K. Taylor and Weems (2011); Wamser-Nanney, Scheeringa, and Weems (2016); Wuthrich, Rapee, Kangas, and Perini (2016)
Eating disorder	Chakraborty and Basu (2010); Dalle Grave, El Ghoch, Sartirana, and Calugi (2016); Fairburn et al. (1995); Hay (2013); Wilson (1999)
Personality disorders	Leichsenring and Leibing (2003)
Substance misuse disorders	Tyrer et al. (2003, 2004)
Marriage and couple problems	Hesser et al. (2017); Macdonald, Pukay-Martin, Wagner, Fredman, and Monson (2016); Waring, Carver, Stalker, Fry, and Schaefer (1990)
Self-injurious behaviors	Gonzales and Bergstrom (2013); Linehan et al. (2015); MacPherson, Weinstein, and West (2018); Neacsiu, Rizvi, and Linehan (2010); B. Stanley, Brodsky, Nelson, and Dulit (2007)
Obsessive-compulsive disorder	Anton et al. (1999); Franklin, Foa, and March (2003); Piacentini et al. (2011); Whittal, Robichaud, Thordarson, and McLean (2008); Williams et al. (2010)
Schizophrenia and schizophrenic symptom reduction	Barrowclough et al. (2001); Bechdolf et al. (2004, 2010); Bechdolf, Kohn, Knost, Pukrop, and Klosterkotter (2005); Cather et al. (2005); Granholm, Holden, Link, McQuaid, and Jeste (2013); Morrison et al. (2016); Rector, Seeman, and Segal (2003); Tarrier et al. (1999, 2004); Turkington et al. (2008); Zimmer, Duncan, Laitano, Ferreira, and Belmonte-de-Abreu (2007)
Health anxiety (hypochondriasis)	Hedman, Ljótsson, and Lindefors (2012); Tyrer et al. (2011); Weck, Nagel, Hofling, and Neng (2017); Weck, Neng, Richtberg, Jakob, and Stangier (2015)
ADHD	Özcan, Oflaz, Türkbay, and Freeman Clevenger (2013)
Borderline personality disorder (using CBT/DBT approach)	Bellino, Zizza, Rinaldi, and Bogetto (2007); Bohus et al. (2004); Kroger, Harbeck, Armbrust, and Kliem (2013); Linehan, Heard, and Armstrong (1993); Linehan, Tutek, Heard, and Armstrong (1994); B. Stanley et al. (2007)

ADHD, attention deficit hyperactivity disorder; CBT, cognitive behavior therapy; DBT, dialectical behavior therapy; PMDD, premenstrual dysphoric disorder; PTSD, posttraumatic stress disorder.

COGNITIVE TECHNIQUES FOR STABILIZATION

The APPN has access to numerous specific psychotherapeutic techniques that have been shown to be effective in changing or modifying the patient's thinking and behaviors. While there are times when it is necessary to be direct and firm, and even confrontive, in general, guided discovery rather than directly challenging the patient's views is more effective. Techniques that are collaborative and allow the patient to find the answers to problems or dilemmas increases the patient's belief in the conclusions, minimizes debate, and increases the sense of mastery and participation.

Socratic Dialogue

The Socratic dialogue (SD) is the hallmark of CBT. It is a technique described as "mutual discovery in which the therapist guides the patient through a series of questions and answers to elicit automatic thoughts and assumptions, and examine the logic and evidence that relates to them" (Leahy, 2001, p. 63). Socratic methods are radically different from psychodynamic schools and nondirective styles of therapy technique (Freeman, 2005). The former synthesizes the patient's information and the therapist interprets it back to the individual encapsulating intentions, motivations, and conflicts (Freeman, 2005). By interpreting for the patient, it is thought that the therapist will lead the person to insight, integration and eventual change. In contrast, SD involves the therapist asking specific questions derived primarily from restatement of the individual's own words as the major technique where the individual is able to self-discover insight, which leads to subsequent changes (Freeman, 2005).

SD consists of a series of well-placed questions that literally guide the person to his or her own conclusions based on the therapist's expected response, rather than simply pointing out the answer to the individual. Mastery of the SD is one of the most difficult of the CBT skills to achieve. A competent therapist is adept at using a wide range of questions to assist the person in discovering his or her own automatic thoughts, conclusions, and patterns. Use of guided discovery using SD appears relaxed and nonconfrontational, with the therapist genuinely listening and reflecting what the patient is saying. The SD process includes seven basic types of questions: memory, translation, interpretation, application, analysis, synthesis, and evaluation. It is a much more powerful technique to have the individual find the answer for him- or herself than to direct the individual. Box 8.1 describes the types of questions used in the SD method of therapeutic interaction (Freeman, 2005).

BOX 8.1 Examples of Question Types in the Socratic Dialogue

1. History questions: *"How many children did you have in your first marriage?"* (non-SD)
2. Memory questions (remembering that the individual's recall is influenced temporally, interference and "facts" being considered inconsequential): *"When did you first notice that your sleep patterns had changed?"*
3. Translation questions (asks the patient how the data refer to the individual): *"When you say you become anxious, explain to me what it feels like to feel anxious to you."*
4. Interpretation (helps the patient identify relationships between facts and experiences): *"How does your sensitivity to criticism play out with your husband?"*
5. Application (asks the individual to apply previously mastered skills to a new situation): *"How can you use what you learned with your boss in your discussion with your son?"*

(continued)

BOX 8.1 Examples of Question Types in the Socratic Dialogue (*continued*)

> 6. Analysis (requires breaking a problem into a number of parts): *"What evidence do you have to support this conclusion?"*
> 7. Evaluation (asks the individual to make decisions/judgments based on data): *"On a scale of 0-10, where would you rate your level of anxiety today?"* *"And how does that compare to 4 months ago?"*

Source: Freeman, A. (2005). Socratic dialogue. In A. Freeman, S. H. Felgoise, A. M. Nezu, C. M. Nezu, & M. A. Reinecke (Eds.), *Encyclopedia of cognitive behavior therapy* (pp. 380–384). New York, NY: Springer.

Box 8.2 illustrates the basic rules for SD adapted from Freeman (2005) used in conjunction with the types of questions described in Box 8.1.

BOX 8.2 Socratic Dialogue Basic Rules

> 1. The techniques are embedded in the collaborative dialogue and are goal-directed and specific.
> 2. The therapist has a problem list that generates the plan of direction that begins the SD process. SD is not a series of drifting questions that "follow the patient." Each question must be strategically placed in order to reach the predefined goal. This is where the concept of "guided discovery" comes from for the therapeutic interaction.
> 3. The questions must be short, focused and targeted. For example, "Do you experience difficulty agreeing with your husband?" "Is this similar to interactions with others?" "How does this play itself out in this situation?" "Can you think of another way to respond that may result in a less defensive response from him?"
> 4. The questions must progress in a manner that keeps anxiety at a minimum for the individual.
> 5. The SD questions should be framed in a way to elicit an affirmative response. For example, in a reluctant individual: "There are probably a lot of places you would rather be than here, right?"
> 6. The additional point to the above is that negative responses to questions mean that the therapist must reframe the question to gain an affirmative response. "Is it your idea to come to therapy today?" "No! I don't want to be here!" "There are probably a lot of things you would rather be doing today than sitting here." "Yeah! That's for sure!"
> 7. The therapist must monitor the patient's reactions and moods on an ongoing basis. If a question increases a reaction, the therapist needs to address it immediately. "What just happened—I noticed a reaction—what was that?"
> 8. The therapist must pace the questions to suit the individual's mood, style, and content of information.
> 9. The questions must be planned and in logical sequence. The therapist must have an internal map for the session and move the session in a planned direction toward the desired goal.
> 10. The therapist must be careful to self-monitor and not "jump in" to offer interpretations or solve the patient's problems. This is not only more respectful to the patient it allows for greater clarity.
> 11. Self-disclosure should be extremely limited and only used with extreme caution and great care as to the motive for the disclosure. Comparing what the therapists did or does with what the patient did or does moves away from SD into discussion and possibly misjudgment.
> 12. The therapist may use everyday experiences as therapeutic metaphors. For example, this author uses Aesop's Fables and other well-known story characters to make a point such as "sour grapes" that can elicit both content and affect.

Source: Freeman, A. (2005). Socratic dialogue. In A. Freeman, S. H. Felgoise, A. M. Nezu, C. M. Nezu, & M. A. Reinecke (Eds.), *Encyclopedia of cognitive behavior therapy* (pp. 380–384). New York, NY: Springer.

Downward Arrow: This technique was first used by Beck in 1979 to refer to the technique of logical sequencing of reasoning. The individual is helped to uncover underlying assumptions in logic and sequence through careful questioning by the therapist asking, "If this is true, then what happens?" For example, Mrs. Jones, a successful attorney, was concerned that a staff member she was having problems with would undermine her practice if she terminated her even after months of disagreements. The APPN asked her what specifically would happen if she fired Jane.

Mrs. Jones:	"I'm sure she would bad mouth me to her friends at the courthouse and that would give me a bad name!"
APPN:	"And how would that affect your practice?"
Mrs. Jones:	"Everyone would believe her. I have a lot of patient that work at the courthouse!"
APPN:	"And how many of those patient do you have at the courthouse?"
Mrs. Jones, thinking:	"I guess about 15."
APPN:	"And how many patient do you have in your practice?"
Mrs. Jones:	"About 250"
APPN:	"And how many of the 15 at the courthouse would believe Jane and drop you?"
Mrs. Jones (laughing):	"OK, about two or three maybe."
APPN:	"So, if you fired Jane, two or three patient out of 250 would possibly drop you."
Mrs. Jones:	"Yes, I guess I do this all the time! I've been making myself nuts over nothing!"

Idiosyncratic Meaning: The therapist assists the patient to clarify statements and terms used so that both the APPN and the patient have a clear understanding of perceived reality.

For example: Mr. Smith says, "When she makes those little faces it just puts me out! You know what I mean." APPN: "No, I don't what you mean. Please explain what you mean by 'puts you out'."

Labeling of Distortions: Individuals are helped to identify automatic thoughts that are "dysfunctional or irrational" as a type of self-monitoring for more accurate description. See Table 8.2 for examples of cognitive distortions (CDs). Patients are initially asked to choose four or five of their "favorite" CDs in their first session and to bring this information to the next session. This information is then integrated into future sessions as educational material as it is noticed in the patient's verbalizations and/or written information. The patient is stopped and asked to "notice" what they have said (thought) and encouraged to reframe the information. Other examples of distorted automatic thoughts are also "caught" and similarly restructured as needed.

Questioning the Evidence: This technique assists the individual in questioning the facts related to their cognitions and conclusions. This procedure investigates whether their information is based on facts or assumptions. For example, Mr. Hanson has been struggling with intimacy issues with his wife and reported that they had "finally" had sexually intercourse after 2 years of abstinence. He was very happy that this had occurred but was upset because he was sure she was not satisfied with the experience.

TABLE 8.2 COGNITIVE DISTORTIONS

Type	Example
All-or-nothing	*"I'm either a success or a failure."*
Mind reading	*"They probably think that I'm incompetent."*
Emotional reasoning	*"Because I feel inadequate I am inadequate."*
Personalization	*"That comment must have been directed toward me."*
Global labeling	*"Everything I do turns out wrong."*
Catastrophizing	*"If I go to the party, there will be terrible consequences."*
Should statements	*"I should be a better daughter."*
Overgeneralization	*"Everything always goes wrong for me."*
Control fallacies	*"If I'm not in complete control all the time, I will go out of control."*
Comparing	*"I am not as competent as my coworkers or supervisors."*
Heaven's reward	*"If I do everything perfectly here, I will be rewarded later."*
Disqualifying the positive	*"Just because one person liked me, it doesn't mean it will happen again."*
Perfectionism	*"I must do this perfectly or I will be criticized and a failure."*
Time tripping	*"I screwed up my past and now I must be vigilant to secure my future."*
Objectifying the subjective	*"I have to be funny to be liked. It is fact."*
Selective abstraction	*"All of the good men are taken or gay."*
Externalization of self-worth	*"My worth depends on what others think of me."*
Fallacy of the change of others	*"If everyone would just follow the rules I would feel happier/feel better."*
Fallacy of worrying	*"If I worry about it enough, it will be resolved."*
Ostrich technique	*"If I ignore it, maybe it will go away."*
Unrealistic expectations	*"I must be the best absolutely all of the time."*
Filtering	*"I tend to focus on the negative details while I ignore and filter out all the positive aspects of a situation."*
Being right	*"I must prove that I am right as being wrong is unthinkable."*
Fallacy of attachment	*"I can't live without a partner." "If I was in a relationship, all of my problems would be solved."*
Fallacy of perfect effect	*"If I do things perfectly, the results will be perfect."*

The APPN stopped him at this point and asked him for his evidence to this fact. He said he just "knew." The APPN saw that Mr. Hanson's statement was his evidence and helped Mr. Hanson review the basis for his conclusion. The APPN asked Mr. Hanson what his wife said to him. Mr. Hanson reported that his wife said that she was happy and felt "good." The APPN said, "So you think she lied to you?" Mr. Hanson said "No." The APPN said, "Well, either she lied to you or she felt happy, which do you think was true?" Mr. Hanson replied, "I guess she was happy." He then smiled.

Examining Options and Alternatives: This technique involves the development of all possible alternative explanations to learn the skills in generating options rather than "only one way" thinking. For example, Mrs. Umber was going to visit her son and daughter-in-law whom she did not get along with very well. She said, "I just can't stand the idea of spending a whole week with them!" The APPN said, "How did you choose to spend the entire week?" Mrs. Umber said, "Well it is clear out on the coast so if we are going clear out there it doesn't make sense to only go for a weekend." The APPN said, "What are your options?" Mrs. Umber replied, "I am not sure what you mean?" "You are going to the coast for a week; do you have to spend the entire week with your son?" "I hadn't thought about that," said Mrs. Umber, "I guess I don't, do I?" With that revelation she began to explore the possibilities of shortening her visit with her son and instead having a brief vacation with her husband in addition with the visit with her son.

Reattribution: In individuals with the habit of accepting all or most of the blame for outcomes, this is an excellent technique for redistribution of responsibility. This is also helpful for individuals with personality disorders that place the blame squarely on the shoulders of others for most outcomes. Mrs. White: "I can't believe he left me! I am such a loser!" APPN: "You were married to him for 22 years and he had five affairs that you knew of. You yourself said that you were more there for him than any other woman would have been. How is that being a loser?" "I know, I just feel like a loser!" APPN: "What was his part in this break up?" Mrs. White: "I guess he had some of it, but maybe if I wasn't such a loser he wouldn't have had all of those affairs." Mrs. White has a way to go here but she has opened the door to the possibility that her husband played a part in the ending of her marriage. The APPN can now work with her in identifying the component parts of her husband's responsibility and hers.

Decatastrophizing: Catastrophic thinking is one of the hallmarks of anxious individuals. These individuals tend to focus on the most negative possible outcome of any given situation. Decatastrophizing allows for balance and realistic focusing by examining the "worst possible outcome" and developing a plan of action. For example, a young woman complains that she can't sleep. "I haven't been able to sleep for 2 months! If I can't get some sleep I won't be able to stand it! I can't live like this!" APPN: "Take a deep breath and tell me what is the worst thing that would happen if you can't sleep." Woman: "I can't live like this!" APPN: "But what would happen if you continue to not sleep?" Woman: "I would walk around like a zombie!" APPN: "Have you been to your doctor for sleeping medication?" Woman: "No! I am worried I would get addicted!" APPN: "What would be worse: not sleeping or getting addicted?" Woman: "Not sleeping." APPN: "Do you think your doctor would let you get addicted?" Woman: "No, she has known me for years. She is really careful." APPN: "Would you let me call from here and get you an appointment today for an evaluation for medication?" Woman: "Yes. I guess I am really overreacting because I am so tired!"

Advantages and Disadvantages: For individuals who appear to be stuck between two options, examination of the advantages and disadvantages of certain situations helps them to develop alternative perspectives. This breaks the "all-or-nothing" mindset and permits a more balanced view of the situation. For example, Mr. Black is wondering whether or not to accept a promotion at work that means more money but more travel and time away from his family. The APPN may help him outline a list of advantages and disadvantages in a cost-benefit analysis similar to what he may do at his job that looks familiar to him so he can "weigh" out his choices by placing points next to each choice and then total the categories to help him decide.

Paradox or Exaggeration: This type of technique should only be used by the very skilled APPN; otherwise, the patient may view this technique as sarcasm or belittling. When used appropriately the APPN takes an issue to the extreme to help the person see the absurdity of the overinflated viewpoints. One APPN had been working with a couple for several months. The couple had originally come in with issues related to his obsessive-compulsive tendencies for neatness and her tendency to be a free spirit. They had reached a few compromises and were now very happy. At one point in the session they were talking about putting in a garden area and were having difficulty deciding how to organize the arrangements. The APPN said to the couple: "Oh my goodness! He wants the plants in rows and to be neat and orderly! Where on earth would he get an idea like that?" The couple, realizing that this exactly matched his style, immediately started laughing.

Turning Adversity to Advantage: This technique is akin to making lemonade out of lemons. The individual is helped to identify how to use what appears to be a negative situation to his or her advantage. For example, being turned down for a job may open the individual up for more attractive possibilities that had not been investigated previously.

Cognitive Rehearsal: Prior to making a behavioral change it is sometimes less threatening to "practice" the new behavior through visualization and discussion. For example, this would include practicing assertiveness in a mirror or "talking through" a confrontation out loud prior to actually following through with the conversation.

Automatic Thought Records: The automatic thought record (ATR) is a key component of CBT. The record was first introduced by Beck in 1979 to capture and analyze automatic thoughts both during and between sessions (Beck et al., 1979). The ATR is used as homework after introducing the process within the therapy session. The individual completes the columns in the ATR identifying a troubling situation, resulting emotion, and thoughts associated with both. The APPN and patient work on clarification and development of "rational" responses to debate or challenge the original reaction. When practiced and repeated, the process of clarification and debate becomes internalized in the individual. See Appendix 8.1 for copy of a form for an ATR.

Thought-Stopping: This is one of the simpler techniques in CBT. Basically, the patient interrupts his or her stream of thoughts with a sudden stimulus such as snapping a rubber band on the wrist, saying "Stop it!" out loud, or some other real or imagined stimulus and then changes his or her stream of thoughts. The technique is most credible when demonstrated to the patient in session and then assigned as homework. Once a patient is given a loud stimulus in a session such as "Stop it!" and then allowed to regain his or her composure and report what his or her thought pattern is after the stimulus, the person realizes that this simple technique is very effective.

Cognitive Restructuring: The process of cognitive restructuring refers to the use of an ATR combined with other cognitive techniques to effect changes in negative thinking patterns. The patient is asked to check in a few times a day at random times and write down what he or she is thinking. After keeping the ATR for a week, the APPN and patient review the log and underline which thoughts are negative and identify the CDs the patient uses. See Table 8.2. The patient then is asked to say the negative thoughts aloud to enhance awareness and to slow down and say out loud to themselves the targeted negative messages whenever they occur during the next week. A list is then generated with the patient that counters those distortions. For example, one patient who

BOX 8.3 Steps in Cognitive Restructuring

1. Tune in . . . keep a thought diary. Identify the upsetting situation. Describe the event or problem that's upsetting you.
2. Focus on the feeling words that are negative and record them. Give each negative feeling word a score on a scale from 1 (for the least) to 100 (for the most).
3. Substitute rational responses in the right-hand column on the automatic thought record and record how strongly you believe each one between 0 (not at all) and 100 (completely).
4. Review the list of rational responses and observe your feelings. Re-rate the scores to see how you have modified negative feelings to more positive feelings.

was anxious about going to an upcoming social event became aware that her negative thoughts reflected her poor self-esteem with this statement, "I will have a terrible time since nobody likes me." The positive comment developed to counter this was, "People usually like me." The patient was asked that whenever she found herself thinking the negative thought in the next week that she practice thought-stopping and substitute her positive statement from her list of positive statements that she carried with her. There are four basic steps in cognitive restructuring (see Box 8.3).

Homework

The hallmark behavioral technique in CBT is the use of homework assignments. Activities, some of which have been described, are designed within the therapy session to be carried outside and practiced in between sessions. The self-help designed assignments reinforce and continue what has been learned and addressed within the therapy framework. This results in a truly collaborative process between patient and APPN. For example, the APPN may develop a homework plan for deep-breathing exercise practice, role-play practice on how to act in a certain social situation, or in cases of alcohol misuse, practice ways to decline an alcoholic beverage. New, redeveloped, or revised rational responses are practiced until they replace previous, unhealthy responses. Homework also allows individuals to "try on" and experiment with new skills in order to give feedback to the APPN on which techniques work and which do not work. Techniques that do not work can then be modified or discarded as needed.

Psychoeducation

Psychoeducation is an integral component of all CBT techniques. In CBT the educational component is skillfully interwoven within the specific therapeutic techniques that the APPN is choosing and supplemented with bibliotherapy if that is appropriate. For example, a couple came for marital therapy following the husband's serial episodes of infidelity. The husband was not sure about whether to remain in the marriage or to leave his wife and two teenage sons, so he could continue to have serial affairs without guilt and restrictions. The APPN assigned two specific books to read, *After the Affair* by Janis Abrahms Spring (1997) and *Not Just Friends* by Shirley Glass (2003). In addition, the APPN used the SD to guide the husband through a cost/benefit analysis of each choice making sure to help him focus on the realities of the cost and benefit to the decision to leave versus the decision to stay. After completing the cost/benefit list the APPN pointed out that he had not identified any costs to his sons as far as lessons learned from him about how men treat women and families with respect to responsibility (education).

The next step was to help the patient self-identify that he had missed this component and discuss how he might be teaching his sons lessons that are unhealthy and explore his thoughts about this consequence. The focus on consequences became a focus of his therapy, not as a "blaming session" but a moment of education and self-identification of behavioral consequences of actions.

BEHAVIORAL TECHNIQUES

APPNs who specialize in CBT are very much attuned to the artistic side of therapy that flows back and forth between cognitive techniques and behavioral techniques. Psychotherapy rarely falls on one side or another between these two domains. Some individuals will require primarily behavioral techniques and others will benefit most from cognitive techniques. The key for the therapy to be successful is choosing the technique based on severity of symptoms and cognitive abilities. For example, a patient with a significant impairment with memory would best benefit from behavioral experiments as would children under the age of 7 or 8 years. Play therapy using behavioral experiments that help a child modify expectations of situations or problems is an example of integrating cognitive and behavioral therapies. See Chapter 21, for how to work with children with CBT. APPNs develop behavioral experiments out of the SD knowing that the salient ingredient in CBT is the dialogue as opposed to individual techniques.

Specific Behavioral Techniques

Assertiveness Training: Assertiveness training involves a combination of cognitive and behavioral practice. Prior to beginning an assertiveness training program, the APPN needs to define the terms "assertive, aggressive, and passive." For example, a person who is demanding, blunt, and self-righteous may perceive their behavior as assertive when in fact it is aggressive. In this type of a situation the therapy starts by educating the individual in the importance of modifying the confrontational style. Most individuals with depressive disorders tend to exhibit more passive behaviors and would require education on assertiveness as opposed to aggressiveness in order to make the idea of assertive changes more appealing. The APPN may for example model assertive behavior, assist the patient within the session with role-play, and finally develop in vivo experiments that increase in complexity over time until the new behavior is internalized. A basic textbook for patients with assertiveness issues is *Mind Over Mood: Change How You Feel by Changing the Way You Think* by Dennis Greenberger and Christine Padesky (1995). It is an excellent general workbook and reviews CBT techniques with helpful homework examples and information.

Behavioral Rehearsal: The behavioral component usually follows the cognitive training component and again includes behavioral experiments to gather more evidence or to develop more effective responses and styles. Rehearsal is usually practiced first in the therapy session itself, often with role-playing, and then as often as possible outside the session. The person then reports back in the following session for modification of the behavior if necessary. For example, Kevin, a 15-year-old male, often gets into arguments with his 6-year-old brother, Galen. The arguments usually stem from Galen "getting into my stuff," according to Kevin. After exploring the purpose of Galen's behavior (obtaining attention from Kevin), Kevin was encouraged to increase positive exchanges when Galen was not expecting it. This was practiced in session until Kevin felt comfortable with the modified exchanges. Initially Kevin stated, "I can't do that, I'd feel dumb being nice to him! He's a kid!" In order to help Kevin feel more comfortable with specific things to say and do, the APPN and Kevin explored possible exchanges and then put them into "play" in the therapy setting. The rehearsal repeated until Kevin reported "Okay, I can do that—that's cool." In situations in which the APPN is assisting the individual using this technique it is important to evaluate for safety as well as understanding of behavioral boundaries. In the preceding example the APPN would problem-solve possible outcomes to prepare Kevin for responses as well as set boundaries with him regarding potential aggressive interchanges.

Contingency Management: Contingency management is based on the systematic application of generally accepted principles of human behavior. An undesirable behavior is more likely to recur if it is immediately followed by some kind of reinforcer that is pleasurable (positive reinforcement). Positive reinforcers or rewards are more effective at changing behaviors than punishment (aversive reinforcement). An example of aversive stimuli is punishing the child who does not behave. Negative reinforcers are those that increase the probability that a behavior will recur by removal of an undesirable reinforcing stimulus. For example, if the child behaves, he does not get scolded. The use of contingency management is very useful for individuals with self-control problems because it provides a self-motivator for internal motivation of control. It generalizes well, which means it can be used in a variety of setting such as home, school, work, and social settings.

For example, in substance misuse settings, reinforcement is usually in the form of vouchers exchangeable in the form of groceries or other goods, services such as self-care, transportation, or healthcare and sometimes local retail services. The reinforcers target abstinence behaviors such as attendance, adherence to treatment goals, compliance with medication, participation in therapy, abstinence from substances and completion of therapy (Stitzer & Petry, 2006). It is important to evaluate the value of the reinforcer to the individual. The likelihood of the reward effectiveness increases with the perceived value of the reward. Lamb et al. discovered that higher payment amounts and the easier target criterion resulted in a higher likelihood of participants meeting the criterion (Lamb, Kirby, Morral, Galbicka, & Iguchi, 2004).

A contingency contract is a more formalized written agreement that is developed in collaboration with the person and/or significant other to explicitly state the positive and negative reinforcers for performing the desired behavior, as well as aversive reinforcers for failure to perform the behavior. Suitable targets are those behaviors that are observable. The negotiated terms of the contract are specific and relatively straightforward with the reinforcing (positive or desirable) contingency being available shortly after the behavior is observed. A common example of a contingency contract is a paycheck given after a set amount of work is completed. See Box 8.4 for a checklist to assist the APPN in developing a contingency contract. The steps in this checklist should be sequential because if secondary gains are not identified (see item 4 in Box 8.4), the individual will not be able to accomplish the desired behavior. Often, secondary gains are unconscious and should be explored with the patient prior to beginning the subsequent steps.

Bibliotherapy: The CBT therapist will often prescribe specific readings related to the individual's difficulties. Readings and references can be given to the patient of the many CBT-based self-help books as an adjunct to in-session work. A full list of readings and CBT-based self-help books can be found on the Academy of Cognitive Therapy website at www.academyofct.org. The website is updated regularly to include the most relevant and up-to-date titles for both clinicians and patients.

BOX 8.4 Checklist of Patient Outcomes for Contingency Contract

1. Identify target behavior.
2. Explore reasons for behavior.
3. Verbalize knowledge of consequences of behavior.
4. Identify secondary gains from behavior (i.e., attention).
5. Keep diary of when problem behavior occurs.
6. Keep log of sequence and pattern of behavior (who, what, when, how, and why).
7. Identify feelings that precede and follow behavior.
8. Keep diary of behavior and feelings.
9. Identify alternatives to behavior.
10. Write conditions under which desired behavior will occur and how behavior will be observed and measured.
11. Select positive reinforcers (i.e., weight loss, rewards).
12. Select aversive consequences for failure of desired behavior (i.e., chores).
13. Carry out plan for 1 week.
14. Practice desired behavior, step-by-step.
15. Keep diary of practice.
16. Involve family/friends in feedback/encouragement.
17. Identify other positive aspects associated with changed behavior.
18. Monitor ongoing weekly progress.

Source: Data from Dykes, P., Wheeler, K., & Boulton, M. (1998). Psychiatric copathways. In P. Dykes (Ed.), *Psychiatric clinical pathways: An interdisciplinary approach* (pp. 265–275). Gaithersburg, MD: Aspen.

Guided Relaxation and Meditation: APPNs often employ behavioral techniques aimed at reduction of autonomic nervous system responses to anxiety. They include deep breathing, relaxation training, meditation, and other exercises. These techniques help the individual to distract him- or herself from the upsetting thoughts and increase awareness of conscious control over breathing, heart rate, and other anxiety symptoms and thoughts. The individual may be assisted in "overbreathing" as a way to demonstrate control over "hyperventilation." This technique should be used only by the experienced APPN. One very brief relaxation exercise is to have the patient breath in deeply for 5 seconds, breath out for 5 seconds while saying: "Relax. . . . . . .relax. . . . . . .relax" in a soothing tone. I recommend that patients practice this easy exercise a minimum of 10 times daily until they find they are able to do it almost automatically.

Social Skills Training: These skills are often taken for granted by many individuals. It is therefore important for the APPN to review and instruct on behaviors that will improve the potential for successful social interactions. For example, a therapist may notice that the patient looks at the floor or the ceiling during conversation or when introducing herself. The APPN may make use of this information by role-playing skills such as maintaining eye contact during an interview, shaking hands assertively, developing techniques for self-expression, and conveying opinions as well as overt changes such as appropriate language in public.

Shame-Attacking Exercises: This technique was first introduced by Albert Ellis, the father of rational emotive therapy (RET). In this type of therapy, the therapist engages the individual in exercises that emphasize their concern for what others think of them. For example, a person who is afraid of drinking soup in public may be assigned the task of going to a restaurant with a friend, ordering soup, and drinking it loudly while the friend makes note of how many people are really interested in what they are doing. The friend would then share the notes on the actual responses of the other diners as a way to disarm the person's irrational belief that others are looking at him or her eat, slurp, etc.

EXPOSURE THERAPY

Exposure therapies are a specific type of CBT that are aimed to reduce distress as a person experiences the sounds, smells, thoughts, and sights of things associated with danger. As the person is exposed to the stimuli, the person become less sensitive to them and fear eases as arousal decreases. Exposure therapies are used for most of the anxiety disorders including posttraumatic stress disorder, specific phobias, and social anxiety disorders. One rapidly expanding type of exposure therapy is virtual reality (VR) therapy that closely mimics the feared environment. Examples of situations that can be duplicated using VR include public speaking, school or social phobia situation, driving situations, combat-related scenarios for military members that simulate the environment without having to travel to another area, flying in an airplane, and a multitude of other situations limited only by imagination. A person is never put in a simulation that is dangerous or unethical or not agreed to by that person in advance. For example, a simulation to recreate a rape would be (at the least) unethical; however, recreating a university parking lot, concert hall, or apartment would be possible exposure options. To introduce the process of exposure therapy, this author uses the example of putting your feet in the water at the beach or pool and discovering that the water is very cold. This is at first very uncomfortable; however, if the person continues to stand there (exposure) they will habituate to the cold sensation. They then gradually enter the water, waiting at each step to habituate to the temperature. If the person states, "I can't go in that cold water! I'm leaving!" when they first step into the water, the person will never be able to enter the water and will be left on the sidelines watching everyone else enjoy the experience.

Exposure therapy then begins with the development of a "fear hierarchy" that consists of 10 to 15 levels of exposure. The hierarchy consists of the feared objects or situations graded or rank-ordered in their level of "subjective units of distress scale," referred to as the SUDS score. The SUDS score ranges from 0 to 10, with 0 reflecting no disturbance at all and 10 reflecting the worst disturbance that the patient feels for that particular situation. It is usually ranked with the lowest scored SUDS items at the bottom and the highest SUDS items at the top (Dobson & Dobson, 2009). Exposure therapy includes temporal components such as:

1. Graded exposure using a fear hierarchy, in which feared objects, activities, or situations are ranked high to low with mildly or moderately difficult exposures at the top progressing to more difficult ones.
2. Flooding also uses a fear hierarchy; however, the exposure begins with the most frightening task (e.g., fear of snakes is conquered by sitting in a container full of snakes).
3. Systematic desensitization in which exposure to an anxiety-producing situation is combined with relaxation exercises to the associated feared objects, activities, or situations with mastery feelings and relaxation.

Processing in exposure includes strategies such as flooding, prolonged exposure, in vivo exposure, directed exposure, interoceptive exposure, and imaginal exposure. Exposure involves confrontation with the feared stimulus with prolonged excitation of the fear response until habituation and then extinction of the fear response in the presence of the trigger occurs. Deciding which exposure component to use depends on the person's presenting problem as various methods for exposure have been developed. If the person suffers from panic anxiety, interoceptive exposure should be considered. This involves exercises such as stair stepping and head shaking that bring on panic-like symptoms. If the person does not suffer from panic, imaginal exposure through writing or talking about the trauma is appropriate.

Exposure or prolonged exposure involves the ongoing systematic activation of the fear response until extinction or desensitization occurs. The process may involve specific or nonspecific environmental cues in reality (in vivo) or through imaging. It can be likened to watching a scary movie repeatedly until it no longer creates hyperarousal and fear. For example, when someone experiences fear of an object, they tend to avoid it. Avoidance or escape from the phobic object results in a temporary reduction in anxiety. As a result the individual's coping choice is reinforced through negative reinforcement. In prolonged exposure, the therapist uses a process of systematically desensitizing the individual to the avoidance pattern by gradually exposing them to the phobic object (either virtually or actually) until it can be tolerated without disabling anxiety.

For severe trauma and phobias it is recommended to teach the patient some relaxation techniques prior to beginning the exposures. If relaxation techniques are taught, it is important to teach the patient when it is acceptable to use relaxation (in between or after exposures, not during the actual exposures conducted with the therapist). Prior to beginning the desensitization process, the APPN and the individual explore alternative cognitive strategies such as distraction to cope with anxiety. This helps the individual build a set of tools to control fear outside the exposures themselves. After the individual has mastered alternative responses the person is gradually exposed to the feared object. In exposure and response prevention practice, the patient is required to keep the fear level as high as possible during the exposure. The person will experience an inability to keep a high level of fear with successful exposure therapy within APPN 10 to 15 minutes. For example, someone who has a fear of contamination would be assisted in developing a fear hierarchy with individual situations rated on a scale of 10 (worst possible exposure) to 1 (very limited exposure). The APPN and the individual practice with increasingly unpleasant situations: a sink at a public restroom to a visibly contaminated or a smelly outhouse, for example. At each step in the progression, the patient is desensitized to the fear by preventing the usual response. The person realizes that nothing bad happens from the exposure, and the fear gradually extinguishes. For example, a person with a fear of attending classes may begin with driving around the school, then gradually moving up to touring a classroom both empty and filled before actually signing up for and attending a class.

Example of Exposure and Response Prevention Session

Exposure and response prevention (ERP) is a guided exposure through fear responses in order to habituate the patient to the perceived threat by preventing the usual response to threat (avoidance). The process begins with an explanation of ERP and the development of a fear hierarchy. The therapist guides the patient through gradual mastery of each level of the hierarchy until the patient is ready to master the actual situation in vivo. Before beginning exposure therapy, make sure that the patient is medically cleared for having elevated heart rates and increased respirations that occur with fear responses.

For example, a psychologist, Dr. J, came to treatment for an inability to drive over bridges without significant anxiety after suffering a seizure while he was driving several friends in the car. Six months previously he had been diagnosed with a brain tumor after suffering a seizure. Dr. J had surgery and the tumor was removed without complications and he had not needed radiation or chemotherapy. He was now on anticonvulsant medication and reported that his surgeon felt he had a good prognosis and suffered no residual neurological deficits. See Box 8.5 for the hierarchy constructed and how this was paired with ratings of distress and imagery.

BOX 8.5 Hierarchy for Driving Fear of Bridges

Thinking about going in the car if he has to go across a bridge.

1. Imagining driving across the bridge (pick a specific bridge)
2. Getting into the car with the idea you are going driving
3. Driving the car for about 2–3 minutes with image of bridge
4. Riding in the car to a bridge with a friend driving, but not driving over the bridge
5. Riding in the car with a friend driving and going over a small bridge
6. Driving the car with a friend and getting off the exit before the small bridge
7. Driving the car with a friend and going across the small bridge
8. Driving the car alone and going across the small bridge
9. Driving the car alone and going over a slightly larger bridge
10. Repeat with larger bridges

For example, in the exposure therapy example above, Dr. J. constructs a hierarchy of feared situations in session 1. At his next session, he was asked to visualize himself at #1 in his hierarchy of fears, thinking about going in a car over a bridge with as much vividness and detail as possible, as if he were "right there." He is asked to stay with all of his "fear thoughts" and to say them out loud while he is imagining. It is important to rate the current SUDS score at the beginning of the exposure, and throughout the exposure. Dr. J states that he has a SUDS rating of 3 at the beginning of the exposure. He reports his thoughts out loud along in detail, with the therapist asking for (a) current SUDS score, (b) what other thoughts he might be having, and (c) the experience of the exposure physically. It is very important that the exposure continue until the SUDS score is at least 50%, or more, lower than the starting SUDS score. This is the body's way of extinguishing the automatic fight/flight response to a stimulus. If the patient does not reach at least a 50% reduction in SUDS score, he or she will accentuate the fear response, as this would be the same as an avoidance response.

He was asked to stay with the fear thoughts and is asked to rate his anxiety on a 1 to 10 scale, with 10 being the worst, and he responded that it was a 3. He was then asked to describe his thoughts regarding his fears ("what is your worst-case scenario in this image?") repeating his SUDS rating. Dr. J stated, "I don't have any distress at all now with this image!" It is explained that this is successful exposure and he is asked to practice this level of the exposure at home daily for 1 week. Then #2 was imaged in the same way repeating the fear and stating automatic thoughts (about a minute each). If the patient experiences greater than a 4 on a 0 to 10 scale with the fear, it is extremely important to continue the exposure until a rating of at least 2 is achieved (although most individuals will find that they cannot stay anxious over a 1). The patient must master the current step (SUDS of 1 or 0 at the beginning of the imagery) before going onto the next one. Dr. J was able to work through this exercise and could then transfer this learning in vivo.

The APPN must remain sensitive to the individual's response pattern in order to prevent traumatization or increasing anxiety. It is strongly suggested that anyone who is considering adding ERP to their toolbox be trained by someone expert in ERP and use the process for one of their own fears to experience how ERP works (e.g., common phobic responses to spiders, snakes, or bugs).

It is beyond the scope of this single chapter to review all of the options that have been adapted and researched in the area of exposure therapy. Please see Table 8.3 for a partial list of research on exposure therapy.

TABLE 8.3 EXPOSURE THERAPY RESEARCH	
Exposure Therapy	**Citation***
VR exposure superior to CBT alone for social anxiety disorder	Anderson, Zimand, Hodges, and Rothbaum (2005); Morina, Brinkman, Hartanto, Kampmann, and Emmelkamp (2015); Price, Mehta, Tone, and Anderson (2011); Safir, Wallach, and Bar-Zvi (2012)
PE	Foa, McLean, Capaldi, and Rosenfield (2013); Nacasch et al. (2011)
CPT	Resick, Nishith, Weaver, Astin, and Feuer (2002); Resick et al. (2015)
SIT	Foa et al. (1999); Meichenbaum and Deffenbacher (1988)
VR	Rothbaum et al., (2006); Rothbaum, Hodges, and Kooper (1997); Rothbaum et al. (1995); Rothbaum, Hodges, Smith, Lee, & Price (2000); Rothbaum, Rizzo, & Difede (2010)
EMDR	Novo et al. (2014); Shapiro (1989, 1996)
ERP	Bolton and Perrin (2008); Lindsay, Crino, and Andrews (1997); Meyer (1966)

CBT, cognitive behavior therapy; CPT, cognitive processing therapy; EMDR, eye movement desensitization and reprocessing; ERP, exposure and response prevention; PE, prolonged exposure; SIT, stress inoculation training; VR, virtual reality.

MODIFICATIONS OF CBT

Schema Therapy

Schemas develop early in life based on an individual's experiences with others and their environment. Schemas are fundamental core beliefs or assumptions and are part of the perceptual filter people use to view the world. People are guided by templates, or schemas, through every action, reaction, and interaction based on our own developmental, personal, religious, familial, cultural, gender, and age-related experiences (Beck, Freeman, & Associates, 1990; Beck, Freeman, Davis, & Associates, 2003; Beck et al., 1979; Freeman & Freeman, 2005). Schemas are in a constant state of change and adaptation and become increasingly complex as one ages. Although schemas are alterable, the process of accommodation and adaptation may serve to help or hinder individuals when they apply their schema to new situations or functions that come their way. For example, those with an abandonment/instability schema would be plagued by thoughts about the unreliability of those available for support and connection and may have borderline personality traits while those with a social/isolation/alienation schema would have thoughts of being different from the rest of the world and might suffer from schizoid traits. Schemas are selected for recall or suppressed in memory; they are used for interpretation of information, generation of affect, motivation, action, and control (Beck et al., 1990; Freeman & Freeman, 2005). Understanding a person's schemas, belief systems, and underlying attitudes is essential in understanding the individual (Freeman & Freeman, 2005). See Table 8.4 for personality disorder diagnoses and corresponding schemas.

Young (1991) proposed that early schemas are more resistant to change than schema that develops later in life. He identified these schemas as early maladaptive schemas.

TABLE 8.4 PERSONALITY DISORDER DIAGNOSES AND CORRESPONDING SCHEMA	
Diagnosis	**Schema**
Paranoid personality disorder	It isn't safe to confide in other people. Other people have hidden motives.
Schizoid personality disorder	It doesn't matter what other people think of me. I enjoy doing things by myself.
Antisocial personality disorder	What others think of me doesn't matter. Rules are meant for others and only fools follow the rules. If someone is hurt or inconvenienced by me, that is their problem.
Borderline personality disorder	It is impossible to control my emotions. I need to be close to someone, but I don't trust that anyone who gets close to me really understands me, or likes me.
Narcissistic personality disorder	I am a very special person entitled to special treatment and privileges. It is very important to get recognition and praise. People have no right to criticize me!
Avoidant personality disorder	I am socially inept and undesirable. I don't fit in. Others are potentially critical, indifferent, demeaning, and rejecting.
Dependent personality disorder	I am helpless when left on my own. I can't make decisions on my own. I can't cope as other people cope.
Obsessive-compulsive personality disorder	I have to depend on myself to see that things get done. It is important to have rules, systems, and order. If I don't perform at the highest level, I have failed.

According to Young et al., in comparison with standard cognitive therapy, schema therapy probes more deeply into the childhood origins of distorted thinking, relies more on imagery and emotion-focused techniques, and is somewhat longer-term and is often combined with traditional cognitive therapy (Young, Klosko, & Weishaar, 2003). For example, Young uses the CBT technique of identifying if the patient is using an emotion that is adaptive or maladaptive to guide decision-making and cognitive processing. He then assists to facilitate the identification of beliefs that block the process of change. Images, according to Young, are powerful forms of cognitions and long before we develop language, we develop memory encoded as pictures, or images. Schema therapy is and has been a critical component of classical CBT.

Young uses many of the CBT techniques of guided imagery, imagery rescripting, imagery substitution, or even cognitive restructuring of images to reframe the view of an image to something more positive, less distressing or even useful for a patient.

Dialectical Behavior Therapy

Dialectical behavior therapy (DBT) is a multimodal cognitive behavioral treatment developed by Dr. Marsha M. Linehan to work with subgroups of those diagnosed with borderline personality disorder (BPD), specifically those who have chronic nonsuicidal self-harm behaviors, or who abuse substances (Linehan, Tutek, Heard, & Armstrong,

1994). DBT works very well in the subset of cluster B personality disordered patients, which includes those viewed as dramatic-emotional such as antisocial, borderline, histrionic, and narcissistic individuals (Linehan, Heard, & Armstrong, 1993). DBT has recently been modified for those who have both BPD and eating disorders (EDs; Linehan & Chen, 2005). A full description of DBT is included in Chapter 18, of this volume and the reader is referred there for additional information.

Acceptance and Commitment Therapy

Acceptance and Commitment Therapy (ACT) is often referred to as a "third wave" of CBT (Hayes, 2016). ACT helps the person to accept the difficulties that come with life and focuses on three areas: (a) accept your reactions and be present; (b) choose a valued direction; and (c) take action. ACT is thus based on acceptance and mindfulness strategies that provide a means of modifying the relationship between thoughts, feelings, and overt actions. It is a behavior and analytically based psychotherapy approach that attempts to undermine emotional avoidance and increase the capacity for behavior change using a theory of language and cognition called relational frame theory (Hayes, Barnes-Holmes, & Roche, 2001). Patients are taught to observe and mindfully watch their thoughts while they fully feel their feelings, rather than trying to change them. They are next taught to focus on overt actions that will move them in valued directions (Hayes et al., 2001).

The process of ACT helps the person to accept undesirable thoughts and feelings, while behaving in a manner that is congruent with his or her values and goals (Hayes, Luoma, Bond, Masuda, & Lillis, 2006). For example, the negative impact of stigmatizing beliefs and attitudes comes from the function of those thoughts, not from the presence of such thoughts. ACT helps people develop a more accepting, mindful relationship with their thoughts and feelings. As acceptance of certain stigmatizing thoughts and feelings is achieved, they are disconnected from the previously acquired overt negative behavior that might obstruct recovery (Hayes et al., 2006). For example, if a person with a substance use disorder thinks "I hurt everyone I love," he will tend to develop avoidance behaviors of family members or loved ones to avoid experiencing the negative attribution of being a hurtful person. ACT helps that person respond in different ways that aim to increase behaviors that expand his or her support systems moving him or her forward in recovery (Hayes & Wilson, 1994).

APPLICATION OF CBT TO COMMON PSYCHIATRIC DISORDERS

There are numerous practice guidelines for therapists who are skilled in CBT based on research outcomes for specific problems such as depression, anxiety, personality disorders, and substance misuse patients. A partial list of practice guidelines is provided in Table 8.5.

Cognitive Model for Depression

The cognitive model of depression emphasizes the *cognitive triad* to illustrate depression generation and maintenance. The premise is that individuals develop and then maintain a negative self-view and this attitude extends to the world, their experiences and on into the future. As a result, they perceive themselves as worthless, abandoned, and inadequate. As depression takes hold, the individual feels overwhelmed with demands and seemingly impenetrable barriers preventing them from realizing their goals. The world takes on a gray cast devoid of pleasure and is viewed pessimistically.

TABLE 8.5   SOURCES OF PRACTICE GUIDELINES FOR USE OF COGNITIVE BEHAVIOR THERAPY FOR SPECIFIC DISORDERS

Disorder	Guideline Resources
Psychiatric disorders (general)	American Psychiatric Association. (2006). *Practice guidelines for the treatment of psychiatric disorders: Compendium 2006.* Washington, DC: Author.
Obsessive-compulsive disorder	Foa, E. B., Elna, Y., & Lichner, T. K. (2012). *Exposure and response (ritual) prevention for obsessive compulsive disorder: Therapist guide.* New York, NY: Oxford University Press.
Posttraumatic stress disorder	Foa, E. B., Keane, T. M., Friedman, M. J., & Cohen, J. A.. (2010). *Effective treatments for PTSD. Practice guidelines from the International Society for Traumatic Stress Studies.* (2nd ed.). New York, NY: Guilford Press.
Psychosis	Hagen, R., Turkington, D., Grawe, R. (2010). *CBT for psychosis: A symptom-based approach.* New York, NY: Routledge.
Depression	Gilson, M., Freeman, A., Yates, M. J., & Freeman, S. M. (2009). *Overcoming depression: A cognitive therapy approach: Therapists guide.* New York, NY: Oxford University Press.
Anxiety	Barlow, D. H., & Craske, M. G. (2006). *Mastery of your anxiety and worry: Therapists guide.* New York, NY: Oxford University Press; Craske, M. G., & Barlow, D. H. (2006). *Mastery of your anxiety and panic: Therapist guide.* New York, NY: Oxford University Press.
Insomnia	Edinger, J. D., & Carney, C. E. (2008). *Overcoming insomnia: A cognitive-behavioral therapy approach: Therapist guide.* New York, NY: Oxford University Press.
Hoarding	Steketee, G., & Frost, R. O. (2006). *Compulsive hoarding and acquiring: Therapist guide.* New York, NY: Oxford University Press.
Eating disorders	Agras, W. S., & Apple, R. F. (2015). *Overcoming eating disorders: A cognitive-behavioral therapy approach for bulimia nervosa and binge-eating disorder. Therapist guide* (2nd ed.). New York, NY: Oxford University Press
Sexual dysfunction	Wincze, J. (2009). *Enhancing sexuality: A problem-solving approach to treating dysfunction: Therapist guide.* New York, NY: Oxford University Press.
Chronic pain	Otis, J. D. (2007). *Managing chronic pain: A cognitive behavioral therapy approach: Therapist guide.* New York, NY: Oxford University Press.

CBT focuses on altering patients' views of themselves, their situations, and the resources around them (Beck et al., 1979). Therapy is structured, active, and reality based as well as time-limited. The individual is taught to take certain specific steps to combat his or her depressive views. These steps include identifying and monitoring automatic thoughts, critical examination of evidence, substitution of objective interpretations for negative, dysfunctional attributions and to recognize connections between thoughts and feelings.

For those who have been traumatized numerous negative cognitions may be present, particularly for those who have suffered from interpersonal violence. These include thoughts about self-blame, guilt, shame, low self-esteem, danger, defectiveness, and unworthiness (Beck, 1989; Briere & Scott, 2006). It is important that patients describe their thoughts and perceptions related to the trauma. This can be accomplished through the narrative as well as through journaling about the event. The journaling can be assigned as homework occasionally during therapy so that the patient writes about a specific topic, recalling in as much detail as possible the event. The person is then asked to read it aloud to the therapist the following week. Using the Socratic method described above, the APPN can ask open-ended questions that allow the patient to examine his or her interpretations about the experience. Briere & Scott (2006) list some typical questions:

> *"Did you have any thoughts while it (the traumatic event) was happening? What were they?"*
> *"Given, the situation, do you think there was anything else you could have done?"*
> *"So, that made you feel that you were to blame/responsible/bad/stupid/seductive. Can we go over what happened and see what made you think that?"*
> *"Did you want him/her/them to rape/beat/abuse/hurt you?" Do you remember ever wanting that?"*
> *"You say that you were hurt/raped/beaten because you asked for it/were deductive/didn't lock the door/were out late. Can we go over the evidence for that conclusion? Maybe it's more complicated than that?"*
> *"If this happened to someone else, would you come to the same conclusion?"*
> *"It sounds like you believe what he/she said about that. Was he/she a person you would believe when he/she said something?"*
> *"Why do you think he/she did that? Did he/she get anything out of it?"*
> *(Briere & Scott, 2006, pp. 112–113)*

Outcome studies of different types of CBT treatments historically used self-report measures of symptom change. More recently, researchers are studying the effect of CBT psychotherapies on brain function using a variety of brain imaging techniques such as functional MRI. In studies that include brain imaging techniques to evaluate both CBT and pharmacological interventions, outcomes reported indicated that there are significant changes in cerebral blood flow in specific brain areas in response to both treatments for depression and anxiety disorders (Furmark, Tillfors, & Marteinsdottir, 2002; Goldapple et al., 2004; Nakatani et al., 2003; Paquette et al., 2003).

Cognitive Model for Anxiety

Anxiety is an adaptive survival strategy. When the body experiences or perceives a threat to survival, it prepares for flight, fight, or fleeing through activation of the autonomic nervous system. The nervous system activation is experienced as increased heartbeat, muscle tension, increased blood flow, and diaphoresis (to cool the body). If there is an actual threat, the individual is prepared to respond adaptively. If there is no threat, the individual interprets the symptoms as anxiety with the accompanying psychological response called "fear." Anxiety symptoms that seem to come out of nowhere cause the individual to fear the onset of this uncomfortable experience (Williams et al., 2010). The individual scans the environment and may or may not locate something to attribute to the symptom activation. As more and more attributions of threat occur (e.g., bridge, heights, public speaking), the person becomes more and more alert to potential activation. This sets the person up for a "fear of fear" response. The anxious individual distorts innocuous events, exaggerates the potential for harm, and develops behaviors that interfere with adaptive coping strategies. As the cycle increases in velocity, the individual believes that he or she is unable to cope and is therefore helpless to alleviate the anxiety symptoms (Williams et al., 2010).

The best illustration of the efficacy of CBT for anxiety comes from the work of Barlow and Clark on the treatment of panic disorders (Adler, Craske, Kirshenbaum, & Barlow, 1989; Barlow, Brown, & Craske, 1994; Craske, Rapee, Jackel, & Barlow, 1989; Rapee, Craske, & Barlow, 1994). They observed the constellation of cognitive symptoms that team with behavioral symptoms to create a panic reaction/response in an individual. Through extensive research they demonstrated that combining cognitive techniques to modify fearful cognitions along with specific behavioral approaches reduced or eliminated the panic response/reaction in most individuals (Hofmann, Barlow, Clark, Hollon, & Mayo-Wilson, 2015; Margraf, Barlow, Clark, & Telch, 1993; Wells et al., 2016).

Cognitive Model for Personality Disorder

One of the hallmark treatments of personality disorders is CBT. Cognitive theorists and psychoanalysts have both agreed that it is imperative to identify and then modify "core" problems when treating individuals with personality disorders. The difference between the two theories lies in the perspective of the structure of personality disorder. Psychoanalysis believes that the structures are unconscious and therefore are mostly unavailable to the individual, while the cognitive theorist believes that the products and processes are within the realm of awareness and therefore more accessible. Dysfunctional behaviors, thoughts, and feelings, according to cognitive theory, are in large part due to the function of certain schemas (rules or patterns we have developed for living). These schemas consistently bias our judgments and create a tendency to skew our views, creating situations in which we tend to make cognitive errors and draw faulty conclusions (Freeman, Davis, & DiTomasso, 1992; Stoffers et al., 2012).

It is rare that someone will seek treatment for their personality disorder traits; instead, they usually come into treatment at the behest of some significant other or other external pressure. They may also come in for treatment of a secondary result of the outcomes of their behavior patterns such as depression, relationship difficulties, anxiety problems, or other issues. Often these individuals will see their problems as independent of their own behavior and describe themselves as a victim with little to no idea as to how they got into these difficulties, how they contribute to their problems, and/or how to change (Brown, Newman, Charlesworth, Crits-Christoph, & Beck, 2004; Davidson, Tyrer, Norrie, Palmer, & Tyrer, 2010; Davidson et al., 2006). Others in their lives are well aware of the self-defeating elements of their behaviors (such as overdependence, lack of empathy, self-centeredness, inhibition, drama) and may express frustration, dismay, or even incredulousness that the individual does not see it himself (Beck et al., 2003; Freeman et al., 1992).

Cognitive Model for Substance Misuse

The community reinforcement approach (CRA) has been developed for use with patients who abuse substances (Miller, Meyers, & Hiller-Sturmhöfel, 1999). Contingency management is a key component and interventions include social, recreational, familial, and vocational reinforcers in order to help the person through the process of abstinence and maintenance. Additional components in CRA include (a) functional analysis of substance use, (b) social and recreational counseling, (c) employment counseling, (d) drug refusal training, (e) relaxation training, (f) behavioral skills training, and (g) reciprocal relationship counseling. The *National Institutes of Drug Addiction Therapy Manual* recommends a reinforcement model that typically includes vouchers for behavioral outcomes such as clean urine drug screens, participation in treatment, and completion of the treatment program (pubs.niaaa.nih.gov/publications/arh23-2/116-121.pdf). Vouchers are used as opposed to cash or saleable items to avoid triggering the individual's craving response to cash (cash is usually associated with ability to purchase substances). See Table 8.6 for therapist resources and websites for specific populations.

TABLE 8.6 CBT WEBSITE RESOURCES FOR SPECIFIC POPULATIONS	
Population	**Specific Approaches and Websites and Links for Additional Information**
Addiction	TIP 34: Brief Interventions and Brief Therapies for Substance Abuse. This manual introduces brief interventions, and includes cognitive behavior therapy for mental illness, substance use disorders, or both. It presents practical methods and case scenarios for implementing shorter forms of treatment for a range of populations and issues. URL: https://store.samhsa.gov/product/TIP-34-Brief-Interventions-and-Brief-Therapies-for-Substance-Abuse/SMA12-3952
Depression	www.psychologyinfo.com/depression/cognitive.htm Brief overview of treating depression by Psychology Information Online developed by Donald J. Franklin, PhD. Reviews the thoughts, feelings, and behaviors common to depressive diseases as well as the therapeutic interventions used in CBT to reverse the depressive cycle. Automatic thoughts are outlined, as are specific ways to cope more effectively.
Child sexual abuse	www.childwelfare.gov/pubPDFs/trauma.pdf and www.samhsa.gov/child-trauma Substance Abuse and Mental Health Services Administration Model Programs: CBT for Child Sexual Abuse Trauma Focused Treatment.
Anxiety and social anxiety	socialanxietyinstitute.org and www.nimh.nih.gov/health/topics/anxiety-disorders/index.shtml Dr. Thomas Richards, Director of the Social Anxiety Institute, has posted several excellent monographs on treating anxiety disorders with CBT on his websites. He discusses the cognitive, behavioral, and physical components common to these disorders in easy-to-understand terms. The reader is "walked" through the guidelines of the CBT process of treatment and referred to additional resources.
Obsessive-compulsive disorder	www.ocdonline.com/cbt-for-ocd and ocdla.com/cognitivebehavioraltherapy These websites outline basic CBT treatment of obsessive-compulsive disorder. The explanation also includes a brief explanation of the integration of behavioral techniques utilized within the CBT framework to augment the total CBT therapeutic armament thereby strengthening the overall treatment effect.

TABLE 8.6 CBT THERAPIST WEBSITE RESOURCES FOR SPECIFIC POPULATIONS (*CONTINUED*)	
Eating disorders	https://medicine.yale.edu/psychiatry/research/programs/clinical_people/power/?locationId=354 https://www.div12.org/treatment/cognitive-behavioral-therapy-for-anorexia-nervosa/ These websites include information on CBT treatment of eating disorders, specifically self-image components, incorrect beliefs about the disorder, behavioral changes that the individual will be making (such as meal diaries), developing mastery over mood and other facets of their lives, and other very important components of the eating disorders spectrum. The outline also discusses expectations of treatment, length of treatment, relapse and follow-up.
Chronic pain	Winterowd, C., Beck, A. T. & Gruener, D. (2003). *Cognitive therapy with chronic pain patients.* New York, NY: Springer Publishing Company. Caudill, M. (2016). *Managing pain before it manages you* (4th ed.). New York, NY: Guilford Press. Both of these volumes are excellent adjuncts to the CBT clinician working with individuals with chronic pain conditions. They contain full explanations of the physiology of pain, the cognitions association with chronic pain as well as behaviors common to chronic pain sufferers. In addition they contain the techniques used in CBT to alter the thoughts, feelings, and behaviors that cripple chronic pain sufferers.
Schizophrenia	www.psychologyinfo.com/schizophrenia/cognitive.htm There is a misconception that CBT cannot be used with persons who are "too dysfunctional." This is incorrect. In fact, CBT is very effective with individuals who are cognitively impaired. The therapist simply uses a greater number of *behavioral* techniques in these cases. In cases with individuals with schizophrenia the therapist is often working with the family members in addition to the patient. Dr. Donald Franklin has a very brief discussion on his website of this type of treatment:
General information	en.wikipedia.org/wiki/Cognitive_behavior_therapy Online encyclopedia definition. The National Library of Medicine online reference book for Cognitive Behavior Therapy: https://www.ncbi.nlm.nih.gov/books/NBK279297/ Wright, J. H., Brown, G. K., Thase, M. E., & Basco, M. R. (2017). *Learning cognitive-behavior therapy: An illustrated guide* (Core competencies in psychotherapy, 2nd ed.). Washington, DC: American Psychiatric Publishing.

CBT, cognitive behavior therapy.

CASE EXAMPLE

Bethany is a 44-year-old woman who has been married for 20 years to her step-uncle who raised her after her parents died and is 40 years her senior. She has no children and works as an attorney. She described her parents as distant, paying minimal attention to her while she was growing up. Mother and father died when she was 15 and the loss was considered "a surprise and shock." She has one brother whom she describes as "distant" and seldom available to her. Her brother lives at a significant distance from her, making contact difficult. She has occasional affairs, but they are less frequent and less pleasurable than they used to be.

Bethany has had more than 10 years of treatment with medications as well as a variety of psychotherapeutic techniques for her self-reported depression and attention deficit disorder. Her Beck Depression Inventory (DPI) score at intake was 51 (out of 63 possible) and her Quick Inventory of Depression Symptomatology (QIDS) was 23 (out of 27 possible), both of which are in the severe range. She denied suicidal ideation or intent. There was no evidence of hallucinations, delusions, or cognitive impairment. She reported significant sleep problems with daytime somnolence. She stated that she used to be very productive, creative, and happy; however, she has not felt that way for a very long time. She was extremely tearful during the interview, reporting feeling overwhelmed, hopeless, and exhausted. She felt extreme guilt that she had not been the kind of wife her husband deserved and wondered why he puts up with her. She was concerned she would lose her job because of her inability to concentrate and low productivity level. She felt unappreciated at work by her supervisor, who told her she was the "least productive" member of the firm. Bethany stated that she had no energy, restless sleep, irritability, and indecisiveness and felt like a "total failure at life." She has only one close female friend, who has been unaware of her affairs.

Bethany is very attractive and maintains good physical condition, although she feels unattractive. She also experiences moderate to severe pain related to fibromyalgia and arthritis. Treatment included several long- and short-acting opiate pain relievers as well as gabapentin (an anticonvulsant used for neuropathic pain relief).

Her diagnosis from previous and current psychiatrists included major depression, recurrent, severe and attention deficit hyperactivity disorder (ADHD), predominantly inattentive type. Medication attempts had included more than 10 different antidepressants (all noneffective) as well as several stimulants for treatment of her ADHD. Laboratory tests completed included thyroid function tests, liver and kidney function tests, vitamin B12 and folate levels, iron panel with percent saturation, electrolytes, and a complete blood count. All of her tests were in normal range.

The initial interview focused on eliciting her current impression of her problems, her view of her treatment history, and underlying beliefs regarding both issues. It was important to determine the psychodynamic impact regarding her lack of improvement over the past decade to evaluate the effect this had on her expectations for change, hope for improvement, and impact on motivation for another type of intervention. Care was taken to create a timeline of symptoms both historically and temporally. Information was documented using her own words whenever possible. Patient-generated metaphor, life rules, and conclusions were noted regarding her perception of her illness and its impact on her function, cognition, and outlook.

For this patient it was clear that several factors could be contributing to her depressive symptomatology. These factors are outlined here:

1. *Chronic pain.* It is well known that patients with chronic pain disorders are susceptible to depression due to feeling trapped in the pain, a lack of hope for improvement, and lack of sleep that disrupts normal sleep architecture. In addition, this patient was being treated with narcotic pain relievers at a significantly high dose. Narcotic pain relievers are notorious for problematic side effects that include somnolence, insomnia, and confusion. Somnolence and insomnia create severe lack of energy and motivation that can be mistaken as depressive symptoms.
2. *Stimulant use for ADHD.* Stimulant use, prescribed or not, has known side effects that include nervousness, insomnia, depression, and drowsiness. These medications can fuel an already existing depression and add an anxious quality.
3. *Chronic severe depression.* The patient's temporal course of severe depression would make it very likely that she would develop the negative cognitive set as described previously. A person's expectation of treatment failure is a significant predictor of

treatment outcome. Her disappointment in previous psychotherapeutic interventions as well as pharmacological interventions makes it likely that she does not trust that treatment, or treatment professionals, will be able to help her.

Formulation and Treatment Plan

The first step in any case formulation and treatment plan is an accurate diagnosis. The evaluation of Bethany's symptoms included exploration of hypomanic episodes to rule out a cyclical mood disorder such as bipolar disorder. Two episodes of spending in excess that included reduced need for sleep were uncovered in the previous 12 years. Each of the episodes was memorable to Bethany but did not create a severe hardship on herself or her husband, thereby meeting the criteria for hypomania, but not full mania. The presence of hypomanic episodes eliminated a diagnosis of major depressive disorder, and her diagnosis was changed to bipolar II disorder. Bipolar II, depressed type does not usually respond to traditional antidepressant therapies. Further questioning determined that Bethany may additionally suffer from a personality disorder; she had mild symptoms of dysfunction and the first depressive episode prior to adolescence . Once the diagnosis was in place, the clinician reviewed her medical history and childhood and family history, along with her current relationships. It was determined that the medications previously prescribed for Bethany had negatively impacted her level of depression as well as increased her feelings of pessimism that she would ever improve. She felt there was no treatment, medication, or healthcare practitioner who could help her. To minimize the impact of narcotic analgesics on her depressive symptoms and energy levels, a consultation was sought with her pain management team with Bethany's consent and cooperation. A narcotic medication taper was agreed to by Bethany, her pain team, and therapist to limit the dose to the lowest effective dose for pain while minimizing cognitive impairment, confusion, lack of concentration, and somnolence. Given that the patient had never experienced symptoms of distraction and lack of concentration prior to the time her depression became severe, it is most likely that her problems were due to hypomania and agitation. Therefore, it was agreed that the medications for ADHD would also gradually be tapered and discontinued.

Finally, she was prescribed a course of lamotrigine, which is indicated for bipolar disorders that are primarily depressive in quality. Patients who are severely incapacitated by depressive cognitions and symptoms are not as likely to respond to cognitive interventions until the depressive symptoms begin to abate. She was educated in the expectations for the new medication for effect and side effect. She was also educated in realistic expectations of medication for control of her symptoms, specifically that the medication would not be a "magic" solution. For her to experience maximum benefit, the APPN felt that she would have to "undo" the automatic thoughts and beliefs that perpetuated the depression. Providing her with a realistic introduction evaluating her thought patterns is the first cognitive intervention in her treatment plan. It says, "This is treatable, this is what to expect, this is what the pill will do, AND this is what you will need to do." (*Note:* these steps are not always contained within the cognitive therapy model of treatment.)

It should be noted that her decision to marry a man 40 years her senior who is/was her father-figure was most likely due to her low self-esteem and need for a father figure after her father's death. Her frequent affairs also point to an underlying personality disorder that is most likely fueled by the hypomania. She gains powerful feelings from attracting men and this gives her short-term relief from her feelings of insecurity about herself. Because stabilization is the most important first goal, these issues should not be addressed immediately as they would push the patient rather quickly out of therapy. If, and when, she wishes to bring these issues up in therapy they can be dealt with, but only at that time. It is important for the therapist to remember that it is the patient's goals, not the therapist's, that set the agenda in therapy.

Course of Therapy

The initial session included the components of assessment, preparation for therapy, introducing the patient to cognitive therapy, problem conceptualization, and initial goal development. The second session reinforced the first and integrated the information obtained from collateral sources, which refined the treatment plan. Medication changes were begun in the second session once it was clear that the patient understood the rationale for each of the changes recommended. Each session subsequent to these two sessions included a medication and symptom check prior to beginning the psychotherapy component of the session. Sessions typically begin with a review of any homework (out of session practice, or experiments). Initial interventions for Bethany were behavioral in content, given the level of cognitive impairment she was suffering. For example, Bethany's level of physical inactivity was affecting her energy, self-concept, and negative cognition. A daily exercise program was negotiated with Bethany that included 20 minutes of walking each morning.

The next set of sessions focused on uncovering specific irrational automatic thoughts as they appeared in the session. Once a thought was identified, the therapist repeated the thought and discussed it with the patient. For example, "Everyone thinks I am such a slug!" Bethany was asked "Everyone? Virtually everyone thinks you are a slug?" Her response was, "Well, no, not everyone, almost everyone." This was explored further, and it was determined that the only one who had complained about Bethany's activity level was her boss. Another example of Bethany's use of overgeneralization was, "There is nothing normal in my life!" and "Why do these things always happen to me?" Bethany was interrupted each time she used an overgeneralization. The thoughts were challenged in a respectful, exploration friendly manner until Bethany was stopping herself in therapy by saying "I don't mean 'always,' I mean most of the time."

Decatastrophizing techniques were used when Bethany began escalating, beginning with a small discrete problem ("I couldn't find my keys for a couple of minutes") to a bigger one ("My mind is a mess! I can't remember anything! I am never going to be able to convince my boss that I can do my job!"). The APPN modeled slowing down and evaluating the pattern of escalation by beginning with the activating event (losing the keys). Another technique that was useful with Bethany was the use of Socratic questioning. For example, asking, "What might be another explanation?" Questions framed in this way helped Bethany to break down errors in thought such as all-or-nothing thinking. Exaggerations in thinking were assessed using a scaling technique when Bethany expressed dichotomous categorical thinking processes. Breaking down categorized variables such as "I didn't get any sleep at all!" into "on a scale of 1 to 100, where would you rate your sleep last night?"

Interruption of Bethany's tearfulness was difficult during the early sessions because of the depth of her depression. For interruption to be considered respectful and helpful as a technique to (a) deescalate and (b) evaluate, Bethany was introduced to the technique early in the relationship. The introduction included the component that "for me to really understand what you are saying, I will be interrupting you at times to ask questions. For me to help I need to make sure I have a clear understanding of what you are telling me." Allowing Bethany to dissolve into tears perpetuates her current method of dealing with her depressive thinking. Interruption coupled with Socratic questions and scaling helped Bethany experience disruption of her escalation, which reinforces her ability to interrupt the process on her own.

Therapy Monitoring and Use of Feedback Information

Bethany's progress was monitored through use of the Beck Depression Inventory (BDI) and the Quick Inventory of Depressive Symptomatology-Clinician Rated (QIDS-C16). Bethany scored 51 (out of a possible 63) on the BDI and 23 (out of a possible 27) on the QIDS-C16 at time of initial assessment. The scores fall into the severe range of depression. Repeat measures were taken at biweekly intervals. Using the standardized instruments was a helpful adjunct to clinical judgment in psychotherapy in that it provided concrete evidence of improvement of symptoms.

Bethany's self-report during her first two return visits included "I am still a mess! I am not any better at all!" Use of the instruments supported the cognitive approaches used including using evidence to challenge her self-defeating thinking patterns. The evidence was introduced in a respectful manner using a method of cooperative inquiry. "Let's look at the scores on your reports. They indicated that your depression is still in the severe range but there are some changes. It looks like you are moving in the right direction." With assistance in evaluating each of her symptoms rather than her overall experience Bethany began to express hesitant optimism that she was improving. During the first month her scores decreased from 51 and 23 to 38 and 15 on the BDI and QIDS-C, respectively.

Once Bethany began to experience an improvement in her mood along with hope for additional improvement, she moved into a more active role in the therapy sessions. The APPN then was much more active during her first four sessions given her severe disabling symptoms and her weight. Her sleep gradually improved and her daytime somnolence began to abate. With the increase in energy she was able to walk 5 minutes a day beginning week 5 of therapy. Initially the exercise increased the pain of her fibromyalgia, which is an expected response. The APPN warned her that this was to be expected and did not indicate that she was harming herself. According to Bethany, several of her healthcare practitioners had told her that the best treatment for fibromyalgia was exercise but she had never felt motivated enough to begin a program.

Getting Bethany to take an active part in her healthcare (via exercise) was a key component in her therapy. Exercise served multiple purposes: (a) it helped reduce the pain experience, (b) it increased her body's tolerance for physical activity, (c) it increased her energy and motivation level, (d) exercise increased release of the body's endorphins and serotonin, both of which improve mood, and finally (e) reduced her weight, which motivated her to continue the program of activity and therapy.

Approximately 3 months into therapy, Bethany was introduced to two other components in her treatment: the daily thought record (DTR) and her activity/mood diary. She was assigned the book *Mind Over Mood* by Greenberger and Padesky (1995) as her resource and for supportive information both in and outside the sessions. Bethany had experienced success in challenging her automatic thoughts in the therapy setting and this information was used to reinforce DTR homework as a productive and helpful adjunct to her sessions. The APRN also used the DTRs suggested by Greenberger and Padesky (1995), including daily written entries indicating the person's (a) situation, (b) current mood rating, (c) automatic thoughts, (d) evidence that supports the hot thoughts, (e) evidence that does not support the hot thoughts, (f) alternative or balanced thoughts, and finally (g) postexercise mood rating.

Bethany's affect remained labile in the sessions with tearfulness during periods when she talked about feeling overwhelmed and useless. She would point this out and dichotomize her perception of the episode as "I am so tired of feeling like this all the time! I am never going to stop crying all the time!" Her expression of "all the time" and "never get better" were highlighted to help her evaluate the tearful episodes rationally. This type of situation lends itself to use of scaling techniques. This technique breaks down "all or nothing" thinking into a continuum to help the patient experience her perception in a more balanced way.

For Bethany this meant asking her "When you say 'all the time,' help me to understand how much of the time is 'all the time.' Is it 100% of the time (holding my hands about 2 feet apart), 50% of the time (moving my hands closer together) or another percentage of time?" Bethany's response was to stop crying, think deeply for a few minutes during which the APRN remained quiet, and then she said, "I am not sure . . . maybe 50%." The perception of all the time was broken down even further now that she was considering that "all the time" didn't mean "100% of the time." To help her evaluate her perception with more data the therapist asked: "When you came in the first day you said you would cry about four to five times a day for an hour or two each time. That means you were crying between 4 and 10 hours a day. Let's take the first variable. How many times a day are you crying?"

Bethany:	Maybe once or twice.
APPN:	So you have reduced the number of times you are crying from four or five to one or two. That is about 60% to 75%. And each time you have a crying episode, how long are you crying?
Bethany:	Oh, only about 10 minutes, sometimes as much as 20 minutes, but never more than that.
APPN:	It sounds like the duration of crying is pretty significantly reduced! As much as 80%. Let's go back and look at what you said earlier: "I cry all the time." What do you think about crying now?
Bethany:	I get it. I am doing it again! (laughs) It is still so easy to bury myself by automatically thinking the worse that can happen. When I stop and look at things realistically I know I am doing much better now. I have to practice stopping myself!

Documented baseline measurements help with the process of examining the evidence. Capturing the patient's own words, especially if there are measurable data points, is critical in the process of examining the evidence of progress when a patient has a bad moment or a bad day. Using the data to confront in a kind and respectful manner reinforces hope of recovery, which is one of the cornerstones of motivation to maintain change.

Concluding Evaluation of the Therapy's Process and Outcome

At this point in treatment Bethany has been in therapy for 6 months beginning with a weekly session for eight sessions tapering to one session a month. She continued to use the DTR for tough times and felt more confident with the process of challenging her automatic thoughts. The most difficult times for Bethany include those times when her pain flares up, usually during periods of unusual activity. Her overall pain ratings have fallen from her initial daily ratings of "8 or 9" to baselines of "4 to 6." A reduction in pain experience of 50% is considered successful in a pain management program. Bethany is happy with the change in baseline and is more functional. She walks twice a day, 10 minutes each time, which is a 100% increase in activity from her first session.

Bethany had a good response to the lamotrigine, which managed her hypomania very well. It is important with patients who have a disruptive underlying psychiatric problem amenable to medication that the medication is integrated into the therapy treatment plan. The APPN reinforced to Bethany that the medication would help stabilize her moods but would have no effect on the automatic thoughts, habits, and other destructive forces that had fueled her severe depression. The first 10 to 15 minutes of each session was devoted to evaluation of medication effectiveness, side effects, and dose response until she stabilized. Again, this is not a usual component of traditional cognitive psychotherapy; however, psychopharmacological education needs to be integrated into the treatment plan if the therapist is also the prescribing practitioner. See Chapters 14 and 15 for further information about integrating prescribing with psychotherapy.

POST-MASTER'S CBT TRAINING AND CERTIFICATION REQUIREMENTS

The American Association of Directors of Psychiatry Residency Training (www.aadprt .org) mandated training competencies in CBT (Sudak, Beck, & Wright, 2003). The National Association of Cognitive-Behavioral Therapists provides four certifications— the Certified Cognitive-Behavioral Therapist (CCBT), the Diplomate in Cognitive-Behavioral Therapy (DCBT), the Certified Cognitive-Behavioral Group Therapist (CBGT), and the Certified Cognitive-Behavioral Group Facilitator (CBGF). Certification at the Diplomat level requires a master's or doctoral degree in psychology, counseling, social work, psychiatry, or related field from a regionally accredited university. In addition, 10 years of postgraduate experience at providing CBT is required along with three letters of recommendation from mental health professionals who are familiar with the applicant's cognitive-behavioral skills. Applicants for the Diplomat certification must successfully complete a certification program in CBT that is recognized by the NACBT, such as Rational Emotive Behavior Therapy, Rational Behavior Therapy, Rational Living Therapy, or Cognitive Therapy. APRNs who wish to pursue certification can find additional information on their website (www.nacbt.org/certifications-htm).

The Academy of Cognitive Therapy offers certification for licensed mental health professionals in CBT and evaluates applicants' knowledge and ability before granting certification. The standards of the academy are designed to identify and credential clinicians with the necessary training, experience, and knowledge to be effective cognitive therapists. The Academy requires 40 hours of course work, completion of a compiled list of assigned readings including at least one core text on CBT theory and methods, a written case formulation, case supervision, and the submission of audio or videotaped sessions that are reviewed and rated by experienced cognitive therapists. In addition, the practitioner must have significant practice experience treating individuals with CBT with a variety of diagnoses. APPNs who wish to pursue CBT certification can find the requirements on their website at www.academyofct.org.

CONCLUDING COMMENTS

CBT is the most widely researched psychotherapeutic model with demonstrated effectiveness in the treatment of a wide range of emotional and behavioral problems. CBT is a "system of psychotherapy based on a theory which maintains that how someone structures his or her experiences largely determines how he or she feels and behaves" (Beck & Weishaar, 1986, p. 43). The underlying premise of CBT is that dysfunctional (or maladaptive) thoughts relating to self, world, and/or others are based on irrational or illogical assumptions. CBT places significant importance on cognitive information processing and behavioral change. Therapy is structured, active, and reality-based as well as time-limited. The individual is taught to take certain specific steps to combat their dysfunctional or maladaptive views. These steps include identifying and monitoring automatic thoughts, critical examination of evidence, substitution of objective interpretations for their negative dysfunctional attributions, and recognizing connections between thoughts and feelings. It would be incorrect to say that severely impaired individuals, such as individuals with schizophrenia, cannot be treated with CBT. For these individuals, the therapist uses a greater number of behavioral techniques, for example, than cognitive techniques. For higher functioning individuals the therapist uses more cognitive techniques. For any individual, therapy is a collaborative process taking schemas, ability, and physiology into account when deciding the plan of action.

DISCUSSION QUESTIONS

1. Discuss the importance of assisting individuals to identify their own cognition, behaviors, and other factors that contribute their problems.
2. What is the role of homework in cognitive therapy? Why is homework important?
3. What are some common types of distorted thinking styles in a person with an anxiety disorder? What techniques would be helpful for this problem?
4. According to cognitive theory, what is the basis for depressive disorders?
5. Would you refer an individual with severe anxiety to a cognitive therapist? Why or why not?
6. Describe two cognitive techniques and two behavioral techniques. In what types of situation would you choose each?
7. Develop a written contingency contract for yourself for a behavior that you would like to change.
8. Fill out the ATR for a recent situation that you found disturbing.

REFERENCES

Adler, C. M., Craske, M. G., Kirshenbaum, S., & Barlow, D. H. (1989). 'Fear of panic': An investigation of its role in panic occurrence, phobic avoidance, and treatment outcome. *Behaviour Research and Therapy*, 27(4), 391–396. doi:10.1016/0005-7967(89)90009-0

Agras, W. S., & Apple, R. F. (2015). *Overcoming eating disorders: A cognitive-behavioral therapy approach for bulimia nervosa and binge-eating disorder. Therapist guide* (2nd ed.). New York, NY: Oxford University Press. doi:10.1093/med:psych/9780195311693.001.0001

American Psychiatric Association. (2006). *Practice guidelines for the treatment of psychiatric disorders: Compendium 2006.* Arlington, VA: American Psychiatric Publishing.

Anderson, P. L., Zimand, E., Hodges, L. F., & Rothbaum, B. O. (2005). Cognitive behavioral therapy for public-speaking anxiety using virtual reality for exposure. *Depression & Anxiety*, 22(3), 156–158. doi:10.1002/da.20090

Andersson, E., Ljótsson, B., Hedman, E., Kaldo, V., Paxling, B., Andersson, G., . . . Rück, C. (2011). Internet-based cognitive behavior therapy for obsessive compulsive disorder: A pilot study. *BMC Psychiatry*, 11, 125. doi:10.1186/1471-244x-11-125

Andersson, G., Cuijpers, P., Carlbring, P., Riper, H., & Hedman, E. (2014). Guided Internet-based vs. face-to-face cognitive behavior therapy for psychiatric and somatic disorders: A systematic review and meta-analysis. *World Psychiatry*, 13(3), 288–295. doi:10.1002/wps.20151

Andersson, G., Hesser, H., Hummerdal, D., Bergman-Nordgren, L., & Carlbring, P. (2013). A 3.5-year follow-up of Internet-delivered cognitive behavior therapy for major depression. *Journal of Mental Health*, 22(2), 155–164. doi:10.3109/09638237.2011.608747

Anton, R. F., Moak, D. H., Waid, L. R., Latham, P. K., Malcolm, R. J., & Dias, J. K. (1999). Naltrexone and cognitive behavioral therapy for the treatment of outpatient alcoholics: Results of a placebo-controlled trial. *American Journal of Psychiatry, 156*(11), 1758–1764. doi:10.1176/ajp.156.11.1758

Barlow, D. H., Brown, T. A., & Craske, M. G. (1994). Definitions of panic attacks and panic disorder in the DSM-IV: Implications for research. *Journal of Abnormal Psychology, 103*(3), 553–564. doi:10.1037/0021-843X.103.3.553

Barrowclough, C., Haddock, G., Tarrier, N., Lewis, S. W., Moring, J., O'Brien, R., . . . McGovern, J. (2001). Randomized controlled trial of motivational interviewing, cognitive behavior therapy, and family intervention for patients with comorbid schizophrenia and substance use disorders. *American Journal of Psychiatry, 158*(10), 1706–1713. doi:10.1176/appi.ajp.158.10.1706

Bechdolf, A., Knost, B., Kuntermann, C., Schiller, S., Klosterkötter, J., Hambrecht, M., & Pukrop, R. (2004). A randomized comparison of group cognitive-behavioural therapy and group psychoeducation in patients with schizophrenia. *Acta Psychiatrica Scandinavica, 110*(1), 21–28. doi:10.1111/j.1600-0447.2004.00300.x

Bechdolf, A., Knost, B., Nelson, B., Schneider, N., Veith, V., Yung, A. R., & Pukrop, R. (2010). Randomized comparison of group cognitive behaviour therapy and group psychoeducation in acute patients with schizophrenia: Effects on subjective quality of life. *Australian and New Zealand Journal of Psychiatry, 44*(2), 144–150. doi:10.3109/00048670903393571

Bechdolf, A., Kohn, D., Knost, B., Pukrop, R., & Klosterkötter, J. (2005). A randomized comparison of group cognitive-behavioural therapy and group psychoeducation in acute patients with schizophrenia: Outcome at 24 months. *Acta Psychiatrica Scandinavica, 112*(3), 173–179. doi:10.1111/j.1600-0447.2005.00581.x

Beck, A. T. (1976). *Cognitive therapy and the emotional disorders.* New York, NY: Meridian Publishers.

Beck, A. T. (1989). Psychiatry: Cognitive therapy for depression and panic disorder. *Western Journal of Medicine, 151*(3), 311–311.

Beck, A. T., Freeman, A., & Associates. (1990). *Cognitive therapy of personality disorders.* New York: Guilford Press.

Beck, A. T., Freeman, A. Davis, D. D., & Associates. (2003). *Cognitive therapy of personality disorders* (2nd ed.). New York, NY: Guilford Press.

Beck, A. T., & Lester, D. (1976). Components of suicidal intent in completed and attempted suicides. *Journal of Psychology, 92*, 35–38. doi:10.1080/00223980.1976.9921330

Beck, A. T., Rush, A. J., Shaw, B. F., & Emery, G. (1979). *Cognitive therapy of depression.* New York, NY: Guilford Press.

Beck, A. T., & Weishaar, M. E. (1986). *Cognitive therapy* (p. 43). Philadelphia, PA: Center for Cognitive Therapy.

Beck, J. S. (2011). *Cognitive behavior therapy: Basics and beyond.* New York, NY: Guilford Press.

Bellino, S., Zizza, M., Rinaldi, C., & Bogetto, F. (2007). Combined therapy of major depression with concomitant borderline personality disorder: Comparison of interpersonal and cognitive psychotherapy. *Canadian Journal of Psychiatry, 52*(11), 718–725. doi:10.1177/070674370705201106

Blom, K., Jernelöv, S., Rück, C., Lindefors, N., & Kaldo, V. (2017). Three-year follow-up comparing cognitive behavioral therapy for depression to cognitive behavioral therapy for insomnia, for patients with both diagnoses. *Sleep, 40*(8), zsx108. doi:10.1093/sleep/zsx108

Bohus, M., Haaf, B., Simms, T., Limberger, M. F., Schmahl, C., Unckel, C., . . . Linehan, M. M. (2004). Effectiveness of inpatient dialectical behavioral therapy for borderline personality disorder: A controlled trial. *Behaviour Research and Therapy, 42*(5), 487–499. doi:10.1016/s0005-7967(03)00174-8

Bolton, D., & Perrin, S. (2008). Evaluation of exposure with response-prevention for obsessive compulsive disorder in childhood and adolescence. *Journal of Behavior Therapy and Experimental Psychiatry, 39*(1), 11–22. doi:10.1016/j.jbtep.2006.11.002

Briere, J., & Scott, C. (2006). *Principles of trauma therapy: A guide to symptoms, evaluation, and treatment.* New York, NY: Sage Publications.

Brotto, L. A., Erskine, Y., Carey, M., Ehlen, T., Finlayson, S., Heywood, M., . . . Miller, D. (2012). A brief mindfulness-based cognitive behavioral intervention improves sexual functioning versus wait-list control in women treated for gynecologic cancer. *Gynecologic Oncology, 125*(2), 320–325. doi:10.1016/j.ygyno.2012.01.035

Brown, G. K., Newman, C. F., Charlesworth, S. E., Crits-Christoph, P., & Beck, A. T. (2004). An open clinical trial of cognitive therapy for borderline personality disorder. *Journal of Personality Disorders, 18*(3), 257–271. doi:10.1521/pedi.18.3.257.35450

Buhrman, M., Syk, M., Burvall, O., Hartig, T., Gordh, T., & Andersson, G. (2015). Individualized guided internet-delivered cognitive-behavior therapy for chronic pain patients with comorbid depression and anxiety: A randomized controlled trial. *Clinical Journal of Pain, 31*(6), 504–516. doi:10.1097/ajp.0000000000000176

Carney, R. M., Blumenthal, J. A., Freedland, K. E., Youngblood, M., Veith, R. C., Burg, M. M., . . . Jaffe, A. S. (2004). Depression and late mortality after myocardial infarction in the Enhancing Recovery in Coronary Heart Disease (ENRICHD) study. *Psychosomatic Medicine, 66*(4), 466–474. doi:10.1097/01.psy.0000133362.75075.a6

Cather, C., Penn, D., Otto, M. W., Yovel, I., Mueser, K. T., & Goff, D. C. (2005). A pilot study of functional cognitive behavioral therapy (fCBT) for schizophrenia. *Schizophrenia Research, 74*(2–3), 201–209. doi:10.1016/j.schres.2004.05.002

Caudle, D. D., Senior, A. C., Wetherell, J. L., Rhoades, H. M., Beck, J. G., Kunik, M. E., . . . Stanley, M. A. (2007). Cognitive errors, symptom severity, and response to cognitive behavior therapy in older adults with generalized anxiety disorder. *American Journal of Geriatric Psychiatry, 15*(8), 680–689. doi:10.1097/JGP.0b013e31803c550d

Chakraborty, K., & Basu, D. (2010). Management of anorexia and bulimia nervosa: An evidence-based review. *Indian Journal of Psychiatry, 52*(2), 174–186. doi:10.4103/0019-5545.64596

Craske, M. G., Rapee, R. M., Jackel, L., & Barlow, D. H. (1989). Qualitative dimensions of worry in DSM-III-R generalized anxiety disorder subjects and nonanxious controls. *Behaviour Research and Therapy, 27*(4), 397–402. doi:10.1016/0005-7967(89)90010-7

Dalle Grave, R., El Ghoch, M., Sartirana, M., & Calugi, S. (2016). Cognitive behavioral therapy for anorexia nervosa: An update. *Current Psychiatry Reports, 18*(1), 2. doi:10.1007/s11920 -015-0643-4

Davidson, K. M., Norrie, J., Tyrer, P., Gumley, A., Tata, P., Murray, H., & Palmer, S. (2006). The effectiveness of cognitive behavior therapy for borderline personality disorder: Results from the borderline personality disorder study of cognitive therapy (BOSCOT) trial. *Journal of Personality Disorders, 20*(5), 450–465. doi:10.1521/pedi.2006.20.5.450

Davidson, K. M., Tyrer, P., Norrie, J., Palmer, S. J., & Tyrer, H. (2010). Cognitive therapy v. usual treatment for borderline personality disorder: Prospective 6-year follow-up. *British Journal of Psychiatry, 197*(6), 456–462. doi:10.1192/bjp.bp.109.074286

Deale, A., Chalder, T., Marks, I., & Wessely, S. (1997). Cognitive behavior therapy for chronic fatigue syndrome: A randomized controlled trial. *American Journal of Psychiatry, 154*(3), 408–414. doi:10.1176/ajp.154.3.408

Deale, A., Husain, K., Chalder, T., & Wessely, S. (2001). Long-term outcome of cognitive behavior therapy versus relaxation therapy for chronic fatigue syndrome: A 5-year follow-up study. *American Journal of Psychiatry, 158*(12), 2038–2042. doi:10.1176/appi.ajp.158.12.2038

DeRubeis, R. J., Hollon, S. D., Evans, M. D., & Bemis, K. M. (1982). Can psychotherapies for depression be discriminated? A systematic investigation of cognitive therapy and interpersonal therapy. *Journal of Consulting and Clinical Psychology, 50*(5), 744–756. doi:10 .1037/0022-006X.50.5.744

Dobson, D., & Dobson, K. S. (2009). *Evidence-based practice of cognitive-behavioral therapy.* New York, NY: Guilford Press.

Dykes, P., Wheeler, K., & Boulton, M. (1998). Psychiatric copathways. in P. Dykes (Ed.), *Psychiatric clinical pathways: An interdisciplinary approach* (pp. 265–275). Gaithersburg, MD: Aspen.

Fairburn, C. G., Norman, P. A., Welch, S. L., O'Connor, M. E., Doll, H. A., & Peveler, R. C. (1995). A prospective study of outcome in bulimia nervosa and the long-term effects of three psychological treatments. *Archives of General Psychiatry, 52*(4), 304–312. doi:10.1001/ archpsyc.1995.03950160054010

Fava, G. A., Ruini, C., Rafanelli, C., Finos, L., Conti, S., & Grandi, S. (2004). Six-year outcome of cognitive behavior therapy for prevention of recurrent depression. *American Journal of Psychiatry, 161*(10), 1872–1876. doi:10.1176/ajp.161.10.1872

Foa, E. B., Dancu, C. V., Hembree, E. A., Jaycox, L. H., Meadows, E. A., & Street, G. P. (1999). A comparison of exposure therapy, stress inoculation training, and their combination for reducing posttraumatic stress disorder in female assault victims. *Journal of Consulting and Clinical Psychology, 67*(2), 194–200. doi:10.1037/0022-006X.67.2.194

Foa, E. B., McLean, C. P., Capaldi, S., & Rosenfield, D. (2013). Prolonged exposure vs supportive counseling for sexual abuse-related PTSD in adolescent girls: A randomized clinical trial. *Journal of the American Medical Association, 310*(24), 2650–2657. doi:10.1001/jama.2013.282829

Forman, E. M., Shaw, J. A., Goetter, E. M., Herbert, J. D., Park, J. A., & Yuen, E. K. (2012). Long-term follow-up of a randomized controlled trial comparing acceptance and commitment therapy and standard cognitive behavior therapy for anxiety and depression. *Behavior Therapy, 43*(4), 801–811. doi:10.1016/j.beth.2012.04.004

Franklin, M., Foa, E., & March, J. S. (2003). The pediatric obsessive-compulsive disorder treatment study: Rationale, design, and methods. *Journal of Child and Adolescent Psychopharmacology, 13*(Suppl. 1), S39–S51. doi:10.1089/104454603322126331

Freedland, K. E., Carney, R. M., Rich, M. W., Steinmeyer, B. C., & Rubin, E. H. (2015). Cognitive behavior therapy for depression and self-care in heart failure patients: A randomized clinical trial. *JAMA Internal Medicine, 175*(11), 1773–1782. doi:10.1001/jamainternmed.2015.5220

Freeman, A. (2005). Socratic dialogue. In A. Freeman, S. H. Felgoise, A. M. Nezu, C. M. Nezu, & M. A. Reinecke (Eds.), *Encyclopedia of cognitive behavior therapy* (pp. 380–384). New York, NY: Springer.

Freeman, A., Davis, D. D., & DiTomasso, R. A. (1992). Cognitive therapy of personality disorders. *Progress in Behavior Modification, 28*, 55–81.

Freeman, A., & Freeman, S. (2005). Understanding schemas. In A. Freeman, S. H. Felgoise, A. M. Nezu, C. M. Nezu, & M. A. Reinecke (Eds.), *Encyclopedia of cognitive behavior therapy* (pp. 421–426). New York, NY: Springer.

Furmark, T., Tillfors, M., & Marteinsdottir, I. (2002). Common changes in cerebral blood flow in patients with social phobia treated with citalopram or cognitive-behavioral therapy. *Archives of General Psychiatry, 59*, 425–433. doi:10.1001/archpsyc.59.5.425

Glass, S. (2003). *Not just friends: Rebuilding trust and recovering your sanity after infidelity.* New York, NY: Free Press.

Goldapple, K., Segal, Z., Garson, C., Lau, M., Bieling, P., Kennedy, S., & Mayberg, H. (2004). Modulation of cortical-limbic pathways in major depression: Treatment-specific effects of cognitive behavior therapy. *Archives of General Psychiatry, 61*(1), 34–41. doi:10.1001/archpsyc .61.1.34

Gonzales, A. H., & Bergstrom, L. (2013). Adolescent non-suicidal self-injury (NSSI) interventions. *Journal of Child and Adolescent Psychiatric Nursing, 26*(2), 124–130. doi:10.1111/ jcap.12035

Granholm, E., Holden, J., Link, P. C., McQuaid, J. R., & Jeste, D. V. (2013). Randomized controlled trial of cognitive behavioral social skills training for older consumers with schizophrenia: Defeatist performance attitudes and functional outcome. *American Journal of Geriatric Psychiatry, 21*(3), 251–262. doi:10.1016/j.jagp.2012.10.014

Greenberger, D., & Padesky, C. A. (1995). *Mind over mood: Change how you feel by changing the way you think.* New York, NY: Guilford Press.

Hay, P. (2013). A systematic review of evidence for psychological treatments in eating disorders: 2005–2012. *International Journal of Eating Disorders, 46*(5), 462–469. doi:10.1002/eat.22103

Hayes, S. C. (2016). Acceptance and commitment therapy, relational frame theory, and the third wave of behavioral and cognitive therapies—Republished article. *Behavior Therapy, 47*(6), 869–885. doi:10.1016/j.beth.2016.11.006

Hayes, S. C., Barnes-Holmes, D., & Roche, B. (2001). *Relational frame theory: A post-Skinnerian account of human language and cognition.* San Diego, CA: Academic Press.

Hayes, S. C., Luoma, J. B., Bond, F. W., Masuda, A., & Lillis, J. (2006). Acceptance and commitment therapy: Model, processes and outcomes. *Behaviour Research and Therapy, 44*(1), 1–25. doi:10.1016/j.brat.2005.06.006

Hayes, S. C., & Wilson, K. G. (1994). Acceptance and commitment therapy: Altering the verbal support for experiential avoidance. *Behavior Analysis, 17*(2), 289–303. doi:10.1007/BF03392677

Hedman, E., Andersson, G., Lindefors, N., Gustavsson, P., Lekander, M., Rück, C., . . . Ljótsson, B. (2014). Personality change following internet-based cognitive behavior therapy for severe health anxiety. *PLoS One, 9*(12), e113871. doi:10.1371/journal.pone.0113871

Hedman, E., Hesser, H., Andersson, E., Axelsson, E., & Ljótsson, B. (2017). The mediating effect of mindful non-reactivity in exposure-based cognitive behavior therapy for severe health anxiety. *Journal of Anxiety Disorders, 50,* 15–22. doi:10.1016/j.janxdis.2017.04.007

Hedman, E., Ljótsson, B., & Lindefors, N. (2012). Cognitive behavior therapy via the Internet: A systematic review of applications, clinical efficacy and cost-effectiveness. *Expert Review of Pharmacoeconomics & Outcomes Research, 12*(6), 745–764. doi:10.1586/erp.12.67

Hendriks, G. J., Kampman, M., Keijsers, G. P., Hoogduin, C. A., & Voshaar, R. C. (2014). Cognitive-behavioral therapy for panic disorder with agoraphobia in older people: A comparison with younger patients. *Depression & Anxiety, 31*(8), 669–677. doi:10.1002/da.22274

Herbert, J. D., Gaudiano, B. A., Rheingold, A. A., Moitra, E., Myers, V. H., Dalrymple, K. L., & Brandsma, L. L. (2009). Cognitive behavior therapy for generalized social anxiety disorder in adolescents: A randomized controlled trial. *Journal of Anxiety Disorders, 23*(2), 167–177. doi:10.1016/j.janxdis.2008.06.004

Hesser, H., Axelsson, S., Backe, V., Engstrand, J., Gustafsson, T., Holmgren, E., . . . Andersson, G. (2017). Preventing intimate partner violence via the Internet: A randomized controlled trial of emotion-regulation and conflict-management training for individuals with aggression problems. *Clinical Psychology & Psychotherapy, 24*(5), 1163–1177. doi:10.1002/cpp.2082

Hofmann, S. G., Barlow, D. H., Clark, D. M., Hollon, S. D., & Mayo-Wilson, E. (2015). Treatments for social anxiety disorder: Considerations regarding psychodynamic therapy findings. *American Journal of Psychiatry, 172*(4), 393. doi:10.1176/appi.ajp.2015.14101347

Hofmeister, S., & Bodden, S. (2016). Premenstrual syndrome and premenstrual dysphoric disorder. *American Family Physician, 94*(3), 236–240.

Hollon, S. D., Stewart, M. O., & Strunk, D. (2006). Enduring effects for cognitive behavior therapy in the treatment of depression and anxiety. *Annual Review of Psychology, 57,* 285–315. doi:10.1146/annurev.psych.57.102904.190044

Hunter, M. S., Ussher, J. M., Browne, S. J., Cariss, M. Jelley, R., & Katz, M. (2002). A randomized comparison of psychological (cognitive behavior therapy), medical (fluoxetine) and combined treatment for women with premenstrual dysphoric disorder. *Journal of Psychosomatic Obstetrics & Gynecology, 23*(3), 193–199. doi:10.3109/01674820209074672

Johansson, R., Nyblom, A., Carlbring, P., Cuijpers, P., & Andersson, G. (2013). Choosing between Internet-based psychodynamic versus cognitive behavioral therapy for depression: A pilot preference study. *BMC Psychiatry, 13,* 268. doi:10.1186/1471-244x-13-268

Johansson, R., Sjoberg, E., Sjogren, M., Johnsson, E., Carlbring, P., Andersson, T., . . . Andersson, G. (2012). Tailored vs. standardized internet-based cognitive behavior therapy for depression and comorbid symptoms: A randomized controlled trial. *PLoS One, 7*(5), e36905. doi:10.1371/journal.pone.0036905

Kaldo, V., Cars, S., Rahnert, M., Larsen, H. C., & Andersson, G. (2007). Use of a self-help book with weekly therapist contact to reduce tinnitus distress: A randomized controlled trial. *Journal of Psychosomatic Research, 63*(2), 195–202. doi:10.1016/j.jpsychores.2007.04.007

Kroger, C., Harbeck, S., Armbrust, M., & Kliem, S. (2013). Effectiveness, response, and dropout of dialectical behavior therapy for borderline personality disorder in an inpatient setting. *Behaviour Research and Therapy, 51*(8), 411–416. doi:10.1016/j.brat.2013.04.008

Lamb, R., Kirby, K., Morral, A., Galbicka, G., & Iguchi, M. (2004). Improving contingency management programs for addiction. *Addictive Behaviors, 29,* 507–523. doi:10.1016/j.addbeh.2003.08.021

Leahy, R. L. (2001). *Overcoming resistance in cognitive therapy.* New York, NY: Guilford Press.

Leichsenring, F., & Leibing, E. (2003). The effectiveness of psychodynamic therapy and cognitive behavior therapy in the treatment of personality disorders: A meta-analysis. *American Journal of Psychiatry, 160*(7), 1223–1232. doi:10.1176/appi.ajp.160.7.1223

Lewinsohn, P. M., Hoberman, H. M., & Teri, L. (1985). An integrative theory of depression. In S. R. R. Bootzin (Ed.), *Theoretical issues in behavior therapy* (pp. 331–359). New York, NY: Academic Press.

Lindsay, M., Crino, R., & Andrews, G. (1997). Controlled trial of exposure and response prevention in obsessive-compulsive disorder. *British Journal of Psychiatry, 171*, 135–139. doi:10.1192/bjp.171.2.135

Linehan, M. M., & Chen, E. Y. (2005). Dialectical behavior therapy for eating disorders. In A. Freeman, S. H. Felgoise, A. M. Nezu, C. M. Nezu, & M. A. Reinecke (Eds.), *Encyclopedia of cognitive behavior therapy* (pp. 168–171). New York, NY: Springer.

Linehan, M. M., Heard, H. L., & Armstrong, H. E. (1993). Naturalistic follow-up of a behavioral treatment for chronically parasuicidal borderline patients. *Archives of General Psychiatry, 50*(12), 971–974. doi:10.1001/archpsyc.1993.01820240055007

Linehan, M. M., Korslund, K. E., Harned, M. S., Gallop, R. J., Lungu, A., Neacsiu, A. D., . . . Murray-Gregory, A. M. (2015). Dialectical behavior therapy for high suicide risk in individuals with borderline personality disorder: A randomized clinical trial and component analysis. *JAMA Psychiatry, 72*(5), 475–482. doi:10.1001/jamapsychiatry.2014.3039

Linehan, M. M., Tutek, D. A., Heard, H. L., & Armstrong, H. E. (1994). Interpersonal outcome of cognitive behavioral treatment for chronically suicidal borderline patients. *American Journal of Psychiatry, 151*(12), 1771–1776. doi:10.1176/ajp.151.12.1771

Lovato, N., Lack, L., Wright, H., & Kennaway, D. J. (2014). Evaluation of a brief treatment program of cognitive behavior therapy for insomnia in older adults. *Sleep, 37*(1), 117–126. doi:10.5665/sleep.3320

Macdonald, A., Pukay-Martin, N. D., Wagner, A. C., Fredman, S. J., & Monson, C. M. (2016). Cognitive-behavioral conjoint therapy for PTSD improves various PTSD symptoms and trauma-related cognitions: Results from a randomized controlled trial. *Journal of Family Psychology, 30*(1), 157–162. doi:10.1037/fam0000177

MacPherson, H. A., Weinstein, S. M., & West, A. E. (2018). Non-suicidal self-injury in pediatric bipolar disorder: Clinical correlates and impact on psychosocial treatment outcomes. *Journal of Abnormal Child Psychology, 46*(4), 857–870. doi:10.1007/s10802-017-0331-4

Mansson, K. N., Salami, A., Frick, A., Carlbring, P., Andersson, G., Furmark, T., & Boraxbekk, C. J. (2016). Neuroplasticity in response to cognitive behavior therapy for social anxiety disorder. *Translational Psychiatry, 6*, e727. doi:10.1038/tp.2015.218

Margraf, J., Barlow, D. H., Clark, D. M., & Telch, M. J. (1993). Psychological treatment of panic: Work in progress on outcome, active ingredients, and follow-up. *Behaviour Research and Therapy, 31*(1), 1–8. doi:10.1016/0005-7967(93)90036-T

McLean, P. D., Whittal, M. L., Thordarson, D. S., Taylor, S., Sochting, I., Koch, W. J., . . . Anderson, K. W. (2001). Cognitive versus behavior therapy in the group treatment of obsessive-compulsive disorder. *Journal of Consulting and Clinical Psychology, 69*(2), 205–214. doi:10.1037/0022-006X.69.2.205

Meichenbaum, D. H. (1977). *Cognitive-behavioral modifications: An integrative approach.* New York, NY: Springer.

Meichenbaum, D. H., & Deffenbacher, J. L. (1988). Stress inoculation training. *The Counseling Psychologist, 16*(1), 69–90. doi:10.1177/0011000088161005

Meyer, V. (1966). Modification of expectations in cases with obsessional rituals. *Behaviour and Research Therapy, 4*(4), 273–280. doi:10.1016/0005-7967(66)90023-4

Miller, W. R., Meyers, R. J., & Hiller-Sturmhöfel, S. (1999). The community-reinforcement approach. *Alcohol Research & Health, 23*, 116–121. Retrieved from https://pubs.niaaa.nih.gov/publications/arh23-2/116-121.pdf

Mohr, D. C., Boudewyn, A. C., Goodkin, D. E., Bostrom, A., & Epstein, L. (2001). Comparative outcomes for individual cognitive-behavior therapy, supportive-expressive group psychotherapy, and sertraline for the treatment of depression in multiple sclerosis. *Journal of Consulting and Clinical Psychology, 69*(6), 942–949. doi:10.1037/0022-006X.69.6.942

Morasco, B. J., Greaves, D. W., Lovejoy, T. I., Turk, D. C., Dobscha, S. K., & Hauser, P. (2016). Development and preliminary evaluation of an integrated cognitive-behavior treatment for chronic pain and substance use disorder in patients with the hepatitis C virus. *Pain Medical, 17*(12), 2280–2290. doi:10.1093/pm/pnw076

Morina, N., Brinkman, W. P., Hartanto, D., Kampmann, I. L., & Emmelkamp, P. M. (2015). Social interactions in virtual reality exposure therapy: A proof-of-concept pilot study. *Technology and Health Care, 23*(5), 581–589. doi:10.3233/thc-151014

Morris, J., Firkins, A., Millings, A., Mohr, C., Redford, P., & Rowe, A. (2016). Internet-delivered cognitive behavior therapy for anxiety and insomnia in a higher education context. *Anxiety Stress Coping, 29*(4), 415–431. doi:10.1080/10615806.2015.1058924

Morrison, A. P., Burke, E., Murphy, E., Pyle, M., Bowe, S., Varese, F., . . . Wood, L. J. (2016). Cognitive therapy for internalised stigma in people experiencing psychosis: A pilot randomised controlled trial. *Psychiatry Research, 240*, 96–102. doi:10.1016/j.psychres.2016 .04.024

Nacasch, N., Foa, E. B., Huppert, J. D., Tzur, D., Fostick, L., Dinstein, Y., . . . Zohar, J. (2011). Prolonged exposure therapy for combat- and terror-related posttraumatic stress disorder: A randomized control comparison with treatment as usual. *Journal of Clinical Psychiatry, 72*(9), 1174–1180. doi:10.4088/JCP.09m05682blu

Nakagawa, A., Sado, M., Mitsuda, D., Fujisawa, D., Kikuchi, T., Abe, T., . . . Ono, Y. (2014). Effectiveness of cognitive behavioural therapy augmentation in major depression treatment (ECAM study): Study protocol for a randomised clinical trial. *BMJ Open, 4*(10), e006359. doi:10.1136/bmjopen-2014-006359

Nakatani, E., Nakgawa, A., Ohara, Y., Goto, S., Uozumi, N., Iwakiri, M., . . . Yamagami, T. (2003). Effects of behavior therapy on regional cerebral blood flow in obsessive-compulsive disorder. *Psychiatry Research, 124*(2), 113–120. doi:10.1016/S0925-4927(03)00069-6

Neacsiu, A. D., Rizvi, S. L., & Linehan, M. M. (2010). Dialectical behavior therapy skills use as a mediator and outcome of treatment for borderline personality disorder. *Behaviour Research and Therapy, 48*(9), 832–839. doi:10.1016/j.brat.2010.05.017

Nixon, R. D. V., Sterk, J., Pearce, A., & Weber, N. (2017). A randomized trial of cognitive behavior therapy and cognitive therapy for children with posttraumatic stress disorder following single-incident trauma: Predictors and outcome at 1-year follow-up. *Psychological Trauma, 9*(4), 471–478. doi:10.1037/tra0000190

Novo, P., Landin-Romero, R., Radua, J., Vicens, V., Fernandez, I., Garcia, F., . . . Amann, B. L. (2014). Eye movement desensitization and reprocessing therapy in subsyndromal bipolar patients with a history of traumatic events: A randomized, controlled pilot-study. *Psychiatry Research, 219*(1), 122–128. doi:10.1016/j.psychres.2014.05.012

Özcan, C. T., Oflaz, F., Türkbay, T., & Freeman Clevenger, S. M. (2013). The effectiveness of an interpersonal cognitive problem-solving strategy on behavior and emotional problems in children with attention deficit hyperactivity. *Noro Psikiyatr Ars, 50*(3), 244–251. doi:10.4274/ npa.y6455

Paquette, V., Lévesque, J., Mensour, B., Leroux, J. M., Beaudoin, G., Bourgouin, P., & Beauregard, M. (2003). "Change the mind and you change the brain": Effects of cognitive-behavioral therapy on the neural correlates of spider phobia. *Neuroimage, 18*(2), 401–409. doi:10.1016/ S1053-8119(02)00030-7

Paunovic, N., & Öst, L.-G. (2001). Cognitive-behavior therapy vs exposure therapy in the treatment of PTSD in refugees. *Behaviour Research and Therapy, 39*(10), 1183–1197. doi:10.1016/ S0005-7967(00)00093-0

Piacentini, J., Bergman, R. L., Chang, S., Langley, A., Peris, T., Wood, J. J., & McCracken, J. (2011). Controlled comparison of family cognitive behavioral therapy and psychoeducation/ relaxation training for child obsessive-compulsive disorder. *Journal of the American Academy of Child and Adolescent Psychiatry, 50*(11), 1149–1161. doi:10.1016/j.jaac.2011.08.003

Price, M., Mehta, N., Tone, E. B., & Anderson, P. L. (2011). Does engagement with exposure yield better outcomes? Components of presence as a predictor of treatment response for virtual reality exposure therapy for social phobia. *Journal of Anxiety Disorders, 25*(6), 763–770. doi:10.1016/j.janxdis.2011.03.004

Rapee, R. M., Craske, M. G., & Barlow, D. H. (1994). Assessment instrument for panic disorder that includes fear of sensation-producing activities: The Albany panic and phobia questionnaire. *Anxiety, 1*(3), 114–122. doi:10.1002/anxi.3070010303

Rector, N. A., Seeman, M. V., & Segal, Z. V. (2003). Cognitive therapy for schizophrenia: A preliminary randomized controlled trial. *Schizophrenia Research, 63*(1–2), 1–11. doi:10.1016/ S0920-9964(02)00308-0

Resick, P. A., Nishith, P., Weaver, T. L., Astin, M. C., & Feuer, C. A. (2002). A comparison of cognitive-processing therapy with prolonged exposure and a waiting condition for the treatment of chronic posttraumatic stress disorder in female rape victims. *Journal of Consulting and Clinical Psychology, 70*(4), 867–879. doi:10.1037/0022-006X.70.4.867

Resick, P. A., Wachen, J. S., Mintz, J., Young-McCaughan, S., Roache, J. D., Borah, A. M., . . . Peterson, A. L. (2015). A randomized clinical trial of group cognitive processing therapy compared with group present-centered therapy for PTSD among active duty military personnel. *Journal of Consulting and Clinical Psychology, 83*(6), 1058–1068. doi:10.1037/ ccp0000016

Ritterband, L. M., Thorndike, F. P., Ingersoll, K. S., Lord, H. R., Gonder-Frederick, L., Frederick, C., . . . Morin, C. M. (2017). Effect of a web-based cognitive behavior therapy for insomnia intervention with 1-year follow-up: A randomized clinical trial. *JAMA Psychiatry, 74*(1), 68–75. doi:10.1001/jamapsychiatry.2016.3249

Robinson, S. K., Viirre, E. S., Bailey, K. A., Kindermann, S., Minassian, A. L., Goldin, P. R., . . . McQuaid, J. R. (2008). A randomized controlled trial of cognitive-behavior therapy for tinnitus. *International Tinnitus Journal, 14*(2), 119–126.

Roest, A. M., Carney, R. M., Freedland, K. E., Martens, E. J., Denollet, J., & de Jonge, P. (2013). Changes in cognitive versus somatic symptoms of depression and event-free survival following acute myocardial infarction in the Enhancing Recovery In Coronary Heart Disease (ENRICHD) study. *Journal of Affective Disorders, 149*(1–3), 335–341. doi:10.1016/j .jad.2013.02.008

Rothbaum, B. O., Anderson, P., Zimand, E., Hodges, L., Lang, D., & Wilson, J. (2006). Virtual reality exposure therapy and standard (in vivo) exposure therapy in the treatment of fear of flying. *Behavior Therapy, 37*(1), 80–90. doi:10.1016/j.beth.2005.04.004

Rothbaum, B. O., Hodges, L., & Kooper, R. (1997). Virtual reality exposure therapy. *The Journal of Psychotherapy Practice and Research, 6*(3), 219–226. Retrieved from https://www.ncbi.nlm.nih .gov/pmc/articles/PMC3330462

Rothbaum, B. O., Hodges, L., Kooper, R., Opdyke, D., Williford, J. S., & North, M. (1995). Effectiveness of computer-generated (virtual reality) graded exposure in the treatment of acrophobia. *American Journal of Psychiatry, 152*(4), 626–628. doi:10.1176/ajp.152.4.626

Rothbaum, B. O., Hodges, L., Smith, S., Lee, J. H., & Price, L. (2000). A controlled study of virtual reality exposure therapy for the fear of flying. *Journal of Consulting and Clinical Psychology, 68*(6), 1020–1026. doi:10.1037/0022-006X.68.6.1020

Rothbaum, B. O., Rizzo, A. S., & Difede, J. (2010). Virtual reality exposure therapy for combat-related posttraumatic stress disorder. *Annals of the New York Academy of Sciences, 1208*, 126–132. doi:10.1111/j.1749-6632.2010.05691.x

Safir, M. P., Wallach, H. S., & Bar-Zvi, M. (2012). Virtual reality cognitive-behavior therapy for public speaking anxiety: One-year follow-up. *Behavior Modification, 36*(2), 235–246. doi:10.1177/0145445511429999

Schienle, A., Schafer, A., Hermann, A., Rohrmann, S., & Vaitl, D. (2007). Symptom provocation and reduction in patients suffering from spider phobia: An fMRI study on exposure therapy. *European Archives of Psychiatry and Clinical Neuroscience, 257*(8), 486–493. doi:10.1007/s00406 -007-0754-y

Shapiro, F. (1989). Eye movement desensitization: A new treatment for post-traumatic stress disorder. *Journal of Behavior Therapy and Experimental Psychiatry, 20*(3), 211–217. doi:10.1016/ 0005-7916(89)90025-6

Shapiro, F. (1996). Eye movement desensitization and reprocessing (EMDR): Evaluation of controlled PTSD research. *Journal of Behavior Therapy and Experimental Psychiatry, 27*(3), 209–218. doi:10.1016/S0005-7916(96)00029-8

Spring, J. A. (1997). *After the affair: Healing the pain and rebuilding trust when a partner has been unfaithful.* New York, NY: HarperCollins.

Stanley, B., Brodsky, B., Nelson, J. D., & Dulit, R. (2007). Brief dialectical behavior therapy (DBT-B) for suicidal behavior and non-suicidal self injury. *Archives of Suicide Research, 11*(4), 337–341. doi:10.1080/13811110701542069

Stanley, M. A., Wilson, N. L., Novy, D. M., Rhoades, H. M., Wagener, P. D., Greisinger, A. J., . . . Kunik, M. E. (2009). Cognitive behavior therapy for generalized anxiety disorder among older adults in primary care: A randomized clinical trial. *Journal of the American Medical Association, 301*(14), 1460–1467. doi:10.1001/jama.2009.458

Steketee, G., Frost, R. O., Tolin, D. F., Rasmussen, J., & Brown, T. A. (2010). Waitlist-controlled trial of cognitive behavior therapy for hoarding disorder. *Depression & Anxiety, 27*(5), 476–484. doi:10.1002/da.20673

Stitzer, M., & Petry, N. (2006). Contingency management for treatment of substance abuse. *Annual Review of Clinical Psychology, 2*(1), 411–434. doi:10.1146/annurev.clinpsy.2.022305 .095219

Stoffers, J. M., Vollm, B. A., Rucker, G., Timmer, A., Huband, N., & Lieb, K. (2012). Psychological therapies for people with borderline personality disorder. *Cochrane Database of Systematic Reviews,* (8), CD005652. doi:10.1002/14651858. CD005652.pub2

Sudak, D. M., Beck, J. S., & Wright , J. (2003). Cognitive behavioral therapy: A blueprint for attaining and assessing psychiatry resident competency. *Academic Psychiatry, 27*(3), 154–159.

Tarrier, N., Lewis, S., Haddock, G., Bentall, R., Drake, R., Kinderman, P., . . . Dunn, G. (2004). Cognitive-behavioural therapy in first-episode and early schizophrenia.18-month follow-up of a randomised controlled trial. *British Journal of Psychiatry, 184,* 231–239. doi:10.1192/bjp .184.3.231

Tarrier, N., Wittkowski, A., Kinney, C., McCarthy, E., Morris, J., & Humphreys, L. (1999). Durability of the effects of cognitive-behavioural therapy in the treatment of chronic schizophrenia: 12-month follow-up. *British Journal of Psychiatry, 174,* 500–504. doi:10.1192/ bjp.174.6.500

Taylor, D. J., Peterson, A. L., Pruiksma, K. E., Young-McCaughan, S., Nicholson, K., & Mintz, J. (2017). Internet and in-person cognitive behavioral therapy for insomnia in military personnel: A randomized clinical trial. *Sleep, 40*(6), zsx075. doi:10.1093/sleep/zsx075

Taylor, L. K., & Weems, C. F. (2011). Cognitive-behavior therapy for disaster-exposed youth with posttraumatic stress: Results from a multiple-baseline examination. *Behavior Therapy, 42*(3), 349–363. doi:10.1016/j.beth.2010.09.001

Turkington, D., Sensky, T., Scott, J., Barnes, T. R., Nur, U., Siddle, R., . . . Kingdon, D. (2008). A randomized controlled trial of cognitive-behavior therapy for persistent symptoms in schizophrenia: A five-year follow-up. *Schizophrenia Research, 98*(1–3), 1–7. doi:10.1016/j .schres.2007.09.026

Tyrer, P., Cooper, S., Tyrer, H., Salkovskis, P., Crawford, M., Green, J., . . . Barrett, B. (2011). CHAMP: Cognitive behaviour therapy for health anxiety in medical patients, a randomised controlled trial. *BMC Psychiatry, 11,* 99. doi:10.1186/1471-244x-11-99

Tyrer, P., Thompson, S., Schmidt, U., Jones, V., Knapp, M., Davidson, K., . . . Wessely, S. (2003). Randomized controlled trial of brief cognitive behaviour therapy *versus* treatment as usual in recurrent deliberate self-harm: The POPMACT study. *Psychological Medicine, 33*(6), 969–976. doi:10.1017/S0033291703008171

Tyrer, P., Tom, B., Byford, S., Schmidt, U., Jones, V., Davidson, K., . . . Catalan, J. (2004). Differential effects of manual assisted cognitive behavior therapy in the treatment of recurrent deliberate self-harm and personality disturbance: The POPMACT study. *Journal of Personality Disorders, 18*(1), 102–116. doi:10.1521/pedi.18.1.102.32770

Wamser-Nanney, R., Scheeringa, M. S., & Weems, C. F. (2016). Early treatment response in children and adolescents receiving CBT for trauma. *Journal of Pediatric Psychology, 41*(1), 128–137. doi:10.1093/jpepsy/jsu096

Waring, E. M., Carver, C., Stalker, C. A., Fry, R., & Schaefer, B. (1990). A randomized clinical trial of cognitive marital therapy. *Journal of Sex & Marital Therapy, 16*(3), 165–180. doi:10.1080/ 00926239008405263

Weck, F., Nagel, L. C., Hofling, V., & Neng, J. M. B. (2017). Cognitive therapy and exposure therapy for hypochondriasis (health anxiety): A 3-year naturalistic follow-up. *Journal of Consulting and Clinical Psychology, 85*(10), 1012–1017. doi:10.1037/ccp0000239

Weck, F., Neng, J. M., Richtberg, S., Jakob, M., & Stangier, U. (2015). Cognitive therapy versus exposure therapy for hypochondriasis (health anxiety): A randomized controlled trial. *Journal of Consulting and Clinical Psychology, 83*(4), 665–676. doi:10.1037/ccp0000013

Wells, A., Clark, D. M., Salkovskis, P., Ludgate, J., Hackmann, A., & Gelder, M. (2016). Social phobia: The role of in-situation safety behaviors in maintaining anxiety and negative beliefs. *Behavior Therapy, 47*(5), 669–674. doi:10.1016/j.beth.2016.08.010. Republished from *Behavior Therapy, 29,* 1998, 357–370. doi:10.1016/S0005-7894(98)80037-3

Whittal, M. L., Robichaud, M., Thordarson, D. S., & McLean, P. D. (2008). Group and individual treatment of obsessive-compulsive disorder using cognitive therapy and exposure plus response prevention: A 2-year follow-up of two randomized trials. *Journal of Consulting and Clinical Psychology, 76*(6), 1003–1014. doi:10.1037/a0013076

Williams, T. I., Salkovskis, P. M., Forrester, L., Turner, S., White, H., & Allsopp, M. A. (2010). A randomised controlled trial of cognitive behavioural treatment for obsessive compulsive disorder in children and adolescents. *European Child & Adolescent Psychiatry, 19*(5), 449–456. doi:10.1007/s00787-009-0077-9

Wilson, G. T. (1999). Cognitive behavior therapy for eating disorders: Progress and problems. *Behaviour Research and Therapy, 37*(Suppl. 1), S79–S95. doi:10.1016/S0005-7967(99)00051-0

Wuthrich, V. M., Rapee, R. M., Kangas, M., & Perini, S. (2016). Randomized controlled trial of group cognitive behavioral therapy compared to a discussion group for co-morbid anxiety and depression in older adults. *Psychological Medicine, 46*(4), 785–795. doi:10.1017/s0033291715002251

Young, J. E. (1991). *Cognitive therapy for personality disorders: A schematic focused approach.* Sarasota, Fl: Professional Resources Press.

Young, J. E., Klosko, J. S., & Weishaar, M. E. (2003). *Schema therapy: A practioner's guide.* New York, NY: Guilford Press.

Zimmer, M., Duncan, A. V., Laitano, D., Ferreira, E. E., & Belmonte-de-Abreu, P. (2007). A twelve-week randomized controlled study of the cognitive-behavioral integrated psychological therapy program: Positive effect on the social functioning of schizophrenic patients. *Revista Brasileira de Psiquiatria, 29*(2), 140–147. doi:10.1590/S1516-44462006005000030

APPENDIX 8.1
Automatic Thought Record

Date	Situation	Emotion (s)	Automatic Thoughts	Rational Response	Outcome
	Describe: 1. Actual event leading to unpleasant emotion, or 2. Stream of thoughts or recollections, leading to unpleasant emotion.	1. Specify sad; anxious; angry; etc. 2. Rate degree of emotion, 1–10	1. Write automatic thought(s) that preceded emotion(s) 2. Rate your belief in the automatic thought(s), 0–10	1. Write rational response to automatic thought(s) 2. Rate belief in rational response, 0–10	1. Re-rate your belief in the automatic thought(s) 2. Specify and re-rate your subsequent emotions, 0–10

Motivational Interviewing

Susie Adams and Edna Hamera

Motivational interviewing is a collaborative person-centered communication process designed to help individuals resolve ambivalence and plan for change. It can be used alone to increase motivation for engaging in psychotherapy or in combination with other forms of therapy when resistance is encountered. This chapter begins with an overview of the guiding principles, the history, and evidence-based research for motivational interviewing. Application of motivation interviewing is discussed within the phases of change outlined by Miller and Rollnick (2013). Motivational interviewing is closely aligned with the Transtheoretical Model developed around the same time (Prochaska, DiClemente, & Norcross, 1992). Although both models concern changing behavior, motivational interviewing puts greater emphasis on getting ready to change. The two approaches are integrated in an evidence-based substance abuse treatment program (Center for Substance Abuse Treatment, 1999), which is discussed in the section on modifications of motivational interviewing. Process recordings from two cases, one in an integrated primary care setting and one during medication services at a community mental health center, illustrate the application of motivational interviewing.

GUIDING PRINCIPLES

The origins of motivational interviewing (MI) emerged from Miller's clinical practice in addictions (1983) and research on therapists' behaviors that elicit motivation. In the latest edition of their book, Miller and Rollnick (2013) elaborate on the values and philosophy of MI. The "spirit" of MI embodies a partnership with patients incorporating the principles of acceptance, belief in individual autonomy, and acknowledgment of the individual's strengths and efforts with empathy and affirmation. The principles of acceptance, conveying accurate empathy, honoring the worth of individuals, affirming their strengths, and respecting their autonomy are adapted from Carl Rogers's person-centered therapy (1965). Miller and Rollnick (2013) added the principles of compassion and evocation. Compassion means therapists give priority to the well-being of patient over their own needs. Evocation is accepting that individuals have within themselves what they need to change and it is the practitioner's job to "draw it out" (Miller & Rollnick, 2013, p. 21).

MI contains elements of other theories that underlie the change process. Festinger's cognitive dissonance theory (Festinger, 1957) focuses on prejudice, asserting that awareness of discrepancies among beliefs and goals and behavior is an incentive for people to reconcile their inconsistencies. MI highlights dissonance between unhealthy behaviors and the person's values and goals. Bem's (1967) self-perception theory is a refinement of cognitive dissonance theory, proposing that hearing oneself argue for change increases desire to change. In MI it is important for individuals to voice the change they desire, which reinforces motivation for change (Amrhein, Miller, Yahne, Palmer, & Fulcher, 2003). Because MI deals with ambivalence and resistance, it resembles reactance theory (Brehm & Brehm, 1981), the belief that some individuals are more defensive when persuasion or coercion is used because their sense of freedom is threatened. Miller and Rollnick (2013) prefer to use the word discord and believe that discord or differences arise in the context of the relationship and are not an individual trait. However, they concur that taking a directive role and using persuasion to encourage change is the antithesis of their philosophy.

HISTORY

W. R. Miller reviewed addiction studies and conducted research that led him to dismiss the idea that denial was a predominant trait of individuals with alcoholism and to question the belief that confrontation was effective (Miller, 1983, 1985; Miller, Andrews, Wilbourne, & Bennett, 1998; Miller, Benefield, & Tonigan, 1993).

The development of MI paralleled that of transtheoretical model of change, which proposed that people go through stages in the process of change (Prochaska & DiClemente, 1983). Miller and Rollnick have continued to define and elaborate MI over time (Miller & Rollnick, 1991, 2002, 2013). As a practice theory it follows a bottom-up approach to theory development, emerging from clinical practice and clinical research. A few studies have examined the elements in the process of MI that are related to outcomes. They indicate that a high frequency of behaviors inconsistent with MI is linked to patient resistance and worse outcomes, whereas the reverse, that is, a lower frequency of behaviors inconsistent with MI, is related to patient engagement and better outcomes (Apodaca & Longabaugh, 2009). Consistent use of reflection versus giving direction increases change talk, and consistent use of MI strengthens commitment to change, leading to change behavior as long as the practitioner does not "get ahead" of the patient (Miller & Rose, 2009).

EVIDENCE-BASED RESEARCH

A number of studies on MI have been captured in systematic reviews and meta-analyses. Initial meta-analyses combined studies across a variety of behaviors including substance abuse, smoking, and health behaviors such as safe sex and weight loss, because there were few randomized controlled studies (RCTs) of each behavior. Outcomes included self-report and objective measures. The results are reported as effect size (Cohen's d or Hedges' g) for continuous variables with larger correlations indicating greater effects. Effect sizes range from 0 to 3.0, with .2 indicating small effect, .5 a medium effect, and .8 a large effect (Cohen, 1992; Hedges & Olkin, 1985). Results may also be reported as level of risk. Relative risk is derived from dividing the risk, for example, relapse, in one group by risk in another, and odds ratio is the number of people in a group with an event (e.g., relapse) divided by the number without an event (Kissling & Davis, 2009). The large ranges in effect sizes indicate that MI has differential effectiveness across behaviors. Many early studies implemented adapted versions of MI, and most did not assess the fidelity of MI (see Table 9.1).

One recent meta-analysis of MI in primary care settings found that mean effect sizes ranged from .07 to .47 with significant effect sizes of .19 (95% CI [confidence interval]: .01 − .37, p = .04) for medication adherence and .18 (95% CI: .03 − .33, p = .02) for all outcomes (blood pressure, substance use, body weight, physical activities, and medication

TABLE 9.1 META-ANALYSES OF MOTIVATIONAL INTERVIEWING WITH SUBSTANCE USE, SMOKING, AND HEALTH-RELATED BEHAVIORS

Author*	Studies	Focus	Comparison Treatment	Effect Size and Relative Risk (RR)
Meta-Analyses Across Behaviors				
Burke, Arkowitz, and Menchola (2003); Burke, Dunn, Atkins, and Phelps (2004)	N = 30	Drug, alcohol, diet, and exercise	No tx	.25–.57
Hettema, Steele, and Miller (2005)	N = 72	Alcohol, smoking, HIV, drugs, and compliance	No tx and standard tx	.11–.77
Lundahl, Kung, Brownell, Tollefson, and Burke (2010)	N = 119	Substance use, health-related behaviors, gambling, and engagement in tx	Weak comparison Specific comparison	.28 .09
Lundahl et al. (2013)	N = 48	Substance use, HIV, health-related behaviors, compliance	Standard tx	.25
VanBuskirk and Wetherell (2014)	N = 12	Patient outcomes in primary care settings	Waitlist and standard tx	.07–.47
Meta-Analyses of Specific Behaviors				
Samson and Tanner-Smith (2015)	N = 73	Alcohol	Single session MET/MI Psychoeducational tx	.18
Tanner-Smith and Lipsey (2015)	N = 185	Alcohol	Brief alcohol interventions, no tx	.27 Consumption Adol .19 Consequences Adol .17 Consumption Yg Adult .11 Consequences Yg Adult

(continued)

TABLE 9.1 META-ANALYSES OF MOTIVATIONAL INTERVIEWING WITH SUBSTANCE USE, SMOKING, AND HEALTH-RELATED BEHAVIORS *(continued)*

Author*	Studies	Focus	Comparison Treatment	Effect Size and Relative Risk (RR)
Tanner-Smith and Risser (2016)	N = 190	Alcohol	Brief alcohol intervention, no tx	.25 Adol .15 Yg Adult
Lai, Cahill, Qin, and Tang (2010)	N = 14	Smoking	Usual care/brief advice	1.27 RR
Hettema and Hendricks (2010)	N = 31	Smoking	No tx, brief advice, and pamphlet	.12 <6 months .17 >6 months
Lindson-Hawley, Thompson, and Begh (2015)	N = 28	Smoking	MI 1–6 sessions Usual care/brief advice	1.16–7.94 RR
Jensen et al. (2011)	N = 21	Adolescent substance abuse	Control	.17
Armstrong et al. (2011)	N = 11	Obesity	No treatment	.51
Smedslund et al. (2011)	N = 59	Substance use	No tx immediate post Short term follow-up	.79 .17
Lenz, Rosenbaum, and Sheperis (2016)	N = 12 N = 19	Substance use	MET vs. no tx MET vs. alternative tx	–.46 –.32
Sayegh, Huey, Zara, and Jhaveri (2017)	N = 82	Substance use (ES for polysubstance abuse)	MI Contingency management	.09 T–1, .14 T–2 .15 T–1, –.06 T–2

*References cited in this table are provided in the references listed at the end of the chapter.

Adol, adolescents; ES, MET, motivational enhancement therapy; MI, motivational interviewing; tx, treatment; Yg Adult, young adults.

adherence; VanBuskirk & Wetherell, 2014). Another meta-analysis by Lundahl et al. (2013) found that MI delivered in primary care settings targeting a variety of health behaviors and outcomes across 48 studies demonstrated modest (OR [odds ratio] = 1.55, $p < .001$, that equates to effect size of .2) advantage over treatment as usual (Lundahl et al., 2013). MI was not effective with eating disorders or self-care behaviors or medical outcomes such as heart rate. These findings suggest that MI provides a moderate advantage over comparison interventions and could be used for a wide range of healthcare issues.

More recent meta-analyses of MI have focused on specific behaviors with most research being done on alcohol and drug abuse and nicotine dependence (see Table 9.1). The meta-analysis by Lenz, Rosenbaum, and Sheperis (2016) found small mean effect sizes for 25 studies evaluating the effect of motivational enhancement therapy (MET) on decreasing the amount of substance use. In the 12 RCTs that compared MET to no treatment, the effect size was $-.46$ (95% CI: $-.60 - -.31, p < .01$). In the 19 RCTs that compared MET to alternative interventions, the effect size was smaller, $-.20$ (95% CI: $-.32 - -.09$, $p < .01$; Lenz et al., 2016). Another meta-analysis of 82 studies evaluated the efficacy of contingency management (CM) with MI across all substance use at 3 and 6 months follow-up (Sayegh, Huey, Zara, & Jhaveri, 2017). CM had significant small and medium effect on multiple substances (i.e., alcohol, tobacco, polysubstances) at 3-month follow-up only. MI had one significant medium effect at 3-month follow-up (i.e., marijuana), but had several significant small effects at 6-month follow-up (i.e., alcohol, tobacco, polysubstance; Sayegh et al., 2017). These results illustrate that extrinsically focused CM may produce medium follow-up effects in the short run, but intrinsically focused MI may produce small but durable follow-up effects (Sayegh et al., 2017).

There has been increasing interest in brief motivational interventions to reduce alcohol and/or drug use among adolescents and young adults who have the highest prevalence of binge drinking and heavy drug use. Samson and Tanner-Smith (2015) found that single session MET and MI had larger effect sizes than cognitive behavioral therapy (CBT) or psychoeducation therapy (PET) modalities (overall mean effect size = .18, 95% CI: .12 – .24). Tanner-Smith and Lipsey (2015) reported that in 185 studies of brief alcohol interventions for adolescents and young adults intervention led to significant reductions in alcohol consumption (Hedges g = .27 for adolescents, .17 for young adults) and significant reductions in alcohol-related consequences (Hedges g = .19 for adolescents, .11 for young adults). These effects lasted up to 1 year after intervention and did not vary across participant demographics, intervention length, or format. While the results are modest, they is noteworthy given their low cost and brevity (Tanner-Smith & Lipsey, 2015). Tanner-Smith and Risser (2016) found significant self-reported reductions in alcohol use following brief alcohol interventions among adolescents (Hedges g = .25, 95% CI: .13 – .37) and young adults (Hedges g = .15, 95% CI: .12 – .18). These modest effects were observed across measures and show promise for interrupting problematic alcohol use among youth (Tanner-Smith & Risser, 2016).

Research on the effectiveness of MI for individuals with serious mental illness is limited. Kelly, Daley, and Douaihy (2012) reviewed RCTs of individuals with comorbid psychiatric and substance abuse disorders. In one study, MI, CBT, and family therapy with individuals who had schizophrenia reduced their substance use over 1 year (Barrowclough et al., 2010). Another study (Bellack & Gearon, 1998) cited by Kelly et al. (2012) examined MI and case management in individuals with comorbid serious and persistent mental illness and substance abuse. The combination of MI and case management was effective in keeping individuals in treatment, and they were 59% more likely to have clean urine compared to 25% in the control group. Steinberg, Ziedonis, Krejci, and Brandon (2004) evaluated an MI session in individuals with schizophrenia who were nicotine dependent to see whether it motivated them to seek treatment for tobacco dependence. A greater proportion of those receiving MI contacted smoking cessation providers and attended the first session compared to those receiving psychoeducational counseling or advice. Hunt, Siegfried,

Morley, Sitharthan, and Cleary (2013) in a Cochrane Review of eight randomized clinical trials found no advantage for MI alone compared with usual treatment in reducing losses to treatment for people with both severe mental illness and substance misuse. They did find that significantly more participants in the MI group reported for their first aftercare appointment. Vanderwaal's systematic review of six studies on the impact of MI on medication adherence for persons with schizophrenia did not find support for its efficacy in medication adherence, decreased rehospitalization rates, or reduced symptoms of psychosis (2015). MI may be beneficial for some patients with schizophrenia, but should not be considered first-line therapy.

Since 2000 MI has been used to motivate individuals diagnosed with anxiety disorders to engage in psychotherapy. Westra and Dozois (2006) examined MI prior to CBT and found that those receiving MI attended more CBT sessions and reported lower anxiety at 6 months post treatment than individuals receiving only CBT. Similar results were found in a subsequent study of individuals with generalized anxiety disorder (Westra, Arkowitz, & Dozois, 2009). More recently Marker and Norton (2018) found that across 12 clinical trials MI plus CBT outperformed standard CBT alone in terms of overall reduction of anxiety symptoms (Hedges $g = .59$), further supporting the use of MI as an adjunct to CBT for anxiety disorders including generalized anxiety disorders, obsessive-compulsive disorders, and posttraumatic stress disorders.

Across studies there are several issues that merit the attention of future research on the efficacy of MI. Given the growing attention to cost effectiveness in healthcare delivery, it is important to clearly describe the role (e.g., physician, nurse practitioner, licensed counselor, health educator) of the person providing MI intervention and his or her level of training in MI. The majority of studies on MI including systematic reviews and meta-analyses did not address clear steps of the MI intervention or whether there was any assessment of treatment fidelity. Thus, variability in who delivers MI and how the MI intervention is delivered may account for the low effect sizes. Additionally, there is limited research to determine the therapeutic mechanism of action of MI.

In one of the early reviews seeking to understand MI's mechanism of action, Apodaca and Longabaugh (2009) found that patient change talk and intention, patient experience of discrepancy, and therapist use of decisional balance exercise all correlated with better outcomes. Therapist MI-inconsistent language/behavior correlated with worse outcomes. A meta-analysis of 12 studies by Magill et al. (2014) found partial support of key causal model wherein therapist-MI consistent skills were correlated with more patient language in favor of behavior change (change talk; $r = .26$, $p < .0001$), but noted patient language against behavior change (sustain talk; $r = .10$, $p = .09$) did not support behavior change. MI-therapist inconsistent skills were associated with less change talk ($r = -.17$, $p = .001$) and more sustain talk ($r = .07$, $p = .009$). Romano and Peters (2015) evaluated 20 studies that explored mechanism of action. They found that while MI did not increase patient motivation more than comparison conditions, MI did have a favorable effect on patient engagement variable, suggesting that as a potential mechanism of action. In a systematic review that included 39 studies, Copeland, McNamara, Kelson, and Simpson (2015) identified MI spirit and motivation as the most promising constructs associated with mechanism of MI and that self-efficacy, the most studied construct, was not identified as a mechanism of MI.

MOTIVATIONAL INTERVIEWING SKILLS

In the latest edition of their book, Miller and Rollnick (2013) introduced phases in the process of change that allows practitioners to tailor communication to the patient's phase of change. The communication skills are captured in the acronym OARS: asking

TABLE 9.2	SIMPLE AND COMPLEX REFLECTIONS
Simple reflections	Example 1: Mother whose adult son took his life "I cry myself to sleep every night, I keep thinking I shouldn't have left and maybe he would still be alive." Content: "You think if you stayed he would still be alive." Feeling: "At night you feel especially sad."
Complex reflections	Adding meaning: "You believe you could have prevented him from taking his life." Adding feeling: "You're feeling overwhelmed with guilt." Double sided: "Part of you feels responsible but another part knows that when he was using drugs he was impulsive."
Simple reflections	Example 2: Man beginning alcohol abstinence "I need to have a bottle of Jack Daniels on hand in case one of my buddies comes by." Content: "You want to have liquor in the house." Feeling: "You feel you gotta have liquor on hand for your buddies."
Complex reflections	Added content: "Offering your buddies a drink is expected." Added feeling: "You'd feel weird if you didn't offer them a drink." Double sided: "You're used to having liquor around but know it is a temptation."

Open questions, **A**ffirming, **R**eflecting, and **S**ummarizing. Open questions are simply questions that cannot be answered yes or no or with short answers. Affirmations are comments on the person's strengths and efforts. Reflections are statements mirroring the content or feelings explicitly or implicitly stated by the person. Reflections are distinguished from questions by voice inflection; inflection goes up at the end of a question and down at the end of a reflective statement. Reflections can be simple, staying with what was said, or complex, adding to the content, feeling, or highlighting discrepancies in behaviors or beliefs. See Table 9.2 for examples of reflective statements. Summaries link together what has been stated or serve in moving from one idea to the next idea. MI consists of detecting what phase the person is in and using OARS skills judiciously to help the person move through the phases toward change.

Phases of the Change Process

Engagement is the phase in which a trusting and respectful relationship is established. Without this there is little hope of facilitating change in behavior. *Focusing* is the process of clarifying the patient's goals and direction. *Evoking* is eliciting motivation for a specific change, and the final stage is *planning* a specific change strategy.

Engagement encompasses patient-centered counseling skill with special emphasis on reflections that convey understanding. Psychiatric nurses have a history of understanding the role of empathy in interpersonal relationships (Peplau, 1952/1991), but like other interpersonal competencies these skills need to be periodically revisited and reaffirmed. Empathic reflections are based on active listening (Klagsbrun, 2001) for both what is not said as well as what is said. If accurate, these reflections are acknowledged by the person's nonverbal behaviors such as shaking the head up and down, sighing and lowering shoulders indicating relaxation, or by verbalizing a feeling of being understood. Listening and reflecting on what is not being said can be difficult; overstepping what the person feels ready to acknowledge can increase suspiciousness. Engagement can be assessed by how responsive the person is in the conversation and by asking yourself how well you understand the person's situation. Table 9.3 show potential OARS communication statements during engagement.

TABLE 9.3 PHASES OF CHANGE AND OARS COMMUNICATION SKILLS	
Phase of Change	**OARS Communication Skills**
Engagement Goal: Establish trust and helping relationship	Open questioning: Tell me more about that. What concerns you most? What led to your decision to come? Affirming: It took effort to come today. You took the first step and are ready to take the next. Reflecting: You are getting tired of helping your mother. Being short with your kids is a warning sign. Summarizing: Your father's death and now pressure from your relatives to get a job are too much.
Focusing Goal: Identify direction/ target of change	Open questioning: What concerns you the most? What aspect of managing your son's behavior is most troublesome to you? Affirming: It is your choice of whether or not to tackle this right now. You have been successful in the past. Reflecting: You are not sure whether individual or group therapy would be most helpful. You feel swimming is the best exercise for you. Summarizing: You have eliminated simple sugar from your diet but are not sure what else to do to prevent diabetes.
Evoking Goal: Bring forth person's motivation for change	Open questioning: What do you see as some of the downsides to your present weight? How do you want things to be different? Affirming: You care that your kids will be happier if you stop smoking. You were successful before in quitting. Reflecting: You know it will be difficult but you worry about your health if you don't lose weight. You feel anxious about not checking whether your door is locked more than two times but are concerned with getting to work on time. Summarizing: You have identified that it will be hard for you to exercise in the morning but are not sure you can fit it in after work.
Planning Goal: Elicit plan that will be followed	Open questioning: What is the first step in making this happen? Have you thought how you might make this change? Affirming: Praying for his success is the best way to support him now. Beginning therapy is a big step, but you have found a way to make it work. Reflecting: Gaining a little weight is a possible pitfall if you stop smoking, but it is worth it if your breathing is easier. Summarizing: You decided to get away when you quit so you don't alienate your roommate. You think that suddenly stopping all sugary drinks is the best way for you to work on your diet.

Focusing is guiding the interaction to identify a direction of change. This may emerge without prompting, but in many cases it is a matter of narrowing the focus and prioritizing the options. Patients may present global issues, and it is difficult guiding them in selecting a focus. Open questions are used to understand what the person knows about the outcomes of not changing. Practitioners instinctively want to share information about the consequences of unhealthy behaviors. Although well intended, these automatic "right" reflexive comments frequently engender resistance, such as "My drinking is not a problem, I have never gotten a DUI." Miller and Moyers (2006) advocate using reflection to diffuse resistance, for example, saying "Your drinking has never caused you to be arrested." Another method of "rolling with resistance" is to convey to patients that changing is their choice. This intervention needs to be stated in a sincere manner because it can easily be misinterpreted as dismissive or as giving permission to continue the behavior. If you discover that the patient may not understand consequences of the behavior, ask permission to relate your understanding of the effects of continuing the behavior; for example, "You mentioned sleep is important to you, and you are only getting about 4 hours a night. I am concerned how your smoking might be related to sleep. I wonder whether that might be something we could talk about?" If there are multiple directions for change, asking patients what aspect is most important to them may be effective. The focusing phase has been achieved when there is a clear direction that is acknowledged by you and the patient. Table 9.3 show potential OARS communication statements during the focusing phase.

Evoking is eliciting and responding to change talk. In moving to the evoking phase, listen for change talk and amplify it with reflective statements in order to develop discrepancy between sustaining and changing the behavior. Sometimes the clues are subtle, such as the patient relating she had a nicotine patch and stopped smoking when she was in the hospital or surviving without a daily Coke on Easter when visiting family. It is easy for practitioners to elicit resistance in the evoking phase. Miller and Rollnick (2013) believe there is a strong pull to continuing the same behavior because it is supported by habits and environmental cues. As with most behavioral and cognitive therapies, resistance emerges from interactions that evoke defensiveness. Change may be elicited by cautiously asking whether there is anything positive about changing behavior: such as "reducing the amount you drink on weekends," "reducing the sugary drinks you consume," or "not eating during the night?" Summarizing the pros and cons of changing, always ending with the pros, can be useful, stating "You know it'll be difficult, but you worry about your health if you don't." Gauging commitment to change can be assessed by asking how important it is to change on a scale of 1 to 10, with 10 being most important. Because you want to support change, follow with what would make changing more important. Listening to see whether change talk is more predominant than sustain talk is the best way to assess whether the patient is ready to move to the planning phase. Table 9.3 show potential OARS communication statements during the evoking phase.

Evoking hope is important when individuals lack confidence that they can change. This is especially true of individuals with serious mental illness who suffer relapses that challenge their motivation to continue working toward recovery. Confidence in changing can be assessed by asking how confident the patient feels on a scale of 1 to 10, with 10 being very confident. Follow up on what would increase confidence. Miller and Rollnick (2013) suggest that breaking change behavior into smaller steps and acknowledging past attempts are helpful methods to increase confidence that change is possible.

Planning is the fourth phase and involves reinforcing commitment and assisting the patient in developing a plan for change. Readiness to begin the planning phase can be detected when patients begin to use verbs like will, begin, do, and plan rather than verbs like need and should (Amrhein et al., 2003). In this phase the automatic "default" is for the practitioner to give the person suggestions about how to proceed with change. This is likely to elicit patient resistance and stall or delay change. Returning to open-ended questions, affirmations, and reflections are most helpful. For example, "What ideas do you have about how to begin changing your drinking/eating/increasing physical activity?" Table 9.3 shows potential OARS communication statements during the planning phase.

MODIFICATIONS OF MOTIVATIONAL INTERVIEWING

MI has been incorporated into a best practice substance abuse treatment based on the transtheoretical five-stage model of change of precontemplation, contemplation, preparation, action, and maintenance combined with MI (Center for Substance Abuse Treatment, 1999). The treatment uses a FRAMES approach that includes (a) personalized **F**eedback on substance use from standard tests, (b) giving the individuals **R**esponsibility for change, (c) presenting **A**dvice with permission in a nonjudgmental manner, (d) offering a **M**enu of change options with (e) **E**mpathy and empowering, and (f) **S**elf-efficacy. MI interventions are tailored to the person's stage of change, and evidence shows that they are helpful with individuals from different cultural backgrounds and socioeconomic levels (Center for Substance Abuse Treatment, 1999). Enhanced motivation for change has been widely adopted in substance abuse programs, and the manual is available from the Substance Abuse and Mental Health Services Administration. Another similarly based program for adolescent cannabis addiction is available at www.motivationalinterview.org (Sampl & Kadden, 2001). It entails a five-session MI enhancement prior to cognitive behavioral treatment for adolescent cannabis use.

CASE EXAMPLES

Two cases from different clinical settings illustrate the spirit and communication skills of MI. In each case the interview is conducted by a psychiatric–mental health nurse practitioner [PMHNP]. Case 1 is a 35-year-old Caucasian woman seen in an integrated primary care office who was referred for counseling on her alcohol use. She had no previous psychiatric services, was married, and had three young children. Because MI is a communication process, a process recording is the best way to illustrate application.

Case Example 1

ENGAGEMENT

PMHNP: I'm a psychiatric nurse practitioner, and your practitioner asked me to see you. Perhaps we could start with what you understand about our meeting.

Sue: I'm not sure. She asked me about my drinking and ordered some tests.

PMHNP: Maybe we could start there. Your lab results look fine except for some elevation in your liver enzymes. I want to explore what might be causing this. You mentioned that you do drink, and alcohol can raise liver enzymes.

Can you tell me more about your drinking? *(open questioning)*

Sue: I don't drink that much.

You have to understand, I stay at home all day. I have three kids—5 years, 3 years, and 9 months old. Do you have any kids? The oldest is in kindergarten now, but getting the 3-year-old down for a nap and now that the baby is crawling and putting everything in her mouth . . .

[pause] I have a drink after lunch. And it helps. A lot.

I'm not sure how I'd handle it otherwise.

PMHNP: You find it stressful being home with three young children and having a drink helps you relax? *(simple reflection)*

Sue: Yes. Yes. Exactly. Because I don't get time off. This is not a "job" I can take a break from. My husband, he leaves, he gets time away. But me? I'm always watching them, feeding them, breaking up fights. And the boys—they FIGHT. My 5-year-old son has real issues with anger.

PMHNP: There's a lot of energy in a house with boys. You don't have the opportunity your husband does to get away. *(simple reflection)*

Sue: And Eric, my husband, has no idea what it's like staying home with small children. He imagines I watch cartoons all day, eat ice cream.

PMHNP: You don't feel supported by him? *(complex reflection)*

Sue: Shakes head yes . . .

PMHNP: Maybe he doesn't recognize the strain you feel caring for the children all day. It sounds like you're drinking during the day to help you handle the stress. *(simple reflection)*

Sue: I guess I am.

FOCUSING

PMHNP: We could go in any number of directions here. I wonder what makes the most sense to you. Your relationship with your husband and the lack of support you feel is an issue. I'm also concerned about how your drinking is affecting your health. What would you like to focus on? *(closed question)*

Sue: I don't know, I . . .

Eric would be so angry if he knew that I drink during the day and when Eric gets angry he doesn't yell—nothing like that—he just shuts down. Completely. Ignores me AND the kids.

PMHNP: If you share that you are drinking, you feel he would shut you out more. *(complex reflection)*

Sue: Yes. Definitely.

EVOKING

PMHNP: What kind of relationship would you like to have with your husband? *(open question)*

Sue: I want to have a relationship where we communicate with each other, where he listens to me, and asks me what my day has been like.

We used to have a relationship like that. We talked much more before Amy was born.

You see, we didn't plan on having more children—she's 9 months now—and I'm happy we have a girl and so is Eric, but I think he feels overwhelmed with the finances. . . .

I didn't drink during the pregnancy but since Amy stopped nursing . . .

PMHNP: You feel Eric might be shutting you out because he is stressed with money. (*complex reflection*)

Sue: Sure. I guess that's possible.

PMHNP: You remember when your relationship with your husband was better and you weren't drinking during the day. (*simple reflection*)

Sue: Yes.

PMHNP: How important is it to you to stop drinking and improve your relationship with your husband? Say on a scale from 1 to 10, with 10 being very important. (*closed question*)

Sue: I'd say at least an 8.

I know we should sit down and talk, but I've been so stressed and angry lately, it'll be hard not to just blow up at him.

PLANNING

PMHNP: You're concerned you won't be able to share how much you miss your time with him. (*complex reflection*)

Sue: I am not sure he misses me.

PMHNP: It is difficult sharing how you feel, particularly if you're concerned about him shutting you out. But perhaps it's a risk worth taking. (*simple reflection*)

Sue: Yes. You're right. I know you're right.

PMHNP: And perhaps if you can clear the air with Eric, you'll feel less anxious and overwhelmed. Soon, you may not need that drink after lunch. (*complex reflection*)

Sue: Yes. Yes. I know.

. . .

I think I'll talk with him tonight.

Analysis of Interaction: Case 1

Using reflection and open questioning revealed that Sue was feeling isolated from her husband, which she related to her alcohol use. If the PMHNP had focused exclusively on her alcohol use, her strained relationship with her husband might not have emerged. It is doubtful Sue would be willing to consider changing her drinking without addressing the issue of her husband as well. Miller and Rollnick (2013) recommend examining the frequency of OARS communication skills to attain competency in MI. In this encounter, the PMHNP offered more open-ended questions than closed questions and more reflections than questions.

Case Example 2

Case 2 is a 20-year-old woman, Melena, who attended a medication visit with her case manager at a community mental health center. She is diagnosed with mood disorder not otherwise specified and borderline personality disorder and is prescribed lamotrigine, trazodone, and citalopram. Melena has just returned from an out-of-state visit to see her boyfriend.

PMHNP: How is it going? *(open questioning)*

Melena: He has another girlfriend; he didn't want to tell me on the phone.

PMHNP: That must be distressing after you traveled to get there. *(complex reflection)*

Melena: When he told me I told him I was going to start cutting.

PMHNP: You were angry with him? *(complex reflection)*

Melena: He told me he would have sex with me if I did not cut on myself.

PMHNP: How did that go? *(open questioning)*

Melena: So I didn't do any cutting, but since I've been back I'm angry about small things. At the airport I just wanted to knock the cowboy hat off a man. Nothing helps. I can't sleep and started drinking four to five shots of whiskey with beer at night.

PMHNP: You're drinking to help you sleep? *(simple reflection)*

Melena: I get to sleep but don't sleep long.

PMHNP: You think that might be related to your drinking? *(simple reflection)*

Melena: I don't know.

PMHNP: If you're willing, I would like to tell you about the effects of alcohol on sleep. *(asking permission to give information)*

Melena: Shakes head positively.

PMHNP: Alcohol initially makes you sleepy, but with large amounts your body begins withdrawal, which disrupts your sleep.

Melena: I didn't know that.

PMHNP: Remind me of the coping skills you have used in the past? *(open questioning)*

Melena: I have a special pillow. I used to listen to my MP3 player, but I haven't got a charger so I can't now.

PMHNP: So music has been helpful. *(simple reflection)*

Case manager: We could see about replacing the charger and look at what other activities you have in your wrap plan.

PMHNP: Is that something you are willing to do? *(closed questioning)*

Melena: Shakes head yes.

Analysis of Interaction: Case 2

This brief MI intervention helped to avert a full relapse into drinking to cope with her anger and disappointment about her boyfriend.

TRAINING IN MOTIVATIONAL INTERVIEWING

No definitive certification for MI exists that is widely recognized. Training programs are designed to prepare a wide range of professionals such as case managers, primary care practitioners, counselors, and therapists from varying disciplines. Online and live programs are usually divided into beginning and advanced MI skills, each lasting 2 to 3 days live or 40 to 50 hours online.

There are three key methods to consider in learning MI:

1. Break down the skills into steps (Miller & Moyers, 2006).
2. Practice the skills in live sessions, taping them if possible.
3. Get coaching and feedback on direct observation of skills.

One of the best resources for training is the Motivational Interviewing Network of Trainers website at www.motivationalinterview.org, which offers videotapes of experts implementing MI, online programs, and a list of live training opportunities. Look for programs that incorporate experiential and practice sessions.

Rosengren's workbook (2009) is excellent for all stages of learning motivational interviewing The book by Naar-King and Suarez (2010) ia a guide to using motivational interviewing with adolescents and young adults.

As with any communication skill, there is drift over time, so a mechanism for follow-up training is important. This can be achieved by creating learning groups that listen and code tapes of real patients and offer consultation with difficult patients. Learning groups are most effective when sanctioned or sponsored by one's workplace. Coding systems used by trainers focus on interviewer responses or examine both interviewer and patient responses and provide feedback on level of mastery of MI. Miller and Rollnick (2013) recommend counting reflections and questions with the goal of having twice as many reflections as questions and identifying the patient's change talk and therapist's responses inconsistent with MI. Inconsistent responses include using confrontation such as, "You will get diabetes if you continue what you are doing," or persuasion, "You will feel so much better if you exercise regularly." Confrontation and persuasion are based on the false belief that denial needs to be directly attacked. This is not supported by research (Miller et al., 1998; Miller et al., 1993).

Motivational Interviewing Network of Trainers (motivationalinterviewing.org/about_mint) is an international organization of trainers in MI, incorporated as a 501(c)(3) tax-exempt nonprofit charitable organization in the state of Virginia. Trainers come from diverse backgrounds and apply MI in a variety of settings. Their central interest is to improve the quality and effectiveness of counseling and consultations with patients about behavior change. Started in 1997 by a small group of trainers trained by William R. Miller and Stephen Rollnick, the organization has since grown to represent 35 countries and is conducted in more than 20 languages.

CONCLUDING COMMENTS

MI facilitates the patient's inherent motivation to change. It is not a therapy but a method of communication that partners with patients through accepting their autonomy and respecting that they have within themselves the knowledge of how to change. MI is an evidence-based person-centered approach that started in addiction counseling coupled with the transtheoretical model of change (Prochaska & DiClemente, 1983). It can be used in helping people engage in lifestyle changes to improve their health. Also, MI can be used to motivate individuals to initiate therapy for anxiety disorders preceding more action-oriented therapy.

Some may see MI as a time-consuming intervention in our fast-paced, cost-conscious healthcare delivery system. However, with the growing focus on patient outcomes and the need for people to embrace healthier lifestyles, there is evidence that using MI is an important and needed skill for all health professionals. Approximately 42.4% of adults (2020) and 18.5% of children and adolescents (2019) are obese in the United States (Centers for Disease Control and Prevention). An estimated 48.3% of U.S. adults don't engage in the minimum recommended physical activity (Robert Wood Johnson Foundation, 2018). Individuals with serious mental illness report less physical activity than the general population, resulting in 15- to 20-year shorter lifespans than the general population, largely attributed to chronic health problems stemming from sedentary lifestyle, obesity, and poor health outcomes (Vancampfort et al., 2017). Physical activity is one of the key modifiable lifestyle habits that can improve overall health. MI offers a person-centered approach to support individuals to both initiate and maintain increased physical activity.

DISCUSSION QUESTIONS

1. Describe differences in implementing MI in an established relationship versus an initial relationship.
2. Discuss the philosophy and principles of MI.
3. Identify situations from your clinical practice in which MI would be applicable.
4. What function is served by asking the patient "How important is it to change your behavior on a scale of 1 to 10, with 10 being very important?"
5. Discuss why offering reflections versus asking questions reduces defensiveness.
6. Describe the approach in "SAMHSA TIP 35: Enhancing Motivation for Change in Substance Use Disorder Treatment."
7. What steps facilitate learning MI?

REFERENCES

Amrhein, P. C., Miller, W. R., Yahne, C. E., Palmer, M., & Fulcher, L. (2003). Client commitment language during motivational interviewing predicts drug use outcome. *Journal of Consulting and Clinical Psychology*, *71*, 862–878. doi:10.1037/0022-006X.71.5.862

Apodaca, T. R., & Longabaugh, R. (2009). Mechanisms of change in motivational interviewing: A review and preliminary evaluation of the evidence. *Addiction*, *104*, 705–715. doi:10.1111/j.1360-0443.2009.02527.x

Armstrong, M. J., Mottershead, T. A., Ronksley, P. E., Signal, R. J., Campbell, T. S., & Hemmelgarn, B. R. (2011). Motivational interviewing to improve weight loss in overweight and/or obese patients: A systematic review and meta-analysis of randomized controlled trials. *International Association for the Study of Obesity*, *12*, 709–723. doi:10.111/j.1467–789X2011.00892.x

Barrowclough, C., Haddock, G., Wykes, T., Beardmore, R., Conrod, P., Craig, T., . . . Tarrier, N. (2010). Integrated motivational interviewing and cognitive behavioural therapy for people with psychosis and comorbid substance misuse: Randomized controlled trial. *British Medical Journal, 341*, c6325. doi:10.1136/bmj.c6325

Bellack, A. S., & Gearon, J. S. (1998). Substance abuse treatment for people with schizophrenia. *Addictive Behaviors, 23*, 749–766. doi:10.1016/S0306-4603(98)00066-5

Bem, D. J. (1967). Self-perception: An alternative interpretation of cognitive dissonance phenomena. *Psychological Review, 74*, 183–200. doi:10.1037/h0024835

Brehm, S. S., & Brehm, J. W. (1981). *Psychological reactance: A theory of freedom and control.* New York, NY: Academic Press.

Burke, B. L., Arkowitz, H., & Menchola, M. (2003). The efficacy of motivational interviewing: A meta-analysis of controlled clinical trials. *Journal of Consulting and Clinical Psychology, 71*, 843–861. doi:10.1037/0022-006X.71.5.843

Burke, B. L., Dunn, C. W., Atkins, D., & Phelps, J. S. (2004). The emerging evidence base for motivational interviewing: A meta-analytic & qualitative inquiry. *Journal of Cognitive Psychotherapy, 18*, 309–322. doi:10.1891/jcop.18.4.309.64002

Center for Substance Abuse Treatment. (1999). *Enhanced motivation for change in substance abuse treatment* [Treatment Improvement Protocol (TIP) Series, No. 35. HHS Publication No. (SMA) 12–4212]. Rockville, MD: Substance Abuse and Mental Health Services Administration. Retrieved from https://www.ncbi.nlm.nih.gov/books/NBK64967

Centers for Disease Control and Prevention. (2019). *Childhood obesity facts.* Retrieved from https://www.cdc.gov/obesity/data/childhood.html.

Centers for Disease Control and Prevention [CDC]. (2020). *Adult obesity facts.* Retrieved from https://www.cdc.gov/obesity/data/adult.html.

Cohen, J. (1992). A power primer. *Psychological Bulletin, 112*, 155–159. doi:10.1037/0033-2909.112.1.155

Copeland, L., McNamara, R., Kelson, M., & Simpson, S. (2015). Mechanisms of change within motivational interviewing in relation to health behaviors outcome: A systematic review. *Patient Education and Counseling, 98*(4), 401–411. doi:10.1016/j.pec.2014.11.022

Festinger, L. (1957). *A theory of cognitive dissonance.* Evanston, IL: Row, Peterson.

Hedges, L. V., & Olkin, I. (1985). *Statistical methods for meta-analysis.* New York, NY: Academic Press.

Hettema, J. E., & Hendricks, P. S. (2010). Motivational interviewing for smoking cessation: A meta-analytic review. *Journal of Clinical and Consulting Psychology, 78*(6), 864–884. doi:10.1037/a0021498

Hettema, J. E., Steele, J., & Miller, W. (2005). Motivational interviewing. *Annual Review of Clinical Psychology, 1*, 91–111. doi:10.1146/annurev.clinpsy.1.102803.143833

Hunt, G. E., Siegfried, N., Morley, K., Sitharthan, T., & Cleary, M. (2013). Psychosocial interventions for people with both severe mental illness and substance misuse. *Cochrane Database of Systematic Reviews*, (10), CD001088. doi:10.1002/14651858.CD001088.pub3

Jensen, C. D., Cushing, E. D., Aylward, B. S., Craig, J. T., Sorell, D. M., & Steele, R. G. (2011). Effectiveness of motivational interviewing interventions for adolescent substance use behavior change: A meta-analytic review. *Journal of Consulting and Clinical Psychology, 79*(4), 433–440. doi:10.1037/a0023992

Kelly, T. M., Daley, D. C., & Douaihy, A. G. (2012). Treatment of substance abusing patients with comorbid psychiatric disorders. *Addictive Behaviors, 37*, 11–24. doi:10.1016/j.addbeh.2011.09.010

Kissling, L. S., & Davis, J. M. (2009). How to read and understand and use systematic reviews and meta-analyses. *Acta Psychiatrica Scandinavica. 119*, 443–450. doi:10.111/j.1600–0447.2009.01388.x

Klagsbrun, J. (2001). Listening and focusing: Holistic health care tools for nurses. *Nursing Clinics of North America, 36*, 115–130.

Lai, D. T., Cahill, K., Qin, Y., & Tang, J. L. (2010). Motivational interviewing for smoking cessation. *Cochrane Database of Systematic Reviews*, (1), CD006936. doi:10.1002/14651858.CD006936.pub2

Lenz, A. S., Rosenbaum, L., & Sheperis, D. (2016). Meta-analysis of randomized controlled trials of motivational enhancement therapy for reducing substance use. *Journal of Addictions & Offender Counseling, 37*(2), 66–86. doi:10.1002/jaoc.12017

Lindson-Hawley, N. K., Thompson, T. P., & Begh, R. (2015). Motivational interviewing for smoking cessation. *Cochrane Database of Systematic Reviews*, (3), CD006936. doi:10.1002/14651858.CD006936.pub3

Lundahl, B. W., Kung, C., Brownell, C., Tollefson, D., & Burke, B. L. (2010). A meta-analysis of motivational interviewing: Twenty-five years of empirical studies. *Research on Social Work Practice*, *20*, 137–160. doi:10.1177/1049731509347850

Lundahl, B. W., Moleni, T., Burke, B. L., Butters, R., Tollefson, D., Butler, C., & Rollnick, S. (2013). Motivational interviewing in medical care settings: A systematic review and meta-analysis of randomized controlled trials. *Patient Education and Counseling*, *93*(2), 157–168. doi:10.1016/j.pec.2013.07.012

Magill, M., Gaume, J., Apodaca, R.R., Walthers, J., Mastroleo, N. R., Borsari, B., & Longabaugh, R. (2014). The technical hypothesis of motivational interviewing: A meta-analysis of MI's key causal model. *Journal of Consulting and Clinical Psychology*, *82*(6), 973–983. doi:10.1037/a0036833

Marker, I., & Norton, P. J. (2018, June). The efficacy of incorporating motivational interviewing to cognitive behavior therapy for anxiety disorders: A review and meta-analysis. *Clinical Psychology Review*, *62*, 1–10. doi:10.1016/j.cpr.2018.04.004

Miller, W. R. (1983). Motivational Interviewing with problem drinkers. *Behavioural Psychotherapy*, *11*, 147–172. doi:10.1017/S0141347300006583

Miller, W. R. (1985). Motivation for treatment: A review with special emphasis on alcoholism. *Psychological Bulletin*, *98*, 84–107. doi:10.1037/0033-2909.98.1.84

Miller, W. R., Andrews, N. R., Wilbourne, P., & Bennett, M. E. (1998). A wealth of alternatives: Effective treatments for alcohol problems. In W. R. Miller & N. Heather (Eds.). *Treating addictive behaviors: Processes of change* (pp. 203–216). New York, NY: Plenum Press.

Miller, W. R., Benefield, R. G., & Tonigan, J. S. (1993). Enhancing motivation for change in problem drinking: A controlled comparison of two therapist styles. *Journal of Consulting and Clinical Psychology*, *61*, 455–461. doi:10.1037/0022-006X.61.3.455

Miller, W. R., & Moyers, T. B. (2006). Eight stages in learning motivational interviewing. *Journal of Teaching in the Addictions*, *5*(1), 3–17. doi:10.1300/J188v05n01_02

Miller, W. R., & Rollnick, S. (1991). *Motivational interviewing: Preparing people to change addictive behaviors*. New York, NY: Guilford Press.

Miller, W. R., & Rollnick, S. (2002). *Motivational interviewing: Preparing people for change* (2nd ed.). New York, NY: Guilford Press.

Miller, W. R., & Rollnick, S. (2013). *Motivational interviewing: Helping people change* (3rd ed.). New York, NY: Guilford Press.

Miller W. R., & Rose, G. S. (2009). Towards a theory of motivational interviewing. *American Psychologists*. *64*(6), 527–537. doi:10.1037/a0016830

Naar-King, S., & Suarez, M. (2010). *Motivational interviewing with adolescents and young adults*. New York, NY: Guilford Press.

Peplau, H. (1991). *Interpersonal relations in nursing*. New York, NY: Springer Publishing Company. (Original work published 1952).

Prochaska, J. O., & DiClemente, C. C. (1983). Stages and processes of self-change of smoking: Towards an integrative model of change. *Journal of Consulting and Clinical Psychology*, *31*, 390–395. doi:10.1037/0022-006X.51.3.390

Prochaska, J. O., DiClemente, C. C., & Norcross, J. C. (1992). In search of how people change: Applications to addictive behaviors. *American Psychologists*, *47*, 1102–1114. doi:10.1037/0003-066X.47.9.1102

Robert Wood Johnson Foundation. (2018). The state of obesity: Better policies for a healthier America. Retrieved from https://www.tfah.org/report-details/the-state-of-obesity-2018/.

Rogers, C. R. (1965). *Client-centered therapy*. New York, NY: Houghton Mifflin.

Romano, M., & Peters, L. (2015). Evaluating the mechanisms of change in motivational interviewing in the treatment of mental health problems: A review and meta-analysis. *Clinical Psychology Review*, *38*, 1–12. doi:10.1016/j.cpr.2015.02.008

Rosengren, D. B. (2009) . *Building motivational interviewing skills: A practitioner workbook*. New York, NY: Guilford Press.

Sampl, S., & Kadden, R. (2001). *Motivational enhancement therapy and cognitive behavioral therapy for adolescent cannabis users: 5 sessions, Cannabis Youth Treatment (CYT) Series* (Vol. 1). Rockville,

MD: Center for Substance Abuse Treatment, Substance Abuse and Mental Health Services Administration. BKD384. Retrieved from http://lib.adai.washington.edu/clearinghouse/downloads/MET-and-CBT-for-Adolescent-Cannabis-Users-CYT-Series-Volume-1-339.pdf

Samson, J. E., & Tanner-Smith, E. E. (2015). Single-session alcohol interventions for heavy drinking college students: A systematic review and meta-analysis. *Journal of Studies on Alcohol and Drugs*, *76*(4), 530–543. doi:10.15288/jsad.2015.76.530

Sayegh, C. S., Huey, S. J., Zara, E. J., & Jhaveri, K. (2017). Follow-up treatment effects of contingency management and motivational interviewing on substance use: A meta-analysis. *Psychology of Addictive Behaviors*, *31*(4), 403–414. doi:10.1037/adb0000277

Smedslund, G., Berg, R. C., Hammerstron, K. T., Steiro, A., Leiknes, K. A., Dahl, H. M., & Karlsen, K. (2011). Motivational interviewing for substance abuse. *Cochrane Database of Systematic Reviews*, (5), CD008063. doi:10.1002/14651858.CD008063.pub2

Steinberg, M. L., Ziedonis, D. M., Krejci, J. A., & Brandon, T. H. (2004). Motivational interviewing with personalized feedback: A brief intervention for motivating smokers with schizophrenia to see treatment for tobacco dependence. *Journal of Consulting and Clinical Psychology*, *72*(4), 723–728. doi:10.1037/0022-006X.72.4.723

Substance Abuse & Mental Health Services Administration (SAMHSA). (2019). *TIP 35: Enhancing motivation for change in substance use disorder treatment. Updated 2019*. SAMHSA Publication No. PEP19-02-01-003 Published 2019.

Tanner-Smith, E. E., & Lipsey, M. W. (2015). Brief alcohol interventions for adolescents and young adults: A systematic review and meta-analysis. *Journal of Substance Abuse Treatment*, *51*, 1–18. doi:10.1016/j.jsat.2014.09.001

Tanner-Smith E. E., & Risser, M. D. (2016). A meta-analysis of brief alcohol interventions for adolescents and young adults: Variability in effects across alcohol measures. *The American Journal of Drug and Alcohol Abuse*, *42*(2), 140–151. doi:10.3109/00952990.2015.1136638

VanBuskirk, K. A., & Wetherell, J. L. (2014). Motivational interviewing with primary care populations: A systematic review and meta-analyses. *Journal of Behavioral Medicine*, *37*(4), 768–780. doi:10.1007/s10865-013-9527-4

Vancampfort, D., Firth, J., Schuch, F. B., Rosenbaum, S., Mugisha, J., Hallgren, M., . . . Stubbs, B. (2017). Sedentary behavior and physical activity levels in people with schizophrenia, bipolar disorder and major depressive disorder: A global systematic review and meta-analysis. *World Psychiatry*, *16*(3), 308–315. doi:10.1002/wps.20458

Vanderwaal, F. M. (2015). Impact of motivational interviewing on medication adherence in schizophrenia. *Issues in Mental Health Nursing*, *36*(11), 900–904. doi:10.3109/01612840.2015.1058445

Westra, H. A., Arkowitz, H., & Dozois, D. J. A. (2009). Adding a motivational interviewing pretreatment to cognitive behavioral therapy for generalized anxiety disorder: A preliminary randomized controlled trial. *Journal of Anxiety Disorders*, *23*(8), 1106–1117. doi:10.1016/j.janxdis.2009.07.014

Westra, H. A., & Dozois, D. J. A. (2006). Preparing clients for cognitive behavioral therapy: A randomized pilot study of motivational interviewing for anxiety. *Cognitive Therapy and Research*. *30*, 481–490. doi:10.1007/s10608–006–9016-y

Interpersonal Psychotherapy

Kathleen Wheeler and Marie Crowe

Interpersonal psychotherapy (IPT) is a brief, structured psychotherapeutic approach based on the operating principle that psychiatric disorders occur within an interpersonal, social context. Symptoms of psychiatric disorders in four specific areas of social functioning create problems in which IPT therapists are trained to intervene: interpersonal disputes, role transitions, grief, and interpersonal deficits.

This chapter provides an overview of IPT theory and techniques by tracing the history of the approach and identifying relevant psychological and nursing theories congruent with the concepts of IPT. The application of IPT to specific populations with depression, perinatal/postpartum depression, adolescent depression, bipolar disorder, and counseling in the medical setting is discussed. Goals and phases of treatment are delineated, and a case example illustrates use of the IPT approach. The chapter ends with a list of websites for information on further training in this treatment modality.

FOUNDATIONS OF IPT

The work of three psychopathology theorists shaped some of the underlying approaches of IPT (Markowitz & Weissman, 2012). Their theories emphasized the importance of the interpersonal environment and the relationships therein as the foundation of personality development. A brief background of the theorists and their theoretical frameworks are described here in relation to the foundational concepts of IPT:

- Harry Stack Sullivan is recognized as one of the major figures in American psychiatry. He became interested in the field in the early 1930s and is widely recognized as a charismatic leader who became a pioneer in the treatment of schizophrenia. Sullivan's view on the development of mental illness was influenced by many other fields including cultural anthropology and political science (Horowitz & Strack, 2011). His central theory is that interpersonal relationships and the communications therein form the basis for psychiatric disorders. He believed that effective communications are interfered with by anxiety. Sullivan also posits that "each person in a two-person relationship is involved as a portion of an interpersonal field, rather than as a separate entity, in processes which affect and are affected by the field" (Sullivan, 1953, p. 12). Sullivan and nurse theorist Hildegard Peplau, who is discussed later in this chapter, are both recognized as pioneer thinkers in the treatment of schizophrenia (Peplau, 1952). Although IPT is not recognized as a treatment model in the treatment of schizophrenia, the humanistic approaches of Sullivan and Peplau are respected as universally applicable in the mental health treatment of individuals in emotional pain.

- Adolf Meyer was a Swiss psychoanalyst who was strongly influenced by the psychobiology and psychopathology theories of Darwin, Freud, and Jung. He became the primary architect in professionalizing the field of psychiatry when he became the first professor of psychiatry at Johns Hopkins University in Baltimore, Maryland. Meyer used the findings and recommendations for the field of clinical psychiatry that appeared in the *Flexner Report*, published early in the 20th century, when he implemented the use of research, professional scholarship, and full-time faculty to improve clinical knowledge in the field of psychiatry. Meyer "viewed mental illness as an attempt by the individual to adapt to the changing environment" (Klerman, Weissman, Rounsaville, & Chevron , 1984, p. 42). Adolf Meyer is recognized as one of the founding fathers of the field of social epidemiology, the field that researches the causes and effective treatment of social and mental ills.
- John Bowlby was an English psychoanalyst who developed the concept of attachment theory. He is recognized as one of the century's most influential theorists on personality development and social relationships (Horowitz & Strack, 2011). When Bowlby worked with infants and children as the head of the Children's Department at the Tavistock Clinic after World War II, he recognized the powerful effects of mother–child separation. Bowlby believed that the attachment of the child to the mother had an evolutionary basis, rather than the oral gratification theoretical approach held by the Freudians. Bowlby is well known as the author of three important texts describing how the mother–child bond affects human responses to attachment, separation, loss, and depression over the life continuum.

NURSING THEORY AND IPT

The IPT model is in strong alignment with the primary themes of nursing. In this section, the approaches of three nursing theorists who have examined the psychosocial dimensions of illness are reviewed to demonstrate the similarity of the values of psychiatric nursing with those of IPT.

Peplau is considered to be the founder of the field of mental health nursing. Hildegard Peplau's model and the fundamental values of psychosocial nursing are congruent with the foundational concepts of IPT. A core concept is the importance of interpersonal relations in nursing. Her clinical model of nursing interaction is outlined in her view of the major themes of nursing:

1. Patient: A unique biopsychosocial being. An organism that lives in an unstable equilibrium.
2. Nursing: The assistance provided to patients to aid their understanding of the course of their health problem and to help them learn from the experience. A significant therapeutic interpersonal process that promotes the health of the individual (defined subsequently).
3. Environment: The psychodynamic milieu. The existing forces outside the person that provide the social context in which psychological healing occurs.
4. Health: Ongoing development of the personality and other developmental processes that lead to full personal development, including constructiveness, creativity, productivity, and self and social fulfillment (Peplau, 1952, 1991).

Martha Rogers's theoretical framework, the Science of Unitary Human Beings, is similar to Sullivan's field theories. Her theories, based on foundations in physics and systems and psychosocial theories, emphasized the power of fields in the maintenance of health and the development of and treatment of disease (Rogers, 1970). Watson's

Transpersonal Caring Theory emphasizes the importance of the therapeutic and healing presence of the nurse who focuses his or her attention on caring, healing, and wholeness, rather than on disease, illness, and pathology. A meaningful nurse–patient relationship is based on caring and the demand for authentic person-to-person exchange (Watson, 2013).

The holistic nursing model outlined in Chapter 1 evolved from these theoretical roots and is consistent with the major themes of nursing identified previously. The individual is embedded in relationships with others that affect and influence all dimensions of the person. Interpersonal interactions reveal the perceptions, feelings, and thoughts unique for a person and give expression to implicit memory networks. IPT focuses on relationships, targeting current social and interpersonal interactions. By understanding the effects of the person's problem on significant relationships and how past and present relationships affect the problem, new relational patterns and roles can be discussed and implemented. Changing the social context and relationships with others reverberates to all dimensions of the person, because all components are interrelated. Through interpersonal change, *right relationship* with others and self occurs.

HISTORY OF IPT

IPT was developed by Myrna Weissman and the late Gerald Klerman in a research setting as a treatment intervention in the early 1980s for a series of studies conducted on the assessment and treatment of depression (Markowitz & Weissman, 2012a). These studies tested whether antidepressants or antidepressants and psychotherapy resulted in better outcomes and less recidivism. The results of these studies guided the development of an IPT treatment manual based on the premise that most psychiatric disorders occur within a social context. The IPT treatment manual addressed the four types of interpersonal problems (interpersonal disputes, role transitions, grief, and interpersonal deficits) described earlier.

Within the different psychiatric disorders studied, including depression, perinatal depression and others mentioned previously, these four types of interpersonal difficulties produced symptom clusters that were uniquely different from each other (Klerman et al., 1984; Weissman, Markowitz, & Klerman, 2000). As the psychiatric disorders were studied, it was found that the assessment and treatment of each disorder required modifications in the original model for depression (Markowitz & Weissman, 2012). These IPT clinical approaches to a variety of psychiatric disorders and treatment settings are described later in the chapter.

Underlying Assumptions of the IPT Model

The work of John Bowlby in describing disruptions in the maternal–child relationship as the source of psychosocial difficulties in adolescence and adulthood is foundational to IPT. Bowlby's research and teaching emphasized the impact of early life issues, with separation and loss as the underlying basis for depression. The development of IPT was based on the theoretical perspectives of Bowlby and on the social interaction theories of Sullivan and Meyer (Markowitz & Weissman, 2012).

IPT recognizes that psychopathology arises from underlying personality issues that will *not* become the focus of treatment. Instead, IPT emphasizes that the problems created by the psychiatric disorder occur interdependently within the conscious social and interpersonal realms. These problems and conscious awareness of the context are the focus of IPT treatment (Markowitz & Weissman, 2012).

In developing the IPT approach, it was thought that earlier depression treatment programs paid too little attention to techniques aimed at reduction of symptoms and easing the patient's current social functioning and interpersonal relations (Klerman et al., 1984). IPT emphasizes the patient's disputes, frustrations, anxieties, and goals in his or her current social and interpersonal environments. The purpose of IPT is to intervene with symptoms and to reduce the risk of additional symptom formation by relieving current problems in interpersonal relations and social adjustment.

Symptoms are described as the development of depressive affect and its accompanying indications that may be the result of psychobiological or psychodynamic mechanisms. Although the IPT founders recognize the presence of unconscious (implicit) personality and character dynamics in the development of depression, the IPT approach, which is a time-limited treatment model, does not intervene directly with these underlying dynamics. *Social and interpersonal relations* are described as interactions in social roles with others. These interactive social problems are addressed with "reassurance, clarification of emotional states, improvement of interpersonal communication, and testing of perceptions and performance through interpersonal contact" (Klerman et al., 1984, p. 7). Related aspects of IPT are addressed in subsequent sections of this chapter.

Contrasts Between Underlying Assumptions of IPT and Psychodynamic Psychotherapy

Weissman and Klerman, the original developers of IPT, were well schooled in the underlying theory of psychodynamically oriented psychotherapy (Markowitz & Weissman, 2012). They recognized the importance of understanding the original foundations of personality difficulties whose origins were based in early and later childhood and acknowledged that these foundations were primarily housed in the unconscious (implicit memory) realms of depressed persons. Because of the many years of treatment usually required for dynamic psychotherapy or psychoanalysis, a new psychotherapy model was created, motivated by the changing worlds of the mental health treatment setting and by healthcare economics, both of which were oriented to a shorter length of mental health treatment than was generally available in the 1970s (Barry, 2002).

During the formative and developmental studies of depression, research models were created to demonstrate the most explicit operational approach to effective depression treatment. The original premises of the research recognized the seminal psychoanalytic and psychodynamic contributions of Freud and his followers. However, new ground was covered by integrating an updated approach to the theory of the causes of depression and empirical evidence about the treatment of depression based on the findings of depression researchers through the 1970s (Barry, 2002; Markowitz & Weissman, 2012).

In addition to the emerging knowledge of the dynamics of depression post–World War II, there had been a significant change in the social face of psychiatry because of increased awareness of gender and race issues, concern about human potential, and increased interest in and striving for personal well-being. There was also an important scientific and professional shift in recognition of the importance of personal development and interpersonal relations over the life span (Barry, 2002; Markowitz & Weissman, 2012).

The result of these important changes in society and the field of psychiatry was that IPT theorists and practitioners recognized that psychodynamic psychotherapy was not a realistic clinical approach to use with the masses of people who were suffering from depression and who required a time-limited and affordable approach to treating psychiatric disorders. IPT practitioners switched the traditional psychodynamic focus on unconscious mental processes and implicit memories to what they called a "purely interpersonal approach," which focuses on social roles and interpersonal interactions in the patient's current and past experiences. The IPT model addresses interpersonal relations, essentially addressing the interactions between self and other, whereas the psychodynamic therapist focuses on object relations, which is an *intrapsychic* formulation of self with others (Barry, 2002; Markowitz & Weissman, 2012).

PRINCIPLES AND GUIDELINES OF IPT

The development of IPT was driven by the belief that progress in creating new clinical interventions should be guided by clinical experience and research evidence. Research evidence is acquired by carefully designed, well-controlled investigative trials (Markowitz & Weissman, 2012). The social roots of depression are the primary focus of IPT so that diagnosis and treatment of depression could occur in a timely manner and expedite the recovery time of depressed individuals to meet the requirements of the up-and-coming managed care insurance world during the late 1970s and subsequent decades. Mental health research during the 20th century pointed strongly to social factors being critical in the development of depression.

The driving force in the development of IPT was to treat and relieve the three primary aspects of depression:

1. Symptom function: how depressive affect and neurovegetative signs and symptoms are affecting the patient personally and in relationships with others
2. Social and interpersonal relations: how a person interacts with others, based on early childhood experiences, current social reinforcement, and the sense of mastery
3. Personality and character problems: characterological traits, such as pessimism, poor self-esteem, resentment, and poor communication with others

IPT actively addresses the first two sources of depression described. Personality and character problems, the third source, are generally viewed as being deep seated and having their origins in unconscious (implicit) memory (Markowitz & Weissman, 2012a). Although IPT does not actively address this aspect of personality and character issues, the active work on the first and second points, the symptom characteristics and interpersonal functioning, supports the development of new social skills that may reduce some of the characteristic personality difficulties.

Weissman et al. (2000) describe IPT as follows:

[IPT is a] focused, time-limited psychotherapy that emphasizes the link between mood and the current interpersonal relations of the depressed patient while recognizing the roles of genetic, biochemical, developmental, and personality factors in the causation of and vulnerability to depression. IPT is not a causal explanation for depression, but a pragmatic treatment for it. (pp. 4—5)

Weissman et al. (2000) explain that it is important for the IPT therapist to recognize clinical depression as described in the *Diagnostic and Statistical Manual of Mental Disorders (DSM)* and to be aware of its social, biological, and medical precipitants. The IPT therapist is then urged to recognize the interpersonal context of the depression and the importance of its underlying roots of difficulties with attachment, bonding, stress, and interpersonal disputes. The prominence and persistence of the depression are also associated with neurovegetative signs of sleep disruption, such as appetite disturbance, changes in weight, and energy level, as well as thought and memory processes, including worthlessness, guilt, helplessness, and thoughts of death and suicide.

IPT was used in research studies that investigated methods to support the early improvement in functioning observed 2 to 4 weeks after inception of antidepressant therapies. Research on depression treatments in the mid-20th century found a consistent and gradual decline in the original clinical improvement of patients. Treatment approaches were identified that built on the theoretical underpinnings of the origins of depression and that would sustain the early improvement related to psychopharmacological interventions. Hundreds of clinical studies have demonstrated success in developing a clinical intervention based on a manual with very specific assessment and treatment criteria. Many of those studies (described later) demonstrated the efficacy of modifications to the original IPT protocol for use with other types of psychiatric populations.

The following features provide a summary of the IPT approach (Weissman et al., 2000) compared with other psychotherapy models:

1. Time limited, not long term
2. Focused, not open ended
3. Based on current, not past, relationships
4. Interpersonal in nature, not intrapsychic
5. Interpersonal, not cognitive or behavioral
6. Aware of personality, but not focused on it

The Role of the Therapist in IPT

The foundation of the role of the therapist is related to the personality style of the therapist. The guidelines of the therapist are to be nonjudgmental, warm, and communicating with unconditional positive regard. The therapist is viewed as an ally fostering the patient's positive expectations about the therapy. Because of the time-limited nature of the therapy and the active, advocating role of the therapist, there are limited issues of transference. Transference is not addressed in the IPT model unless the patient's feelings toward the therapist are clearly disrupting the therapeutic relationship and progress of therapy.

The IPT model is one in which the therapist is able to be interpersonally open with the patient when the therapist's experience can be used to illustrate a point in the discussion. Activities between the therapist and patient that do not relate directly to the therapy should not be engaged. The therapist is active and proactive in the relationship, while at the same time recognizing that change is the responsibility of the patient. The therapist usually does not make active suggestions for change. Rather, change is viewed as the desired outcome of the interactions of the patient and therapist in IPT. Homework is not assigned in IPT. It is expected, however, that the results of clinical sessions will bring about gradual change that is reported in subsequent sessions (Weissman et al., 2000).

Table 10.1 shows examples of interactive statements used by an IPT therapist based on the principles of the IPT therapeutic protocol.

Establishing the Therapeutic Alliance in IPT

Because the therapy process is strongly guided by adherence to goals and principles outlined in the IPT instruction manual, the therapy process is strongly influenced by the model itself, an essential aspect for the outcome of IPT efficacy. Another significant factor in the course of therapy is the quality of the therapeutic relationship established between

TABLE 10.1 INTERACTIVE DIALOGUE: EVIDENCE OF ABNORMAL GRIEF TASK

Task	Therapist's Questions
Multiple losses	What else was going on in your life around the time of the death? Has anyone else died or left? What has reminded you of it since it happened? Has anyone died in a similar fashion or when your circumstances were similar?
Inadequate grief in the bereavement period	In the months after the death, how did you feel? Did you have trouble sleeping? Could you carry on as usual? Were you beyond tears?
Avoidance behavior about the death	Did you avoid going to the funeral? Did you avoid visiting the grave?
Symptoms around a significant date	When did the person die? What was the date? Did you start having problems around the same time?
Fear of the illness that caused the death	What did the person die of? What were the symptoms? Are you afraid of having the same illness?
History of preserving the environment as it was when the loved one died	What did you do with the possessions? What did you do with the room? Were the possessions left the same as when the person died?
Absence of family or other social supports during the bereavement period	Who could you count on when the person died? Who helped you? Who did you turn to? Who could you confide in?

Source. Data from Klerman, G., Weissman, M., Rounsaville, B., & Chevron, E. (1984). *Interpersonal psychotherapy of depression* (pp. 7, 42). New York, NY: Basic Books.

the therapist and patient. The findings reported in this section have been summarized from a number of studies on the therapeutic alliance in a variety of therapy approaches.

An important aspect of the therapeutic alliance is that therapists can be well trained in therapeutic skills and treatment models, but there are essential factors that cannot be gained through training. These factors include the personality and emotional styles of the therapist. These factors usually have been operative in therapists long before they became therapists. As the result of their studies on the effects of training in therapists, Strupp and Anderson (1997) concluded that the effects of the training were filtered through the therapists' preexisting personality dispositions. They found that although therapists were trained to use a therapy following a specific manual that directed all aspects of patient–therapist interactions, the therapy results were strongly colored by the underlying personality characteristics of the therapists.

There were additional findings related to the use of training manuals by therapists. Although therapists demonstrated compliance with the recommended approaches of the manual, there were unanticipated consequences of manual-based therapies. In general, Henry, Strupp, Butler, Schacht, and Binder. (1993) found that many therapists delivered the therapy in a "fairly forced mechanical fashion" (Safran & Muran, 2000, p. 4). Therapists with a style that was identified as self-controlling and self-blaming were more inclined to astutely follow the treatment manual and showed more hostility and a lack of warmth and friendliness with their patients. One of the questions in the conclusions of this study was how to avoid the possibility of the manual approach becoming an external standard that had to be conformed to, rather than a personally integrated way of being present with patients (Safran & Muran, 2000). A challenge for therapists who are using a manual approach to IPT is to remain open and be aware of their interpersonal style with patients and to create a social environment for the therapy that is human to human in its interpersonal style.

GOALS AND PHASES OF IPT

Specific strategies have been identified in the IPT model. The therapist uses an IPT treatment manual as a guide in the treatment process that outlines the specific goals and strategies to use in IPT treatment. These strategies occur within three phases of treatment:

1. The initial sessions: assessment phase (sessions 1 through 4); the therapist and patient deal with the depression.
    • In this stage of IPT, the patient is assessed for the presence of depressive symptoms. The therapist gives the depression a name. The nature of depression and its treatment are explained to the patient. The effects of depression on the person are explained. Depressive symptoms are evaluated to determine the possible benefit of medication.
    • The effects of depression on interpersonal relationships are clearly identified. The results of the depression are discussed with regard to prior interpersonal relationship patterns and the effects of the depression on current relationships. Significant relationships and the interpersonal expectations and mutual needs of the patient and significant persons are discussed as they are affected by the current depression. The satisfying and unsatisfying aspects of these relationships are also addressed. The patient is assisted to verbalize the changes she or he desires in the relationship.
    • The patient's sick role is discussed, with an expectation of the patient's responsibility to work toward recovery.
    • The major problem area in interpersonal relations that the depression is impacting is identified. The primary problem is clarified. Treatment goals associated with this problem and its interconnection with the depression are determined.
    • The effects of the depression on the significant relationship and the steps toward resolution of this interpersonal problem are formulated and built into the treatment plan and treatment contract.
2. The middle sessions: active treatment phase (sessions 5 through 12); the IPT model delineates specific goals for the identified problem area affected by the depression and how the problem should be addressed by the therapist. The treatment focus agreed on by the therapist and patient is the main topic for each session. Concerns of the patient are discussed with an eye to the use of specific strategies to address the concerns.
    • This phase of IPT treatment offers the opportunity for the patient to create new relational patterns in established relationships and to develop interest in new

relationships and roles. This process involves grieving what has been lost in old relationship patterns related to the depression.

- In this phase of treatment, the patient is asked to discuss experiences occurring between the weekly sessions as they relate to the specific problem identified as the focus for treatment. The therapist guides the patient to connect the symptoms described in the weekly meeting with the identified interpersonal issue.
- The therapist greets the patient during each session with a general question about what has been happening. The focus is on the here and now concerns and events. Strategies appropriate to the initial treatment contract and the stage of therapy are discussed.
- The patient's experiences are discussed, with the therapist leading the patient to understand the experience within the framework of the identified problem and its intended focus.
- As the therapy progresses, the patient is encouraged to use alternative strategies if and when the originally identified strategies are not successful in reducing the distress surrounding the focus problem.

3. The final sessions: termination phase (sessions 14 through 16); the work of the final sessions overlaps with the final sessions of the middle phase of treatment. The focus of this stage is the ending of treatment, working with the grief of the loss of therapy and the relationship with the therapist, and attending to the issues of relapse prevention. One of the aspects of IPT is that there is purposeful discussion about which number the session is in the overall total of 16 sessions throughout the treatment process. This enables the patient to deal with the upcoming loss and not to avoid it until the final therapy sessions.

Follow-up research after the conclusion of IPT shows that the beneficial outcomes of the therapy are increasingly demonstrated during the months following IPT treatment (Markowitz & Weissman, 2012). These findings support the importance of addressing ways in which the patient is able to continue the work of the therapy independently. An IPT maintenance model was developed to work specifically with individuals who were at higher risk for relapse after conclusion of traditional IPT (Klerman et al., 1984). The following aspects of the termination phase of treatment support the potential for effective outcomes of IPT:

- Engage in frank discussion about the end of therapy, particularly during the final three sessions, as well as during the earlier sessions if the patient demonstrates distress when the therapist discusses the number of sessions that have been completed.
- Acknowledge the patient's reaction to the end of therapy, and initiate discussion about the patient's reaction.
- Allow that the ending of therapy is a time of grieving.
- Recognize the patient's movement during therapy to independent compliance and success in mastering strategies to change original relationship patterns.
- Assess the treatment, and review future needs.
- Examine early warning signs of relapse, and discuss strategies to address them.
  - Discuss self-assessment criteria to indicate the need to reenter treatment.

THE EVIDENCE BASE FOR USE OF IPT

IPT is an evidence-based psychotherapy and is recommended as either a stand-alone or adjunctive treatment to medication in international clinical practice guidelines for the treatment of depression (see American Psychiatric Association, 2010; Australian

Psychological Society (2018). National Institute for Health and Care Excellence, 2009). There is evidence to support its use in both the acute and maintenance phases of depression. IPT is one of two psychotherapies (the other is cognitive behavioral therapy [CBT]) with evidence to support its use as a sole treatment for mild to moderate depression and in combination with medication for moderate to severe depression (Malhi et al, 2015). The evidence suggests that a combination of an evidence-based psychotherapy and medication is more effective than medication alone.

There is also convincing evidence that the adaptation of IPT for bipolar disorder (BD; borderline personality disorder (Bozzatello & Bellino (2016); interpersonal and social rhythm therapy [IPSRT]) as an adjunctive therapy to medication is effective in reducing relapse; longer term efficacy for binge eating disorder than those in the CBT group; improving functioning, reducing suicidal and self-harm behavior in BD and decreasing delusions (Andreou et al., 2017; Crowe, Beaglehole & Inder, 2016; Frank, 2005; Frank, 2008; Hilbert et al., 2012; Inder et al., 2015; Inder, 2016; Miklowitz & Scott, 2009). The evidence to support the use of interpersonal counselling is not as robust, but some studies have demonstrated effectiveness.

Treating Depression With IPT

Depression is posited to arise in the context of losses, role transitions, role disputes, or social isolation that serve as the treatment focus. IPT does not focus on cognition but on emotions and interpersonal interactions. Thus, there is no specific homework and IPT is less prescriptive than CBT. The focus is on the person's current life rather than on the past causes of the problem. Social supports are stabilized and the therapist is warm, hopeful, and positive.

A seminal study demonstrating the efficacy of IPT was completed in the early 1980s using sites at Harvard and Yale Universities–affiliated mental health centers that serviced patients from a wide range of social backgrounds. The initial IPT study was considered advanced for its time because the mental health clinicians who participated in the study adhered to a treatment manual (Weissman et al., 2000). The treatment manual eventually became the basis for IPT training (Weissman et al., 2000). There were four groups of depressed individuals in the study: persons who received IPT intervention; persons who had IPT and antidepressant therapy; persons treated with antidepressant therapy with no psychotherapy; and persons who had unscheduled treatment, which involved each participant being assigned to a psychiatrist and being told to call the psychiatrist and talk whenever he or she needed to do so. The patients could also schedule an appointment with a psychiatrist for a 50-minute session no more than once per month if their symptoms were of a certain level of intensity. All study participants were assessed on a regular basis by a clinician who did not know the group to which the patient had been assigned.

At the end of the study, the participants who were in the groups that consisted of IPT alone or IPT with antidepressant medication were significantly improved compared with the individuals who were in the nonscheduled treatment group. Those who were treated with antidepressant medication alone also improved compared with the nonscheduled treatment group. There were important differences, however, in the outcomes of the IPT groups and the group that received only the antidepressant medication. IPT recipients had improvements in mood, improved work performance and interest, and decreased suicidal ideation and guilt. These improvements were statistically significant after the initial 4 to 8 weeks of treatment. In contrast, those who received medication alone showed improvement only in decreased neurovegetative signs of depression sleep, appetite disturbance, and somatic complaints (DiMascio et al., 1979).

There have been numerous studies demonstrating the beneficial outcomes of IPT treatment of depressed individuals since the original studies that brought optimism to the treatment of depression (Blanco, Lipsitz, & Caligor, 2001; Dowrick et al., 2000; Klein & Ross, 1993; Klerman, 1988; Reay, Stuart, & Owen, 2003; Shea et al., 1992; Ward et al., 2000). The primary method used in these studies to demonstrate improvement in depressive symptoms was a statistical difference in the mean scores on depression scales of IPT recipients at the beginning of IPT and the mean scores on completion of the therapy (Blanco et al., 2001; Dowrick et al., 2000; Klein & Ross, 1993; Klerman, 1988; Klerman et al., 1984; Reay et al., 2003; Shea et al., 1992; Ward et al., 2000; Weissman et al., 2000).

A meta-analysis (Karyotaki et al., 2016) of trials of psychotherapy for depression (25% of which were IPT) found that psychotherapy in combination with antidepressants was more effective than medication alone and maintained this superiority for at least 6 months. This combination of antidepressants and psychotherapy is also more effective than placebo alone and psychotherapy plus placebo (Cuijpers, de Wit, Weitz, Andersson, & Huibers, 2015). A meta-analysis of IPT for any mental health problem (Cuijpers, Donker, Weissman, Ravitz, & Cristea, 2016) confirmed findings from a previous meta-analysis (Cuijpers et al., 2011) that it was effective in the acute phase of treatment for depression and there were indications it may be effective in preventing relapse and new depressive disorders.

Perinatal and Postpartum

The term *perinatal* refers to the gestation period beginning at 20 to 28 weeks of pregnancy and extending to 1 to 4 weeks after delivery. A longitudinal study of 14,000 prenatal immigrant women from the Dominican Republic found that 13.5% scored in the range of probable depression at 32 weeks of pregnancy (Evans, Heron, Francomb, Oke, & Golding, 2001). To add credence to these findings of depression incidence in pregnant women, a study done at two intervals with impoverished, single, inner-city, and pregnant women found that they had depression rates of 27.5% and 24.5% during the two periods of measurement (Hobfoll, Ritter, Lavin, Hulsizer, & Cameron, 1995).

Evans et al. (2001) conducted a study that involved a perinatal 6-week, 16-session research methodology for one IPT group and one group of parenting education. Both groups improved in mood over the course of therapy. The IPT group improved by 33.3%, and the parenting education group showed an improved change of 11.8% (Evans et al., 2001). Spinelli and Endicott (2003) conducted a 16-week and 16-session study of depressed antepartum women who were placed in a parenting education group or an IPT group. The IPT group showed a significant improvement in mood on three different measures compared with the parent education group.

Because of the specific focus of IPT on interpersonal dynamics, IPT has been used as an intervention with mothers who develop depression after delivery. One of the great concerns for women who develop this condition is the impact it has on their social role and interpersonal functioning, particularly the mother–infant bond, and also relationships with their spouses and other children (Stuart, 2012). The period after birth is particularly challenging, because it requires an almost immediate need to redefine relationships with family members and friends. Another demand that many new mothers experience is the sudden change in their work role as they assume the care of a new infant. Most women who become depressed during this postpartum period are averse to the use of medication, primarily because many of them are breastfeeding. Accordingly, IPT is often a welcome intervention for new mothers.

Several meta-analyses provide empirical support for the use of IPT for postpartum depression (Cuijpers, Brannmark, & van Straten, 2008; Sockel, Epperson, & Barber, 2011). A number of randomized clinical trials have found a significant decrease in the depression scores of IPT recipients compared with depressed postpartum women who were placed in a group waiting for treatment (Grote et al., 2009; O'Hara, Stuart, Gorman, & Wenzel, 2000; Reay et al., 2003). Positive outcomes have also been demonstrated for IPT used within a group setting (Klier, Muzik, Rosenblum, & Lenz, 2001; Mulcahy, Reay, Wilkinson, & Owen, 2010; Reay et al., 2006).

Adolescent Depression

Modifications were made in the original IPT model when treating depressed adolescents (Morris, 2012). Mufson and her colleagues (1994; Mufson, Moreau, Weissman, & Klerman, 1993; Mufson, Weissman, Moreau, & Garfinkel, 1999) reported on the adaptation of the original IPT manual to research the efficacy of IPT with adolescents (IPT-A). The findings of their study recommended shortening the traditional 16-week IPT protocol used with adults to a 12-session model for adolescents. A study comparing 12 weeks of IPT with sertraline in the treatment of 49 adolescents with major depressive disorder found that both treatments led to improvement but that IPT was superior across all measures (Santor & Kusumakar, 2001). More recent studies using this IPT model with inner-city adolescents reported good results for those with depression (Gunlicks-Stoessel, Mufson, Jekal, & Turner, 2010; Miller, Gur, Shanok, & Weissman, 2008).

In the revised treatment manual for adolescents, use of the terms sick and sick role, which were used more actively with adults, was minimized with adolescents. A final modification in the protocol was the addition of parents in the adolescents' treatment. Parents' involvement in the IPT model includes psychoeducation for the parents and teen about the following:

- Recognizing the symptoms of depression
- Emphasizing the importance of family involvement in treating the depression
- If there is a communication problem with one family member, asking the family member to participate in the active treatment phase of IPT so that communication issues can be addressed and improved
- Modifying home and school expectations of the adolescent while the depression symptoms are active
- Clarifying the original expectations at home and school as the depression lifts

Problem areas of adolescent functioning contributing to depression have been identified as separation from parents, exploration of authority in relation to parents, development of dyadic relationships with members of the opposite sex, initial experience with death of a family member or friend, and peer pressures (Mufson et al., 1999). IPT has been significantly more effective than other psychotherapies in decreasing depressive symptoms in adolescents, accompanied by general improvement in overall social functioning. The typical course of treatment and further discussion of this model are provided by Morris (2012).

A meta-analysis of studies of IPT-A (Pu et al., 2017) identified seven published studies and found that the overall polled standardized mean difference indicated a significant advantage to IPT compared to control conditions.

Treating Bipolar Disorder With Interpersonal and Social Rhythm Therapy

While medication is considered the first line of treatment in BD, there is increasing evidence that the course of BD can be further modified by interventions targeted at the social and environmental context. A meta-analysis of eight adjunctive psychotherapy studies demonstrated a significant reduction in relapse rates (of about 40%) compared with standard treatment alone (Scott, Colom, & Vieta, 2007). Ellen Frank and Holly Swartz from University of Pittsburgh have led the development of IPSRT for BD. Their work in adapting IPT involved addressing the three factors associated with relapse in BD: stressful life events, medication nonadherence, and disruptions in social rhythms (Jamison, Goodwin, Ghaemi, 2007). Post and Leverich (2006) found there were a variety of critical junctures at which psychosocial stress may exert profound effects on the onset and course of illness; and Malkoff-Schwartz et al. (1998) identified that serious life events are associated with the onset of a BD episode. Medication nonadherence can also influence the timing of mood episodes; however, the adverse effects of lithium, anticonvulsants, and antipsychotic medication contribute to illness burden, comorbidity, and nonadherence (Malhi, Adams, Cahill, Dodd, & Berk, 2009). It also needs to be noted that nonadherence is not specific to BD and that adherence rates in BD are similar to those of people with other long-term physical conditions (Horne & Weinman, 1999).

Social rhythms entrain a cascade of neurohormonal events such as diurnal patterns of cortisol and melatonin secretion, which are key components of circadian physiology (Frank, Swartz, & Boland, 2007). Disruption to social rhythms can cause significant disruptions to circadian rhythms (most noticeable in the sleep/wake cycle). People who have BD are generally more susceptible to the cognitive and somatic effects of social rhythm disruption (Boland et al., 2012). IPSRT combines the principles of IPT with social rhythm therapy. There are some modifications to the IPT components (e.g., inclusion of the problem area "loss of healthy self" or "development of sense of self"). Other modifications included attention to the impact of social rhythms on IPT problem areas, regulation of social rhythms, emotion regulation, regulation of levels of stimulation, and evaluation of comorbid substance abuse. The social rhythm component involves the use of social rhythm matrices to identify the stability and regularity of daily rhythms such as sleep/wake times, interactions with others and eating, and the relationship of these rhythms to mood. These social rhythms are regarded as the architecture underpinning circadian physiology. Disruption or instability in social rhythms can lead to disruption in circadian rhythms, which can precipitate mood episodes in BD.

Attending to the social rhythms provides an opportunity to regulate and stabilize the patient's functioning so that interpersonal relationships are less threatened; the patient feels more secure with self and others; and the vulnerability created by the social stress activation of the bipolar episodes is decreased (Schwartz, Levenson, & Frank, 2012).

The first studies of effectiveness of IPSRT for BD were conducted as part of the Systematic Treatment Enhancement Program for Bipolar Disorder, a 22-site randomized controlled trial of treatments for BD involving 4,360 participants from 1998 to 2005 (Sachs et al., 2003). IPSRT was found to increase social rhythm regularity, which was associated with reduced likelihood of recurrence during maintenance phase (Frank et al., 2005). Subsequent trials have continued to support the effectiveness of IPSRT in reducing time to relapse and improving functioning (Inder, 2015). A follow-up study of young people who received IPSRT found that this effect was maintained over a 3-year period (Inder et al., 2017).

While IPSRT has mostly been delivered in a one-to-one format, there is also evidence to support its use in a group therapy format (IPSRT-G). (Hogberg, Ponto, Nelson, & Frye, 2013). There is also some preliminary evidence of the superiority of IPSRT in relation to quetiapine (Schwartz, Frank, & Cheng, 2012).

Interpersonal Counseling in Medical Settings

The traditional IPT protocol was modified so that it could be used more effectively with persons in medical settings who did not have a preexisting psychiatric disorder but were experiencing adaptive challenges to current stressors in their lives in addition to their medical conditions. The counseling model is used in six or fewer sessions of 15 to 20 minutes each. This counseling approach can be utilized well by medical clinicians who are not mental health specialists and who are provided with an 8-hour training program in interpersonal counseling (IPC). (Weissman et al., 2000).

The types of problems addressed in this counseling intervention include stressors at home, in the workplace, in the extended family, or in friendships. In general, the counseling is intended to relieve distress in interpersonal relationships. Its efficacy has been demonstrated in two medical settings in studies with medical personnel who had a master's degree or higher educational preparation in a medical, rather than psychiatric, clinical discipline, administering the therapy (Klerman et al., 1987; Mossey, Knott, & Craig, 1990).

Although there have been few studies of IPC subsequent to these early studies, some evidence has suggested that it may be effective for treating previously untreated mild to moderate depression in primary care (Kontunen, Timonen, Muotka, & Liukkonen, 2016). Another study identified that in primary care settings patients had a preference for IPC (51.2%) over antidepressants (48.8%) for treating their mild to moderate depression (Magnani et. al., 2016).

The case example in this chapter illustrates the four interpersonal difficulties that are the primary criteria recommended when considering using IPT as a psychotherapy choice: interpersonal disputes, role transitions, grief, and interpersonal deficits.

CASE EXAMPLE

Sarah was a 28-year-old single woman who had been referred to IPT by her general practitioner after he had diagnosed depression and she did not want to use antidepressants. She participated in 12 IPT sessions, over which time her mood was initially rated by Beck Depression Inventory-II (BDI-II; Beck et al., 1961) and *Structured Clinical Interview for DSM-III-R* (SCID-D). (American Psychiatric Association, 1994) as moderately depressed. At the conclusion of the IPT sessions, Sarah was no longer experiencing depressive symptoms. Ethical approval and consent had been obtained for the analysis of these sessions.

Assessment Phase

The first stage of IPT involved conducting an interpersonal inventory in which Sarah was asked to identify all the people who were significant in her life and then she was prompted with these questions: (a) What is your boyfriend like as a person? (b) How often do you see him? (c) What kind of things do you do together? (d) Do you ever clash at all? and (e) Would you want the relationship to be different? Sarah described her relationships with family members and friends and also identified a pattern of avoidance when faced with conflicts, "I do try to avoid as much [conflict] as I can." The completion of the interpersonal inventory was followed by completion of a timeline of significant events and mood episodes in order to help identify connections between the two. This was Sarah's first depressive episode and she was unable to identify significant events that could have contributed to the episode.

Following the interpersonal inventory and timeline there was a negotiation about which IPT problem area should be the focus of treatment—interpersonal disputes, role transitions, grief, or interpersonal deficits. It was agreed that interpersonal disputes would be the focus for Sarah as this area was impacting most on her mood symptoms. In interpersonal disputes the focus is on examining relationship expectations, patterns of relating, and communication style within relationships. Sarah initially expressed some uncertainty about relationship expectations, "I don't know what I expect from my friends, I don't know if what I expect is realistic." The nature of Sarah's equivocal relationship with her friends was also a source of distress that she opted to avoid. Rather than explore the nature of these friendships, she opted to take on increasing responsibility. Sarah avoided addressing relationship issues, which may be regarded as a fear of addressing or challenging the subject positions she had engaged with in the past. Sarah described how she had learned avoidance as a child: "Most of our childhood was just spent trying to not be seen essentially, . . . all we heard was lots of yelling and screaming and the less you were noticed the better." She described avoiding being seen as a way of avoiding being caught up in family conflicts. Avoidance became a pattern throughout her life for dealing with situations with which she felt uncomfortable. Sarah saw what was happening but avoided involvement by learning not to be seen. Sarah also revealed a number of significant losses that she had experienced over the previous 2 years, including the deaths of both parents and a close friend. She described responding with an absence of feeling as a way of managing the cumulative effect of the losses. She avoided any feeling rather than be overwhelmed by feelings of grief. "Before I always managed to survive but just recently I stopped [being able to survive], it is such a struggle." Sarah was encouraged to explore her feelings and make connections between them and her relationships with others. She identified that she found this difficult because it felt that attending to her own feelings was selfish. She was able to identify how she had struggled with an ideal of womanhood to be selfless and considering own needs felt selfish.

Sarah was encouraged to think about experiences that might be construed as selfish by others and to explore her feelings associated with this. This exploration enabled Sarah to identify times when she had felt good about herself and how this had improved her mood. A connection was made between feeling good about herself and her mood. This appeared to be a meaningful point for Sarah as she identified the factors that had contributed to her feeling good. Throughout this phase in psychotherapy, Sarah made connections between what had been happening in her relationships and her mood, while being gently challenged to consider the continued use of avoidance as a relationship tactic.

Middle Phase

During the middle sessions of psychotherapy Sarah identified trust as a significant issue for her and made the connection that if she was unable to trust herself then it was difficult for her to trust others. During this phase she was also exploring what type of relationship she wanted with a male friend and the frustration she felt in regard to her indecisiveness. She identified how in the past she had often avoided making decisions and gone along with what others wanted as an easier option. As a result she often found herself in situations in which she assumed a placatory role. Despite her perception of herself as indecisive, Sarah described a choice she did make about committing to psychotherapy rather than giving into feelings of hopelessness. This acknowledgment of commitment to change appeared to be a significant therapeutic moment for Sarah, and she seemed to have shifted from not wanting to be regarded as selfish to wanting to focus on addressing her own needs. She was able to recognize that change was possible and had constructed a personal axiom of being true to herself. When her progress was acknowledged and supported, Sarah's response revealed a shift in her perception of herself as having options.

After experiencing a more hopeful view of her future Sarah described how she had addressed a number of relationship issues that she had previously felt unable to deal with: "So I actually just said no, look I can't cope, I can't do it, I have other things to do, she was really nice, so that was all right." Sarah described how by expressing her feelings in a direct manner she was able to achieve the outcome she wanted. She also described how she was able to feel less responsible for the behavior of others when previously she would have felt compelled to help fix the problem. She was able to recognize the ambivalent feelings she has about putting other people's needs ahead of her own—she felt wanted and needed, but she also felt as though she lost her sense of control self in the process. Sarah also identified a similar ambivalence about a relationship she was having with a male friend: "I just don't really know whether I want to be by myself at this stage." However, as she explored this she was able to come to a decision: "I am going to try and say no; I really want to be by myself . . . I am just not ready for a relationship." As she continued with the psychotherapy Sarah was able to identify what she wanted at the same time as affirming herself as worthwhile; she was able to articulate what she wanted without feeling as though she was being selfish, which was a significant point in the psychotherapy process because it was associated with a significant improvement in mood. She suggested that the improvement may have been because she was no longer taking a position of a critical external observer but was more accepting of herself.

Termination Phase

In the termination phase of psychotherapy Sarah described a shift in her feelings which she described as promoted by a shift in her perception: "Yeah I feel better, I was just thinking today, the situation hasn't changed, I just don't feel as bad about it." As a consequence of feeling better she had been able to communicate her needs to the male friend she had been equivocating over. Sarah described how she felt more able to think through and consider options for her future. A sense of hope in her future was a significant feature of Sarah's improvement in mood. Sarah described the effect of psychotherapy as helping her to see things more clearly and employed the metaphor of a guide dog to describe her experience of psychotherapy. "Now that I am feeling better I might actually be able to see where the opportunities are, whereas I was just so wound up, I just couldn't see anything. I just couldn't see a damn thing. I needed a guide dog." The sessions during this phase focused on the new skills Sarah had developed and exploring how these may be used across a range of situations into the future.

It was the interpersonal context of Sarah's experience of depression that provided the focus for psychotherapy. The interpersonal context enabled Sarah to develop a sense of self that was both more rewarding and less likely to contribute to future depressive episodes. By focusing on herself in relation to others the focus shifted from attributing the depression to faulty individual functioning to considering the context within which it had emerged. It was the exploration of this context that enabled Sarah to move from quite passive positions and avoidance of conflict to a more active subject position. Sarah was able to identify how she saw her role as placating within relationships and the effect of this was that she appeared avoidant and passive in describing her responses.

When she became aware of the patterns in her relationships, Sarah was able to explore what she wanted from a relationship, which contrasted with how she initially saw this as an either/or situation—either she became involved in a relationship that did not really meet her needs or she remained on her own. A significant shift occurred when Sarah reconstructed what it meant to be "selfish" and reevaluated her desire to be in an intimate relationship at that point in time. The process involved trusting herself and exploring what "being me" meant to her. Through the IPT process, much of Sarah's focus was on addressing these issues of self-assertion in relationships. As she was able to practice self-assertion responses and have them received favorably, she was more able to redirect the energy previously expended on maintaining dissatisfying relationships to asserting her own needs to others and identifying how she wanted to live her life.

POST-MASTER'S IPT TRAINING AND CERTIFICATION REQUIREMENTS

There is no single standard for training and competency in IPT. Although no certifying body exists, the International Society of Interpersonal Therapy (ISIPT, 2006) oversees the certification and training standards for this particular IPT clinical approach. See https://interpersonalpsychotherapy.org. The UK IPT organization proposes guidelines for certification, but whether these become adopted universally is doubtful. Relevant websites for information on IPT are shown in Table 10.2

CONCLUDING COMMENTS

IPT is a psychotherapy approach developed during the 1970s, is responsive to medical economics and societal changes, and focuses primarily on a protocol for treating depression. This model has been tested in multiple settings in randomized clinical trials and is efficacious compared with behavioral, cognitive, and pharmacological interventions. Efficacy of IPT is documented in a number of other clinical conditions, such as dysthymia, adolescent depression, substance misuse, BD, eating disorders, and medical settings as a short-term counseling intervention (Klerman et al., 1984; Markowitz & Weissman, 2012). The validity and efficacy of IPT with a variety of mental health

---

TABLE 10.2   WEBSITES RELATED TO INTERPERSONAL PSYCHOTHERAPY (IPT)

Scott Stuart's group (based in the University of Iowa, Iowa City) has regular IPT courses planned throughout the year (www.iptinstitute.com/ipt-training/ipt-institute-training-events).

Dr. Paula Ravitz can be contacted directly (Paula.Ravitz@sinaihealthsystem.ca).

Kenneth Kobak reports the availability of a new, on-line self-study course for IPT (telepsychology.net/IPT_Default.aspx).

Courses are also provided by the Institute for Interpersonal Psychotherapy (www.interpersonalpsychotherapy.org).

The official IPT website offers further information (www.interpersonalpsychotherapy.org/trainings/training-by-region).

This website supplies information about the interpersonal psychotherapy method and about related training protocol and standards (www.interpersonalpsychotherapy.org).

An excellent online course of interpersonal and social rhythm therapy (IPSRT) is available at www.ipsrt.org/training.

disorders offer promise and may prove to be worthwhile for both patients and therapists. The ongoing changes in the delivery of healthcare in an increasingly restrictive economic environment value brevity of care, often at the expense of quality of care. IPT meets the challenge of short-term treatment without sacrificing effective outcomes.

DISCUSSION QUESTIONS

1. What are the differences in approach when using IPT compared with psychodynamic psychotherapy?
2. Discuss the rationale for using a time-limited structured approach such as IPT with the problem focus areas that IPT was created to address. These focus areas are interpersonal disputes, role transitions, grief, and interpersonal deficits.
3. What are the potential benefits to using IPT for depression in antepartum and postpartum women?
4. What adaptations have been made to IPT for special groups?
5. Discuss the advantages and disadvantages of using a protocol-driven psychotherapy intervention such as IPT with depressed patients.
6. Name the types of psychiatric disorders that can be treated effectively with IPT. What are your ideas about why this type of intervention is successful with these clinical conditions?
7. What do you think it is about the problem-focused approach of IPT that makes it most successful with depressed patients?
8. What are the primary interpersonal values incorporated in the IPT approach? How do they compare with the interpersonal model of Hildegard Peplau?

REFERENCES

Andreou, C., Wittekind, C. E., Fieker, M., Heitz, U., Veckenstedt, R., Bohn, F., & Moritz, S. (2017). *Journal of Behavior Therapy and Experimental Psychiatry*, 56, 144–151.

American Psychiatric Association (2010). Practice guideline for treatment of patients with major depressive disorder (3rd ed.). Retrieved from www.psychiatry.org

Barry, P. (2002). *Mental health and mental illness* (7th ed.). Philadelphia: J. B. Lippincott Company.

Blanco, C., Lipsitz, J., & Caligor, E. (2001). Clinical case conference: Treatment of chronic depression with a 12-week program of interpersonal psychotherapy. *American Journal of Psychiatry*, 158, 371–375.

Boland, E. M., Bender, R. E., Alloy, L. B., Conner, B. T., Labelle, D. R., & Abramson, L. Y. (2012) Life events and social rhythms in bipolar spectrum disorders: an examination of social rhythm sensitivity. *Journal of affective disorders*, 139(3), 264–272.

Bozzatello, P., & Bellino, S. (2016). Combined therapy with interpersonal psychotherapy adapted for borderline personality disorder: A 2-years follow-up. *Psychiatry Research*, 240, 151–156.

Cuijpers, P., Brannmark, J. G., & van Straten, A. (2008). Psychological treatment of postpartum depression: A meta-analysis. *The Journal of Clinical Psychiatry*, 64, 103–118.

Cuijpers, P., de Wit, L. M., Weitz, E. S., Andersson, G., & Huibers, M. J. H. (2015). The combination of psychotherapy and pharmacotherapy in the treatment of adult depression: A comprehensive meta-analysis. *Journal of Evidence-Based Psychotherapies*, 15(2), 147–168.

Cuijpers, P., Donker, T., Weissman, M. M., Ravitz, P., & Cristea, I. A., (2016). Interpersonal Psychotherapy for Mental Health Problems: A Comprehensive Meta-Analysis. *The American journal of psychiatry*, 173(7), 680–687.

Cuijpers, P., Geraedts, A. S., van Oppen, P., Andersson, G., Markowitz, J. C., & van Straten, A., (2011). Interpersonal psychotherapy for depression: a meta-analysis. *The American journal of psychiatry*, 168(6), 581–592.

Crowe, M., Beaglehole, B., & Inder, M. (2016). Social rhythm interventions for bipolar disorder: a systematic review and rationale for practice. *Journal of psychiatric and mental health nursing, 23*(1), 3–11.

DiMascio, A., Weissman, M., Prusoff, B., Neu, C., Zwilling, M., & Klerman, G. (1979). Differential symptom reduction by drugs and psychotherapy in acute depression. *Archives of General Psychiatry, 36,* 1450–1456.

Dowrick, C., Dunn, G., Ayuso-Mateos, J. L., Dalgard, O. S., Page, H., Lehtinen, V., Casey, P., Wilkinson, C., Vazquez-Barquero, J. L., & Wilkinson, G. (2000). Problem solving treatment and group psychoeducation for depression: Multicentre randomized controlled trial. Outcomes of Depression International Network (ODIN) Group. *British Medical Journal, 321,* 1450–1454.

Evans, J., Heron, J., Francomb, H., Oke, S., & Golding, J. (2001). Cohort study of depressed mood during pregnancy and after childbirth. *British Medical Journal of Psychiatry, 323,* 257–260. [Abstract/Free Full Text].

Frank, E., Kupfer, D. J., Thase, M. E., Mallinger, A. G., Swartz, H. A., Fagiolini, A. M., Grochocinski, V., Houck, P., Scott, J., Thompson, W., & Monk, T. H. (2005). Two-year outcomes for inter-personal and social rhythm therapy in individuals with bipolar I disorder. *Archives of General Psychiatry, 62,* 996–1004. doi: 10.1001/archpsyc.62.9.996

Frank, E., Soreca, I., Swartz, H. A., Fagiolini, A. M., Mallinger, A. G., Thase, M. E., Grochocinski, V. J., Houck, P. R., & Kupfer, D. J. (2008). The role of interpersonal and social rhythm therapy in improving occupational functioning in patients with bipolar I disorder. *The American journal of psychiatry, 165*(12), 1559–1565.

Frank, E., Swartz, H. A., & Boland, E. (2007). Interpersonal and social rhythm therapy: an intervention addressing rhythm dysregulation in bipolar disorder. *Dialogues in clinical neuroscience, 9*(3), 325–332.

Grote, N. K., Swartz, H. A., Geibel, S. L., Zuckoff, A., Houck, P. R., & Frank, E. (2009). A randomized controlled trial of culturally relevant, brief interpersonal psychotherapy for perinatal depression. *Psychiatric Services, 60*(3), 313–321.

Gunlicks-Stoessel, M., Mufson, L., Jekal, A., & Turner J. B. (2010). The impact of perceived interpersonal functioning on treatment for adolescent depression: IPT-A versus treatment as usual in school-based health clinics. *Journal of Consulting and Clinical Psychology, 78*(2), 260–267.

Henry, W., Strupp, H., Butler, S., Schacht, T., & Binder, J. (1993). Effects of training in time-limited psychotherapy: Changes in therapist behavior. *Journal of Consulting and Clinical Psychology, 61,* 434–440.

Hilbert, A., Bishop, M. E., Stein, R. I., Tanofsky-Kraff, M., Swenson, A. K., Welch, R. R., & Wilfley, D. E. (2012). Long-term efficacy of *psychological treatments for binge eating disorder The British Journal of Psychiatry, 200,* 232–237.

Hoberg, A. A., Ponto, J., Nelson, P. J., & Frye, M. A., (2013). Group interpersonal and social rhythm therapy for bipolar depression. *Perspectives in psychiatric care, 49*(4), 226–234.

Hobfoll, S., Ritter, C., Lavin, J., Hulsizer, M., & Cameron, R. (1995). Depression prevalence and incidence among inner-city pregnant and postpartum women. *Journal of Consulting and Clinical Psychology, 63*(3), 445–453.

Horne, R., & Weinman, J., (1999). Patients' beliefs about prescribed medicines and their role in adherence to treatment in chronic physical illness. *Journal of Psychosomatic Research, 47*(6), 555–567.

Horowitz, L. M., & Strack, S. (2011). Introduction. In *Handbook of interpersonal psychology: Theory, research, assessment & therapeutic intervention* (pp. 1–15). Hoboken, NJ: John Wiley & Sons.

Inder, M. L., Crowe, M. T., Luty, S. E., Carter, J. D., Moor, S., Frampton, C. M., & Joyce, P. R. (2015). Randomized, controlled trial of Interpersonal and Social Rhythm Therapy for young people with bipolar disorder. *Bipolar disorders, 17*(2), 128–138.

Inder, M. L., Crowe, M. T., Moor, S., Carter, J. D., Luty, S. E., Frampton, C. M., & Joyce, P. R. (2017). Three-year follow-up after psychotherapy for young people with bipolar disorder. *Bipolar disorders,* 10.1111/bdi.12582. Advance online publication.

International Society for Interpersonal Psychotherapy. (2006). Retrieved from http://www.interpersonalpsychotherapy.org/adolescent_depression.htm

Jamison, K. R., Goodwin, F. K., Ghaemi, S. N. (2007). Manic-Depressive Illness: Bipolar Disorders and Recurrent Depression. United Kingdom: Oxford University Press, USA.

Karyotaki, E., Smit, Y., Holdt Henningsen, K., Huibers, M. J., Robays, J., de Beurs, D., & Cuijpers, P. (2016). Combining pharmacotherapy and psychotherapy or monotherapy for major depression? A meta-analysis on the long-term effects. *Journal of affective disorders, 194*, 144–152.

Klein, D., & Ross, D. (1993). Reanalysis of the National Institute of Mental Health Treatment of Depression Collaborative Research Program general effectiveness report. *Neuropsychopharmacology, 8*, 241–251.

Klerman, G. (1988). The current age of youthful melancholia. *British Journal of Psychiatry, 152*, 4–14.

Klerman, G. L., Budman, S., Berwick, D., Weissman, M. M., Damico-White, J., Demby, A., & Feldstein, M. (1987). Efficacy of a brief psychosocial intervention for symptoms of stress and distress among patients in primary care. *Medical Care, 25*(11), 1078–1088.

Klerman, G., Weissman, M., Rounsaville, B., & Chevron, E. (1984). *Interpersonal psychotherapy of depression* (pp. 7, 42). New York, NY: Basic Books.

Klier, C. M., Muzik, M., Rosenblum, K. L., & Lenz, G. (2001). Interpersonal psychotherapy adapted for the group setting in the treatment of postpartum depression. *The Journal of Psychotherapy Practice and Research, 10*, 124–131.

Kontunen, J., Timonen, M., Muotka, J., & Liukkonen, T. (2016). Is interpersonal counseling (IPC) sufficient treatment for depression in primary care patients? A pilot study comparing IPC and interpersonal psychotherapy (IPT). *Journal of affective disorders, 189*, 89–93.

Magnani, M., Sasdelli, A., Bellino, S., Bellomo, A., Carpiniello, B., Politi, P., Menchetti, M., & Berardi, D. (2016). Treating Depression: What Patients Want; Findings from a Randomizd Controlled Trial in Primary Care. *Psychosomatics, 57*(6), 616–623.

Malhi, G. S., Adams, D., Cahill, C. M., Dodd, S., & Berk, M. (2009) The management of individuals with bipolar Disorder: A review of the evidence and its integration into clinical practice. *Drugs, 69*(15), 2063–2101.

Malhi, G. S., Bassett, D., Boyce, P., Bryant, R., Fitzgerald, P. B., Fritz, K., Hopwood, M., Lyndon, B., Mulder, R., Murray, G., Porter, R., & Singh, A. B. (2015). Royal Australian and New Zealand College of Psychiatrists clinical practice guidelines for mood disorders. *The Australian and New Zealand journal of psychiatry, 49*(12), 1087–1206.

Malkoff-Schwartz, S., Frank, E., Anderson, B., Sherrill, J. T., Siegel, L., Patterson, D., & Kupfer, D. J. (1998). Stressful life events and social rhythm disruption in the onset of manic and depressive bipolar episodes: a preliminary investigation. *Archives of general psychiatry, 55*(8), 702–707.

Markowitz, J. C., & Weissman, M. M. (2012). Interpersonal psychotherapy: Past, present and future. *Clinical Psychology and Psychotherapy 19*, 99–105. doi: 10.1002/cpp.1774

Miklowitz, D., & Scott, J. (2009). Psychosocial treatments for bipolar disorder: cost-effectiveness, mediating mechanisms, and future directions. *Bipolar disorders, 11 Suppl 2*, 110–122.

Miller, L., Gur, M., Shanok, A., & Weissman, M. (2008). Interpersonal psychotherapy with pregnant adolescents: Two pilot studies. *Journal of Child Psychology and Psychiatry and Allied Disciplines, 49*(7), 733–742.

Morris, J. (2012). Interpersonal psychotherapy in child and adolescent mental health services. In J. Safran & J. Muran (Eds.). (2000). *Negotiating the therapeutic alliance: A relational treatment guide* (p. 4). New York, NY: Guilford Press.

Mossey, J., Knott, K., & Craig, R. (1990). The effects of persistent depressive symptoms on hip fracture recovery. *Journal of Gerontology, 45*(5), M163–M168.

Mufson, L., Moreau, D., Weissman, M., & Klerman, G. (1993). Interpersonal psychotherapy for depressed adolescents. In G. Klerman & M. Weissman (Eds.), *New applications of interpersonal psychotherapy*. Washington, DC: American Psychiatric Press.

Mufson, L., Moreau, D., Weissman, M., Wickramaratne, P., Martin, J., & Samoilov, A. (1994). The modification of interpersonal psychotherapy with depressed adolescents (IPT-A): Phase I and II studies. *Journal of the American Academy of Child and Adolescent Psychiatry, 33*(5), 695–705.

Mufson, L., Weissman, M., Moreau, D., & Garfinkel, R. (1999). Efficacy of interpersonal psychotherapy for depressed adolescents. *Archives of General Psychiatry, 56*, 573–579.

Mulcahy, R., Reay, R. E., Wilkinson, R. B., & Owen, C. (2010). A randomised control trial for the effectiveness of group interpersonal psychotherapy for postnatal depression. *Archives of Women's Mental Health, 13*(2), 125–139.

National Institute for Health and Care Excellence (NICE). (2009). Depression in adults: recognition and management. London (UK): National Institute for Health and Care Excellence (NICE). (Clinical guideline; no. 90). Retrieved from: https://www.nice.org.uk/guidance/cg90/ifp/chapter/Treatments-for-mild-to-moderate-depression

O'Hara, M., Stuart, S., Gorman, L., & Wenzel, A. (2000). Efficacy of interpersonal psychotherapy for postpartum depression. *Archives of General Psychiatry, 57,* 1039.

Peplau, H. (1991). *Interpersonal relations in nursing: A conceptual frame of reference for psychodynamic nursing.* New York, NY: Springer Publishing Company.

Peplau, H. (1952). *Interpersonal relations in nursing.* New York, NY: Springer Publishing Company.

Post, R. M., & Leverich, G. S. (2006). The role of psychosocial stress in the onset and progression of bipolar disorder and its comorbidities: the need for earlier and alternative modes of therapeutic intervention. *Development and psychopathology, 18*(4), 1181–1211.

Pu, J., Zhou, X., Liu, L., Zhang, Y., Yang, L., Yuan, S., Zhang, H., Han, Y., Zou, D., & Xie, P. (2017). Efficacy and acceptability of interpersonal psychotherapy for depression in adolescents: A meta-analysis of randomizd controlled trials. *Psychiatry Research, 253,* 226–232.

Reay, R., Stuart, S., & Owen, C. (2003). Implementation and effectiveness of interpersonal psychotherapy in a community mental health service. *Australasian Psychiatry, 11*(3), 284.

Reay, R., Fisher, Y., Robertson, M., Adams, E., Owen, C., & Kumar, R. (2006). Group interpersonal psychotherapy for postnatal depression: A pilot study. *Archives of Womens Mental Health, 9*(1), 31–39.

Rogers, M. (1970). *An introduction to the theoretical basis of nursing.* Philadelphia, PA: F. A. Davis.

Sachs, G. S., Thase, M. E., Otto, M. W., Bauer, M., Miklowitz, D., Wisniewski, S. R., Lavori, P., Lebowitz, B., Rudorfer, M., Frank, E., Nierenberg A. A., Fava, M., Bowden, C., Ketter, T., Marangell, L., Calabrese, J., Kupfer, D., & Rosenbaum, J. F. (2003). Rationale, design, and methods of the systematic treatment enhancement program for bipolar disorder (STEP-BD). *Biological psychiatry, 53*(11), 1028–1042.

Safran, J., & Muran, J. (2000). *Negotiating the therapeutic alliance: A relational treatment guide* (p. 4). New York, NY: Guilford Press.

Santor, D. A., & Kusumakar, V. (2001). Open trial interpersonal therapy in adolescents with moderate to severe major depression: Effectiveness of novice IPT therapists. *Journal of the American Academy of Child and Adolescent Psychiatry, 40,* 236–240.

Scott, J., Colom, F., & Vieta, E. (2007). A meta-analysis of relapse rates with adjunctive psychological therapies compared to usual psychiatric treatment for bipolar disorders. *The international journal of neuropsychopharmacology, 10*(1), 123–129.

Shea, M. T., Elkin, I., Imber, S. D., Sotsky, S. M., Watkins, J. F., Collins, J. F., Pilkonis, P. A., Beckham, E., Glass, D. R., Dolan, R. T. (1992). Course of depressive symptoms over follow-up. Findings from the National Institute of Mental Health Treatment of Depression Collaborative Research Program. *Archives of General Psychiatry, 49*(10), 782–787.

Sockel, L., Epperson, C. N., & Barber, J. (2011). A meta analysis of treatments for perinatal depression. *Clinical Psychology Review, 31,* 839–849.

Spinelli, M., & Endicott, J. (2003). Controlled clinical trial of interpersonal psychotherapy versus parenting education program for depressed pregnant women. *American Journal of Psychiatry, 160,* 555–562.

Strupp, H., & Anderson, T. (1997). On the limitations of treatment manuals. *Clinical Psychology Science and Practice, 4,* 76–82.

Stuart, S. (2012). Interpersonal psychotherapy for postpartum depression. *Clinical Psychology and Psychotherapy, 19,* 134–140. doi: 10.1002/cpp.1778

Sullivan, H. (1953). *The interpersonal theory of psychiatry* (p. xii). New York, NY: W. W. Norton & Company.

Swartz, H. A., Frank, E., & Cheng, Y. (2012). A randomized pilot study of psychotherapy and quetiapine for the acute treatment of bipolar II depression. *Bipolar disorders, 14*(2), 211–216.

Swartz, H. A., Levenson, J. C., & Frank, E. (2012). Psychotherapy for bipolar II disorder: The role of interpersonal and social rhythm therapy. *Clinical Psychology and Psychotherapy, 19*, 145–153. doi: 10.1037/0027671

Ward, E., King, M., Lloyd, M., Bower, P., Sibbald, B., Farrelly, S., Gabbay, M., Tarrier, N., & Addington-Hall, J. (2000). Randomised controlled trial of non-directive counseling, cognitive-behaviour therapy, and usual general practitioner care for patients with depression. I: Clinical effectiveness. *British Medical Journal, 321*, 1383–1388.

Watson, J. (2013). Jean Watson's theory of caring. Retrieved from http://currentnursing.com/nursing_theory/Watson.html

Weissman, M., Markowitz, J., & Klerman, G. (2000). *Comprehensive Guide to Interpersonal Psychotherapy*, 4–5.

Trauma Resiliency Model® Therapy

Linda Grabbe

Trauma, violence, and betrayal are intolerable events that by definition supersede our ability to cope. Such experiences may leave an indelible mark on our being through the intricate and interconnected pathways of mind and body, and may cause lifelong changes in our ability to function well, and to have relationships and good health. For many trauma survivors, the capacity to experience pleasure in ordinary living, deal with common stressors, and preserve emotional stability are compromised; longevity itself is affected. When trauma is left unprocessed and untreated, patients may be vulnerable to reactivation of trauma memories triggered by all manner of stimuli and may experience emotional distress, dissociation, or disconnection with the present. Such distress may elicit unhealthy behaviors as a default means of coping, particularly use of substances, self-harm, and other risky behaviors.

The burden of childhood trauma is in fact borne by the body, in a child's growth and development, at the level of cells and synapses, neural circuitry, stress hormones, and neurotransmitters, and even at the molecular level. A series of publications illustrate dynamic changes in the understanding of the mind-body interaction, how trauma impacts the body, and how people can heal from experiences that scar the soul, interfering with the ability to live fully. The Body Bears the Burden (Scaer, 2001), The Body Remembers (Rothschild, 2011), The Body Keeps the Score (van der Kolk, 1994, 2014), and other scholarly works (Heller & LaPierre, 2012; Levine, 1997, 2003, 2010; Ogden & Fisher, 2015; Ogden, Minton, & Pain, 2006; Steele, Boon, & van der Hart, 2017) herald a fundamental shift toward body-based or somatic approaches to help patients understand trauma and restore their mental well-being. This chapter describes a body-based psychotherapy model, the Trauma Resiliency Model.

THE TRAUMA RESILIENCY MODEL

Trauma Resiliency Model (TRM) therapy is an example of a "bottom-up" or biologically based psychotherapy method (Miller-Karas, 2015). The TRM posits that physical sensations precede and underlie emotions, and TRM therapy facilitates a patient's awareness of pleasant, unpleasant, and neutral body sensations as a way to regulate one's emotional state and achieve equilibrium. TRM acknowledges negative affect and its accompanying unpleasant physical sensations and teaches patients techniques to intentionally modulate negative affect, altering one's emotional state by shifting away from unpleasant bodily sensations to pleasant or neutral sensations. TRM is used to process acute or cumulative trauma once patients have learned preliminary stabilization skills. The TRM therapist gently guides a patient through understanding trauma and its impact and teaches several concepts and skills that the patient can access in therapy and then apply in daily life. Stabilization skills consist of the ability to recognize the sensations associated with negative and positive emotions and the use of these body-based techniques to bring the body back to a regulated state.

Preliminary psychoeducation includes types of trauma and normal responses to such experiences, the parts of the brain, and how the autonomic nervous system works. TRM uses a graphic model, the Resilient Zone, to describe the experience of mind-body balance or resilience, and how experiences of trauma, stress, and triggers can cause us to move into a state of dysregulation. Patients learn to recognize their own dysregulation and use specific skills to shift to a more regulated state by consciously tapping into the autonomic nervous system. The patient's capacity for emotion regulation and for mental wellness self-care is critical to trauma processing in TRM therapy.

The stabilization skills and concepts that form the foundation of TRM stand alone as a model in and of itself and are called the Community Resiliency Model® (CRM). CRM can be taught to groups or individuals in any setting but does not constitute therapy and is not for trauma processing; however, individuals who regularly practice CRM's body awareness skills may experience relief from chronic traumatic stress. It may be that by incorporating a habit of sensory awareness, there is a gradual release of some of the stress- and trauma-related toxicity caught in the body and imprinted in the mind. Practicing body awareness and reequilibrating the nervous system may be a means of bolstering positive, resilient neural networks and pathways to better mental health.

It is of note that Bessel van der Kolk (2014) identifies three modes of treating trauma: "top-down" therapy, medications, and "bottom-up" therapy. These three methods respectively involve processing or treating trauma experiences as a means of changing behavioral responses through (a) cognitive processes ("top-down"); (b) interrupting or dampening the overactive alarm response in trauma survivors through psychopharmacological agents (medications); and (c) regaining self-mastery by "allowing the body to have experiences which deeply and viscerally contradict the helplessness, rage, or collapse that result from trauma" ("bottom-up"; van der Kolk, 2014, p. 3). According to van der Kolk, many persons with complex developmental trauma or posttraumatic stress disorder (PTSD) do best with a blend of these three approaches.

Origins of TRM

Developed by Elaine Miller-Karas, Geneie Everett, and Laurie Leitch (Miller-Karas, 2015), TRM emerged from a well-established body-based psychotherapy tradition that used sensory awareness as a healing modality for trauma survivors. The psychotherapy pioneer Peter Levine founded Somatic Experiencing (SE) in which the perception of body sensations are used to treat symptoms of PTSD and other trauma-related problems (Levine, 1997, 2003, 2010; Payne, Levine, & Crane-Godreau, 2015). In SE, patients attend to their internal impulses and sensations; the therapist guides but does not interpret. Other psychotherapists have also developed innovative biological models for trauma in a shift away from cognitive-behavioral models. These include Heller and LaPierre's NeuroAffective Relational Model (2012), Ogden's Sensorimotor Psychotherapy (Ogden & Fisher, 2015; Ogden et al., 2006), Rothschild's Somatic Trauma Therapy (2010, 2011, 2017), and Steele, Boon, and van der Hart's (2017) integrative therapy for complex trauma and structural dissociation.

The developers of TRM were schooled in Peter Levine's SE Model, which focuses on the biology of the trauma response and somatic techniques linked to cognitive and emotional processing. The concepts for TRM and its antecedents began to be created when SE-trained psychotherapists participated in humanitarian efforts after the Asian tsunami in Thailand (M. L. Leitch, 2007; Parker, Doctor, & Selvam, 2008). In these settings, lengthy psychotherapy was impossible. As TRM was developed and interventions were used in interactions with trauma survivors in Haiti and China subsequent to their respective earthquakes, the TRM-trained therapists realized that teaching stabilization and self-regulation techniques to the distressed survivors were effective in alleviating suffering. CRM emerged as a brief intervention as trauma survivors were helped to find sources of strength, resiliency, and hope from within, by accessing pleasant or neutral body sensations. CRM was developed from these experiences and Elaine Miller-Karas' background as a teacher of family medicine, providing time-limited interventions in primary care clinics. In the United States, CRM was taught to survivors of chronic or cumulative trauma as a wellness, self-care strategy and demonstrated effectiveness for improving mental well-being (Citron & Miller-Karas, 2013).

EVIDENCE BASE

There is a limited amount of research on body-based approaches in psychotherapy for many reasons. Funding streams tend to favor therapies that are already evidence-based and manualized, disadvantaging novel interventions such as body-based therapy. In addition, persons with the complex presentations of trauma, who often do not have clear-cut psychiatric diagnoses or who have significant comorbidity, are often excluded from research studies (Corrigan & Hull, 2015). Further, understanding and acknowledging the extensive and long-lasting impacts of adverse childhood experiences (ACEs) and traumas have only occurred over the last 20 years.

In spite of a paucity of research on body-based psychotherapy or body awareness as a self-care modality, there is strong neuroscientific evidence for why it may present a good fit for persons with trauma (Haase et al., 2015, 2016; Szyf, Tang, Hill, & Musci, 2016), or offer a mental wellness model as a means to enhance resiliency. Corrigan and Hull (2015) suggest that for "bottom-up" body-based processing psychotherapy, neuroscientific plausibility should be considered as "evidence" as a rationale for treatment. CRM's first randomized controlled trial was with nurses and found significant improvement in well-being and resiliency, with reduced secondary stress and physical symptoms after a 3-hour class; these benefits were sustained one year after the class (Grabbe, Higgins, Baird, Craven, & San Fratello, 2019). Existing research on TRM and SE is presented in Table 11.1

UNDERLYING ASSUMPTIONS OF TRM

TRM's approach is based on the following assumptions:

- Human responses to threat are biological, primitive, instinctual, and physiological, that is, subcortical in nature. Threat, stress, and trauma may overwhelm the normal cognitive processes that allow for reasoned decision-making and reflection. Body-based, noncognitive approaches as preventive or healing modalities focus on conscious awareness of the autonomic nervous system responses to stress, that is, subcortical brain centers.
- The response to trauma can be deeply etched and persistently lodged in the mind and body, to the extent that emotion regulation may not be possible. Serious mental conditions, for example, PTSD, major depressive disorder, and dissociative disorders, may

TABLE 11.1   RESEARCH ON TRM AND SE INTERVENTIONS FOR EMOTION REGULATION AND STABILIZATION

Authors (Year)*	Study Design, Population, Setting, Follow-Up	Intervention	Measures	Results
M. L. Leitch (2007)	Study design: Single group pretest/posttest N: 53 adults and children Population/Setting: Tsunami survivors in Thailand Follow-up: 1 year	1 or 2 sessions (40-60 minute) of SE/trauma first aid	Observed and reported Post-traumatic symptoms: Pain, headaches, sleep problems, worry, anxiety, fear, agitation, flat affect, flashbacks, sadness, hypervigilance, muscle tension, shallow breathing, trouble concentrating	90% of participants reported full or partial recovery from posttraumatic symptoms
Parker, Doctor, and Selvam (2008)	Study design: Uncontrolled field study N: 150 Population/Setting: Tsunami survivors with trauma symptoms in Southern India Follow-up: 8 months	75 minutes of SE self-regulation skills	Post-traumatic symptoms: intrusion, arousal, and avoidance	Significant improvement or resolution of PTSD symptoms in 90% of participants
M. L. Leitch, Vanslyke, and Allen (2009)	Study design: RCT N: 142 Population/Setting: Social service workers during Hurricanes Katrina and Rita efforts Follow-up: 3–4 months	1 or 2 sessions of TRM stabilization skills	17-item PTSD Checklist-Civilian; 7-item resilience scale: frequency of experiencing sense of humor, relaxed breathing, feeling hopeful, feeling peaceful, being well-rested, a positive mood, and smiling	Statistically lower PTSD symptoms and increased resilience compared with a control group

(continued)

Authors (Year)*	Study Design, Population, Setting, Follow-Up	Intervention	Measures	Results
L. Leitch and Miller-Karas (2009)	Study design: Single group pretest/posttest N: 350 Population/Setting: Front-line providers after Sichuan Province earthquake (nurse, doctors, teachers, counselors) Follow-up:18 months	TRM stabilization skills (CRM) training in six cities	Training Relevance, Use, and Satisfaction Scale	97% of participants found skills relevant to their work; 88% applied the skills in their work; 60% used skills for their own self-care
Citron and Miller-Karas (2013)	Study design: Single group pretest/ posttest N: 155 Population/Setting: Groups of persons with cumulative trauma in San Bernardino, California (racism, homophobia, poverty, untreated posttraumatic stress from combat) Follow-up: 3 to 6 months	CRM as a mental wellness self-care intervention	Calgary Symptoms of Stress Inventory (56 items)	Statistically significant decreases in depression, hostility, anxiety, and somatic symptoms; significant increases in relaxation, contentedness, and somatic well-being Over 95% of the participants used the stabilization skills of CRM daily to manage stress
Grabbe et al. (2019)	Study design: RCT, pretest/posttests N: 77 Population/Setting: Hospital nurses Follow-up: 1 week, and 3 months, and 1 year	A 3-hour CRM training	WHO Well-Being Index Connor-Davidson Resilience Scale Somatic Symptoms Scale-8 Secondary Traumatic Stress Scale Copenhagen Burnout Inventory— Work-Related subscale	The CRM group demonstrated significant increases in well-being and resilience, and decreases in secondary traumatic stress and somatic symptoms

*These authors are listed in the references at the end of the chapter.

CRM, Community Resiliency Model; PTSD, posttraumatic stress disorder; RCT, randomized controlled trial; SE, somatic experiencing; TRM, Trauma Resiliency Model.

result (van der Kolk, 2014). Trauma may also lead to somatization, substance abuse, compulsions, and cognitive, mood, and identity disturbances (Courtois & Ford, 2014).

- Current psychiatric concepts do not yet account for the impact of multiple or long-term traumas. Instead, patients are given an array of diagnoses. Developmental trauma disorder has been proposed as a new diagnosis for many years but has not yet gained mainstream acceptance by the American Psychiatric Association (van der Kolk, 2014). However, complex PTSD was included in the *International Classification of Diseases,* 11th revision *(ICD-11)*.

- When dysfunctional adaptations to stress and trauma occur, the resultant distress can derail the sense of well-being and present-moment awareness. Many of the default mechanisms in which trauma survivors engage are attempts to deal with trauma triggers and mood instability. These attempts to cope include maladaptive, self-injurious behaviors such as cutting, eating disorders, violence, and using drugs and alcohol.

- Even in cases of severe and long-lasting abuse and neglect, resilient individuals may survive and thrive. Positive biological functional adaptations in the brain are a feature of resilience and depend on genetic, epigenetic, neural, and environmental factors (Groger et al., 2016); these factors are mediated by adaptations in neural circuits, neurotransmitters, and molecular pathways (Horn, Charney, & Feder, 2016).

- People readily recognize and respond to uncomfortable sensations such as fatigue, pain, or hunger, but neutral or pleasant body sensations are rarely brought to awareness. The awareness of internal sensations, termed "interoception" or "felt sense," passes unrecognized and unarticulated, but sensory awareness to internal states has been shown to be the key to high resiliency levels under conditions of stress (Haase et al., 2015, 2016).

- The mind has a natural negativity bias, that is, we make sense of the world in an asymmetrical manner, with a tendency to remember negative rather than positive information (Vaish, Grossmann, & Woodward, 2008). Highly emotionally charged negative experiences are quickly stored in memory for their protective survival value. The premise of new, healthy neural connections is based on the concept that "neurons that fire together wire together" (Hebb, 1949; Shatz, 1992). Establishing resilient neural circuitry may counteract the mind's natural negativity bias.

- Felt-sense, or awareness of internal sensations, may offer options for preventing and treating stress and trauma disorders (van der Werff, Pannekoek, Stein, & van der Wee, 2013; van der Werff, van den Berg, Pannekoek, Elzinga, & van der Wee, 2013). Somatic or "body-based" therapy gives individuals a chance to strengthen connections in their nervous system, learning more adaptive ways to deal with stress and traumatic triggers with resources from within that are unique to the individual.

- Somatic techniques may help survivors understand their trauma responses and regain their sense of self in the most tangible way, through body awareness. Miller-Karas (2015) posits that the body has an inherent but unarticulated healing capacity if we can learn how to draw on it. Resilient sensations, when accessed purposefully and articulated, are a key to recovery from trauma (Miller-Karas, 2015).

Rationale for a Body-Based Psychotherapy Approach

Over the past 20 years, a sea change has occurred in our understanding of the life-long impact of childhood trauma (Centers for Disease Control and Prevention, n.d.) supported by research on the neurobiology of trauma and resilience. Simultaneously, mindfulness is emerging as a new modality for mental wellness and for multiple mental health problems (Grant et al., 2017; Lang, 2017; Rodrigues, Nardi, & Levitan, 2017; Williams, Teasdale, Segal, & Kabat-Zinn, 2007), with research into its neurobiological underpinnings (Black & Slavich, 2016; Haase et al., 2016; Tang, Holzel, & Posner, 2015). Although standard or mainstream psychotherapies have been modified by becoming "trauma-informed" or "mindfulness-based," innovative, alternative, and body-based or somatic therapy approaches have been quietly gaining evidence and momentum and seem to make intuitive sense for trauma survivors who live with implicit body memories of trauma.

In the landmark Adverse Childhood Experiences (ACE) study of 17,000 insured, working adults (Felitti et al., 1998), 10% of participants had witnessed domestic violence, 20% had been molested, and 30% had been physically abused before age 18. Replicated many times since, 64% had had at least one type of ACE; among the 25.5% with three or more of these events, the impact of these ACEs on health later in life was startling. Dramatically increased rates of mental health problems and a host of ailments including cancer, heart disease, addiction, diabetes, and earlier death occurred for those with high ACE scores. This relationship was dose-related; that is, the more ACEs, the greater the likelihood of health disorders. Considering that 23% of this population had three or more ACEs, one can infer that many of those individuals experienced complex developmental trauma and that posttrauma sequelae are rife in the general population.

Because the ACE study only examined working and insured Kaiser Permanente patients who were mostly college-educated and White, recent ACE research has included more diverse and representative samples; a higher rate (73%) of ACEs was found in a more representative sample in Philadelphia (Cronholm et al., 2015). As a further contribution to our understanding of ACEs, Cronholm and colleagues also expanded the definition of ACEs to include witnessing violence, living in an unsafe neighborhood, and experiencing discrimination or bullying. In their study, accounting for both conventional and this expanded definition of ACEs, 83% of persons had experienced childhood adversity. This underscores the need for well-founded trauma therapies for a large portion of our population.

Early life traumas leave their imprint on the anatomy and physiology of the brain (De Bellis & Zisk, 2014) and are associated with the development of dysfunctional neural circuits, behavioral dysfunction, and mental disorders, essentially leaving functional "scars" in emotional control, learning, and memory (Groger et al., 2016). Trauma's impact reaches virtually all body systems, including persistent biological alterations in neuroendocrine and neurotransmitter systems, proinflammatory cytokines, and alterations in brain areas associated with mood regulation; these lead to psychiatric and medical vulnerability (Nemeroff, 2016). Telomeres, the protective covering at the tips of chromosomes, are damaged by childhood adversity, mediating cell aging and early disease (Puterman et al., 2016; Shalev et al., 2013). Chronic stress leaves its mark through DNA methylation of genes in the brain and peripheral tissues, and these changes are associated with adverse gene expression, that is, health disorders, but are potentially preventable and reversible (Szyf et al., 2016). Calculations of population attributable risk demonstrate that the bulk of social and psychological problems are accounted for by ACEs. For example, if ACEs could have been prevented, serious persistent mental illness would be diminished 65%, alcoholism by 65%, and incarceration by 61% (Anda & Brown, 2010).

Explanatory Mechanisms of Action for TRM

Although the neural mechanisms and structural brain changes due to sensory awareness practice are not yet completely understood, work in the area of mindfulness meditation illuminates mechanisms of action. TRM involves sensory mindfulness, a component of other mindfulness practices. The core components of such practices appear to be attention control (anterior cingulate cortex and the striatum), emotion regulation (prefrontal areas and striatum), and self-awareness (insula, medial prefrontal cortex, and posterior cingulate cortex/precuneus). Mindfulness meditation techniques affect these areas and support stress reduction, control of emotions, and sense of well-being (Tang et al., 2015). Although there is often a focus on nonjudgmental acceptance of thoughts and emotions in mindfulness and meditation practices, CRM and TRM seem to bypass these more cognitive processes, and instead, focus most purely on noticing body sensations and using them as a therapeutic modality. Interoception (awareness of internal body sensations) and exteroception (awareness of external body sensations) occur in the insular cortex and its tracts to other cortical regions (Haase et al., 2015, 2016; van der Werff, Pannekoek, et al., 2013; van der Werff, van den Berg, et al., 2013). Studies of mindfulness practice demonstrate a shift from self-referential processing toward a more objective, detached view (Farb et al., 2007). Such a shift would possibly support a changed narrative in psychotherapy regarding traumatic experience through TRM (i.e., a shift from a trauma narrative to a tale of survival and resiliency).

In a review of the neuroscience of mindfulness, Tang and coauthors (2015) suggest multiple reasons why brain structure and function might change with mindfulness practice. These include induced branching of dendrites, synaptogenesis, myelinogenesis, and neurogenesis; alternatively, positive autonomic regulation and immune activity might result in neuronal changes. Awareness of body sensations appears to provide increased autonomic nervous system control by inducing parasympathetic dominance and reducing the sympathetic discharge that elicits agitation, irritability, and anxiety. Stress symptoms abate, thereby altering activity in the sympathetic-adrenal-medullary and hypothalamic-pituitary-adrenal axes.

Long, myelinated neurons are located in the insula and adjoining structures and are thought to be the seat of the social brain responsible for empathy, social interaction skill, and the sense of self (Cauda, Geminiani, & Vercelli, 2014). These deep brain structures demonstrate sharply reduced activity in persons who have experienced cumulative trauma, making awareness of physical sensations and personal meaning of information input challenging (van der Kolk, 2014). These same networks in the brain are affected in acute trauma exposure, with subsequent posttraumatic stress symptoms and diminished volume in the insula and associated structures (Herringa, Phillips, Almeida, Insana, & Germain, 2012). Sense of self may be lost in acute trauma or never fully developed in developmental trauma, but under the gentle guidance of a skilled therapist, the intentional awareness of internal sensations may be learned, leading to enhanced self-regulation and access to positive internal resources. These can be a portal to healing from trauma, a richer sense of being, improved interpersonal relationships, and better control of emotions.

THE TRAUMA RESILIENCY MODEL SKILLS

TRM therapy includes a set of nine skills, the first six of which are stabilization skills. These stabilization skills are also a standalone model of self-care called the CRM. These stabilization skills are a critical part of TRM's trauma-processing psychotherapy. Patients learn grounding and tracking techniques to calm themselves when distress occurs in the therapy context. They also reach within themselves to retrieve comforting memories or thoughts that, when elaborated, become a resource for emotion regulation and stress tolerance during therapy and in daily life. Once the first six self-care stabilizing skills are firmly established, there are three additional therapy components: titration, pendulation and completion of survival response, which are trauma-processing techniques adapted from Levine's SE psychotherapy model.

These latter skills require advanced training in psychotherapy because of the potential to destabilize the patient when they experience distressing triggers or traumatic memories. The CRM skills training is available to both licensed and nonlicensed individuals who wish to help community members.

Patients and professionals alike can use the set of six CRM wellness skills to enhance resiliency and a sense of well-being through sensory awareness. It should be noted that therapists and other front-line providers of care are at particular risk for vicarious trauma and may themselves have trauma histories. Clinicians and other human services providers can develop symptoms of secondary traumatic stress and burnout that impair their ability to help others effectively and could cause them to leave their professions (Figley, 1999). CRM may be preventive self-care or simply "good medicine" for mental health or social service professionals, healthcare providers, public safety officers, first responders, shelter or corrections staff, and community workers.

TRM Concepts

TRM's cornerstone concept is the resilient zone (RZ), which represents the natural rhythm or balanced flow of energy and human vitality; it is also the bandwidth of stress tolerance (Figure 11.1). The rise of the waving line corresponds to the activation of the sympathetic nervous system with its increased heart and respiratory rate in response to environmental or internal demands; the downslope of the wave represents parasympathetic activation, with its reduced heart and respiratory rate as the body recharges its energy. All persons have a RZ (or zone of well-being) where they have the greatest sense of balance, capacity to work with others, learn, think clearly, and function at their best. The RZ is a felt-sense experience and ability to function where one can handle the ups and downs of daily experiences, even if somewhat distressed, sad, or irritable. One of the goals of TRM is to help patients recognize and identify sensations connected to their RZ and to actively access them.

Patients learn that with stress and trauma, they may experience too much sympathetic discharge and can be pushed out of the RZ into a state of hyperarousal called the "high zone;" alternatively such experiences may elicit too much parasympathetic discharge and we are pushed out of the RZ into a state of hypoarousal called the "low zone" (See Figure 1.3 in Chapter 1). Excess sympathetic or parasympathetic nervous stimulation will cause anyone to feel uncomfortable and distressed because of accompanying physical changes. When people are outside their RZ, TRM skills can help them be aware of body sensations that accompany anger and irritability in the high zone (excess sympathetic activation) or sluggishness and sadness in the low zone (excess parasympathetic activation). Because teaching about the RZ emphasizes the physiology of stress reactions, most patients respond positively to the concept, feeling validated that their emotions and behaviors are explainable, normal, and nonpathological. Reassuringly,

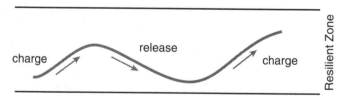

FIGURE 11.1 The Resilient Zone. When functioning within one's Resilient Zone, flexibility and adaptability in body, mind, and spirit can be achieved at highest capacity. Community Resiliency Model skills help widen the resilient zone.

Source: Reprinted with permission from the Trauma Resource Institute, Claremont, CA.

uncomfortable symptoms are viewed as biological responses to stress. Patients learn that all persons (even the therapist) are sometimes "bumped-out" of the RZ and that these responses are about biology, not moral or psychological weakness and failure. As traumatic stress symptoms are normalized, feelings of shame and self-blame are reduced or eliminated.

Some individuals, because of temperament or life challenges, may have an innately narrow RZ, while others have a naturally wide RZ. We all have narrowed RZs when we are hungry, angry, tired, bored, lonely, or in pain, and the narrowed RZ increases the likelihood of being bounced out of the RZ. The RZ concept normalizes stress responses, explains the biology of symptoms, and offers hope to patients that they themselves can widen their RZ or return to it when they sense that they are outside the RZ. Merely visualizing the RZ is part of patients' ability to anchor themselves in the present moment. The RZ concept is derived from the work of Dan Siegel (1999), who described a "window of tolerance" and states of arousal to describe normal brain/body reactions to adversity. In TRM, the RZ is seen as a state of stability, well-being, and resilience; the notions of hyper- and hypoarousal are key tools for patients to understand their stress and trauma responses.

Basic psychoeducation in TRM involves understanding types of trauma. The concepts of "Big T" trauma (e.g., natural disasters, assault, injury, abuse), "little t" trauma (e.g., medical procedures, fender-benders), and cumulative "C" trauma (e.g., racism, vicarious trauma, microaggression, poverty) help individuals understand the uniqueness of their perception of what is traumatic. This trauma conceptualization frames further education about responses to stress and trauma. Spiritual, emotional, physical, behavioral, cognitive, and relational traumatic responses are discussed as common reactions (e.g., not sleeping, trouble concentrating, cutting, drinking) and explained as efforts (albeit maladaptive) to get back to the RZ. TRM uses a simple "triune" or three-part brain model so that patients understand the work of the survival (brainstem), emotional (limbic system), and thinking (cortex) parts of the brain—how they support us, but also how, when out of the RZ, the subcortical parts of the brain dominate, making reasoned decision-making impossible. TRM's sensory mindfulness skills allow for coordination of all parts of the brain and controlled responses to traumatic or stressful experiences. Dan Siegel's "hand-model" of the brain, taught in TRM, serves as anchor for present moment awareness and autonomic regulation (Siegel, 1999).

Using CRM Skills in TRM Therapy

TRM's goals are to stabilize the nervous system, reduce or prevent the symptoms of traumatic stress, and process traumatic experiences. The first six self-regulation skills of TRM are used throughout TRM therapy; three additional techniques are used by the therapist for processing traumatic experiences or memories. Psychoeducation begins with an explanation of the RZ; the nature of trauma; types of responses to stress and trauma; simplified explanations of the nervous system's symptoms of hyperarousal and hypoarousal; the autonomic nervous system responses to threat and fear; trauma and memory (explicit vs. implicit); and the three-part brain model (Miller-Karas, 2015).

The basics of TRM's six self-care skills for patients are described here briefly. These skills, also called CRM, are used in any order or independently; they may be taught to groups or in individual sessions. CRM has been used in group settings with high-risk, incarcerated, and homeless youth with beneficial effects (Grabbe & Miller-Karas, 2018). Note that CRM is always taught by two CRM teachers in the event that a participant responds to CRM skills by becoming emotionally dysregulated. The free app, "ichill," provides excellent reinforcement for the self-care, stabilization skills. Please note that in order to teach the CRM skills, therapists should be adept at using the skills themselves.

Skill 1: Tracking

In tracking, the patient describes the "felt-sense" of internal or external body sensations. These sensations are noticed and named; by naming sensations (e.g., fuzzy, heavy, open), patients are engaging all three parts of the brain. This is Dan Siegel's "if you name it, you can tame it" concept. The patient pays attention to the physical reactions to stress and well-being, and is able to distinguish these and identify and name sensations of distress versus those of well-being. Patients learn the sensations associated with resilience (relaxed muscles, easy breathing), stress (muscle tension, rapid heart rate), and release (shaking, yawning). Release sensations are autonomic, involuntary responses that occur as the body shifts back into an equilibrated state, reentering the RZ. The clinician may inquire about observed movements or reported sensations, but without interpretation: "What are you aware of now?" and "Is the sensation pleasant, unpleasant, or neutral?" It is well known that trauma survivors are sometimes cut off from body awareness and therapists must be sensitive to body awareness as a trigger for distress. For this reason, it is critical that TRM be used with a gentle, understanding manner.

Skill 2: Resourcing and Resource Intensification

The patient is asked to identify a person, animal, place, memory, activity, belief, or personal strength that brings a sense of comfort, safety, peacefulness, or joy. The clinician invites the patient to describe the resource and then intensifies it by asking for more description, particularly sensory details. As the patient responds with a fuller description, the clinician asks what the patient is noticing currently in his or her body, and if the sensation is unpleasant, pleasant, or neutral. If pleasant or neutral, the patient is asked to simply experience the sensations for some moments. These sensations need to be held in awareness for a dozen or more seconds to transfer from short-term memory to long-term storage (Hanson, 2010). This effort is made to develop positive neural pathways to counteract the brain's natural tendency to dwell on the negative.

Resource questions can be used to shift from thoughts or feelings of stress or trauma to a resilience narrative. For example, "What is it about you that helped you get through that?" allows the patient to recognize internal strengths. Resilience-focused questions help shift away from distress, amplifying resources that are often otherwise side-lined. Note that sometimes patients select a resource related to an unhealthy behavior. In this case, another resource should be selected, or some healthy aspect of it can be elaborated. For example, one patient identified "smoking weed" as a resource, but was able to focus on and describe a screened-in porch at his aunt's house where he felt safe and secure.

Skill 3: Grounding

Grounding is present-moment awareness of body contact with surfaces, i.e., the floor, a table top, a chair, or one's own clothing or skin. This felt-sense of contact in the present moment provides gravitational security and a sense of safety and control. Sometimes drawing attention to the body in the present moment can activate uncomfortable sensations or even flashbacks. For this reason, resourcing and tracking are taught before grounding. For some patients who have difficulty with this technique and experience a floating, dissociative sensation, a weighted pillow or blanket may facilitate grounding.

Skill 4: Gesturing

Spontaneous expressions beneath conscious awareness can be healing and self-soothing, adding to the patient's toolbox for self-regulation. The TRM therapist may identify and mirror open or soothing gestures so that patients can themselves initiate the gesture as a form of self-regulation. The therapist may ask to do the movement together with the patient, slowing it down and repeating it, noticing and naming accompanying sensations in the body.

Skill 5: Help Now!

The 10 Help Now! strategies decrease or raise activation within the nervous system when a person is hyper- or hypoaroused, and may be used during or outside the therapy session. Explained as a kind of emotional "CPR" when the therapist or patient recognizes signs or symptoms of being outside the RZ, the strategies help the patients focus on something other than the distress and the sense of being overwhelmed. Examples are counting steps, identifying objects or colors, or pushing against a wall. See Box 11.1 for a list Help Now! skills. Patients can use the strategies when they recognize they are out of their RZ, or to help another person who is emotionally dysregulated. In a therapeutic session, the clinician can invite the patient to try one of the strategies and to do it together, again noticing sensations and reporting them as pleasant, unpleasant, or neutral. Mindful attention to a sensory input may have a calming effect.

Skill 6: Shift and Stay

Internal and external triggers of trauma can create fear, anxiety, anger, sadness, and isolation. When consciously aware of symptoms of distress, the patient has a choice of what might work best to relieve the distress by shifting awareness from the distressing sensations to tracking, a resource, grounding, a gesture, or a Help Now! strategy. The mindful awareness of the more pleasant or neutral sensations is consciously held in the mind for about 15 seconds until stabilization occurs.

BOX 11.1 HELP NOW! Skills

If you are stuck in the high and/or low zones the strategies below can help you get back to your Resilient Zone. Some will work better for you than others. Use the one(s) that fit the best for you. It can be beneficial to share this information with someone close to you who can assist you with the strategies if you need help or you can offer to help another person in an invitational way.

1. Open and close your eyes.
2. Drink a glass of water, tea, or juice.
3. Look around the room or wherever you are, paying attention to anything that catches your attention.
4. Name six colors you see in the room (or outside).
5. Count backward from 20 as you walk around the room.
6. If you're inside, notice the furniture, and touch the surface, noticing if it is hard, soft, rough, etc. . . . .
7. Notice the temperature in the room.
8. Notice the sounds within the room and outside.
9. Push your back against the wall or push your hands against the wall or door slowly and notice your muscles.
10. If you're outside or inside, walk and pay attention to the movement in your arms and legs and how your feet are making contact with the ground.

These strategies are options for you to use; there may be others you may want to add to the list.

CASE EXAMPLE: USING CRM SKILLS FOR STABILIZATION

Ms. C is a 39-year-old woman who experienced extensive trauma during childhood, including neglect and physical and emotional abuse over many years. Her mother had untreated schizophrenia. The patient is in transitional housing related to serious mental illness and homelessness. Her psychiatric diagnoses include complex PTSD and bipolar disorder. The advanced practice psychiatric nurse (APPN) has seen her for supportive therapy for several years. She has a good understanding of the above concepts and the RZ. She uses CRM sensory awareness skills in her daily life and has shared it with others at her treatment center. We start the session with creating a new resource.

APPN:	I'd like you to think of something that brings you a sense of peace and calm, and safety, and maybe joy. So it could be a place, or a person, or a memory. Or something about yourself that you feel is a strength. It could be physical or it could be part of your personality.
Ms. C:	(long pause) Hmm. There's only two things that I can think of really and that's two people who are in my life: Jim who I've been seeing for like 6 months, and the other is another friend, Tracy, who I've known for 26 years, that I reconnected with.
APPN:	So were you with either of those people for a moment that felt really special? That might be a way you could pick one.
Ms. C:	Okay, I'd have to say my old friend, Tracy. We've got a lot of memories together.
APPN:	Can you tell me more about Tracy?
Ms. C:	I don't know, we could just talk about anything and everything, and we don't pass judgment on each other. You know it's a totally different construct as far as a relationship goes. . . I mean, you know there's no judgments, she's never throwed anything up in my face. We have never had an argument the whole 26 years that we've known each other. Never gotten into an argument. Never had a falling out. We've, you know, lost contact with each other and everything but, um, other than that there's been nothing. You know it's just like we're sisters. You know there ain't nothing different except we don't have the same blood.
APPN:	So how did you find her?
Ms. C:	She found me on Instagram.
APPN:	Okay.
Ms. C:	We've been on Facebook together and everything for years but I don't know why that didn't click, but all of a sudden, you know, I decided to get an Instagram account a few months ago and all of a sudden she popped up and she goes "Oh my god, I found you." And I'm going "like shit I've been right here. (laughing) Where have you been, you know?" And we've just been talking and texting and sending each other pictures and laughing and, you know it's just like, you know, the time that we were apart and everything doesn't even matter.
APPN:	How long had it been?

Ms. C:	Oh my god, about 2005. About when I got my divorce and everything.... I don't have a car so I can't go see her. She lives up around _____. And she says as soon as she gets a chance to get a car or get some transportation or anything she's going to come see me.
APPN:	Okay. So if you think back to when you were together with Tracy, and you knew her around the time you got divorced, can you think of a certain time that was special, where you were with her that was even a lot of fun or just very relaxed and calm?
Ms. C:	Well, we're always laughing together. (laughs) Um, I don't know it's just being comfortable with somebody.
APPN:	Um-hm.
Ms. C:	And having that safety thing with that person. Cause like I said I don't have to worry about being judged or attacked and everything.
APPN:	Um-hm. And so when you think about Tracy, what do you notice happening on the inside?
Ms. C:	Well, it just makes me happy, because you know even though I lost a connection with somebody that I thought that was, you know, close enough to be a sister, I turned around and found, or found again, the sister that I always had that I thought I had lost and everything. So, um, I mean I'm thankful to have her and I know she feels that way about me and everything.
APPN:	Hm.
Ms. C:	She's like, back where I was 2 or 3 years ago, and everything. And she's in that stuck mode and everything. And she's not up here where I'm at and I can see all these things in her and everything. And I've tried, oh believe me I've tried, you know throwing hints out there and right out coming out well you need to do this. And she's like, are you kidding me? That's not going to ever work. And I'm going like if you give it halfway a chance and be open-minded about it will. You know, I mean she's gone through a *lot* of trauma, and everything. She was molested, her daddy's a drunk. Um, you know just that in itself. And then the time that we were apart and everything her best friend, that she thought that she had, slept with her daddy. And then, um, her other best friend, you know her first love, he died. And then there was a huge stink and everything that went on there and everything and it just got, everything just came to a head, and she just kind of just blanked out and did some things that she didn't even realize that she did, and everything. And she said that she started cutting, and all this stuff, and I'm going like "girl you need to go see a doctor." And she goes, well she's got some physical issues, some really *bad* physical issues, and she said her neurologist told her to go to a psychiatrist because they can prescribe things that a regular doctor can't, or something like that? So she's supposed to be going to see a doctor but she hasn't went yet. And I'm going like, Tracy, "you *need to go*."
APPN:	Well you know, people are afraid. You said one thing that sort of stuck out for me and that's was something like "she's negative" and she's sort of stuck, but you're way out here, and can you describe that strength in you?

Ms. C: I used to feel that way. I used to feel like yeah. I was that girl. You know the one that always stayed in the room and wanted to grab the covers over her head. You know the one that was always searching for that one and everything and always making the wrong decisions and the wrong choices and then wind up getting pissed off and angry and hurt because they turned out to be abusive or using me and everything, you know. And being depressed all the time, and negative. You know, what's wrong with me? Nothing's ever going to work. You know, why can't I do this? or why can't I have that? And, she's got so much potential because she's a wonderful person. She's got a huge heart, and you know, we wouldn't be friends if we hadn't clicked a long time ago at some kind of level and everything, and we just complement each other. I mean I'm Christian and she claims to be a witch. So I mean we're on opposite ends of the spectrum as far as that goes, and everything. I understand why she gave up Christianity. You know she felt because of everything she went through as a child and everything that God wasn't there. He didn't help her so, F. . . it, I'm not going to believe any more. I get that. I understand that. She just has never been in the situation where she's allowed herself to be touched, by God or anything like that. To be changed. So, I don't judge her for the way she feels. I don't hold it against her. We don't push our beliefs off on each other, nothing like that. We've always had that respect. Um, I'd just like to see more for her.

APPN: Okay, so let's focus on Tracy. It sounds like Tracy's definitely your peace person.

Ms. C: Yeah.

APPN: Okay. So can you just describe Tracy to me? Will you tell me about her appearance?

Ms. C: (deep sigh) Well, knowing her like I do, she to me she always looks sad. Even though we can laugh and cut up and have a good time and everything I know she's always hurting.

APPN: Um-hm. I noticed your deep sigh.

Ms. C: And it's because of all the shit that she's went through. Um, she definitely needs to find somebody to help her get through that and everything so she can move out of that hole that's she's in. Um, and I've tried to give her some of the tips that they made *me* go through (in my program) and everything to get through it. But she's just, no. I don't think she's ready. I can't remember how old I was when I met her. It was 1993 I think. She was 17. She was just fixing to graduate high school. I went to her graduation party.

APPN: Okay.

Ms. C: And I had some friends and everything and we used to cruise around and go to the hangout spots and things in ____. And I think that's where we met. And everything was through mutual friends. We got drunk together. It was a blast. Um, we've just been friends ever since. . . I think it took years before she ever really opened up to me and told me how bad it was.

APPN: Um-hm. So she—

Ms. C: She grew, you know grazed over it a little bit you know, talked about being molested and stuff like that. She just did never really go into a lot of details. Um, like I said, you know smiling through the tears type scenario. And I get that; I've been there. I know, I know how bad it hurts. I know what she's going through and there's nothing I can do for her to make it any better. She has to do it herself.

APPN: Except the—

Ms. C: Except for being there for her.

APPN: Exactly. Exactly. So when you think about her and, you know it sounds like it's not that just you guys understand each other very well and are—

Ms.C: Oh it's almost like we could read each other's minds.

APPN: So really connected. And so when you think about that connection, tell me what you notice happening on the inside.

Ms. C: Well, like I said it makes me happy. I mean it's—

APPN: Where do you feel the happiness?

Ms. C: Right in through here (pats chest). I mean I just feel, it's almost like a joyful feeling. You know to have, to know that I've still got that connection with somebody.

APPN: So um—

Ms. C: You know I'm not isolated anymore. I've still got that, you know, that person.

APPN: Yes, so that's so important for both of you. So when you touch here, on your chest, is there a temperature change that you notice when you think about that?

Ms. C: Yeah, I probably get a little warmer.

APPN: Warmer? Okay. Is there any other sensation?

Ms. C: Probably excitement.

APPN: Excitement, okay. Where do you feel that excitement in your body?

Ms. C: Hmm. Probably all over and everything.

APPN: Mm-hm, okay. All over.

Ms. C: It would be anticipation and everything because you never know what's going to come out of her mouth. (laughingly) And she really cracks me up sometimes. Um, we're the, like Thelma and Louise. Never know what we're going to do. Or how we're going to do it when we get together. So, um, it's that kind of—it's that kind of, kind of relationship that, like I said, you never know what's going to come out of it.

APPN: Okay, so it's a little unpredictable and, but good surprises.

Ms. C: Yeah.

APPN: Yes, okay. So just stay with those sensations and some thoughts and feelings for like 10 or 15 seconds. (20-second pause) And is there any difference in your breathing or your heart rate?

Ms. C:	(long pause) Well sometimes it will speed up, and everything because I'll think of some of the stupid shit we've done or some of the stuff that we say to each other. But then again, you know at the same time there's that calmness.
APPN:	Okay.
Ms. C:	And everything because of the comfort, being comfortable and everything with her.
APPN:	Yeah. So, and then what about muscle tension?
Ms. C:	I don't feel any of that.
APPN:	Okay. Or relaxation?
Ms. C:	Mm-hm.
APPN:	All right. So, when you do have stress, or a trigger, or a bad mood or anxiety, you know the CRM skills are there for you. So you can do some kind of immediate thing like get up and count your steps, count colors. And you know, name the colors in the room, push up against a wall. That might help when you know you're outside your zone. But if you're in a bad mood or you just feel real irritable then you could go to your resource, which is Tracy and just remember that connection. That sense of connection. That somebody understands you, somebody cares about you. And then re-sense that warmth in your chest, and you said you sort of feel excited through your body. Maybe some activation I guess you call it in your body.
Ms. C:	Um-hm.
APPN:	And just try to stay with that if you can. If you're in a place where you can do that. But again, hang in there for about 15 seconds to sort of re-create in your body that joy and excitement and happiness. Those are the words that you described to just think about having a friend who is so understanding.

TRAUMA PROCESSING IN TRM

Once patients have learned and practiced the six wellness skills for self-care and emotion regulation, the clinician can move forward to the extent desired by the patient to address trauma. The approach is gentle and invitational, and patients may not choose to recount details of their trauma, but rather, can go to the "edge" of sensation related to any thoughts of the trauma. Patients can regulate their own nervous system during moments of distress during therapy, and the advanced practitioner can focus on working with them to reprocess traumatic experiences by helping them shift awareness of sensations of discomfort to sensations of well-being. This can change the sensory experience of the traumatic memory in the present moment.

It is important that patients understand the difference between implicit and explicit memory, and that some of their cues or triggers for emotion dysregulation are related to the nonchronologic, nonintegrated nature of implicit memory. External senses are used therapeutically if a patient is triggered by a visual or auditory stimulus and the therapist can make suggestions to reduce the intensity or volume of a sensory trigger, for example, by bringing awareness to some piece or edge of the image or imagining a distancing from the trigger. With distress, pleasant or neutral sensations can be accessed and reinforced. Sensations related to emotional pain are never explored nor deepened because these already have formed deep grooves in the nervous system, and the goal is to establish the sense of safety and strength.

The therapeutic relationship in TRM may be a departure from other models the therapist has used. The therapist serves as a guide, providing the necessary concepts to establish a common vocabulary and framework for thinking, but is essentially helping patients to find their own resources from within. The therapist allows for time and stays "one step behind" the patient, following that lead and making few inferences. The approach is gentle and highly trauma-sensitive, with the knowledge that trauma history may have caused a long-term shutdown of body awareness and that awareness of body sensations may be triggering for trauma survivors. Patients are always offered the option of not tracking internal sensations, but are usually able to notice their own breathing, heart rate, or muscle tone, which can be a first step to greater awareness of self. Whatever level of body awareness is possible can be a vehicle for therapy. Use of the six CRM stabilization skills is called "scaffolding" in TRM's trauma-processing steps. Therapists also need to be aware of their own body sensations during the session. If the therapist is in a parasympathetic restorative state through tracking sensations in the body, the patient is likely to attune or co-regulate with the therapist.

Trauma survivors may have difficulty distinguishing between safe or dangerous situations or people. Cues may be misread and there can be either a hypersensitivity or a hyposensitivity to danger, that is, a lack of trust when there should be or, alternatively, a failure to detect danger in risky situations. The therapist can help patients to use the scaffolding skills so that they are more aware of their own innate ability to create safety. External sensory perceptions can serve as anchors and internal senses such as breathing, heart rate, or noticing hunger or other body needs may help to develop a sense of safety.

Throughout therapy sessions, the therapist is finely attuned to patients' voluntary and involuntary movements and emotional expressions, and can reinforce self-calming or protective movements or expressions. Tiny micromovements of the extremities may be indicative of nonverbal impulses and these often precede gross movements. The therapist can ask, "What would you like to do?" or "What do your feet want to do?" If there appears to be an impulse to complete the survival response, this opens an avenue to process the trauma. If the patient's distress is aggravated, the scaffolding skills are used to guide the patient to self-regulate.

The therapist asks about any positive or negative thoughts or any new meanings that are experienced by the patient during the session. Although in TRM there is no interpretation of the patient's experience, when someone is stuck in negative beliefs, it is possible to help the patient explore any alternative meanings that might be more positive. For example, a patient who says, "I am never safe," could come to a different conclusion, such as "I am safe in this moment, even though the world is not always safe." New understandings or meanings can be transformational, and offer a portal to healing from trauma. When there is a shift to new meanings, insights, or healthier beliefs, it is important to help the patient bring awareness to the internal sensations that are experienced as part of that new understanding. Body sensations connected to transformational meaning or thinking are explored and are a way to save the new discovery to the "hard drive" of the brain, thereby developing a template of resiliency. Three trauma-processing techniques form the core of TRM psychotherapy: titration, pendulation, and completion of survival response. These three trauma-processing techniques are used in a fluid manner, sometimes together, with the first six stabilization (scaffolding) skills as needed for anchors through the therapeutic session.

Skill 7: Titration

The skill of titration refers to the focus on small, manageable sensations associated with a traumatic experience. The TRM clinician gently asks the patient about sensations when the patient recalls a painful memory, and invites the patient to concretize and describe the sensation. For example, with a chance to reflect, the patient might report a "block" or a "ball" sensation, and describe its size, weight, and color. This purposeful focus on description helps the patient manage sensations of distress without becoming overwhelmed. The patient is asked to bring awareness to a small bit of activation within the body: "Can you sense a tiny edge of that distress (block/ball)?" As a small part of the sensation is concretized, the intensity of the experience is generally diminished, with a release of tension. The TRM clinician observes and comments on body movements and appearance, while the patient reports subjective sensations in the body, as well as heart rate, breathing, and muscle tone.

Skill 8: Pendulation

The skills of titration and pendulation are used together. When a sensation is titrated, a natural shifting occurs, and the patient may notice the distressing sensation lessening. Pendulation is the shifting back and forth between sensations of distress (pain, muscle tension, or autonomic nervous system dysregulation symptoms) and sensations of greater well-being (comfortable, neutral, or less uncomfortable sensations). If patients report sensations of distress, they are invited to bring awareness to places within the body that are less tense, less painful, or neutral or pleasant. This shift, accomplished by the patient, should diminish the intensity of the unpleasant sensations. While titrating and pendulating the sensations connected to the traumatic experience, the patient may become aware of release sensations such as heat, trembling, burping, yawning, and tingling. The patient is then simply invited to notice the sensations of release, which are natural biological responses, as shifting occurs away from sensations of distress. Sensations of release occur as the body returns to the RZ and will have been explained as part of the stabilization training earlier in therapy.

Skill 9: Completion of Survival Response

Following a traumatic event, a person can be triggered by almost anything reminiscent of the event. It is helpful for patients to understand that the nervous system response to triggers is meant to be protective, and does not indicate weakness. Levine (1997) conceptualized the body's responses to threat as massive amounts of energy mobilized for self-defense. In a therapy session, the patient may be invited to respond to internal stimuli related to a trauma, for example, the urge to strike out or run. The patient might stand and carry out the urge in the therapist's presence, or verbally describe it. If the patient can complete the defensive response that had not been completed at the time of the trauma, there may be a natural release of toxic energy.

TRM accounts for four phases of the survival response, and the clinician who understands these phases can guide the patient to reprocess the traumatic experience. As patients describe the traumatic event or as they are aware of the sensations connected to the trauma experience, the clinician can assess what phase was not completed during the event. Four survival response phases are part of Skill 9: (a) the orienting response, (b) mobilization of fight or flight, (c) completion of survival responses, and (d) return to RZ. Each phase is part of the autonomic nervous system's effort to assess, respond, and recover from threat; the patient's body urges can be tracked by the patient and therapist together. Those somatic sensations that could not be completed at the time of the trauma may be carried out in vivo or mentally and may be critical to resolution of trauma symptoms.

It is important to note that when the patient is feels unsafe, some degree of safety needs to be established prior to attempting trauma processing. Further cautions include when the patient does not have the capacity to attend to interoceptive stimuli or when attention to it is highly dysregulating. In addition, if a stable therapeutic alliance cannot be established, TRM should not be used. Many sequelae of trauma need further interventions, and TRM is basically meant to regulate the nervous system and to resolve some traumatic memory, which can be a foundation for further work.

CASE EXAMPLE: USING TRM SKILLS FOR PROCESSING

The APPN asks Ms. C what is going on with her currently that is stressful. She does not have custody of her daughter and has rarely been able to see her because of the instability of her living situation and conflict with the girl's father.

Ms. C: The only thing I can think of is my situation with Kate, my 5-year-old.

APPN: Please tell me more about that.

Ms. C: That's the only hard thing I've had to deal with. Now I can't see her at all. He (father) won't even let me talk to her on the phone. He's left the state with her. They're now in _____, supposedly. Um, so, talking to him or, you know (sighs) basically begging him to let me talk to my daughter or see her and everything and then have him come up with his smart-ass remarks and stuff and everything. You know it pisses me off. I get really, really angry at him because he's not being fair to Kate.

APPN: When was the last time you saw her?

Ms. C: Last April. This coming up April will be 2 years.

APPN: So it's been over a year and a half, or almost a year and a half.

Ms. C: And I still have the court order saying I'm supposed to see her every weekend, and he's still in contempt. But yet he thinks that he can do whatever he wants to. And he *supposedly* has talked to his lawyer and it's okay for him to move out of the state. He doesn't have to uphold the court order. From my understanding, from what I've researched on laws and the lawyers I've talked to, that's a crock of shit.

APPN: Hm.

Ms. C: Just putting it straight and everything. You know he's in contempt.

APPN: Okay. So when you're talking about this very emotional topic, what do you notice in your body. Are there places in your body where you register that stress?

Ms. C: How I saw it, I noticed that I get real agitated. I tense up. My heart rate goes up, probably my blood pressure, too.

APPN: Now when you say you tense up, where in your body do you feel that?

Ms. C: I feel it in my shoulders and my arms.

APPN:	Okay. Now let's try this shift, okay. So I want you to, right now, shift to some place in your body that feels less tension. Is there anywhere in your body that you feel less of that tension?
Ms. C:	(laughs) That's so funny. I guess the only place I can feel less tension is my toes. (laughs)
APPN:	Hm.
Ms. C:	(laughing) Everything is like wanting to just, you know I've told everybody ever since he's done this and everything that it's a good thing I don't win the lottery or I can't have the money and get a gun and everything because you wouldn't have to worry about him anymore. And we laugh it off and everything, but deep down in a way I'm serious about it, and everything. It's just like I say, I can't figure out how to do it and get away with it, where I don't wind up in prison. So therefore I'm not going to do that because I'm not going to take myself completely away from K. To where I can never see her at all ever again like that.
APPN:	Right.
APPN:	Okay. Can you tell me what you notice in your toes.
Ms. C:	They just feel different from the rest of me.
APPN:	Okay. Do they feel—
Ms. C:	Like I don't feel like they're cramping or, um, I don't know, they just feel like toes. (laughingly)
APPN:	So do they feel like pleasant, unpleasant, or neutral?
Ms. C:	Mm, probably neutral to pleasant.
APPN:	Okay. Now let's shift back to you saying you felt that tension in your shoulders. Does that feel any different now?
Ms. C:	A little bit.
APPN:	Okay. Then let's go to your toes again. So you said either pleasant or neutral. Any other words come to mind to describe what you feel in your toes?
Ms. C:	The only thing that pops in my head is "indifferent."
APPN:	Uh-huh. You can make up a word.
Ms. C:	What's a feeling word? (laughs) Um, let's see. (long pause) I don't want to say anxious, but the feeling that's there is like, you know, kind of like I want to—
APPN:	Like what?
Ms. C:	Like I want to run away from what I am feeling . . . if that makes any sense.
APPN:	Oh! So your toes want you to run away, is that what you're saying?
Ms. C:	(nods head)
APPN:	Okay.

Ms. C: You know, I have those conflict issues and everything from way back, and I don't like conflict and everything, so therefore I don't like feeling that way. I don't like feeling the helplessness, the anger, the um, (sighs) the being pissed off. You know, frustrated. . . everything that goes along with that. Everything that you can think of that's negative and everything that I think of when I think of (the father) and everything, it's there. And, I don't like feeling that way cause that's not who I am.

APPN: Mm-mm. I can see you have tears in your eyes.

Ms. C: Well, you know I'm not that person. (tearfully)

APPN: Mm-mm.

Ms. C: I would never in a million years be one of these people like out on the street where I'd take a gun and just blow somebody away just to make myself feel better (crying and sniffing). I would never do anything like that. I don't think of things like that. But when it comes to him and what he's doing, it's like my mind just goes there, and sometimes it scares me.

APPN: Mm-mm. And I think that any person who's had severe trauma can do things, can go to things that aren't them. Trauma reactions like you said; Tracy was cutting, you know, and doing unhealthy things. And you feel murderous toward him and it's not you to feel that way. Is that what you're saying?

Ms. C: (nods head)

APPN: Yes.

Ms. C: Yeah, I had somebody tell me a long time ago, around the time I started the process of going into therapy and everything, cause I never did that when I was a teenager, it was after my dad died. And I mentioned, or tried to talk about some of the stuff that happened growing up and everything, and told them that I was having dreams about a shotgun and wanting to blow my mother away. And they just kind of like, oh, you know brushed it off and said well that's just your mind, you know, processing things and your subconscious way of dealing with it and everything. It doesn't mean nothing and I'm like really? You know cause it just, I just thought of that again, talking about it now and everything. About the consequences of trauma and everything, there's so many people out there that something happens and they snap. They can't control their actions.

APPN: They get dominated by the lower parts of the brain, and when you're so overwhelmed with emotion, the thinking part of the brain is offline. And it happens to everybody. So that's why CRM can be helpful, because there are these other techniques. Grounding for example, or going to a resource, or starting to track sensations even if in your toes, you know, it's a way to bring your heart rate down and your blood pressure down and pull yourself back from that instinctive response of fight or flight. So it gives you some control. But it comes from inside. I'm sorry you're going through that.

Ms. C: It's not been easy.

APPN: Yeah. But and what's remarkable is that even though this is a bad time from the perspective of, you know, being without your daughter and seeing her grow up, it sounds like she is being cared for. He cares about her enough to take her with him when he had to leave, and *you*, in the meantime, are really moving forward, in a lot of ways. It sounds like you've made decisions to protect yourself from people who are toxic to you. You've reconnected with this person with whom you have such a strong connection. It sounds like you both can help each other because you've been through some of the same stuff. And you're getting on top of your health situation, too. So it seems like it's a good time and a bad time, too. What do you think?

Ms. C: Oh, if it wasn't for some of the good things going on and everything I probably would lose it. It's being on track and really trying to cope.

TRAINING FOR CRM AND TRM

Training for TRM psychotherapy involves attending two 3-day courses (Levels 1 and 2) offered by the Trauma Resource Institute (TRI), which is based in Claremont, California, with follow-up supervision. The course prerequisite is a master's degree or equivalent in counseling or therapy. TRM is meant to be practiced as one-to-one psychotherapy and training courses are held by Master TRM Trainers from TRI in different locations throughout the year. TRM teaching tools and manuals come with the training, and Elaine Miller-Karas's book provides in-depth descriptions of both CRM and TRM. Information is available at the TRI website. The first 3-day course explores the biology of fear and threat and the automatic, natural defensive responses; the concept of resiliency and how to restore balance to the body and the mind after traumatic experiences. The second 3-day course further explores the concept of resiliency and the restoration of balance to the body and mind and working with trauma reprocessing in light of survival responses.

Training to become a certified CRM teacher is also available from TRI. In order to teach CRM, a 5-day training is available through TRI, with follow-up certification requirements to ensure fidelity to the model. CRM teacher training is conducted only by TRI-certified CRM Master Trainers and requires an application elaborating the purpose in taking the training. CRM teachers do not need to be mental health providers: paramedics, peer counselors, teachers, nurses, physicians, and persons in recovery can teach CRM. Once certified, CRM teachers can target diverse audiences in a group or one-on-one format, for example, school children, public safety officers, first responders, healthcare and social service providers, cancer patients, persons with addiction or mental health disorders, and prisoners. CRM teachers can lead 1- or 2-day classes to teach skills and knowledge for students to apply CRM for self-mental wellness care and to share with family, friends, or patients. Brief trainings as short as 3 hours have also demonstrated benefit (Grabbe et al., 2019), and for one-to-one situations, CRM may be even be taught in less time. Reinforcement through the "ichill" app and ongoing consultation through TRI are ideal. See Box 11.2 for Resources for CRM and TRM.

BOX 11.2 Resources for CRM and TRM

Trauma Resource Institute: www.traumaresourceinstitute.com

CRM self-care skills: "ichill," app or www.ichillapp.com (also in Spanish)

Trauma-informed care: www.acesconnection.com

Hand model of the brain: www.youtube.com/watch?v=gm9CIJ74Oxw

National Center for Trauma-Informed Care: www.samhsa.gov/nctic

CONCLUDING COMMENTS

TRM provides APPNs with a "bottom-up" trauma-processing model that is consistent with nursing's mind-body orientation. A large portion of patient-therapist work draws on the foundational stabilizing, emotion regulation skills of CRM. TRM is unique, as it offers two models in one. CRM can stand alone as a preventive mental wellness intervention for individuals and to help those who struggle with common mental health issues, such as anxiety, depression, or substance abuse issues in a support or psychoeducational group setting.

As a trauma-processing modality, TRM explains, normalizes, and de-pathologizes human responses to stress or trauma and gives people simple tools for self-regulation and self-care. Stress and trauma and their associated symptoms and responses are explained in biological terms, and the stabilizing self-regulation skills are themselves biological tools, that is, drawn from one's own internal and external sensory perceptions. Because of its non-pathologizing framework and the emphasis on biology, this therapeutic approach may be acceptable to individuals who might otherwise resist psychological support. Individuals can be taught to use the skills for emotional self-regulation, starting with the ability to distinguish between sensations of distress and well-being, and then how to intentionally move from sensations of distress to sensations of well-being and strength. Finally, through skilled use of advanced TRM trauma-processing techniques, patients can engage in the processing of fragmented memories, triggers, and cues of distress that can haunt trauma survivors.

TRM's trauma-processing tools integrate the patient's self-regulation skills to handle the symptoms of distress that can occur during therapy and in daily life. Then, and with TRM's gentle and oblique manner of addressing trauma, therapy can proceed at a pace unique to the patient, drawing from their own strengths, and using resources found organically from within. Relief of symptoms and resolution of conflicts and deep-seated wounds may ensue. Trauma, particularly in childhood, leaves its legacy of hurt and psychological impairment, but TRM, with its strengths-based, positive strategies, may be a valuable approach for many patients.

DISCUSSION QUESTIONS

1. Discuss your understanding of how patients function when they are in the RZ, related to the autonomic nervous system.
2. Discuss potential triggers that can cause an individual to be "bounced out" of the RZ and possible signs or symptoms of being stuck on high or low.
3. Identify common physical, emotional, behavioral, relational, spiritual, and cognitive responsive to stress and trauma that are maladaptive.
4. Discuss techniques used by the therapist and the patient for their own self-regulation.
5. Discuss how titration and pendulation are used together to process trauma.
6. Explain how tracking internal sensations may reinforce patients' new understandings of trauma experiences as therapy progresses.
7. Explain the phases of the survival response that, if uncompleted, may lead to traumatic stress responses.
8. Discuss how TRM concepts apply with your clinical population or to specific mental health problems you are interested in.
9. Discuss how APRNs can reinforce safety for themselves and patients in therapeutic sessions.

REFERENCES

Anda, R. F., & Brown, D. B. (2010). *Adverse childhood experiences & population health in Washington: The face of a chronic public health disaster. Results from the 2009 Behavioral Risk Factor Surveillance System*. Olympia, WA: Washington State Family Policy Council. Retrieved from http://www.wvlegislature.gov/Senate1/majority/poverty/ACEsinWashington2009BRFSSFinalReport%20-%20Crittenton.pdf

Black, D. S., & Slavich, G. M. (2016). Mindfulness meditation and the immune system: A systematic review of randomized controlled trials. *Annals of the New York Academy of Sciences, 1373*(1), 13–24. doi:10.1111/nyas.12998

Cauda, F., Geminiani, G. C., & Vercelli, A. (2014). Evolutionary appearance of von Economo's neurons in the mammalian cerebral cortex. *Frontiers in Human Neuroscience, 8*, 104. doi:10.3389/fnhum.2014.00104

Centers for Disease Control and Prevention, National Center for Injury Prevention and Control, Division of Violence Prevention. (n.d.). *Adverse childhood experiences (ACEs)*. Retrieved from https://www.cdc.gov/violenceprevention/acestudy/index.html

Citron, S., & Miller-Karas, E. (2013). *Community resilience training innovation project: Final CRM innovation evaluation report*. San Bernardino, CA: San Bernardino County Department of Behavioral Health.

Corrigan, F. M., & Hull, A. M. (2015). Neglect of the complex: Why psychotherapy for post-traumatic clinical presentations is often ineffective. *BJPsych Bulletin, 39*(2), 86–89. doi:10.1192/pb.bp.114.046995

Courtois, C. A., & Ford, J. D. (Eds.). (2014). *Treating complex traumatic stress disorders: Scientific foundations and therapeutic models*. New York, NY: Guilford Press.

Cronholm, P. F., Forke, C. M., Wade, R., Bair-Merritt, M. H., Davis, M., Harkins-Schwarz, M., . . . Fein, J. A. (2015). Adverse childhood experiences: Expanding the concept of adversity. *American Journal of Preventive Medicine, 49*(3), 354–361. doi:10.1016/j.amepre.2015.02.001

De Bellis, M. D., & Zisk, A. (2014). The biological effects of childhood trauma. *Child and Adolescent Psychiatric Clinics of North America, 23*(2), 185–222, vii. doi:10.1016/j.chc.2014.01.002

Farb, N.A., Segal, Z. V., Mayberg, H., Bean, J., McKeon, D., Fatima, Z., & Anderson, A. K. (2007). Attending to the present: Mindfulness meditation reveals distinct neural modes of self-reference. *Social Cognitive and Affective Neuroscience, 2*, 313–322. doi:10.1093/scan/nsm030

Figley, C. R. (1999). Compassion fatigue: Toward a new understanding of the costs of caring. In B. H. Stamm (Ed.), *Secondary traumatic stress: Self-care issues for clinicians, researchers, and educators* (2nd ed., pp. 3–28). Lutherville, MD: Sidran Press.

Felitti, V. J., Anda, R. F., Nordenberg, D., Williamson, D. F., Spitz, A. M., Edwards, V., . . . Marks, J. S. (1998). Relationship of childhood abuse and household dysfunction to many of the leading causes of death in adults. The adverse childhood experiences (ACE) study. *American Journal of Preventive Medicine, 14*(4), 245–258. doi:10.1016/s0749-3797(98)00017-8

Gogolla, N. (2017). The insular cortex. *Current Biology, 27*(12), R580–R586. doi:10.1016/j.cub.2017.05.010

Grabbe, L., Higgins, M. K., Baird, M., Craven, P. A., & San Fratello, S. (2019).The Community Resiliency Model to promote nurse well-being. *Nursing Outlook*. doi:10.1016/j.outlook.2019.11.002

Grabbe, L.,& Miller-Karas, E. (2018). The trauma resiliency model: A "bottom-up" intervention for trauma psychotherapy. *Journal of the American Psychiatric Nurses Association, 24*(1) 76–84. doi:10.1177/1078390317745133

Grant, S., Colaiaco, B., Motala, A., Shanman, R., Booth, M., Sorbero, M., & Hempel, S. (2017). Mindfulness-based relapse prevention for substance use disorders: A systematic review and meta-analysis. *Journal of Addiction Medicine, 11*, 386–396. doi:10.1097/adm.0000000000000338

Groger, N., Matas, E., Gos, T., Lesse, A., Poeggel, G., Braun, K., & Bock, J. (2016). The transgenerational transmission of childhood adversity: Behavioral, cellular, and epigenetic correlates. *Journal of Neural Transmission (Vienna), 123*(9), 1037–1052. doi:10.1007/s00702-016-1570-1

Haase, L., May, A. C., Falahpour, M., Isakovic, S., Simmons, A. N., Hickman, S. D., . . . Paulus, M. P. (2015). A pilot study investigating changes in neural processing after mindfulness training in elite athletes. *Frontiers in Behavioral Neuroscience, 9*, 229. doi:10.3389/fnbeh.2015.00229

Haase, L., Stewart, J. L., Youssef, B., May, A. C., Isakovic, S., Simmons, A. N., . . . Paulus, M. P. (2016). When the brain does not adequately feel the body: Links between low resilience and interception. *Biological Psychology, 113*, 37–45. doi:10.1016/j.biopsycho.2015.11.004

Hanson, R. (2010, October 26). *Confronting the negativity bias* [Online Newsletter]. Retrieved from http://www.rickhanson.net/your-wise-brain-/how-your-brain-makes-you-easily -intimidated

Hebb, D. O. (1949). *The organization of behavior*. New York, NY: Wiley & Sons.

Heller, L., & LaPierre, A. (2012). *Healing developmental trauma: How early trauma affects self-regulation, self-image, and the capacity for relationship*. Berkeley, CA: North Atlantic Books.

Herringa, R., Phillips, M., Almeida, J., Insana, S., & Germain, A. (2012). Post-traumatic stress symptoms correlate with smaller subgenual cingulate, caudate, and insula volumes in unmedicated combat veterans. *Psychiatry Research, 203*(2–3), 139–145. doi:10.1016/j.pscychresns.2012.02.005

Horn, S. R., Charney, D. S., & Feder, A. (2016). Understanding resilience: New approaches for preventing and treating PTSD. *Experimental Neurology, 284*(Pt. B), 119–132. doi:10.1016/j.expneurol.2016.07.002

Khalsa, S. S., Adolphs, R., Cameron, O. G., Critchley, H. D., Davenport, P. W., Feinstein, J. S., . . . Paulus, M. P. (2018). Interoception and mental health: A roadmap. *Biological Psychiatry. Cognitive Neuroscience and Neuroimaging, 3*(6), 501–513. doi:10.1016/j.bpsc.2017.12.004

Khoury, N. M., Lutz, J., & Schuman-Olivier, Z. (2018). Interoception in psychiatric disorders: A review of randomized, controlled trials with interoception-based interventions. *Harvard Review of Psychiatry, 26*(5), 250–263. doi:10.1097/HRP.0000000000000170

Lang, A. J. (2017). Mindfulness in PTSD treatment. *Current Opinions in Psychology, 14*, 40–43. doi:10.1016/j.copsyc.2016.10.005

Leitch, L., & Miller-Karas, E. (2009). A case for using biologically-based mental health intervention in post-earthquake China: Evaluation of training in the trauma resiliency model. *International Journal of Emergency Mental Health, 11*(4), 221–233. Retrieved from https://www.omicsonline.org/open-access-pdfs/a-study-of-stress-affecting-police-officers-in-lithuania.pdf

Leitch, M. L. (2007). Somatic experiencing treatment with tsunami survivors in Thailand: Broadening the scope of early intervention. *Traumatology, 13*, 11–20. doi:10.1177/1534765607305439

Leitch, M. L., Vanslyke, J., & Allen, M. (2009). Somatic experiencing treatment with social service workers following hurricanes Katrina and Rita. *Social Work, 54*(1), 9–18. doi:10.1093/sw/54.1.9

Levine, P. A. (1997). *Waking the tiger: Healing trauma*. Berkeley, CA: North Atlantic Books.

Levine, P. A. (2003). Panic, biology and reason: Giving the body its due. *The USA Body Psychotherapy Journal, 2*, 5–21. Retrieved from https://www.ibpj.org/issues/usabpj-articles/(1)_Levine__P._A._Panic__Biology__and_Reason._USABPJ_2.2__2003.pdf

Levine, P. (2010). *In an unspoken voice: How the body releases trauma and restores goodness*. Berkeley, CA: North Atlantic Books.

Miller-Karas, E. (2015). *Building resilience to trauma: The trauma and community resiliency models*. New York, NY: Routledge Press.

Nemeroff, C. B. (2016). Paradise lost: The neurobiological and clinical consequences of child abuse and neglect. *Neuron, 89*(5), 892–909. doi:10.1016/j.neuron.2016.01.019

Ogden, P., & Fisher, J. (2015). *Sensorimotor psychotherapy: Interventions for trauma and attachment*. New York, NY: W. W. Norton.

Ogden, P., Minton, K., & Pain, C. (2006). *Trauma and the body: A sensorimotor approach to psychotherapy*. New York, NY: W. W. Norton.

Parker, C., Doctor, R. M., & Selvam, R. (2008). Somatic therapy treatment effects with tsunami survivors. *Traumatology, 14*, 103–109. doi:10.1177/1534765608319080

Payne, P., Levine, P. A., & Crane-Godreau, M. A. (2015). Somatic experiencing: Using interoception and proprioception as core elements of trauma therapy. *Frontiers in Psychology, 6*, 93. doi:10.3389/fpsyg.2015.00093

Puterman, E., Gemmill, A., Karasek, D., Weir, D., Adler, N. E., Prather, A. A., & Epel, E. S. (2016). Lifespan adversity and later adulthood telomere length in the nationally representative US

Health and Retirement Study. *Proceedings of the National Academy of Sciences of the United States of America, 113*(42), E6335–E6342. doi:10.1073/pnas.1525602113

Rodrigues, M. F., Nardi, A. E., & Levitan, M. (2017). Mindfulness in mood and anxiety disorders: A review of the literature. *Trends in Psychiatry and Psychotherapy, 39*, 207–215. doi:10.1590/2237-6089-2016-0051

Rothschild, B. (2010). *8 keys to safe trauma recovery*. New York, NY: W. W. Norton.

Rothschild, B. (2011). *The body remembers: The psychophysiology of trauma and trauma treatment*. New York, NY: W. W. Norton.

Rothschild, B. (2017). *The body remembers: Volume 2: Revolutionizing trauma treatment*. New York, NY: W. W. Norton.

Scaer, R. C. (2001). *The body bears the burden: Trauma, dissociation, and disease*. Binghamton, NY: Hawthorn Medical Press.

Shalev, I., Entringer, S., Wadhwa, P. D., Wolkowitz, O. M., Puterman, E., Lin, J., & Epel, E. S. (2013). Stress and telomere biology: A lifespan perspective. *Psychoneuroendocrinology, 38*(9), 1835–1842. doi: 10.1016/j.psyneuen.2013.03.010

Shatz, C. J. (1992). The developing brain. *Scientific American, 267*(3), 60–67. doi:10.1038/scientificamerican0992-60

Siegel, D. (1999). *The developing mind*. New York, NY: Guilford Press.

Steele, K., Boon, S., & van der Hart, O. (2017). *Treating trauma-related dissociation: A practical, integrative approach*. New York, NY: W. W. Norton.

Szyf, M., Tang, Y. Y., Hill, K. G., & Musci, R. (2016). The dynamic epigenome and its implications for behavioral interventions: A role for epigenetics to inform disorder prevention and health promotion. *Translational Behavioral Medicine, 6*(1), 55–62. doi:10.1007/s13142-016-0387-7

Tang, Y. Y., Holzel, B. K., & Posner, M. I. (2015). The neuroscience of mindfulness meditation. *Nature Reviews Neuroscience, 16*(4), 213–225. doi:10.1038/nrn3916

Vaish, A., Grossmann, T., & Woodward, A. (2008). Not all emotions are created equal: The negativity bias in social-emotional development. *Psychological Bulletin, 134*(3), 383. doi: 10.1037/0033-2909.134.3.383

van der Kolk, B. (1994). The body keeps the score: Memory and the evolving psychobiology of posttraumatic stress. *Harvard Review of Psychiatry, 1*(5). 253–265. doi:10.3109/10673229409017088

van der Kolk, B. (2014). *The body keeps the score: Brain, mind, and body in the healing of trauma*. New York, NY: Penguin.

van der Werff, S. J., Pannekoek, J. N., Stein, D. J., & van der Wee, N. J. (2013). Neuroimaging of resilience to stress: Current state of affairs. *Human Psychopharmacology, 28*(5), 529–532. doi:10.1002/hup.2336

van der Werff, S. J., van den Berg, S. M., Pannekoek, J. N., Elzinga, B. M., & van der Wee, N. J. (2013). Neuroimaging resilience to stress: A review. *Frontiers in Behavioral Neuroscience, 7*, 39. doi:10.3389/fnbeh.2013.00039

Williams, J. M. G., Teasdale, J. D., Segal, Z. V., & Kabat-Zinn, J. (2007). *The mindful way through depression: Freeing yourself from chronic unhappiness*. New York, NY: Guilford Press.

Group Therapy

Richard Pessagno

In one of the very first systematic reviews of what was then the relatively new clinical method of group psychotherapy, Raymond Corsini and Bini Rosenberg (1955/1992) identified a number of crucial "mechanisms" (pp. 146–147) that appeared to be essential for the efficacy of all of the group psychotherapies, irrespective of their formal theoretical allegiances. Their concept of mechanisms for change, the intragroup processes that appeared to bring about beneficial change and growth whatever the overt theoretical orientation of the group, was to inspire one of the most prodigious theorists and practitioners in the field of group psychotherapy, the existential psychoanalyst Irvin Yalom. He elaborated on these processes and has described 11 core elements or therapeutic factors in his still widely used textbook (Yalom & Leszcz, 2005; for the fifth edition, Yalom was joined for the first time by a coauthor, group psychotherapist Molyn Leszcz).

These core elements or therapeutic factors of group psychotherapy are highlighted after a history of group psychotherapy in the United States is presented. Types of groups and the benefits of groups are discussed. The evidence-based research supporting group psychotherapy for a range of different mental disorders follows. Phases of group development are delineated and strategies for integrating group work into advanced practice psychiatric nurse (APPN) practice are identified. The chapter ends with a case example illustrating group psychotherapy interventions and guidelines on how to obtain post-master's training and certification.

THE HISTORY OF GROUP PSYCHOTHERAPY

Human beings have been discussing mysteries and dilemmas, collaborating, and arguing in groups since the dawn of hominid time (Fehr, 2003). Yet, group therapy as a formalized practice did not really begin to take off until the 1940s, just after World War II, when emerging clinical literature began to appear. Under-resourced military physicians during wartime found themselves swamped by psychiatrically disturbed soldiers recoiling from the horrors of war, and these physicians resorted to group work as the most efficient means of trying to treat large groups of soldiers at the same time (Scheidlinger, 2004).

Around this time, Joseph Moreno, a physician, brought a radical new method into the group psychotherapy arsenal: psychodrama. Disagreeing sharply with the Freudian psychoanalysis of his time, which he felt evaded the pressing realities of the here and now in favor of an unreachable distant past, he used an observation of Aristotle as his inspiration: Spectators in a theater often identify passively with the predicaments of the actors they are watching. Moreno concluded that much psychopathology was the product of massively internalized behavioral and emotional controls, which were far in excess of necessity. He devised methods of role reversal in improvised group dramatizations, wherein patients could reenact, in role play, powerful scenarios from their lives, current as well as past, and learn to outface their fears and handle anxiety-laden situations less self-defeatingly or destructively. His view, essentially, was that patients needed practice in releasing their suppressed emotions (catharsis) and their creative potential in the here and now (Moreno, 1940/1992, 1966/1992).

Wilfred Bion managed the rehabilitation of traumatized soldiers as a physician in the British army and had noticed that some of them were able to work well together in groups while others were not, despite sharing similar experiences (Bion, 1959). He focused on collective group processes, rather than on the individuals making up the group, and noticed three fundamental patterns, which could undermine the rational, primary task of the group. According to Bion (1959), the "work group" is a term that describes the group's focus on what is supposed to be achieved by the group. The fundamental patterns or "basic assumptions" are primitive, unconscious beliefs that powerfully influenced and sabotaged conscious activity and action in the group. The first pattern is "dependency," wherein a group feels hopelessly lost as to how it should achieve its task and craves a magic solution from a charismatic leader. In the "fight or flight" pattern a change in the group, such as the introduction of a new member or a new idea, upsets the previously established equilibrium and generates powerful anxieties, which get deflected or projected onto an enemy (which could be a new thought). The enemy must be fought or fled from: mutual antagonisms and hostilities or a determination to fight an external enemy constitute the fight reaction, while changing the subject of discussion to a less disturbing one constitutes an example of a flight reaction (see Vinogradov & Yalom, 1989, pp. 65–69, for further examples). Finally, Bion described "pairing," a process that frequently occurs as a group is coming toward its termination; group members tend to pair up with one another in the hope of identifying or creating a Messianic new leader who will solve all of the group's problems, save it, and perpetuate it. However, the aim is the postponement of salvation, and the endless perpetuation of an imaginary hopefulness; any new leader will rapidly be attacked and neutralized by the group as soon as he or she is proved not to be the wished-for (impossible) Messiah figure (for a useful summary, see Riosch, 1970).

In the United States, a major figure in the emerging group psychotherapy discipline was Samuel Slavson, a founding father of the American Group Psychotherapy Association (AGPA), who practiced group therapeutic methods derived from psychoanalysis with disturbed children and adolescents between 1934 and 1956. As Fehr (2003) notes, Slavson believed that when engaged in a group task, participants could develop a strong sense of common purpose and solidarity, bringing out dimensions to their personalities that they rarely used, or perhaps did not even know about previously. He directed his interventions to the encouragement and cementing of group cohesion.

By the 1950s, group therapy was becoming increasingly multivocal, with a range of different theoretical backgrounds informing different approaches (Scheidlinger, 2004). As Scheidlinger (2004) notes, in the 1960s and 1970s the climate became distinctly fractious, with disputes not only among the various analytic groups (Freudians, followers of Adler, and neo-Freudians such as the disciples of Harry Stack Sullivan and Karen Horney) but also among group therapists and the emerging new approaches. These included, among others, Berne's (1961) transactional analysis method of group therapy, the Gestalt approach pioneered by Peris (1969), existential group psychotherapy (see Mullan, 1992, for an overview), and group applications of Rogers's person-centered approach. By the 1980s, cognitive behavioral therapy (CBT; see Beck, Rush,

Shaw, & Emory [1979] for the classic text introducing cognitive therapy, and Beck [2011] for an updated overview of contemporary CBT practice) was making the transition from an individual therapy to a group intervention. Although the literature on cognitive behavioral group psychotherapy is now voluminous, there are few works outlining comprehensive models for the technique's application in groups. An exception remains the fusion between rational-emotive therapy and CBT outlined by Ellis (1992) and Ellis and Ellis (2011).

Despite the diversity of different approaches currently available in group psychotherapy, the fractiousness, rivalry, and mutual antagonisms alluded to earlier have given way to a remarkable willingness among practitioners from different schools to learn from one another and incorporate pragmatic strategies from one another into their methods. Both Scheidlinger (2004) and Yalom and Leszcz (2005) believe that the threat to psychotherapy of all kinds posed by the introduction of managed healthcare systems in the 1990s, which emphasized cost-effective and brief treatments, appears to have made such disunity an unaffordable luxury.

THE PRINCIPLES OF GROUP PSYCHOTHERAPY

Despite the array of different theoretical schools of group psychotherapy today, they have some core principles and underlying assumptions in common. Yalom has argued (Yalom & Leszcz, 2005) that these assumptions are crucial to all modalities if therapeutic progress is to be made. These are the basic mechanisms of change; Yalom's massive review of the literature on group psychotherapy and change led him to conclude that 11 central factors will be at work in any therapeutically effective group, regardless of overt theoretical allegiances. Primary theoretical models include psychodynamic, cognitive behavioral, interpersonal, solution focused, and person centered (see Table 12.1).

It seems wisest to adopt Yalom's approach: although there are many more short-term groups with a homogeneous composition today (groups targeted at specific symptoms or problems, such as eating disorders, panic disorders, acute or chronic depression, and so on), they are of comparatively effective. Knowledge can be obtained from the far more long-standing research into (and clinical observations of) long-term, heterogeneous group psychotherapy is of considerable relevance to all psychotherapy groups.

The 11 Therapeutic Factors of Group Psychotherapy

All groups, whether based on psychoeducation, solution-focused approaches, or CBT, attempt to bring about beneficial change even if the group techniques are a formulaic application. For any form of beneficent progress to occur, however, Yalom and Leszcz argue, therapists need to engage sensitively in the here and now of every group session with the intricacies, ambiguities, and subtleties of interpersonal interaction. Managed-care health delivery systems may be pushing for the setting up of "cost-effective," short-term groups aimed at relieving specific symptoms, but it would be a mistake to believe that change occurs simply because of a particular technique (e.g., CBT). How those techniques are practiced, how group psychotherapists enable group members to interact freely and safely so that patients can discover how their customary interactions may backfire or cause unhappiness, and how to change these patterns—all require sensitive attention to and careful stewardship of group process and the nuanced, interpersonal

TABLE 12.1   EXAMPLES OF THEORETICAL APPROACHES AND FOCUS OF APPROACH

Theoretical Orientation	Focus of Approach	Example of Approach
Psychodynamic	Examine interactions among and between group members and the group leader. Group work focuses on assisting each group member to increase awareness of his or her unconscious motivations and unconscious needs. Group membership is founded on providing a deeper understanding of both themselves and their relationships under the guidance of the group leader.	Group member Mary has been consistently late the past three sessions and then becomes very irritable with other group members when the group topic has focused on the issue of death of a parent. **Group leader:** Mary, you have been late the last three sessions and then when you have come to group, you seemed irritated with other group members. Have you noticed this? **Group member Mary:** Traffic has been bad for the past several weeks. **Group member Bob:** Mary, I know your mom died 13 months ago; this topic must be difficult for you. **Group leader:** Thanks for acknowledging that, Bob. Mary, do you think your lateness and irritability might be related to your feelings around your mom's death? **Group member Mary:** Maybe. It's still very difficult for me to deal with the fact that she is gone. I know it's hard to come to group because when I talk about my mom's death it makes me upset. And I don't like everyone talking about her death; it's painful when other bring it up. **Group leader:** Do you think coming late might be a way of avoiding the topic of your mom's death? **Group member Mary:** Yes, that might be why I am late. **Group leader:** As a group let's talk about how this might happen to each of you when you want to avoid something painful.
Cognitive behavioral	Focus on identifying cognitive distortions and how thinking or thoughts influence feelings and emotions, and then identify the behaviors that evolved as a result of these factors.	**Group leader:** Bob, I notice that you didn't participate much last week after Tom brought up his concern about your lateness to group. Can we take a moment to talk about your response? What type of automatic thoughts you were having about that interaction? **Group member Bob:** I am thinking Tom thought I am stupid for being late which caused me to shut down and not want to participate or even come to group. **Group leader:** Okay, so you are thinking that the Tom thought you are stupid when you came to group late. Can you tell me what Tom did or said that led to you thinking Tom believed that you are stupid?

(continued)

Theoretical Orientation	Focus of Approach	Example of Approach
		Group member Bob: Well, Tom seemed angry at me, when I was late for our last group. I believe Tom thought I was stupid. **Group leader:** So let's check in with Tom to see if he was angry with you last week when you were late for group. **Group member Bob:** Tom were you angry with me and did you think I was stupid? **Group member Tom:** I wasn't angry with you and I'm sorry you felt I was attacking you. I don't think you are stupid for being late. I just wanted you to understand that I think it's important to come to group on time **Group leader:** Bob, I would encourage you to ask other group members if how they're responding to you matches what you think their response really means. I think sometimes you have told yourself the response you get from others means something other then what is meant. You thought Tom was angry with you when he brought up your lateness to group, you then felt Tom thought you were stupid, which then caused you to not want to participate or even not come to group. If you check in with Tom, you can then evaluate if what you thought matches what in fact Tom was thinking or what Tom meant. Your believing that Tom was angry and he thought you were stupid then led to shutting down and not participating. If you check in with Tom, that could help you make sure what you are thinking matches what Tom was conveying. **Group member Bob:** That makes sense. I see how that could help me not think that Tom was angry and then thought I was stupid for being late. **Group leader:** Changing your thoughts can help change your feelings, which then can lead to you responding or behaving in a certain way. Does that make sense? **Group member Bob:** Yes, it does. I need to do that more so I don't let my negative thoughts get in the way of me responding in a way that causes me to shut down with others.

(continued)

TABLE 12.1   EXAMPLES OF THEORETICAL APPROACHES AND FOCUS OF APPROACH (CONTINUED)

Theoretical Orientation	Focus of Approach	Example of Approach
Person centered	Focus of healing comes from group members; group therapist provides unconditional positive regard for the group members; group leader creates a trusting environment and honest feedback is provided to and among group members; group leader shows empathy and authenticity toward group members.	**Group member June:** I am having a very difficult time dealing with the fact that my divorce is final next week, my 16-year-old daughter has been sick with mono, and my scheduled vacation has been canceled because of increased work demands. **Group leader:** June, I can understand why you are having such a difficult time. **Group member June:** Thanks … it has been very tiring. I feel all alone. **Group leader:** I appreciate your sharing your feelings … let's ask the group to share about June's experience of feeling all alone. **Group member John:** June, we are here to support you. We cannot take away the stress you are under right now, but we can listen and provide support to you. **Group leader:** John, thanks for acknowledging that the group is a source of support for June. It's important to remember the support that group members do get from one another.

communication patterns, both spoken and nonspoken. The following therapeutic factors or principles, formerly termed curative factors, can be applied to all groups:

PRINCIPLE 1: THE INSTILLATION OF HOPE

By the time people come to group psychotherapy, the problems they have been struggling with have usually defeated them; seeking help can often be experienced as an admission of personal defeat and despair. A key feature of successful group psychotherapy is therefore the instillation of hope (Yalom & Leszcz, 2005), which means the promotion of a belief that, with one another's shared resources, progress is possible. Without this, little else can be achieved. The therapist's strong belief in the therapeutic process, coupled with the emerging evidence that group members are indeed beginning to transform as the group progresses, are important sources of this realistic, therapeutic hope.

PRINCIPLE 2: UNIVERSALITY

No matter how idiosyncratic, or even shameful, a patient may consider his or her difficulty to be, a major factor in group psychotherapy is the cultivation of a belief among all members in universality—essentially, that they are not alone. As Yalom and Leszcz state: "There is no human deed or thought that is fully outside the experience of other people" (2005, p. 6). Many people have felt forced into isolation and fear intimacy because of their difficulties, and this process of nonjudgmental group acceptance can help dissolve chronic feelings of shame and estrangement.

PRINCIPLE 3: IMPARTING INFORMATION

This principle involves essentially intervening to obstruct the course of destructive thought processes by imparting established knowledge concerning, for example, a particular mental illness, and how it can manifest itself. Although it is often implicit, embodied in the therapist's comments or queries about a particular belief, for instance, it is sometimes didactic in nature. An example given by Yalom and Leszcz is of a patient believing he is about to die whenever he suffers a panic attack. Great benefits can accrue from describing the physiological foundations of panic attacks, such as the hyperventilation and dizziness stimulated by elevated adrenaline, and by the didactic description of relaxation methods that can easily be practiced to bring the event back under control (Yalom & Leszcz, 2005).

PRINCIPLE 4: ALTRUISM

To give is to receive. Yalom and Leszcz (2005) cite the example of a depressed man who was beginning to confound other group members by constantly rebuffing their suggestions and ideas. Another group member, a depressed woman who had struggled with substance abuse, explained to him that she, too, used to refuse the help offered by others. She thought she was unworthy, but when she realized that people felt hurt by her rebuttals, she made a concerted effort to receive what was given graciously and began to feel enormously better as a result. Receiving with gratitude appears to bring to life one's own generosity and desire to help others in need, developments that are intrinsically therapeutic, and even beneficial, to the survival of the species (Phillips & Taylor, 2009).

PRINCIPLE 5: THE CORRECTIVE RECAPITULATION OF THE PRIMARY FAMILY GROUP

Yalom's clinical experience and extensive research led him to conclude that most patients seeking group psychotherapy have suffered toxic and harmful experiences in the first group they ever encountered—their original families. Members frequently find that they start to replicate patterns from these original group experiences in the context of the therapy group, transferring unfinished business with parents onto the group leaders, or unresolved issues with siblings onto other group members. The therapeutic group is the ideal setting for such recapitulations, offering a safe and compassionately corrective environment.

PRINCIPLE 6: DEVELOPMENT OF SOCIALIZING TECHNIQUES

Partly through the corrective recapitulation of primary group scenarios and partly through the inevitability of misunderstandings, group members learn from each other about how to correct chronic and maladaptive social tendencies. One man, cited by Yalom & Leszcz (2005), suddenly became aware in a group meeting of a lifelong habit of obsessively including irrelevant details in all his conversations, something that others found exceptionally off-putting. The group helped him to notice this without condemning or humiliating him. Tactful and compassionate feedback from group members can help patients to process complex emotions and develop better social skills, as well as to learn how to resolve conflicts safely, and become more empathic.

PRINCIPLE 7: IMITATIVE BEHAVIOR

Isolated people frequently learn to expand their repertoire of coping skills and become more accepting of themselves and others in group psychotherapy by "trying out" other people's behavior and seeing whether it suits them. Both therapists and other group members can be mirrored in this way by patients eager to grow and change; they may adopt physical postures and styles of talking similar to the therapist's, for example, and even try to think like him or her (Yalom & Leszcz, 2005). Similar to the socializing techniques described earlier, imitative behavior can be an occasion for rich, new learning.

PRINCIPLE 8: INTERPERSONAL LEARNING

Interdependence is not a weakness but a great strength for the human animal and, much like the capacity for altruism, has played a part in species survival (Yalom & Leszcz, 2005). The need for human contact appears to be fundamental and part of our evolutionary makeup. The group environment can enhance the value of interpersonal connectedness—self-disclosure in groups always implies the overcoming of fears, and the corrective, intelligent emotional responses of group members can help restore (or even create for the first time) a hurt and withdrawn member's faith in the value of human fellowship for facing life's adversities. Learning from one another greatly facilitates therapeutic change and personal growth. As a result of interpersonal learning, self-understanding and the achievement of greater levels of insight into the origins and underlying motivation of one's behavior occurs.

PRINCIPLE 9: GROUP COHESIVENESS

Group cohesiveness occurs when members start to feel that they belong, that they can draw comfort and warmth from their peers in the group, and that they are unconditionally accepted by the other group members. Yalom considers this the primary therapeutic factor in group therapy, facilitating improved self-esteem, hope, and well-being. Group cohesiveness is the indispensable precondition for therapeutic change, enabling the personal exploration and self-disclosure on which effective therapy hinges (Steen, Vasserman-Stokes, & Vannatta, 2014).

PRINCIPLE 10: CATHARSIS

Catharsis occurs when group members become able to express deep emotional feeling states, a process that appears to foster profound feelings of release and recovery. As with the other factors, it depends on strong group cohesiveness for maximum therapeutic effect; but other group members appear to benefit and grow from witnessing a peer in emotional catharsis.

PRINCIPLE 11: EXISTENTIAL FACTORS

As an existential psychotherapist, Yalom is profoundly aware that there are occasions when human beings cannot escape from pain; we are mortal and will suffer losses during life, no matter how close and intimate we become with others. These are the ineluctable truths of human existence. The existential factors that Yalom and Leszcz describe essentially refer to the capacity to face these truths, to be with one another in a group with a deep awareness of these truths without taking flight into trivialities. Life is enriched by such awareness, as indeed it is by the existentialist axiom that each individual is ultimately responsible for how he or she lives life (Frankl, 1969/1988).

TYPES OF GROUPS

There are a wide variety of groups, with both varying purposes and functions. Psychoeducational groups are one of the most commonplace groups to most practicing nurses. These groups primarily function to facilitate education or information to patients and/or families about various psychiatric-mental topics. Psychoeducational groups can mediate an educational process and promote knowledge about a multitude of topics such as psychiatric diagnosis, addictions, medication, self-care, and recovery issues. Groups such as these reinforce information, augment knowledge, and improve wellness. Psychoeducational groups are often time limited with a specified number of sessions being offered. The content of the psychoeducational group lends itself to be structured where group members can assign specific topics for discussion during each session. Psychoeducational groups can be facilitated by either a professional (such as an RN, health educator, social worker, or licensed professional counselor) or nonprofessional (peer specialist or family member) group leader.

Support groups are another type of group that focuses on providing group members with an environment that they share with others who are experiencing a common type of experience (such as grief, cancer, multiple sclerosis, and diabetes). Support groups typically allow group members to share their individual experiences, listen to others, provide information to one another, and provide sympathetic understanding to one another. Support groups often have a specified number of sessions. The structure of these groups can be more formal with specific topics that are covered each week, or the groups can be more fluid and allow group members to direct the formation of topics. These types of groups can be led by nonprofessional or professional group leaders.

Self-help groups are formed in order to provide mutual support to their members. These groups come together because of shared experiences such as substance use disorders in order for group members to help each other deal with this specified experience. Self-help groups provide a medium for group members to share their individual stories and to share struggles and successes with others in order to allow members to feel that they are not alone. Well-known self-help groups include Alcoholics Anonymous and Narcotics Anonymous. Self-help groups are not time-limited groups, and participation in groups can continue for months to years. For groups that focus on recovery, such as Alcoholics Anonymous, participation and fellowship are seen as an integral parts of continued sobriety. The shared community experience is viewed as the medium for change. The self-help group focuses on having a veteran member guiding and supporting newer group members. The self-help group model does not use professional group leaders; all group members take responsibility for group leadership.

Benefits of Groups

Treatments for psychiatric disorders are varied and can include psychotherapy, psychoeducation, support groups, and pharmacotherapy. Treatment choices for patients depend on multiple factors, including availability, cost, convenience, and accessibility. Group psychotherapy can be an ideal treatment option for many reasons for both the therapist and the patient. Two of the most important factors in today's healthcare landscape are cost and cost-effectiveness. The cost-effectiveness of group psychotherapy has made this an ideal choice for many patients (Burlingame, Fuhriman, & Mosier, 2003; McRoberts, Burlingame, & Hoag, 1998). Cost-effectiveness is articulated as a significant factor in providing group psychotherapy as an alternative treatment to individual therapy in a study comparing the two types of interventions over an 18-month period.

Patients with and without insurance coverage for mental health services may find group psychotherapy an affordable treatment option. For the therapist, group psychotherapy affords group-trained clinicians the opportunity to offer treatment to several patients at once, allowing for greater access to treatment for the patient and providing the therapist the ability to see larger numbers of patients at one time. Group psychotherapy also provides the therapist with the option to diversify his or her practice, providing patients with a wide array of services from which to choose. Additionally, from a time management perspective, a group therapist typically can see six to 10 patients in a group therapy session using the traditional 90-minute group psychotherapy session. Yet treating each of the same six to 10 patients within the confines of an individual psychotherapy session would require the same therapist to dedicate six to 10 individual sessions, requiring many hours of treatment.

In addition, accessibility to group psychotherapy can increase the quantity of psychotherapy visits compared to individual psychotherapy. Additionally the increased quantity of group psychotherapy sessions has been more closely linked to improved sense of treatment adequacy than for patients in individual therapy (Sripada et al., 2016). As Yalom and Leszcz note (2005, p. 12), today there are tried-and-tested group psychotherapy interventions available for a vast range of conditions.

Groups exist for anxiety disorders such as panic disorder, depression, perinatal mood disorders, eating disorders such as anorexia and bulimia nervosa; there are groups for people suffering with HIV/AIDS or cancer, or other conditions such as rheumatoid arthritis, obesity, multiple sclerosis, bone marrow transplant, renal failure, diabetic blindness, paraplegia, myocardial infarction, Parkinson disease, irritable bowel syndrome, and for people with a genetic predisposition to cancer. There are also groups for victims of sexual abuse, for parents of sexually abused children, for victims of domestic violence, for people recovering from a first episode of schizophrenia, for people with chronic schizophrenia, for adult children of alcoholic parents, for self-harmers, for the bereaved, for troubled families and couples, and for divorcees. This is by no means an exhaustive list and does not include self-help groups such as Alcoholics Anonymous or Narcotics Anonymous. The scope of group psychotherapy is vast.

The literature further notes that the homogeneity of psychotherapy groups related to the specific diagnostic similarity of participants can positively influence the group's outcome and efficacy (Kösters, Burlingame, Nachtigall, & Strauss, 2006). These same researchers also noted that psychotherapy groups with a limited size of six to 10 participants also positively influenced outcomes and efficacy. Patients grouped together based on similar diagnoses, such as cancer, bereavement, or depression, do better than those in groups with divergent diagnoses among group members (Leszcz & Goodwin, 1997). The greater the commonality among group participants, the greater the opportunity that exists for abatement of symptoms. Another meta-analysis of 45 studies evaluated a variety of homogeneous psychotherapy groups that segregated depressed patients, schizophrenic patients, and anxious patients. The psychotherapy groups that were homogeneous or segregated based on diagnosis outperformed psychotherapy groups of patient cohorts that were mixed based on diagnoses (Burlingame et al., 2003).

Group psychotherapy does afford some benefits to the patient that are not afforded to patients who seek out and use individual psychotherapy. These benefits include the fact that the therapeutic value of working within a group provides members with the opportunity to share common experiences with others. This ability to share experiences with others has been positively linked to symptom resolution, particularly among depressed and anxious patients (McRoberts et al., 1998). Group psychotherapy also creates a forum for patients to work on relational issues with other individuals within a structured environment. Individual therapy does not provide this benefit. McRoberts et al. (1998) also commented that patients engaged in group psychotherapy saw more rapid resolution of symptoms compared to individual therapy participants, which might support using group psychotherapy interventions.

Group psychotherapy via telehealth is a possible psychotherapeutic options for patients. Providing an array of psychiatric-mental health services including group and individual psychotherapy via a teleconferencing has been in existence in the United States since 1959 (Von Hafften, n.d.ation Video). See Chapter 4, for a thorough discussion of telemental health. The research that has been done relative to using group psychotherapy through a telemedicine platform has mainly come out of the Veterans Administration. It has been noted that veterans with posttraumatic stress disorder (PTSD) who were treated using a group therapy intervention suggested that providing group psychotherapy via telepsychiatry is an acceptable means of providing this service (Green et al., 2010; Morland, Hynes, Mackintosh, Resick, & Chard, 2011).

EVIDENCE-BASED RESEARCH

Participating in psychotherapeutic group interventions such group therapy, support groups, and psychoeducational groups can have a positive impact on a variety of human responses such as depression, anxiety, self-esteem, stress, and grief, to name a few. Research has articulated how group therapy can influence positive change for patients facing a variety of physical health issues. For example, cancer survivors participating in group work have been shown to have enhanced personal growth, an increased sense of personal well-being, and improvement in identifying purpose in life (van der Spek et al., 2017). Group therapy has also been linked to successfully reducing core symptom clusters related to PTSD including hyperarousal, reexperiencing, and avoidance (Lubin, Loris, Burt, & Johnson, 1998). Additionally, group therapy has been linked to reducing grief symptoms among those with complicated grief (Rosner, Lumbeck, & Geissner, 2010).

While more research is needed to further articulate how specific neurophysiological mechanisms are responsible for the creating the positive responses that are appreciated in individuals participating in group therapy, a possible explanation may lie in the neuroplasticity of the brain. Flores (2010) noted the neuroplasticity of brain has correlations to attachment theory and group therapy. It is suggested that the early development of the human brain is influenced and molded by the attachments to other human beings that occur early in life and that as the individual matures and grows, those relationships or attachments to others continue to create neuronal and structural changes within the brain. This framework provides a means to hypothesize that the use of group psychotherapy can further enhance and provide a positive influence in the development of brain through the initiation of human connection and attachment to others through a psychotherapeutic group experience.

A review of 107 clinical studies and 14 meta-analyses by Burlingame, MacKenzie, and Strauss (2004) concluded that, for outpatient populations, group therapy was equal in effectiveness to individual therapy, whether it was used as the primary treatment or as an adjunct to a more multimodal treatment program. Group therapy was also found by these authors to be effective for patients suffering with severe mental illnesses such as bipolar disorders and schizophrenia. An earlier meta-analysis by Burlingame et al. (2003), comparing the effectiveness of outpatient and inpatient group psychotherapy, found that, in comparison to waiting-list control groups, outpatient groups significantly outperformed inpatient groups; however, a limitation was that only six inpatient studies were included, which is considered a small number.. A more recent meta-analysis of the effectiveness of group psychotherapy in inpatient settings, however, found marked improvements postintervention (Kösters et al., 2006). The authors analyzed 46 studies with pre-post measures and 24 controlled studies, all of which had been published between 1980 and 2004. Patients with mood disorders improved considerably more after group psychotherapy interventions than those with mixed diagnoses or with PTSD, schizophrenia, or psychosomatic illness, although all groups showed measurable improvements.

These studies suggest that, theoretical orientations aside, group psychotherapy as a treatment modality is as effective as individual psychotherapy, and that it may well be considerably more cost-effective. As mentioned earlier, it has been shown to be an effective intervention for patients suffering with physical as well as mental health conditions. For example, the systematic review and meta-analysis conducted by Himelhoch, Medoff, and Oyeniyi (2007) into the effects of group psychotherapy on depressive symptoms among male, HIV-infected individuals showed that it significantly reduced depression ratings. Eight randomized, controlled, double-blinded studies encompassing 655 patients were used in the review; five of the studies used CBT as the theoretical basis for group therapy, two used supportive therapy, and one used a psychoeducational approach involving coping-effectiveness training. The strongest improvements occurred in the CBT groups.

Spiegel's groundbreaking work on group psychotherapy with cancer patients was the first to bring cancer patients together to address the terrors, pain, and depression associated with cancer diagnosis and treatment. His research furnishes compelling evidence that both their survival times and quality of life were substantially enhanced as a result of group psychotherapy (see Spiegel & Classen [2000] for a comprehensive review and abundant clinical illustrations). For patients with advanced terminal cancer, a relatively new group psychotherapy modality, meaning-centered group psychotherapy (based on Victor Frankl's work on logotherapy, see Frankl, 1969/1988), substantially improved measures of spiritual well-being, optimism/pessimism, desire for death, hopelessness, anxiety, and depression in just 8 weeks of treatment (Breitbart et al., 2015). Follow-up assessment showed that the improvements were maintained 2 months after the cessation of treatment.

Even in a challenging subgroup, such as those with substance use disorders, compelling evidence is emerging that group psychotherapy can be an effective treatment intervention. A systematic review of 24 treatment outcome studies in relation to patients with substance use disorders found that group psychotherapy was as effective as individual psychotherapy in the treatment of addiction, although no single modality of group therapy proved any more efficacious than the other group orientations (Weiss, Jaffee, de Menil, & Cogley, 2004). Moreover, in a study by Scherbaum et al. (2005), a 20-session CBT group proved considerably more effective in reducing substance use among opiate use disorder patients than a routine methadone maintenance treatment (MMT) alone. Both cohorts of patients received MMT, but one received CBT group therapy in addition. Moreover, the reductions were still in evidence 6 months after the cessation of treatment and were much more poorly sustained among the MMT-only patients.

These are only a few samples of the voluminous, peer-reviewed research supporting the use of group psychotherapy as an effective treatment modality across an enormous span of different conditions and illnesses (Table 12.2).

TABLE 12.2 SELECTED EVIDENCE-BASED RESEARCH FOR GROUP PSYCHOTHERAPY			
Study*	**Population**	**Type of Group**	**Outcome**
Breitbart et al. (2015)	Patients with cancer	Meaning center group therapy	Meaning centered group therapy highly useful treatment option for those with cancer in advanced disease and those with palliative care needs.
Grenon et al. (2017)	Individuals with eating disorder	Varied group modalities	Group psychotherapy is recommended as a primary treatment for compulsive overeating
Hartig and Viola (2015)	Bereaved individuals	Support group communities	Participation in online support group community reduces psychological distress
Ivezic, Sesar, and Muzinic (2017)	Individuals with schizophrenia	Psychoeducation groups	Psychoeducation groups lower self-stigma of those with schizophrenia

(continued)

TABLE 12.2 SELECTED EVIDENCE-BASED RESEARCH FOR GROUP PSYCHOTHERAPY (*CONTINUED*)			
Study*	Population	Type of Group	Outcome
Lorentzen, Ruud, Fjeldstad, and Hoglend (2015)	Individuals with personality disorders	Analytic group psychotherapy	Long-term group therapy is effective for personality disorders
Mulcahy, Reay, Wilkinson, and Owen (2010)	Women with depression	Interpersonal group psychotherapy	Group psychotherapy has less depression and better mother-infant bonding than treatment as usual (TAU)
Schwartz, Nickow, Arseneau, and Gisslow (2015)	Individuals with compulsive overeating	Psychodyanmic groups	Group psychotherapy is recommended as a primary treatment for compulsive overeating
Sripada et al. (2016)	Veterans with posttraumatic stress disorder	Cognitive behavioral groups	Groups increase access to care and improve treatment adequacy
van der Spek et al. (2017)	Individuals with cancer	Meaning-centered groups	Members had increased sense of personal growth

*Studies in this table are listed in the references given at the end of the chapter.

THE DEVELOPMENT OF A GROUP

How does a group develop over time? This may seem like a relatively straightforward question, but research by Arrow, Poole, Henry, Wheelan, and Moreland (2004) provides ample reasons to explain why it is not necessarily straightforward. For one thing, what version of time is being employed? Beyond the commonsense, everyday notion of time, matters start getting seriously complicated. This research suggests that in many collective human endeavors, such as the work of psychotherapeutic groups, time is socially constructed: how group members think about time, and the meanings they attribute to it, will profoundly affect how they handle temporal issues.

These researchers draw on work by Ancona, Okhuysen, and Perlow (2001), which identified five models of time. They are clock time, cyclical time (e.g., the annual cycle of the seasons), time as punctuated by predictable events (e.g., birthdays, paydays, and so on), time as punctuated by unpredictable events (e.g., accidents, natural disasters such as floods or earthquakes, or terrorist atrocities), and life cycle time, which refers to development within a finite life span.

Any one human being will experience and contribute to each of these different social constructs of time depending on which of them seems most pressing to the particular group task and group culture in which he or she is engaged. Time can also be experienced as a kind of currency or resource, with people not wishing to "waste" it or expecting a return on their "investment." These considerations complicate certain research assumptions, such as the belief that groups develop systematically as time unfolds, or that groups exhibit discernible temporal patterns in their development. The inconsistent empirical findings in relation to these expectations have led to the development of more complex theorizations about the development of small group systems, including the assumption that groups may be more effectively conceptualized and thus governed by nonlinear dynamics, summating that groups are complex systems (Arrow et al., 2004).

Arrow et al. (2004) call for the development of a more adequate "complex theory" of group development, which takes account of the fact that group systems are not "well behaved" (i.e., they do not conform to simple models of linear causality and often show discontinuities and unexpected novelties in their developmental path). Such complex theories should also take account of the fact that group systems interact at multiple levels, both within each group, and in relation to external environmental influences.

MacKenzie (1995) presented a rather striking statistic: more than 80% of patients attending mental health services are seen for no more than eight sessions, and fewer than 15% remain in treatment for 6 months or longer. MacKenzie argues for a creative approach to the impact of managed care, honing skills to assess which patients will require longer-term treatments as accurately as possible in the earliest stages of intervention. This is where clinical acumen is clearly relevant; moreover, being able to judge who will benefit from short-term crisis intervention only, who will require time-limited therapy of between 8 and 26 sessions, and who will need longer-term, group psychotherapy of more than 6 months, can empower clinicians to provide the right help to the right patients in a climate of scarce resources and finite provision.

With these provisos in mind, at the level of clinical stewardship of a group, Yalom and Leszcz (2005) suggest that, while nothing is predictable, much can be gained by having a fundamental clinical awareness of certain necessary transitions in the life of an effective psychotherapeutic group. Four broad phases or stages of group psychotherapy formation or development are identified, and these phases appear to be consistent across a broad range of theoretical modalities (Yalom & Leszcz, 2005).

Psychotherapy groups all seem to begin with an orientation or the forming (Tuckerman, 1965) phase or stage, when members feel somewhat lost and search for structures and goals, feeling exceptionally dependent on the therapist for leadership and guidance in the midst of their uncertainty. This phase eventually transmutes into a period of conflict or storming phase or stage, when issues of interpersonal dominance, rebellion, or submission take center stage similar, in fact, to the descriptions given earlier of the recapitulation of primary family group dynamics. Provided the therapist is able to ensure a corrective emotional experience (Jacobs, 1990) in the group, so that damaging original family dynamics can emerge and be ameliorated without being simply replicated, the group appears to move into a phase of internal harmony and warmth, when group cohesiveness takes center stage, and when interpersonal differences are downplayed or ignored. This appears to be a necessary step in the creation of a shared sense of safety, the belief that the group is a secure base for exploration and growth, as attachment theorist John Bowlby (1988) would describe it. See Table 12.3 for the phases of group development.

As group cohesiveness is consolidated, a process that can take a considerable period, another spontaneous evolution appears to take place: the emergence of the mature work group—highly cohesive, but willing to explore, investigate, and analyze with a very high degree of commitment to the group as a whole, its primary task, and to the individual members who constitute it. The importance of group cohesion cannot be underestimated. Cohesion within the group is a foundational element, which needs to

TABLE 12.3 PHASES OF GROUP FORMATION/DEVELOPMENT	
Group Phase/Stage	**Characteristic of Phase/Stage**
Orientation or forming	Group members are adapting to being in the group; members will seek out guidance and approval from the group leader about appropriate boundaries, limits, and behaviors; limited personal disclosure is done by group members; some group members may experience anxiety and apprehension.
Storming	Group members are attempting to find their place within the group; group members may experience conflict among themselves; group members exchange ideas, which can cause group members to experience conflict; group members begin to notice differences among themselves; this stage/phase is necessary in order for the group to mature and grow.
Norming	Group members become more aligned as a whole, and identify and work to a common goal. This stage/phase allows members to experience a great sense of trust among themselves.
Performing	Group members are more autonomous and independent; group members feel ownership of group experience. Deeper sense of work is accomplished. Group members are able to be more honest with one another, and a deeper sense of sharing occurs among members.
Adjourning	Members have appreciation for other group members. It is during this phase/stage that the termination is addressed and occurs. Group members may experience more difficult emotional responses and emotions to the group ending.

Source: Tuckerman, B. (1965). Development sequence in small groups. *Psychological Bulletin, 63*(6), 384–399. doi:10.1037/h0022100

be present for a group in order for members to fully appreciate the progression of the group through the phases of group development. Group cohension is the foundation for members to establish trust, to explore sensitive issues, and to enhance their ability to become more authentic and vulnerable with others. It is the group leader who is responsible for initiating and developing this sense of group cohesion within the group (Burlingame, McClendon, & Alonso, 2011). It been found that establishing a sense of group cohesion among members is a strong predictor relative to whether members will tolerate conflict, feedback, and change within the group (Budman, Soldz, Demby, Davis, & Merry, 1993).

INTEGRATING GROUP TREATMENT INTO APPN PRACTICE

Exploring the idea of starting a group within one's practice can be a daunting task. APPNs may feel that their skill level, relative to leading and facilitating a group, may be inadequate. There may also be concerns about the process one must undertake in order to start a group. Questions can arise about how to identify the most appropriate type of group, how to screen and select appropriate patients, how to establish a fee schedule, how to implement an advertising strategy, and whether to use a co-therapist leader. Although there are multiple steps one must take in order to initiate a psychotherapeutic group into one's practice, this can be an exciting and challenging way to invigorate and diversify one's practice, no matter what the practice setting.

Yalom and Leszcz (2005) provide a lucid overview of the pros and cons of running groups as a solo therapist or as a co-therapist. The decision to lead a group as an individual group therapist or to have co-therapists is dependent on many factors. Many group psychotherapists are comfortable with leading groups individually, but often co-leading adds to the dynamics of the group and can aid the management of the group, especially among adolescent groups. Co-leading groups provides the opportunity to process group issues with the other therapist, to learn from a colleague, and at times make the group process more enjoyable. Varying styles among therapists, as well as differing theoretical orientations, can create challenges in identifying a co-leader, yet it can also lead to developing a greater sense of collaboration and the opportunity to explore new approaches to working with patients.

There are multiple benefits from co-leading a group. There are so many forms of communication, process, and dynamics occurring in a group psychotherapy session, even in prolonged periods of silence, that two heads are often better than one. When working with a co-therapist, one therapist, typically, concentrates on the content of interpersonal communication, while the other focuses on the process. Group members often benefit from watching and learning how the co-therapists interact with one another to resolve differences or conflicts. This modeling behavior can be a great medium for group members to witness healthy communication and positive relationship skills. Therapeutic styles, theoretical and clinical resources, and the wisdom of the group leaders are multiplied by having two therapists. Additionally, having a competent colleague in the room helps to diminish the inevitable therapist anxieties when running a group psychotherapy session. Using a co-therapist provides a medium to access, discuss, and debrief clinical issues before and after each group session.

However, there are also drawbacks. Co-therapists who simply do not get along with each other will have a formidable task in managing their own differences therapeutically when they are also managing immensely complex group differences and conflicts. It is also possible for parent–child dynamics to arise if one therapist is more skilled and experienced than the other. Given that group members are likely to recapitulate dynamics originating in their families, it is also very likely that forms of splitting may arise, with one therapist apparently idealized, while the other becomes devalued or denigrated. Finally, group members may feel coerced by co-therapists who become adamant in promoting a particular therapeutic message, a phenomenon that can set off underground dynamics of resistance and rebellion.

The first step in starting a group is to identify the purpose of the group and the types of patients who will benefit from the group. An APPN working within an acute inpatient setting should explore what types of psychotherapy or process groups are currently being provided within the institution. Often, partnering with the hospital-based licensed clinical social workers or psychologists, who may be engaged in leading psychotherapy groups, may prove to be beneficial. Owing to the limited time that patients are hospitalized groups that have a broad appeal and that can be more inclusive will afford more patients the opportunity to participate in inpatient psychotherapy groups. For the APPN working within an outpatient setting (such as in private practice, community mental health centers, substance abuse programs, or homeless shelters), using the same process is beneficial.

When starting a group, it is often best to identify a target population. The APPN might notice, for example, that his or her current caseload includes several patients with the same psychiatric diagnosis, or several patients who share the same issues (such as divorce, new onset of a cancer diagnosis, or gender identity issues). Using a group intervention or starting a therapy group can allow the APPN to expand the caseload of patients, diversify treatment options for patients, provide cost savings to patients, possibly improve revenues for the APPN practice, and potentially improve productivity. Finding a commonality among patients will be helpful in identifying those individuals who might work well together within a group.

After identifying a target population, the APPN needs to identify the type of group to be offered. Will the group be time limited (i.e., offering 8 to 12 sessions) or will the group be longer term (i.e., requiring a patient to commit to 3 months to a year)? It is also important to identify whether the group will be an open or a closed group. Open groups allow new members to join as space permits, and closed groups allow no new members once the group begins. It is also important for the APPN to decide the number of group members. Typical therapy groups will include six to eight members. Groups that are larger than this can minimize both the effectiveness and quality of the group. Education groups can have more members or be larger, as the focus of these types of group do not require the same attention to group process or group dynamics as other types of group might. The theoretical orientation of the provider often will dictate the type of framework used within the group. As noted earlier, various theoretical orientations fit well when using group psychotherapy.

The next step is to decide whether the group will be led by one or two group leaders. For APPNs who have limited group therapy experience, using a co-therapist can be an effective path to becoming more comfortable with the role of group leader, as well as provide a means of sharing the responsibility of group treatment. When offering mixed-gender groups, having a male and a female group leader can provide a means of offering a varying gender approach as well as provide a suitable means for modeling adaptive male–female interaction and behavior. On the other hand, when working with female sexual abuse survivors, the group may prove to be more productive if led by two female co-therapists. The same may be true if a therapy group is offered for gay men; two male co-therapists may create an enhanced therapeutic balance within the group. Regardless of the gender of the co-therapist, having the right fit, relative to skill, interests, alignment of group philosophy and theoretical approach, and ability to create a therapeutic bond within a group environment, is critical to selecting a compatible co-therapist. Remember, selecting a co-therapist who is a good fit for the APPN's temperament, style, theoretical orientation, and personality is a vital part of building a successful group.

Fees for the group will typically be based on several factors including insurance reimbursement and geographic location. Group psychotherapy fees vary from region to region. Fees are often market driven and dependent on the skill level, education, and experience of the group psychotherapist. For the patient, group psychotherapy can be a more affordable alternative to individual psychotherapy.

Marketing and advertising a new group presents another set of challenges. Often, networking with colleagues can be a very effective way of identifying potential group members. Inform colleagues that a new group is being offered and tell them what types of patients are being sought. Ask colleagues to refer potential patients. Also remember that maintaining regular contact with other mental health professionals in the community is a way to enhance visibility as a provider. Making referrals to other therapists who have specific treatment expertise with patients is also a way to increase a referral base. Other providers are more likely to refer patients when reciprocal referrals occur. Advertising in local publications, church bulletins, schools, hospitals, community centers, and on appropriate social media sites can also improve visibility of the new group. Using professional websites for psychotherapists and for other mental health professionals, or designing your own personal website may also be effective means of advertising.

Patient selection will largely depend on the setting. For outpatient settings, it is often beneficial for the group therapist(s) to interview each potential group member to determine if the group being formed would be a good fit for the patient. Patient goals, group goals, motivation, ability to attend weekly sessions, past psychiatric history, intellectual functioning, past experience with psychotherapy, and personality characteristics may all be factors in determining whether a patient is the right fit for the therapy group. If patients are not the right fit for a group, offering alternative treatment options is very important. It is essential to assure that patients are connected to other mental treatment services. The therapist can offer to see the patient for individual therapy, or make referral to another provider who might better suited to meet the patient's needs.

When setting up the schedule for the group, it can be beneficial to hold the group sessions on the same day and time each week, as well as to have the same established space that can be utilized for all group sessions in order to maintain consistency. As with individual sessions, starting and ending on time is important to establish structure for the group sessions and to provide a pattern so that patients can develop an expectation of reliabilty relative to the group. These factors can enhance a sense of trust, for patients as well as members appreciate established norms and consistency. This structure will also allow group members to plan ahead, which can improve success relative to attendance. Many therapy groups typically run for 90 minutes.

At the start of the first group session, the group leader reviews the group's ground rules and articulates the expectations for group members. It is important to articulate the importance of attending all sessions and arriving on time, how and when to notify the group leader if a member cannot attend a session, and the frequency and length of sessions. The start of the group also provides an opportunity to ask each group member to sign a consent for treatment that serves as a contract if this has not been competed prior to the first session. This consent for treatment should also include the focus of the group; the type of group being offered; expectations; the dates, time, and location of the group sessions; confidentiality; and how and when payment is expected. It should be stated that certain socially accepted norms are expected to be upheld by group members; when participating in the group, members are expected be civil and to show respect for all group members, even if there is disagreement or a conflict among them. It is also important to ask group members not to socialize with one another outside group sessions, as this can cause alliances to be formed that can cause an imbalance to the group dynamics for all members of the group.

A discussion about confidentiality is important so that group members understand that they can only talk about their own personal experience outside the group. Group members are told that giving the names of other groups members or making reference to other people outside the group is not acceptable. Additionally, talking about other group members, either directly or indirectly, or disclosing what other members have discussed in group breaks confidentiality. It is important to stress that maintaining group confidentiality lies with each group member and is not solely the responsibility of the group leader. Asking each member of the group to agree to this ground rule begins to establish a basis for cohesion and trust among members.

CASE EXAMPLE

This case example illustrates the four phases of group psychotherapy and process, as noted over the course of an outpatient, structured, 8-week, short-term psychotherapy group for first-time mothers at risk of postpartum depression. The group is composed of eight women, all of whom had given birth within 1 month of the start of the group. The women were all screened by the APPN prior to the beginning of the group to assess their appropriateness for group treatment including the absence of suicidality and psychosis, as well as each participant's ability and willingness to attend all eight, 90-minute group sessions. Prior to participating, each woman had completed the Edinburgh Postnatal Depression Scale (EPDS), a publicly available tool that is used to detect depressive symptoms among women during the postpartum period. Each woman had scored an 11 or higher on the EPDS, indicating a risk for postpartum depression. The purpose of the group was to decrease the risk for postpartum depression as evidenced by a decrease in the EPDS after the completion of an 8-week group psychotherapy intervention. An interpersonal psychotherapy orientation was used for the group.

The first group session was spent articulating ground rules for the group. Each participant was asked to maintain confidentiality of the communication within the group by agreeing not to disclose any specific information revealed by other participants. This is a standard ground rule for any psychotherapy group. In addition, during the first session, participants were asked to agree to come to the group sessions on time and not to intentionally miss any sessions. If a participant had to miss a group session, she agreed to call the group leader beforehand to notify him or her of the reason for her absence. This session also addressed the issue of emergency psychiatric services. Participants were instructed that if any emergent psychiatric needs surfaced (such as suicidal or homicidal thoughts, hallucinations, or other thought disturbances) while participating in the group, they were immediately to contact the group leader and/ or seek services at the nearest ED or crisis center. Emergent psychiatric symptoms were not anticipated, because all of the participants had been deemed safe and stable through the psychiatric evaluation and mental health clearance provided by the group leader and which were conducted individually with the group leader before the start of the group. Group members were also provided with the 24-hour answering service number for the group leader as well as the phone number for the hospital's ED and the local crisis center.

The first two sessions were structured around introducing participants to one another and allowing participants to get to know each other. Participants discussed their birth experiences, the catalyst that made them decide to participate in the group, the types of depressive symptoms the participants were experiencing, and the expectations each participant had for the group. These processes are illustrative of the orientation stage in the group process. In this phase, the group leader provides more leadership and guidance.

The third and fourth sessions provided time for each group member to check in with one another, providing the opportunity for each participant to share how she had been feeling over the preceding week. The group, during this storming phase or conflict phase, processed the issues and feelings regarding role adjustment and discussed strategies for improving individual coping. During these 2 weeks, group members noted some interpersonal conflict in the form of minor disagreements centering on parenting styles and parenting roles. During these sessions, each group member attempted to find her place within the group and evaluated other members within the group relative to issues of trust and relationship building. During these sessions, the group leader provided guidance and assisted group members as they addressed issues of conflict as well as helped to clarify statements and issues being identified in the group. The fifth session again followed the same check-in format, allowing each member to talk briefly about her week. During this phase, or the norming stage, group members further developed a sense of belonging to the group as a whole. The focus of these sessions was to address how their depression may have influenced or impacted their relationships, primarily with their significant others and their newborns. This session also served as a check-in for participants regarding the progress they were making in the group as well as identified whether the group was meeting the participants' expectations at the halfway point in the process. In these sessions, the group leader focused on solidifying the group and assisting members to work together on identifying and pointing out when group members were working cohesively toward the goals of the group.

The sixth and seventh sessions followed the same check-in format with discussion on how participants felt over the past week and then refocusing at a deeper level on their interpersonal relationships; examining how their relationships were now changing as new mothers; and examining how each member's communication traits and styles were impacting their relationships and their ability to discuss their current issues and symptoms with others. The group processed issues and feelings related to interpersonal relationships, and identified ways to strengthen interpersonal relationships to better manage depression. These sessions also addressed means of strengthening participants' child care behaviors when the mothers were feeling depressed. Time during the seventh session was also dedicated to beginning to address termination of the group, linking other types of endings in the participants' own lives. During this session, the therapist focused on allowing the group members to lead themselves, providing guidance and encouragement when needed but allowing members autonomy over the processes occurring within the group.

The eighth group session followed the same check-in format, and served as a foundation for participants to examine their progress in the group as well as to identify how the group had helped them individually. The last session also served as an opportunity to terminate with one another and to examine how each member's mental health needs were met or not met now that the group was ending. Participants were given an opportunity to explore whether they needed more treatment or support and how those needs might be met. Participants were also asked to complete the second EPDS, which would be compared to the first EPDS in order to determine whether the intervention was effective. During this session, the group leader guided the members through termination, identifying any issues that surfaced that indicated members may be having difficulty with the group ending. The therapist also clearly articulated the successes and the challenges faced by the group as well as the accomplishments of the group.

At the end of group therapy, EPDS scores for participants did decrease, suggesting a decrease in a risk for postpartum depression. Six of the participants ended treatment with the completion of the group. Two participants decided to begin individual therapy with a previous therapist with whom they had worked in the past.

POST-MASTER'S GROUP PSYCHOTHERAPY TRAINING AND CERTIFICATION REQUIREMENTS

The American Group Psychotherapy Association (AGPA) has established the competency standards for group psychotherapy. These standards and resources for the group psychotherapist can be found online (www.agpa.org/group/index.html). Various training sessions and postgraduate education for both seasoned practitioners and new graduates are available through the AGPA during its annual meeting as well as through various regional chapters nationwide that are affiliated with the organization.

The International Board for Certification of Group Psychotherapists (IBCGP; www. agpa.org/stdnt/certindex.html) also offers a means for those interested in credentialing as a group psychotherapist to achieve professional certification. Certification as a Certified Group Psychotherapist (CGP) is available to licensed mental health practitioners with current malpractice coverage and who hold a minimum of a master's degree in their respective discipline. This intraprofessional international certification is open to psychiatrists, psychologists, APPNs, social workers, expressive therapists, drug and alcohol counselors, pastoral counselors, professional licensed counselors, and marriage and family therapists. APPNs seeking national board certification as either a psychiatric mental health clinical nurse specialist (adult or child and adolescent designation) or a psychiatric nurse practitioner are eligible for the CGP designation. Further requirements for all candidates include completion of 300 hours of group psychotherapy experience during graduate training or postgraduate, documentation of a minimum of 75 hours of group psychotherapy supervision either during graduate training or after graduation; completion and submission of two references verifying completion of practice and supervision requirements; submission of proof of malpractice coverage; and an active professional licensure in an approved discipline. Recertification requirements include ongoing clinical practice and completion of continuing education requirements. Recertification must be maintained every 2 years.

CONCLUDING COMMENTS

Group psychotherapy is well established and has been showed to be effective for a wide range of both acute and chronic psychiatric conditions. Groups help individuals improve interpersonal skills, reduce a wide range of psychiatric symptoms, and provide positive outcomes for those individuals facing an array of co-morbid medical issues. For the APPN, group psychotherapy offers the ability to increase access to care for patients, and to diversify one's practice by offering services other than individual, couples, or family therapy, while at the same time affording patients a cost-effective and evidence-based intervention for addressing mental health issues. This chapter reviewed the core underlying principles informing all theoretical approaches to group psychotherapy and the principles on which the beneficial effects hinge. However, the mechanical application of a theoretical approach will not succeed unless the interpersonal, here-and-now therapeutic factors are handled adroitly and sensitively by a competent and trained group therapist. Recent literature posits that group psychotherapeutic interventions may provide a means of further enhancing brain development through the interpersonal relationships and bonds that are created through participating in a group experience.

Even though many of the group interventions available today are relatively short term, there is a rich research base pertaining to long-term group therapies extending back many decades, which shorter interventions can draw from and adapt. Proficiency in a specific theoretical orientation is a necessity for all practicing group psychotherapists, but awareness of the nuances, ambiguities, and subtleties of interpersonal interaction, and how to handle them in the immediacy of the clinical encounter to therapeutic effect are indispensable.

DISCUSSION QUESTIONS

1. What are the benefits and the challenges of offering group psychotherapy services within both inpatient and outpatient clinical environments?
2. Discuss key components of group process that occur during all phases of group development, giving examples of patient-focused activity that occurs during each phase.
3. Describe how various theoretical orientations could be used when leading short-term group psychotherapy. What patient populations or clinical presentations would be best served by each theoretical framework.

4. Discuss the benefits and challenges of using one or two group therapists during a psychotherapeutic intervention.
5. Discuss the importance of identifying ground rules, especially in relation to confidentiality for group psychotherapy services.
6. Describe how group psychotherapy differs from individual psychotherapy and describe the types of patients who might be better served by group psychotherapy.
7. Identify a specific group you would like to lead in your practice and discuss the purpose, your target population, how you would screen and recruit participants, establishing a fee schedule, the time frame (open or closed), number of participants, theoretical orientation for the group, selection of a co-therapist or why you do not want a co-therapist, marketing and advertising, and length of each session.

REFERENCES

Ancona, D. G., Okhuysen, G. A., & Perlow, L. A. (2001). Taking time to integrate temporal research. *Academy of Management Review, 26*(4), 512–529. doi:10.5465/amr.2001.5393887

Arrow, H., Poole, M. S., Henry, K. B., Wheelan, S., & Moreland, R. (2004). Time, change and development: The temporal perspective on groups. *Small Group Research, 20*(10), 1–133. doi:10.1177/1046496403259757

Beck, A. T., Rush, A. J., Shaw, B. F., & Emory, G. (1979). *Cognitive therapy of depression*. New York, NY: Guilford Press.

Beck, J. S. (2011). *Cognitive behavior therapy: Basics and beyond* (2nd ed.). New York, NY: Guilford Press.

Berne, E. (1961). *Transactional analysis in psychotherapy*. New York, NY: Grove.

Bion, W. R. (1959). *Experiences in groups and other papers*. New York, NY: Basic Books.

Bowlby, J. (1988). *A secure base: Parent–child attachment and healthy human development*. New York, NY: Basic Books.

Breitbart, W., Rosenfeld, B., Pessin, H., Applebaum, A., Kulikowski, J., & Lichtenthal, W. (2015). Meaning-centered group psychotherapy: An effective intervention for improving psychological well-being in patients with advanced cancer. *Journal of Clinical Oncology, 33*(7), 749–754. doi:10.1200/JCO.2014.57.2198

Budman, S. H., Soldz, S., Demby, A., Davis, M., & Merry, J. (1993). What is coehesiveness: An empirical examination. *Small Group Research, 24*(2), 199–216. doi:10.1177/1046496493242003

Burlingame, G. M., Fuhriman, A., & Mosier, J. (2003). The differential effectiveness of group psychotherapy: A meta-analytic perspective. *Group Dynamics: Theory, Research, and Practice, 7*(1), 3–12. doi:10.1037/1089-2699.7.1.3

Burlingame, G. M., MacKenzie, K. R., & Strauss, B. (2004). Small group treatment: Evidence for effectiveness and mechanisms of change. In M. J. Lambert (Ed.), *Bergin and Garfield's handbook of psychotherapy and behavior change* (5th ed., pp. 647–696). New York, NY: Wiley.

Burlingame, G. M., McClendon, D. T., & Alonso, J. (2011). Cohesion in group therapy. In J. Norcross (Ed.), *Psychotheapy relationships that work: Evidence based responsiveness* (pp. 110–131). New York, NY: Oxford University Press.

Corsini, R. J., & Rosenberg, B. (1992). Mechanisms of group psychotherapy: Processes and dynamics. In K. R. MacKenzie (Ed.), Classics in group psychotherapy (pp. 144–153). New York,NY: Guildford Press. (Reprinted from *Journal of Abnormal and Social Psychology*, 15, 1955, 406–41. (Reprinted in MacKenzie, K. R. (Ed.). (1992). *Classics in group psychotherapy* (pp. 144–153). New York, NY: Guildford Press)1. doi:10.1037/h0048439)

Ellis, A. (1992). Group rational-emotive and cognitive-behavior therapy. *International Journal of Group Psychotherapy, 42*(1), 63–80. doi:10.1080/00207284.1992.11732580

Ellis, A., & Ellis, D. J. (2011). *Rational emotive behavior therapy*. Washington, DC: American Psychological Association.

Fehr, S. S. (2003). *Introduction to group psychotherapy: A practical guide*. New York, NY: The Haworth Press.

Flores, P. J. (2010). Group therapy and neuroplasticity: An attachment theory perspective. *International Journal of Group Psychotherapy, 60*(4), 547–570. doi:10.1521/ijgp.2010.60.4.546

Frankl, V. F. (1988). *The will to meaning: Foundations and applications of logotherapy* (expanded ed.). New York, NY: Penguin Books. (Original work published 1969)

Green, C., Morland, L., MacDonald, A., Frueh, B. C., Grubbs, K., Rosen, C. (2010). How does tele-mental health affect group therapy process? Secondary analysis of a noninferiority trial. *Journal of Consulting and Clinical Psychology, 78*(5), 746–750. doi:10.1037/a0020158

Grenon, R., Schwartze, D., Hammond, N., Ivanova, I., Mcquaid, N., Proulx, G., & Tasca, G. (2017). Group psychotherapy for eating disorder: A meta-analysis. *International Journal of Eating Disorders, 50*(9), 997–1013. doi:10.1002/eat.22744

Hartig, J., & Viola, J. (2015). Online grief support communities: Therapeutic benefits of membership. *Journal of Death and Dying, 73*(1), 24–41. doi:10.1177/0030222815575698

Himelhoch, D., Medoff, D. R., & Oyeniyi, G. (2007). Efficacy of group psychotherapy to reduce depressive symptoms among HIV-infected individuals: A systematic review and meta-analysis. *AIDS Patient Care and STDs, 21*(10), 732–739. doi:10.1089/apc.2007.0012

Jacobs, T. J. (1990). The corrective emotional experience: Its place in current technique. *Psychoanalytic Inquiry, 10*(3), 433–545. doi:10.1080/07351690.1990.10399617

Ivezic, S. S., Sesar, M. A., & Muzinic, L. (2017). Effects of a group psychoeducation program on self-stigma, empowerment and perceived discrimination of persons with schizophrenia. *Psychiatria Danubina, 29*(1), 66–73. doi:10.24869/psyd.2017.66

Kösters, M., Burlingame, G. M., Nachtigall, C., & Strauss, B. (2006). A meta-analytic review of the effectiveness of inpatient group psychotherapy. *Group Dynamics: Theory, Research, and Practice, 10*(2), 146–163. doi:10.1037/1089-2699.10.2.146

Leszcz, M., & Goodwin, P. (1997). The rationale and foundations of group psychotherapy for women with metastatic breast cancer. *International Journal of Group Psychotherapy, 48*(2), 245–273. doi:10.1080/00207284.1998.11491538

Lorentzen, S., Ruud, T., Fjeldstad, A., & Hoglend, P. A. (2015). Personality disorder moderates outcome in short- and long-term group analytic psychotherapy: A randomized clinical trial. *British Journal of Clinical Psychology, 54*(2), 129–146. doi:10.1111/bjc.12065

Lubin, M. D., Loris, M., Burt, J., & Johnson, D. R. (1998). Effiacy of psychoeducational group therapy in reducing symptoms of posttraumatic stress disorder among multiple traumatized women. *The American Journal of Psychiatry, 155*(9), 1172–1177. doi:10.1176/ajp.155.9.1172

MacKenzie, R. (1995). *Effective use of group therapy in managed care*. Washington, DC: American Psychiatric Press.

McRoberts, C., Burlingame, G., & Hoag, M. (1998). Comparative efficacy of individual and group psychotherapy: A meta-analysis. *Group Dynamics: Theory, Research, and Practice, 2*(2), 101–107. doi:10.1037/1089-2699.2.2.101

Moreno, J. L. (1992). Mental catharsis and psychodrama. In K. R. MacKenzie (Ed.), *Classics in group psychotherapy* (pp. 47–55). New York, NY: Guildford Press. (Reprinted from *Sociometry, 3*, 1940, 208–244. doi:10.2307/2785151)

Moreno, J. L. (1992). Psychiatry of the twentieth century. Function of the universalia: Time, space, reality and cosmos. In K. R. MacKenzie (Ed.). *Classics in group psychotherapy* (pp. 55–60). New York, NY: Guildford Press. (Reprinted from *Group Psychotherapy, 19*, 1966, 146–158.)

Morland, L. A., Hynes, A. K., Mackintosh, M. A., Resick, P. A., & Chard. K. M. (2011). Group cognitive processing therapy delivered to veterans via telehealth: A pilot cohort. *Journal of Traumatic Stress, 24*(4), 465–469. doi:10.1002/jts.20661

Mulcahy, R., Reay, R. E., Wilkinson, R. B., & Owen, C. (2010). A randomized control trial for group effectiveness of group interpersonal psychotherapy for postnatal depression. *Archives of Women's Mental Health, 13*(2), 125–139. doi:10.1007/s00737-009-0101-6

Mullan, H. (1992). "Existential" therapists and their practice. *International Journal of Group Psychotherapy, 42*(4), 453–468. doi:10.1080/00207284.1992.11490718

Peris, F. S. (1969). *Gestalt therapy verbatim*. Lafayette, CA: Real People Press.

Phillips, A., & Taylor, B. (2009). *On kindness*. London, UK: Hamish Hamilton.

Riosch, M. J. (1970). The work of Wilfred Bion on groups. *Journal for the Study Interpersonal Processes, 1*(33), 56–66. doi:10.1080/00332747.1970.11023613

Rosner, R., Lumbeck, G., & Geissner, E. (2010). Effectiveness of an inpatient group therapy for comorbid complicated grief. *Psychotherapy Research*, *21*(2), 210–218. doi:10.1080/10503307.2010.545839

Scheidlinger, S. (2004). Group psychotherapy and related helping groups today: An overview. *American Journal of Psychotherapy*, *58*(3), 265–280. doi:10.1176/appi.psychotherapy.2004.58.3.265

Scherbaum, N., Kluwig, J., Specka, M., Krause, D., Merget, B., Finkbeiner, T., & Gastpar, M. (2005). Group psychotherapy for opiate addicts in methadone maintence treatment—A controlled trial. *European Addiction Research*, *11*(4), 163–171. doi:10.1159/000086397

Schwartz, D. C., Nickow, M. S, Arseneau, R., & Gisslow, M. T. (2015). A substance called food: Long-term psychodynamic group treatment for compulsive overeating. *International Journal of Group Psychotherapy*, *65*(3), 386–409. doi:10.1521/ijgp.2015.65.3.386

Spiegel, D., & Classen, C. (2000). *Group therapy for cancer patients: A research-based handbook of psychosocial care*. New York, NY: Basic Books.

Sripada, R., Bohnert, K., Ganoczy, D., Blow, F., Valenstein, M., & Pfeiffer, P. (2016). Initial group versus individual therapy for post traumatic stress disorder and subsequent follow-up treatment adequacy. *Psychologic Services*, *13*(4), 349–355. doi:10.1037/ser0000077

Steen, S., Vasserman-Stokes, E., & Vannatta, R. (2014). Group cohesion in experiential growth groups. *The Journal for Specialists in Group Work*, *39*(3), 236–256. doi:10.1080/01933922.2014.924343

Tuckerman, B. (1965). Development sequence in small groups. *Psychological Bulletin*, *63*(6), 384–399. doi:10.1037/h0022100

van der Spek, N., Vos, J., van Uden-Kraan, C. F., Breitbart, W., Cuijpers, P., Holtmaat, K., … Verdonck-de Leeuw, I. M. (2017). Efficacy of meaning-centered group psychotherapy for cancer survivors: A randomized controlled trial. *Psychological Medicine*, *47*(1), 1990–2001. doi:10.1017/S0033291717000447

Vinogradov, S., & Yalom, I. D. (1989). *A concise guide to group psychotherapy*. Washington, DC: American Psychiatric Press.

Von Hafften, A. (n.d.). *History of telepsychiatry: The history of synchronous videoconferencing in telepsychiatry* [Video file]. Retrieved from http://psychiatry.org/psychiatrists/practice/telepsychiatry/history-of-telepsychiatry

Weiss, R. D., Jaffee, W. B., de Menil, V. P., & Cogley, C. B. (2004). Group therapy for substance use disorder: What do we know? *Harvard Review Psychiatry*, *12*(6), 339–350. doi:10.1080/10673220490905723

Yalom, I. D., & Leszcz, M. (2005). *The theory and practice of group psychotherapy* (5th ed.). New York, NY: Basic Books.

Family Therapy

Candice Knight

This chapter provides an overview of family therapy for the advanced practice psychiatric nurse (APPN). Highlighting the importance of this therapeutic approach, this chapter defines the family in contemporary society and traces the historical evolution of family therapy, identifying its seminal leaders. Four major family therapy approaches are described in detail, explicating their key concepts, goals, and therapeutic interventions. They are systemic, structural, strategic, and emotionally focused family therapies. Attention is then focused on the practical aspects of conducting family therapy, which includes identifying assessment strategies, developing case conceptualizations, determining common diagnoses, and delivering therapeutic interventions that a beginning-level APPN would be able to employ. Case examples are provided to illustrate conceptualization and intervention. Evidence-based research in family therapy is presented and the chapter concludes with a description of post-master's training and certification programs for family therapy.

WHY IS KNOWLEDGE OF FAMILY THERAPY IMPORTANT FOR THE APPN?

The first master's degree in psychiatric–mental health nursing, inaugurated at Rutgers University in 1952, viewed the primary role of the APPN as providing individual, group, and family therapy. For the next four decades, APPNs became certified as psychiatric clinical nurse specialists (CNSs), gained legitimacy, and honed their skills as psychotherapists (American Nurses Association [ANA], American Psychiatric Nurses Association [APNA], and the International Society of Psychiatric-Mental Health Nurses [ISPN], 2007). With new discoveries in neuroscience in the 1990s, APPNs incorporated the role of prescriptive authority, necessitating more knowledge in pathophysiology, health assessment, and pharmacology. As educational programs added content in these basic sciences, psychotherapy content began to be jettisoned, particularly content in family therapy. Although some programs maintained coursework and practicum experience in family therapy, others diminished family therapy by relegating it to cursory lectures or eliminated the content entirely.

By the late 1990s, the role of the psychiatric nurse practitioner (NP) emerged. Leaders in the field debated whether psychiatric NPs should focus on the biological and psychopharmacological aspects of care while retaining the psychosocial and individual, group, and family psychotherapy aspects of care for the CNS (Knight, 1997a, 1997b, 1998). Eventually, in response to the mental health needs of society as well as the requirements reflected in the *Essentials of Master's Education for Advanced Practice Nursing* document (American Association of Colleges of Nursing [AACN], 1996), the curricula of psychiatric NP and psychiatric CNS programs became more similar than different, with both incorporating a holistic, biopsychosocial model of care. In 2011, a decision was made to have one entry-level role for the APPN, with preparation across the life span. This decision, endorsed by the major professional organizations, essentially combines the best of the psychiatric CNS role and the psychiatric NP role for all new APPNs. By the end of 2014, only one certification existed for all newly certified APPNs, the psychiatric-mental health nurse practitioner (PMHNP-BC; American Nurses Credentialing Center [ANCC], 2012).

With these changes, it is essential to ensure a prominent place for family therapy in the curriculum of programs that educate new APPNs. Family therapy is an important theoretical and psychotherapeutic approach, especially when working with patients across the life span. In the Scope and Standards of Practice for APPNs (ANA, APNA, & ISPN, 2012), family therapy retains its place of importance. In particular, when working with children and adolescents, it is essential for the APPN to consider patients within their family systems. APPNs need to know how to do a comprehensive family assessment, well beyond a basic genogram, as well as know how to assess functional and dysfunctional family patterns, develop accurate family case conceptualizations, and conduct competent family therapy.

An article by Bloch, Sharpe, and Allman (1991) notes that teaching and training in family therapy are required in psychiatry residency programs and integrated into the routine work of child and adolescent psychiatrists. They strongly suggest that family therapy be integrated into the routine work of adult psychiatrists as well. In their study of 50 families, a significant number of identified patients with diverse diagnoses had an underlying issue primarily associated with family dysfunction. These issues encompassed four main categories: (a) separation and individuation issues of young adults who failed to develop, and which were linked to dysfunctional family relational patterns; (b) family difficulties revolving around dysfunctional parental relationships with one or more of the children deeply involved in parental conflict; (c) family structural issues related to poor role differentiation of parents or children and/or inappropriate relational dyads such as a coalition between mother and children with the exclusion of father; and (d) unresolved grief of family members. As with psychiatry, education and training in family therapy are essential for APPN students and need to be included in education and practicum experiences.

Although it is clear that patients' symptoms and problems are caused by many factors, including biological and intrapsychic/interpersonal dynamics, a significant cause also emerges from dysfunctional family patterns. It is essential that APPNs use a multidimensional approach when working with patients, especially children and adolescents. The APPN needs to be able to determine how much of the patient's symptoms and dysfunction have their origin in the family system and how much are caused by other factors. Without knowledge of family therapy, the treatment of patients by the APPN would be extremely narrow in scope, which could have deleterious consequences for the patient.

Family therapy should not be confused with *family-based treatment*, an umbrella term used to characterize a broad range of approaches. Although family-based treatment includes family therapy, it also includes supportive (e.g., groups for families having a mentally ill member), psychoeducational (e.g., parenting skill building), and community-based approaches (e.g., crisis intervention and in-home support services; Diamond & Josephson, 2005). All of these family-based treatment approaches have merit as part of an APPN's knowledge base. In psychiatric nursing education, however, supportive, psychoeducational, and community-based approaches are commonly taught on an undergraduate level. Family therapy, a more difficult and complex therapeutic intervention, is reserved for the APPN and is taught on the graduate level.

Practicing family therapy at a beginning level of competence is not only possible, but necessary for an APPN. Yet, becoming an expert in family therapy takes a great deal of training beyond that which can be provided in a basic APPN program. In-depth training occurs after graduation at training institutes and professional workshops. A recent case example from my private practice illuminates the importance of family therapy for the APPN.

CASE EXAMPLE

Sarah, an adopted, 16-year-old teen, was brought to an outpatient private practice by her parents, who were concerned about their daughter's behavior. Sarah had begun "cutting" 6 months earlier and did not know why she engaged in self-harming behavior. A detailed family assessment revealed that Sarah and her parents had been experiencing a great deal of conflict since Sarah, according to her parents, transformed from being their "nice little girl" to being a difficult, oppositional adolescent who shunned their company, frequented social networking sites, and demanded total independence. The parents, fearful of these changes, began to set stricter limits, believing that they needed to protect Sarah. The parents had little knowledge of adolescent development and felt exceedingly rejected by their daughter and anxious for her safety.

Sarah's mother had a difficult adolescence and as a result of parental neglect, "ran wild," and consequently blundered into significant trauma due to early dating, coupled with the use of alcohol and drugs. Her fear for Sarah was out of proportion to the reality of the situation, and she wanted to control Sarah and protect her from potential harm. Sarah's father, in contrast, came from an inordinately rigid, controlling family system, which allowed little expression of feelings, especially anger. He was very compliant during his adolescence and spent most of his time in academic and athletic pursuits. He had great difficulty with what he viewed as Sarah's lack of respect for her parents. After the first two assessment sessions were completed, Sarah's problems were conceptualized by the APPN from a systems perspective and family therapy was initiated.

Different session configurations were used, that is, initially two sessions were held with the parents to teach them normal adolescent development and help them work through some of their own adolescent issues, followed by two sessions with Sarah to help her develop awareness of her feelings and appropriate feeling management skills. Then followed six family sessions with the focus on developing positive family communication, helping the parents begin the process of "letting go" of Sarah, and helping Sarah express love and anger toward her parents and reattach to them in a healthy, adolescent fashion. Toward the end of therapy, Sarah's self-harming behavior ceased. At the twelfth, termination session, Sarah stated, "When I think about cutting, I just can't imagine that I did that—it seems so ridiculous now."

This case study illustrates the necessity for the APPN to possess knowledge and skills in family therapy. Assessment and intervention would have been incomplete without an in-depth understanding of the family system's role in contributing to the dysfunction exhibited by Sarah. Goldenberg and Goldenberg (2012) take the position that clinicians need to view all symptoms and dysfunctional behavior expressed by an individual patient within the context of the family system. A systems approach certainly does not prohibit the APPN from employing other approaches, but broadens the traditional emphasis from one that is exclusively focused on the individual.

Family therapy is decidedly not a panacea, yet it is a significant theoretical and therapeutic intervention that APPNs need to master in order to practice competently. Without family therapy, understanding patients would necessarily be limited to individual case conceptualization and treatment comprising prescription of psychopharmaceutical agents and/or employing individual psychotherapy approaches. An approach devoid of family therapy would be counterproductive and detrimental to the patient's well-being when the family system is a major piece in the mosaic of the presenting problem.

THE FAMILY IN CONTEMPORARY SOCIETY

The family is the basic unit of structure in social organizations and can be viewed as a unique relational system with complex, well-entrenched interactional patterns. These patterns are determined by many variables, including the parents' values and beliefs, the personalities of its members, and the influence of the extended family and society at large. Families are united by blood or bond, have a shared history and future, and consist of diverse configurations. These configurations include the traditional nuclear family as well as the single-parent, blended, extended, alternative, and institutional family.

The family is the main structure in which children learn what it means to be human within a particular culture. The family transmits cultural values, attitudes, and norms, and serves as a mediator between the needs of its members and the demands of society. It provides nurturance and support and is responsible for developing aspects of the child's personality and socialization skills including how to learn, express thoughts and feelings, behave, adapt to change, and cope with stress.

Although all families are unique, most experts would agree that functional families are characterized by having a solid structure, clear roles, and open communication patterns. They support differentiation and individuation of its members. As families grow and develop, they are flexible and able to adapt to change. Family members love, support, and encourage each other throughout their lives and live together in relative harmony. Dysfunctional families, in contrast, have a paucity of these characteristics. They express their dysfunction in various ways, such as displaying an excessive amount of conflict and mental health problems. These ineffective patterns may be passed down through generations (Beavers & Hampson, 1990; Nichols, 2012).

FAMILY THERAPY

Family therapy, like individual therapy, comprises a diverse group of approaches, each having specific concepts and therapeutic interventions. While individual psychotherapy approaches seek to understand the patient from an intrapsychic, interpersonal, humanistic–existential, or cognitive behavioral perspective, family therapy strives to understand the patient in the context of a system. Individuals are born into families, grow and develop in families, and live most of their lives in families. Therefore, it makes sense that patients are best understood within the context of the family system. A philosophy that unites the various family therapy approaches posits that the source of dysfunction and the unit for change are located within the family. Common underlying assumptions of family therapy can be found in Box 13.1.

In general, family therapy is a brief form of therapy that takes place within eight to 20 sessions. Working directly with the family system usually stimulates rapid change. The main focus in family therapy is on here-and-now interactions within the family system and how these interactions contribute to the development and maintenance of symptoms and dysfunctional patterns. The concepts, goals, and therapeutic techniques are

BOX 13.1 Underlying Assumptions of Family Therapy

- Individuals are best understood in the context of their family system.
- The family as a whole is viewed as the patient rather than the identified patient.
- The family is a unique social system with its own structure and patterns of interaction.
- The behavior of a family member inexorably influences all family members.
- The behavior of the family influences each family member.
- Symptoms are viewed as an expression of dysfunction within the family.
- A family member's problematic behavior may serve a purpose for the family.
- A family member's problematic behavior may be unintentionally maintained by the family.
- Attempts at change are best facilitated by working with the family as a whole.
- Treatment may address the identified patient but the focus is on the family system.
- Gender, race, ethnicity, sexual orientation, and socioeconomic/cultural factors all influence the family system and play an important role in family therapy treatment.

determined by the specific family therapy approach as well as by the needs of the family, which are determined collaboratively.

Family therapy is a viable solution when dysfunction occurs in families and when symptoms occur in one or more family members. The family and its members will greatly benefit when dysfunctional patterns are changed during family therapy. It is common for one family member, usually the healthier member of the adult dyad, to recognize there is a problem and seek psychotherapy. If both adults are willing to enter psychotherapy, the system has a better chance of flourishing. If one member is resistant and unwilling to work on the issues, the system usually will not endure. The resistant member, fearful or incapable of change, commonly will create the same dysfunctional patterns in future family configurations.

Although there are many family therapy approaches that offer a wealth of knowledge for the APPN, this chapter focuses on four popular approaches. These four approaches all use a family systems perspective and view an individual's symptoms and dysfunctional behaviors as a manifestation of a dysfunctional family system. They are systemic family therapy, structural family therapy, strategic family therapy, and emotionally focused family therapy.

EVOLUTION OF FAMILY THERAPY

The family has long been acknowledged as a significant factor in the emotional functioning of its individual members. Theory development and research studies on dysfunctional families date back to Sigmund Freud. In fact, Guerin and Chabot (1997) note that many of Freud's published case studies illustrated dynamic family formulations and treatment approaches such as the phobic problems of Little Hans, who Freud treated by coaching his father. Alfred Adler's emphasis on the importance of the family in the diagnosis and treatment of emotional problems in children led to the Child Guidance Movement in the United States during the 1920s under the influence of Rudolph Dreikurs, a student of Adler (Adler, 1931). Nathan Ackerman, a psychoanalyst and child psychiatrist, published a paper in 1937 on the importance of family-caused mental illness in children and emphasized the need to take both individual and family dynamics into account (Ackerman, 1958). These early pioneers in the family therapy movement were psychoanalysts who modified psychoanalytic theory to include family concepts and experimented with various types of family interventions.

In the late 1940s, a major change in conceptualizing systems was ushered in by Karl Ludwig von Bertalanffy's general system theory (von Bertalanffy, 1968). His theory referred to the self-regulating system found in nature and was applied to many fields including physics, anthropology, biology, and psychology. When applied specifically to mental health problems, individual dynamics were deemphasized and problems were viewed as an expression of dysfunction in family dynamics. By the 1950s, the family therapy movement emerged (Becvar & Becvar, 2008). During this time, psychodynamic, behavioral, and humanistic–existential approaches dominated the field of psychotherapy. They were considered the first, second, and third forces of psychotherapy, respectively. As researchers and clinicians turned their attention to the family as the unit of change, family therapy became recognized as the fourth force of psychotherapy (Corey, 2011).

Early approaches to family therapy were the communication and the contextual approaches. The communications approach was developed in the 1950s by Gregory Bateson, a well-known anthropologist and a group of psychiatrists and psychologists at the Mental Research Institute (MRI) in Palo Alto, CA, including Don Jackson, Jay Haley, John Weakland, and Paul Watzlawick. Their well-known research on feedback loops and cybernetics; double-bind communication in schizophrenic families; and the oft-cited idea that when the identified patient improves, another family member becomes symptomatic, were highly regarded and influenced the early development of family therapy (Guerin & Chabot, 1997).

On the East Coast, at the Eastern Pennsylvania Psychiatric Institute (EPPI) in Philadelphia, Ivan Boszormenyi-Nagi and Paul Framo developed the contextual approach to family therapy in the late 1950s. Their comprehensive model of family therapy integrated individual, interpersonal, existential, and systemic aspects and proposed four dimensions for conducting therapy: (a) genetics, physical health, and historical events; (b) individual psychology; (c) systemic transactions of family rules, power, alignments, and triangles; and (d) relational ethics of trust, justice, reciprocity, fairness, and loyalty (Nichols, 2012).

By the 1960s and 1970s, the family therapy movement became a major treatment modality. New family therapies developed, which are still prominent today, including systemic, structural, strategic, and emotionally focused family therapies. The individuals who developed these approaches became revered leaders in the family therapy movement. Their approaches emerged from working with specific populations such as families with a schizophrenic member (e.g., systems) or acting-out juveniles (e.g., structural). Later, they were adapted to fit many different types of family problems. These four approaches continue to develop conceptually and empirically. The next section describes them in depth.

SYSTEMIC FAMILY THERAPY APPROACH

Overview

Murray Bowen (1913–1990), an American psychiatrist, is the founder of the systemic family therapy approach. He originally trained at the psychoanalytically oriented Menninger Clinic. While there, he experienced much success with patients when he began bringing their families into sessions. In 1954, he became the first director of the Family Division of the National Institute of Mental Health and led a research project in which he studied 18 families having a schizophrenic member over a 5-year period. From 1959 to 1990, as an academician and clinician at Georgetown University, he developed and refined Bowen Family Systems Theory. In 1969, he started the Bowen Family Systems Therapy Family Program, working with families and training therapists in his systemic approach. A transformative paper he presented at a professional meeting in 1967 explicated the emotional processes in his own family, which recognized the need for clinicians to work through the dysfunction in their own families if they were to be effective family therapists (Bowen, 1972). Bowen's theory and therapeutic approach are clearly outlined in his book, *Family Therapy in Clinical Practice* (Bowen, 1978).

Many of Bowen's students became leaders in the field and skillful trainers including Phillip Guerin and Thomas Fogarty of The Center for Family Learning in New Rochelle, NY, known for their work on family triangles (Guerin, Fogarty, Fay, & Kautto, 1996); Monica McGoldrick of the Multicultural Family Institute in Highland Park, NJ, known for her work on gender, ethnicity, and genograms (McGoldrick, 1995; McGoldrick, Gerson, & Petry, 2008; McGoldrick, Pearce, & Giordano, 1982); and Betty Carter of the Family Institute of Westchester, NY, known for her work on feminism, family life cycle, and stages of divorce and remarriage (Carter & McGoldrick, 1980).

With the systems approach, the family is understood when examined within a multi-generational framework. It describes the family as a complex, self-regulating, emotional unit that strives to maintain homeostasis. Accordingly, a change in the functioning of one family member is predictably followed by a reciprocal change in the functioning of other family members. Family systems therapy proposes that dysfunctional systemic factors maintain problems within the family and seek to promote functioning by changing the systemic factors that produce the dysfunction (Bowen, 1978). It represents a combination of the psychodynamic approaches that emphasizes the significance of the past and self-development with systems approaches that focus on intergenerational issues and dysfunctional interacting patterns. Bowen's theory is composed of eight interlocking concepts, six of them addressing emotional processes within the nuclear and extended families and two later concepts addressing processes across generations and in society (Goldenberg & Goldenberg, 2012; Kerr & Bowen, 1988).

Key Concepts

DIFFERENTIATION OF SELF

A person's sense of self, or degree of wholeness, is demonstrated by the ability to separate one's intellectual and emotional functioning. The greater the degree of differentiation, the less a person will be drawn into dysfunctional patterns with other family members. Scales to measure levels of differentiation have been developed (Anderson & Sabatelli, 1992; Skowron & Friedlander, 1998). A differentiated person has a firm sense of self and is individuated from the family, yet in contact with them. He or she has clear values and beliefs and is flexible, goal directed, secure, capable of handling stress, and less reactive to praise or criticism, and can decide important issues deliberately rather than with emotional reactivity and impulsivity. An undifferentiated person has little or no self and is susceptible to family influence, dependent on others for approval, emotionally reactive, impulsive, and vulnerable to stress, and has difficulty maintaining his or her emotional equilibrium.

An *undifferentiated ego mass* is described as a family system with members possessing low levels of differentiation who are "stuck together" in symbiotic relationships. Members have great difficulty individuating, for they are unable to function independently. *Fusion* indicates a blurring between self and other that occurs when two undifferentiated people form a dysfunctional interaction pattern and function as a single emotional system, such as an overfunctioning/underfunctioning pattern (Goldenberg & Goldenberg, 2012).

TRIANGLES

Triangles are three-person systems that manage tension between two people by bringing in a third person. Dyads are inherently unstable, as two people will vacillate between closeness and distance; a triangle can manage more tension (Nichols, 2012). An example would be a couple who has a highly emotional, unresolved argument. Afterward, one person calls his or her best friend to talk about the fight, blaming the partner. Tension is reduced through diversion, yet, the problem between the couple goes unresolved. Undifferentiated people and families with high levels of fusion are likely to triangulate others and be triangulated as well. Family triangles contribute significantly to clinical problems, especially when a child is triangulated by a parent.

MULTIGENERATIONAL TRANSMISSION PROCESS

In this process the transfer of dysfunctional family patterns occurs from one generation to the next. For example, the repeated message to a young girl, "You're just like your grandmother, irresponsible and unable to care for yourself," will transmit this behavioral pattern to the girl and shape her developing sense of self. Genograms are used to elucidate these patterns (Nichols, 2012).

NUCLEAR FAMILY EMOTIONAL SYSTEM

In this system ineffective patterns are used in fused families to cope with family problems and stress. Bowen contends that people select partners with equivalent levels of differentiation; thus, an undifferentiated person will select a spouse who is equally fused to his or her family of origin and attempt to reduce anxiety in one of three ways: (a) overt, chronic, marital conflict with dysfunctional patterns such as overfunctioning/underfunctioning (family anxiety absorbed by husband and wife); (b) emotional dysfunctioning of one partner (anxiety absorbed by a symptomatic partner); or (c) psychological impairment in a child (banding together to focus attention on the child; Bowen, 1978). The novice therapist often focuses on the underfunctioning spouse, the dysfunctional spouse, or the impaired child rather than recognize it is a problem with differentiation for both spouses.

FAMILY PROJECTION PROCESS

In this process parental undifferentiation is transmitted to the children. The child, serving as an emotional extension of the parents, is fused and triangulated to the parents, has a low level of differentiation, and has difficulty separating from the parents. Usually the child targeted is the most emotionally vulnerable and unprotected, regardless of birth order. Other children in the family may have higher levels of differentiation.

EMOTIONAL CUTOFF

This process involves reducing or cutting off emotional contact with family members in order to manage anxiety and conflict. As an adult, the person may cut off completely, separate geographically (moving far distances), or put up psychological barriers (superficial, inauthentic, brief contact). He or she may appear to be independent from family members, but is arrested emotionally at the time of the cutoff. Emotional cutoff reduces anxiety but creates isolation and undue emotional significance to subsequent relationships. Reattachment to one's family of origin must occur in order to become a healthy, differentiated adult (Bowen, 1978).

SIBLING POSITION

The sibling position is the functional position in the family hierarchy that each child holds, which predicts certain roles, functions, and personality characteristics. This may reflect the order of birth but is more related to the person's functional position in the family. Bowen wrote of 10 positions and suggested that the more closely a marriage duplicates one's sibling place in childhood, the more successful it will be. For example, an oldest child who marries a youngest will feel comfortable taking on more responsibility and decision-making. Two youngest children who marry may both feel overburdened by responsibility, while two oldest children may be overly competitive because each will want to be in charge (Bowen, 1978).

Goals of Therapy

The most important goal of family systems therapy is to help family members increase their level of self-differentiation, especially the adult couple. Differentiation results in rewarding emotional contact within the family and across generations. Undifferentiation results in emotional fusion, cutoffs, and transmission of dysfunctional patterns. Other goals are to reduce emotional turmoil in the family as well as detriangulate three-person systems (Nichols, 2012).

Psychotherapeutic Interventions: Assessment

In a systems approach, the therapist begins the session by asking each member his or her perception of the problem. The therapist assumes a neutral and objective role. In this approach, it is crucial for the therapist to be differentiated from his or her own family system; otherwise, the therapist may be triangulated into family conflicts, take sides, and project his or her unresolved issues onto family members. The therapist assesses the degree of emotional functioning and intensity of emotional processes. What is the degree of dysfunction? What are the stressors? How differentiated are the members? Do triangles exist? Are emotional cutoffs operating? Is one spouse more dysfunctional? What are the multigenerational patterns?

An important tool used by systemic therapists is the genogram, a three-generational, graphic diagram of family processes that is constructed during the assessment phase of therapy. It is an interpretive tool used to identify patterns, generate hypotheses, and obtain a significant amount of information about the evolution of family problems in a condensed period. A joint family genogram or separate genogram on each family member (common in couple therapy) can be drawn on a sheet of paper or drawn on a flip chart. The flip chart allows everyone in the family to observe the construction of the genogram and begin to understand the dysfunctional processes and how they are handed down from generation to generation. Standard symbols are used to depict gender, dates (e.g., birth, separation, marriage, and death), important life events, illnesses, and occupational roles as well as emotional processes among family members such as conflict, closeness, coalitions, cutoffs, and triangles. A picture of a basic genogram can be found in Chapter 3, Assessment and Diagnosis, of this text. An in-depth look at constructing genograms can be found in the text *Genograms: Assessment and Intervention* by McGoldrick et al. (2008). Several online software programs are also available to assist in creating a genogram. See www.smartdraw.com/downloads or www.genopro.com/genogram/how-to-create. Some sample questions that are commonly asked by system therapists in constructing the genogram are included in Box 13.2.

BOX 13.2 Comments and Sample Questions for Constructing a Genogram

- It would be helpful to take some time to learn who the people are in your family in order to better understand your family and the current problems. What I like to do is diagram the family over three generations.
- Who are the members of your family?
- What are their ages and birth and/or death dates?
- What are other characteristics (e.g., marriage/divorce, ethnicity, occupation, key events)?
- Give two or three adjectives for each member.
- What is your relationship with each family member? Has it changed over time?
- Who are you closest to and most distant from?
- Are there any members who are emotionally cut off from each other?
- How and when did emotional cutoffs occur?
- Are there any family secrets?
- What are the family scripts (messages given to members)?

The therapist also assesses the level of differentiation of each family member and identifies family triangles and multigenerational transmission processes as well as dysfunctional emotional processes and interactional patterns. The therapist offers feedback during this process (e.g., "I notice that what attracted you to each other are Jim's solid, responsible qualities and Megan's warm, emotional qualities, which are similar to parental patterns in your respective families of origin").

Psychotherapeutic Interventions: Psychotherapy Techniques

Once the genogram is complete, session configurations are determined. The therapist may choose to meet with individual family members, different dyads, or the entire family. It is common in this approach to meet with the adult dyad or the most differentiated family member for a period of time. Bowen believed that if one person is motivated to work on differentiation, the other family members will inevitably improve. There is less attention focused on the presenting problem and more on increasing levels of differentiation and decreasing emotional turmoil (Kerr & Bowen, 1988). The following are interventions used in this approach.

PROMOTE SELF-STATEMENTS

Assist members to differentiate by helping them identify their own beliefs by using first-person pronouns. The therapist encourages family members to use self-defining "I-position" statements to help separate their own emotions and beliefs from the family. When even one person begins to take "I-stands," other members inevitably do so as well.

TRANSFORM DYSFUNCTIONAL GENERATIONAL PATTERNS

Identify and change dysfunctional multigenerational patterns. For example, the therapist who is working with the adult female of the dyad may say, "I notice that the women in your family overfunction and marry men who are irresponsible and underfunction." The therapist would begin to question ways in which these patterns can be changed and would begin a line of questioning, "Would you like to change this pattern in your marriage? How does this pattern affect you? What could you do differently?"

DECREASE ANXIETY AND INTERRUPT CONFLICT

Reduce high anxiety and high levels of conflict, for they prevent differentiation and cause more emotional fusion. Sessions are controlled and cerebral. Each family member talks to the therapist rather than directly to each other. The therapist minimizes blame and interrupts confrontation while modeling skills of problem-solving and conflict resolution. Family members are encouraged to listen, think about the situation, externalize what they are thinking, and control their emotional reactivity. Calm questioning is used by the therapist to defuse emotion and force the partners to think about the issues causing their difficulty. The therapist may ask, "What part do you think you may play in this pattern?"

DETRIANGULATE

Neutralize triangles by having family members speak directly to one another, rather than a third person. For example, the therapist might direct a member to speak directly to another by stating, "Can you tell him that directly?" A therapist might attempt to remove an adult patient from an intense, emotional triangle with his or her parents by arranging a solo visit by the patient to the parents' home but with a very structured plan of detriangulation.

REPAIR CUTOFFS

Reestablish connection with other family members and repair cutoffs. This is crucial in this approach. The therapist may also invite a cutoff member to attend a session in order to bring the person back into the family.

DISRUPT NUCLEAR FAMILY EMOTIONAL PROCESSES

Use process questions to interrupt dysfunctional patterns. For example, the therapist may use a statement such as, "I notice you do the tasks that your husband agreed to do but has not, and this frustrates you." The therapist may ask members to try out different interactional patterns (Goldenberg & Goldenberg, 2012).

STRUCTURAL FAMILY THERAPY APPROACH

Overview

The structural family therapy approach was developed by Salvadore Minuchin (1921–2017), an extremely creative, much loved therapist, known for his mastery of technique. Minuchin was originally a psychoanalytically trained psychiatrist who studied with Nathan Ackerman; received psychoanalytic training at the Alanson White Institute; and worked with troubled youths at the Wiltwyck School for Boys in New York City in the late 1950s and early 1960s. Realizing the limitations of psychoanalytic methods for treating these disadvantaged boys, he and a group of colleagues developed new methods of working with the boys and their families, which later evolved into structural family therapy. After becoming the director of the Philadelphia Child Guidance Clinic in 1965, he and his colleagues published the groundbreaking text, *Families of the Slums: An Exploration of Their Structure and Treatment* (Minuchin, Montalvo, Guerney, Rosman, & Schumer, 1967), and later his classic text, *Families and Family Therapy* (Minuchin, 1974). Under Minuchin's direction, the Philadelphia Child Guidance Clinic became one of the world's foremost family therapy training centers. In 1976, Minuchin stepped down as director of the clinic and started his own center in New York City, where he continued to practice and train family therapists until 1996. Although recently deceased, the legacy of his work continues by well-known structural family therapists including Harry Aponte, Michael Nichols, and Braulio Montalvo (Nichols, 2012).

The structural family therapy approach believes that symptoms and family problems are embedded in a dysfunctional family organization. It offers a framework to address problems by focusing on the structure and substructure as well as the imperceptible rules, coalitions, power structures, communication patterns, and boundaries that operate within a dysfunctional system. Minuchin believed that what distinguishes a functional family is not the absence of problems, but lack of an effective organizational structure to handle problems when they arise (Minuchin, 1974).

Key Concepts

FAMILY STRUCTURE

An invisible set of functional, recurrent patterns that organize the way family members relate to one another, structure defines and stabilizes the family. It includes aspects such as family roles and rules, hierarchy and power structures, communication patterns, and decision-making functions.

SUBSYSTEMS

These smaller units carry out necessary tasks for the functioning of the overall family system. They are determined by generation, age, sex, spousal relationship, interest, and function. They may include the spousal subsystem (wife and husband), parental subsystem (mother and father), sibling subsystem (children), and extended family subsystem (grandparents and other relatives). Family members belong to a number of different subsystems that help in the process of individuation and organize the way members relate to one another.

BOUNDARIES

Boundaries are physical or invisible emotional barriers that protect the integrity of individual members, subsystems, and families. They function to regulate contact, maintain individual identity, modulate emotional closeness, define rules of relating, and regulate the flow of resources and information within the family and the outside environment. Boundaries should be clear and flexible, allowing members to attain a sense of personal identity and connection within the family, without undue interference (Minuchin, 1974).

ENMESHED FAMILY

In this extreme pattern of family organization boundaries are diffuse and permeable, resulting in a denial of differences and loss of personal autonomy. Family members are overly dependent on one another. Interactions among members are intense with an overload of communication and emotions and a great deal of bickering. Parents are overly intrusive and protective, hindering the competency development of their children. Family conflicts revolve around issues of power and control with parents fearful of losing control and children vying for more control. Some examples include (a) excessive involvement in children's minor conflict, not allowing them the opportunity to solve their own problems; (b) a family becoming overwrought because a child brings home a poor grade; (c) a mother who tells her 9-year-old daughter the details of her marital problems and asks for advice; and (d) a parent reading a child's text messages. As families grow, boundaries for closeness and distance change.

DISENGAGED FAMILY

In this extreme pattern of family organization boundaries are rigid and impermeable, resulting in a heightened sense of personal autonomy and independence. Family members are so disconnected that they seem unaware of their impact on each other. There is usually a scarcity of communication, limited support, and interpersonal isolation. Family structure and parental authority are weak. Parents are often immature and overwhelmed with the parental role. Family members are oblivious to the effects of their actions on one another. It is common for members to be dependent on outside systems with little interpersonal engagement within the family. An example would be little involvement with a child who has a serious academic problem or a significant psychological problem.

COALITION

A coalition is a dysfunctional alliance between two family members against a third. There are several types of coalitions. A cross-generational coalition exists when a parent and child side against a third member of the family. A schism coalition exists when a child joins one parent of two warring spouses and the joined parent devalues the other parent to the child. In a skewed coalition one spouse overfunctions for an underfunctioning spouse in order to preserve the marriage and family.

PARENTIFICATION

Parentification is a form of role reversal wherein a child is given the power and authority that appropriately belong to the parents. The child is put in a position of meeting the emotional or physical needs of the parent or other children. This can occur in many types of situations such as when a parent is irresponsible or neglectful. It is common with addiction or other forms of mental illness. The child willingly accepts the role because it brings with it power and status; however, it is very detrimental to the child. Ultimately, the child is unable to perform the role adequately, increasing his or her anxiety and guilt as well as lowering self-esteem. The child also cannot develop normal peer relationships, resulting in social deprivation (Nichols, 2012).

Goals of Therapy

The most important goal of structural family therapy is to create an effective family structure with functional subsystems and clear boundaries. A strong parental hierarchy is stressed with parents having the necessary power and control. Communication is open and direct, rules are fair, roles are flexible, and decision-making is productive. In this way, the family has the capacity to handle problems when they arise (Minuchin, 1974).

Psychotherapeutic Interventions: Assessment

In a structural approach, the focus is not on the presenting problem but on assessing dysfunction in overall structure, subsystems, boundaries, power structures, and communication patterns. The therapist begins by first asking the parents what they believe the problem to be, respecting the parental hierarchy. Each person is encouraged to participate, but without insistence of a response. The therapist joins, accommodates, and affiliates with the family. Joining is a process of uniting empathically with the family, temporarily becoming part of the system, and forming a therapeutic system in which each family member accepts the therapist as someone who is influential and can bring about change. Accommodating is adjusting and adapting to the family's affective style, language patterns, and interactive style by actually emulating these aspects of the family to solidify the alliance. Affiliating is connecting to family members by making positive, confirming statements to help build self-esteem and allow others to see that person in a new light as well as by making negative statements about a family member while absolving that person of responsibility for the behavior. Minuchin and Fishman (1981) give the following examples of affiliating:

> To a child, the therapist might say: "You seem to be quite childish. How did your parents manage to keep you so young?" To an adult, the therapist could say: "You act very dependent on your spouse. What does she do to keep you incompetent?" (p. 34)

Psychotherapeutic Interventions: Psychotherapy Techniques

After joining with family members, the therapist continues to work with the entire family. He or she rarely sees individual members alone or in separate dyads.

ENACTMENTS

Enactments involve acting out dysfunctional transactional patterns within the family therapy session. Families are directed by the therapist to demonstrate how they have dealt with a particular problem. This spotlights the structural dysfunctions in the family. For example, if the family identifies a great deal of fighting in their structure, the therapist might ask the family to choose a recent issue they fought about at home and demonstrate how it unfolded in the session. With the enactment, the therapist may notice a weak parental hierarchy, a child with too much power, or a couple involved in a pursuer/distancer pattern.

Videotaping an enactment and watching the tape together give the family a chance to see how they interact and come up with possible solutions. Viewing a family snapshot and placing the family in the same dysfunctional positions and then changing them to a healthy configuration in the session is another example. Another technique is to have the family plan an event, noticing the dysfunctional patterns and then modifying them (Minuchin, 1974).

STRUCTURAL MAPPING

Commenting on what went wrong within the enactment and reframing the problem in the context of the family's structure, the therapist maps the family structure with simple symbols and helps the family broaden the problem from the identified patient to an inadequate structure. These diagrams are useful in hypothesizing family functioning and forming goals for structural change. For example, boundaries are often mapped as follows:

Rigid boundary (disengagement) _____
Diffuse boundary (enmeshment) ....
Clear boundary (normal range) _ _ _ _ _ _ _ _ _ _

For a complete understanding of family mapping, examples can be found in Minuchin's text, *Families and Family Therapy* (Minuchin, 1974).

MODIFYING PROBLEMATIC INTERACTIONS

This process involves restructuring the system and modifying the dysfunctional interactions observed during an enactment by using forceful interventions. The therapist, as the architect of the interventions, creates intense interventions, while not provoking or shaming family members. Some interventions to modify interactions are:

- **Boundary making.** The therapist tries to change the distance between enmeshed or disengaged subsystems. Two examples are:
  - An enmeshed father and daughter sit next to each other and frequently exchange looks and laughter, while ignoring the mother, who asks them frequently, "What did you just say?" The therapist asks the mother and father to change seats so that the mother is next to the daughter and the enmeshed father and daughter have more distance.
  - A disengaged family attempts to deal with their 12-year-old daughter who failed three courses by shrugging and saying, "What can we do? It's her life." The parents are challenged to come up with three possible solutions to the problem that would create conflict.
- **Unbalancing.** The therapist tries to change the hierarchical relationships of a subsystem. Two examples are:
  - A 15-year-old male patient requests an extended curfew and each time he begins to speak, the mother interrupts, attempting to convince the boy that his request is unreasonable, while the father sits there uninvolved. The therapist sets a 3-minute timer and tells the boy to argue his point for 3 minutes without any interruptions. He is then asked to leave the room while the parents are instructed to come up with a solution together. After 10 minutes, the son returns to the session and the father is asked to inform the son of their joint decision.
  - Two school-age children, ages 7 and 9, refuse to pay attention to their parents' requests that they comport themselves in a less unruly fashion in session. The children are asked to leave the room while the therapist helps to strengthen the parental subsystem, which is very weak.
- **Tracking.** The therapist follows a theme identified from communication and uses it deliberately in conversation with the family. An example is a phrase a 10-year-old boy stated early in the assessment, which was, "I don't want to receive any *low blows* in here." Tracking the phrase, the therapist discovers that a common way the family communicates is by humiliating comments. The therapist closely tracks these undermining comments and when they occur, helps members communicate kindly.
- **Reframing.** The therapist recasts the problem in a new light in order to modify interactions and provide a different perspective. For example, a 12-year-old daughter is described by her parents as difficult. After listening to them squabble, the therapist said, "Is this what happens when the three of you try to communicate with each other?" The problem is reframed as a systems problem rather than as an individual problem within the daughter.
- **Shaping competence.** The therapist reinforces new, desirable patterns by praising the family members for their success. For example, the therapist states, "That was terrific that you were able to work together and present a united front to your child."

The therapist recognizes the dysfunctional structure in this approach and intervenes in a directive fashion to modify the problematic interactions. Further structural techniques can be found in the text *Family Therapy Techniques* by Minuchin and Fishman (1981).

STRATEGIC FAMILY THERAPY APPROACH

Overview

The strategic family therapy movement is derived from the work on feedback loops, double binds, cybernetics, homeostasis, and circular causality by Bateson and his colleagues at the Mental Research Institute (MRI) when they studied faulty communication patterns in families with schizophrenic members (Nichols, 2012). Their classic text, *Pragmatics of Human Communication* (Watzlawick, Beavin, & Jackson, 1967), focused on the study of pragmatics (the behavioral consequences of communication). They came up with a number of axioms regarding the interpersonal nature of communication including: (a) all behavior is communication; (b) communication occurs simultaneously at the metacommunication level (gesture, body language, tone of voice, posture, and intensity) and the content (surface) level; and (c) problems develop and are maintained within the context of dysfunctional interactive patterns and recursive feedback loops. The model emphasized that the solutions people use in attempting to alleviate a problem often contribute to the problem's maintenance or even its exacerbation.

In the 1980s, the strategic family therapy approach took center stage. Its leaders were Jay Haley and Cloe Madanes at the Family Therapy Institute in Washington, DC (Madanes, 1981) and later Mara Selvini Palazzoli, Luigi Boscolo, Gianfranco Cecchin, and Guliana Prata of the Milan, Italy group (Selvini Palazzoli, Boscolo, Cecchin, & Prata, 1978).

In addition to cybernetics, it also incorporated Milton Erickson's work with paradoxical and solution-generating interventions and structural family therapy's emphasis on family organization. Jay Haley integrated the Communication Theory of MRI with the work of structural family therapy and Ericksonian hypnosis.

Strategic family therapy believes that dysfunctional family patterns of behavior are deeply embedded within the family. Families maintain and perpetuate these patterns by their own actions, which are misguided attempts to solve the problem. The therapist identifies the sequence that keeps the repetitive patterns deeply entrenched within the system and uses provocative, strategic interventions to change the dysfunctional patterns (Haley, 1976).

Key Concepts

CYBERNETICS

Cybernetics is the theoretical study of control processes in a system, especially the analysis of the flow of information in a system through feedback loops and how it regulates a system.

HOMEOSTASIS

Homeostasis is a dynamic state of equilibrium or balance within a system. Families are believed to seek such a state in an effort to ensure a stable environment.

FEEDBACK LOOPS

Feedback loops are circular processes by which information about a system's output is continuously reintroduced back into the system, initiating a chain of subsequent events.

CIRCULAR CAUSALITY

In this view causality is nonlinear, occurring instead within a relationship context and by means of a network of interacting loops; any cause is thus seen as an effect of a prior cause. All families encounter difficulties, but whether they become problematic depends on the response of family members. Families often make cogent but misguided attempts to solve their problems, and when they persist they apply more of the same erroneous solutions. This produces an escalation of the problem and more of the same repeating cycles (Nichols, 2012).

FIRST-ORDER CHANGES

These changes are superficial behavioral changes within a system that do not change the structure of the system itself. For example, suppose the family makes a decision to stop shouting at each another. The underlying systemic rules governing the interaction between them have not changed, so the attempt to stop shouting will be violated sooner or later.

SECOND-ORDER CHANGES

These in-depth behavioral changes require a fundamental revision of the system's structure and function. An example would be changing the rules of the family system and reorganizing the system so that it reaches a different level of functioning rather than just calling a stop to shouting (Goldenberg & Goldenberg, 2012).

Goals of Therapy

The goal in strategic family therapy is to alter problematic patterns of behavior that maintain the family dysfunction by using strategic directives, also known as behavioral tasks. The belief is that the problem-maintaining sequences and cycles can be disrupted and extinguished by these strategic directives and replaced by functional sequences (Haley, 1976).

Psychotherapeutic Interventions: Assessment

The therapeutic relationship in this approach is empathic and collaborative. The therapist poses questions to help define the problem completely. Each member is asked to articulate a description of the problem in great detail. The therapist may say, "If we had a videotape of the problem, what would it look like?" The assessment stage demands a complete understanding of the problem by the therapist and the family members. The therapist then determines how the family has attempted a solution, recognizing that the attempted solution more than likely has contributed to maintaining and worsening the problem. The therapist, in collaboration with the family, determines goals to solve the problem.

Psychotherapeutic Interventions: Psychotherapy Technique

The intervention is known as the task-setting stage of therapy and is brief. Here, the therapist concludes the session by suggesting a directive, which is a concrete, tailored, behavioral task the family can do outside of therapy to break their entrenched dysfunctional cycle and outmaneuver resistance. The therapist is collaborative and compassionate in giving the directive and frequently asks, "Is this okay?" "Are you willing to do this?" The therapy is viewed as a staging area with directives typically taking place outside the session in the family's real-life situation. The directives are often provocative and paradoxical. Further therapy sessions seek to determine the outcome of the given directive, gain further understanding of the family's problems and their maintaining sequences, and develop further directives. The following are examples of common directives used in this approach.

PLACE THE PROBLEM UNDER THE FAMILY'S CONTROL

Have the family control the problem rather than have the problem control the family. The therapist gives a specific directive as to how long family members are to discuss the problem, whom they are to discuss it with, and how long these discussions should last. As members carry out the directive, they develop a sense of control over the problem, which helps them deal with it effectively.

PARADOXICAL TECHNIQUE

Do a seemingly illogical intervention that runs counter to common sense. The directive entails a maneuver that is in apparent contradiction to the goals of therapy, yet is designed to bring about positive change (Haley & Richeport-Haley, 2007). Major types include prescribing the symptom or problem, restraining change, and exaggerating the problem. An example of prescribing the symptom would be to ask the patient to do more of the symptom or problem such as to fight more or be more negative. In restraining change, an example would be for the therapist to ask the couple or family not to change. In exaggerating the problem, an example would be for the therapist to ask the patient to amplify the problem.

PRETEND TECHNIQUES

Ask a symptomatic person to pretend to exhibit symptoms, reclassifying them as voluntary and not genuine. An example would be to ask an anxious patient to pretend to be anxious. This in turn alters the family's response, for they do not know whether the symptoms are real when the symptomatic person expresses them. Another pretend technique is to ask the patient to do something he or she would not ordinarily do. An example would be to ask someone very neat and compulsive to pretend that he or she is messy.

ORDEALS

Direct patient to engage in mildly noxious activities if they engage in the symptomatic or problematic behavior. The consequences for the behavior become more difficult and time consuming than they are worth. For example, a teenager who has a very disrespectful attitude will have to, after each episode of disrespect, engage in a lengthy process with the family, where everyone, in great detail, expresses how they feel about his or her behavior.

RITUALS

Perform a series of actions according to a prescribed order that gives members a sense of belonging and togetherness. For example, the family is directed to exaggerate a family ritual such as preparing and eating a meal together in a specific order.

INVARIANT PRESCRIPTION

Break up existing dysfunctional interactional sequences with a new sequence. For example, in a family with an unhealthy coalition, the parents are encouraged to form a secret alliance and sneak away, without informing the children of their departure or return. This new pattern unites the parents and helps the children relinquish inappropriate roles.

EMOTIONALLY FOCUSED FAMILY THERAPY APPROACH

Overview

Emotionally focused family therapy (EFT) is a short-term (10–15 sessions), experiential, evidence-based approach to couple and family therapy, rooted in the humanistic–existential school. It was developed by Leslie Greenberg and Sue Johnson, two Canadian psychologists, in the mid-1980s. EFT was derived from emotion-focused therapy, an individual approach to psychotherapy. Although it has many similarities to emotion-focused therapy, this therapy also includes systems theory and attachment theory and works predominantly with helping couples and families communicate from an in-depth emotional level and fully connect with each other.

As a doctoral student of Leslie Greenberg, Sue Johnson worked with couples in distress. She realized these couples were caught in negative cycles of interactions that kept them stuck and unable to resolve their conflicts. Using theories of attachment and theories of emotions, Greenberg and Johnson developed a treatment to help distressed couples. They believed that basic attachment issues and interrupted emotions were underneath these negative cycles of interactions. Later, the approach was applied to families.

EFT has become immensely popular in the past few years and has revitalized the central role of emotion in couple and family psychotherapy. Greenberg and Johnson and others have carried out extensive evidence-based process and outcome research studies. EFT is currently the most empirically validated couple and family therapy to date. The approach has been manualized, which is useful for beginning-level practitioners (Greenberg & Johnson, 1988; Johnson & Greenberg, 1995).

Experiential couple and family therapy emerged in the 1960s, preceding Greenberg and Johnson. The early founders were Carl Whitaker (1912–1995) and Virginia Satir (1916–1988), two enormously engaging and intuitive clinicians lauded as the most influential early leaders of the family therapy movement. Whitaker's Symbolic-Experiential Family Therapy Model and Satir's Human Validation Process Model saw the family as a dynamic, interactive system that could be reshaped to achieve deep levels of intimacy. Experiential interventions focused on the expression of feelings and authentic communication and included role plays, Gestalt experiments, guided awareness, psychodrama, creative arts, and communication training (Napier & Whitaker, 1966; Satir, 1964; Satir & Baldwin, 1983; Whitaker & Bumberry, 1988). Whitaker and Satir were criticized for their lack of conceptual and therapeutic precision as well as lack of empirical research. Nevertheless, they continue to be praised today for their extraordinary presence, inspirational brilliance, and unique contributions to the field. Gus Napier continues to train therapists in Whitaker's approach in Atlanta, Georgia. Satir's work lives on in her numerous writings, training institutes, and DVDs.

During the 1970s, Walter Kempler, Sonia Nevis, and Joseph Zinker of the Gestalt Institute of Cleveland expanded Gestalt therapy to include couples and families and developed a Gestalt Family Therapy Model that integrated family systems therapy with Gestalt therapy. Their experiential approach helps families experience issues in the here and now, release blocked emotions, and increase awareness and contact within and among family members. Gestalt family therapy, although rich in theory, was also criticized for its lack of therapeutic precision.

EFT is a humanistic–existential, structured approach to working with couples and families that integrates attachment theory, person-centered therapy, Gestalt therapy, systems theory, and neuroscience theory of emotions. EFT emphasizes helping couples and families explore their moment-to-moment inner experiences in order to strengthen their emotional attachments. The therapy helps couples and families connect with their primary, core emotions, viewed as central to the development of secure attachment bonds.

EFT believes that couples and families in distress are caught in negative interaction patterns (e.g., pursuing–distancing, attacking–withdrawing, dominance–submission, and rage–shame) that limit contact with one another and create emotional distance. Couples and families conceal their primary emotions (genuine, authentic) and rather display secondary emotions (defensive, reactive), which serve to create the negative interaction patterns. Over time, members fear revealing their primary emotions and attachment bonds are further weakened. In this approach, an empathically attuned therapeutic relationship is used to help couples access primary emotions, strengthen attachment bonds, and change their negative interactional patterns (Greenberg & Johnson, 1988).

Key Concepts

EMOTIONS

Emotion is an affective state of information processing that informs a person of important needs, prepares the self for action, and creates strong attachment bonds. Emotions may be primary or secondary. Primary emotions are the fundamental, initial emotional reactions in response to a situation, such as sadness in response to a loss or anger in response to an attack. Secondary emotions are emotional reactions to thoughts or feelings, rather than to the situation itself, such as feeling guilty about feeling angry. The therapist particularly focuses on emotions because they so potently organize key responses in intimate relationships. Negative emotional responses, such as frustration, if not attended to and restructured, undermine the repair of a couple's relationship, whereas softer emotions, such as expressions of vulnerability, can be used to create new patterns of interaction. From a systemic point of view, emotions are viewed as the primary element in the organization of the couple's relationship (Johnson, 1996).

ATTACHMENT STYLES

These styles involve emotional bonds in relationships that are maintained by responsiveness, accessibility, and engagement. Secure attachment occurs when people can express primary emotions, while insecure attachment occurs when primary emotions cannot be accessed. Insecure attachment occurs when people conceal their primary emotions and display secondary emotions. Four attachment styles have been described by Johnson and Sims (2000):

1. Secure attachment—People who are secure perceive themselves as lovable. They are able to trust self and others in relationships. They are able to be vulnerable and express their needs and feelings in relationships.
2. Insecure attachment—People who have a diminished ability to express their needs and feelings and tend to discount their need for attachment. They tend to adopt a position of safe distance and solve problems by themselves without understanding the effect they have on their partners.
3. Anxious attachment—People who are psychologically reactive exhibit anxious attachment and are inclined to demand reassurance in an aggressive and controlling way, frequently blaming and manipulating in order to engage their partner.
4. Vacillating attachment—People who have been traumatized frequently fluctuate between attachment and hostility. They are typically reactive and they vacillate with frequency.

ATTACHMENT INJURIES

An attachment injury is an emotional injury that is experienced in a couple relationship. The injury is generally characterized as abandonment, betrayal, or violation of trust

(Johnson & Whiffen, 1999). An attachment injury can range from infidelity to feelings of abandonment, such as when one partner is unresponsive to the other for the kind of support that is expected of attachment figures during a time of need, life transition, illness, or loss. These injuries, if unresolved, damage the nature of the attachment bond and sometimes prevent the repair of the bond. Some partners may have endured insecure attachment bonds over a period of years and then one incident exacerbates this distress and acts as a symbolic marker of insecure attachment for the injured partner. Other couples may have a relatively secure bond and this kind of incident marks the beginning of their relational distress. Much depends on how the injured partner interprets the injury and how the other spouse responds to expressions of hurt by the injured party. When the other spouse discounts, denies, or dismisses the injury, this prevents the processing of the event in the relationship and compounds the injury. The unresolved event may be the topic of constant bickering or it may lay dormant and unexpressed for a period of time until it reemerges in the here and now when a current incident evokes an emotional response related to the initial injury. A sudden increase in the emotional intensity of the couple's interaction is a marker that alerts the therapist that the couple is dealing with an attachment injury (Johnson, Makinen, & Makinen, 2001).

Goals of Therapy

The primary goals of EFT are to expand constricted emotional responses that create negative interaction patterns, restructure interactions so that partners become more accessible and responsive to each other, and foster positive cycles of comfort and caring. Couples are helped to access their authentic emotions, transform negative interactional patterns, and strengthen attachment bonds. This is achieved within an empathically attuned therapeutic relationship (Greenberg & Johnson, 1988).

Assessment

Assessment is described as the first phase of therapy and usually takes two sessions. There are no genograms or other tools used in EFT. During this phase, the therapist creates a comfortable and supportive environment for the couple to have an open discussion about any hesitations they may have about therapy. A strong therapeutic relationship is developed based on the patient-centered work of Carl Rogers, emphasizing empathy, congruence, and authenticity. The problematic interactional patterns that maintain attachment insecurity and relationship distress are identified as well as the primary emotions underlying these patterns. There is a reframing and summarizing of the problematic interactional patterns and the attachment needs so that the couple is no longer victim of the patterns but allies against them in the pursuit of positive attachment patterns (Greenberg, 2002, 2010; Greenberg & Johnson, 1988).

Psychotherapy Techniques

A central belief in EFT is the premise that positive interaction patterns follow from the attainment of an experience of emotional bonding between the partners during therapy. This occurs when primary emotions can be expressed and responded to during the therapeutic relationship. Change is achieved through the facilitation of three sequential movements:

- Deescalation of the conflict between the partners involves the progressive unfolding of the experience that each partner has in the relationship and the clarification of the interactive cycle between them.

- Reengagement of the withdrawing or submissive partner in the relationship involves that partner identifying and owning, in the presence of the other, his or her primary emotional experience in the relationship.
- Softening involves dominant or pursuing partners owning and expressing their primary vulnerability such as the experience of being unlovable or the shame that lies beneath the controlling behavior or critical demands.

Interventions used in EFT are for the purpose of accessing core emotions and developing positive attachment patterns (Johnson, 2002, 2004).

EMPATHIC ATTUNEMENT

Throughout therapy, the therapist attempts to empathically attune to each partner and connect on a deep personal level. The therapist is concerned not with evaluating the patient's comments as they relate to truth, but to make contact with the patient's subjective world. Each member's experience is closely followed empathically. The therapist speaks slowly, calmly, and patiently, checking frequently with the patient to make sure he or she is understood and engaged (Johnson, 1996).

REFLECTIVE STATEMENTS

These statements reflect the deeper, primary emotions that a person possibly experiences based on a comment made by another. For example, a wife makes a comment, "A part of me wants a divorce." The husband is silent and looks afraid and the therapist comments to him, "It seems you are feeling terribly scared by the comment your spouse made. Is that correct?" This helps the husband access the primary emotion and for the wife to understand his emotional response.

EVOCATIVE QUESTIONS

These questions are used to evoke deeper, primary emotions that are not experienced directly. For example, a husband states, "She is never home. She always is working or out with her friends." The therapist comments, "What's happening *now for you as you say that?*" This draws attention to the deeper emotions.

CREATIVE IMAGES AND METAPHORS

These representations are evoked to capture an elusive emotional experience. For example, a patient states that she cannot speak when her husband voices anger toward her. The therapist comments, "It feels like a noose around your throat that is strangling you."

ENCOURAGING ACCEPTANCE

When a family member begins to express deeper emotions and needs, the therapist encourages other family members to be supportive and receptive to this new openness. For example, a husband expresses deep sadness about a job loss. The wife perceives him in a new way, "I didn't know how *sad* you are, for I've only seen your anger. I see you need my caring."

CREATING INTIMATE ATTACHMENTS

The couple recognizes and expresses their attachment and consolidates a new emotional position. In the example above, the husband states, "I do need your love and caring for I am going through a rough time." And, she states, "I am able to do this for I see I am needed by you." At times, the therapist needs to assist the couple in creating new attachment patterns.

PRACTICAL ASPECTS OF FAMILY THERAPY FOR THE APPN

Four approaches to family therapy have been described in this chapter. Systemic, structural, strategic, and emotionally focused family therapies all use a family systems perspective and view an individual's symptoms and dysfunctional behaviors as a manifestation of a dysfunctional family system. Table 13.1 compares these four approaches, articulating their leaders, key concepts, and key interventions. The reader is referred to original texts as well as research articles in these approaches in the references listed at the end of the chapter.

The following section gives practical information for the beginning-level APPN. These suggestions are drawn from the literature and years of experience with the four approaches.

TABLE 13.1 FOUR MAJOR FAMILY THERAPY APPROACHES

Family Therapy Founder(s)	Key Concepts	Key Interventions
Systemic family therapy—Murray Bowen	Family as an emotional unit Differentiation of self Triangles Multigenerational transmission Nuclear family emotional processes Family projection process Emotional cutoff	Genogram Self-statements Transform generational patterns Anxiety and conflict interruption Detriangulation Cutoff repair Nuclear family process disruption
Structural family therapy—Salvadore Minuchin	Family structure Subsystems Boundaries Enmeshment Disengagement Coalitions Parentification	Joining and accommodating Enactments Family mapping Modifying problem interactions – Boundary making – Unbalancing – Reframing
Strategic family therapy—Jay Haley and Milton Erickson	Cybernetics Homeostasis Feedback loops Circular causality First-order change Second-order change	Directives Paradoxical interventions Pretend techniques Ordeals Rituals Invariant prescription
Emotionally focused family therapy—Leslie Greenberg and Sue Johnson	Emotions Primary and secondary emotions Attachment styles Attachment injuries	Empathic attunement Reflective statements Evocative questions Creative images and metaphor Encouraging acceptance Creating intimate attachments

Forming a Relationship

Warmth, empathy, and joining with each family member are important in relationship building, from the beginning contact with the family and throughout the therapy. The APPN also needs to have a spirit of collaboration when working with families.

The initial phone contact is very important and gives the APPN a beginning notion of the family problem and dynamics. It may influence who the APPN decides to see for the first session. For example, consider the following three phone contacts:

- My 14-year-old son is depressed, doing poorly in school, and I am overwhelmed with fear. I have not slept for the past few days.
- My husband and I are going through a divorce and my 14-year-old son is having a rough time of it, doing poorly in school and having symptoms of depression.
- My 14-year-old son is being discharged from an inpatient unit for depression and needs someone to prescribe his medication.

With this available information, the APPN might choose to see the mother alone in the first case scenario, the family as a unit in the second, and the dyad of mother and son in the third.

Beginning the Session

Often the novice APPN has difficulty beginning a session. With family therapy, it is very important to set clear rules and ask effective opening questions.

SET CLEAR RULES

Setting rules is very important for safety especially when working with chaotic or abusive families. At the beginning of the first session, it is imperative to give a clear message that this is your office and you, as the APPN, are in charge and have certain rules and expectations. These may be written on a flip chart or a handout. With more structured, contained families, setting rules may not be as essential to safety, but in general, it is a good idea to have a few rules even with these families. Box 13.3 gives some rule-setting suggestions.

STARTING THE SESSION

Starting the session is very important. The initial phone contact as well as the first meeting in the waiting room and on entering the therapy room will provide clues and preliminary ideas as to how to proceed and tailor opening statements and questions. For example, does the family seem resistant? Do they seem scared? Do certain members not want to be there? Does one member seem to have a major psychiatric problem?

BOX 13.3 Initial Rule Setting

- No name calling or other forms of disrespect
- No physical violence
- No interrupting—only one person may speak at a time
- No speaking for another person
- No blaming or evoking guilt
- No consequences for what is said during the session after leaving the session
- No continuation of the session after it is over
- No unproductive communication such as why, should, or can't

BOX 13.4 Effective Opening Statements and Questions

- To start with, I would like to go over a few rules so we are all on the same page.
- How do you all feel about coming here today?
- I believe that you are the experts on your family and I am here to help.
- Today, we will be clarifying problems and seeing what changes need to occur.
- What happened in your family for you to seek help now?
- What would each of you like to see changed in your family?
- I'd like each of you to describe what you consider the problem to be.
- If you were to awaken tomorrow and magically, your family was exactly how you would like it to be, how would it be different?
- What part of the problem does each of you think you play?

Where do family members sit when they come into the consultation room? Some beginning statements and questions are included in Box 13.4.

Some of these statements and questions are better for certain types of families. For example, with a difficult, resistant family, a solution-oriented lead question might be more effective than a problem-oriented question. A solution-oriented question typically decreases tension as well as provides clues to family interactional problems. In the following dialogue, the initial solution-oriented question gives clues to excessive family conflict with possible enmeshment, without actually talking about problems:

APPN: If you were to awaken tomorrow and magically, your family was exactly how you would like it to be, how would it be different?

Mother: The family would be calm and peaceful.

Daughter: My room would be a safe haven.

With a family that strongly identifies one member as the patient when it is clear that it is a family problem, the question, "What part of the problem does each of you think you play?" is an effective question. This begins to take the focus of the illness off the identified patient and sends a message that everyone most likely plays a role in contributing to the problem.

Conducting the Assessment

The assessment, as stated previously, begins at the initial phone contact. However, a more formal assessment is carried out during the first session with select family members or the entire family system. The official guidelines of the American Academy of Child and Adolescent Psychiatry (AACAP) state that a family assessment is standard procedure and always indicated in the psychiatric evaluation of a child or adolescent (Josephson, 2007). A genogram, structural mapping, or observation may be used, depending on the approach and the needs of the family. As with individual therapy, the assessment is ongoing and information is further collected as the therapy progresses.

When working with children and adolescents, it is important to ascertain the degree of influence of the family on the child's problems and the child's influence on the family. For example, in an unstructured family with inadequate boundaries, the degree of family effect on the child is probably more significant in both influencing and maintaining clinical problems. In contrast, in a case of a child with a developmental disability, the influence of the child on the family may be more significant to the clinical problems. A thorough assessment will result in an accurate case conceptualization and determine the best course of action. Important aspects to assess that are informed from all four family therapy approaches include the following.

DIFFERENTIATION

Are members differentiated or undifferentiated? Is there fusion? Are there triangles? Is there emotional reactivity? Are there emotional cutoffs?

MULTIGENERATIONAL TRANSMISSION

What patterns are passed on from one generation to the next?

EMOTIONAL ATMOSPHERE

What is the general atmosphere? Do members feel proud to belong or are they reluctant to be associated with the family? Is the atmosphere conflictual and emotionally reactive or is it happy and loving? Do members feel safe?

STRUCTURE

Is the structure solid? Who has the power in the system? Are the parents at the top tier of the hierarchy? Do they work together? Is the parental coalition weak or strong? Is the parental power equal or unequal? Does the hierarchy change with adolescents?

BOUNDARIES

Are there adequate boundaries or is there an excess or dearth of emotions, communication, and concern? Are they enmeshed or disengaged? Are boundaries appropriate to age and circumstance? Are they isolated or invasive?

SUBSYSTEMS

What are the subsystems and are they functional? Are there coalitions or parentification? Who is close to whom?

DECISION-MAKING AND PROBLEM-SOLVING

How are decisions made and problems solved? Do all family members share in the decision-making, or do one or both parents make all decisions? Do family members have a chance to say how they feel about decisions that directly affect them? Who has the power? Does the family move toward resolution or just blame each other? Is decision-making effective or ineffective, rigid or adaptable?

CONFLICT RESOLUTION

How does the family handle disagreement? Can they fight with each other? How do they fight? Do they fight fairly?

ROLES IN THE FAMILY

Are the roles clearly defined? Are they flexible or rigid? Are they balanced or imbalanced? Are they prescribed or negotiable? Who deals with school problems and household finances? How are tasks distributed?

FAMILY RULES

What are the rules? Are they fair, consistent, and appropriate? Are they vague or clear, fixed or flexible? How are they modified? What are the consequences for breaking the rules?

STRESS AND COPING

Are there developmental (e.g., birth of a baby and retirement) or situational stressors (e.g., loss of a job)? Do the adults recognize normal developmental changes? Are members at the appropriate stages of development? How is stress handled? Are there effective coping mechanisms?

RELATIONSHIP OF THE FAMILY TO THE LARGER COMMUNITY

Are the parents involved in the outside community? Is the family insulated or involved?

MENTAL ILLNESS

Are there signs of psychopathology? Are there addictions, abuse, eating disorders, suicidal ideation, psychosis, or physiological disorders?

RELATIONSHIPS

What is the relationship like between the parents? Are they able to be caring and intimate? Or do they fight to make contact? Are the attachment bonds effective? Does one pursue sexually and the other push away for not getting emotional needs met?

COMMUNICATION PATTERNS

Is communication sensitive, responsive, stifled, spontaneous, confused, clear? Do people listen to one another? Do people give clear messages of their wishes, thoughts, needs, and feelings, or do they expect others to magically know? Can people speak freely? Are some or all family members interrupted? Who interrupts? Who talks to whom? Does one person act as the switchboard? Do they take the message in and think about it? Are perceptions accurate? Can members repeat what they have heard?

DYSFUNCTIONAL FAMILY PATTERNS

Are there dysfunctional patterns deeply embedded within the family? Do families maintain and perpetuate these dysfunctional patterns by their own actions? What are the sequences that keep the repetitive patterns deeply entrenched?

EMOTIONS

How are emotions expressed and dealt with? Can everyone express feelings? Who handles emotional needs? How are anger and love expressed? Is there unresolved anger? Does one person want to talk about feelings and the other not? What is the general feeling tone of the family? Are feelings primary or secondary? Are they adaptive or maladaptive?

Conceptualizing the Problem

Out of the assessment emerges a case conceptualization, also known as a case formulation. This is a theoretical understanding of the causation of the family dysfunction, which is based on an analysis of the assessment data. The conceptualization guides the APPN in determining a diagnosis and developing interventions. When it is determined that the family's interactions have precipitated and maintained the problem, the formulation indicates interventions that will alter patterns of family interaction. When it is determined that the family's interactions are responses to a child's biologically mediated condition, a supportive, psychoeducational treatment approach may be employed. The family's formulation of the problem as well as what they want to change is equally important.

The APPN provides an acceptable family systems explanation for the family distress that leads to some action. A plan consistent with the explanation should be provided for the family.

Diagnosing the Problem

Diagnosing in family therapy uses process diagnoses that address dysfunctional patterns of interaction between or among members. Concepts described previously such as fusion, disengagement, differentiation, structure, triangles, coalitions, maladaptive emotions, and ineffective attachment are used to describe family functioning.

Diagnoses may also be used from the Z codes of the *Diagnostic and Statistical Manual* (5th ed.; *DSM-5*; American Psychiatric Association, 2013). These include various relational units associated with clinically significant impairment in functioning among one or more members of the unit or the functioning of the unit itself. These diagnoses are included in Box 13.5.

Facilitating Change

Facilitating change includes two parts. The first part is contracting with the family and the second is working on the problems to bring about change.

CONTRACTING

A plan needs to be made with the family regarding frequency, length, and number of sessions as well as attendance. Family therapy sessions are generally weekly and last for 1 hour. Family therapy usually lasts for approximately eight to 20 sessions. Depending on the type of family therapy, families may meet as a group or in various configurations. Expectations for work outside sessions such as homework assignments should be addressed. An APPN practicing from an EFT model will commonly work exclusively within the session while the APPN practicing from a strategic therapy model will give homework assignments.

WORKING ON PROBLEMS

The interventions used to work on problems depend on the family therapy approach and the needs of the family as well as the creativity and skill of the APPN. To follow are some examples of interventions, reflective of specific problems:

- **Enmeshed family.** If an interaction problem is enmeshment, with a great deal of bickering and parental intrusiveness, the APPN might set up an experiment in which the parents have to listen to the children without asking questions, lecturing, or giving advice. Each child is given 10 minutes to talk without any interruptions.
- **Disengaged family.** If a problem interaction is disengagement, in which members give limited support and are isolated from each other, the APPN might give a family homework assignment of instructing each family member to spend a minimum of 1 hour with each other family member and learn about his or her interests. Each child

BOX 13.5 *DSM-5* Code Diagnoses Specific to Relational Problems

- Z63.0 Relational Distress with Spouse or Intimate Partner
- Z63.5 Disruption of Family by Separation or Divorce
- Z63.8 High Expressed Emotion Level within Family
- Z62.820 Parent–Child Relational Problem
- Z62.891 Sibling Relational Problem
- Z62.898 Child Affected by Parental Relationship Distress

DSM-5, Diagnostic and Statistical Manual, Fifth Edition.

Source: American Psychiatric Association. (2013). *Diagnostic and statistical manual of mental disorders* (5th ed.). Arlington, VA: American Psychiatric Publishing.

is to learn something about each parent's interests, and each parent is to learn something about each child's interest.

- **Coalition.** When a dysfunctional alliance is identified, changing the dynamics is suggested. For example, if the APPN identifies an alliance between a father and daughter who side together against the mother, an experiment might be for the daughter and mother to spend several blocks of time together during the week and for the father and daughter to limit their communication. The APPN might ask the parents to go out together and spend quality time together.
- **Triangulation.** When two people manage tension by bringing in a third person, the APPN may ask the original dyad to speak to one another. "Why don't you tell him directly how you feel?"
- **Ineffective communication.** When family members are indirect, the APPN should help them be more direct. Family members may inaccurately perceive each other and the APPN will notice these inaccuracies and help members correct them. For example, an inaccurate perception is obvious in the following dialogue:

Daughter:	Hi Dad.
Dad:	Can't talk now. [Dad had a bad day and needs space]
Daughter:	[Withdraws believing that Dad is mad at her]
APPN:	What did you just hear? [APPN to daughter]
Daughter:	That Dad is mad at me.
APPN:	Is that what you meant? [APPN to Dad]

TERMINATION

During termination, the APPN and the family look back on the work that has been completed. Were the goals accomplished? What did each person learn? What helped or did not help? Termination with family therapy is similar to individual therapy and may bring up a variety of issues for the family including grief and loss issues as well as anger and resistance.

EVIDENCE-BASED RESEARCH

The research regarding the effectiveness of family therapy is extensive and reveals that two-thirds of patient in any kind of family therapy get better, which is similar to individual psychotherapy. Meta-analytic studies have concluded that couple and family therapies are significantly more effective than no treatment and at least as effective as other forms of psychotherapy, with an overall effect size of 0.53 (Sexton et al., 2011; Shadish & Baldwin, 2002). The literature also shows that one family therapy approach is no better than another, even when applied to specific problems (Liddle, Santisteban, Levant, & Bray, 2001). More gains are found, however, when the therapist is skillful and active in the early phases of therapy (Gurman, 2008, 2011).

Family therapy is effective for treating child and adolescent psychiatric disorders. It has proved effective with a range of problems including anxiety, depression, conduct disorders, school behavior problems, trauma, eating disorders, attention-deficit hyperactivity disorder (ADHD), and substance abuse disorders, among others (Sheeber, Hops, Stanton, & Shadish, 1997).

All four therapies mentioned in this chapter have a strong research base. Systemic family therapy has made notable contributions in family theory development such as

McGoldrick's work with diversity (McGoldrick et al., 1982) and Betty Carter's work with the family life cycle (Carter & McGoldrick, 1980). Systemic family therapy has also been in the forefront in testing concepts (Nichols, 2012). Instruments to measure differentiation of self have been correlated with many psychological constructs such as marital satisfaction, intimacy, triangulation, and marital distress. Couples with higher levels of differentiation have higher levels of marital satisfaction (Skowron, 2000), greater intimacy (Protinsky & Gilkey, 1996), greater psychological adjustment (Skowron, Wester, & Azen, 2004), more effective coping skills in stressful situations (Murdock & Gore, 2004), less anxiety (Skowron & Friedlander, 1998), and less psychological reactance (Johnson & Buboltz, 2000). Differentiated adults also have a significantly greater therapeutic alliance (Friedlander, Heatherington, Escudero, & Diamond, 2011; Lambert & Friedlander, 2008). Families with lower levels of differentiation have higher levels of triangulation and marital distress (Gehring & Marti, 1993). Multigenerational transmission research has found that parents' and children's beliefs are highly correlated (Troll & Bengston, 1979) and that family violence (Alexander, Moore, & Alexander, 1991), eating disorders (Whitehouse & Harris, 1998), and alcoholism (Sher, Gershuny, Peterson, & Raskin, 1997) are highly transmitted from one generation to the next.

Attention has been placed in more recent years on applying systemic family therapy to working with couples. Cook and Poulsen (2011) utilized photographs with genograms to enhance growth in couple therapy, and Yektatalab, Oskouee, and Sodani (2017) found systemic couple therapy to be very effective with those in highly conflicted relationships. Systemic family therapy has also integrated neurobiology and trauma theory, developing interventions to work with adults who were abused as children (MacKay, 2012). A number of studies have focused on vicarious trauma among therapists, concluding that improving differentiation of self protects against secondary traumatic stress and burnout (MacKay, 2017) and serves as a resiliency factor protecting against vicarious trauma (Halevi & Idisis, 2017). Research has also emphasized using systemic family therapy to work effectively with pediatric obesity (Kaplan, Arnold, Irby, Boles, & Skelton, 2014) and appetite self-regulation (Saltzman, Fiese, Bost, & McBride, 2018).

A great deal of research has been published on the effectiveness of structural family with poorly structured, low socioeconomic families (Minuchin et al., 1967). Studies have shown its effectiveness with families with drug abusers (Stanton & Todd, 1982), physical disorders (Minuchin, Rosman, & Baker, 1978), eating disorders (Campbell & Patterson, 1995), obesity (Jones, Lettenberger, & Wickel, 2011), ADHD (Barkley, Guevremont, Anastopoulos, & Fletcher, 1992), conduct disorder (Szapocznik et al., 1989), and acculturation difficulties (Kim, 2003). More recently attention has been placed on using structural family therapy to work effectively with couples battling pornography addiction (Ford, Durtschi, & Franklin, 2012) and social media addiction (Méndez, Qureshi, Carnerio, & Hort, 2014). Structural family therapy has been successful with low-income families with gang involvement (McNeil, Herschberger, & Nedela, 2013) as well as incarcerated families (Tadros & Finney, 2018) and death row families (Long, 2011). A number of articles have been published using structural family therapy for managing problems in children with autism spectrum disorders (Brockman, Hussain, Sanchez, & Turns, 2016; Parker & Molteni, 2017) and intermittent explosive disorder (Fisher, 2017).

Early research in strategic family therapy was case reports illustrating successful, strategic directives. Later, empirical research has revealed its effectiveness in treating adolescent behavior problems and substance abuse (Santisteban et al., 2003), heroin addicts (Stanton & Todd, 1982), Hispanic youths with drug abuse and behavioral problems (Szapocznik & Williams, 2000), conduct disorders (Coatsworth, Santisteban, McBride, & Szapocznik, 2001), and eating disorders (Castelnuovo, Manzoni, Villa, Cesa, & Molinari, 2011). It has also been effective in reducing bullying behavior, risk-taking, and aggression in bullying girls (Nickel et al., 2006). Robbins et al. (2008) found that successful therapy cases have a high level of positive alliance. More recent research has continued to focus on using strategic family therapy to effectively deal with adolescence substance use disorders (Horigian et al., 2015; Lindstrom, Filges, & Jørgensen, 2015). Strategic family therapy has also proved to be effective with adolescents with gang involvement (Valdez, Cepeda, Parrish, Horowitz, & Kaplan, 2013) and gaming addiction (Yu & Park, 2016).

There has been significant research on EFT revealing that it is highly effective with couples and families. In general, 90% of families show significant improvement with this approach (Elliott, Greenberg, & Lietaer, 2004; Johnson, Hunsley, Greenberg, & Schindler, 1999; MacIntosh & Johnson, 2008). EFT has been recognized as one of only two empirically validated couple interventions (Baucom, Shoham, Mueser, Daiuto, & Stickle, 1998). It is effective with diverse families, families experiencing chronic stress, and families coping with a chronically ill child (Gordon, Johnson, Manion, & Cloutier, 1996). It has also been effective for couples who have experienced sexual abuse as children (MacIntosh & Johnson, 2008), distressed couples dealing with forms of traumatic stress (Johnson, 2002), and couples in which one partner has symptoms of posttraumatic stress disorder (PTSD; Johnson & Williams-Keeler, 1998). EFT continues to show evidence of effectiveness in dealing with families with trauma and PTSD (Roundy, 2017; Weissman et al., 2018). Specific couple problems such as separation and divorce (Allan, 2016) and sexual desire discrepancy (Girard & Wolley, 2017) have been successfully helped with EFT. There has been a great deal of research in the effectiveness of EFT with families dealing with eating disorders (Robinson, Dolhanty, & Greenberg, 2015; Robinson, Dolhanty, Stillar, Henderson, & Mayman, 2016); Strahan et al., 2017). EFT has been applied to working with children using emotion-focused play therapy (Willis, Haslam, & Bermudez, 2016). Process interventions have been developed such as in heightening emotion in couple therapy (Hinkle, Radomski, & Decker, 2015) and emotional processing for unresolved anger (Diamond, Shahar, Sabo, & Tsvieli, 2016). An excellent article by Wiebe and Johnson (2016) explicates the research in EFT since its development in the 1980s as well as future research trends in areas such cultural diversity and physical illness and is highly recommended. See Table 13.2 for selected family therapy research studies.

TABLE 13.2 SELECTED FAMILY THERAPY RESEARCH	
Description of Study	**Authors**
Multiple studies of family therapy vs. other forms of therapy and therapeutic gain	Gurman (2008, 2011); Sexton et al. (2011); Shadish and Baldwin (2002)
Comparison of family therapy types with specific problems	Liddle, Santisteban, Levant, and Bray (2001)
Family and couple therapy for drug abuse	Sheeber, Hops, Stanton, and Shadish (1997)
Systemic therapy with diverse families	McGoldrick, Pearce, and Giordano (1982)
Systemic therapy with the family life cycle	Carter and McGoldrick (1980)
Concepts in systemic family therapy	Nichols (2012)
Differentiation of self and marital satisfaction, intimacy, adjustment, coping, anxiety, reactance, therapeutic alliance, triangulation, and marital distress	Friedlander, Heatherington, Escudero, and Diamond (2011); Gehring and Marti (1993); Johnson and Buboltz (2000); Lambert and Friedlander (2008); Murdock and Gore (2004); Protinsky and Gilkey (1996); Skowron (2000); Skowron and Friedlander (1998); Skowron, Wester, and Azen (2004)

(continued)

TABLE 13.2   SELECTED FAMILY THERAPY RESEARCH (*CONTINUED*)

Description of Study	Authors
Multigenerational transmission and beliefs of family members, family violence, eating disorders, and alcoholism	Alexander, Moore, and Alexander (1991); Sher, Gershuny, Peterson, and Raskin (1997); Troll and Bengston (1979); Whitehouse and Harris (1998)
Using photographs with genograms to enhance growth in systemic couple therapy	Cook and Poulsen (2011)
Systemic couple therapy with highly conflicted couples	Yektatalab, Oskouee, and Sodani (2017)
Systemic family therapy and relational trauma, secondary trauma, and vicarious trauma	Halevi and Idisis (2017); MacKay (2012); MacKay (2017)
Systemic therapy with obesity	Jones, Lettenberger, and Wickel (2011); Kaplan, Arnold, Irby, Boles, and Skelton (2014)
Systemic therapy and appetite self-regulation	Saltzman, Fiese, Bost, and McBride (2018)
Structural family therapy with low-income families	Minuchin, Montalvo, Guerney, Rosman, and Schumer (1967)
Structural family therapy with drug abusers	Stanton et al. (1982)
Structural family therapy with physical disorders	Campbell and Patterson (1995); Minuchin, Rosman, and Baker (1978)
Structural family therapy with attention-deficit hyperactivity disorder	Barkley, Guevremont, Anastopoulos, and Fletcher (1992)
Structural family therapy for problematic Hispanic boys	Szapocznik et al. (1989)
Structural family therapy for Asian families with acculturation difficulties	Kim (2003)
Structural couple therapy with pornography addiction	Ford, Durtschi, and Franklin (2012)
Structural couple therapy with social media addiction	Méndez, Qureshi, Carnerio, and Hort (2014)
Structural family therapy with gang involvement	McNeil, Herschberger, and Nedela (2013)
Structural family therapy with incarcerated and death row families	Tadros and Finney (2018); Long (2011)
Structural family therapy for managing problems in children with autism spectrum disorders	Brockman, Hussain, Sanchez, and Turns (2016); Parker and Molteni (2017)
Structural family therapy with members with intermittent explosive disorder	Fisher (2017)

(continued)

TABLE 13.2   SELECTED FAMILY THERAPY RESEARCH (*CONTINUED*)

Description of Study	Authors
Strategic family therapy with substance abuse	Coatsworth,Santisteban, McBride, and Szapocznik (2001); Horigian et al. (2015); Lindstrom, Filges, and Jø (2015); Santisteban et al. (2003); Stanton et al. (1982); Szapocznik and Williams (2000);
Strategic family therapy vs. cognitive behavioral therapy with adolescents with binge eating disorders	Castelnuovo, Manzoni, Villa, Cesa, and Molinari (2011)
Strategic family therapy with reducing bullying behavior, risk-taking, and aggression in bullying girls	Nickel et al. (2006)
Strategic therapy and positive parent alliances	Robbins et al. (2008)
Strategic family therapy with adolescents with gang involvement	Valdez, Cepeda, Parrish, Horowitz, and Kaplan (2013)
Strategic family therapy and game addiction	Yu and Park (2016)
Overview of research in emotion-focused therapy and its effectiveness with couples and families	Elliott, Greenberg, and Lietaer (2004); Johnson, Hunsley, Greenberg, and Schindler (1999); Baucom, Shoham, Mueser, Daiuto, and Stickle (1998); Wiebe and Johnson (2016)
Emotion-focused therapy and its effec-tiveness with families coping with a chronically ill child	Gordon, Johnson, Manion, and Cloutier (1996)
Emotion-focused therapy and its effec-tiveness with couples and families with posttraumatic stress disorder and other trauma-related disorders including sexual abuse	Johnson (2002); Johnson and Williams-Keeler (1998); MacIntosh and Johnson (2008); Roundy (2017); Weissman et al. (2018)
Emotion-focused therapy and its effec-tiveness with separated and divorced couples	Allan (2016)
Emotion-focused therapy and its effec-tiveness with couples experiencing sexual disorders	Girard and Wolley (2017)
Emotion-focused therapy and its effec-tiveness with families dealing with eating disorders	Robinson, Dolhanty, and Greenberg (2015); Robinson, Dolhanty, Stillar, Henderson, and Mayman (2016); Strahan et al. (2017)
Emotion-focused play therapy and its effec-tiveness with children	Willis, Haslam, and Bermudez (2016)
Heightening emotion in emotion-focused couple therapy	Hinkle, Radomski, and Decker (2015)
Emotion-focused therapy for unresolved anger	Diamond, Shahar, Sabo, and Tsvieli (2016)

Note: Authors listed in this table can be found in the references at the end of the chapter.

CASE EXAMPLE

Assessment

Robert, a 42-year-old attorney, and Keira, a 39-year-old social worker, have been married for 14 years. They have two children, Brendan, age 12, and Jenna, age 10. Keira has been in individual therapy for the past 6 months. Recently, her therapist recommended a course of family therapy because issues related to her marriage and children were encroaching on her individual sessions.

A family assessment revealed that Robert, an emotionally unsupportive, demanding man, works long 14-hour days, underfunctions in the home, and is disengaged from his children. Robert smokes marijuana on a daily basis to relax. Keira, a warm, dependent woman, who overfunctions in the home, is enmeshed with the children. Keira has acquiesced to Robert over the years, letting him make most of the decisions and control the finances. Keira abused alcohol on a daily basis until 2 months ago, then stopped drinking, and began attending Alcoholics Anonymous (AA) meetings. Since she stopped drinking, the tension and conflict in the home have increased. Keira is now more inclined to fight with Robert than to go along with his demands. Robert's marijuana use has increased over the past few months. A genogram revealed male domination and addictions in Robert's family as well as parental divorce. Submission, anxiety, and addictions were prominent in Keira's family. Keira's mother became very bitter as she grew older. Communication patterns between Robert and Keira consist of an abundance of blame with little primary communication.

The children react to the tension in the home by making excessive demands on their mother. Brendan has symptoms of anxiety and difficulty getting along with his peers. He is irritable with his father but is supportive of his mother, often taking her side in marital disputes. Brendan also takes on many adult responsibilities at home. He also feels somewhat responsible for his mother's well-being. Jenna recently began experiencing nausea and stomachaches in the morning and sometimes resists going to school. Each parent colludes with Jenna, trying to get her take his or her side in the marital conflict.

Conceptualization

The parents have a low level of self-differentiation. They do not have appropriate parental authority nor work together in rule-setting. A number of dysfunctional patterns include cross-generational coalition between the mother and son, parentification of the son by the mother, and triangulation of the daughter by both parents. The parents have an insecure attachment with each other and do not communicate on a primary adaptive feeling level and, thus, do not express their needs or authentic feelings. The parents fight unfairly, blaming each other for the family problems. The family roles are undefined and tasks are not evenly distributed. Parents have a deeply embedded overfunctioning–underfunctioning pattern. Attachment bonds are weak between the parents.

Facilitating Change and Working on Problems

The APPN had an early session with the spousal dyad. Examples of some dialogue follows:

APPN: Do you notice anything about the genogram? [to Robert and Keira]

Robert: Well, the men all worked very hard in my family and many died very young. They all seem to be addicted to work or some substance.

Keira:	I notice that many of the women had alcohol problems and seemed to be angry and bitter. I don't want to be like that, which is why I recently stopped drinking.
APPN:	I know that you have stopped drinking 2 months ago and are attending AA.
Robert:	Now that Keira has stopped drinking, she spends so much time at AA meetings and is rarely at home to take care of the kids. The kids are falling apart. She needs to be at home.
APPN:	And, when Keira spends time away from home, you feel angry that she isn't there for the family and scared that the children are not being taken care of.
Keira:	Well, I'm no longer going to assume all the responsibility for the house while he just lounges around. It's over for me. He needs to take some responsibility, too.
APPN:	Can you say that to Robert?
Keira:	I am no longer going to take all the responsibility in the home!
Robert:	I would like to do that, but she doesn't know how difficult my job is and how much stress I am under.
APPN:	Can you tell her that?
Robert:	I am under so much stress and pressure at work. When I come home and find you not there, I feel terribly alone and scared that you are going to leave me.
APPN:	It seems you are feeling terribly scared by that.
Robert:	I would like you to be at home more for I feel scared and abandoned.
APPN:	What's happening now for you as you say that?
Robert:	Uh, uh . . . [he begins to cry]. My mother left my father and I don't want that to happen. I feel very scared.

A later session was held with the entire family. The APPN asked the children to draw their family. Jenna drew herself in the middle of the page with her parents on opposite sides of the paper. Her arms were abnormally long, in an exaggerated extension toward each parent.

APPN:	I notice that your arms are pulled very long. They look a little like stretched silly putty. I wonder what that is like for you.
Jenna:	It's scary. Sometimes I feel like I'm going to be pulled apart.
APPN:	What do you think about that? [APPN to parents]
Robert:	Well, I guess I do try to get her on my side when I'm arguing with Keira.
Keira:	I do the same.
APPN:	What do you think you can do, Jenna, to get yourself out of that position of being in the middle?
Jenna:	I don't know.

APPN:	How about if you say to Mom and Dad that you will not listen to them complain to you about the other parent. Can you do that?
Jenna:	Umm, I think so.
APPN:	Can you try that now?
Jenna:	[to Mom] If you tell me anything bad about Dad, I will not listen and will tell you to talk to him. [to Dad] If you tell me anything bad about Mom, I will not listen and I will tell you to talk to her.

Brendan drew the family in a row. On the left was he and his mother drawn very close, then Jenna in the middle of the page, and then his father on the right side of the page, drawn very small and not close to anyone. It was clear that the relationship between Brendan and his mother was enmeshed and that he was engaged in a parentified role with her, giving her emotional support. Brendan had too much responsibility, which was thwarting his own emotional needs.

APPN:	I notice that you are very close to your mother.
Brendan:	Yes, I am. She needs me.
APPN:	Could you, Mom, tell Brendan, that you can take care of yourself?
Keira:	Brendan, I am able to take care of my own needs. You need to look after yourself.
APPN:	[The APPN gave everyone a directive.] How about for this week Brendan and Dad will spend two nights together. Mom and Dad will go out by themselves one night and have fun. Jenna will enjoy some time by herself working on some of her art projects.

These session dialogues with this family illuminate some examples of how the APPN could work with a family having numerous dysfunctional patterns and attachment problems. The therapy utilizes techniques from the four major types of family therapy and demonstrates how these approaches can be integrated when conducting family therapy.

POST-MASTER'S FAMILY THERAPY TRAINING AND CERTIFICATION REQUIREMENTS

There are national certifying exams in family therapy. The Association of Marital and Family Therapy Regulatory Board (AMFTRB) examination in marital and family therapy is provided to assist state boards of examiners in evaluating the knowledge of applicants for licensure or certification. Although there are a number of APPNs who have a national certification, most APPNs do not pursue this route, because the APPN license allows practitioners to practice family therapy if they are competent in the area. There are many comprehensive postgraduate family therapy training programs throughout the United States. Most of these are 3 years in length, but weekend workshops and shorter programs are available. Some leading couple and family therapy institutes are listed in Box 13.6, and organizations that offer workshops and post-master's training in couple and family therapy are listed in Box 13.7.

BOX13.6 Leading Couple and Family Therapy Institutes

- Ackerman Institute for the Family, New York, NY, www.ackerman.org
- Bowen Center for the Study of the Family, Washington, DC, www.thebowencenter.org
- Minuchin Center for the Family, Oaklyn, NJ, www.minuchincenter.org
- Philadelphia Child & Family Therapy Training Center, Philadelphia, PA, www.philafamily.com
- Family Institute of Westchester, White Plains, NY, www.fiwny.org
- Mental Research Institute for Strategic Family Therapy, Palo Alto, CA, www.mri.org/strategic_family_therapy.html
- International Centre for Emotionally Focused Therapy, Ottawa, Ont., Canada, www.iceeft.com
- Emotion-Focused Therapy Clinic, Toronto, Ont., Canada, www.emotionfocusedclinic.org/training

BOX 13.7 Organizations That Provide Workshops and Post-Master's Training

- American Association for Marriage and Family Therapy (AAMFT), www.aamft.org
- American Family Therapy Association (AFTA), www.afta.org
- International Family Therapy Association (IFTA), www.ifta-familytherapy.org
- International Association of Marriage and Family Counselors (IAMFC), www.iamfconline.org

CONCLUDING COMMENTS

This chapter provides an overview of family therapy for the APPN, highlighting the importance of this approach for the practicing APPN. It explicates four major approaches (systems, structural, strategic, and emotionally focused family therapies), describing their key concepts, goals, and interventions. The chapter describes the practical aspects of conducting family therapy. It includes evidence-based family therapy research, a case study, and information on how to receive postgraduate certification and training. It is hoped that the chapter gives the reader enough of an introduction to the diverse field of family therapy that he or she will want to learn more and continue training in family therapy.

There are other approaches to family therapy not mentioned in this chapter such as psychodynamic, cognitive behavioral, solution-focused, narrative, and feminist family therapy. These approaches, although very valuable, are not considered to be a family systems approach. In general, they apply basic concepts of individual therapy to the family. Nevertheless, it is suggested that the APPN explore these other types of family therapy as well. For a comprehensive compilation of family therapy approaches, the two texts, *Family Therapy: An Overview* by Goldenberg and Goldenberg (2012) and *Family Therapy: Concepts and Methods* by Nichols (2012) are recommended for the APPN student and beginning practitioner. Original texts are highly recommended for advanced practitioners and can be found in the reference list.

DISCUSSION QUESTIONS

1. Why is it important for the APPN to have basic competence in family therapy?
2. What are the similarities and differences among the four major approaches to family therapy (e.g., systemic, structural, strategic, and emotionally focused) discussed in this chapter?

3. Draw a three-generation genogram of your family. How do you think your family has contributed to your development and self-definition?
4. Structural family therapy emphasizes the importance of a structure with a clear parental hierarchy. What problems emerge when this organization does not occur?
5. Strategic therapy emphasizes issuing directives as its major intervention. Give an example of a directive that you might use in a specific family situation.
6. Develop a brief couple dialogue that illuminates empathic attunement as used in EFT.
7. Which family therapy approach do you find the most interesting and hope to further explore? Why?

REFERENCES

Ackerman, N. (1958). *The psychodynamics of family life*. New York, NY: Basic Books.

Adler, A. (1931). *Guiding the child*. New York, NY: Greenberg.

Alexander, P. C., Moore, S., & Alexander, E. R. (1991). Intergenerational transmission of violence. *Journal of Marriage and the Family, 53*, 657–667. doi:10.2307/352741

Allan, R. (2016). The use of emotionally focused therapy with separated or divorced couples. *Canadian Journal of Counselling and Psychotherapy, 50*(Suppl. 3), S62–S79. Retrieved from https://cjc-rcc.ucalgary.ca/article/view/61069/pdf

American Association of Colleges of Nursing. (1996). *The essentials of master's education for advanced practice nursing education*. Washington, DC: Author. Retrieved from https://files.eric.ed.gov/fulltext/ED435321.pdf

American Nurses Association, American Psychiatric Nurses Association, International Society of Psychiatric-Mental Health Nurses. (2012). *Psychiatric-mental health nursing: Scope and standards of practice, draft*. Silver Spring, MD: Author. Retrieved from https://www.apna.org/files/public/12-11-20-PMH_Nursing_Scope_and_Standards_for_Public_Comment.pdf

American Nurses Credentialing Center. (n.d.). *Frequently asked question abut the APRN Consensus Model for APRN Regulation*. Retrieved from https://www.aacn.org/certification/advanced-practice/np-and-cns-educational-program-resources/frequently-asked-questions-about-aprn-consensus-model-for-np-programs

American Psychiatric Association. (2013). *Diagnostic and statistical manual of mental disorders* (5th ed.). Arlington, VA: American Psychiatric Publishing.

Anderson, S. A., & Sabatelli, R. M. (1992). The differentiation in the family system scale (DIFS). *American Journal of Family Therapy, 20*(1), 77–89. doi:10.1080/01926189208250878

Barkley, R., Guevremont, D., Anastopoulos, A., & Fletcher, K. (1992). A comparison of three family therapy programs for treating family conflicts in adolescents with attention-deficit hyperactivity disorder. *Journal of Consulting and Clinical Psychology, 60*, 450–463. doi:10.1037/0022-006X.60.3.450

Baucom, D., Shoham, V., Mueser, K. T., Daiuto, A. D., & Stickle, T. R. (1998). Empirically supported couple and family interventions for marital distress and adult mental health problems. *Journal of Consulting and Clinical Psychology, 66*, 53–88. doi:10.1037/0022-006X.66.1.53

Beavers, W. R., & Hampson, R. B. (1990). *Successful families: Assessment and intervention*. New York, NY: Jason Aronson.

Becvar, D. S., & Becvar, R. J. (2008). *Family therapy: A systemic integration* (7th ed.). Boston, MA: Allyn & Bacon.

Bloch, S., Sharpe, M., & Allman, P. (1991). Systemic family therapy in adult psychiatry. A review of 50 families. *British Journal of Psychiatry, 159*, 357–364. doi:10.1192/bjp.159.3.357

Bowen, M. (1972). Towards a differentiation of self in one's family. In J. L. Framo (Ed.), *Family interaction: A dialogue between family researchers and family therapists* (pp. 111–173). New York, NY: Springer Publishing Company.

Bowen, M. (1978). *Family therapy in clinical practice*. New York, NY: Jason Aronson.

Brockman, M., Hussain, K., Sanchez, B., & Turns, B. (2016). Managing child behavior problems in children with autism spectrum disorders. *The American Journal of Family Therapy, 44*(1), 1–10. doi:10.1080/01926187.2015.1099414

Campbell, T., & Patterson, J. (1995). The effectiveness of family interventions in the treatment of physical illness. *Journal of Marital and Family Therapy, 21*, 545–584. doi:10.1111/j.1752-0606.1995 .tb00178.x

Carter, B., & McGoldrick, M. (1980). *The family life cycle: A framework for family therapy.* New York, NY: Gardner Press.

Castelnuovo, G., Manzoni, G. M., Villa, V., Cesa, G. L., & Molinari, E. (2011). Brief strategic therapy vs cognitive behavioral therapy for the inpatient and telephone-based outpatient treatment of binge eating disorder: The STRATOB randomized controlled clinical trial. *Clinical Practice and Epidemiology in Mental Health, 7*, 29–37. doi:10.2174/1745017901107010029

Coatsworth, J. D., Santisteban, D. A., McBride, C. K., & Szapocznik, J. (2001). Brief strategic family therapy versus community control: Engagement, retention, and an exploration of the moderating role of adolescent symptom severity. *Family Process, 40*(3), 313–332. doi:10.1111/ j.1545-5300.2001.4030100313.x

Cook, J. M., & Poulsen, S. S. (2011). Utilizing photographs with the genogram: A technique for enhancing couple therapy. *Journal of Systemic Therapies, 30*(1), 14–23. doi:10.1521/jsyt .2011.30.1.14

Corey, G. (2011). *Theory and practice of counseling and psychotherapy* (9th ed.). Belmont, CA: Brooks/Cole.

Diamond, G., & Josephson, A. (2005). Family-based treatment research: A 10-year update. *Journal of the American Academy of Child and Adolescent Psychiatry, 44*(9), 872–887. doi:10.1097/01.chi .0000169010.96783.4e

Diamond, G., M., Shahar, B., Sabo, D., & Tsvieli, N. (2016). Attachment-based family therapy and emotion-focused therapy for unresolved anger: The role of productive emotional processing. *Psychotherapy, 53*(1), 34–44. doi:10.1037/pst0000025

Elliott, R., Greenberg, L., & Lietaer, G. (2004). Research on experiential psychotherapy. In A. E. Bergin & S. L. Garfield (Eds.), *Handbook of psychotherapy and behavior change* (4th ed., pp. 493–539). New York, NY: Wiley.

Fisher, U. (2017). Use of structural family therapy with an individual client diagnosed with intermittent explosive disorder: A case study. *Journal of Family Psychotherapy, 28*(2), 150–169. doi:10.1080/08975353.2017.1288989

Ford, J. J., Durtschi, J. A., & Franklin, D. L. (2012). Structural therapy with a couple battling pornography addiction. *The American Journal of Family Therapy, 40*, 336–348. doi:10.1080/ 01926187.2012.685003

Friedlander, M. L., Heatherington, L., Escudero, V., & Diamond, G. M. (2011). Alliance in couple and family therapy. *Psychotherapy, 48*(1), 25–33. doi:10.1037/a0022060

Gehring, T. M., & Marti, D. (1993). The family system test: Differences in perception of family structures between nonclinical and clinical children. *Journal of Child Psychology and Psychiatry, 34*, 363–377. doi:10.1111/j.1469-7610.1993.tb00998.x

Girard, A. & Woolley, S. R. (2017). Using emotionally focused therapy to treat sexual desire discrepancy in couples. *Journal of Sex & Marital Therapy, 43*(8), 720–735. doi:10.1080/0092623X .2016.1263703

Goldenberg, H., & Goldenberg, I. (2012). *Family therapy: An overview* (8th ed.). Belmont, CA: Brooks/Cole.

Gordon, W. J., Johnson, S. M., Manion, L., & Cloutier, P. (1996). Emotionally focused marital interventions for couples with chronically ill children. *Journal of Consulting and Clinical Psychology, 64*, 1029–1036. doi:10.1037/0022-006X.64.5.1029

Greenberg, L. (2002). *Emotion-focused therapy: Coaching clients to work through feelings.* Washington, DC: American Psychological Association.

Greenberg, L. S. (2010). Emotion-focused therapy: A clinical synthesis. *Focus: Journal of Lifelong Learning in Psychiatry, 3*(1), 32–42. doi:10.1176/foc.8.1.foc32

Greenberg, L., & Johnson, S. M. (1988). *Emotionally focused therapy for couples.* New York, NY: Guilford Press.

Guerin, P. J., & Chabot, D. R. (1997). Development of family systems theory. In P. Wachtel & S. B. Messer (Eds.), *Theories of psychotherapy: Origins and evolution* (pp. 181–225). Washington, DC: American Psychological Association.

Guerin, P. J., Fogarty, T. F., Fay, L. F., & Kautto, J. G. (1996). *Working with relationship triangles: The one-two-three of psychotherapy.* New York, NY: Guilford Press.

Gurman, A. S. (Ed.). (2008). *Clinical handbook of couple therapy* (4th ed.). New York, NY: Guilford Press.

Gurman, A. S. (2011). Couple therapy research and the practice of couple therapy: Can we talk? *Family Process, 50*(3), 280–292. doi:10.1111/j.1545-5300.2011.01360.x

Halevi, E., & Idisis, Y. (2017). Who helps the helper? Differentiation of self as an indicator for resisting vicarious traumatization. *Psychological Trauma: Theory, Research, Practice, and Policy, 10*(6), 698–705. doi:10.1037/tra0000318

Haley, J. (1976). *Problem-solving therapy: New strategies for effective family therapy.* San Francisco, CA: Jossey-Bass.

Haley, J., & Richeport-Haley, M. (2007). *Directive family therapy.* New York, NY: Haworth Press.

Hinkle, M. S., Radomski, J. G., & Decker, K. M. (2015). Creative experiential interventions to heighten emotion and process in emotionally focused couples therapy. *The Family Journal: Counselling and Therapy for Couples and Families, 23*(3), 239–246. doi:10.1177/1066480715572964

Horigian, V. E., Feaster, D. J., Robbins, M. S., Brincks, A. M., Ucha, J., Rohrbaugh, M. J., . . . Szapocznik, J. (2015). A cross-sectional assessment of the long term effects of brief strategic family therapy for adolescent substance use. *The American Journal on Addictions, 24,* 637–645. doi:10.1111/ajad.12278

Johnson, S. M. (1996). *Creating connections: The practice of emotionally focused marital therapy.* Philadelphia, PA: Brunner/Mazel.

Johnson, S. M. (2002). *Emotionally focused couple therapy with trauma survivors: Strengthening attachment bonds.* New York, NY: Guilford Press.

Johnson, S. M. (2004). *The process of emotionally focused couple therapy.* New York, NY: Brunner-Routledge.

Johnson, P., & Buboltz, W. C. (2000). Differentiation of self and psychological reactance. *Contemporary Family Therapy, 22,* 91–102. doi:10.1023/A:1007774600764

Johnson, S. M., & Greenberg, L. S. (1995). The emotionally-focused approach to problems in adult attachment. In N. S. Jacobson & A. S. Gurman (Eds.), *Clinical handbook of couple therapy* (pp. 121–141). New York, NY: Guilford Press.

Johnson, S. M., Hunsley, J. I., Greenberg, L., & Schindler, D. (1999). Emotionally focused couples therapy: Status and challenges. *Journal of Clinical Psychology: Science & Practice, 6,* 67–79. doi:10.1093/clipsy.6.1.67

Johnson, S. M., Makinen, J. A., & Makinen, J. W. (2001). Attachment injuries in couple relationships: A new perspective on impasses in couples therapy. *Journal of Marital and Family Therapy, 27,* 145–155. doi:10.1111/j.1752-0606.2001.tb01152.x

Johnson, S. M., & Sims, A. (2000). Attachment theory: A map for couples. In T. Levy (Ed.), *Handbook of attachment interventions* (pp. 169–191). San Diego, CA: Academic Press.

Johnson, S. M., & Whiffen, V. E. (1999). Made to measure: Adapting emotionally focused couples therapy to partner's attachment styles. *Clinical Psychology: Science and Practice, 6,* 366–381. doi:10.1093/clipsy.6.4.366

Johnson, S. M., & Williams-Keeler, L. (1998). Creating healing relationships for couples dealing with trauma: The use of emotionally focused marital therapy. *Journal of Marital and Family Therapy, 24,* 25–40. doi:10.1111/j.1752-0606.1998.tb01061.x

Jones, K. E., Lettenberger, C. L., & Wickel, K. (2011). A structural/strategic lens in the treatment of children with obesity. *The Family Journal, 19,* 340–346. doi:10.1177/1066480711408787

Josephson, A. M. (2007). Practice parameter for the assessment of the family. *Journal of the American Academy of Child & Adolescent Psychiatry, 46*(7), 922–937. doi:10.1097/chi.0b013e318054e713

Kaplan, S. G., Arnold, E. M., Irby, M. B., Boles, K. A., & Skelton, J. A. (2014). Family systems theory and obesity treatment: Applications for clinicians. *ICAN: Infant, Child, & Adolescent Nutrition, 6*(1), 24–29. doi:10.1177/1941406413516001

Kerr, M. E., & Bowen, M. (1988). *Family evaluation: An approach based on Bowen theory.* New York, NY: W. W. Norton.

Kim, J. M. (2003). Structural family therapy and its implications for the Asian American family. *The Family Journal, 11,* 388–392. doi:10.1177/1066480703255387

Knight, C. (1997a). The future of clinical nurse specialists in psychiatric-mental health nursing. *New Jersey Nurse, 27,* 1–2.

Knight, C. (1997b). The future of clinical nurse specialists in psychiatric-mental health nursing. *New Jersey Nurse, 27*(1), 10.

Knight, C. (1998). The future of clinical nurse specialists in psychiatric-mental health nursing. *New Jersey Nurse, 28*(1), 12–13.

Lambert, J. E., & Friedlander, M. (2008). Relationship of differentiation of self to adult client's perceptions of the alliance in brief family therapy. *Psychotherapy Research, 18*(2), 160–166. doi:10.1080/10503300701255924

Liddle, H. A., Santisteban, D. A., Levant, R. F., & Bray, J. H. (2001). *Family psychology: Science-based interventions.* Washington, DC: American Psychological Association.

Lindstrom, M., Filges, T., & Jørgensen, A. K. (2015). Brief strategic family therapy for young people in treatment for drug use. *Research on Social Work Practice, 25*(1), 61–80. doi:10.1177/1049731514530003

Long, W. C. (2011). Trauma therapy for death row families. *Journal of Trauma and Dissociation, 12,* 482–494. doi:10.1080/15299732.2011.593258

MacIntosh, H. B., & Johnson, S. (2008). Emotionally focused therapy for couples and childhood sexual abuse survivors. *Journal of Marital and Family Therapy, 34*(3), 298–315. doi:10.1111/j.1752-0606.2008.00074.x

MacKay, L. M. (2012). Trauma and Bowen family systems theory: Working with adults who were abused as children. *The Australian and New Zealand Journal of Family Therapy, 33*(3), 232–241. doi:10.1017/aft.2012.28

MacKay, L. M. (2017). Differentiation of self: Enhancing therapist resilience when working with relational trauma. *The Australian and New Zealand Journal of Family Therapy, 38,* 637–656. doi:10.1002/anzf.1276

Madanes, C. (1981). *Strategic family therapy.* San Francisco, CA: Jossey-Bass.

McGoldrick, M. (1995). *You can go home again: Reconnecting with your family.* New York, NY: W. W. Norton.

McGoldrick, M., Gerson, R., & Petry, S. (2008). *Genograms: Assessment and intervention* (3rd ed.). New York, NY: W. W. Norton.

McGoldrick, M., Pearce, J. K., & Giordano, J. (Eds.). (1982). *Ethnicity and family therapy.* New York, NY: Guilford Press.

McNeil, S. N., Herschberger, J. K., & Nedela, M. N. (2013). Low-income families with potential adolescent gang involvement: A structural community family therapy integration model. *The American Journal of Family Therapy, 41*(2), 110–120. doi:10.1080/01926187.2011.649110

Méndez, N. A., Qureshi, M. E., Carnerio, R., & Hort, F. (2014). The intersection of facebook and structural family therapy. *The American Journal of Family Therapy, 42,* 167–174. doi:10.1080/01926187.2013.794046

Minuchin, S. (1974). *Families and family therapy.* Cambridge, MA: Harvard University Press.

Minuchin, S., & Fishman, H. C. (1981). *Family therapy techniques.* Cambridge, MA: Harvard University Press.

Minuchin, S., Rosman, B. L., & Baker, L. (1978). The psychosomatic family. In *Psychosomatic families* (pp. 23–50). Cambridge, MA: Harvard University Press.

Minuchin, S., Montalvo, B., Guerney, B., Rosman, B., & Schumer, F. (1967). *Families of the slums.* New York, NY: Basic Books.

Murdock, N. L., & Gore, P. A. (2004). Stress, coping, and differentiation of self: A test of Bowen's theory. *Contemporary Family Therapy, 26,* 319–335. doi:10.1023/B:COFT.0000037918.53929.18

Napier, A., & Whitaker, C. (1966). *The family crucible: The intense experience of family therapy.* New York, NY: Harper & Row.

Nichols, M. P. (2012). *Family therapy: Concepts and methods* (10th ed.). Upper Saddle River, NJ: Prentice Hall.

Nickel, M., Luley, J., Krawczyk, J., Nickel, C., Widermann, C., Lahmann, C., . . . Loew, T. (2006). Bullying girls—Changes after brief strategic family therapy: A randomized, prospective, controlled trial with one-year follow-up. *Psychotherapy and Psychosomatics, 75,* 47–55. doi:10.1159/000089226

Parker, M. L., & Molteni, J. (2017). Structural family therapy and autism spectrum disorder: Bridging the disciplinary divide. *The American Journal of Family Therapy, 45*(3), 135–148. doi:10.1080/01926187.2017.1303653

Protinsky, H., & Gilkey, J. K. (1996). An empirical investigation of the construct of personality authority in late adolescent women and their level of college adjustment. *Adolescence, 31*, 291–296.

Robbins, M. S., Mayorga, C. C., Mitrani, V. B., Szapocznik, J., Turner, C. W., & Alexander, J. F. (2008). Adolescent and parent alliances with therapists in brief strategic family therapy with drug-using hispanic adolescents. *Journal of Marital and Family Therapy, 34*(3), 316–328. doi:10.1111/j.1752-0606.2008.00075.x

Robinson, A. L., Dolhanty, J., & Greenberg, L. (2015). Emotion-focused family therapy for eating disorders in children and adolescents. *Clinical Psychology and Psychotherapy, 22*, 75–82. doi:10.1002/cpp.1861

Robinson, A. L., Dolhanty, J., Stillar, A., Henderson, K., & Mayman, S. (2016). Emotion-focused family therapy for eating disorders across the lifespan. *Clinical Psychology and Psychotherapy, 23*, 14–23. doi:10.1002/cpp.1933

Roundy, G. T., (2017). Phase-based emotionally focused couple therapy for adults with complex posttraumatic stress disorder. *Journal of Couple & Relationship Therapy, 16*(4), 306–324. doi:10.1080/15332691.2016.1253519

Saltzman, J. A., Fiese, B., Bost, K. K. F., & McBride, B. A. (2018). Development of appetite self-regulation: Integrating perspectives from attachment and family systems theory. *Child Development Perspectives, 12*(1), 51–57. doi:10.1111/cdep.12254

Santisteban, D., Coatsworth, J., Perez-Vidal, A., Kurtines, W., Schwartz, S., LaPerriere, A., & Szapocznik, J. (2003). The efficacy of brief strategic family therapy in modifying Hispanic adolescent behavior problems and substance use. *Journal of Family Psychology 17*(1), 123–133. doi:10.1037/0893-3200.17.1.121

Satir, V. M. (1964). *Conjoint family therapy*. Palo Alto, CA: Science and Behavior Books.

Satir, V. M., & Baldwin, M. (1983). *Satir step by step: A guide to creating change in families*. Palo Alto, CA: Science and Behavior Books.

Selvini Palazzoli, M., Boscolo, L., Cecchin, F. G., & Prata, G. (1978). *Paradox and counterparadox*. Northvale, NJ: Aronson.

Sexton, T., Gordon, K. C., Gurman, A., Lebow, J., Holtzworth-Munroe, A., & Johnson, S. (2011). Guidelines for classifying evidence-based treatments in couple and family therapy. *Family Process, 50*(3), 377–392. doi:10.1111/j.1545-5300.2011.01363.x

Shadish, W. R., & Baldwin, S. A. (2002). Meta-analysis of MFT interventions. In D. H. Sprenkle (Ed.), *Effectiveness research in marriage and family therapy* (pp. 339–370). Alexandria, VA: American Association for Marital and Family Therapy.

Sheeber, L., Hops, H., Stanton, M. D., & Shadish, W. R. (1997). Outcome, attrition, and family-couples treatment for drug abuse: A meta-analysis and review of controlled, comparative studies. *Psychological Bulletin, 122*, 170–191. doi:10.1037/0033-2909.122.2.170

Sher, K. J., Gershuny, B. S., Peterson, L., & Raskin, G. (1997). The role of childhood stressors in the intergenerational transmission of alcohol use disorders. *Journal of Studies on Alcohol, 58*, 414–427. doi:10.15288/jsa.1997.58.414

Skowron, E. A. (2000). The role of differentiation of self in marital adjustment. *Journal of Counseling Psychology, 47*, 229–237. doi:10.1037/0022-0167.47.2.229

Skowron, E. A., & Friedlander, M. L. (1998). The differentiation of self inventory: Development and initial validation. *Journal of Counseling Psychology, 45*, 1–11. doi:10.1037/0022-0167.45.3.235

Skowron, E. A., Wester, S., & Azen, R. (2004). Differentiation of self mediates college stress and adjustment in late adolescence. *Journal of Counseling & Development, 82*, 69–78. doi:10.1002/j.1556-6678.2004.tb00287

Stanton, M. D., Todd, T. C., & Associates. (1982). *The family therapy of drug abuse and addiction*. New York, NY: Guilford Press.

Strahan, E. J., Stillar, A., Files, N., Nash, P., Scarborough, J., Connors, L., ... Lafrance, A. (2017). Increasing parental self-efficacy with emotion-focused family therapy for eating disorders: A process model. *Person-Centered & Experiential Psychotherapies, 16*(3), 256–269. doi:10.1080/14779757.2017.1330703

Szapocznik, J., Rio, A., Murray, E., Cohen, R., Scopetta, M., Hervis, A., ... Kurtines, W. (1989). Structural family versus psychodynamic child therapy for problematic Hispanic boys. *Journal of Consulting and Clinical Psychology, 57*, 571–578. doi:10.1037/0022-006X.57.5.571

Szapocznik, J., & Williams, R. A. (2000). Brief strategic family therapy: Twenty-five years of interplay among theory, research and practice in adolescent behavior problems and drug abuse. *Clinical Child and Family Psychology Review, 3*(2), 117–134. doi:10.1023/A:1009512719808

Tadros, E., & Finney, N. (2018). Structural family therapy with incarcerated families. *The Family Journal: Counseling and Therapy for Couples and Families, 26*(2), 253–261. doi:10.1177/1066480718777409

Troll, L., & Bengston, V. L. (1979). Generations in the family. In W. R. Burr, R. Hill, F. I. Nye, & I. L. Reiss (Eds.), *Contemporary theories about the family* (pp. 127–161). New York, NY: Free Press.

Valdez, A., Cepeda, A., Parrish, D., Horowitz, R., & Kaplan, C. (2013). An adapted brief strategic family therapy for gang-affiliated Mexican American adolescents. *Research on Social Work Practice, 23*(4), 383–396. doi:10.1177/1049731513481389

von Bertalanffy, K. L. (1968). *General system theory: Foundations, development, applications.* New York, NY: George Braziller.

Watzlawick, P., Beavin, J. H., & Jackson, D. D. (1967). *Pragmatics of human communication.* New York, NY: W. W. Norton.

Weissman, N., Batten, S. V., Rheem, K. D., Wiebe, S. A., Pasillas, R. M., Potts, W., ... Dixon, L. B. (2018). The effectiveness of emotionally focused couples therapy with veterans with PTSD: A pilot study. *Journal of Couple & Relationship Therapy, 17*(1), 25–41. doi:10.1080/15332691.2017.1285261

Whitaker, C. A., & Bumberry, W. M. (1988). *Dancing with the family: A symbolic-experiential approach.* New York, NY: Bruner/Mazel.

Whitehouse, P. J., & Harris, G. (1998). The inter-generational transmission of eating disorders. *European Eating Disorders Review, 6*, 238–254. doi:10.1002/(SICI)1099-0968(199812)6:4<238::AID-ERV208>3.0.CO;2-Y

Wiebe, S. A., & Johnson, S. M. (2016). A review of the research in emotionally focused therapy for couples. *Family Process, 55*(3), 390–407. doi:10.1111/famp.12229

Willis, A. B., Haslam, D. R., & Bermudez, J. M. (2016). Harnessing the power of play in emotionally focused family therapy with preschool children. *Journal of Marital and Family Therapy, 42*(4), 673–687. doi:10.1111/jmft.12160

Yektatalab, S., Oskouee, F. S., & Sodani, M. (2017). Efficacy of Bowen theory on marital conflict in the family nursing practice: A randomized controlled trial. *Issues in Mental Health Nursing, 38*(3), 253–260. doi:10.1080/01612840.2016.1261210

Yu, J.-H., & Park, T.-Y. (2016). Family therapy for an adult child experiencing bullying and game addiction: An application of Bowenian and MRI theories. *Contemporary Family Therapy, 38*, 318–327. doi:10.1007/s10591-016-9382-x doi:10.1007/s10591-016-9382-x

Integrating Medication and Complementary Modalities into Psychotherapy

Psychotherapeutics: Reuniting Psychotherapy and Pharmacotherapy

Barbara J. Limandri and
Mary D. Moller

Have you had a patient come to a session asking you to prescribe a certain medication they saw advertised on television? How does the advanced practice psychiatric nurse (APPN) respond? Our culture is focused on finding a quick fix and the ability to "find an app for that" rather than addressing the complex layers of the psychosocial and economic factors that we face on a daily basis. No doubt, the APPN is drawn into finding simple solutions that take the least amount of time or resources. Unfortunately, the psychiatric and mental health issues our patients bring to us are not easily resolved with just a single medication or therapeutic strategy.

Patients, in their struggle to improve their situation, are seeking answers. They seek professional help for a prescription often after trying several of the literally hundreds of available psychotherapy approaches, reading several published self-help books, and spending large sums of money on a plethora of alternative and complementary treatments guaranteed to relieve symptoms. The holistic approach of the APPN is well suited to guide the person in an organized way through the maze of available "solutions" to the present needs they have. The terminology, "full scope of the role" refers to the reclamation by the APPN of the incorporation of a comprehensive psychotherapeutic approach to care that includes both pharmacotherapy and psychotherapy.

The fracture in service delivery that exists in the current healthcare system perpetuates a split in the ability to implement the full scope of the role, resulting in the inability of the APPN to provide total patient care in an effective and cost-efficient manner. In this chapter we present the evidence of the efficacy of uniting the various treatment approaches compared to the common practice of splitting the delivery of psychotherapy and pharmacotherapy. We present the argument for returning to a full scope of practice in providing services for our patients.

Full scope of practice is based on the understanding that pharmacological therapy is psychotherapy. That is, prescribing should always be done with psychotherapeutic goals in mind. This means that (a) regardless of the source of the referral, the APPN assesses the therapeutic needs and goals of the patient, and (b) in deciding on a medication, describing it, and telling the patient the expected benefits and effects, the practitioner does this with psychotherapeutic goals in mind. This creates expectations about medication effects and is referred to as the "placebo talk." The placebo effect is likely to bring some relief of symptoms without an active ingredient (Fava, Guidi, Rafanelli, & Rickels, 2017; Friesen, 2019).

There is little question placebos enhance the benefits of prescribed medication. Evidence exists that the therapeutic effects of medications such as SSRIs (selective serotonin reuptake inhibitors) are not statistically better than placebo (Hengartner & Pioden, 2018; Kirsch, 2010), and therefore it is likely that most patients can benefit from the expectation that the medication will be helpful. With neuroleptics, the effects and side effects are so general (largely sedating and numbing) that indicating to the patient specifically what to expect from the medication is essential, and of course that expectation relates to the person's goals in therapy. For these reasons, medication considerations need to arise out of some familiarity with the patient, history, context, and therapeutic need; and the APPN who is also the psychotherapist also has the advantage of knowing the patient, progress, and needs.

PRACTICE MODELS

Currently APPNs use several models for their practice: (a) psychotherapy only, (b) pharmacotherapy only, (c) psychotherapy and pharmacotherapy but not both with the same patient, and (d) psychotherapy and pharmacotherapy as needed for all their patients. Additionally, state practice acts differentially authorize autonomous practice, collaborative practice with physician oversight, and transition to practice with time-limited supervisory oversight. See www.aanp.org/advocacy/state/state-practice-environment for state practice acts. Each APPN decides on the practice model to use based on his or her competency, role confidence, clinical setting, community needs, and likely other variables, whereas the state practice act provides the authority of the scope of practice.

Authorized scope of practice. The National Council of State Boards of Nursing (NCSBN) proposed the Model Act in 2012 that identified the title of Advance Practice Registered Nurse (APRN), although individual states may authorize slightly different titles. Having completed an accredited graduate level education program in nursing, the scope of practice includes conducting advanced assessment, requesting and interpreting diagnostic procedures, identifying primary and differential diagnoses, and prescribing therapeutic measures. Licensure for APRN includes an RN license as well as certification by some national accrediting body, in psychiatric nursing that is solely the American Nurses Credentialing Center (ANCC). The Consensus Model is model legislation for states to bring about consistency in advanced practice, and the extent to which states modify their practice acts varies (APRN Joint Dialogue Group & NCSTN APRN Advisory Committee, 2008). Although the APRN Contract recommends autonomous independent practice, as of January 2019 only 21 states grant all APRN roles full practice authority and 29 states maintain some kind of written collaborative practice agreement for supervision by a physician. Not only does such practice restriction create an economic burden on APPNs, it also implies that physicians can practice nursing as well as nurses (or better if supervising) even without meeting the statutory educational requirements. It maintains that nursing is a subset of medicine instead of being a separate healthcare discipline. For states with collaborative practice agreements, changing to full scope of practice may mean opening the Nurse Practice Act completely, which many find daunting and potentially threatening by the medical community.

Collaborative practice agreement. When a collaborative practice agreement (CPA) is required, the APPN will need to negotiate with a physician (or APPN if permitted by the state practice act) for ongoing consultation and case reviews. Such an agreement, however, does not shift responsibility or liability for prescribing to the physician. The CPA must be written and signed by both the collaborative physician and the APRN, submitted to the state board of nursing, and reviewed annually. The collaborating physician must be readily available, although the extent of that availability differs across states. It can be within a mileage limitation, frequency of consultation, number of other APPNs also under the CPA with same physician, etc. (Bell, Hughes, & Lòpez-De Fede, 2018; Kazer, O'Sullivan, & Leonard, 2018). The CPA likely will contain financial agreements for collaborative services, no compete provisions upon termination, conditions of oversight and consultation, confidentiality limitations, and any other business agreements. The noncompete clause can be problematic for an APPN terminating from a contract position by limiting the ability to set up a clinical practice within a set mileage radius of the former employment. Depending on the state in which the APPN resides (banned in California, Montana, North Dakota, and Oklahoma), the noncompete clause may not be enforceable. The purpose of the noncompete clause ostensibly is to protect an employer from losing clientele or "trade secrets." However, it limits employees' ability to pursue a livelihood, lowers wages, and removes professional skills from the free labor market. APPNs in suburban and rural areas have been burdened by noncompete clauses by the inability to leave a contracted position to set up a private practice in the vicinity, even to the extent of having to leave the state (Funk, Weaver, Benbenek, & Anderson, 2019). See Appendix 14.1 for sample collaborative agreements. It is advisable for the APPN to have a separate attorney who is experienced in health practice law to review the agreement prior to signing, especially if there is a noncompete clause upon termination.

PRESCRIBING PROCESS

Prescribing medication is a decision the APPN makes based on additional assessment beyond the full mental health assessment and diagnostic formulation. Basic physical assessment includes measured height and weight (not self-reported), pulse, and blood pressure. Box 14.1 identifies specific factors that need to be considered in establishing the course of treatment. Assessment for medications needs to also include detailed history of previous psychotropic medications (both prescribed and over the counter), reasons for the taking the medication, beneficial effects and adverse effects, length of time taking the medication, and reasons for discontinuing it. The assessment results in a treatment plan that may or may not result in prescribing a medication, that is, just because a patient is referred for medication evaluation does not mean the nurse must prescribe.

APPNs are often referred patients who the patient's psychotherapist feels would benefit from medication but that does not always mean that medication is indicated. It is important for the APPN to understand the psychotherapeutic process in that frequently

BOX 14.1 Neuropsychosocial and Psychopharmacological Assessment

1. Patient's identifying data
2. Patient's identified problem
3. History of the current problem
4. Symptoms that the medications target
5. History of treatment
6. Response and adverse effects to prior medications
7. Family and social history, including ethnicity and culture
8. Personality structure and coping style
9. Medical history and current treatments
10. Drug and other allergies
11. History and current status of substance abuse or dependence and treatment
12. Mental status examination

as the patient gets better, there may be a temporary increase in anxiety or depression. A gain or change in functioning can be experienced as a loss. Chapters 1 and 2, explain the neurophysiological basis of these phenomena as a basic biological principle: "There is no reorganization without disorganization" (Scott, 1979, p. 233). This is especially true for those patients who do not have many adaptive memory networks and are likely to be uncomfortable with positive experiences until the reorganized neural circuitry becomes reinforced and stabilized. As a prescriber, the APPN often assumes a designated or implied leadership role in a group practice with therapists; it is incumbent upon the APPN to understand dynamically what is happening in the therapy process through consultation with the referral source. That is, the APPN needs to discuss with the referring therapist and then the patient that the setback may be a temporary state with suggestions for physiological regulation and increasing resources while staying the therapeutic course. Skilled prescriber APPNs often begin a thorough psychiatric evaluation during the first session and then ask the person to come back in a week or more often before deciding whether medication is indicated. Such a thoughtful and thorough evaluation builds trust with both the patient and the referral source and may even potentiate the likelihood that the medication, if prescribed, will be helpful. Of course, there are always exceptions to this deliberative approach of evaluation over several sessions, including patients in acute distress who are actively psychotic or suffering from panic anxiety or intractable insomnia.

Prior or simultaneous to prescribing, the APPN will likely get diagnostic testing as shown in Table 14.1. Finally, the APPN collaborates with the patient by educating the patient about options for treatment, the mechanisms of action of any proposed medications, anticipated time frame for achieving therapeutic effects, risks and benefits of medication, and duration of treatment. It is this educational component that provides

TABLE 14.1 DIAGNOSTIC ASSESSMENT TOOLS	
Initial laboratory studies	Complete blood count with differential Comprehensive metabolic panel Lipid panel: high-density lipoproteins, low-density lipoproteins, total cholesterol, triglycerides Liver function: albumin, total protein, ALT, AST, ALP, GGT, bilirubin, prothrombin Thyroid panel: triiodothyronine, thyroxine, thyroid-stimulating hormone Hemoglobin A_{1c} β-Human gonadotropin (in women of reproductive age)
Laboratory studies if clinical indicated	Prolactin level (specify if adult or child) Any medication levels (e.g., lithium, valproic acid) Epstein-Barr virus titer HIV titer Serum or urine toxicology: amphetamines, barbiturates, benzodiazepines, cocaine, methamphetamine, opiates, phencyclidine, cannabinoids, alcohol
Other studies	EKG with QT correction Polysomnography Electroencephalogram

ALP, alkaline phosphatase; ALT, alanine aminotransferase; AST, aspartate transaminase; GGT, gamma-glutamyl transferase

some balance in power by virtue of freely sharing knowledge about the medications and how they work neurologically, possible side effects and how the patient can mitigate them, and how to report to the APPN concerns about the medicating process. The best practice is to provide written instructions for each medication prescribed including what and when to report to the APPN. At the conclusion of the initial evaluation, the APPN may ask the patient to sign an agreement that describes in simple terms what to expect from pharmacological treatment, how to get refills, and any specific policies for schedule 2 and 3 prescriptions (e.g., state prescription drug monitoring programs). See Appendix 14.2 for an example prescription practice policy.

Drug selection. Research on pharmacotherapies for specific symptomatology and/or diagnosis is ambiguous and controversial. The underlying assumption that a particular class of drugs can definitively treat a psychiatric diagnosis conflicts with the expressed atheoretical nature of the *Diagnostic and Statistical Manual of Mental Disorders* (5th ed.; *DSM-5;* American Psychiatric Association, 2013). Because psychotropic drugs target specific neurotransmitters, neuroreceptors, or neurotransporters, they can only be associated with neurological functions or dysfunctions. Ghaemi (2019) advocates revising the psychopharmacology nomenclature based on clinical efficacy and scientific basis. Psychiatric diagnoses embodied in the *DSM-5,* however, are a compilation of symptoms that are correlated with a label that best conceptualizes the disorder and are unrelated to putative neurobiology. The diagnosis and the neurobiological processes are loosely related, for example, antipsychotics were originally classified as *neuroleptics,* which are defined as any drug that affects nerve functions.

There are two broad classes of antipsychotics: the dopamine antagonists or first-generation antipsychotics (FGAs) and the serotonin dopamine antagonists or the second-generation antipsychotics (SGAs). These two classes specifically close the dopamine receptor (antagonize). The SGAs have a brief occupancy (receptor blockade) of dopamine receptors and at the same time close the serotonin 2A receptor subtype with a net effect of indirectly causing the nearby dopamine receptor to release dopamine forward to the frontal cortex. These neurobiological events result in decreased anxiety, improved impulse control, and to a lesser extent improved cognitive reasoning regardless of the psychiatric diagnoses. Consequently, the SGAs have shown effectiveness with symptoms related to psychosis, including schizophrenia and bipolar disorders as well as treatment resistant depression, obsessive-compulsive disorders, and borderline personality disorder that manifest as anxiety, mood dysregulation, impulsivity, and poor decision-making (Dold & Kasper, 2017; Lindström, Lindström, Nilsson, & Hoistad, 2017; Nielsen, Hessellund, Valentin, & Licht, 2018; Smith, Leucht, & Davis, 2019; Starcevic & Janca, 2018).

Similar studies show effective use of antiepileptic drugs to treat mood instability of personality disorders as well as bipolar disorders and schizoaffective disorder (Bartoli et al., 2018; Chen et al., 2019; Crawford et al., 2018). Because the antiepileptic drugs target GABA (gamma-amino butyric acid) or glutamate receptors or the sodium and calcium channels that contribute to the vesicular release of those neurotransmitters, they also slow down neural firing that influences impulse control centers (Stahl, 2018). Adrenergic antagonists (alpha and beta blockers) are used to treat anxiety disorders (Rasmussen, Kincaid, & Froehlich, 2017; Sagar-Ouriaghli, Lievesley, & Santosh, 2018; Steenen et al., 2016), nightmares, and posttraumatic stress disorder (Khouzam, 2013; Limandri, 2018a) even though they are Food and Drug Administration (FDA) approved to treat hypertension or benign prostatic hypertrophy. By blocking noradrenergic firing in certain areas of the brain during stress, there is a reduction in anxiety behaviors (Stahl, 2018).

To prescribe effectively and safely the APPN needs to understand the neurobiology of mental disorders and symptoms and the pharmacodynamics of psychotropic medications as well as the pharmacokinetics. Otherwise prescribing is by algorithm, which is overly simplistic and not individualized to the specific patient. It is inviting for a new APPN to rely on decision trees and algorithms as guidelines for practice. In addition, however, consulting with experienced prescribers in clarifying the relationship between symptoms, behaviors, neurobiology, recent research evidence, and patient preferences and needs provides a thoughtful and professional approach to prescribing. Attending professional conferences on psychopharmacology and psychotherapy, regularly reading professional journals, using online educational offerings, and maintaining a colleague consultation group are ways the APPN can maintain and improve knowledge and skill. Evidence-based practice requires the APPN to stay current in research, which further necessitates time (usually not reimbursed) and expertise in reading and critiquing complex literature. An expeditious way of reviewing the literature is to seek meta-analyses that combine many studies of similar levels of quality and reanalyzing the data with a higher effect size. These studies can be found through the Cochrane Database online (Limandri, 2019; Lundh, 2017).

In using medications as part of the total treatment plan, the APPN monitors the patient's progress including therapeutic response to medications, counterbalanced with adverse or side effects. Because side effects usually precede therapeutic effects, it is tempting to prescribe additional medications to alleviate side effects. This approach, however, often leads to polypharmacy and exposes the patient to negative drug interactions. A more cautious and restrained approach would be to recommend nonpharmacological means of mediating side effects or ways for the patient to cope with them until they dissipate, for example, using sugarless gum to reduce dry mouth or taking a sedating medication at bedtime. Frequently, side effects go away within 2–4 weeks as the more therapeutic effects start.

When the patient responds partially to a medication, the APPN needs to consider first how the patient is taking the medication (taking daily as prescribed) before increasing the dosage for complete reduction of target symptoms or augmenting with another medication or treatment strategy. Augmenting with another medication in a different class (e.g., adding a noradrenergic drug to a serotonergic) or a different drug to target another related symptom (insomnia with depression) is a common tactic, even though nonpharmacological augmentation strategies may serve the purpose with less risk of drug-drug interactions. For example, adding a hypnotic (e.g., zolpidem) to a drug regimen may give short-term relief while exposing the patient to possible drug dependence and altered sleep architecture. Adding a 6-week course of cognitive behavior therapy for insomnia (CBT-I), however, will provide a long-term benefit to the patient in managing sleep disturbances. Another strategy when the patient does not get full relief of target symptoms is to change to a different medication in the same class or better yet another class. Reassess with the patient what relief is valued and benefits the patient is seeking is essential in making changes in medication. The more fully informed the patient, the greater chance for following a treatment regimen and getting full response.

A similar concern in prescribing is de-prescribing, that is, when and how to discontinue medications. When a patient comes to the APPN on a medication regimen, there needs to be discussion about how the regimen is contributing to the patient's mental health, including if there are medications that may be contradictory. A common situation is the patient who has been prescribed a benzodiazepine and/or sleeping aid beyond the recommended 3- to 4-week time period, even for many years of refilled prescriptions without reevaluation of the effects or possible detriments. Such a circumstance may place a strain on the therapeutic alliance by suggesting that the patient may have a dependency with rebound exacerbation of symptoms that feels counter to the patient's expressed concerns. Because depression, sleep disturbances, dependency, and tolerance develop over time with benzodiazepines and hypnotics, the patient who has been taking them for an extended time will be resistant to the suggestion that they be discontinued. It is essential that the APPN explain the need for discontinuation in a nonjudgmental manner and describe a slow gradual process that will include substitution of medications and adjunctive therapies to help the patient withdrawal comfortably (Limandri, 2018b). In a similar way, if a patient has been taking medications for depression for an extended period with remission of symptoms, the APPN will need to discuss a tapering plan and schedule because it may no longer be necessary. The tapering process, however, may result in some temporary rebound of symptoms that the APPN needs to explain to the patient and reassure the patient to help with treatment. Older patients may also need medication adjustments because of change in metabolism, comorbid conditions, and additional nonpsychiatric medications.

REUNITING PSYCHOTHERAPY AND PHARMACOTHERAPY

Whether the APPN chooses to provide psychotherapy alone, pharmacotherapy alone, or some combination, the service provided is always in the context of the whole person. The mind and the brain cannot be considered separately, that is, the brain creates the mind and the mind influences brain function. Therefore, treating the patient requires the APPN to understand and treat the neurobiological changes that influence symptoms and whole person reaction just as the APPN needs to address the patient's psychological and environmental concerns when prescribing medications. Psychotropic medications can aid and hasten psychotherapy, and psychotherapy can assist the patient to be open to medication treating neurobiological changes while making psychosocial changes to improve the quality of living.

In the evolution of psychiatry and mental health services there has been a shift in viewing mental illness as character flaw to the recognition that mental illness is a brain disorder that manifests in behavioral and emotional symptoms and influences relationships with others. Psychological treatments have shown efficacy in symptom reduction in major depressive disorders (Cuijpers, Cristea, Karyotaki, Reijnders, & Hollon, 2019; Gajic-Veljanoski et al., 2018; Zhang et al., 2019), anxiety disorders (Beutel, Greenberg, Lane, & Subic, 2019; Timulak, 2018; Zhou et al., 2019), substance use disorders (Baldus et al., 2018; Kim, Brook, & Akin, 2018; Lo Coco et al., 2019;), schizophrenia (Ashcroft, Kim, Elefant, Benson, & Carter, 2018; Juntapim & Nuntaboot, 2018; Rosenbaum, 2018), bipolar disorders (Chatterton et al., 2017; Lovas & Schuman-Oliver, 2018; Wilson, Crowe, Scott, & Lacey, 2018), and personality disorders (Kvarstein et al., 2019; Sachse & Kramer, 2019; Oud, Arntz, Hermens, Verhoef, & Kendall, 2018). However, full remission from a diagnosed serious psychiatric disorder such as schizophrenia or bipolar disorder rarely occurs through psychotherapy alone.

When symptoms meet the criteria established in the *DSM-5* (APA, 2013), the APPN diagnoses a psychiatric disorder. Prescribing medications implies that the symptoms are evidence of an illness, which to some extent indicates brain dysfunction. Therefore, it is reasonable to assume that best treatment would focus on both the brain dysfunction and the behavioral and interpersonal consequences of that brain dysfunction. The brain, however, heals slowly and most medications take weeks to months to show significant therapeutic effect. Unfortunately, our culture reinforces immediacy in treating any kind of illness, and patients want quick solutions. The media promotes pills, yet talk therapy is decried as slow and arduous. In fact, research shows that best outcomes occur when pharmacotherapy, if indicated, is combined with psychotherapy in the treatment plan (Karyotaki et al., 2016).

Even if the APPN is only prescribing, psychosocial and interpersonal interventions are necessary to resolving individual emotional distress and family disturbance (Greenberg,

2016). Meta-analyses of randomized clinical trials demonstrate that the combined effects of pharmacotherapy and psychotherapy are necessary for social and occupational functioning and quality of life with long-term benefits (Kamenov, Twomey, Cabello, Prina, & Ayuso-Mateos, 2017; Karyotaki et al., 2016). Intensive psychotherapy of any kind may not provide sufficient dose-effect benefits as does the combined pharmacotherapy and brief psychotherapy in treating severe depression, bipolar disorder, and some anxiety disorders (Leichsenring & Hoyer, 2019; Miklowitz et al., 2014; Molenaar et al., 2011). Other studies have compared psychotherapy alone and pharmacotherapy alone with combining the two in terms of length of treatment and duration of benefits for posttraumatic stress disorders, eating disorders, and substance use disorders to conclude that the combination of treatments produces the most effective outcomes with enduring remission of symptoms (Grasser & Javanbakht, 2019; Kelly & Daley, 2013).

A major difficulty in researching the benefits of psychotherapy is controlling for the effects of the interpersonal relationship with the therapist and relating to specific therapeutic strategies or variables. Stahl refers to psychotherapy as the new epigenetic drug (Stahl, 2012). One randomized controlled study focused on the therapeutic alliance in relation to symptomatic relief and antidepressant treatment. This study found that the therapeutic alliance and symptom change were intricately entangled regardless of specific medications and that the alliance was essential for symptom improvement. In fact, early symptom change predicted a therapeutic alliance developing but the therapeutic alliance alone did not predict symptom change (Zilcha-Mano, 2015). Therefore, it is reasonable to conclude that the key ingredient to treatment is the therapeutic relationship. Even if the APPN is prescribing medications as the sole treatment strategy, the benefits of treatment are enhanced by developing an alliance with the patient, which requires active and deliberate psychotherapy approaches. Maintaining separate roles of prescribing or psychotherapy is not evidence-based. Yes, each have their benefits but best practice requires unifying the roles.

BARRIERS TO FULL SCOPE OF PRACTICE

What are the barriers to unifying prescriptive and psychotherapy roles? Some argue that prescribing is a power position that interferes with the therapeutic alliance; however, the psychotherapist also has significant albeit subtle authority over the patient. In the early stages of any therapeutic exchange, the APPN establishes the boundaries of the relationship as well as the need for shared decision-making (Ross, 2010). Managing treatment resistance and medication adherence is less onerous when the APPN and patient openly discuss not just what medications to take or specific therapeutic strategies but also the risks and benefits, how to minimize risks, and when there needs to be alteration in the treatment plan. It is that shared decision-making that forms the basis of any therapeutic alliance (Morant, Kaminskly, & Ramon, 2015).

The belief that power in the prescribing role is contradictory to combining psychotherapy and prescribing is based on theoretical assumptions without substantiation by robust research. In fact, there is limited research on the effect on the patient of the prescribing role. Is the notion of imbalance of power in the prescribing role a historical artifact of paternalism of physicians? Could it be that nurse prescribers come from a different tradition and culture than that of physicians and therefore they enact the role differently? Could it be that patient characteristics interact with the prescriber role, such as opposition or submission, to contribute to power imbalance? Two qualitative studies and one meta-synthesis of qualitative studies out of the United Kingdom shed some light on the interaction involved in nurse prescribing. Fisher (2010) analyzed his interviews with APRNs, physician general practitioners, and pharmacists using the theories of power and domination by Foucault and Weber to describe three elements of the prescribing interaction: how professional knowledge is incorporated in practice; how professional roles are negotiated and constructed within and across organizational boundaries; and how the clinician creates and maintains a role in systems of value and power (Fisher, 2010).

From a different perspective Ross (2015) included the perceptions of patients as well as nurse and physician prescribers and pharmacists with a focus on the mental health setting. She found that patients preferred the consistency of maintaining a therapy relationship with their nurse who also prescribed their medications and understood the patient and the condition. Nurse prescribers were seen as those who negotiated treatment based on informed decision-making with a different style than those of the medical profession. The theme of power was dominant in this study in terms of the nurse feeling empowered to provide a full range of care and involve the patient in that care (Ross, 2015).

A meta-synthesis study of nurse prescribing in primary care included qualitative literature from Spain, Norway, Finland, Sweden, Ireland, The Netherlands, New Zealand, South Africa, Columbia, Australia, Canada, and the United States (Nuttall, 2018). Although not specific to mental health or combination of prescribing and psychotherapy, the study provided an exhaustive research base. The conclusions were that nurse prescribers provide patient-centered care that improves overall service and is well received by patients. This study identified a power shift in interprofessional relationships with a lack of understanding and misperceptions of expectations by other professionals of the nurse role. Such a power shift required renegotiation of role boundaries with physicians and pharmacists. Although not mentioned in this study, in the mental health setting psychologists and social workers would also be included in those with which the nurse prescribers need to clarify role boundaries. Ultimately, this study emphasized the importance of building a relationship with patients and other professionals and clarifying the culture of prescribing within the total context of service to the patient.

At an individual level the APPN decides on the extent of the scope of practice and negotiates it with the organization or agency or maintains an independent practice within the legal parameters of the state practice act. Practicing within the full scope of the advanced practice role includes both prescribing and providing therapy for patients. How one enacts the role requires thoughtfulness and flexible decision-making. Some guidelines for the clinician are:

1. Clearly state what you include in your practice in writing and verbally at first contact. This may be variable, however, based on your assessment of each patient. Discussing this early in treatment and inviting the patient's preferences and needs will help establish the therapeutic alliance.
2. Discuss options for enacting these roles including specific allotment per session for medication issues separate from therapy issues, separating medication sessions from therapy sessions throughout the week or month; discuss referrals to other clinicians for elements you decide to carve out of your role with the patient.
3. Provide brief, simple written instructions regarding contacts outside the appointment times for medication questions, refills, emergencies, cancellations, rescheduling, and DEA (Drug Enforcement Agency) scheduled drugs.
4. Reflect on your own preferences, skills, knowledge, and attitudes about patient situations that influence your ability to provide both services for patients.
5. Engage the patient in specifically and openly discussing boundaries and conditions of treatment over time. If there are problems with staying within the boundaries, discuss in a neutral way and engage in collaborative problem-solving.

APPLICATION TO PRACTICE

In a shared decision model based on a holistic approach to determination of priority needs and development of a mutually agreed upon treatment plan we have developed a chart incorporating major areas of consideration including common symptom clusters, identification of adverse childhood events (ACEs), and the social determinants of health (Box 14.2).

Depending on the nurse practice act in the state in which you are practicing, you will have the ability to independently or collaboratively determine the focus and direction of care. Functioning within the full scope of the role whether prescribing alone or in conjunction with psychotherapy or psychotherapy alone or in conjunction with medication facilitates fulfillment in practice. See Box 14.3 for resources for additional education about psychopharmacology.

BOX 14.2 Factors that Need to be Considered in Establishing the Course of Treatment

Diagnostic Symptom Clusters	Adverse Childhood Events	Social Determinants of Health
Anxiety	Physical abuse	Availability of resources to meet daily needs (e.g., safe housing and local food markets)
Attentional	Verbal abuse	Access to educational, economic, and job opportunities
Bipolar spectrum	Sexual abuse	Access to healthcare services
Depression	Physical neglect	Public safety
Disruptive/impulse control	Emotional neglect	Availability of community-based resources in support of family and community living.
Dissociative disorders	Parental alcoholism	Transportation options
Feeding/eating disorders	Intimate partner violence	Quality of education and job training
Intellectual	Family member in jail	Social support
Neurocognitive	Family member diagnosed with mental illness	Social norms and attitudes (e.g., discrimination, racism, and distrust of government)
Obsessive-compulsive	Disappearance of a parent through divorce, death, abandonment	Exposure to crime, violence, and social disorder (e.g., presence of trash and lack of cooperation in a community)

(continued)

BOX 14.2 Factors that Need to be Considered in Establishing the Course of Treatmen (*continued*)

Diagnostic Symptom Clusters	Adverse Childhood Events	Social Determinants of Health
Paraphilias		Socioeconomic conditions (e.g., concentrated poverty and the stressful conditions that accompany it)
Personality		Residential segregation
Schizophrenia spectrum		Language/literacy
Sexual/gender dysphoria		Access to mass media and emerging technologies (e.g., cell phones, the Internet, and social media)
Sleep/wake		Culture
Somatic		Opportunities for recreational and leisure-time activities
Substance use disorders		Access to healthcare services (addiction services)
Trauma and stressor-related		Access to health care services (trauma therapy)

BOX 14.3 Resources for Additional Education

Electronic Resources
- American Psychiatric Nurses Association (APNA) website, Continuing Education (CE; www .apna.org/i4a/pages/index.cfm?pageid=3824), offers low-cost and even free CE content from the APNA annual conferences and annual Clinical Psychopharmacology Institute as well as courses developed specifically by APNA.
- Neuroscience Education Institute has a full website that includes many resources (www. neiglobal.com/Home/tabid/55/Default.aspx) by subscription for $249/year. Included in the benefits are discounts to many of the educational conferences, Stephen Stahl books, the *CNS Spectrums* journal, CE podcasts, mobile applications, and other things.
- PsychU (www.psychu.org/resource-library/collections/psychopharmacology) is a free subscription service with an extensive resource library including psychotherapy and pharmacotherapy.

Organizational Resources
- American Psychiatric Nurses Association (www.apna.org) provides an annual conference for all psychiatric-mental health nurses and two annual clinical psychopharmacology conferences (one on West coast, one on East coast), mentorship opportunities with experienced nurse leaders, online continuing education offerings, and networking via member bridge website. The APNA also publishes a journal *The Journal of the American Psychiatric Nurses Association*.
- International Society of Psychiatric-Mental Health Nurses (www.ispn-psych.org) is an organization specific to advanced practice psychiatric mental health nurses that

CASE EXAMPLE

A 36-year-old woman was referred by her primary care provider (PCP) because of persistent feelings of depression and anxiety. She scored 16/27 on the Patient Health Questionnaire-9 (PHQ-9) in her PCP's screening. In her intake questionnaire she described feeling sad, worried, and unmotivated for at least 3 months with vague thoughts of wishing she were dead but without specific thoughts or plans to kill herself. She is uncertain about any particular situations that preceded these feelings and reports no previous psychiatric hospitalizations or outpatient treatments. She acknowledges a prolonged period of depression when she was completing college and starting employment, at which time she thought she was depressed but did not seek help at that time. She improved over time, has had two committed relationships, and married 3 years ago. She is employed full time as a systems analyst for a large technological company, a job she describes as stressful but fulfilling. Her husband is supportive; he works full time as a construction contractor. They have no children and participate in activities with their families and friendship network.

Medical history: She denies any drug or food allergies. Two years ago, she developed menstrual irregularities and was treated by a gynecologist for endometriosis with oral contraceptives. She was diagnosed hypothyroid at age 28 years and has continued with a prescription of Iiothyronine (Cytomel) 25 mcg daily. She has occasional migraine headaches treated with sumatriptan as needed. Otherwise she has regular preventive health appointments annually.

Substance use history: Drinks two or three glasses of wine per week irregularly. Smoked marijuana occasionally in college but none recently. Denies any other drug use.

Family history: Raised by an intact family with a younger sister who has episodes of anxiety and is a "worrisome" person. Father died in an automotive accident when the patient was in college. Mother has remained single and is active in church and community theater.

Personal history: Full-term birth. No known complications. Uneventful childhood. Very active in school activities and above average student. Graduated from state college with some postbaccalaureate classes for her occupation. Sexually assaulted 2 years after graduating from college when working nights as a barista in a café. Saw a rape counselor through the district attorney's office while crime was adjudicated and assailant was convicted. Denies current trauma symptoms are related to that event.

Mental health assessment: Mental status examination was all within normal limits with the exception of depressed and anxious mood most of the day, and nearly every day loss of motivation and interest in pleasurable activities. Difficulty falling asleep most nights and not feeling rested in the morning. Feels tired most of the time as well as agitated and restless more days than not. Acknowledges low self-esteem and not striving to her potential. Difficulty thinking and concentrating at work. Was surprised by thinking about dying and that her husband would grieve briefly but move on with his life. Denied a specific plan to kill herself "but I've thought it might be nice to not wake up in the morning." Stated that she has had no previous suicide attempts or hospitalizations for suicidal ideation. She noted that she is anxious about not performing well at work and losing her job, even though she has had yearly high-performance evaluations. Worried that her husband will get tired of her and want to have an affair but is afraid to talk to him about this.

Current medications prescribed by PCP:

1. Norgestimate/ethinyl estradiol one tab daily × 2 years for birth control
2. Sumatriptan 50 mg tab as needed for migraine headaches
3. Liothyronine 25 mcg daily for hypothyroidism
4. Sertraline 75 mg daily × 4 weeks for depression
5. Zolpidem 5 mg hs × 2 weeks for sleep

This woman clearly meets criteria for major depressive disorder (MDD) with anxious features; and MDD is a recurrent event for her. The current stresses in her life makes her more vulnerable to a return of depressive symptoms with the counterbalancing factors of a supportive support system (may be too sparse for her situation) and fulfilling job that adequately provides for her and her husband. Her medical conditions both add to her anxiety symptoms and serve as background stressors.

Her developmental history adds the element of resiliency related to early family losses and her mother apparently modeling coping strategies. However, there may be some genetic disposition for anxiety. What remains a significant trauma was the sexual assault she experienced and resolved through both the criminal prosecution (finding justice?) and the support of a rape counselor. Still that may present background triggering for her in some situations and also places her in a neurophysiologically vulnerable state. Both the death of her father and the sexual assault in her young adulthood may be seen as ACEs. This woman seems to have protective factors of access to education, job, economic, food, housing, and health resources.

Additional important information and considerations:

- What other persons are available to her for social support? Women and men friends, co-workers, other family members?
- How willing is she to seek therapy and does she see this as a value right now?
- How has she managed the thoughts about her self-image and esteem, job, her husband, and her thoughts of dying? What does she do and how does she feel when she has these thoughts?
- Describe more about her sleep difficulties. How long does she take to fall asleep? What does she do while awake at night? What thoughts does she have? How does she manage these? What has she tried to help her sleep better?
- Explore her thoughts about dying in greater detail. What is she thinking? How often does she have these thoughts? How long do they persist and what does she do to manage them? Has she ever actively or passively acted on these thoughts. Conduct a full Columbia Suicide Severity Rating Scale (CSSR) with her and explain the rationale behind this test.
- How does she take her medications? How often does she miss doses? How has the sertraline affected her, that is, improvement of symptoms, side effects, specific adverse effects, for example, suicidal thoughts since initiation, sexual arousal changes. How has the zolpidem affected her? Any side effects, for example, sleep walking or eating?

Explain her diagnosis and treatment plan in relation to her presentation. What treatment options are recommended and why?

- First ask her what she knows about her diagnosis from the PCP and what she thinks about that diagnosis.
- Show her the *DSM-5* diagnosis criteria for MDD and the anxious features and ask if this best describes her. Also show her PTSD (posttraumatic stress disorder) criteria to be sure to rule out additional symptoms that she may not have endorsed but experiences.
- Also consider the neurological traumagenic cascade that may influence her experience of anxiety connected with loss and sadness.
- Review the CSSR results and ask what she thinks and feels about these results. Clarify that it is not a judgment but a way to measure the assessment and be able to reassess at a later date to see changes.

A suggested initial approach in negotiating treatment for this patient:

- Recommend psychotherapy with preference for CBT approach to help with her thinking symptoms, interpersonal therapy to help her develop relational and coping skills and insight, or EMDR if triggering symptoms are more bothersome.
- CBT-I course to replace sleeping medication for more long-term effective treatment of her sleep disturbance. Explain that zolpidem is recommended for short-term treatment of 3–4 weeks only and CBT-I is the standard of care. Discuss gradual tapering of zolpidem as she becomes more skilled with CBT-I.
- Inquire how she would like to involve her husband in treatment, both as a collateral information source and as supportive care. Explain how important it is to have him involved but that it is her choice.
- Create with her a safety plan (using Stanley and Brown Suicide Safety Implementation template [suicidepreventionlifeline.org/wp-content/uploads/2016/08/Brown_StanleySafetyPlanTemplate.pdf]). Explain that as her APPN, you would like to review with her at the next appointment and encourage her to share with her husband.
- Ask what she thinks about these ideas, what other ideas she has, what she feels about these plans, and what her preferences are. Also ask how she feels about working with you as her APPN and what she would like to change or add.

Discuss medication plan:

- Discuss increasing medications, specifically dosage of sertraline, for better symptomatic relief. Explain the treatment lag time related to serotonin receptor upregulation. Explain possible increase in suicidal thinking related to improved energy without full depressive symptom relief.
- Assess alternative medication choices including a less activating medication, for example, citalopram or escitalopram if anxiety remains a major concern.
- Discuss the need to taper off the zolpidem over time and replace with CBT-I. Explain reasons for taper and how it would be done.
- Explain how you will communicate medication regimen with PCP.

Time frame for plan:

It is important to explain that her symptoms are recurrent and that she is vulnerable for future episodes. This vulnerability may be reduced by fully treating not just the symptoms but also underlying psychosocial issues and learning coping strategies. This takes time to learn and for the brain to reestablish functioning. Explain neurotransmission theories of depression and anxiety and the process of neurogenesis in healing the brain at a level she will understand. Explain the role of insight and coping skills development as helpful in resiliency and sense of self-efficacy. Discuss the importance of developing a therapeutic relationship together that includes trust and confidence. Recommend 6-week trial of combined psychotherapy and pharmacotherapy.

Coordination of care with the other providers:

- Explain the importance of coordination of care with PCP and value of the PCP's referral to mental health care for this situation.
- Suggest that husband and family are important players in overall care and ask how she would like to involve them, with an option that she discusses with them and/or invite them in for a session with you.
- It is not necessary to get a release of information to share with the PCP because it is within standard of care, but it is certainly important that the APPN convey to the patient what she is sharing with the PCP. This can be in writing or verbally and needs to be documented in the chart that the APPN has informed the patient. Any communication with the PCP needs to be documented in the chart as well.

After initial stabilization:

- Suggest continuation of effective medication dosage for at least 1 year of complete remission of symptoms then taper off the medication as symptoms permit. If symptoms recur, may need to reinstitute dosage for additional 3 to 6 months and try to taper off again. PCP can manage medications if patient would like to return to PCP for medications.
- Communicate medication transitions to PCP.
- Recommend tapering off psychotherapy as well with transition from weekly to every other week for 1 to 2 months, then monthly check-ins for 2 months, then check-in at 6 months if patient wishes.
- Leave the door open for return visits if symptoms return, other symptoms develop, or just for refresher in therapeutic effects.

CONCLUDING COMMENTS

Advanced practice psychiatric nursing continues to evolve and develop as a significant contribution to overall mental health care. From the beginning under Hildegard Peplau's direction the central focus of psychiatric mental health nursing has been the interpersonal relationship between the patient and the nurse. Until the 1980s the role has solidly involved psychotherapy from a wide array of therapeutic modalities and theories. As the prescribing role was added, schools of nursing shifted focus to the more technical aspects of prescribing to the loss of emphasis on psychotherapy knowledge and skills. It is time for the pendulum to swing back to center and reincorporate psychotherapy and psychopharmacology into the holistic paradigm of advanced practice. For some this may require reschooling, collegial consultation, continuing education and mentorship, and reinvestment in clinical time. In organizations this may require renegotiating practice roles and job assignments, reviewing and rewriting policies, and engaging colleagues in other disciplines in understanding the scope of our practice. Most importantly, however, psychiatric mental health nursing as a discipline and each of us as individuals must examine our commitment to the future place of advanced psychiatric mental health nursing in the mental healthcare system.

DISCUSSION QUESTIONS

Answer the following questions for the following two case examples. The information provided may not be sufficient but it is what is available for you to analyze and conceptualize how you might proceed with the following patients, Case Example A and Case Example B. After reviewing each vignette discuss with colleagues the following questions. There are no single correct answers to the questions, just different approaches to take.

1. In reviewing this chapter, which factors are important to consider for this patient?
2. What additional information would you like to have to be more comfortable in working with this patient?
3. How will you explain your diagnosis and treatment plan in relation to the patient presentation? What treatment options will you recommend and why?
4. What is your initial approach in negotiating treatment for this patient?
5. What medication changes would you want to discuss with the patient and how will you negotiate that with her or him?
6. What time frame do you propose for this plan and how will you transition with the patient?
7. How will you coordinate care with the other providers working with this patient?
8. After stabilization, which psychotherapeutic approach would you take?

CASE EXAMPLE A

Campus security was called to the dormitory to assess a 19-year-old man who barricaded himself in his room and covered the windows with aluminum foil. His roommate reported that this man hasn't been attending classes for the past week, hasn't bathed or eaten, and has been mumbling that the FBI is monitoring all his communications. Security removed the door and took the man into custody and to the community mental health center for evaluation.

History of current episode: Information obtained by interview with the patient and with collateral telephone interviews with each of his parents, his college roommate, and his English professors. This is the first year away from home for this young man, who has been described as an "odd and reserved" person since teen years. Academically he did well his first semester at college, although he has made few friends and does not participate in any social or extracurricular events. His teachers describe him as a bright and quiet student. His parents, who live in a small town over 70 miles away from the college, expressed sadness but not surprise at his behavioral deterioration because they didn't expect him to be able to cope with the discrepancy of the large college campus compared to his small-town previous experience.

Psychiatric history: Although he has never been hospitalized or had outpatient psychiatric treatment, this young man has been showing signs of emotional and cognitive disorganization since his early teens. During his high school years the patient became more and more aloof, and strange with both his family and friends. At times he would be mute for days at a time, remained in his room and refused to bathe. He said he did not have control over his thoughts and he believed he was possessed. In his junior year of high school his counselor recommended he attend a breakout group to help him learn interpersonal skills and make friends, but he never attended. The summer before going to college his parents asked if he wanted to see a therapist or counselor to talk about transitions but he said he didn't want to do that and that he wasn't concerned about living away from his family for the first time.

Medical history: Has had regular preventive care and immunizations through local family practice. In good health, weight proportion to height, denies smoking or alcohol or drug consumption. Broke his left wrist at age 7 years when he fell off his bike. Moderate acne in late teens treated with oral doxycycline for several months. No drug or food allergies. Allergic reaction to bee sting when 10 years old with swelling, shortness of breath, now carries EpiPen.

Family history: Has an older brother, 23 years old, who graduated from college and is now attending graduate school in business administration. Younger sister is 15 years old and in good health. Father is a business executive, has chronic obstructive pulmonary disease (COPD) related to long-standing cigarette smoking. Mother is an Episcopal priest and is in good health. Maternal uncle died at age 49, diagnosed with schizophrenia.

Personal history: Normal pregnancy and uncomplicated childbirth. Was an active and creative child who enjoyed reading, art, and cooking with his mother and grandmother. Parents said he started to become reserved and shy in middle school for no apparent reason. By early teens he seemed socially inept, had few friends, and preferred solitary play. Never interested in romantic relationships or dating in high school and spent most of his time studying or reading fantasy novels. Seemed to be withdrawn and serious, although denied feeling sad, or depressed.

Trauma/abuse history: Mild bullying in middle school, otherwise no apparent trauma.

Mental status examination: Well groomed, neatly attired, cooperative. Polite without motor abnormalities or gait. Moderate eye contact when directly addressed. Alert, mildly sedated, oriented to time, place, person. Attentive during interview and provided accurate albeit minimal history that was corroborated by family members. Based on fund of knowledge seemed of average intelligence. Speech is normal rate and soft spoken and at times mumbled responses to questions. Stated that he hears a soft voice in his head that tells him to "be careful" but offered no other explanation of voices. Denied visual or other perceptual hallucinations. Thought processes are linear and coherent. Reports that he believes people talk about him behind his back and that he is being controlled by unseen forces. Refused to elaborate on these thoughts. Stated that he has never thought of killing himself or anyone else. Described his mood as "fine" and refused to elaborate. Affect is flat. Demonstrates impulse control and alludes to feeling like an automaton. Judgment is reasonable in terms of recognizing consequences of actions.

Current medications: No regularly prescribed medications. Given lorazepam 1.0 mg orally in urgent care when brought in by campus security because of his extreme agitation. Slept for an hour after administration while waiting to be interviewed.

Differential diagnosis: Brief Psychotic Disorder versus First Episode of Schizophrenia. The duration of the episode is greater than 1 day but uncertain if longer than 1 month, and no previous psychiatric hospitalization. Teen years are suggestive of prodromal period of schizophrenia that may be precipitated by stress of independence from family and college experience.

CASE EXAMPLE B

John B. is a 15-year-old man of Sudanese descent who resides with his mother, grandmother, 23-year-old brother, and his brother's wife. They are all asylum seekers to the United States, having arrived from South Sudan 2 years prior to this. He is seen in this mental health clinic after discharge from an inpatient stay following a suicide attempt by hanging.

Brother found patient hanging by a rope tied to the clothes rod in the closet. Patient was cyanotic with slow pulse and taken to the hospital by ambulance. He was treated in the inpatient adolescent unit for 1 week and discharged to this clinic for an assessment and follow-up treatment. He reported that he has been feeling depressed "for as long as I can remember" with low self-esteem, feelings of hopelessness and being a burden to his family, guilt, and self-hatred. He said he had been thinking about killing himself for several months and has been cutting on his arms in practicing for this. His brother came home from work unexpectedly to find him. He described not fitting in at school and not feeling comfortable in his new home. His brother arranged to bring his mother and grandmother to the United States to flee from the war. His brother was brought to the United States when he was 14 years old under the UNICEF program for rehabilitation of child soldiers, and believes the patient was being recruited to be a soldier before coming here. Patient sleeps less than 4 hours/night with frequent nightmares and refuses to sleep in bed, prefers to sleep under the bed. Has poor appetite. Teachers report he has difficulty concentrating in school and has to take frequent breaks to sit in quiet room with soft music. He has made few friends and gets into fights, both physical and verbal, with other boys. Easily upset by loud noises or changes in routine at school or at home.

Medical history: Patient has no known drug or food allergies. He was treated for malnutrition upon arrival to the United States and remains underweight. He was diagnosed with mild intermittent asthma, triggered by exercise and seasonal allergies. Physical exam also revealed several horizontal scars on the inner surfaces of his left forearm.

Substance use history: Denies alcohol or drug use.

Family history: Father died in war in South Sudan when patient was 4 years old. Raised by mother and maternal grandmother with older brother. Older sister killed in village raid when patient was 5 years old. Unknown paternal history. Mother is 42 years old with unknown health history.

Personal history: Full-term birth without known complications. Attended school intermittently in South Sudan due to civil war. Currently attending special school and mostly fluent in English. Has had behavioral problems in school due to inattentiveness, anger, poor impulse control, and low frustration tolerance. Mother and grandmother do not speak English and are unable to provide description of patient's behavior at home. Brother works two jobs, as does brother's wife.

Trauma history: Witnessed his sister and mother being raped and sister's death. Possible torture prior to coming to United States.

Mental status examination: Thin, lanky young man with multiple scars on arms and back. Clean, casually attired with close-cropped hair. Cooperative and sullen during the assessment. Sits in chair with legs pulled up on the chair and gripping his knees with his arms. Makes moderate eye contact. Alert, oriented to time, place, and person. Memory not formally assessed but appears to be intact based on his ability to accurately relate details from his recent experience. Hypervigilant to the environment and interviewer's behavior. Linear thinking with abstract reasoning and seems to be of average to above average intelligence based on fund of knowledge. Speech is soft with pronounced accent, regular rate and rhythm. Comprehends English sufficiently to not need interpreter. Thinking process is coherent and goal directed. Thought content is focused on distress of hospitalization. Acknowledges wanting to die but without current plan to kill self and feeling remorseful that he upset his family with his recent attempt. Described his current mood as scared and depressed. Affect is fearful, tearful, and angry. Impulsive previous behavior with poor judgment and belief in limited future. Insight is reasonable in terms of understanding why he is referred to treatment.

Current medications prescribed at last hospitalization:

1. Prazosin 5 mg bid for nightmares and daytime stress
2. Vortioxetine 10 mg daily for depression and anxiety
3. Fluticasone-salmeterol inhaler qd for asthma
4. Theophylline 300 mg qd for asthma

Differential diagnosis: Major depressive disorder with suicidal thinking. Posttraumatic stress disorder.

REFERENCES

American Psychiatric Association. (2013). *Diagnostic and statistical manual of mental disorders.* (5th ed.). Arlington, VA: American Psychiatric Publishing.

APRN Joint Dialogue Group & National Council of State Boards of Nursing APRN Advisory Committee. (2008). *Consensus model for APRN regulation: Licensure, accreditation, certification & education.* Chicago: National Council of State Boards of Nursing. Retrieved from https://www.ncsbn.org/Consensus_Model_for_APRN_Regulation_July_2008.pdf

Ashcroft, K., Kim, E., Elefant, E., Benson, C., & Carter, J. A. (2018). Meta-analysis of caregiver-directed psychosocial interventions for schizophrenia. *Community Mental Health Journal, 54*(7), 983–991. doi:10.1007/s10597-018-0289-x

Baldus, C., Mokros, L., Daubmann, A., Arnaud, N., Holtmann, M., Thomasius, R., & Legenbauer, T. (2018). Treatment effectiveness of a mindfulness-based inpatient group psychotherapy in adolescent substance use disorder: Study protocol for a randomized controlled trial. *Trials, 19*(1), 706. doi:10.1186/s13063-018-3048-y

Bartoli, F., Clerici, M., Di Brita, C., Riboldi, I., Crocamo, C., & Carrà, G. (2018). Effect of clinical response to active drugs and placebo on antipsychotics and moods stabilizers relative efficacy for bipolar depression and mania: A meta-regression analysis. *Journal of Psychopharmacology, 32*(4), 416–424. doi:10.1177/0269881117749851

Bell, N., Hughes, R., & Lòpez-De Fede, A. (2018). Collaborative practice agreements and their geographic impact on where nurse practitioners can practice. *Journal of Nursing Regulations, 9*(3), 5–14. doi:10.1016/S2155-8256(18)30149-2

Beutel, M. E., Greenberg, L., Lane, R. D., & Subic, W. C. (2019). Treating anxiety disorders by emotion-focused psychodynamic psychotherapy (EFPP)—An integrative, transdiagnostic approach. *Clinical Psychology and Psychotherapy, 26*(1), 1–13. doi:10.1002/cpp.2325

Chatterton, M. L., Stockings, E., Berk, M., Barendregt, J. J., Carter, R., & Mihalopoulos, C. (2017). Psychosocial therapies for the adjunctive treatment of bipolar disorder in adults: Network meta-analysis. *British Journal of Psychiatry, 210*(5), 333–341. doi:10.1192/bjp.bp.116.195321

Chen, T.-Y., Kamali, M., Chu, C.-S., Yeh, C.-B., Huang, S.-Y., Mao, W.-C., . . . Hsu, C.-Y. (2019). Divalproex and its effect on suicide risk in bipolar disorder: A systematic review and meta-analysis of international observational studies. *Journal of Affective Disorders, 245*, 812–818. doi:10.1016/j.jad.2018.11.093

Crawford, M. J., Sanatinia, R., Barrett, B., Cunningham, G., Dale, O., Ganguli, P., . . . Reilly, J. G. (2018). The clinical effectiveness and cost-effectiveness of lamotrigine in borderline personality disorder: A randomized placebo-controlled trial. *American Journal of Psychiatry, 175*(8), 756–764. doi:10.1176/appi.ajp.2018.17091006

Cuijpers, P., Cristea, I. A., Karyotaki, E., Reijnders, M., & Hollon, S. D. (2019). Component studies of psychological treatments of adult depression: A systematic review and meta-analysis. *Psychotherapy Research: Journal of the Society for Psychotherapy Research, 29*(1), 15–29. doi:10.1080/10503307.2017.1395922

Dold, M., & Kasper, S. (2017). Evidence-based pharmacotherapy of treatment-resistant unipolar depression. *International Journal of Psychiatry in Clinical Practice, 21*(1), 13–23. doi:10.1080/13651501.2016.1248852

Fava, G., Guidi, J., Rafanelli, C., & Rickels, K. (2017). The clinical inadequacy of the placebo model and the development of an alternative conceptual framework. *Psychotherapy & Psychosomatics, 86*(6), 332–340. doi:10.1159/000480038

Fisher, R. (2010). Nurse prescribing: A vehicle for improved collaboration, or a stumbling block to inter-professional working? *International Journal of Nursing Practice, 16*(6), 579–585. doi:10.1111/j.1440-172X.2010.01884.x

Friesen, P. (2019). Mesmer, the placebo effect, and the efficacy paradox: Lessons for evidence based medicine and complementary and alternative medicine. *Critical Public Health, 29*(4), 435–447. doi:10.1080/09581596.2019.1597967

Funk, K. A., Weaver, K. K., Benbenek, M., & Anderson, J. K. (2019). Collaborative practice agreements between nurse practitioners and pharmacists. *Journal for Nurse Practitioners, 15*(7), e139–e141. doi:10.1016/j.nurpra.2019.03.006

Gajic-Veljanoski, O., Sanyal, C., McMartin, K., Xuanqian, X., Walter, M., Higgins, C., . . . Ng, V. (2018). Economic evaluations of commonly used structured psychotherapies for major depressive disorder and generalized anxiety disorder. *Canadian Psychology, 59*(4), 301–314. doi:10.1037/cap0000155

Ghaemi, S. (2019). *Clinical psychopharmacology: Principles and practice.* New York, NY: Oxford University Press.

Grasser, L., & Javanbakht, A. (2019). Treatments of posttraumatic stress disorder in civilian populations. *Current Psychiatry Reports, 21*(2), 11. doi:10.1007/s11920-019-0994-3

Greenberg, R. P. (2016). The rebirth of psychosocial importance in a drug-filled world. *American Psychologist, 71*(8), 781–791. doi:10.1037/amp0000054

Hengartner, M. P., & Pioden, M. (2018). Statistically significant antidepressant-placebo differences on subjective symptom-rating scales do not prove that the drugs work: Effect size and method bias matter! *Frontiers in Psychiatry, 9*, 517. doi:10.3389/fpsyt.2018.00517

Juntapim, S., & Nuntaboot, K. (2018). Care of patients with schizophrenia in the community. *Archives of Psychiatric Nursing, 32*(6), 855–860. doi:10.1016/j.apnu.2018.06.011

Kamenov, K., Twomey, C., Cabello, M., Prina, A. M., & Ayuso-Mateos, J. L. (2017). The efficacy of psychotherapy, pharmacotherapy and their combination on functioning and quality of life in deperssion: A meta-analysis. *Psychological Medicine, 47*(3), 414–425. doi:10.1017/S0033291716002774

Karyotaki, E., Smit, Y., Holdt Henningsen, K., Huibers, M. J. H., Robays, J., de Beurs, D., & Cuijpers, P. (2016). Combining pharmacotherapy and psychotherapy or monotherapy for major depression? A meta-analysis on the long-term effects. *Journal of Affective Disorders, 194*, 144–152. doi:10.1016/j.jad.2016.01.036

Kazer, M. W., O'Sullivan, C. K., & Leonard, M. (2018). Examining changes to statewide NP practice in Connecticut. *The Nurse Practitioner, 43*(2), 37–41. doi:10.1097/01.NPR.0000529669.54564.f0

Kelly, T., & Daley, D. C. (2013). Integrated treatment of substance use and psychiatric disorders. *Social Work in Public Health, 28*(3/4), 388–406. doi:10.1080/19371918.2013.774673

Khouzam, H. R. (2013). Pharmacotherapy for posttraumatic stress disorder. *Journal of Clinical Outcomes Management, 20*(1), 21–33. doi:10.1177/1049731516650517

Kim, J. S., Brook, J., & Akin, B. A. (2018). Solution-focused brief therapy with substance-using individuals. *Research in Social Work Practice, 28*(4), 452–462. doi:10.1177/1049731516650517

Kirsch, I. (2010). Review: Benefits of antidepressants over placebo limited except in very severe depression. *Evidence Based Mental Health, 13*(2), 49. doi:10.1136/ebmh.13.2.49

Kvarstein, E. H., Pedersen, G., Folmo, E., Urnes, Ø., Johansen, M. S., Hummelen, B., . . . Karterud, S. (2019). Mentalization-based treatment or psychodynamic treatment programmes for patients with borderline personality disorders. *Psychology & Psychotherapy: Theory, Research & Practice, 92*(1), 91–111. doi:10.1111/papt.12179

Leichsenring, F., & Hoyer, J. (2019). Does pharmacotherapy really have as enduring effects as psychotherapy in anxiety disorders? Some doubts. *British Journal of Psychiatry, 214*(1), 53. doi:10.1192/bjp.2018.225

Limandri, B. (2018a). Benzodiazepine use: The underbelly of the opioid epidemic. *Journal of Psychosocial Nursing and Mental Health Services, 56*(6), 11–16. doi:10.3928/02793695-20180723-02

Limandri, B. (2018b). Prescribing with a trauma-informed perspective. *Journal of Psychosocial Nursing & Mental Health Services, 56*(8), 7–10. doi:10.3928/02793695-20180723-02

Limandri, B. (2019). Evidence-based prescribing in mental health nursing. *Journal of Psychosocial Nursing and Mental Health Services*, *57*(6), 9–13. doi:10.3928/02793695-20190517-02

Lindström, L., Lindström, E., Nilsson, M., & Höistad, M. (2017). Maintenance therapy with second generation antipsychotics for bipolar disorder: A systematic review and meta-analysis. *Journal of Affective Disorders*, *213*, 138–150. doi:10.1016/j.jad.2017.02.012

Lo Coco, G., Melchiori, F., Oieni, V., Infurna, M. R., Strauss, B., Schwartze, D., . . . Gullo, S. (2019). Group treatment for substance use disorder in adults: A systematic review and meta-analysis of randomized-controlled trials. *Journal of Substance Abuse Treatment*, *99*, 104–116. doi:10.1016/j.jsat.2019.01.016

Lovas, D. A., & Schuman-Olivier, Z. (2018). Mindfulness-based cognitive therapy for bipolar disorder: A systemic review. *Journal of Affective Disorders*, *240*, 247–261. doi:10.1016/j.jad.2018.06.017

Lundh, A. L. (2017). Industry sponsorship and research outcome. *Cochrane Database of Systematic Reviews*, (2), MR000033. doi:10.1002/14651858.MR000033.pub3

Miklowitz, D. J., Schneck, C. D., George, E. L., Taylor, D. O., Sugar, C. A., Birmaher, B., . . . Axelson, D. (2014). Pharmacotherapy and family-focused treatment for adolescents with bipolar I and II disorders: A 2-year randomized trial. *American Journal of Psychiatry*, *171*(6), 658–667. doi:10.1176/appi.ajp.2014.13081130

Molenaar, P. J., Boom, Y., Peen, J., Schoevers, R. A., Van, R., & Dekker, J. J. (2011). Is there a dose-effect relationship between the number of psychotherapy sessions and improvement in social functioning? *British Journal of Clinical Psychology*, *50*(3), 268–282. doi:10.1348/014466510X516975

Morant, N., Kaminskly, E., & Ramon, S. (2015). Shared decision making for psychiatric medication management: Beyond the micro-social. *Health Expectations*, *19*, 1002–1014. doi:10.1111/hex.12392

Nielsen, R. E., Hessellund, K. B., Valentin, J. B., & Licht, R. W. (2018). Second generation LAI are associated to favorable outcome in a cohort of incident patients diagnosed with schizophrenia. *Schizophrenia Research*, *202*, 234–240. doi:10.1016/j.schres.2018.07.020

Nuttall, D. (2018). Nurse prescribing in primary care: A metasynthesis of the literature. *Primary Health Care Research & Development*, *19*(1), 7–22. doi:10.1017/S1463423617000500

Oud, M., Arntz, A., Hermens, M. L. M., Verhoef, R., & Kendall, T. (2018). Specialized psychotherapies for adults with borderline personality disorder: A systematic review and meta-analysis. *Australian & New Zealand Journal of Psychiatry*, *52*(10), 949–961. doi:10.1177/0004867418791257

Rasmussen, D. D., Kincaid, C. L., & Froehlich, J. C. (2017). Prazosin prevents increased anxiety behavior that occurs in response to stress during alcohol deprivations. *Alcohol & Alcoholism*, *52*(1), 5–11. doi:10.1093/alcalc/agw082

Rosenbaum, B. (2018). Psychotherapy for people diagnosed with schizophrenia. *Psychoanalytic Psychotherapy*, *32*(3), 321–325. doi:10.1080/02668734.2018.1447280

Ross, J. C. (2010). Mental health nurse prescribing: Using a constructivist approach to investigate the nurse-patient relationship. *Journal of Psychiatric Mental Health Nursing*, *21*(1), 1–10. doi:10.1111/jpm.12039

Ross, J. D. (2015). Mental health nurse prescribing: The emerging impact. *Journal of Psychiatric and Mental Health Nursing*, *22*(7), 529–542. doi:10.1111/jpm.12207

Sachse, R., & Kramer, U. (2019). Clarification-oriented psychotherapy of dependent personality disorder. *Journal of Contemporary Psychotherapy*, *49*(1), 15–25. doi:10.1007/s10879-018-9397-8

Sagar-Ouriaghli, I., Lievesley, K., & Santosh, P. J. (2018). Propranolol for treating emotional, behavioural, autonomic dysregulation in children and adolescents with autism spectrum disorders. *Journal of Psychopharmacology*, *32*(6), 641–653. doi:10.1177/0269881118756245

Scott, J. (1979). Critical periods in organizational processes. In F. Falker & J. Tanner (Eds.), *Human growth* (Vol. 3). *Neurobiology and nutrition* (pp. 223–243). New York, NY: Plenum Press.

Sebas, M. (1994). Developing a collaborative practice agreement for the primary care setting. *Nurse Practitioner*, *19*(3), 49–51. doi:10.1097/00006205-199403000-00012

Smith, R. C., Leucht, S., & Davis, J. M. (2019). Maximizing response to first-line antipsychotics in schizophrenia: A review focused on finding from meta-analysis. *Psychopharmacology*, *236*(2), 545–559. doi:10.1007/s00213-018-5133-z

Snowden, A., & Martin, C. R. (2010). Mental health nurse prescribing: A difficult pill to swallow? *Journal of Psychiatric and Mental Health Nursing, 17*(6), 543–553. doi:10.1111/j.1365-2850.2010.01561.x

Stahl, S. M. (2012). Psychotherapy as an epigenetic 'drug': Psychiatric therapeutics target symptoms linked to malfunctioning brain circuits with psychotherapy as well as with drugs. *Journal of Clinical Pharmacy and Therapeutics, 37*, 249–253. doi:10.1111/j.1365-2710.2011.01301.x

Stahl, S. M. (2018). Comparing pharmacologic mechanism of action for the vesicular monamine transporter 2 (VMAT2) inhibitors valbenazine and deutetrabenazine in treating tardive dyskinesia: Does one have advantages over the other? *CNS Spectrums, 23*, 239–247. doi:10.1017/S1092852918001219

Starcevic, V., & Janca, A. (2018). Pharmacotherapy of borderline personality disorder: Replacing confusion with prudent pragmatism. *Current Opinion in Psychiatry, 31*(1), 69–73. doi:10.1097/YCO.0000000000000373

Steenen, S. A., van Wijk, A. J., van der Heijden, G. J. M. G., van Westrhenen, R., de Lange, J., & de Jongh, A. (2016). Propranolol for the treatment of anxiety disorders: Systematic review and meta-analysis. *Journal of Psychopharmacology, 30*(2), 128–139. doi:10.1177/0269881115612236

Timulak, L. (2018). Humanistic-experiential therapies in the treatment of generalized anxiety: A perspective. *Counseling & Psychotherapy Research, 18*(3), 233–236. doi:10.1002/capr.12172

Wilson, L., Crowe, M., Scott, A., & Lacey, C. (2018). Psychoeducation for bipolar disorder: A discourse analysis. *International Journal of Mental Health Nursing, 27*(1), 349–357. doi:10.1111/inm.12328

Zhang, A., Franklin, C., Jing, S., Bornheimer, L. A., Hai, A. H., Himle, J. A., . . . Ji, Q. (2019). The effectiveness of four empirically supported psychotherapies for primary care depression and anxiety: A systematic review and meta-analysis. *Journal of Affective Disorders, 245*, 1168–1186. doi:10.1016/j.jad.2018.12.008

Zhou, X., Zhang, Y., Furukawa, T. A., Cuijpers, P., Pu, J., Weisz, J. R., . . . Xie, P. (2019). Different types and acceptability of psychotherapies for acute anxiety disorders in children and adolescents: A network meta-analysis. *JAMA Psychiatry, 76*(1), 45–50. doi:10.1001/jamapsychiatry.2018.3070

Zilcha-Mano, S. R. (2015). Therapeutic alliance in antidepresant treatment: Cause or effect of symptomatic levels? *Psychotherapy & Psychosomatics, 84*(3), 177–182. doi:10.1159/000379756

APPENDIX 14.1
Collaborative Agreement

The following mutually agreed on collaborative agreement shall form the basis of a prescribing relationship between _____ APRN and _____ MD, wherein the APRN may prescribe and administer medical therapeutics and corrective measures, and may dispense drugs in the form of professional samples.

1. The categories of medical therapeutics, corrective measures, laboratory tests, and other diagnostic procedures, which may be prescribed, dispensed, or administered by the advanced practice registered nurse (APRN) are as follows:
   a. Medications, which may include but are not limited to antidepressants, antipsychotics, anxiolytics/hypnotics, mood stabilizers, antihistamines, and antiparkinsonian drugs.
   b. Laboratory tests, medical therapeutics, diagnostic procedures, and treatment that are commonly performed in the assessment and treatment of psychiatric disorders.

2. Periodically, the APRN will randomly select cases for review with the collaborating physician. The purpose will be to review patient outcomes including a review of medical therapeutics, corrective measures, laboratory tests, and other diagnostic procedures that may be prescribed, dispensed, and administered by the APRN.

3. Schedule II and III drugs may be prescribed by the APRN. Patients receiving these medications will be reviewed in the same manner as in Section 2.

4. A registered nurse may take orders for medical therapeutics, corrective measures, laboratory tests, and other diagnostic procedures from an APRN under the supervision of a collaborating physician.

_____APRN   Date: _____

_____MD   Date: _____

APPENDIX 14.1
Collaborative Agreement (Optional Language Added)

Advanced practice registered nurse (APRN) collaborative agreement for the outpatient setting.

This form is proposed as a guideline for advanced practice registered nurses in developing a collaborative agreement for their prescribing practices. It is not an authorized standard of practice, nor is it a legal document. The Connecticut Society of Nurse Psychotherapists bears no responsibility for its use.

The following mutually agreed on collaborative agreement shall form the basis of a prescribing relationship between _____ APRN and _____ MD, wherein the APRN may prescribe and administer medical therapeutics and corrective measures, and may dispense drugs in the form of professional samples.

1. The categories of medical therapeutics, corrective measures, laboratory tests, and other diagnostic procedures, which may be prescribed, dispensed, or administered by the APRN, are as follows:
   a. Medications, which may include but are not limited to antidepressants, antipsychotics, anxiolytics/hypnotics, mood stabilizers, antihistamines, and antiparkinsonian drugs.
   b. Laboratory tests, medical therapeutics, diagnostic procedures, and treatment that are commonly performed in the assessment and treatment of psychiatric disorders.
2. Periodically, the APRN will randomly select cases for review with the collaborating physician. The purpose will be to review patient outcomes, including a review of medical therapeutics, corrective measures, laboratory tests, and other diagnostic procedures that may be prescribed, dispensed, and administered by the APRN.
3. Schedule II and III drugs may be prescribed by the APRN. Patients receiving these medications will be reviewed in the same manner as in Section 2.
4. A registered nurse may take orders for medical therapeutics, corrective measures, laboratory tests, and other diagnostic procedures from an APRN under the supervision of a collaborating physician.
5. Consultation and referral shall be on a case-by-case basis as deemed appropriate by the APRN.
6. Coverage for patients during non-office hours and vacations will be arranged by the APRN.
7. There will be a method of disclosure to the patient of the MD–APRN collaboration.

_____APRN   Date: _____
_____MD   Date: _____

Connecticut Society of Nurse Psychotherapists (2000).

APPENDIX 14.2
Sample Prescribing Practice Policy

To provide thorough services to all patients we have developed this policy for prescribing medications to patients receiving care. This policy is based on the state nursing practice act and current standards for clinical practice.

1. Introduction
   a. All patients who are registered with this clinic and receiving care from a therapist have access to a prescriber. Some therapists are also qualified as prescribers (psychiatrists and psychiatric mental health nurse practitioners) and may prescribe for their therapy patients or refer to another prescriber if the situation warrants.
   b. Medications are prescribed after a full assessment that includes health history, focused physical assessment such as vital signs and weight, and history of previous care. The initial prescription may be provided at that initial assessment or require a follow-up appointment pending medical records and/or laboratory assessments.
   c. Prior to prescribing all medications are reviewed with the patient (and family if a minor) regarding risks and benefits, reason for the medication being prescribed, and manner in which the medication will help. Patients will receive written instructions for taking the medication, and will sign a consent that they understand the medication and agree to take it.
   d. Repeat prescribing is a partnership between patient and prescriber that allows the prescriber to authorize

a prescription so it can be repeatedly issued at agreed intervals, without the patient having to consult the prescriber at each issue. The community pharmacy may order the repeat on behalf of the patient under the managed prescription service.
   e. All prescriptions are sent to the pharmacy through the electronic health record only. There will be no hard copy (written) prescriptions issued except under unique circumstances or as required by the Drug Enforcement Agency (DEA).
2. Renewal of prescriptions
   a. After an initial trial of medication that includes gradual tapering of the dosage to achieve likely effectiveness, a medication can be renewed for no more than 90 days at a time unless a shorter time is required by DEA regulations.
   b. Patients need to monitor the supply of medications available and request refill within no less than 7 workdays prior to running out.
   c. To request a refill, the patient will call the pharmacy. The pharmacy will seek renewal from the prescriber as necessary. Although pharmacies vary, most require at least 4 days to refill a prescription.
   d. Controlled substances (e.g., benzodiazepines, stimulants) can be prescribed for 30 days only without refill. Therefore, all refills require a direct prescription from the prescriber
   e. to the pharmacy as opposed to automatic refills.

(continued)

APPENDIX 14.2
Sample Prescribing Practice Policy (Continued)

3. Preauthorization with third-party payers
   a. Some medications require a preauthorization with third-party payers. Commonly these include relatively new medications, expensive medications, and controlled substances.
   b. The insurance company or pharmacy will notify the prescriber of the need for preauthorization. This requires the prescriber to complete additional documents and sometimes appeal documents. Completing the preauthorization requires at least 5 workdays that will likely delay receipt of medication. The patient may call the insurance company to request an expedited review.
   c. If the preauthorization is denied, the prescriber may appeal the decision or develop an alternative treatment plan in collaboration with the patient.
4. Controlled substances
   a. Medications controlled by the DEA require special consideration. These medications include benzodiazepines, stimulants, and pain medications.
   b. This clinic does not provide pain management and will not prescribe these medications. Patients who need pain medications will be referred to a primary care provider (PCP) and/ or a pain management clinic.
   c. Benzodiazepines are indicated for the treatment of anxiety; however, they are limited to short-term (no more than 4 weeks) use due to their high

potential for tolerance and dependency. Benzodiazepines will be prescribed within these clinical standards only and uses beyond the 4-week limit require a written plan for tapering and discontinuing the medication as soon as clinically reasonable. The plan will include the schedule for tapering and be signed by both the patient and the prescriber. Deviation from the plan may result in termination of treatment.
   d. Stimulants such as amphetamines and methylphenidates are indicated for treatment of attentional disorders that require extensive assessment for diagnosis. When prescribed for the first time, the dosage needs to be modified based on effects until the therapeutic level is achieved. Therapeutic doses may vary widely depending on individual patient variables. Once the patient achieves the therapeutic effect, that dose will remain unaltered until further assessed. Refills require a direct prescription to the pharmacy and cannot be ordered early or additional doses authorized without a separate prescription. This usually requires an appointment with the prescriber.
   e. Prior to refilling any controlled substance, the prescriber will review the Prescription Drug Monitoring Program (PDMP), a statewide online tool that provides information about prescriptions and medication

(continued)

dispensing of all schedule II–IV controlled substances. Prescription refills can be denied if the PDMP shows that the patient has received a prescription for the requested drug or related drug by anyone other than this prescriber.

5. Laboratory assessments

   a. Since medications affect changes in the body overall, it may be necessary for the prescriber to request laboratory assessments prior to prescribing medications and monitoring the effects of medications. The prescriber will explain these assessments prior to requesting these and inform the patient of how to get the assessments.

   b. Laboratory assessments are done at other locations not affiliated with this clinic, and the patient is responsible for insurance coverage. The prescriber will provide referrals to the appropriate laboratories or outpatient services, including the PCP.

   c. The patient is responsible for getting all necessary laboratory assessments within a week of the request. If this cannot be done, the patient needs to inform the prescriber to make other arrangements.

   d. Occasionally random urine samples are necessary to assure appropriate treatment plans. When this is needed, the patient will provide the sample.

6. Treatment adherence monitoring

   a. The treatment plans, including prescribed medications, are negotiated collaboratively between the patient and all the involved providers at this clinic. Additionally, collaboration with the PCP and any other medical providers is essential for quality coordinated care.

   b. Upon admission to this clinic the patient will sign for permission to gather necessary medical records. The patient is responsible for communicating with the PCP regarding medications provided by this clinic. The prescriber may also collaborate with the PCP regarding medication changes and laboratory tests needed for assessment of medication effects. The prescriber will inform the patient of any communication with other providers as needed for continuity of care.

   c. It is the patient's responsibility to take medications as prescribed and to communicate with the prescriber any adverse or side effects experienced or difficulty in taking the medication. Usually side effects can be managed with time and dosage adjustments that your prescriber can help you find.

   d. At every contact with the patient, the prescriber will review all the medications the patient is taking, the dosages, and frequencies. This is to clarify any drug-drug interactions, duplications, and contradictions.

   e. If a patient is significantly over- or underusing medication, the prescriber will discuss with the patient and may not refill further prescriptions.

The patient will receive a copy of these policies. Signature indicates receipt and understanding of the contents.

Signature of the patient _____
Date _____
Printed name of the patient: _____

Trauma-Informed Medication Management

Kathryn Kieran

Awareness of trauma's effects in the world, our patients, and ourselves helps us be more empathic and responsive medication prescribers. Trauma-informed care (TIC) practice is central in treating patients with histories of trauma. Patients overwhelmingly struggle with polypharmacy due to increased medical illness, comorbid mood, and substance use disorders. Vulnerability to somatization, and self-neglect due to dissociative or avoidant symptoms, increase provider-patient misunderstanding. Patients with trauma histories experience accentuated power dynamics, and contact with an authority figure can cause defensive anger or intense fearfulness. The prescribing advanced practice psychiatric nurse (APPN) will need to assess and validate traumatic beliefs, sensations, and thoughts, while remaining present-focused. Compassion and patient choice must be interwoven with firm boundaries, and clearly outlined treatment goals and plans.

This chapter begins with an introduction to TIC and describes how to integrate a trauma-informed approach in medication management. Using a holistic approach and therapeutic use of self, the meaning of medications for both the patient and the APPN is examined. Maintaining rational pharmacotherapy in the face of obstacles is addressed. Guidelines for addressing nonadherence are provided. Psychodynamic prescribing, the situational briefing model and the deprescribing model are discussed as useful strategies. The chapter ends with examples of how to apply principles of TIC in a medication management practice.

INTRODUCTION

Traumatic experiences are pervasive, including our own experiences of caring for others' pain. TIC provides a framework to investigate the current state of care and conceive of new ways of being with our patients to co-create a new narrative. If we do not stay alert, we can unknowingly replicate abusive or neglectful dynamics in our prescribing relationships. There are a variety of ways we can assess and respond when trauma sensations, thoughts, and beliefs present. To do this well, we practice universal precautions, provide education about trauma responses and nonmedication options, and treat target symptoms with medication. Scrutinizing or probing trauma is not the role of the prescribing APPN and can do harm. A genuine stance of openness to patients' whole stories and whole selves, however, can be healing and supportive. Humility is necessary when addressing cultural and spiritual dimensions of care. Psychodynamic prescribing;

situation, background, assessment, and recommendation (SBAR) communication methods; and a deprescribing model provide techniques and skills to supplement our standard good nursing practices.

The APPN may be providing therapy or may be in a split treatment program, providing medication management while another clinician provides the therapy. This may also shift over the course of treatment, as a patient may be referred by us or another clinician to trauma-focused therapy or other brief treatments or adjunct modalities we may not administer. Split treatment has much to recommend it, including a broader base of evaluation, opportunities for collaboration, and often more frequent visits. It requires increased communication, which can be taxing at times, and carries risks of missed information (Gitlin & Milkowitz, 2016). It is wise to find out, before starting medication management, if the patient is currently in or planning to start in any adjunctive therapy, or if the prescribing APPN is expected to provide the therapy. Each APPN has limits, boundaries, and requirements around split or integrated treatment. Releases of information should be signed between all care providers, including medical providers, such as a primary care provider, and relevant specialists. It is important to clearly communicate expectations about treatment and communication at the outset, to avoid reactivation of traumatic scripts around abandonment, loss of control over information transfer, or unworthiness (see Chapter 14, for more information on split and integrated treatment).

As clinicians, we are not immune to trauma exposure and trauma responses. Nothing in this chapter will share explicit trauma details, but terms and examples may have resonance for some of us. Acknowledging that, I want to encourage anyone who needs to take space or take care of themselves around these issues to do so. A recent shift toward exploring vicarious resiliency and the use of vicarious trauma to do good clinical work through self-reflection has emerged in the literature (Boulanger, 2018; Cohen & Collens, 2013). Vicarious trauma is no longer discussed solely as something to avoid, but as unavoidable and to be monitored. Monitoring vicarious responses guides our practices of self-care as well as our clinical practices more broadly, and our decision-making moment by moment. Therefore, I offer not a trauma or trigger warning, as important as those can be, but a moment to reflect on how we may take care of our responses to whatever we have heard today, this week, this month, this year, and whatever might spark recognition as we read.

This approach is in alignment with TIC guidelines, which recommend considering how all of us may have experiences of trauma and responses formed in traumatic contexts. TIC is increasingly recognized by all specialties as central to successful care of patients with histories of trauma (Antai-Otong, 2016; Reeves, 2015). The principles of TIC are not standardized across the available research base. At a national level the Substance Abuse and Mental Health Services Administration (SAMHSA) defines TIC approaches as understanding the existence of trauma and its impacts for everyone who encounters the services, as well as ways to recover from trauma (SAMHSA, 2015). This necessitates creating agile policies that incorporate the existing database on trauma and recovery, as well as working to avoid retraumatization of all those who experience the services or system (SAMHSA, 2015). Largely, the implementation of TIC has focused on limiting or eliminating seclusion, restraint, and other obvious sources of potential retraumatization (Muskett, 2013). Gains in this area can be easily measured and quantified. However, envisioning relationships that acknowledge and attempt to minimize dynamics of power and control in other ways has been a persistent challenge. Criticism of TIC suggests that a renewed engagement with justice is a needed corrective; at this moment a new paradigm has not yet emerged (Birnbaum, 2019).

Of the remaining SAMHSA TIC guidelines, the most modifiable by individual APPNs during medication visits with individual patients include: safety, trustworthiness and transparency, and collaboration and mutuality. If we attend to these guidelines, we will center patient empowerment in our practice, and offer opportunities to strengthen voice and increase choice. Assessing at intervals for cultural, historical, and gender issues as well as assessing level of family and peer support are crucial (SAMHSA, 2015). We must keep in mind that patients who have experienced trauma in a family or partnered context may be safest setting some stringent boundaries with anyone still in contact with their perpetrators.

Trauma is unfortunately common. The Diagnostic and Statistical Manual of Mental Disorders, (5th ed.; DSM-5; American Psychiatric Association [APA], 2013b) identifies the criteria for trauma as "death, serious injury, or sexual violence" that is directed toward us, that we witness directly, or that we learn affected a close family member or friend. Occupational exposures to these events in vivo or through electronic or traditional media such as pictures are also considered criteria for development of posttraumatic stress disorder (PTSD). We also know that other forms of danger and abuse have profound and lifelong effects on individuals.

The 1998 Adverse Childhood Experiences (ACE) study of chaos and upheaval in a young child's home; the mental illness, suicidality, or imprisonment of caregivers; and psychological abuse found significant relationships with psychological and physical illness (Felitti et al., 1998). Attachment researchers have abundant evidence that insecure or disorganized attachments formed by a chronic mismatch of temperament, subtly frightened or frightening behavior, or unresolved grief and loss in primary caregivers in early childhood is a vulnerability factor (Granqvist et al., 2017). Changes in the amygdala, which coordinates responses to threat among other functions, have been observed after traumatic experience, lack of supportive early-life environments, and/or the development of disorganized attachment to a primary caregiver (Lyons-Ruth, Pechtel, Yoon, Anderson, & Teicher, 2016; Sheynin & Liberzon, 2017). Childhood trauma or maltreatment is often compounded by adult experiences of trauma and loss. Our patients have often experienced multiple forms of trauma (Contractor, Caldas, Fletcher, Shea, & Armour, 2018; Hughes et al., 2017). To be trauma-informed, we must ask all patients if they have experienced trauma, and what they would want us to know about how it affects their daily life and healthcare treatment. To do this work, we must be willing to "face evil," as well as our own fears of incompetence or inadequacy; we must develop a layered and complex view of human nature, just as our patients who are able to metabolize their traumas do (Albaek, Kinn, & Milde, 2018).

Sensations, thoughts, beliefs, and emotional regulation are all affected by trauma in the normal course of recovery. If posttraumatic changes became life-limiting and more enduring, mental health issues may arise. PTSD may be the most well-known mental health diagnosis but it is not the only outcome of traumatic experience. Culture-bound syndromes or cultural concepts of distress such as Khyâl and Hwa-Byung, "wind" illnesses in Asian cultures, have been widely described but remain incompletely mapped onto, or differentiated from, disease models of treatment (Kohrt et al., 2014). Depression, anxiety disorders, personality disorders, dissociative disorders, and partial PTSD, which does not meet full criteria for PTSD, are common and have lifelong effects (Kessler, Sonnega, Bromet, Hughes, & Nelson, 1995; Raposo, Mackenzie, Henriksen, & Afifi, 2014). Older adults are much more likely to suffer from partial PTSD than meet criteria for the full disorder, but still carry a significant symptom burden that affects physical and mental health (Pietrzak, Goldstein, Southwick, & Grant, 2012). The stage model of recovery from trauma supports TIC (Herman, 1997). Being informed about trauma's effects is central. Reestablishing safety, externally and then, ideally, internally, is the first priority (Herman, 1997).

TRAUMA-INFORMED CONCEPTS AND PSYCHOPHARMACOLOGY

Safety and Stabilization

Safety is primary. It is not sensible to initiate a discussion of the finer points of pharmacology if someone is not willing to stay alive to experience the medication's benefits. Assessing for suicidality and safety at every visit can feel awkward, especially in patients who consistently report a lack of a history of suicidal ideation or attempts, but assessment is an unavoidable duty. Suicidal thoughts can occur at any stage of treatment. Patients may be reluctant to disclose suicidal thoughts "cold" without questioning, as they carry a great deal of stigma (Parcesepe & Cabassa, 2013). Normalizing statements such as "changing medications can cause new-onset suicidal thoughts, have you noticed anything like this?" can go a long way to maintaining an alliance. So can acknowledgment such as: "I know you've said you have never thought of suicide and you would never do so, that it is against your moral code, but I will keep checking in with you because suicidal thoughts can occur suddenly and catch us off guard. I would never want to miss something when I could be helping." Providing education around the range of suicidal thoughts, and that ego-dystonic thoughts or intrusive images are still symptoms worth reporting and tracking, can lower defensiveness. Many patients are familiar with screens for suicide and self-harm and appreciate the opportunity to share their experiences.

Medications can feel unsafe to patients for many reasons, including traumatizing experiences that are primarily experienced as somatization. James Chu (1998) writes compellingly of the ways that somatic reexperiencing of trauma can be a powerful form of communication. Medical evaluation should never be withheld, but any possible contribution of traumatic reexperiencing should be explored before any invasive, unnecessary medical procedure may cause physical or psychological harm (Chu, 1998). Exploring the experience by wondering aloud with a patient if the sensation is familiar, or more generally about their experiences of illness in childhood, can be illuminating and bring some relief of the symptom. For example, some patients were highly medically neglected in childhood and punished for reporting physical symptoms. In adulthood these patients can be highly avoidant of healthcare, or conversely highly care-seeking, or vacillate between strategies. They may reenact childhood patterns, or seek to demolish them, to establish a sense of safety internally. They may use both strategies simultaneously; treating certain conditions with high motivation while exhibiting significant self-neglect around others.

Some patients will report histories of a lessening of abuse when ill. These patients may speak fondly of a hospitalization where they received a full reprieve from the chaos and violence at home, such as an appendectomy, tonsillectomy, or even a grave illness. The link to an adult experience of hospitalizations and surgical care seeking can be slowly, gently discussed over time, while offering the patient a chance to choose alternative self-soothing methods (Loewenstein & Goodwin, 1999). At times healthcare providers may disagree with the patient's priorities. Remembering that trauma makes some experiences feel unbearable, and others easily avoided or dissociated, within the same person, can help us remain collaborative.

Body or somatic memories, or as we can consider them, partial sensory flashbacks, are a common experience among trauma survivors, and can be confused with medical illness or medication side effect. In the literature they are sometimes discussed as historical syndromes such as "hysteria," while noting their presence today as "embodied memories" (van der Kolk, 2014, p. 179). We often think of flashbacks as multisensory experiences, and in the classic sense they are. There has been a shift since the introduction of the *DSM-5* to viewing intrusive memories accompanied by a sense that they are occurring in the present as a salient indicator of PTSD (Brewin, 2015). Brewin (2015) reviews compelling research into the identification of flashbacks, including partial flashbacks, as distinct from other intrusive autobiographical memory at a physiological and emotional level, with good validity and specificity for PTSD. Individuals quite often will have partial flashbacks, with only one sense involved. They will repeatedly hear the expletive their rapist whispered in their ear during an assault, for example; or feel the brush of a hand on their arm, or the squeezing sensation of a hand around their neck; feel diffuse or specific pains; they may smell the perfume of an enraged parent, or the taste of a drink they were having before the trauma. These limited, repeatedly intrusive experiences might be elicited in screening for hallucinations. They are best understood, discussed, and treated as partial flashbacks.

Emotional safety in the treatment room is paramount. When we feel rushed or uncomfortable with trauma content, we can communicate this to patients in harmful ways, verbally, through body language, and through our prescribing practices. Richard Chefetz, in his powerful 2015 book *Intensive Psychotherapy for Persistent Dissociative Processes: The Fear of Feeling Real*, warns against dismissiveness in working with people with histories of trauma. "Avoiding responding has potential serious negative consequences in a repetition of past neglect or dismissiveness" (Chefetz, 2015, p. 131). Dismissiveness can, of course, be communicated via withholding care or medications. Giving medications too readily without willingness to hear the story behind the symptoms and acknowledge the source of the distress as trauma communicates dismissiveness. This may reactivate neural networks of relationship trauma and feelings of "I'm not important." Nursing often upholds the role of relationship in the treatment team. As the representatives of the science of caring, we can often bridge gaps between biological, psychological, and social needs. This does not mean we are responsible for excavating trauma so we can "prove" it to others, even if patients are telling us they are eager to "get over" trauma and want to talk about it in great detail upon our first meeting.

Safety and trust go hand in hand; the person may need a reminder that there is no fast track to trust. Some patients need active help with pacing and containment. Pacing treatment may include gentle interruptions, redirection to the present moment or to a coping skill when patients become flooded with traumatic material in sessions. The balance of disclosure and tolerance of traumatic information is delicate and one that we relearn differently with each patient we see. Eye movement desensitization and reprocessing (EMDR) therapy is an evidence-based psychotherapy for PTSD (Department of Veterans Affairs & Department of Defense, 2017; International Society for Traumatic Stress Studies, 2018), and allows the person to confront the traumatic material in a supportive, structured way with a trusted therapist. In addition, cognitive therapies such as prolonged exposure (PE) and Cognitive Processing Therapy (CPT) are effective (Kaczkurkin & Foa, 2015). The most salient feature of processed traumatic memories occurs when the person is no longer triggered in the present and the memories are experienced as in the past. The person learns to establish and maintain a sense of safety, a feature of all effective trauma therapy (Craske, Liao, Brown, & Vervliet, 2012).

Those who have experienced repeated early life traumas by trusted caregivers may have a hard time forming a trusting relationship with the therapist, particularly in short-term treatments. Attachment style and realistic safety fears, given their historical experiences, as well as the sheer amount of traumatic experiences with which they contend, may contribute to feelings of fear in relationship. Evidence has shown that ruptures in the treatment alliance during PE predict worse outcome, and more significant scores on PTSD scales, while a repaired rupture did not predict worse outcomes (McLaughlin, Keller, Feeny, Youngstrom, & Zoellner, 2014). Participants who experienced childhood abuse overall had a more variable treatment alliance, suggesting that perception of the treatment was more unstable for these individuals, but outcomes were not significantly affected by this variability (McLaughlin et al., 2014). Foa and Rausch note that there are issues with both what they term "underengagement" in these therapies as well as "overengagement" (Foa & Rauch, 2006, p. 61). Studies of "flooding" treatment also provide insight into benefits and risks, as well as Lisa Najavits's review of dropout in trauma therapies (Najavits, 2015; Pitman et al., 1991). Notably, the predictive factors beforehand and risks afterward of treatment failing the patient are not well understood, and mostly clinically observed. Further investigation into augmentation strategies and variant applications of treatment are well underway (Hendriks, de Kleine, Broekman, Hendriks, & van Minnen, 2018; Craske et al., 2012).

Power and Control

The prescription pad, our education, and our knowledge base all confer power. Unexamined power dynamics are quite problematic in therapeutic contexts. We need to know our limits and boundaries and communicate them clearly. We need to check in with our patients frequently, to avoid taking our assumptions and biases at face value. When we are overeager to help, we may inadvertently disempower our patients. Chefetz (2015) reports that he is reluctant to intervene with medication if a patient appears to be able to manage distress with emotional support alone. This is congruent with recommendations from SAMHSA (2015) about empowerment. Giving the fanciest, best, newest treatments may cause individuals to worry, and feel and act worse, emotionally and physically, as in the case of individuals given sham DNA testing (Turnwald et al., 2019).

Similarly, knowledge of *APOE* genotype caused worsening of both performance on cognitive testing, and perception of performance, when older adults were told that this genotype put them at risk for dementia (Lineweaver, Bondi, Galasko, & Salmon, 2014). Direct-to-consumer genetic testing is a burgeoning field with little research to guide our recommendations. Boeldt, Schork, Topol, and Bloss (2015) found increased anxiety and distress, though not diagnosable illness, in individuals who perceived less control over their risk and severity of the illness tested, most notably myocardial infarction and Alzheimer disease. Patient populations already struggling with mental health concerns that predispose them to hopelessness and negative appraisals may be problematically affected, especially if they receive results with limited guidance or support. Wang and colleagues (2016), studying obesity, suggest awareness of both genetic and lifestyle risks may influence intent to change behavior, possibly a first step in effecting behavior change. Our understanding of the delineations between helpful educational outreach and potentially damaging disclosure will likely evolve over time.

Believing that we have less control in our lives, either because someone else holds the control, or because circumstances are biologically determined, may bring about a higher risk of reducing or neglecting self-care practices. Individuals with traumatic backgrounds and histories of interpersonal trauma carry the lived experience of being controlled by someone else. Activating those memories and feelings in the healing relationship can be devastating. Jennifer Freyd first proposed "betrayal trauma" and "institutional trauma" as important factors that may perpetuate relational difficulty and forgetting after traumas (Freyd, 1994; Freyd & Smith, 2014). Freyd and her colleagues specifically note that betrayal has the side effect of silencing survivors. The betrayer has power over the survivor and the maintenance of the relationship with the abuser/betrayer is important. This can mean symptoms that we might consider self-silencing, such as forgetting, or dissociation, may be more prominent when betrayal is present. Cultural, interpersonal, and family factors may also lead to an experience of feeling silenced by one's community, identity group, friends, or family. This silencing naturally leads to a complicated relationship with one's own identity after the trauma (Freyd, 1994; Freyd & Smith, 2014).

IDENTITY, STIGMA AND SELF-STIGMA

Stigma within society; within racial, ethnic, or religious groups; and within individuals about a diagnosis, a medication, or mental health treatment in general has significant effects on healing and wellness. Racial and ethnic discrimination is an additive burden to adversities and traumas in childhood and adulthood (Myers et al., 2015). Both perceiving stigma subjectively and belonging to groups that are objectively rated by experts and the public as stigmatized within the culture increase vulnerability (Wang, Burton, & Pachankis, 2018). Stigma becomes more problematic the more we believe and identify ourselves with stigma-laden statements about groups with which we are aligned (Al-Khouja & Corrigan, 2017). Of course, an individual may not agree with the traditions or norms of his or her culture but awareness alone has an impact. It may create a stigma within ourselves, or the group. Women and individuals who do not identify as ethnically White experience higher levels of self-stigma in general. Study of stigma has suggested that high affiliation with a stigmatized group is more protective than low affiliation, including self-identification as a member of a cohort with mental illness (Al-Khouja & Corrigan, 2017). Co-occurring substance use disorders may reduce the protective effects of identifying as a member of a group (Al-Khouja & Corrigan, 2017). Belonging is deeply primal, a human need. This need becomes disrupted and distorted through trauma.

Individuals who have limited or terminated relationships with abusive or unsupportive family members may especially experience a sense of loss around engaging with mental health care if this is not accepted in their culture of origin. By choosing to reject family and subcultural or cultural beliefs about silence after trauma, or loyalty above individualism, there can be considerable losses in identity along with potential symptom relief. Conflicting beliefs about what mental health is and is not; what medications do and are for; and who is allowed to seek care, and for what reasons, may be held at the level of individual, family, subculture, or culture. Medication and health beliefs may be in conflict within the same individual. It is important to acknowledge that experiences vary widely. While reconnecting with traditional modes of healing may be beneficial for some, other individuals with trauma may align with another group than the one in which they were abused and with values that oppose the dominant group in which they were raised, to individuate and provide relief. For example, some people raised within an Evangelical Christian subculture in which they were abused may find great healing from reconnecting with spirituality on their own terms; others may oppose the beliefs of their youth as a way to heal from the abuse. There is no one correct path through healing.

Ethnic groups may carry historical and collective trauma, in addition to daily experiences of discrimination. Reengagement with cultural heritage and identity offers a pathway for some to engage collectively, rather than suffering in isolation (Hinton & Kirkmayer, 2013). Healing rituals within a culture often seek to offer resolution of the feelings of rejection and shame that occur after trauma. This process invites the individual back into the cultural or religious group through acknowledging the benefits and the "work" of suffering. The individual's experience may be compared to the trials of a revered figure, for example, imparting a greater meaning to the suffering and status to the sufferer (Hinton & Kirkmayer, 2013). There may be physiological benefits to rituals that alter biological rhythms like heart rate, promote togetherness within the group, and provide a relaxation response (Hinton & Kirkmayer, 2013). Additionally, there are culture-bound syndromes as well as common features associated with certain ethnic groups or subgroups of individuals affected by trauma. Orthostatic panic in traumatized Cambodian refugees provides one well-documented example (Hinton, Hofmann, Pitman, Pollack, & Barlow, 2008).

Distinct syndromes and features can be identified through prior knowledge of their existence, or by careful, attuned questioning (Dixon, Holoshitz, & Nossel, 2016; Lewis-Fernández & Aggarwal, 2013). Using the Cultural Formulation Interview in the *DSM-5* can assist the assessment of beliefs pertaining to mental health and traditional modes of healing (APA, 2013a). The Cultural Formulation Interview consists of an 11-item, clinician-administered scale that elicits information from the patient about background and identity, beliefs about care-seeking, and past experiences of feeling misunderstood by providers.

The fear of becoming one's perpetrator, resembling them in any way, evokes a strongly fearful, at times phobic, response. Diagnosis with the same illness process as a perpetrator can result in complicated feelings and gut-level revulsion. Patients who remember the medications their perpetrators were taking may have strong opinions, beliefs, and physical responses when considering taking the same medication. This complicates some of the heuristics of medication treatment. We know that some illnesses have a heritable component, and that at times medications given to family members may aid our patient. We need to be aware of the emotional landscape of the family when asking about family mental health history and known medication trials, especially when we suspect or are aware of abusive dynamics. Simply asking about personal and familial beliefs about medication can yield a great deal of information about intergenerational patterns of medication misuse, avoidance, or stigma. Acknowledging that complicated relationships create complicated feelings can communicate understanding. We may need to clearly state our willingness to avoid medications that may hold meanings that our patients fear. Unlinking mental health from pure heritability and biology, which is not supported by evidence anyway, helps our patients differentiate their fears of losing their family, culture, and identity, being shunned from it, or replicating it in the ways that harmed them.

MEANING OF SYMPTOMS, MEANING OF WELLNESS

Part of being trustworthy and transparent as an APPN is being predictable, genuine, and up front about our biases, limits, and theoretical orientation. Once this is established, remaining open to exploring multiple causes for behavior, symptoms, and somatic experiences allows patients to share, knowing they will not be preemptively labeled or stigmatized. Openly acknowledging placebo and nocebo effects with patients while prescribing is an important part of this role. We know that pills or tablets can have effects independently of *any* psychoactive properties, referred to as placebo effects when beneficial, and nocebo effects when deleterious. Research on placebo, the beneficial effects of the "rituals, symbols, and interactions" of therapeutic contact, including inert pills and sham procedures, has been limited (Kapchuk & Miller, 2015, p. 8).

The psychiatric nursing field has long recognized the therapeutic use of self, as well as the patient's self-concept and narrative, as important ingredients in healing (McAllister, Robert, Tsianakas, & McCrae, 2019). Placebo is widely considered an irritant and confounder in studies of medication efficacy (Crum, Leibowitz, & Verghese, 2017). Nocebo effects are even less well studied and appreciated. Widely understood as sensitivity to the ground state of sensation, nocebo effects create very real, measurable distress, and even pain (Colloca, 2017). Nocebo experiences cluster around the administration of an inert pill or sham procedure, or even through warnings about potential side effects (Kapchuk & Miller, 2015). We must share information about the risks and benefits of everything we prescribe. Awareness of the possibility of placebo and nocebo effects, and that trauma may accentuate these processes, helps APPNs rise to meet these challenges.

Each symptom may have multiple meanings, and amelioration of each symptom has meaning. Loewenstein and Goodwin offer us a glimpse into the power of symptoms for individuals with traumatic histories when they write that "symptoms serve many functions: to substitute for missing memories, to communicate distress, to symbolize crucial relationships, to contain internal conflicts, to manage interpersonal issues" (1999, p. 83). The use of prazosin to treat trauma-related nightmares provides a vivid example of the many functions of symptoms. It can be a startling revelation to have an experience as physically and emotionally exhausting and activating as a full-blown nightmare, often accompanied by restlessness, calling out, crying, or even punching or hitting, significantly reduced or eliminated by taking a capsule at bedtime (Simon & Rousseau, 2017). For trauma survivors, who often tangle with the nature of memory and its malleability in a way that feels like torture, it can shake their faith in their experience. If it can go away with a pill, was it ever that important? Was it ever truly real? If the nightmares can subside in this way, are they justified in the steps they may have taken to protect themselves from further abuse? Relief is welcome, but self-doubt raised by confronting the potential vulnerability of their experience to outside influence can make it a mixed blessing.

Rushing to silence symptoms can paradoxically worsen distress. Mintz and Belnap (2011) note how symptoms can both "create painful difficulties" as they "solve other problems" (p. 45). The "sick role," as it is often termed, can be powerful, especially for a trauma survivor, who often has experienced very little in the way of familial or institutional power (Mik-Meyer & Obling, 2012). Twinned with medically unexplained symptoms, the sick role can become the arena where the arc of the trauma is revisited, relived, and repeated (Mik-Meyer & Obling, 2012). For example, the adult, whose parents were routinely neglectful, failing to notice or respond to cues that the child sent while being abused, may now, through the sick role, have a powerful way to be seen, if not by parents, then by treaters. If the parents continue to refuse to acknowledge the trauma, they can be made to pay—literally and figuratively—through out-of-pocket expenses for therapists, brand name medications, and novel treatments; time spent in waiting rooms and EDs, and so forth. When families refuse to talk, or think, about the trauma, they may be more willing to attend to a third party. The patient's struggle with mental illness can become a proxy. Providers are often caught in the middle of arbitrating which of a trauma patient's symptoms are valid or real, when the truth is that distress is valid no matter what, and the brain, a part of the body, will forever be inextricably intertwined with every symptom. Some family members may only perceive the trauma as "bad" if it results in a diagnosable condition that requires medication management. Medication, therefore, mediates the relationship between APPN, patient, family or societal messaging, and the trauma.

Finances

It is important to ask patients whose families or partner may be paying for treatment about a crisis plan if family members who may be abusive and capricious stop paying for medications or therapy. Some family members may suddenly demand treatment details or trauma details to continue to fund treatments. Painfully underdiscussed, economic abuse is a common tactic in abusive homes, and is compounded by marginalized identities (Kutin, Russell & Reid, 2017). Although few scholarly articles address money and therapy, and most study economic abuse in intimate partner relationships, a group of therapists developed a manualized course of financial therapy for families, and tackled head-on the weighty transference issues involved in communications about money (Smith, Richards, Panisch, & Wilson, 2017). These authors note that competing values about money can represent "unfinished business between parents and their children" and "an effort to resolve past hurts and disputes" (p. 259). These conflicts can also intersect in abusive family or partnered contexts with themes of neglect and denial of needed mental or physical health care.

Neglect may be presented under the guise of a survivor being wasteful or malingering, or undeserving of the basic human right to healthcare. It can be yet another way of keeping a survivor off-balance, unsure if their healthcare providers or insurance copays will be paid or denied. At the same time their perpetrator, who controls the purse strings in the relationship, may also be actively working to prevent the survivor from achieving financial independence. In fact, denying the survivor healthcare may serve multiple functions of control: keeping the survivor fighting partially or untreated symptoms, worried sick about money, and unable to work due to symptoms and stress, as well as possibly lack of access to reliable transportation, and so forth. Abuse stacks upon neglect and control in an exhausting pile of intersecting gambits. The provider as well as the patient must work to stay motivated in the face of many ongoing challenges, and to avoid the pitfall of assigning all the hope and expectation to the medication portion of the equation of healing.

Comorbidity

At times, comorbid mood, substance, psychotic and voice-hearing experiences, anxiety symptoms or disorders can mask trauma symptoms. Treating the comorbidity can cause an escalation in distress until the trauma is also treated. The observation that decreased substance use or sobriety can expose underlying trauma symptoms such as nightmares, flashbacks, and so on is a common example. Individuals with comorbid dissociative disorders may describe "blackouts without drinking." Perceptual and time distortion symptoms, as well as sudden mood changes, may become more noticeable to them, and to their friends and loved ones. Without the explanation of substance use, the trauma sequelae become harder to ignore. With comorbid mood symptoms, we may see paradoxical responses. Reducing depression symptoms with medications and therapy may cause an increase in self-harm behaviors, if trauma-based cognitive distortions and state-dependent somatic memories are driving the patient to self-punish. Feelings of pleasure may result in worsened self-harm, danger-seeking, or impulsive behavior, due to underlying feelings of worthlessness and self-loathing.

When obsessive-compulsive symptoms are treated, intrusive memories may resurface. Some patients may be resistant to taking antipsychotic medications because their trauma symptoms worsen when their positive symptoms are more under control. When hypersexuality, impulsive spending, and hypomania or mania are modulated by mood stabilizers, the underlying avoidance of sexual intimacy and reexperiencing symptoms during attempts at intimacy become more obvious to our patients and their sexual partners, often causing embarrassment or shame, and partner conflict. Trauma symptoms complicate treatment (Ojserkis et al., 2017). Treating trauma symptoms benefits patients with comorbid conditions in most cases. It is unclear if concurrent or sequential treatment is more beneficial (Banerjee & Spry, 2017; de Bont et al., 2019). Treating the whole person, using a holistic framework as described in Chapter 1, provides the best care.

THE MEANINGS OF MEDICATION

Transference, Placebo, and Nocebo

Medication elicits potent transference responses. David Karp, a long-time professor of sociology at Boston College, addressed the transferential relationships between individuals and their medications in an insightful 2006 book, *Is It Me or My Meds?* Based on extensive qualitative interviews, the book asks, Is wellness in the form of a pill truly wellness? Is it weakness? Many people struggle with these concerns. Asking about how people think and what they believe about their medications is a form of universal precaution, just like asking all patients whether they have a trauma history they are willing to share. Asking about past overdoses or underdosing, suddenly stopping, or misusing medications provides an important window into a patient's risk. It is also a way to join with our patients and build an alliance. By showing we understand, without preemptively providing advice, prescription, or proscription, we develop into a true ally. We can then talk openly with the person receiving mental health care about all the potential good and bad that can come from medications.

Psychodynamic prescribing provides one way forward throughout this process, as it actively links the patient and provider transference to one another, and to the medication (Mintz & Belnap, 2011). Mintz and Belnap (2011) refer to these "symbolic aspects" of the medication experience, including willingness to be active in treatment, the stage of change, treatment alliance with the prescriber, and the experience of the medication. The authors distinguish between treatment resistance *to* medication, having powerful side effects to extremely low doses, for example; and resistance *from* medication, when benefit is derived but it is limited and overall does not improve the patient's life (Mintz & Belnap, 2011).

When we prescribe using the available evidence, which ideally involves large, randomized controlled trials (RCTs) of many thousands of people, we play the odds in the patient's best interest, statistically and biologically speaking. We count on the bell curve. When we sit with individuals and ask specific questions about what their medications mean to them, we are providing a complementary modality, one that considers what a large study cannot: the highly divergent social history, beliefs, experiences, culture, subculture, and trauma experiences of the individual. If we neglect the scientific literature, we are not providing best practice. If we neglect the individual's system of meaning about medications, we are not using a whole other data set that can often help explain treatment resistance, and problematic medication behaviors such as overuse, underuse, and suddenly stopping medications.

Part of medication effectiveness is driven by how the mind makes sense of the medication. Nocebo and placebo effects are affected by learning, which is impaired by trauma; expectations, which are affected by trauma; and misattribution, a prominent feature of trauma-based thinking when misapplied outside a crisis (Webster et al., 2016). It is difficult to learn when hypervigilance and avoidance are high; it is difficult not to expect the worst after the worst has happened; and cognitive distortions regarding the cause of the traumatic events are quite common. Placebo and nocebo effects can be due to learning acquired in early life experience, such as seeing pills cause harm or pills bring relief for members of our household. Expectation effects can also accrete after a single incident trauma. When someone with both physical and emotional injury obtains relief from pain medications, that association can be enduring. Similarly, if after an injury one takes a pain medication and vomits all night, that memory will likewise be quite durable, and may affect future medication experiences. If the pill that caused the all-night vomiting was blue, and then a blue antidepressant is prescribed, it makes sense that our patient comes in and reports extreme nausea to the dose, though most tolerate this dose quite well. Misattribution is a similar common experience, as when a patient will begin noticing a new sensation in the body after starting a medication, though in fact, it had been there all along, ignored. The event of taking a new medication can touch off introspection that highlights sensations, thoughts, or belief patterns that have been dormant (Barsky, 2017).

Sometimes those who have been traumatized have heightened somatization and hypervigilance and are hypersensitive to bodily changes and sensations so that an event like starting a medication can heighten self-vigilance. This can set the stage for abundant side effects or positive effects. It is not surprising to hear from patients about a transient, immediate few days to a few weeks of bliss after starting a selective serotonin reuptake inhibitor (SSRI). While some would call them early responders, with "high metabolization" to explain repeated positive effects followed by a crash back to reality, or worsened dysphoria, we can also always hold open the power of a relationship to transmit a robust placebo effect. Similarly, someone who tells us about horrific responses to paroxetine 5 mg, when they have tolerated other SSRIs without difficulty, can spur curiosity about the meaning that medication and its effects holds. What was happening in life when that paroxetine was started? Did it remind them of anyone, or anything?

One way to assess these experiences is the validated five-item Perceived Sensitivity to Medicines Scale (Horne et al., 2012). Simply asking about past experiences often yields sufficient information to predict sensitivities. The five-point Likert scale offers a high level of detail regarding beliefs about physical responses to medication such as: "My body is very sensitive to medicines. . . . I have had a bad reaction to medicines in the past; even very small amounts of medicines can upset my body" (Horne et al., 2012, p. 3). Education about misattribution during medication trials and validating how anxiety-provoking starting a new medication can be may be beneficial (Barsky, 2017). Validation and being heard, after past experiences of feeling harmed and often unheard in experiences of medication taking, can be a healing experience.

It may be that after trauma, placebo and nocebo effects are even more potent. Hodgkins and associates compared an active agent head to head with placebo in an RCT in a sample of women with PTSD, and found a very robust placebo effect (Hodgkins et al., 2018). The authors hypothesized that the structure and support of a clinical trial (none of the women were in therapy relationships), and the repetition of performing a CAPS (Clinician-Administered PTSD Scale) screen, may have been therapeutic in and of itself. What we do as clinicians, what we say, may likewise have a significant effect on how our patients experience medication, for good or for ill (Webster, Weinman, & Rubin, 2016).

Colloca (2017), in a special issue of *Science* on placebo and nocebo effects, suggests that we need to balance truth-telling by illuminating not just side effects, but expected benefit. Discussions of risks and benefits are often, due to possibly our own discomforts, legal concerns, or time pressures, weighted on the side of sharing each possible risk. Colloca (2017) stresses the importance of finding out beliefs about medications, particularly any difficult experiences with medication, and setting expectations for treatment as well as noting things that are known to affect perceived potency, or to cause risk of treatment dropout, like price.

When talking about potential side effects, centering what is possible to control may help to reduce nocebo effects and potentially retraumatizing hopeless or helpless internal scripts. When sharing information about serious side effects or adverse events such as Stevens-Johnson syndrome (SJS), it is important to try to explain incidence in a way the patient can understand information. For example, the incidence of SJS is estimated at 8 of 18,698 patients taking lamotrigine for any reason, more commonly in the very young, older adults, and those with comorbid cancers, HIV, and autoimmune illnesses (Lerch, Mainetti, Beretta-Piccoli, & Harr, 2018). Educating that SJS is associated with other medications such as antibiotics, corticosteroids, and nonsteroidal anti-inflammatory drugs (NSAIDs) helps to demystify the side effect and locate it in a wider healthcare context, not a risk only to patients receiving mental health treatment (Lerch et al., 2018). Stressing the patient's role in early identification and early presentation for treatment helps to center the locus of control within. Clearly describing that if a mucosal rash presents and rapidly spreads, the ED is the next stop, contextualizes the information and empowers the patient to advocate for his or her health, rather than passively await someone else's determination of risk. The patient is, ultimately, choosing to take the medication. Therefore, the patient has the most power over potential risk mitigation, such as taking the medication very regularly, and reporting any lapses in adherence so retitration versus alternative trials can be discussed and managed. Even when reviewing the occurrence of mild headache or gastrointestinal upset, framing the discussion in terms of safe and effective treatment can help. We can recommend taking over-the-counter (OTC) ibuprofen or acetaminophen, antacids, etc., giving a sense of control to the patient. This approach also conveys a sense of trust by assuming that the patient is actively involved in self-care. Asking about a preferred OTC or herbal remedy for nausea, for example, engages problem-solving and communicates trust and respect for the patient's autonomy and capability.

DEPRESCRIBING

The gerontological literature on polypharmacy notes that older adults and trauma survivors share commonalities that make accessing and maintaining rational, evidence-based medication regimens challenging. Both trauma survivors (Kessler et al., 1995) and older adults (Karlamangla et al., 2007) experience increased risk of comorbidity. Both groups also have increased risk of cognitive challenges: older adults, due to normal age-related cognitive decline and increased risk of cognitive impairment, and trauma survivors, due to symptoms related to trauma exposure, especially cognitive distortions related to trauma (Keshet, Foa, & Gilboa-Schechtman, 2018; Kimble, Shripad, Fowler, Sobolewski, & Fleming, 2018; Sanford, 2017). These physical, emotional, and cognitive challenges may result in self-care deficits, including missed appointments, or confusion about the (polypharmeceutical) regimen, and possibly further polypharmacy due to confounding symptoms versus side effect. Trauma survivors and older adults also experience a well-documented predisposition to somatization, which can increase risk for overdiagnosis and polypharmacy (Cook, McCarthy, & Thorp, 2017; Resnick, Acierno, & Kilpatrick, 1997; see Figure 15.1).

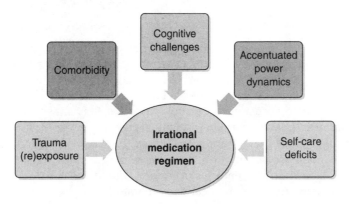

FIGURE 15.1 Older adult and trauma survivor irrational medication regimen diagram.

Power dynamics are also challenging in both groups. Older adults can be infantilized by others and are vulnerable to abuse by family members or caretakers. Individuals with trauma histories can be vulnerable to retraumatization in relationships. Fearfulness or defensive reactivity to authority figures may result in miscommunication and polypharmacy in the prescribing relationship. There is a strong cultural pull toward polypharmacy, but patients who are highly resistant to medications will present for treatment. When themes of fear of medication are woven throughout the patient's narrative, think of assessing for trauma. The field of gerontology has developed a model for patients who are more sensitive to medication side effects, and more at risk for polypharmacy: deprescribing (Gupta & Cahill, 2016). It can be a very effective model for working with patients who continue to experience symptoms arising from their traumatic experiences, whatever their diagnosis. Because in deprescribing you are focused first on relationship, a target medication is identified in collaboration with the patient to increase or to decrease (Bruyère Research Institute, 2019). It can be reasonable, when taking an individual situation into account, to start at low doses: sertraline 6.25 mg, fluvoxamine 12.5 mg, and paroxetine 2.5 mg. Going slower does not mean giving up your ethics or responsibilities. Patients still must be informed about the risks of undertreating their conditions at subtherapeutic dosing, and it is important to continue to discuss all aspects of care, including the evidence base for dosing recommendations. But it is an example of a paradox; the more we strive for rational pharmacotherapy, in the absence of attending to the transference and the relationship, the more irrational the regimen becomes. When we collaborate, with frequent review and support, choosing medication targets together, outcomes improve.

There is no one correct way to proceed in managing medication discontinuation. The emerging practice of shared decision-making in healthcare provides a model to follow. The patient and the nurse confer, but the patient ultimately decides to implement or not implement the recommendations of the nurse (Truglio-Londrigan & Slyer, 2018). At times the APPN will have to act on an ethical obligation. For example, the APPN may need to cease prescribing a substance unilaterally in the case of substance use disorder or repeated misuse, or when it has become clear side effects overwhelmingly outweigh benefit. These are still conversations that can be held with respect. In most cases education is bidirectional; patients are the experts on their own experiences, while the APPN has expertise in medication and treatment options. At times the lack of easily accessible, quality, affordable, evidence-based psychotherapy in our communities may tempt us to attempt to use additional medication to treat a problem we know is best treated with therapy. In these cases, it is best to continue to seek referrals, and consider whether telehealth, travel, or support groups may be necessary to connect the patient with effective therapy.

ADHERENCE

Adherence issues may reflect avoidance as an unseen cluster of behaviors and symptoms. Adherence is challenging to assess because we do not often question people about what they are not doing, or what emotions consciously or unconsciously are avoided. Our patients may be so accustomed to avoidance that they may have neatly hidden even the fact of the avoidance from themselves. As Jennifer Freyd noted in her research on betrayal trauma, abuse that occurs when our survival and/or source of human connection depends upon pretending nothing is happening is more likely to produce forgetfulness and lack or loss of memories of trauma (Freyd, 1994; Freyd & Smith, 2014). Avoidance and nonadherence to medications is common and exploring the meaning of missed medication can be quite fruitful, whether we decide to discontinue, decrease, or discuss a plan for adherence if the medication is helpful. Some patient with trauma histories will discontinue helpful medications because they feel unworthy of feeling better.

The rituals of taking medication, such as a glass of water, opening the pill container, and so forth, can be calming or soothing if the individual's associations are of relief, or terrifying if pretrauma drugging has been a part of their experience. Common in human trafficking scenarios (Deshpande & Nour, 2013), many people who experienced family sexual trauma report use of sedating medications to keep them quiet or compliant during abuse, or during a period of neglect, such as a parent leaving him or her unattended. In the literature, this can also be referred to as "drug-facilitated sexual assault," and "malicious use of pharmaceuticals" (Yin, 2010). Common medications used to harm children, often concurrently with physical or sexual abuse include analgesics, street drugs, sedatives, cough and cold preparations, alcohol, and antihistamines (Yin, 2010). If a patient expresses a strong reaction against or preference for a particular OTC medication, or a class of medication, we may wonder together with the patient about a traumatic reaction or response. Repeated overdoses on the same medication can also contain meaningful information.

Many individuals with histories of trauma readily acknowledge they have problems with controlling their experiences. This can include attempts to control symptoms, affects, body sensations, avoiding or controlling a very particular sensation, mood state, or type of experience. Patients with complex trauma most likely have a very narrow window of tolerance or resilient zone and APPNs might notice the person "titrating to experience" with medications. On a day with few trauma reminders, the person might not take any of their prescribed medications. On a tough day with many reminders, the individual may take many times the prescribed dose. This can develop into a diagnosable substance use disorder, a common comorbidity and experience for those with trauma histories, or it can remain a subclinical treatment-interfering issue that both patient and treaters can find challenging to work on in a healing framework (Dworkin, Ojalehto, Bedard-Gilligan, Cadigan, & Kaysen, 2018; Gilpin & Weiner, 2017).

APPNs are taught about the prescription as a contract between patient and provider; however, only some patients we treat have the same education and assumptions. If we want to make our intentions truly clear, we need to talk about exactly what a prescription means and the responsibilities it entails. See Box 15.1 for a brief outline of the assumptions of the prescription contract. We can work to preempt medication nonadherence by having an up-front discussion about when to call before stopping, lowering, or increasing a dose. There may be times when it would be okay to do so and call after or come to the next appointment to discuss. Sharing our decision-making process openly guides our patients and leaves less room for misinterpretation. A lack of communication about nonadherence can result in inadvertent or purposeful stockpiling of medications, which places the patient at increased risk of death by intentional overdose. Excess amounts of unused medications pose a risk to the patient's entire household. It is uncomfortable to acknowledge our positions of privilege and power in relation to our patients. If we proceed in prescribing without doing so, we can increase our patients' risk factors, despite the best of intentions.

BOX 15.1 Assumptions of the Prescription Contract

The APPN communicates the following expectations:
- Medication will not be used to harm self or others, or be shared with others.
- You will do everything in your power to take medication as prescribed.
- If you are not going to take medication as prescribed, please call first.
- If you don't call first, please reach out as soon as you possibly can.

Reflective practice offers us the chance to notice our countertransference and our physiological responses and pour them back into our work in a useful way (Griffiths, 2017). If someone has "violated" the often unwritten, undiscussed contract of the prescription, we have responses to that as prescribers as well. We can overprescribe or underprescribe to "rescue," as a "victim," and as a "bystander" (Davies & Frawley, 1994). These common responses to trauma in family systems can pull us into behavior we would not consider with other patients that might include longer sessions, giving out our private phone number, starting or increasing medications without due consideration and referral for psychotherapy or medical workup, or offering to allow the patient to text us, for example. Whenever we deviate from our usual responses to patients it can be helpful to seek supervision, and spend some time reflecting on our choices. Nurses' attitudes and stigma about psychiatric diagnoses by and large reflect the society they live in (de Jacq, Norful, & Larson, 2016). Reflecting on our work as nurses at the micro and macro level helps us elevate our care beyond stereotypes and assumptions, and create healing relationships with our patients (Griffiths, 2017).

APPLICATION OF TRAUMA-INFORMED MEDICATION MANAGEMENT

The Situational Briefing Model

The situational briefing model, consisting of situation, background, assessment, and recommendation, or SBAR, was specifically developed in a healthcare context (Leonard, Graham, & Bonacum, 2004). Adapted from systems used in airline traffic control and applied to medical situations and surgery, it is helpful in psychiatric treatment to standardize questioning and ensure collaboration and mutuality.

Patient SBAR

To elicit SITUATION, APPN asks:

> Can you share with me your goal for sleep medication and the reason for the goal?

Patient: I want to stop my sleep medication. It makes me groggy in the morning and I don't feel safe overnight.

To elicit BACKGROUND, APPN asks:

> Can you tell me more about any safety fears at nighttime? A lot of people have more fear at night.

Patient: For years after my assault I would check all the windows and doors. Now I can't do that, and with my children in the home, it doesn't feel safe while my partner is away; he recently has needed to do more travel for work.

To elicit ASSESSMENT APPN asks:

> What are your main concerns about the medication?

Patient: I think I'm overmedicated and I want to stop my sleep medication. It's been my goal for a long time to not need sleep medication every night.

To elicit RECOMMENDATION, APPN asks:

What would you think a solution could be? What do you want to do?

Patient: I would like to stop it today.

APPN SBAR

SITUATION:

- I hear you loud and clear, this situation is making you feel scared and unprotected. Your partner is traveling more and it's bringing up more symptoms and urges for hypervigilance.

BACKGROUND:

- What I'm remembering is last summer, when you stopped your medication suddenly and you felt so terrible.

ASSESSMENT:

- I wonder if we could decrease the dose or change the medication to an as needed medication? How many nights a week have you taken the sleep medication in the last month?
- Have you tried cutting it back? How did that go?
- Have you ever been on a different medication that didn't cause you to feel groggy?

RECOMMENDATION:

- I would like us to work to reduce the medication on a trial basis, with the goal of taking it only when you really need it or eliminating it entirely over the next 3 to 6 months. What do you think about that?

IF NO: ELICIT COUNTER-RECOMMENDATION:

- What are you willing to do? Offer options: as needed (prn), 1-week trial and reassess, wait until further data has been collected (offer a mood monitoring sheet, sleep log, etc.), complete a pros/cons list, etc.

PRACTICALITIES

Upon intake is an especially good time to weave in the deprescribing model in a trauma-informed way. Discussions about practicalities are important, as survivors of chronic interpersonal trauma may downplay their own needs out of fear of retaliation.

Questions That Show a Sensitivity to Practicalities

- Can you afford this medication?
- Do you have a pill splitter at home?
- How do you get to your pharmacy?
- Have you ever had someone helping you with your medication? A spouse, family member, or home care nurse, anyone else?

STARTING NEW MEDICATIONS

Upon ordering a new medication, education around side effects, expected benefits, and duration of time expected to titrate medication as well as see full effects is always important orienting information. Assessing beliefs around medication at this time can yield helpful information.

Example of Assessment of Past Experiences With Medications

- What kinds of side effects have you experienced with other medications?
- Is there anything that caused such a problem for you that you would never want to take it again?
- Is there anything you took for a while and it was helpful, but it stopped helping?

Consider use of the Perceived Sensitivity to Medicines scale (Horne et al., 2013).

Examples of Educational Statements About New Medications

- This medication is processed through your liver, so other medications, and alcohol, which are also processed through your liver, may be processed at different speeds when taken in the same time frame. This can mean feeling more intoxicated, or more suddenly intoxicated, if you drink alcohol while taking this medication.
- Would you like a printout of your current medication interactions? You can also always ask a pharmacist before purchasing any OTC medications; the pharmacist will be able to tell you if it may cause any issues with your medications.
- Some people experience this medication as drying, so they get dry mouth, constipation, things like that, especially at first. It can help to stay well hydrated, carry a water bottle everywhere with you, and chew sugar-free gum. Do you have something you usually take for constipation? Do you like prunes?

DISCUSSING SIDE EFFECTS

At each appointment, reviewing potential side effects or referencing identified concerns about each medication will help to frame the discussion so effects on motivation and adherence can be addressed directly. Patients with symptomatic trauma histories may have symptoms (such as dissociation) that make them less likely to notice or volunteer symptoms, and issues with power and control (e.g., accentuated fear of authority figures) may cause discomfort initiating discussions about side effects.

Examples of Questions to Ask About Side Effects

- You mentioned you've gained weight on SSRIs before. Have you checked your waist circumference or weight since our last appointment?
- Any dry mouth, dry eye, or constipation since we started the olanzapine?
- Sexual side effects can be common with this medication. Any loss of libido, or inability to orgasm?

CLARIFYING COMMUNICATION

Similarly, trauma-based cognitive distortions may inhibit survivors from asking clarifying questions, and cause misunderstandings, if not frequently ventilated and gently challenged. Discussing the communication in an open, un-self-conscious way can help to build a strong treatment alliance. When we feel blind-sided, confused by a patient interaction, we need to train ourselves to be curious about trauma.

Example Questions About Communication

- Do you feel we have worked well together today?
- Do you feel I have heard your concerns?
- Is there anything I am missing?
- Is what is happening between us familiar to you? Is this kind of experience a pattern in your life?
- Did my question cause you pain?

REORIENTING TO THE GOALS OF TREATMENT

Trauma survivors may be distracted and symptomatic in session. Frequent reorientation to the goals of treatment helps increase feelings of safety and the willingness to disclose.

Examples of Reorienting to Goals of Treatment with a Theme of Empowerment

- You're the expert on your body, so you'll have to tell me if you feel the increased sleep outweighs that groggy feeling.
- Some people feel a lot better taking this at night, and sometimes vivid dreams can happen, and then we could just switch it to daytime. I'd like a call from you letting me know if you change it from night to morning, to keep me updated, and I'd like you to wait for a call back before stopping it, so we could talk about the best way to come off it safely and without making your sleep problems worse.
- Do you want a handout about the medication we're thinking about starting?

TREATMENT-INTERFERING BEHAVIOR

Straightforward discussions of treatment-interfering behaviors can help to normalize struggles, connect them to trauma symptoms, and provide psychoeducation and empowerment while transparently communicating the APPN's expectations. Provider concerns about behaviors such as prescription misuse, missing appointments, or limited disclosure should be addressed early and often, rather than left to fester.

Examples of Communication about Treatment-Interfering Behaviors

- Many individuals with trauma symptoms have trouble taking medications as prescribed and may use them to numb symptoms in a way that can make avoidance worse for them. Thank you so much for sharing with me today that this has been a pattern for you. I am concerned we will fall into old patterns together, and I know you are, too. Can we agree that if I notice any pills missing from your medication organizer at any of your follow-up appointments, we will call your (identified support, case worker, therapist) together to make a plan?

- At this clinic we have a policy about discharge after three missed appointments. You shared today that in the past, you have missed appointments and been discharged from treatment because bad nightmares mean you haven't been able to get up and going to get to appointments. I hope our plan for night medications will help with that. What else could be helpful to you? Do you think later afternoon appointments would be more successful?

ASSESSING FOR MEDICATION SAFETY, SUICIDE PLANS

Extensive regimens, infrequently used prescriptions, and/or stockpiling medications are common, and can be dangerous. Access to the means to commit suicide increases the risk of completed suicide considerably (Milner, Witt, Maheen, & LaMontagne, 2017; Turecki & Brent, 2017). Asking about the presence of excess medication, and making a plan together, helps work toward safety.

Examples of Assessing for Excess Medications and Medication Safety

- What do you do with expired or discontinued medication?
- Have you ever needed help from a family member, nurse, or someone else in keeping track of your medications?
- Sometimes when people are thinking of suicide, they hold on to medications somewhere in their home. Do you have medications in your home that you could bring in for us to look at, and dispose of if they aren't necessary anymore, to help keep you safe?
- Looks like you've had a lot of recent medication changes. Do you have old medications you need to bring to be destroyed? Let's look and see where in town may take them.

COLLABORATION AND MUTUALITY

Collaboration ensures a greater likelihood of motivating the patient, and shared documentation of the plan helps keep provider and patient on track.

Examples of Collaboration

- Do you want to write that down, or should I type it up for you?
- Can you call me if the pharmacy says the medication requires a prior authorization? I want to get right on this.

EMPOWERMENT, VOICE, AND CHOICE

Patients with ongoing trauma symptoms may need frequently scheduled visits or calls, either to encourage trust and disclosure when that has not been the pattern, or to preempt frequent calls for reassurance, or requests for additional appointments. Calls can be a mid-range source of connection that feels less threatening.

Examples of Check-ins

- We agreed you would call me every week and leave a brief message, to reduce the fear of calling me in a potential emergency. How is this working for you?
- Thank you for your message! I was glad to hear that the sleep medication was eventually helpful at the new dose, after those rocky first few weeks.

CASE EXAMPLE

Ms. P, a 58-year-old woman is establishing care with the APPN in a community mental health clinic. She has been in long-term psychiatric treatment since a sexual assault in her first semester of freshman year of college caused her to drop out, as she states she could not face being in the same course as her perpetrator. She has been hospitalized psychiatrically five times in her lifetime, first at age 19 after the assault and three additional times that year. She has since been hospitalized once more last year after the death of her father, a childhood perpetrator of verbal, emotional, and sexual abuse. She has prior diagnoses of bipolar type II and PTSD, fibromyalgia, migraines, chronic low back pain, endometriosis, sleep apnea, and a surgical history significant for adenoidectomy and hysterectomy. She reports new-onset choking sensations in the daytime, not near meals, and pelvic pain worsening at nighttime for the past 3 months. Ms. P is following up with her primary care office regarding both these concerns and has a swallow study scheduled and an appointment with an OB/GYN. Of note, she reports a history of missing/skipping OB/GYN appointments in the past after her hysterectomy, though she is aware her cervix is intact and her OB/GYN would like her to continue to follow up with Pap smears. See Box 15.2 for Ms. P's current medications.

Ms. P reports she had been doing well while she raised her children, but since her father's death 1 year ago, with the anniversary looming on the calendar, and her youngest daughter's transition to college this fall she has felt "at sea." She reports her chief complaint as "I don't think my meds are working." Regarding past trials, she reports Provigil "made me anxious" and "lithium made me fat and feel bad. Depakote made me a zombie." When asked about anything that worked well, Ms. P states "my body doesn't work well with medicines, they don't agree with me." Upon careful questioning, Ms. P notes she was diagnosed with bipolar affective disorder due to "rages when my kids didn't come home on time" during their teens, as well as significant postpartum depressions, seasonal affective disorder, and "mood swings" when her children were separated from her, as when her youngest went to summer camp. Reports Ms. P, "I cried all day, every day, the whole time she was gone. I was

BOX 15.2 Ms. P's Medications

Cymbalta 120 mg oral qAM
Wellbutrin SR 200 mg oral qAM
Abilify 15 mg oral qAM
Lyrica 300 mg oral BID
buspirone 15 mg oral TID
Seroquel 100 mg oral qhs
Fioricet 2 tabs oral q6h prn, for migraines
Imitrex 25 mg oral daily prn, for migraine, may repeat x1 in 1 hour
Oxycodone 5 mg TID and daily prn, for chronic low back pain

convinced someone at the camp would hurt her or run off with her." This raised the APPN's suspicion for PTSD and comorbid depression. Collateral contacts with Ms. P's partner and former therapist corroborate a lack of any clear sleepless episodes or euphoria, reckless behavior, fast speech and movement, or anything that points to a hypomanic or manic episode. They report tearfulness and angry outbursts, often fueled by safety fears, have been stable for many years regardless of what medications have been tried.

Today, Ms. P reports for a second appointment to evaluate the need for any medication changes.

Ms. P:	These medications really aren't working.
APPN:	Tell me about that; what symptoms are unmanageable for you right now?
Ms. P:	The pain is way out of control, I'm crying all the time, I can't sleep. None of them work!
APPN:	That does sounds awful. Making sure that everything is okay is a good idea and you are already doing that with the tests your primary care provider is ordering and keeping your OB/GYN visits. Also, your pain and swallowing problems may be due to body memories of your past trauma, so it would be helpful to get trauma psychotherapy. Has your therapy helped you with the childhood and adult traumas you have suffered?
Ms. P:	No, not really. I have been in the hospital many times before and see a therapist now once in a while but I don't think I have had trauma psychotherapy.
APPN:	When a disturbing event occurs, it can get locked in the brain with all the feelings and body sensations and then these can come up later. How do you feel about going to someone who specializes in helping people to process past traumas?
Ms. P:	I'm pretty desperate right now, so I will try anything.
APPN:	Okay, before you leave today, I will give you a name and number of someone who I think is good and has helped people in the past who I have sent to her. Now, let's talk more about your sleep problems as that is something I may be able to help you with. Is the pain keeping you awake? Can you not fall asleep, or not stay asleep, or both?
Ms. P:	Oh, I can fall asleep. But I wake up at 3 a.m. every day with pain and I feel awful all over. Then I lie awake thinking about my kids.
APPN:	So you fall asleep, but then pain, wakes you. A lot of people have nightmares, or body memories at night that make it harder to wind down and sleep. I know you said you have a history of sexual trauma, and that absolutely happens for a lot of women I work with who have that history.
Ms. P:	Well. I do feel like it's happening all over again. I feel pain, and I feel so scared. And then I feel stupid, because there's nothing to be scared of in my house.

APPN:	That makes so much sense to me, actually. Thank you so much for sharing that. I hear a lot from women whose kids have gone away to college, too, that the anxiety can be really difficult, worrying about them. Do you mind sharing the kind of worries you're having?
Ms. P:	Well, I worry about K, she's my youngest, I worry she's going to go to a party, and be stupid and get hurt like I did, and leave school.
APPN:	It's so scary, not knowing she's safe. Was it this bad when the first two went off to college?
Ms. P:	You know it was for a while. I had kind of forgotten how bad it feels!
APPN:	Are you waking from nightmares?
Ms. P:	Sometimes.
APPN:	How many times per night, or per week?
Ms. P:	Oh. . . it might be three times a night or three times a week. Lately. Lately three times a night.
APPN:	Since we last met, or even before?
Ms. P:	Oh, since she went back after the long weekend.
APPN:	Oh, so around 2 months?
Ms. P:	Yes, I suppose it was 2 months or so.
APPN:	How many times a week are you missing the Seroquel?
Ms. P:	Well, since it doesn't seem to be doing much, I stopped it about a month ago.
APPN:	About a month ago. Did things get any worse, any better?
Ms. P:	Maybe a little less sleep. But the nightmares are exactly the same.
APPN:	Have you ever tried anything specifically for nightmares?
Ms. P:	Nope.
APPN:	Have any of your other medications made nightmares better, or worse?
Ms. P:	Well, for a while after I started the Cymbalta I was taking it twice a day, and wow! Those were the worst of my life. They are not that bad yet. I hope they never get that bad again! One time I kicked my partner so hard he fell out of bed and got all bruised up.
APPN:	Thank you so much, this is really helpful information. I'm wondering if before we change anything, we should talk a bit more about the symptoms we're seeing, and goals of treatment. I agree with you we should talk about your current medications and think about some changes. I would really like you to call your primary care office today about your increased pain and see if they have suggestions and to get an appointment with a trauma psychotherapist. For today, I have a few ideas about sleep I would like to run by you, and I'd like to talk with you about the diagnosis of PTSD. Is that okay?
Ms. P:	Yes.

APPN: You are experiencing repeated thoughts about your past traumatic experiences, nightmares about them, and it's disrupting your mood, sleep, and relationships. It makes total sense that your symptoms are increased. After someone who has harmed us dies, sometimes our mind and our body feel like it's safe enough to let some of the memories out. It feels awful, but it's normal, and I think it's extra hard because your youngest daughter is away at school and you wish you could be keeping her safe 24/7.

Ms. P: I guess that makes sense. I have been so keyed up. But I'm scared to start a new sleep medication.

APPN: Absolutely! Let's make sure you feel more comfortable before we would start anything. Let me print out some information about the three things I'm considering. Your input will make the decision, and if you end up feeling like it's not helpful, or it's causing you a problem, I'd like us to agree today that you'll call me before you stop any medication to give me a heads up and a chance to be helpful. Okay?

Ms. P and the APPN can now discuss options for sleep or nightmare prophylaxis with the current symptom presentation centered and clarified. If there were still concerns for a bipolar illness, the discussion could also have screened further for mood concerns, while centering the current source of most distress as sleep disruption and safety fears that are interrelated and related to traumatic experiences. Medical workup is still ongoing around the pelvic pain, and it may be a contributing factor to worsened nightmares and body memories, and/or a result of worsened PTSD symptoms. The throat tightness and difficulty swallowing may have an organic cause that is worsening anxiety or may be related to past oral trauma and worsening Ms. P's nighttime fears and reexperiencing symptoms. Given Ms. P's concerns that her "body doesn't work well with medicines," the APPN may consider lowering a dose, or changing the timing of doses to benefit sleep rather than starting a new medication today. Her avoidance of Seroquel may be due to feeling demoralized, or she may be fearful of sleeping too heavily and not being able to wake from nightmares, an experience and fear that it is worth exploring. Giving her a chance to reflect on other experiences of sleep medications may help her ultimately decide to try a lower dose, or stay off for now while trying a sleep hygiene protocol or nightmare protocol alone, or try an alternative sleep agent while using a protocol or sleep diary to better understand the thoughts, beliefs, emotions, and sensations that are inhibiting restful sleep.

Since the APPN is the prescriber only for Ms. P in her current setting, it is important that Ms P was referred for trauma therapy unless the APPN has the expertise and the time to provide trauma psychotherapy in addition to medication management. Ms. P's multiple childhood and adult traumas most likely are driving her current emotional and somatic symptoms. Considering her long history of medical and psychiatric diagnoses, Ms. P should be screened for a dissociative disorder. Practice guidelines for PTSD state that trauma psychotherapies, such as EMDR therapy or CPT, are evidence-based treatments with medication an adjunct to ameliorate current symptoms. The APPN continued to work with Ms. P to assist her with stabilization skills and building resources during her medication management sessions. See Chapters 1, The Nurse Psychotherapist and a Framework for Practice, and 17, Stabilization for Trauma and Dissociation, for stabilization strategies. As Ms. P's traumas are processed in psychotherapy, ongoing monitoring and adjustment of her medications are essential.

FURTHER EDUCATIONAL OPPORTUNITIES

For those APPNs who wish to further their knowledge and skill in working with those with trauma, the following trainings and resources are helpful:

- The International Society for the Study of Traumatic Dissociation offers learning opportunities about trauma and dissociation, including a certificate program. More information can be found at www.isst-d.org.
- The Veterans Health Administration offers clinical practice guidelines on medications in PTSD treatment, as well as continuing education units (CEUs) in PTSD therapy treatments at the National Center for PTSD website: www.ptsd.va.gov/professional/continuing_ed/index.asp.
- Collaborative prescribing owes much to the principles and practices of the recovery movement. Patricia Deegan's work at recoverylibrary.com and www.commongroundprogram.com is valuable for all populations and includes many suggestions and practices highly congruent with the approaches outlined above.
- Researchers at the Bruyère Research Institute (2019) in Ottawa and the Université de Montréal have collaborated on developing deprescribing guidelines focused on elder care. Their website provides excellent background on the rationale and principles of deprescribing: deprescribing.org/what-is-deprescribing.

CONCLUDING COMMENTS

All medications have meaning. Assessing for meaning at every opportunity is holistic and responsive treatment. It can be healing to offer interventions that are clear, with scheduled check-ins to ventilate concerns and future goals. Taking a thorough history of past experiences of medication will help to determine personalized titration schedules. When starting medications, normalizing nocebo, placebo, and side effects, while offering guidance about warning signs to seek further care, will help to build trust and establish expectations. When giving a prescription, make the medication contract explicit, and discuss harm-reduction plans in anyone who has a history of overtaking, undertaking, or suddenly stopping medications. Awareness that historical trauma beliefs may be guiding current behavior, and mis-taking medications may have been important ways of coping in the past, help the APPN and patient to understand behavior that may not match stated goals. Scheduling a "state of the state" discussion at 3- or 6-month intervals can help to preempt or to readily identify self-discontinuation or misuse patterns.

Medications can serve so many functions, and in patients with trauma those themes can be buried under minutiae if we are not careful. Themes that come up repeatedly in medication meetings can often be covert communication about trauma. Many individuals with trauma experience numbing and flooding cycles of emotions, and physical experiences. Medications can accentuate or dull physical sensations and affects in ways that help fuel these cycles, and thus avoidance of traumatic content and experience. There are many paths to hold space for these difficult cycles to be slowed down; no one technique will be sufficient for all patients. Just as trauma is a layered experience that affects our patients' biology, psychology, and sense of meaning and place in the world, healing and wellness require addressing the whole person.

The stance of curiosity, the domain of the scientist and the artist, when paired with caring, is an effective combination to build a strong alliance with trauma survivors. Safety, pacing, and containment of symptoms must be prioritized to maintain that alliance. Rushing through a medication management session is potentially disastrous, as it can re-create reminders of coercion or disregard. Even within this cultural moment, with all its distractions and pressures, the stabilization of the treatment of trauma can be maintained if we bring ourselves fully to the task.

DISCUSSION QUESTIONS

1. Write a brief reflection on a time when you experienced or witnessed a medication reaction or side effect such as rash, diarrhea, etc., that caused a difficult emotion such as fear, shame, or disgust. Think back and see what you recall about the medication itself, if anything. Close with a brief body scan and note down any body sensations you are feeling after writing about that experience.
2. What seems like the most challenging aspect of implementing trauma-informed medication education?
3. Define placebo, and nocebo. Think of some examples of each that would be likely, or that you have encountered in practice.
4. Split into pairs and choose roles as provider and patient. Using materials at hand, walk through the steps of filling a medication organizer together. The partner acting as the provider will want to focus on a few assessment questions while doing so, with particular attention to motivation and the patient's perception of the regimen. Debrief with the whole group afterward.
5. Select one of the following symptoms, and brainstorm how it could be related to a trauma background, affect trauma symptoms, or mimic trauma symptoms.
   a. bruising at injection site
   b. swallowing liquids
   c. sexual side effects
   d. changes to libido
   e. tremor
   f. nausea
   g. jitteriness
   h. headaches
   i. vivid dreams
   j. cognitive dulling
   k. can't swallow medications
   l. sensations in mouth
   m. feel controlled
   n. shape of pills
   o. insomnia
   p. color of pills or liquid
   q. sedation
   r. weight loss.
   For example, consider weight gain: Secondary sex characteristics returning, dissociation and its relationship to feeling dis-embodied, and medications' contribution to those sensations, or to sensations of having less dissociation and that being uncomfortable; family beliefs about weight, food, morality, and worth: weight gain may bring up old wounds from verbal and/or emotional abuse related to weight or personal appearance. Buying new clothes may bring up beliefs about not being worth new clothes, or "wasting" money on oneself, which might increase ideas about being deserving of punishment, and increase self-harm or self-neglect behaviors. Clothes feeling tighter may increase body memories and awareness of the fact of having a body.

6. View maketheconnection.net/stories/642, or search the site for another video of a veteran's personal experiences of trauma (U.S. Department of Veteran's Affairs, n.d.). Write a brief reflection, six to eight sentences, on what questions you would want to make sure to ask the veteran, if you were treating the veteran as the psychopharmacologist.

7. Consider reasons why someone would act like they trust you, when they do not, or cannot yet. Why would they have needed to act that way in the past, with an abusive parent, or someone else who may have held power over them, such as a human trafficker or abusive intimate partner?

8. Read over the descriptions of Reactive Attachment Disorder (APA, 2013b, 313.89, F94.1) and Disinhibited Social Engagement Disorder (APA, 2013b, 313.89, F94.2). Imagine what the behaviors described might look like in a child and write down three to five examples.

9. Write out a conversation between a patient and yourself in which you are hoping to start a prn medication for anxiety. List some of the fears, past experiences, and questions the patient may have. List all the information you need to convey, and then craft normalizing, validating sentences to communicate that information while honoring the patient's lived experience.

REFERENCES

Albaek, A. U., Kinn, L. G., & Milde, A. M. (2018). Walking children through a minefield: How professionals experience exploring adverse childhood experiences. *Qualitative Health Research*, 28(2), 231–244. doi:10.1177/1049732317734828

Al-Khouja, M. A., & Corrigan, P. W. (2017). Self-stigma, identity, and co-occurring disorders. *Israel Journal of Psychiatry and Related Sciences*, 54(1), 56–61. Retrieved from https://cdn.doctorsonly.co.il/2017/08/09_Self-Stigma-Identity.pdf

American Psychiatric Association. (2013a). *Cultural formulation interview*. Retrieved from https://www.psychiatry.org/File%20Library/Psychiatrists/Practice/DSM/APA_DSM5_Cultural-Formulation-Interview.pdf

American Psychiatric Association. (2013b). *Diagnostic and statistical manual of mental disorders* (5th ed.). Arlington, VA: American Psychiatric Publishing.

Antai-Otong, D. (2016). Caring for trauma survivors. *The Nursing Clinics of North America*, 51(2), 323–333. doi:10.1016/j.cnur.2016.01.014

Banerjee, S., & Spry, C. (2017). *Concurrent treatment for substance use disorder and trauma-related comorbidities: A review of clinical effectiveness and guidelines*. Ottawa, ON, Canada: Canadian Agency for Drugs and Technologies in Health.

Barsky, A. J. (2017). The iatrogenic potential of the physician's words. *Journal of the American Medical Association*, 318(24), 2425–2426. doi:10.1001/jama.2017.16216

Birnbaum, S. (2019). Confronting the social determinants of health: Has the language of trauma informed care become a defense mechanism? *Issues in Mental Health Nursing*, 40(6), 476–481. doi:10.1080/01612840.2018.1563256

Boeldt, D. L., Schork, N. J., Topol, E. J., & Bloss, C. S. (2015). Influence of individual differences in disease perception on consumer response to direct-to-consumer genomic testing. *Clinical Genetics*, 87(3), 225–232. doi:10.1111/cge.12419

Boulanger, G. (2018). When is vicarious trauma a necessary therapeutic tool? *Psychoanalytic Psychiatry*, 35(1), 60–69. doi:10.1037/pap0000089

Brewin, C. R. (2015). Re-experiencing traumatic events in PTSD: New avenues in research on intrusive memories and flashbacks. *European Journal of Psychotraumatology*, 6(1), 27180. doi:10.3402/ejpt.v6.27180

Bruyère Research Institute. (2019). *What is deprescribing?* Retrieved from https://deprescribing.org/what-is-deprescribing

Chefetz, R. (2015). *Intensive psychotherapy for persistent dissociative processes: The fear of feeling real*. New York, NY: W. W. Norton.

Chu, J. (1998). *Rebuilding shattered lives: The responsible treatment of complex post-traumatic and dissociative disorders*. New York, NY: John Wiley & Sons.

Cohen, K., & Collens, P. (2013). The impact of trauma work on trauma workers: A metasynthesis on vicarious trauma and vicarious posttraumatic growth. *Psychological Trauma: Theory, Research, Practice and Policy, 5*(6), 570–580. doi:10.1037/a0030388

Colloca, L. (2017). Nocebo effects can make you feel pain. *Science, 358*(6359), 44. doi:10.1126/science.aap8488

Contractor, A. A., Caldas, S., Fletcher, S., Shea, M. T., & Armour, C. (2018). Empirically derived lifespan polytraumatization typologies: A systematic review. *Journal of Clinical Psychology, 74*(7), 1137–1159. doi:10.1002/jclp.22586

Cook, J. M., McCarthy, E., & Thorp, S. R. (2017). Older adults with PTSD: Brief state of research and evidence-based psychotherapy case illustration. *American Journal of Geriatric Psychiatry, 25*, 522–530. doi:10.1016/j.jagp.2016.12.016

Craske, M. G., Liao, B., Brown, L., & Vervliet, B. (2012). Role of inhibition in exposure therapy. *Journal of Experimental Psychopathology, 3*, 322–345. doi:10.5127/jep.026511

Crum, A., Leibowitz, K. A., & Verghese, A. (2017). Making mindset matter. *British Medical Journal, 356*, j674. doi:10.1136/bmj.j674

Davies, J. M., & Frawley, M. G. (1994). *Treating the adult survivor of childhood sexual abuse: A psychoanalytic perspective*. New York, NY: Basic Books.

de Bont, P. A. J. M., van der Vleugel, B. M., van den Berg, D. P. G., de Roos, C., Lokkerbol, J., Smit, F., . . . van Minnen, A. (2019). Health-economic benefits of treating trauma in psychosis. *European Journal of Psychotraumatology, 10*(1), 1565032. doi:10.1080/20008198.2018.1565032

de Jacq, K., Norful, A. A., & Larson, E. (2016). The variability of nursing attitudes toward mental illness: An integrative review. *Archives of Psychiatric Nursing, 30*(6), 788–796. doi:10.1016/j.apnu.2016.07.004

Department of Veterans Affairs & Department of Defense. (2017). *VA/DoD clinical practice guideline for the management of post-traumatic stress disorder and acute stress disorder*. Retrieved from https://www.healthquality.va.gov/guidelines/MH/ptsd/VADoDPTSDCPGFinal.pdf

Deshpande, N. A., & Nour, N. M. (2013). Sex trafficking of women and girls. *Reviews in Obstetrics and Gynecology, 6*(1), e22–e27. Retrieved from https://www.ncbi.nlm.nih.gov/pmc/articles/PMC3651545

Dixon, L. B., Holoshitz, Y., & Nossel, I. (2016). Treatment engagement of individuals experiencing mental illness: Review and update. *World Psychiatry, 15*(1), 13–20. doi:10.1002/wps.20306

Dworkin, E. R., Ojalehto, H., Bedard-Gilligan, M. A., Cadigan, J. M., & Kaysen, D. (2018). Social support predicts reductions in PTSD symptoms when substances are not used to cope: A longitudinal study of sexual assault survivors. *Journal of Affective Disorders, 229*, 135–140. doi:10.1016/j.jad.2017.12.042

Felitti, V. J., Anda, R. F., Nordenberg, D., Williamson, D. F., Spitz, A. M., Edwards, V., . . . Marks, J. S. (1998). Relationship of childhood abuse and household dysfunction to many of the leading causes of death in adults. The adverse childhood experiences (ACE) study. *American Journal of Preventive Medicine, 14*(4), 245–258.

Foa, E., & Rauch, S. (2006). Emotional processing theory (EPT) and exposure therapy for PTSD. *Journal of Contemporary Psychotherapy, 36*, 61–65. doi:10.1007/s10879-006-9008-y

Freyd, J. J. (1994). Betrayal trauma: Traumatic amnesia as an adaptive response to childhood abuse. *Ethics & Behavior, 4*(4), 307–329. doi:10.1207/s15327019eb0404_1

Freyd, J. J., & Smith, C. P. (2014). Institutional trauma. *American Psychologist, 69*(6), 575–587. doi:10.1037/a0037564

Gilpin, N. W., & Weiner, J. L. (2017). Neurobiology of comorbid post-traumatic stress disorder and alcohol-use disorder. *Genes, Brain and Behavior, 16*(1), 15–43. doi:10.1111/gbb.12349

Gitlin, M. J., & Milkowitz, D. J. (2016). Split treatment: Recommendations for optimal use in the care of psychiatric patients. *Annals of Clinical Psychiatry, 28*(2), 132–137. Retrieved from https://www.aacp.com/article/buy_now/?id=248

Granqvist, P., Sroufe, L. A., Dozier, M., Hesse, E., Steele, M., van Ijzendoorn, M., . . . Duschinsky, R. (2017). Disorganized attachment in infancy: A review of the phenomenon and its implications for clinicians and policy-makers. *Attachment and Human Development, 19*(6), 534–558. doi:10.1080/14616734.2017.1354040

Griffiths, C. (2017). Deep nursing: A thoughtful, co-created nursing process. *Nursing Management, 24*(1), 27–30. doi:10.7748/nm.2017.e1573

Gupta, S., & Cahill, J. D. (2016). A prescription for "deprescribing" in psychiatry. *Psychiatric Services, 67*(8), 904–907. doi:10.1176/appi.ps.201500359

Hendriks, L., de Kleine, R. A., Broekman, T. G., Hendriks, G., & van Minnen, A. (2018). Intensive prolonged exposure therapy for chronic PTSD patients following multiple trauma and multiple treatment attempts. *European Journal of Psychotraumatology, 9*(1), 1425574. doi:10.1080/20008198.2018.1425574

Herman, J. (1997). *Trauma and recovery: The aftermath of violence–from domestic abuse to political terror* (2nd ed). New York, NY: Basic Books.

Hinton, D. E., Hofmann, S. G., Pitman, R. K., Pollack, M. H., & Barlow, D. H. (2008). The panic attack-PTSD model: Applicability to orthostatic panic among Cambodian refugees. *Cognitive Behavior Therapy, 37*(2), 101–116. doi:10.1080/16506070801969062

Hinton, D. E., & Kirmayer, L. J. (2013). Local responses to trauma: Symptom, affect, and healing. *Transcultural Psychiatry, 50*(5), 607–621. doi:10.1177/1363461513506529

Hodgkins, G. E., Blommel, J. G., Dunlop, B. W., Iosifescu, D., Mathew, S. J., Neylan, T. C., . . . Harvey, P. D. (2018). Placebo effects across self-report, clinician rating, and objective performance tasks among women with post-traumatic stress disorder: Investigation of placebo response in a pharmacological treatment study of post-traumatic stress disorder. *Journal of Clinical Psychopharmacology, 38*, 200–206. doi:10.1097/JCP.0000000000000858

Horne, R., Faasse, K., Cooper, V., Diefenback, M. A., Leventhal, H., Leventhal, E., & Petrie, K. J. (2013). The perceived sensitivity to medicines (PSM) scale: An evaluation of validity and reliability. *British Journal of Health Psychology, 18*(1), 18–30. doi:10.1111/j.2044-8287.2012.02071.x

Hughes, K., Bellis, M. A., Hardcastle, K. A., Sethi, D., Butchart, A., Mikton, C., . . . Dunne, M. P. (2017). The effect of multiple adverse childhood experiences on health: A systematic review and meta-analysis. *Lancet Public Health, 2*, e356–e366. doi:10.1016/S2468-2667(17)30118-4

International Society for Traumatic Stress Studies. (2018). *Posttraumatic stress disorder prevention and treatment: Methodology and recommendations*. Retrieved from http://www.istss.org/getattachment/Treating-Trauma/New-ISTSS-Prevention-and-Treatment-Guidelines/ISTSS_PreventionTreatmentGuidelines_FNL-March-19-2019.pdf.aspx

Kaczkurkin, A. N., & Foa, E. B. (2015). Cognitive-behavioral therapy for anxiety disorders: An update on empirical evidence. *Dialogues in Clinical Neuroscience, 17*(3), 337–346. Retrieved from https://www.ncbi.nlm.nih.gov/pmc/articles/PMC4610618

Kapchuk, T. J., & Miller, F. G. (2015). Placebo effects in medicine. *New England Journal of Medicine, 373*(1), 8–9. doi:10.1056/NEJMp1504023

Karlamangla, A., Tinetti, M., Guralnik, J., Studenski, S., Wetle, T., & Reuben, D. (2007). Comorbidity in older adults: Nosology of impairment, diseases, and conditions. *Journals of Gerontology. Series A, Biological Sciences and Medical Sciences, 62*(3), 296–300. doi:10.1093/gerona/62.3.296

Karp, D. (2006). *Is it me or my meds?* Cambridge, MA: Harvard University Press.

Keshet, H., Foa, E. B., & Gilboa-Schechtman, E. (2018). Women's self-perceptions in the aftermath of trauma: The role of trauma-centrality and trauma-type. *Psychological Trauma, 11*(5): 542–550. doi:10.1037/tra0000393

Kessler, R. C., Sonnega, A., Bromet, E., Hughes, M., & Nelson, C. B. (1995). Posttraumatic stress disorder in the national comorbidity survey. *Archives of General Psychiatry, 52*(12), 1048–1060. doi:10.1001/archpsyc.1995.03950240066012

Kimble, M., Shripad, A., Fowler, R., Sobolewski, S., & Fleming, K. (2018). Negative world views after trauma: Neurophysiological evidence for negative expectancies. *Psychological Trauma: Theory, Research, Practice and Policy, 10*(5), 576–584. doi:10.1037/tra0000324

Kohrt, B. A., Rasmussen, A., Kaiser, B. N., Haroz, E. E., Maharjan, S. M., Mutamba, B. B., . . . Hinton, D. E. (2014). Cultural concepts of distress and psychiatric disorders: Literature review and research recommendations for global mental health epidemiology. *International Journal of Epidemiology, 43*(2), 365–406. doi:10.1093/ije/dyt227

Kutin, J., Russell, R., & Reid, M. (2017). Economic abuse between intimate partners in Australia: Prevalence, health status, disability and financial stress. *Australian and New Zealand Journal of Public Health, 41*(3), 269–274. doi:10.1111/1753-6405.12651

Leonard, M., Graham, S., & Bonacum, D. (2004). The human factor: The critical importance of effective teamwork and communication in providing safe care. *Quality and Safety in Health Care, 13*(Suppl. 1), i85–i90. doi:10.1136/qhc.13.suppl_1.i85

Lerch, M., Mainetti, C., Beretta-Piccoli, B. T., & Harr, T. (2018). Current perspectives on Stevens-Johnson syndrome and toxic epidermal necrolysis. *Clinical Reviews in Allergy and Immunology, 54*, 147–176. doi:10.1007/s12016-017-8654-z

Lewis-Fernández, R., & Aggarwal, N. K. (2013). Culture and psychiatric diagnosis. *Advances in Psychosomatic Medicine, 33*, 15–30. doi:10.1159/000348725

Lineweaver, T. T., Bondi, M. W., Galasko, D., & Salmon, D. P. (2014). Effect of knowledge of APOE genotype on subjective and objective memory performance in healthy older adults. *American Journal of Psychiatry, 171*(2), 201–208. doi:10.1176/appi.ajp.2013.12121590

Loewenstein, R. J., & Goodwin, J. (1999). Assessment and management of somatoform symptoms in traumatized patients: Conceptual overview and pragmatic guide. In J. Goodwin & R. Attias (Eds.), *Splintered reflections: Images of the body in trauma* (pp. 67–86). New York, NY: Basic Books.

Lyons-Ruth, K., Pechtel, P., Yoon, S. A., Anderson, C. M., & Teicher, M. H. (2016). Disorganized attachment in infancy predicts greater amygdala volume in adulthood. *Behavioural Brain Research, 308*, 83–93. doi:10.1016/j.bbr.2016.03.050

McAllister, S., Robert, G., Tsianakas, V., & McCrae, N. (2019). Conceptualising nurse-patient therapeutic engagement on acute mental health wards: An integrative review. *International Journal of Nursing Studies, 93*, 106–118. doi:10.1016/j.ijnurstu.2019.02.013

McLaughlin, A. A., Keller, S. M., Feeny, N. C., Youngstrom, E. A., & Zoellner, L. A. (2014). Patterns of therapeutic alliance: Rupture-repair episodes in prolonged exposure for PTSD. *Journal of Consulting and Clinical Psychology, 62*(4), 568–578. doi:10.1037/cou0000106

Mik-Meyer, N., & Obling, A. R. (2012). The negotiation of the sick role: General practitioners' classification of patients with medically unexplained symptoms. *Sociology of Health and Illness, 34*(7), 1025–1038. doi:10.1111/j.1467-9566.2011.01448.x

Milner, A., Witt, K., Maheen, H., & LaMontagne, A. D. (2017). Access to means of suicide, occupation and the risk of suicide: A national study over 12 years of coronial data. *BMC Psychiatry, 17*, Article 125. doi:10.1186/s12888-017-1288-0

Mintz, D., & Belnap, B. A. (2011). What is psychodynamic psychopharmacology? An approach to pharmacological treatment resistance. In E. M. Plakun (Ed.), *Treatment resistance and patient authority: The Austen Riggs reader* (pp. 42–65). New York, NY: W. W. Norton.

Muskett, C. (2013). Trauma-informed care in inpatient mental health settings: A review of the literature. *International Journal of Mental Health Nursing, 23*(1), 51–59. doi:10.1111/inm.12012

Myers, H. F., Wyatt, G. E., Ullman, J. B., Loeb, T. B., Chin, D., Prause, N., . . . Liu, H. (2015). Cumulative burden of lifetime adversities: Trauma and mental health in low-SES African Americans and Latino/as. *Psychological Trauma, 7*(3), 243–251. doi:10.1037/a0039077

Najavits, L. M. (2015). The problem of dropout from "gold standard" PTSD therapies. *F1000PrimeReports, 7*, 43. doi:10.12703/P7-43

Ojserkis, R., Boisseau, C. L., Reddy, M. K., Mancebo, M. C., Eisen, J. L., & Rasmussen, S. A. (2017). The impact of lifetime PTSD on the seven-year course and clinical characteristics of OCD. *Psychiatry Research, 258*, 78–82. doi:10.1016/j.psychres.2017.09.042

Parcesepe, A. M., & Cabassa, L. J. (2013). Public stigma of mental illness in the United States: A systematic literature review. *Administration and Policy in Mental Health and Mental Health Research, 40*(5), 1–22. doi:10.1007/s10488-012-0430-z

Pietrzak, R. H., Goldstein, R. B., Southwick, S. M., & Grant, B. F. (2012). Psychiatric comorbidity of full and partial posttraumatic stress disorder among older adults in the United States: Results from wave 2 of the national epidemiologic survey on alcohol and related conditions. *American Journal of Geriatric Psychiatry, 20*(5), 380–390. doi:10.1097/JGP.0b013e31820d92e7

Pitman, R. K., Altman, B., Greenwald, E., Longpre, R. E., Macklin, M. L., Poiré, R. E., & Steketee, G. S. (1991). Psychiatric complications during flooding therapy for posttraumatic stress disorder. *Journal of Clinical Psychiatry, 52*(1), 17–20.

Raposo, S. M., Mackenzie, C. S., Henriksen, C. A., & Afifi, T. O. (2014). Time does not heal all wounds: Older adults who experienced childhood adversities have higher odds of mood, anxiety, and personality disorders. *American Journal of Geriatric Psychiatry, 22*, 1241–1250. doi:10.1016/j.jagp.2013.04.009

Reeves, E. (2015). A synthesis of the literature on trauma-informed care. *Mental Health Nursing,* *36*(9), 698–709. doi:10.3109/01612840.2015.1025319

Resnick, H. S., Acierno, R., & Kilpatrick, D. G. (1997). Health impact of interpersonal violence 2: Medical and mental health outcomes. *Behavioral Medicine, 23*(2), 65–78. doi:10.1080/08964289709596730

Substance Abuse and Mental Health Services Administration. (2015). *Trauma-informed care in* *behavioral health services: Quick guide for clinicians based on TIP 57.* Retrieved from https:// store.samhsa.gov/sites/default/files/d7/priv/sma15-4912.pdf

Sanford, A. (2017). Mild cognitive impairment. *Clinics in Geriatric Medicine, 33,* 325–337. doi:10.1016/j.cger.2017.02.005

Simon, P. Y. R., & Rousseau, P. (2017). Treatment of post-traumatic stress disorders with the alpha-1 adrenergic antagonist prazosin: A review of outcome studies. *Canadian Journal of* *Psychiatry, 62*(3), 186–198. doi:10.1177/0706743716659275

Sheynin, H., & Liberzon, I. (2017). Circuit dysregulation and circuit-based treatments in posttraumatic stress disorder. *Neuroscience Letters, 10*(649), 133–138. doi:10.1016/ j.neulet.2016.11.014

Truglio-Londrigan, M., & Slyer, J. (2018). Shared decision-making for nursing practice: An integrative review. *The Open Nursing Journal, 12,* 1–14. doi:10.2174/1874434601812010001

Turecki, G., & Brent, D. A. (2017). Suicide and suicidal behavior. *Lancet, 387*(10024), 1227–1239. doi:10.1016/S0140-6736(15)00234-2

Turnwald, B. P., Goyer, J. P., Boles, D. Z., Silder, A., Delp, S. L., & Crum, A. J. (2019). Learning one's genetic risk changes physiology independent of actual genetic risk. *Nature, 3,* 48–56. doi:10.1038/s41562-018-0483-4

U.S. Department of Veteran's Affairs. (n.d.). *Misty found healing for MST in a women's group* [Video file]. Retrieved from https://maketheconnection.net/stories/642

van der Kolk, B. (2014). *The body keeps the score: Brain, mind, and body in the healing of trauma.* New York, NY: Penguin Books.

Wang, C., Gordon, E. S., Norkunas, T., Wawak, L., Liu, C. T., Winter, M., . . . Bowen, D. J. (2016). A randomized trial examining the impact of communicating genetic and lifestyle risks for obesity. *Obesity, 24*(12), 2481–2490. doi:10.1002/oby.21661

Wang, K., Burton, C. L., & Pachankis, J. E. (2018). Depression and substance use: Towards the development of an emotion regulation model of stigma coping. *Substance Use and Misuse,* *53*(5), 859–866. doi:10.1080/10826084.2017.1391011

Webster, R. K., Weinman, J., & Rubin, G. J. (2016). A systematic review of factors that contribute to nocebo effects. *Health Psychology, 35*(12), 1334–1355. doi:10.1037/hea0000416

Yin, S. (2010). Malicious use of pharmaceuticals in children. *The Journal of Pediatrics, 157*(5), 832–836. doi:10.1016/j.jpeds.2010.05.040

Integrative Medicine and Psychotherapy

Sharon M. Freeman Clevenger

Neuropsychiatric and mental health symptoms affect an estimated 37% of the U.S. population. Adults with more than one neuropsychiatric symptom, such as depression, anxiety, insomnia, attention deficits, headaches, excessive sleepiness, and memory loss, are disproportionally more likely to seek complementary and alternative medicine (CAM) options for their symptoms. Many of these symptoms are often refractory to standard, conventional medical treatment. Despite the growing popularity of CAM usage (estimated at more than 30% of all adults by the National Centers on Complementary and Integrative Healthcare (NCCIH), many mental health practitioners including APRNs report limited knowledge and understanding about CAM practices. Integrated means to bring all parts together, to unify. Integrative means to merge all appropriate therapies, both conventional and alternative (National Institutes of Health [NIH], 2018).

Psychiatric practitioners are uniquely positioned to use psychotherapeutic skills to understand, utilize, and communicate about full-body health and nutrition as part of their scope of practice to help their patients achieve optimal functioning. This chapter will take you on a journey that will expand the boundaries of treatment options available for helping your patient feel better quickly and for longer periods of time, while you prevent further illness in many cases. Along the way, we will briefly discuss terminology and ways to integrate psychotherapy, CAM, and pharmacotherapy in mental health settings.

BACKGROUND

A cursory review of complementary treatment options approved of by The National Center for Complementary and Integrative Health (NCCIH) at the NIH opens up hundreds, if not thousands, of inexpensive natural treatments for symptoms and syndromes (NIH, 2018). However, how does one decide if a treatment is safe, effective, and available for your patient? Practitioners in general sometimes assume that "complementary" treatments are not science-based, and even dangerous. In addition, there can be confusion regarding definitions of complementary, alternative, functional, and integrative medical healthcare. Table 16.1 defines terminology that may be helpful as you start, or continue, your journey into the realm of integrating treatment options.

Integrative medicine in healthcare combines modern (mainstream) medical protocols with CAM treatments borrowed from other disciplines. Integrative practitioners

TABLE 16.1   DEFINITIONS OF TERMINOLOGY IN INTEGRATIVE HEALTHCARE

Term	Definition
Complementary healthcare	"Non-mainstream practice used together with, or "in addition to," conventional medicine"
Alternative healthcare	"Non-mainstream practice used "instead of," or in place of, conventional medicine" (National Institutes of Health, 2018)
Complementary and alternative healthcare	Combination of complementary and alternative medicines (CAMs)
Integrated treatments	To bring all parts together; to unify; holistic
Integrative medicine	Approaches that are used in conjunction with (integrated with) CAM approaches in mainstream healthcare (Andreatini, Sartori, Seabra, & Leite, 2002)
Functional medicine	The practice of evaluation and treatment of "upstream" processes (why did this happen?) in addition to current processes (Jones, Bland, & Quinn, 2005/2010)
Integrative functional healthcare	Using a functional approach and integrating all available options for treatment
Mainstream or modern medicine	Treatments, medications, and procedures that are taught as part of approved medical curricula and/or relate to U.S. Food and Drug Administration (FDA) approved pharmacological and medical interventions

are trained in systems approaches for how the body functions as a complex, interwoven connected system rather than traditional single focused approaches (Jones, Bland, & Quinn, 2005/2010). "Functional" medicine is yet another conceptual approach to healthcare and refers to the practice of evaluation and treatment of "upstream" processes in addition to current processes (Jones et al., 2005/2010). Functional practitioners know that the body is an interconnected dynamic system with individual biovariability. In other words, instead of simply treating a disorder, the functional practitioner seeks to determine *why* the person developed that disorder or symptom in the first place, and then seeks to repair the causative issue to restore the system to balance. An example is the patient who is fatigued and determined to be suffering from vitamin B12 deficiency anemia. Current modern medical protocol is to replace the vitamin B12 (usually with cobalamin injections) until the symptoms are gone. The functional medicine practitioner will replace cobalamin (vitamin B12) as well; however, they will seek to determine *why* the person developed the vitamin B12 deficiency. Functional evaluation of cobalamin deficiency would begin with a thorough examination of nutrition/diet, medications that can deplete cobalamin, potential malabsorption problems, and lifestyle issues related to nutrients.

The correct terminology is "integrative functional medicine" (because you are using a functional approach and integrating all options for treatment); however, it is often shortened to integrative medicine, or Integrative healthcare. Regardless of which terminology is used, the integrative functional medicine model includes evaluation and treatment of causality of disease, modern medical practices, CAM, and knowledge of how the body functions as an integrated, connected system rather than traditional single focused approaches (Jones et al., 2005/2010). For purposes of this chapter, integrative functional medicine will be abbreviated FM.

An estimated 37% of the U.S. population are refractory to standard, conventional medical treatment. Adults with more than one neuropsychiatric symptom, such as depression, anxiety, insomnia, attention or concentration problems, headaches, excessive sleepiness, and memory loss, are disproportionly more likely to seek CAM options for their symptoms (Clevenger, 2018). A recent survey of 295 mental health practitioners (MHPs) from multiple disciplines was conducted to investigate knowledge of, and attitudes toward, utilizing CAM treatments. Surprisingly, the results suggested that many MHP's, including advanced practice psychiatric nurses (APPNs), were unaware that they were using CAM approaches. In addition, many practitioners acknowledged a lack of education and training regarding evidence for the use of CAM for mental health symptoms (Clevenger, 2018). Generally, healthcare practitioners, including APPNs, are more likely to recommend treatments that they are familiar with, have confidence in regarding risk/benefit, and feel competent about when explaining the procedures. Another point for consideration is that lack of knowledge or understanding about CAM options may limit potentially helpful treatments to individuals with mental health problems. Practitioners in general should be familiar with potential risks associated with combining herbal or supplement CAM treatments with pharmaceutical treatments, especially potential serious side effects and drug interaction effects, including CAM options that their patients may be using with or without the practitioner's knowledge (U.S. Food and Drug Administration [FDA], 2016).

Integrative Psychiatric Healthcare: Conceptualization

Current modern medical practice can be thought of as "fire extinguisher" medicine (wait for a fire, hit it with the extinguisher, walk away congratulating yourself). Fire extinguisher medicine does not seek to understand what caused the fire, if there are structural consequences from the fire, and whether the fire is completely extinguished or is smoldering elsewhere in the body. The body is not a set of individual organs that function independently. Each system depends on other systems for full, effective, and healthy functioning. Diet, immune responses, life stress, gastrointestinal (GI) health and function, structural components, energy production, waste removal, hormone and neurotransmitter function, and emotions all work together to maintain a healthy body.

This chapter describes a discipline and a model for treating some of the consequences that the dysregulation of traumatic experiences sets in motion. Chapter 2, provides the underlying neurophysiology and theoretical underpinnings for systems dysregulation while this chapter illustrates the complexity and physiological consequences set in motion by adverse experiences. Treatment strategies are discussed that the APPN can consider integrating into a comprehensive plan of care.

The Gut

At the core of a healthy healing environment for both physical and mental function is the intestinal tract. This is why FM practitioners often begin their assessments at the level of the GI tract, or gut (Liska, 20052010). The GI tract is a complex, multitasking organ providing a mucosal structure that performs numerous functions for the entire body. The GI tract prevents pathogens from entering systemic circulation, creates a system for absorption (uptake) of nutrients ingested, and contains an enormous amount of immune functions (Vasquez, 2005/2010). Imbalances of any degree within the GI tract create a domino effect of changes that can lead to eventual organ dysfunction, damage, and even full system breakdown (Lombard, 2005/2010).

The multiple processes involved in digestion include numerous check and balance systems that effectively break down food components into carbohydrates, fats, and proteins (Sult, 2005/2010). However, in addition to reducing food particles into usable molecules, the GI tract selectively chooses what is useful (to be absorbed) and what is potentially harmful (to be neutralized and eliminated; Sult, 2005/2010). Effective digestion begins with ingestion, mastication (chewing), propulsion, mechanical or physical digestion, chemical (acid or alkali) digestion, absorption, and finally, defecation. Enzymes and microorganisms cooperate with the host's gut to protect the mucosa, bind to effectors, and disable harmful organisms. This is a miraculous feat for an estimated 2 to 9 lb of these living, interdependent bacteria and other microorganisms that largely go unnoticed in their daily work (Sult, 2005/2010).

What does digestion and gut health have to do with psychiatry? All physical and biological functions are dependent upon a working GI tract. The delicate system of checks and balances related to GI function provide us with the building blocks for neurotransmitters, enzymes, DNA replication, immune function, and so much more (Arrieta, Bistritz, & Meddings, 2006). You may have heard of "leaky gut syndrome," which is basically an intestinal malabsorption due to permeability caused by inflammation of the mucosal lining. When the lining is inflamed, tight junctions open, permitting larger molecules to pass through into systemic circulation. The most common cause of intestinal permeability is "dysbiosis" (overgrowth of unhealthy bacteria or biota; Arrieta et al., 2006; Bourre, 2006; Rapin & Wiernsperger, 2010).

Many patients presenting with depression or anxiety often have problems with gut function. In the past, we may have interpreted GI symptoms as an expression of inner turmoil and conflicts; but what if the symptoms are much simpler? Foods we eat create the fuel for our cells to function, grow, and repair. An assessment of mineral or vitamin levels provides only one small piece of the puzzle of making a human. We know that vitamin D deficiency is correlated with bone loss, and vitamin B12 deficiency is associated with pernicious anemia. However, evaluating vitamin levels for only these two illnesses illustrates a basic lack of understanding about human biochemistry; as we delve deeper into the integrated human, we discover that correction of deficiencies varies tremendously when you add in genetic variabilities that may alter a person's individual nutritional needs.

Nutrition: The Making of a Human

Humans eat to satisfy hunger and to ingest foods that we need to repair and replace products in our body for healthy function. Ingested nutrients are generally divided into two groups: essential and nonessential. Essential nutrients include those food products that humans cannot manufacture in sufficient quantity for normal biochemical function; therefore, essential nutrients must be ingested. Essential nutrients include amino acids, vitamins, minerals, and many components. Table 16.2 shows essential and nonessential amino acids that form the skeleton for proteins.

All vitamins are essential (Table 16.3) and must be ingested, absorbed, and then transformed into a bioavailable form for processing into numerous products and for utilization in the citric acid energy cycle (Kreb's cycle). These vitamins include:

1. Riboflavin (vitamin B2): flavin adenine dinucleotide (FAD)
2. Niacin (vitamin B3): nicotinamide adenine dinucleotide (NAD$^+$)
3. Thiamine (vitamin B1): thiamine diphosphate
4. Pantothenic acid (vitamin B5; part of coenzyme A)
5. Ascorbic acid (vitamin C): enables energy release called the electron transfer chain (Bender, 2012)

TABLE 16.2 AMINO ACIDS (MAKES PROTEINS)	
Essential (we have to eat these)	**Nonessential (we make these)**
• Leucine • Isoleucine • Valine • Histidine • Lysine • Methionine • Phenylalanine • Threonine • Tryptophan	• Alanine • Arginine • Asparagine • Aspartic acid • Cysteine • Glutamic acid • Glutamine • Glycine • Proline • Serine • Tyrosine

TABLE 16.3 ESSENTIAL VITAMINS (CANNOT BE MADE IN THE BODY)	
Fat Loving (Fat Soluble)	**Water Loving (Water Soluble)**
• Vitamin A (retinol) • Vitamin K • Vitamin E • Vitamin D	• B vitamins • Vitamin C (ascorbic acid)

All minerals are also essential as the body cannot manufacture any of them, and they include trace minerals such as iron, zinc, copper, selenium, iodine, fluoride, and chromium. Major minerals include sodium, potassium, calcium, phosphorus, magnesium, manganese, sulfur, cobalt, and chlorine (Akhondzadeh, Gerbarg, & Brown, 2013; Bourre, 2006).

B vitamins have been implicated in psychiatric mental health care for decades. Most practitioners are familiar with the development of Wernicke encephalopathy and Korsakoff syndrome, which are dementias related to thiamine (vitamin B1) deficiency due to chronic alcohol ingestion that disrupts the ability of the gut to absorb this and other nutrients. Vitamin B12 replacement is available as methylcobalamin or cyanocobalamin. Figure 16.1 shows options for replacing vitamin B12 along with the steps required by the body to process cobalamin (vitamin B12) into its bioavailable form methylcobalamin. Methylcobalamin is essential for normal manufacture of healthy red blood cells and is also critical for neurological function and synthesis and replication of DNA, RNA, and numerous nerve-related components (Bourre, 2006).

Folate (vitamin B9) in its bioavailable form, L-5-methylfolate, is facilitated by vitamin B12 to act as a methyl-group (CH_3–) donor to convert homocysteine to methionine. Methionine combines with adenosine triphosphate (ATP) to form another compound, S-adenosylmethionine (SAMe). Methylation processes require readily available compounds such as SAMe to convert products into active compounds or to inert compounds for elimination from the body. Of all methylating compounds, SAMe is the universal methyl group donor (a carbon atom with three hydrogen atoms attached) for numerous processes including DNA/RNA replication and synthesis of neurotransmitters, hormones, proteins, and lipids (Ames, 1999; Bourre, 2006). See Box 16.1 for the process of methylation.

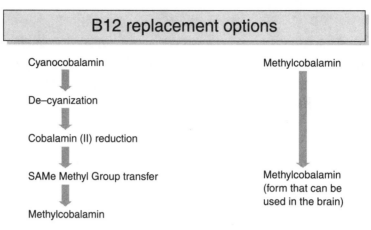

FIGURE 16.1 Vitamin B12 replacement options. SAMe, *S*-adenosylmethionine.

BOX 16.1 Methylation at a Glance

Vitamin B9 (folic acid) (synthetic) → Dihydrofolate (dietary) → Tetrahydrofolate + vitamin B12 → Methylene tetrahydrofolate → (MTHFR) → L-5-methylfolate (biologically active).
Methylcobalamin (vitamin B12) is the form needed to make red blood cells and for normal neurological function and DNA synthesis.
L-Methylfolate needs methylcobalamin to convert homocysteine to methionine.
Methionine combines with adenosine triphosphate (ATP) to form *S*-adenosylmethionine (SAMe).
SAMe is the universal methyl donor for numerous processes including DNA/RNA replication, synthesis of neurotransmitters, hormones, proteins, and lipids.

An assessment of sufficient bioavailability of essential and nonessential nutrient components required for synthesis of neurochemicals should be a basic starting point when assessing a patient with mental health symptoms. Sufficient amounts of essential nutrients are required to manufacture neurotransmitters; therefore, before replacing neurotransmitters with medications we may be able to support the body to increase manufacture of endogenous neurotransmitters. For example, Figure 16.2 shows the components and processes required for biosynthesis of the neurotransmitter serotonin, and Figure 16.3 shows the components and processes required for biosynthesis of the catecholamines.

Let's review the check and balance systems that maintain neurotransmitter homeostasis. Normal function of the brain's cortex reflects a balance between excitation and inhibition. For example, excitatory neurotransmitters will rebalance each other to prevent overactivation. One excitatory neurotransmitter, norepinephrine (NE), will be balanced by reducing acetylcholine (Ach). This is why medications that increase NE have anticholinergic side effects (Fernstrom & Fernstrom, 2007). Another rebalancing process involves gamma-aminobutyric acid (GABA) and glutamate synthesis and metabolism (Petroff, 2002). In the brain, GABA is the main inhibitory neurotransmitter and glutamate is the main excitatory neurotransmitter. It should be noted that the excitatory neurotransmitter, glutamate, is required to synthesize (manufacture) the main inhibitory

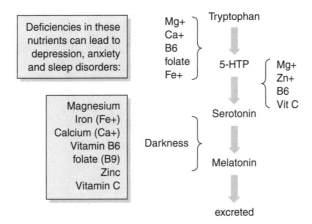

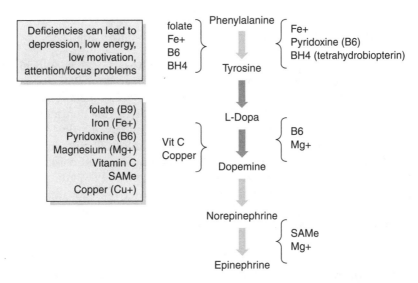

FIGURE 16.2 Synthesis sequence for serotonin from tryptophan.

FIGURE 16.3 Synthesis sequence of catecholamines from phenylalanine/tyrosine.

neurotransmitter, GABA (Petroff, 2002). Synthesis and balance of these two major neurotransmitters depend on the body's ability to synthesize certain enzymes that require adequate amounts of vitamin B6 (pyridoxine; Vonder Haar, Peterson, Martens, & Hoane, 2016). GABA is "recycled" using tricarboxylic acid, which in turn, synthesizes glutamate, which in turn forms GABA, and so on (Vonder Haar et al., 2016). GABA synthesis is unique among neurotransmitters because of coding on two separate gene alleles for separate isoforms of the rate-controlling enzyme glutamic acid decarboxylase (Vonder Haar et al., 2016). Figure 16.4 contains a diagram that shows the GABA-glutamate processing system and the interaction with this system and the citric acid cycle. GABA is available in supplement form (discussed later in this chapter).

General Guidelines for Laboratory Testing in Integrative Psychiatry

Most medical practitioners are trained to evaluate for disease states that mimic psychiatric illnesses such as hypothyroidism and anemia. Other reasons for ordering lab testing in psychiatry is to monitor for side effects of medications based on protocols and

> ● Balances alertness and drowsiness.
> ● Vitamin B6 (pyridoxine) deficiencies can lead to fatigue, irritability, anxiety, insomnia and cell damage.

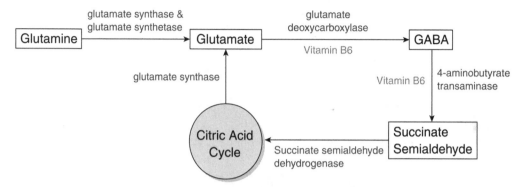

FIGURE 16.4 Gamma-aminobutyric acid (GABA) and glutamate diagram.

guidelines. For example, patients taking atypical antipsychotics should be monitored for increased fasting glucose, weight gain, and lipid elevations. Patients on lithium are monitored for changes in white blood cell count and thyroid function. Basic labs usually include a complete blood count (CBC), electrolytes, liver function tests, thyroid tests, pregnancy test if indicated, and a lipid panel (American Psychiatric Association [APA], 2016; Sadock, Sadock, & Ruiz, 2015). FM practitioners follow all guidelines and protocols as their colleagues; however, additional testing is often ordered based on biochemical properties of neurotransmitter synthesis and metabolism, and FM guidelines for treating the hypothalamic-pituitary-adrenal axis versus only thyroid. In addition, FM interpretation guidelines are different from basic medical guidelines. Commonly ordered tests in FM psychiatric practice are listed in Table 16.4.

GENETIC TESTING

Another tool that is becoming more and more important in psychiatric practice is the availability of genetic assays that provide the practitioner with information on the body's ability to synthesize, utilize, or metabolize certain products. It is well beyond the scope of this chapter to completely review and discuss the proper use of genetic assays in psychiatry; however, a brief overview highlighting genetic testing is necessary for understanding the use of this amazing tool in FM psychiatry.

We know that all living things are made of cells: small, membrane-enclosed units filled with the fundamental molecules of life and of which all living things are composed. Cells are endowed with the miraculous ability to create exact duplicates of themselves by growing and then dividing in two. Despite their apparent diversity, living things are fundamentally similar on the inside. Owing to a now deciphered common molecular code, it is possible to read, measure, and achieve a coherent understanding of all the forms of life, from the smallest to the greatest (Alberts et al., 2015). Within the nucleus of a cell lies the grouping of amino acids, known as DNA. A group of three bases forms a "codon" that codes for a specific amino acid. Proteins are manufactured in the cell nucleus based on the sequence of codons, and therefore the sequence of amino acids. Amino acid "strings" are formed by duplicating the sequence of amino acids and then binding the strings together with chemical "peptide bonds" to create a "chain" of amino

TABLE 16.4 STANDARD LAB TESTS IN FM PSYCHIATRY

Level tested	Functional Lab Test	Implications	Reference
Cobalamin (vitamin B12)	Serum vitamin B12 and methylmalonic acid	In preventive studies on dementia, "normal" levels of vitamin B12 are listed as >500 pg/mL, ideal level is 1,000 pg/mL; methylmalonic acid is a more sensitive measure of chronic deficiency of vitamin B12, normal range >0.4 μmol/mL	Allen, Stabler, Savage, and Lindenbaum, 1993; Grober, Kisters, and Schmidt, 2013; Morris, Jacques, Rosenberg, and Selhub, 2010
Folate (vitamin B9)	Serum homocysteine; folate levels only provide circulating levels of this nutrient; a person with a MTHFR SNP cannot use folate biologically and therefore can be functionally deficient in folate with normal levels	Homocysteine serum levels are a more sensitive marker of chronic folate deficiency; normal range >15 nmoL/mL serum	Allen et al., 1993; Grober et al., 2013; Morris et al., 2010
Vitamin D	25-Hydroxy vitamin D; activation of cholecalciferol and ergocalciferol into 25(OH)D and 1,25(OH)2D occurs in the liver; vitamin D then interacts with vitamin D receptors (VDRs) in target tissues, leading to physiological actions	Serum level should be >50 ng/mL; lower levels of vitamin D 25-OH are associated with both musculoskeletal and neurocognitive dysfunction including balance, migraine, depression, autism, chronic pain, memory impairment, and demyelinating diseases	Fernandes de Abreu, Eyles, and Feron, 2009; Kalueff and Tuohimaa, 2007; Kilpinen-Loisa, Nenonen, Pihko, & Makitie, 2007; Ushiroyama, Ikeda, and Ueki, 2002
Ferritin	Storage form of iron; most sensitive test of iron deficiency anemia; however, levels may be falsely normal/low in many inflammatory conditions; serum ferritin increases with inflammation	>30 ng/mL (30–200 ng/mL) and transferrin saturation >20% (20%–50%)	Massoumi, 2016

(continued)

TABLE 16.4 STANDARD LAB TESTS IN FM PSYCHIATRY (CONTINUED)

Level tested	Functional Lab Test	Implications	Reference
RBC magnesium and zinc levels (intracellular magnesium)	RBC levels of magnesium and zinc are better indicators of the status of these minerals than standard serum levels	RBC magnesium level in the upper half of normal, or >5 mg/dL; low Mg$^+$ is associated with migraines and mood disorders; RBC zinc level (intracellular zinc) >11 mg/L; may mimic ADHD symptoms if low	Al Alawi, Majoni, and Falhammar, 2018; Hariri and Azadbakht, 2015; Lord & Redmond, 2012
CBC with differential	Follow normal guidelines		Lord & Redmond, 2012
Comprehensive metabolic profile that includes electrolytes, fasting blood sugar, liver and kidney function	Follow normal guidelines		APA, 2016; Lord & Redmond, 2012
Liver function tests that include GGT if on pain relievers or heavy alcohol use	Follow normal guidelines		APA, 2016; Lord and Redmond, 2012
Thyroid function panel	RBC iodine level, TSH, T4 free, T3 total, T3 reverse, T3 uptake; if patient is significantly symptomatic, thyroid antibodies and/or thyroid peridoxase may be tested to rule out Hashimoto thyroiditis or other autoimmune thyroid disorders	TSH is not a reliable indicator of many thyroid disorders; some psychiatric medications (lithium) can adversely affect thyroid function, so a baseline is a good idea; thyroid dysfunction can mimic many psychiatric disorders including anxiety, depression and chronic fatigue	Brooks and Post, 2014; Hennessey, Garber, Woeber, Cobin, and Klein, 2016; Mullur, Liu, and Brent, 2014; Pizzorno & Ferril, 2005/2010

Level tested	Functional Lab Test	Implications	Reference
Lipid panel	A baseline and follow-up cholesterol/lipid panel	Some medications, such as atypical antipsychotics, can increase lipid/cholesterol levels	APA, 2016
High sensitivity *C-reactive protein (hsCRP)*	hsCRP	Measures degree of inflammation in blood vessels; some patients with mood disorder may respond to anti-inflammatory agents	Rosenblat and McIntyre, 2017
Iron profile with saturation percent	Serum iron, total iron binding capacity (TIBC), transferrin saturation % (TSat)	Iron is a cofactor for synthesis of catecholamines; low Fe^+ can cause restless leg syndrome, ADHD-like symptoms, and mood disorders; transferrin is the transport protein of iron; TSat is the percentage transferrin bound to iron	Adisetiyo & Helpern, 2015; Ghorayeb, Gamas, Mazurie, and Mayo, 2017; Hariri and Azadbakht, 2015; Hurt, Arnold, and Lofthouse, 2011; Wang, Huang, Zhang, Qu, and Mu, 2017
Cortisol levels and ACTH	Follow normal guidelines	*Cortisol levels and ACTH* are initial tests for adrenal fatigue, which is caused by dysfunction of the HPA axis as a result of chronic stress, resulting in exhaustion; "adrenal fatigue" is an abbreviated descriptor	de Vente, van Amsterdam, Olff, Kamphuis, and Emmelkamp, 2015; Lumpkin, 2005/2010

ACTH, adrenocorticotropic hormone; ADHD, attention deficit hyperactivity disorder; APA, American Psychiatric Association; CBC, complete blood count; FM, functional medicine; GGT, gamma-glutamyl transferase; HPA, hypothalamic-pituitary-adrenal; RBC, red blood cell; SNP, single nucleotide polymorphism; T3, triiodothyronine; T4, thyroxine; TSH, thyroid-stimulating hormone.

Resource for additional information about Integrative and functional lab testing: Lord, R. & Bralley, J. A. (Eds). (2012). Laboratory evaluations for integrative and functional medicine (2nd ed.). Duluth, GA: Metametrix Institute.

acids. Each amino acid has an electrical charge, positive or negative, that influences how the string "folds" up to creates a protein with specific function. The bonds, based on the electrical charge, are referred to as "peptide bonds," which form a "polypeptide" (Weil, 2012a, 2012b). Polypeptides are proteins. To form a new polypeptide, a message is created beginning at the site of the DNA in the nucleus of a cell. Messenger ribonucleic acid (mRNA) creates a template off DNA when the DNA strand "unzips." This allows mRNA to create a mirrored replicate of the sequence of base pairs from the original pattern (Alberts et al., 2015; Weil, 2012c). There are four nucleotides in the "language" of DNA/RNA; however, there are 20 amino acids that form the language of proteins. The full set of codons represents the "genetic code." The genetic code has 64 possible permutations of three nucleotide sequences (codons) made from the four nucleotides. Of the 64 codon combination possibilities, 61 of them represent amino acids and the remaining three represent a signal to "stop" coding (Alberts et al., 2015; Chatterjea & Shinde, 2012).

Variations in human genetic information are referred to as single nucleotide polymorphisms (SNPs; Chatterjea & Shinde, 2012). A SNP refers to a change in sequence within a specific allele where the nucleotide differs from the normal or expected genetic sequence. Genetic variations are considered SNPs, which are "common" if at least 1% of the population has the same genetic variant. Considering that a SNP occurs approximately once every 300 nucleotides or so and given that there are 3 billion nucleotides in a human genome, that translates into about 10 million SNPs per person. Variation among individuals is based on the presence, or absence of these SNPs, making the vast majority of humans 99% identical with less than 1% of their genome, making them individually unique (Weil, 2012a).

A variation in nucleotide sequencing can range from having no consequences on the translated protein up to catastrophic consequences, depending on the function of the coded protein. For example, a single nucleotide alteration changing one amino acid in a protein that codes for the oxygen-carrying beta chain of hemoglobin results in a protein that turns normal hemoglobin into a sickle cell shape, which has lifelong life-threatening consequences in the person with this particular alteration (Clancy, 2008). To have the process of replication run relatively smoothly, DNA interrupters that can trigger mutations, or polymorphisms, need to be kept to a minimum, if possible. Environmentally ingested DNA interrupters include preservatives, pesticides, artificial sweeteners or colorants, and heavy metals, for example. High stress levels that result in chronically elevated levels of cortisol, especially in the brain, increase the likelihood of transcriptional errors. Consumption of nonfood toxins and underconsumption of essential nutrient components increase the possibility of DNA replication errors, causing mutations that are associated with diseases such as depression, anxiety, insomnia, pain, and even cancer (Clancy, 2008).

Some variations in genetic transcription are common (SNPs) and can be tested for affordably and are modifiable with nutrition-based interventions (e.g., the methylene-tetrahydrofolate reductase [MTHFR; Box X.1] genetic SNP that is important for folate metabolism). Many physiological functions depend on the carbon transfer capability of L-5-methylfolate created when a methyl group is donated from methylcobalamin using the MTHFR enzyme. Genetic variants of the MTHFR gene limit "downstream" production of numerous products, causing illnesses related to high homocysteine levels. Elevated homocysteine exerts direct toxic effects on both the vascular and nervous system and is associated with accelerated brain atrophy, atherosclerosis, myocardial infarction, stroke, minimal cognitive impairment, dementia, Parkinson disease, multiple sclerosis, epilepsy and eclampsia (Ansari, Mahta, Mallack, & Luo, 2014; SNPedia, 2019). Some of the cofactors required in the synthesis of SAMe include zinc, pyridoxal 5'-phosphate (vitamin B6), riboflavin 5'-phosphate (vitamin B2), magnesium, zinc, betaine (trimethylglycine), and vitamin D (Moore, Le, & Fan, 2013).

Deficiencies of any of the cofactor nutrients can result in impaired methylation cycles, and therefore increased potential for eventual disease. Another genetic polymorphism interest in psychiatry is of the thiamine transporter gene (*SLC19A3*), which is associated with decreased intestinal absorption of thiamine that mimics Wernicke encephalopathy and can include fever, confusion, seizure, ophthalmoplegia, dysphagia, and in severe cases, coma or death (Ortigoza-Escobar et al., 2014).

Folate

Let's dive a little deeper into folate and its importance in psychiatry. Folate, as dihydrofolate, is a water-soluble B vitamin (vitamin B9) critical for normal growth and repair of nerve tissues. Folate in the synthetic form of folic acid was mandated by the U.S. government in 1998 to be added to grain products when it was found that low levels were associated with severe neural tube birth defects (brain and spinal column; Bottiglieri, 2013). Folic acid is not bioavailable and is therefore unusable by the body in this form. People who have one of the *MTHFR* genetic SNPs (specifically the C677T and/or the 1298C) are not able to convert sufficient amounts of THF from folic acid, or dihydrofolate. The C677T enzyme conducts the lion's share of the work in the body, while the 1298C SNP, although less prevalent, does the majority of the work in the brain. A C677T partial variant (C/T) reduces activity of the enzyme by about 30% to 40%, while a person with the full SNP variant (T/T) has a 60% to 70% reduction of the enzyme activity. Individuals who have either variant will benefit from adequate intake of foods that are rich in B vitamins such as the dark-green leafy vegetables (Minich, 2016). Both synthetic folic acid and dietary dihydrofolate must be reduced with the same enzyme, dihydrofolate reductase (DHFR). When there is a high concentration of folic acid (FA), both folic acid and DHF compete for the same binding site on DHFR. When this happens, folic acid will build up, resulting in the body producing less of the bioavailable DHFR, further reducing the amount of available L-5-methylfolate (Strickland, Krupenko, & Krupenko, 2013). Therefore, previous recommendations to increase folic acid for those with the MTHFR SNP may have been misguided since folic acid supplementation requires greater use of enzymes and cofactors resulting in reduced synthesis of bioavailable folate. MTHFR is also required to synthesize methionine (for SAMe production) from homocysteine; a similar problem is encountered when cobalamin (vitamin B12) is supplemented with cyanocobalamin instead of methylcobalamin (Figure 16.1).

Nutrigenomics is the study of the molecular effects of food constituents and other dietary bioactives on gene expression (Ferguson, 2014). Nutrigenomic evaluation studies the effect of the molecular components of food and dietary constituents on gene expression throughout the body, rather than on a single gene. Therefore, nutrigenomics is focused on the relationship between specific nutrients and gene expression and the potential of this interaction to cause, or prevent, diet-related diseases. Nutrigenetics refers to the response of individual genetic variations or SNPs to nutrients (Minich, 2016).

The catechol-*O*-methyltransferase (COMT) enzyme catalyzes the movement of a methyl group from SAMe to a catecholamine. Catecholamines include various neurotransmitters of great importance and are also significant in sex hormone synthesis and metabolism (Minich, 2016). The COMT enzyme decreases circulating catecholamines such as dopamine (DA) and NE. When there is a genetic variant where methionine is substituted for valine (COMT Met/Met), the person may develop high NE and/or DA symptoms such as anxiety, poor concentration, obsessive worry, irritability, insomnia, depression, and memory disruption (Minich, 2016). Nutrigenomic treatment options would include supplemental SAMe (to force the enzyme to work faster) along with options including vitamin B6, vitamin B12, folate, magnesium, and possibly betaine (Minich, 2016). Nutrigenomics is the study of the molecular effects of food constituents and other dietary bioactives on gene expression (Ferguson, 2014). Nutrigenomic evaluation studies the effect of the molecular components of food and dietary constituents on gene expression throughout the body, rather than on a single gene. Therefore, nutrigenomics is focused on the relationship between specific nutrients and gene expression and the potential of this interaction to cause, or prevent, diet-related diseases. Nutrigenetics refers to the response of individual genetic variation or SNPs to nutrients.

Ordering and Interpreting Genetic Assays

Just because you can order genetic assays doesn't mean you should order genetic assays because (a) specialized training is required to interpret the results, (b) there are inherent ethical and legal risks is releasing someone's entire DNA genome to third parties, and (c) most direct-to-consumer marketing companies provide advice on interpretation that is significantly inaccurate or overly simplistic. When discussing ethical considerations in genetic testing, one must first understand the difference between ethical and legal implications of the information under review. Legally, "genetic information" refers to "any individual, information about—(i) such individual's genetic tests, (ii) the genetic tests of family members of such individual, and (iii) the manifestation of a disease or disorder in family members of such individual" (The Public Health and Welfare, 2018, 42 U.S.C. § 300gg–91(d)(16)). Legal standards are set forth in governmental laws, but ethical standards are based on human principles of right and wrong. It is therefore possible to violate ethical standards without breaking the law.

The following genetic case example describes inaccurate interpretation of a genetic assay. DNA testing for the most part will provide "likelihoods" and odds ratios for disease outcome as shown in the test results. Very few alleles tested can be directly shown to be related to disease states, especially in psychiatry. Clinicians should never replace nutrients or neurotransmitters based solely on a single genetic variant because the variants, SNPs and individual biology (epigenetic) factors, environment, symptom constellation, and so on must be considered. "Epigenetics" refers to mediation interactions between environment, the genome, and disease pathogenesis. Epigenetic factors have been shown to modulate immune responses potentially counteracting inflammatory processes (Aleksandrova, Romero-Mosquera, & Hernandez, 2017). A very important set of epigenetic modifiers includes nutrition and dietary factors associated with gene expression pattern alteration during periods of immune system activation (Choi & Friso, 2010). Remember, genetic testing provides the recipe file for making that person; however, it does not provide information on what the body actually makes. Many genes are suppressed, others are expressed and active. In many cases, something as simple as a methyl group may have attached to an allele signaling a "stop" code for expressing that gene.

Case Example of Genetic Assay Interpretation Gone Wrong

Jean, a 36-year-old woman presented to the clinic with severe anxiety, insomnia, and irritability that she had never before experienced. Jean reported that she saw her family practitioner for depression, and she had run Jean's genetic assay for medication recommendations. The practitioner had noted that there were no gene-drug interactions for bupropion as an antidepressant and started her on that medication. Jean gradually developed side effects that worsened over time. A review of the genetic assay showed a variant for the COMT enzyme with a Met/Met result. The *COMT* gene codes for an enzyme to metabolize (breaks down) dopamine once released into the synapse. The Met/Met variant codes for an inactive COMT enzyme. While it was true that her CYP enzymes were neutral for bupropion, the presence of the COMT variant should have been a red flag that she would eventually develop high levels of dopamine due to an inability to clear it from the synapses. Jean was tapered off bupropion and placed on supplemental SAMe (one option for a COMT Met/Met variant that forces the COMT enzyme to work faster) and her symptoms cleared up in less than a month.

If a practitioner is interested in learning about how to interpret and utilize genetic testing, this author strongly recommends additional formal training in nutrigenetics, nutrigenomics, and genetic testing in general. A glossary of genomic terminology can be found at www.cdc.gov/genomics/about/glossary.htm. See Box 16.2 for resources on genetics.

The Centers for Disease Control and Prevention (CDC) has listed basic competencies that should be met for healthcare professionals who utilize genomic testing in their practice (CDC, 2010). These competencies are included in Box 16.3, and Table 16.5 provides sites for training in genetic testing.

BOX 16.2 Resources for More Information on Genetic Testing and Interpretation of Genetic Assays

1. Learn genetics: www.learn.genetics.utah.edu/content/basics
2. Genetic testing registry: www.ncbi.nlm.nih.gov/gtr/tests/523653
3. The National Center for Biotechnology Information:
   www.ncbi.nlm.nih.gov/genbank

BOX 16.3 Genomic Competencies for Health Professionals

1. Apply basic genomic concepts including patterns of inheritance, gene-environment interactions, role of genes in health and disease, and implications for health promotion programs to relevant clinical services.
2. Demonstrate understanding of the indications for, components of, and resources for genetic testing and/or genomic-based interventions.
3. Describe ethical, legal, social, and financial issues related to genetic testing and recording of genomic information.
4. Explain basic concepts of probability and risk and benefits of genomics in health and disease assessment in the context of the clinical practice.
5. Deliver genomic information, recommendations, and care without patient or family coercion within an appropriate informed-consent process.

TABLE 16.5 TRAINING IN GENETIC TESTING	
Location	**Information**
The Johns Hopkins University/National Human Genome Research Institute Genetic Counseling Training Program	A joint effort combining resources of two outstanding research institutions, the National Human Genome Research Institute (NHGRI) at the National Institutes of Health (NIH) and the Department of Health, Behavior and Society at the Johns Hopkins Bloomberg School of Public Health. These organizations have collaborated to develop a unique genetic counseling graduate program that addresses the growing need for genetic counseling services: www.genome.gov/10001156
Centers for Disease Control and Prevention's Office of Public Health Genomics (OPHG)	Conducts and supports workshops, courses, and other training activities in public health genomics, family history, and human genome epidemiology. OPHG was also involved in developing genomics competencies for public health professionals.

OFF-LABEL DRUG USE AND CAM

Most prescribers are acutely aware of, and concerned about, liability when it comes to treatments or procedures that have not been approved by the FDA. The terminology used is "off-label use" (OLU), which means prescribing a currently available and marketed medication for a disease or a symptom that has never received FDA approval (Wittich, Burkle, & Lanier, 2012). The use of OLU medications in psychiatry is much more prevalent than in other specialties owing to difficulties in obtaining FDA approval for treatments often considered standard of care practice. Clinical trials for a new indication through FDA approved clinical trials can be extremely costly in terms of both time and financial investment. Additional indications for an already approved medication require the manufacturer or owner of the patent to file a supplemental drug application, obtain approval for clinical trials, and even if the already approved medication is given an additional indication, they may never recoup the financial investment for the new indication (Wittich et al., 2012). Medications, nutrients, or supplements that are generically available, and extremely inexpensive (less than $5 USD), do not have financial backers that would support the process required for initial, or additional, FDA-approved clinical trials. A common example is the use of tricyclic antidepressants for neuropathic pain. The tricyclic category is considered a first-line treatment option; however, none of the medications in this class have ever undergone an FDA-approved clinical trial and all are considered off-label for pain indications (Dworkin et al., 2010). Given the hurdles pharmaceutically prepared medications must conquer to be granted approval by the FDA, it is not surprising that nutraceuticals will likely never receive FDA approval for any indication despite clear, compelling, and scientifically supported evidence (often by the NIH) for their use in medicine.

The use of non-FDA approved medication and supplement (biological) use is motivated by several factors. First, a biological agent may have been shown to be safe and effective in the most commonly studied population (adults ages 18 to 65 with no comorbid conditions); however, it might not have been studied and approved for other populations (e.g., pediatric, geriatric, or pregnant patients; Lin, Phan, & Lin, 2006). Second, in some cases, urgent medical conditions may motivate a medical professional to provide treatments that are logical and available, whether approved by the FDA or not (Wittich et al., 2012). Third, medications from one class of drugs such as selective serotoninergic reuptake inhibitors (SSRIs) that have FDA approval, and are effective for one of a group of disorders (such as anxiety or depression) lack specific FDA approval for similar conditions(e.g., generalized anxiety disorder vs. social anxiety disorder). However, these medications have become commonly used standards of care (Stafford, 2008). Fourth, if the biophysiological pathways and features of the conditions are similar, practitioners may use a medication that has received FDA approval for one condition to treat another condition (e.g., diabetes and metabolic syndrome; psychiatric diseases such as anxiety and posttraumatic stress disorder; Lin et al., 2006; Stafford, 2008; Wittich et al., 2012). Despite the quagmire of hoops, hurdles, and navigational difficulties posed by regulating agencies, the APPN must rely on standards of care and FDA approval, when appropriate, and professional recommendations and guidelines in addition to legal counsel to practice safely.

COMPLEMENTARY MODALITIES IN PSYCHIATRIC NURSING PRACTICE

APPNs who specialize in psychotherapy and pharmacotherapy may find themselves in unfamiliar territory if their patient asks for an opinion about a treatment outside mainstream medicine. In many cases, treatments that are complementary are familiar to the APPN; however, the APPN may not realize they are well studied and approved of by the NIH. For example, healthy lifestyle and healthy nutrition are familiar areas for health-care practitioners, but how many practitioners are expertly trained in nutrition science? A good starting point is the general guidelines for overall healthy eating and being familiar with the location of authoritative resources that provide in-depth scientific knowledge and information. This information should be shared with your patient. APPNs should be aware of their own limitations regarding information, education, and recommendations that would be best addressed by an expert (dietitian, nutritionist, etc.). Nutrition-based interventions in psychiatric practice has its underpinnings in biochemistry, molecular biology, and nutrigenomics; therefore, each decision point requires significant understanding of the sequence of events impacted when pathways are modified.

Nutrients and functional bioactive components from foods can influence epigenetic expression through two major pathways: (1) by directly inhibiting enzymes that catalyze DNA methylation or histone modifications, or (2) by altering the availability of substrates necessary for those enzymatic reactions (Choi & Friso, 2010). The ability to modify genetic material, without altering heritable markers that hold genetic information, allows the organism to adapt to changing environments and evolve accordingly (Barnett, Bassett, & Bermingham, 2014). For example, an infant developing in utero in a nutrient-deprived environment may adapt to that environment, and later may thrive in a similar nutrient-poor environment or, in contrast, develop metabolic health-related problems if in nutrient-rich or nutrient-excessive environments. Genetic modification can occur due to deficiencies, or excesses, of common nutrients. Some pathways are biochemical and bioelectrical, as in brain and nervous system function. Treatments that target bioelectrical pathways may be primarily electrical (e.g., electroconvulsive therapy [ECT], repetitive transcranial magnetic stimulation [rTMS], transcutaneous electrical nerve stimulation [TENS]), or may include modification of ions and/or ion channels at the level of individual cellular function. The NCCIH divides CAM treatments into three types: natural, mind-body, and "other" (NIH, 2018). This chapter further divides these categories into several subcategories, as shown in Table 16.6, that separate herbals and nutrients, lifestyle, manipulative, and electrochemical modalities. Treatments for APPNs who are interested in adding CAM to their practice are outlined in this chapter, in brief, with recommendations for resources and additional training and education.

TABLE 16.6 CATEGORIES OF COMPLEMENTARY AND ALTERNATIVE MEDICINE MODALITIES IN PSYCHIATRIC PRACTICE

Category	Description	Examples
Natural	1. Nutraceuticals 2. Herbals	Vitamins, minerals, and amino acids. Probiotics Fish oil products (omega-3 fatty acids) Herbals (capsules, teas, essential oils)
Lifestyle	1. Behavioral 2. Psychotherapy 3. Exercise	Healthy diet and exercise; avoidance of toxins such as substances of abuse, heavy metals, high fat/high sugar diets; counseling, coaching and psychotherapy; yoga, tai chi, qigong, meditation
Manipulative	Practitioner applied	Massage, acupuncture, spinal manipulation (chiropractic/osteopathic)
Electromagnetic	Use of electrical or magnetic devices	Repetitive transcranial magnetic stimulation (rTMS), transcutaneous electrical nerve stimulation (TENS), biofeedback or neurofeedback

Nutraceuticals

Nutraceuticals include essential and nonessential micronutrients, which are those vitamins and minerals required in small, or trace, amounts to complete biological, chemical, and physiological processes throughout the body. Essential nutrients are defined as those products that must be consumed as they cannot be manufactured by the body, at least in adequate amounts. Both essential and nonessential nutrients are required for the synthesis of enzymes, metabolism processes, replication of DNA including modification of gene expression, manufacture of receptors, transporters, ion channels, pump mechanisms, membrane function, mitochondrial function, immune system function, drug metabolism, and a host of other processes.

It is generally assumed that people who live in developed countries have access to adequate nutrition; however, estimates of the general U.S. population show that more than 50% fail to meet estimated average requirements for at least one micronutrient (Popper, 2014). Some examples of deficiency rates of micronutrients related to brain function and mood in the United States includes vitamin B6 (10.5%), iron (9.5%), vitamin D (8.1%), and vitamin C (6%; Popper, 2014). Severe micronutrient deficiencies are relatively rare; however, insufficiency is prevalent and less clinically obvious, especially in psychiatric settings.

Suboptimal levels of micronutrients can compromise and damage physiological processes through numerous biochemical mechanisms. In addition, there are at least 50 known genetic variants or single nucleotide polymorphisms (SNPs) that structurally change binding affinity for cofactors that can easily be treated with dietary supplementation of micronutrient components (Ames, Elson-Schwab, & Silver, 2002). Deficiencies of common micronutrients such as vitamins B12, B6, B9, C, and E; iron; and zinc cause damage to nuclear DNA and other micronutrient deficiencies (in biotin and iron) can damage mitochondrial function (Ames et al., 2002). Alteration of function at the microbiological level causes slow, chronic, insidious damage leading to multisystem metabolic and organ damage, which in turn accelerates aging of cells and neuronal dysfunction (Ames et al., 2002; Wahls, Rubenstein, Hall, & Snetselaar, 2014). Severe micronutrient deficiencies, causing such diseases as pellagra, scurvy, beriberi, and anemias, are known to produce psychiatric symptoms, but have not been associated with mood disorders until the past 50–70 years. Nutrient insufficiencies correlated with mental health symptoms have been demonstrated for B vitamins and vitamins C, D, and E, minerals (calcium, lithium, chromium, iron, magnesium, zinc, copper, and selenium), and vitamin-like compounds (choline; Kaplan, Crawford, Field, & Simpson, 2007). Even though it is known that the body builds nervous tissues, including the brain, from ingested substances from the diet (vitamins, minerals, essential amino acids, and essential fatty acids, including omega-3 polyunsaturated fatty acids), it escapes many psychiatric practitioners that deficiencies or absence of these same nutrients may cause organ dysfunction and symptoms (Bourre, 2006).

While it makes logical sense that a person must eat certain nutrients for neurobiological functioning, research assessing microdeficiencies has been lacking. Studies describing the relationship between nutrient intake and psychiatric functioning in adults with confirmed mood disorders demonstrate significant correlations between generalized assessments of functioning (GAF) scores and energy (kilocalories), carbohydrates, fiber, total fat, linoleic acid, riboflavin, niacin, folate, vitamin B6, vitamin B12, pantothenic acid, calcium, phosphorus, potassium, and iron (all P values <0.05), as well as magnesium and zinc (Davison & Kaplan, 2012). Subsequent reports noted that in populations with confirmed diagnosis of a mental health condition, there is an association with nutrient insufficiency (Davison & Kaplan, 2012). It should also be noted that it is rare for a person to have a single micronutrient insufficiency, and therefore, the practitioner who uncovers a deficiency or insufficiency should assess for additional nutrient problems. Several of the B vitamins have demonstrated roles in development and continued function of the central nervous system. Severe deficiencies or genetic disorders that impair uptake

BOX 16.4 Nutraceuticals in Psychiatric Mental Health Treatment

S-Adenosylmethionine (SAMe) has been shown to dose-dependently increase concentrations of central nervous system monoamine neurotransmitters serotonin and norepinephrine, increase dopaminergic tone in brain regions, including the striatum, and increases CNS beta-adrenergic receptor density and activity (Bottiglieri, 2013). Clinical guidelines recommend taking SAMe on an empty stomach to increase absorption beginning with 400 mg daily, gradually increasing the dose to 800–1600 mg daily in divided doses (Bottiglieri, 2013).

Gamma-aminobutyric acid (GABA) is the main inhibitory neurotransmitter in the human cortex (Boonstra et al., 2015; Petroff, 2002). Research has not fully explained the mechanism of action, if any, of supplementing GABA orally because it had previously been thought that exogenously supplemented GABA did not cross the blood-brain barrier (Boonstra et al., 2015).

L-Theanine is an amino acid and is found in green tea. It is known to have a calming effect without sedation (Alramadhan et al., 2012). Theanine crosses the blood-brain barrier and increases the production of both GABA and dopamine (Kakuda, 2011).

Melatonin is a natural neurochemical produced and released by the pineal gland in response to decreasing levels of daylight. Melatonin is a metabolite of serotonin and is associated with functioning of the clock gene; therefore, people who have low levels of serotonin will likely produce lower levels of melatonin and have sleep onset problems (Emet et al., 2016). Melatonin levels increase in the early to mid-part of the night and begin to decline about 3 to 4 hours before wakening. As a sleep aid, melatonin is available in immediate-release and extended release forms, as well as in combination with products that have other calming ingredients such as theanine, hops, chamomile, passionflower, valerian, and/or lavender (Benke et al., 2009; de Sousa, de Almeida Soares Hocayen, Andrade, & Andreatini, 2015; Schuwald et al., 2013). Therapeutic dose ranges from 0.3 mg to 5 mg. Melatonin is an antioxidant and does not work like benzodiazepine medications (alprazolam or zolpidem) and may take up to 2 weeks for effects to be noticeable (Massoumi, 2016).

N-Acetylcysteine (NAC) has been utilized in medical settings as a U.S. Food and Drug Administration approved emergency treatment of acetaminophen overdose to protect the liver (Johnson, McCammon, Mullins, & Halcomb, 2011) and as an inhaled mucolytic mist to reduce viscosity of secretions in the lungs of individuals with cystic fibrosis (Noone et al., 2001). The mechanism of action for NAC lies in its ability to modulate serotonin, glutamate, and dopamine (Dean, Giorlando, & Berk, 2011).

and metabolism of the B vitamins can result in mental retardation, psychiatric disorders, seizures, and myopathies, to name a few (Bourre, 2006). See Box 16.4 for Nutraceuticals used in mental health treatment and Table 16.7 for Research on Nutraceuticals used in this capacity as well.

PLANT-BASED MEDICINES

Adaptogens are neutraceutical herbals that increase our ability to adapt to stress associated with regulation of homeostasis via mechanisms to the hypothalamic-pituitary-adrenal axis (HPA) along with regulation of key mediators of the stress response, including cortisol, nitric oxide, neuropeptide Y, and others (Panossian & Wikman, 2010). The clinical result is increased energy or a feeling of psychological and physical well-being. Thus, adaptogens may help with fatigue or depression. They also appear to be neuroprotective. Clinical research supports the use of adaptogens to decrease akathisia and parkinsonian symptoms from antipsychotics (Massoumi, 2016; Muskin, Gerberg, & Brown, 2013). See Box 16.5 for adaptogens and their uses and Table 16.8 for plant-based adaptogen research.

TABLE 16.7 RESEARCH USING NUTRACEUTICALS FOR MENTAL HEALTH DISORDERS

Nutraceutical	Type of Study	Results	Reference
SAMe	Depression	Greater response rate compared to placebo; and comparable tolerability and efficacy to imipramine with fewer side effects	Bressa, 1994
SAMe	1,600 mg PO or 400 mg IM SAMe compared to 150 mg imipramine	Multicenter double-blinded trial showed SAMe was comparable to imipramine with fewer adverse effects on the HAM-D and CGI	Delle Chiaie, Pancheri, and Scapicchio, 2002
GABA, 300 mg daily	Prospective, randomized, double-blind, and placebo-controlled chronic insomnia	Test/retest using polysomnography showed GABA improved subjective and objective sleep without severe adverse events	Byun, Shin, Chung, and Shin, 2018
GABA	Effect on EEG wave patterns	Increased alpha waves (associated with relaxed alertness) and decreased beta waves (associated with high stress and difficulty concentrating)	Akhondzadeh, Gerbarg, and Brown, 2013
L-Theanine	Randomized double-blind placebo-controlled repeated measures trial of L-theanine (200 mg) compared to alprazolam 1 mg or placebo.	Neitherl L-theanine nor alprazolam had any significant anxiolytic effects during the experimentally induced anxiety state; however, the L-theanine group had greater relaxing effects under resting conditions	Lu et al., 2004
Melatonin	Numerous	Shown to be effective for insomnia, night terrors, and parasomnias; use a higher dose for parasomnias, up to 6 mg, with full effect taking 2–3 months	McGrane, Leung, St Louis, and Boeve, 2015

Nutraceutical	Type of Study	Results	Reference
N-acetylcysteine (NAC)	Anxiety disorders, specifically obsessive-compulsive disorder	Effective in double-blind randomized clinical trials	Costa et al., 2017; Sarris et al., 2015
NAC	Skin-picking and hair-pulling disorder, 1,200–3,000 mg in divided doses daily	Positive result in randomized, double-blind trial; positive case reports	Barroso, Sternberg, Souza, and Nunes, 2017; Grant et al., 2016
NAC	Cannabis cravings	Increased abstinence in a randomized controlled study among cannabis users	McClure et al., 2014
NAC	Review of the effects of NAC in psychiatry	NAC demonstrated significant effects for cocaine, cannabis, and smoking addictions, Alzheimer and Parkinson diseases, autism, compulsive and grooming disorders, schizophrenia, depression, and bipolar disorder	Berk, Malhi, Gray, & Dean, 2013
Omega-3 fatty acids	Review of use of omega-3 fatty acids in brain function	Omega-3 fatty acids, particularly DHA, may improve the hippocampal neurogenesis, and act similar to mood-stabilizing medications that exert inhibitory effects on neuronal signal transduction systems; large doses (9,600 mg) are associated with a general dampening of signal transduction pathways associated with phosphatidylinositol, arachidonic acid, and other systems	Massoumi, 2016; Mischoulon and Freeman; Perica, and Delas, 2011

CGI, Clinical Global Impression; DHA, docosahexaenoic acid; GABA, gamma-aminobutyric acid; HAM-D, Hamilton Rating Scale for Depression; IM, intramuscular; PO, oral (per os); SAMe, S-adenosylmethionine.

BOX 16.5 Adaptogens

Ashwagandha (*Withania somnifera***)** is an anti-inflammatory herbal used for anxiety, sleep, memory, cognitive function and subclinical hypothyroidism.

Rhodiola rosea is a botanical adaptogen with putative antistress and antidepressant properties (Mao et al., 2015) as well as improved libido (Fintelmann & Gruenwald, 2007). The mechanism for its effectiveness is thought to be related to its ability to increase norepinephrine and dopamine without increased anxiety or irritability (Olsson, von Scheele, & Panossian, 2009).

Valerian root activates glutamic acid decarboxylase, an enzyme involved in the synthesis of gamma-aminobutyric acid (GABA; Ortiz, Nieves-Natal, & Chavez, 1999). Valerian root components have been shown to both increase GABA synthesis and decrease synaptic GABA reuptake, and valerian acts as a GABA agonist by binding to GABA receptors in cell culture systems (Ortiz et al., 1999).

St. John's Wort (*Hypericum perforatum***)** is a flowering plant that has been found to be a weak inhibitor of monoamine oxidase A and B and a reuptake inhibitor at the synaptosomal receptors for serotonin, dopamine, and norepinephrine (Butterweck, 2003). It has been difficult to study owing to extreme variation in the amount of hypericin in different parts of the plant, under different growth conditions, and at different times of the year (Henderson, Yue, Bergquist, Gerden, & Arlett, 2002). Some in vitro binding assays carried out using St. John's wort demonstrated significant affinity for adenosine, GABA(A), GABA(B), and glutamate receptors (Butterweck, 2003). It is thought that hypericum may downregulate beta-adrenergic receptors and upregulate serotonin 5-HT(2) receptors in the frontal cortex, resulting in changes in neurotransmitter concentrations in brain areas implicated in depression (Butterweck, 2003).

Ginkgo biloba is a tree that yields a plant extract preparation that has been used for improvement in cognitive functioning and has been thought to prevent, or reduce, symptoms of dementia (H.-F. Zhang et al., 2016). The mechanisms of action for ginkgo is thought to include increasing cerebral blood flow, antioxidant and anti-inflammatory effects, with antiplatelet effects attributed to flavone and terpene lactones (Diamond & Bailey, 2013). Some authors have cautioned about potential interactions with monoamine oxidase inhibitors, alprazolam, haloperidol, warfarin, and nifedipine, which have been reported in the literature (Diamond & Bailey, 2013; Gauthier & Schlaefke, 2014; Hashiguchi, Ohta, Shimizu, Maruyama, & Mochizuki, 2015).

Kava is a South Pacific medicinal plant (*Piper methysticum*) that is a nonaddictive, nonhypnotic anxiolytic with the potential to treat anxiety disorders (Savage et al., 2015). The evidence for the efficacy of kava for treating anxiety is robust, based on randomized clinical trials and meta-analyses; however, it was banned in some countries as a supplement due to hepatotoxicity (Savage et al., 2015). Evaluation of the cause of the liver damage was found to be related to a solvent used to prepare the herbal supplement rather than the kava itself (Teschke, Sarris, & Lebot, 2011, 2013).

Cannabidiol, often referred to as CBD oil, is the nonpsychoactive constituent ingredient in *Cannabis sativa*. The psychoactive component in *Cannabis sativa* is Δ9-tetrahydrocannabinol (THC). Reported neurological uses of CBD include adjunctive treatment for malignant brain tumors, Parkinson disease, Alzheimer disease, multiple sclerosis, neuropathic pain (Devinsky, Whalley, & Di Marzo, 2015), and the childhood seizure disorders Lennox-Gastaut and Dravet syndromes, for which Epidiolex (a brand of CBD oil) has been approved by the U.S. Food and Drug Administration (Devinsky et al., 2015; Maroon & Bost, 2018). Uses in psychiatric and mood disorders include schizophrenia, anxiety, depression, addiction, postconcussion syndrome, and posttraumatic stress disorders (Maroon & Bost, 2018). Caution should be exercised in prescribing CBD for treatment of any condition due to extreme variability in constituent ingredients, contaminants, and quality control. There are currently an estimated 850 brands of marijuana-derived CBD products and 150 hemp-derived products in the marketplace, making universal dosing recommendations nearly impossible (Maroon & Bost, 2018).

TABLE 16.8 PLANT-BASED ADAPTOGEN RESEARCH

Plant-Based Adaptogen	Type of Study	Results	Reference
Ashwagandha	Randomized clinical trials of anxiety disorder compared to placebo or psychotherapy	Reduced anxiety without tolerance or withdrawal associated with benzodiazepines; comparable results compared to psychotherapy alone	Alramadhan et al., 2012
Ashwaganda	Prospective, randomized, double-blind, placebo-controlled study was conducted in 50 adults (300 mg twice daily) for mood, memory, and cognition	Significant improvement in both immediate and general memory in people with MCI as well as improving executive function, attention, and information processing speed	Choudhary, Bhattacharyya, and Bose, 2017
Ashwaganda	Systematic review of randomized clinical trials	Significant improvement on both anxiety and stress scales	Pratte, Nanavati, Young, and Morley, 2014
Rhodiola	12-week randomized clinical trials for depression, dosing 500 mg to 1,500 mg daily in divided doses	Improvements in symptoms comparable to sertralineand much fewer side effects	Darbinyan et al., 2007; Mao, Li, Soeller, Xie, and Amsterdam, 2014; Mao et al., 2015
Rhodiola	Randomized, double-blind, placebo-controlled study with parallel groups	Significant antifatigue effect with increased mental performance, concentration, with decreased cortisol response to awakening stress in burnout patients with fatigue syndrome	Olsson, von Scheele, and Panossian, 2009
Rhodiola	Open trial, drug monitoring study of effect on exhaustion, decreased motivation, daytime sleepiness, decreased libido, sleep disturbances, and cognitive complaints	Improvement on both physical and cognitive measures	Fintelmann and Gruenwald, 2007

(continued)

TABLE 16.8   PLANT-BASED ADAPTOGEN RESEARCH *(CONTINUED)*

Plant-Based Adaptogen	Type of Study	Results	Reference
Valerian	Pilot study of valerian 400–900 mg daily for anxiety compared to diazepam	As effective as diazepam in reducing anxiety	Andreatini, Sartori, Seabra, and Leite, 2002
Valerian	Systematic review of efficacy for insomnia	Valerian might improve sleep quality without producing side effects	Bent, Padula, Moore, Patterson, and Mehling, 2006
Hypericum (St. John's Wort)	125–900 mg concentrated extract daily for symptoms of mild to moderate major depression.	More effective than placebo, possibly as effective as standard prescription antidepressants with fewer side effects	Linde, Berner, and Kriston, 2008
Hypericum	Evaluation of potential significant interactions with 125 mg and 900 mg of standardized extract of at least 0.3% hypericin and/or 1% to 3% hyperforin	Clinically significant interactions with medicines such as warfarin, phenprocoumon, cyclosporin, HIV protease inhibitors, theophylline, digoxin, and oral contraceptives resulting in a decrease in concentration or effect of the medicines Interactions may be due to the induction of cytochrome P450 isoenzymes CYP3A4, CYP2C9, CYP1A2 and the transport protein P-glycoprotein by constituent(s) in hypericum preparations	Henderson, Yue, Bergquist, Gerden, and Arlett, 2002
Ginkgo	Systematic reviews for improvement of mild cognitive impairment, dementia	Dose-dependent improvement in symptoms only with high daily dose (240 mg); dosages for most clinical trials ranged from 80 to 720 mg daily for 2 weeks to 2 years	Hashiguchi, Ohta, Shimizu, Maruyama, and Mochizuki, 2015; H.-F. Zhang et al., 2016

Ginkgo	Double-blind placebo-controlled trial for dyskinesias	Majority of patients had improvement on AIMS scores greater than 30% compared to placebo over 12 weeks; long-term benefits were also uncovered with G. *biloba* treatment, with no deterioration of the AIMS scores 12 weeks from the end of treatment	W.-F. Zhang et al., 2011
Kava	Multisite two-arm double-blind placebo-controlled clinical trial in Australia	Superior to placebo in the treatment of GAD, and was also shown to be safe, and recommended kava as a first-line treatment	Savage et al., 2015
Cannabidiol	Preliminary open-label trial 100 to 600 mg/day over a 6-week period with treatment as usual for dyskinesia	Dose-related improvement in dystonia and ranged from 20% to 50%; side effects were mild and included hypotension, dry mouth, psychomotor slowing, lightheadedness, and sedation In two patients with coexisting parkinsonian features, doses over 300 mg/day exacerbated the hypokinesia and resting tremor	Consroe, Sandyk, and Snider, 1986

Omega-3 fatty acids provide numerous health benefits to all organisms. Alterations outside of the body's normal concentration has been shown to improve a variety of psychiatric symptoms and disorders, including stress, anxiety, cognitive impairment, mood disorders, and schizophrenia (Perica & Delas, 2011). The use of omega-3 fatty acids in psychiatric treatment is proving to be effective for prevention and treatment of major depressive disorders, attention deficit hyperactivity disorder (ADHD), and other psychiatric disorders as an adjunctive treatment, or a standalone treatment for mild symptoms (Lakhan & Vieira, 2008; Massoumi, 2016; Mischoulon & Freeman, 2013; Perica & Delas, 2011; Wani, Bhat, & Ara, 2015). Dosing ranges for omega-3 supplementation is based on severity of symptoms; however, a general dose range is 1,200 mg two to four times daily with food (Massoumi, 2016).

PROBIOTICS

The interest in probiotic use in psychiatry highlights increasing interest in the gut-brain connection, specifically related to microbiota within the gut (L. Liu & Zhu, 2018). Studies have shown that imbalances in the gut microbiome can greatly influence many physiological parameters, including cognitive functions, such as learning, memory and decision-making processes (Montiel-Castro, Gonzalez-Cervantes, Bravo-Ruiseco, & Pacheco-Lopez, 2013). The gut microbiome is the body's largest immune system organ composed of over 100 trillion bacteria that protect the host against pathogens and act to metabolize complex lipids and polysaccharides that otherwise would be inaccessible nutrients (Montiel-Castro et al., 2013). The microbiota have been shown to secrete neurotransmitters; for example, *Lactobacillus* subspecies can secrete acetylcholine (regulating memory, attention, learning, and mood); *Candida, Streptococcus, Escherichia coli,* and *Enterococcus* can secrete serotonin; and *Bacillus* and *Serratia* can secrete dopamine (Vitetta, Bambling, & Alford, 2014). *Lactobacillus acidophilus, Bifidobacterium infantis, Candida, and Streptococcus* are associated with therapeutic effects on mental health symptoms related to their secretion of GABA, serotonin, glycine, and some catecholamines (Vitetta et al., 2014).

Neuroactive molecules secreted by intestinal microbiota are associated with nerve signaling that affects neuropsychiatric parameters such as sleep, appetite, mood, and cognition (Kali, 2016). There is evidence of a bidirectional signaling system between the GI tract and the brain, mainly through the vagus nerve (microbiota-gut-vagus-brain axis), that is an important system for maintaining homeostasis in addition to aiding in metabolic and mental function (Montiel-Castro et al., 2013). Studies have shown that the intestinal microbiota is associated with the neuroendocrine-immune pathways associated with various mood disorders (L. Liu & Zhu, 2018). Two randomized controlled trials showed improvement of autism spectrum disorder (ASD) behaviors, and three open trials exhibited a trend of improvement (J. Liu et al., 2019). See Table 16.9 for online resources for supplements.

MIND-BODY PRACTICES

Yoga, Qigong, Tai Chi, Meditation

A systematic review of the health outcomes of practicing yoga, tai chi, or qigong showed benefits on bone density, cardiopulmonary effects, physical function, reduced falls, improved overall quality of life measures, self-efficacy, psychological symptoms, and immune function (Jahnke, Larkey, Rogers, Etnier, & Lin, 2010). Tai chi and qigong practiced regularly for wellness and disease prevention resulted in improved energy, immune function, athletic performance, and memory/concentration abilities (Lauche, Wayne, Dobos, & Cramer, 2016).

TABLE 16.9 ONLINE RESOURCES FOR SUPPLEMENTS	
Examine.com	Based in Canada this group of multidisciplinary practitioners evaluates and synthesizes published research on supplements. The site provides a concise table called the "Human Effect Matrix" that outlines each supplement. They provide unbiased information about the quality of the evidence with effect sizes. The table is searchable and will bring up a "pop-up" when clicking within the table with links to PubMed and additional information.
Consumerlab.com	Independent testing lab that evaluates chemical content of many supplements and compares labeling to what is actually in the supplement, including contaminants. Human and animal products are tested. Excellent information about the research behind use of different supplement products is also available. Requires a subscription annually (approximately US$45).

A Cochrane collaboration review of different types of meditation therapy for anxiety disorders found very few studies that were robust enough to form conclusions on efficacy (Krisanaprakornkit, Sriraj, Piyavhatkul, & Laopaiboon, 2006). Only two studies met the criteria for review out of 50 clinical trials, and they included active control comparisons (alternative meditation, biofeedback, or relaxation; Krisanaprakornkit et al., 2006). One of these studies, which used transcendental meditation, showed a reduction in anxiety and electromyography score comparable with biofeedback and relaxation therapy (Raskin, Bali, & Peeke, 1980). The second study compared Kundalini yoga with relaxation/mindfulness meditation and concluded that there was no significant difference between groups (Krisanaprakornkit et al., 2006). A more recent pilot study of yoga-enhanced cognitive behavioral therapy (Y-CBT) showed promising results compared to treatment as usual. After the Y-CBT intervention, pre- and post-comparisons showed statistically significant improvements in state and trait anxiety, depression, panic, sleep, and quality of life (Khalsa, Greiner-Ferris, Hofmann, & Khalsa,2015). Another systematic literature review and meta-analysis of the effects of yoga on positive mental health found weak evidence that yoga improves positive mental health (Hendriks, de Jong, & Cramer, 2017). While the authors concluded that yoga contributed to a significant increase in psychological well-being when compared to no intervention, it did not improve well-being when compared to physical activity (Hendriks et al., 2017). On measures of life satisfaction (emotional well-being), social relationships (social well-being), and mindfulness, there were no significant effects for yoga found over active or nonactive control subjects (Hendriks et al., 2017). The authors reported that the lack of evidence supporting improvement with yoga was likely due to an extremely limited number of available studies that were designed in a way to draw clear conclusions on outcomes.

PUTTING IT TOGETHER: CASE EXAMPLE

Katie, a 37-year-old married woman, was referred by her therapist for evaluation of severe sadness and hopelessness for 3 years. She reported feeling general malaise, fatigue, depression with sadness, tearfulness, hopelessness, despondency, and insomnia with night sweats and nightmares. She stated that she is unable to walk for more than a few minutes at a time owing to severe fatigue. She reported that her fatigue is so severe that she is "unable to make a milkshake without having to sit down and recuperate for a few minutes." Katie reported that her symptoms began shortly after suffering from a respiratory infection that turned into pneumonia. She was hospitalized and underwent a minor procedure requiring insertion of a chest tube; she reported that the "chest tube became infected" and she developed "fungal empyema" in her lungs. According to a review, the diagnosis of *fungal empyema thoracis* is made when there is "(1) observation of a fungal species from thoracentesis fluid belonging to exudates category, (2) signs of infection including fever or leukocytosis and (3) isolation of the same fungus identified in the pleural fluid in other specimens, such as blood, sputum or surgical wounds with evidence of tissue invasion" (Baradkar, Mathur, Kulkarni, & Kumar, 2008, p. 286). Records were requested from the hospital, confirming her report that during a thoracotomy, the physician noted that her lung as "full of pus," which was cultured and found positive for candidiasis.

Following the thoracotomy and hospitalization, she was "bed bound" for 9 months, and then underwent months of rehabilitation; however, she reports that she has never recovered completely. She further reported that during her hospitalization she lost "most of her blood supply" and due to her religious beliefs, she could not receive a blood transfusion. She remembered that her medical team was "extremely angry with her" for refusing the blood transfusion, but she did not agree with them, was not transfused, and was treated with replacement fluids intravenously.

Katie indicated that she lost approximately 80 lb as a result of general loss of appetite and gastroparesis secondary to an injury to her stomach wall during insertion of a chest tube. Gastroparesis is the inability of the stomach to contract and expand normally, resulting in decreased motility and decreased ability to process foods normally (Bharucha, 2015). It is a chronic disorder characterized by impaired gastric emptying and altered motility in the upper GI tract in the absence of mechanical obstruction. Gastroparesis can interfere with normal digestion, cause nausea and vomiting, and cause problems with blood sugar levels and nutrition (Bharucha, 2015). The most common symptoms are early satiation, nausea, emesis, bloating, abdominal pain, heartburn, anorexia, and weight loss (Stevens, Jones, Rayner, & Horowitz, 2013). Katie described vomiting if she eats more than a few tablespoons of preprocessed foods, usually baby food consistency. She craves sugar and carbohydrates and given her weight loss, hunger, and inability to retain foods, she frequently eats milkshakes, ice cream, yogurts, and prepared nutrition drinks. Despite the gastroparesis, she says she is back to her preillness weight and her body mass index (BMI) is 39, which means she (a) is underestimating what she eats or (b) was extremely morbidly obese prior to her illness. Her hospital records indicate that she was slightly more obese prior to becoming ill, with an estimated BMI of 40.5.

At her initial appointment, her medications included mirtazapine 30 mg nightly, prazosin 1 mg for nightmares, and fentanyl patches for pain. She was previously prescribed metoclopramide but developed an allergy to it. Metoclopramide is the only FDA-approved treatment for gastroparesis in diabetics (Stevens et al., 2013). The effect of metoclopramide is enhancement of gastric motility through dopamine-2 (D2) receptor antagonism, stimulation of the serotonin-4 (5-HT4) receptors, and antagonism of the muscarinic receptors. The combination promotes gastric emptying, has antiemetic effects via central pathways, normalizes gastric slow wave dysrhythmias, and modulates visceral hypersensitivity (Stevens et al., 2013).

Following her surgery and subsequent fungal infection of her lungs, and entire body, she developed medication allergies to metoclopramide, sulfa antibiotics, betadine, fluconazole, penicillin, paroxetine, gabapentin, and others she cannot remember. At her first appointment, she was experiencing severe muscle pain and weakness with a low-grade fever ranging from 99.2° to 99.6°F, constant headaches, joint pain, and moderate depression. In addition, she was diagnosed with fibromyalgia approximately a year earlier and is not able to take the usual treatments for the pain due to the development of allergic reactions to the medications.

Her evaluation began with an assessment for myalgic encephalomyelitis/chronic fatigue syndrome (ME/CFS) and chronic systemic *Candida* infection. Katie met 9 of 11 criteria and two of three signs for ME/CFS according to the CDC screening guidelines (Ungeret al., 2016). She does not experience pharyngitis, but has tender lymph nodes to palpation. According to the literature, fungal elements may not always be visible in tissue samples and mycological cultures are frequently negative, making the evidence for proven fungal disease difficult (Fleischhacker et al., 2012). In severely ill patients, *Candida* species, particularly *Candida albicans*, can cause life-threatening systemic infections that are difficult to diagnose and have symptoms similar to those of systemic bacterial infections. These difficulties can lead to delays in initiation in antifungal therapy, which contributes to the high mortality rates (>40%) associated with these infections (Szabo & MacCallum, 2011).

Owing to the complexity of Katie's presentation, a consultation was sought from an integrative medicine (IM) medical practitioner for direction and eventual referral of care. The waiting time for an appointment to IM ranges from 6 to 12 months; therefore, it was imperative to begin treatment as soon as possible. Routine lab tests were ordered according to the protocols discussed previously in this chapter with additional labs at the direction of the IM specialist who was concerned that there could be an additional adrenal fatigue syndrome in addition to the ME/CFS and chronic candidiasis diagnosis. Adrenal fatigue is a disruption of the HPA axis due to chronic stress hormone elevations that eventually fail, resulting in a deficiency of catecholamine production (Lumpkin, 2005/2010). The usual tests for adrenal fatigue were added, including adrenocorticotropic hormone (ACTH) stimulation tests and sequential salivary cortisol levels.

Katie's treatment plan was based on an adaptation to the "4R" program for a patient with GI complaints. The first R is "remove" the offending agent; which was the *Candida*. The second R is "replace" general gut health support including digestive enzymes, glutamine, potassium, zinc, and magnesium. The third R is "reinoculate," referring to dysbiosis of her gut and the need for probiotics, and the fourth R is "repair" the mucosal layer with healthy, viscous, fermentable fiber as well as the glutamine, potassium, zinc, and magnesium already listed (Lukaczer, 2005/2010). An added fifth R was "reprocessing" her traumatic experience in the hospital with trauma-focused cognitive behavior therapy (TF-CBT). With TF-CBT, it is critical to discuss and address her anxiety about her experience in order to help her integrate her "now" reactions into healthier responses. As a result of this work, her views of the traumatic experience in the hospital became a growth experience and she was able to be assertive in getting her needs met in her treatment.

Treatment for systemic *Candida* infection included the following:

1. No sugar including fruits, juices, etc.
2. No yeast products including nuts, breads, cheeses, fermented alcohols, etc.
3. Elimination of milk and other dairy products
4. Begin a daily high-potency bioavailable multivitamin that is bariatric friendly to increase absorption through her damaged GI tract. The vitamin included an antioxidant blend (to replace fruits and juices).
5. Because of her allergy to pharmaceutical antifungals, Katie was begun on a combination treatment that included herbal antifungals (oregano volatile oil and *Melaleuca alternifolia*; Bhat et al., 2018; Rohilla, Bhatt, & Gupta, 2018).

6. A pharmaceutical grade broad-spectrum probiotic was added to be taken daily that included various strains of *Bifidobacterium, Lactobacillus,* and *Saccharomyces boulardii* (to begin recolonizing her gut with healthy flora).

7. Katie also increased her dietary fiber choice to increase volume, and viscosity of food, increase the sensation of satiety, and delay gastric emptying, which is intended to result in fewer calories being consumed. The fiber supplement must be the type to form a viscous gel matrix, which is correlated with reduced postprandial glycemic responses, decreased serum cholesterol levels, and weight loss. Fiber is also thought to contribute to the protection of the gut mucosa and goblet cell health. A fermentable prebiotic polyglycoplex (PGX) includes all of these features and can be added as a powder to smoothies that are dairy and sugar free. PGX fibers also help with waste elimination, increase production of short-chain fatty acids, support enterocytes, and promote probiotic growth.

8. A glutamine supplement and green tea daily were suggested to increase GABA synthesis.

9. She began a program of replacing digestive enzymes with each meal to both correct digestive issues and to mediate food allergies by more fully digesting proteins.

10. After her blood tests confirmed that she had low-normal potassium and magnesium levels, she began a magnesium, zinc, and potassium supplement of 200 mg twice a day.

Katie was continued on mirtazapine, which is one of the only antidepressants she did not develop an allergic reaction to; however, she was changed to the oral disintegrating tablet to improve absorption. Mirtazapine is a strong antagonist of 5-HT2 and 5-HT3 receptors, with weak 5-HT1A and 5-HT1B receptors (Malamood, Roberts, Kataria, Parkman, & Schey, 2017). 5-HT3 antagonist can be given to treat nausea without blocking peristalsis and prevents activation of the 5-HT visceral afferent nerves in the gut (Malamood et al., 2017).

Katie's treatment included psychotherapeutic interventions using a CBT approach that integrated medication management as a component of her sessions. She was seen weekly for eight appointments due to the complexity of her situation, and biweekly for 12 sessions. Her symptoms started to abate beginning with the eighth week of treatment and were largely eliminated about a year later. She was able to return to work part-time, although she was cautioned to remain on her treatment protocol for at least an additional year to continue to provide neurobiological support to her exhausted system. This was an extremely complex and difficult case; however, the key to her treatment was a full assessment that integrated modern medical science, psychological treatment, and CAM science-based treatments that offered alternative options for her medical problems.

POST-MASTERS TRAINING IN INTEGRATIVE MEDICINE

According to the National Centers for Complimentary and Integrative Healthcare, complementary and integrative health approaches include a wide variety of modalities and specializations, and therefore training strategies include innovative approaches that incorporate an understanding of this diversity to ensure that future workforce needs are met. In particular, NCCIH focuses on three main areas:

1. Clinician-scientists, including conventionally trained physicians, complementary health practitioners, and other healthcare professionals (e.g., clinical psychologists,

nurses) who conduct research across a wide range of complementary and integrative health approaches.
2. Scientists trained in key biomedical and behavioral research disciplines necessary for rigorous, state-of-the-art scientific investigation of complementary and integrative health interventions, practices, and disciplines.
3. Individuals from groups who are underrepresented in scientific research (e.g., racial and ethnic minority populations) and are interested in careers in complementary and integrative health research (NIH, 2018).

There are a variety of ways to become trained and certified in integrative healthcare. My training program was a Doctor of Science in Integrative Healthcare through Huntington University of Health Sciences in Knoxville, TN (www.HUHS.edu). Huntington offered an intensive program of study in nutrition, genetics, microbiology, and biochemistry that was outstanding and immediately applicable to practice. To obtain certification after completion of the D.Sc. program, graduates meet the core education requirements for the Certified Clinical Nutritionist exam through the Clinical Nutrition Certification Board (CNCB; see www.cncb.org for eligibility requirements).

The American Nurses Credentialing Center (ANCC) does not offer certification in integrative healthcare at the time of this publication. Many APRNs are being trained in integrative healthcare by their place of employment. One should note that integrative healthcare is already within the scope of the APPN given that the scope of practice includes complementary and alternative options such as nutrition, mindfulness, psychotherapy, pharmacotherapy, and other options. Integrative services are increasingly being provided within hospitals and/or outpatient integrative care settings. In many cases, the individual healthcare organizations are developing and standardizing their procedures for deciding which practitioners are qualified to practice integrative healthcare. Requirements vary across organizations and may include establishing competency (such as proof of training), licensure or certification, background checks, continuing education hours, proof of malpractice insurance coverage, and experience working in the field or specifically in a hospital or research setting (NIH, 2018). Table 16.10 includes a listing of agencies that offer training and/or certifications in integrative healthcare. *Note: The author is not responsible for the content or authenticity of any of the following programs as learners are charged with evaluating each resource for their own learning needs.*

CONCLUDING COMMENTS

Complementary and integrative healthcare is rapidly becoming the norm rather than the exception. Practitioners utilize the science of modern medicine, in addition to knowledge of how the body functions as an integrated, connected system, rather than traditional single focused approaches (Jones et al., 2005/2010). The body is not a set of individual organs that function independently. Each system depends on other systems for full, effective, and healthy functioning. It is extremely important to utilize a holistic approach that examines how nutrition, activity (exercise), immune responses, GI health and function, structural components, energy production, waste removal, hormone and neurotransmitter function, and emotions all work together to maintain a healthy body.

Functional practitioners know that the body is an interconnected dynamic system with individual biovariability. In other words, instead of simply treating a disorder, the functional practitioner seeks to determine *why* the person developed that disorder or symptom in the first place, and then seeks to repair the causative issue to restore the system to balance. An adequate supply of nutrients is critical for healthy brain function

TABLE 16.10 RESOURCES FOR TRAINING AND CERTIFICATION IN INTEGRATIVE HEALTHCARE

Agency	Type of Program	Contact Information
Academy of Integrative Health and Medicine	Fellowship in Integrative Medicine	www.aihm.org/page/fellowship
College of Integrative Medicine	CIHP (Certified Integrative Healthcare Practitioner) Certification Program	www.collegeofintegrativemedicine.org/about-us
Duke University Integrative Medicine	Integrative Health Coach Professional Training Certification	dukeintegrativemedicine.org/integrative-health-coach-training/about-the-certification-course
George Washington University	Master of Science in Health Science in Integrative Medicine	healthsciencesprograms.gwu.edu/program
Huntington University of Health Sciences	Doctor of Science in Integrative Healthcare	www.huhs.edu
Maryland University of Integrative Health	Post-Masters certificate in Nutrition and Integrative Health	www.muih.edu/academics/academic-certificates/post-masters-certificate-nutrition-integrative-health
The University of Kansas	Dietetics and Integrative Medicine Graduate Certificate	www.kumc.edu/school-of-health-professions.html
University of Massachusetts School of Nursing	Graduate Certificate in Complementary and Integrative Modalities (CIM)	www.umass.edu/nursing/academic-programs/graduate-certificate-complementary-and-integrative-modalities-cim
University of Minnesota School of Nursing	The Integrative Health and Healing specialty of the Doctor of Nursing Practice	www.nursing.umn.edu/degrees-programs/doctor-nursing-practice/post-baccalaureate/integrative-health-and-healing
University of Vermont	Certificate Program in Integrative Healthcare	learn.uvm.edu/program/integrative-healthcare-certificate

and that depends on a fully functioning GI system. Psychiatric practitioners are uniquely positioned to use psychotherapeutic skills to understand, utilize, and communicate about full body health and nutrition as part of their scope of practice to help their patients achieve optimal functioning.

DISCUSSION QUESTIONS

1. Compare and contrast the following healthcare models: integrative, complementary, modern mainstream, alternative, functional.
2. What nutrients are associated with healthy brain function and neurotransmitter synthesis?
3. What are some of the ethical responsibilities of a clinician when ordering and interpreting genetic testing?
4. How does the GI system affect the brain?
5. Your patient tells you he ordered several supplements online because his aunt does a lot of health research and said he should take these things for his depression. How do you approach this with your patient? How do you determine if the patient is ingesting safe supplements?
6. Which of your psychotherapeutic tools integrate best with nutrition education, evaluation, and treatment?

REFERENCES

Adisetiyo, V., & Helpern, J. A. (2015). Brain iron: A promising noninvasive biomarker of attention-deficit/hyperactivity disorder that warrants further investigation. *Biomarkers in Medicine*, 9(5), 403–406. doi:10.2217/bmm.15.9

Akhondzadeh, S., Gerbarg, P. L., & Brown, R. P. (2013). Nutrients for prevention and treatment of mental health disorders. *Psychiatric Clinics of North America*, 36(1), 25–36. doi:10.1016/j.psc.2012.12.003

Al Alawi, A. M., Majoni, S. W., & Falhammar, H. (2018). Magnesium and human health: Perspectives and research directions. *International Journal of Endocrinology*. 2018, 9041694. doi:10.1155/2018/9041694

Alberts, B., Johnson, A., Lewis, J., Morgan, D., Raff, M., Roberts, K., & Walter, P. (2015). *Molecular biology of the cell* (6th ed.8).
New York, NY: Garland Science/Taylor & Francis.

Aleksandrova, K., Romero-Mosquera, B., & Hernandez, V. (2017). Diet, gut microbiome and epigenetics: Emerging links with inflammatory bowel diseases and prospects for management and prevention. *Nutrients*, 9(9), 962. doi:10.3390/nu9090962

Allen, R. H., Stabler, S. P., Savage, D. G., & Lindenbaum, J. (1993). Metabolic abnormalities in cobalamin (vitamin B12) and folate deficiency. *The FASEB Journal*, 7(14), 1344–1353. doi:10.1096/fasebj.7.14.7901104

Alramadhan, E., Hanna, M. S., Hanna, M. S., Goldstein, T. A., Avila, S. M., & Weeks, B. S. (2012). Dietary and botanical anxiolytics. *Medical Science Monitor: International Medical Journal of Experimental and Clinical Research*, 18(4), RA40–RA48. doi:10.12659/MSM.882608

American Psychiatric Association. (2016). *The American Psychiatric Association practice guidelines for the psychiatric evaluation of adults* (3rd ed.). Arlington, VA: American Psychiatric Publishing. Retrieved from https://www.appi.org/Products/APA-Practice-Guidelines/American-Psychiatric-Association-Practice-Guid-(4)

Ames, B. N. (1999). Micronutrient deficiencies. A major cause of DNA damage. *Annals of the New York Academy of Sciences*, 889, 87–106. doi:10.1111/j.1749-6632.1999.tb08727.x

Ames, B. N., Elson-Schwab, I., & Silver, E. A. (2002). High-dose vitamin therapy stimulates variant enzymes with decreased coenzyme binding affinity (increased K(m)): Relevance to genetic disease and polymorphisms. *The American Journal of Clinical Nutrition, 75*(4), 616–658. doi:10.1093/ajcn/75.4.616

Andreatini, R., Sartori, V. A., Seabra, M. L., & Leite, J. R. (2002). Effect of valepotriates (valerian extract) in generalized anxiety disorder: A randomized placebo-controlled pilot study. *Phytotherapy Research, 16*(7), 650–654. doi:10.1002/ptr.1027

Ansari, R., Mahta, A., Mallack, E., & Luo, J. J. (2014). Hyperhomocysteinemia and neurologic disorders: A review. *Journal of Clinical Neurology, 10*(4), 281–288. doi:10.3988/jcn.2014.10.4.281

Arrieta, M. C., Bistritz, L., & Meddings, J. B. (2006). Alterations in intestinal permeability. *Gut, 55*(10), 1512–1520. doi:10.1136/gut.2005.085373

Baradkar, V. P., Mathur, M., Kulkarni, S. D., & Kumar, S. (2008). Thoracic empyema due to *Candida albicans*. *Indian Journal of Pathology & Microbiology, 51*(2), 286–288. doi:10.4103/0377-4929.41699

Barnett, M., Bassett, S., & Bermingham, E. (2014). Epigenetics—What role could this play in functional foods and personalized nutrition? In L. R. Ferguson (Ed.), *Nutrigenomics and nutrigenetics in functional foods and personalized nutrition* (pp. 243–260). Boca Raton, FL: Taylor & Francis.

Barroso, L. A. L., Sternberg, F., Souza, M., & Nunes, G. J. B. (2017). Trichotillomania: A good response to treatment with N-acetylcysteine. *Anais Brasileiros de Dermatologia, 92*(4), 537–539. doi:10.1590/abd1806-4841.20175435

Bender, D. M. P. A. (2012). The citric acid cycle: The catabolism of acetyl-CoA. In B. D. R. K. Murray, P. J. Kennelly, V. W. Rodwell, & P. A. Weil (Eds.), *Harper's illustrated biochemistry* (pp. 163–169). Philadelphia, PA: McGraw-Hill.

Benke, D., Barberis, A., Kopp, S., Altmann, K. H., Schubiger, M., Vogt, K. E., . . . Mohler, H. (2009). GABA A receptors as in vivo substrate for the anxiolytic action of valerenic acid, a major constituent of valerian root extracts. *Neuropharmacology, 56*(1), 174–181. doi:10.1016/j.neuropharm.2008.06.013

Bent, S., Padula, A., Moore, D., Patterson, M., & Mehling, W. (2006). Valerian for sleep: A systematic review and meta-analysis. *The American Journal of Medicine, 119*(12), 1005–1012. doi:10.1016/j.amjmed.2006.02.026

Berk, M., Malhi, G. S., Gray, L. J., & Dean, O. M. (2013). The promise of N-acetylcysteine in neuropsychiatry. *Trends in Pharmacological Sciences, 34*(3), 167–177. doi:10.1016/j.tips.2013.01.001

Bharucha, A. E. (2015). Epidemiology and natural history of gastroparesis. *Gastroenterology Clinics of North America, 44*(1), 9–19. doi:10.1016/j.gtc.2014.11.002

Bhat, V., Sharma, S. M., Shetty, V., Shastry, C. S., Rao, C. V., Shenoy, S., . . . Balaji, S. (2018). Characterization of herbal antifungal agent, *Origanum vulgare* against oral *Candida* spp. isolated from patients with *Candida*-associated denture stomatitis: An in vitro study. *Contemporary Clinical Dentistry, 9*(Suppl. 1), S3–S10. doi:10.4103/ccd.ccd_537_17

Boonstra, E., de Kleijn, R., Colzato, L. S., Alkemade, A., Forstmann, B. U., & Nieuwenhuis, S. (2015). Neurotransmitters as food supplements: The effects of GABA on brain and behavior. *Frontiers in Psychology, 6*, 1520. doi:10.3389/fpsyg.2015.01520

Bottiglieri, T. (2013). Folate, vitamin B12, and S-adenosylmethionine. *Psychiatric Clinics of North America, 36*(1), 1–13. doi:10.1016/j.psc.2012.12.001

Bourre, J. M. (2006). Effects of nutrients (in food) on the structure and function of the nervous system: Update on dietary requirements for brain. Part 1: Micronutrients. *The Journal of Nutrition, Health and Aging, 10*(5), 377–385.

Bressa, G. M. (1994). S-adenosyl-l-methionine (SAMe) as antidepressant: Meta-analysis of clinical studies. *Acta Neurologica Scandinavica Supplementum, 154*, 7–14. doi:10.1111/j.1600-0404.1994.tb05403.x

Brooks, M. J., & Post, E. M. (2014). Acquired hypothyroidism due to iodine deficiency in an American child. *Journal of Pediatric Endocrinology and Metabolism, 27*(11–12), 1233–1235. doi:10.1515/jpem-2014-0226

Butterweck, V. (2003). Mechanism of action of St John's wort in depression: What is known? *CNS Drugs, 17*, 539–562. doi:10.2165/00023210-200317080-00001

Byun, J.-I., Shin, Y. Y., Chung, S.-E., & Shin, W. C. (2018). Safety and efficacy of gamma-aminobutyric acid from fermented rice germ in patients with insomnia symptoms: A randomized, double-blind trial. *Journal of Clinical Neurology (Seoul, Korea), 14*(3), 291–295. doi:10.3988/jcn.2018.14.3.291

Centers for Disease Control and Prevention, Office of Genomics and Precision Public Health. (2010). *Genomics competencies*. Atlanta, GA: Author. Retrieved from https://www.cdc.gov/genomics/translation/competencies/index.htm

Chatterjea, M. N., & Shinde, R. (2012). Chemistry of nucleic acids, DNA replication and DNA repair. In
M. N. Chatterjea & R. Shinde (Eds.), *Textbook of medical biochemistry* (8th ed., pp. 239–258). London, UK: Jaypee Brothers Medical Publishers.

Choi, S. W., & Friso, S. (2010). Epigenetics: A new bridge between nutrition and health. *Advances in Nutrition, 1*(1), 8–16. doi:10.3945/an.110.1004

Choudhary, D., Bhattacharyya, S., & Bose, S. (2017). Efficacy and safety of ashwagandha (Withania somnifera (L.) dunal) root extract in improving memory and cognitive functions. *Journal of Dietary Supplements, 14*(6), 599–612. doi:10.1080/19390211.2017.1284970

Clancy, S. (2008). Genetic mutation. *Nature Education, 1*(1), 187. Retrieved from https://www.nature.com/scitable/topicpage/genetic-mutation-441

Clevenger, S. F. (2018). Knowledge and attitudes towards utilizing complementary and alternative medical (CAM) treatments by mental health practitioner from various disciplines. *Journal of Traditional and Complementary Medicine*. Advance online publication. doi:10.1016/j.jtcme.2017.08.015

Consroe, P., Sandyk, R., & Snider, S. R. (1986). Open label evaluation of cannabidiol in dystonic movement disorders. *The International Journal of Neuroscience, 30*(4), 277–282. doi:10.3109/00207458608985678

Costa, D. L. C., Diniz, J. B., Requena, G., Joaquim, M. A., Pittenger, C., Bloch, M. H., . . . Shavitt, R. G. (2017). Randomized, double-blind, placebo-controlled trial of N-acetylcysteine augmentation for treatment-resistant obsessive-compulsive disorder. *The Journal of Clinical Psychiatry, 78*(7), e766–e773. doi:10.4088/JCP.16m11101

Darbinyan, V., Aslanyan, G., Amroyan, E., Gabrielyan, E., Malmstrom, C., & Panossian, A. (2007). Clinical trial of Rhodiola rosea L. extract SHR-5 in the treatment of mild to moderate depression. *Nordic Journal of Psychiatry, 61*(5), 343–348. doi:10.1080/08039480701643290

Davison, K. M., & Kaplan, B. J. (2012). Nutrient intakes are correlated with overall psychiatric functioning in adults with mood disorders. *The Canadian Journal of Psychiatry, 57*(2), 85–92. doi:10.1177/070674371205700205

Dean, O., Giorlando, F., & Berk, M. (2011). N-acetylcysteine in psychiatry: Current therapeutic evidence and potential mechanisms of action. *Journal of Psychiatry & Neuroscience: JPN, 36*(2), 78–86. doi:10.1503/jpn.100057

Delle Chiaie, R., Pancheri, P., & Scapicchio, P. (2002). Efficacy and tolerability of oral and intramuscular S-adenosyl-L-methionine 1,4-butanedisulfonate (SAMe) in the treatment of major depression: Comparison with imipramine in 2 multicenter studies. *The American Journal of Clinical Nutrition, 76*(5), 1172s–1176s. doi:10.1093/ajcn/76.5.1172S

de Sousa, D. P., de Almeida Soares Hocayen, P., Andrade, L. N., & Andreatini, R. (2015). A systematic review of the anxiolytic-like effects of essential oils in animal models. *Molecules, 20*(10), 18620–18660. doi:10.3390/molecules201018620

de Vente, W., van Amsterdam, J. G., Olff, M., Kamphuis, J. H., & Emmelkamp, P. M. (2015). Burnout is associated with reduced parasympathetic activity and reduced HPA axis responsiveness, predominantly in males. *BioMed Research International, 2015*, 1–13. doi:10.1155/2015/431725

Devinsky, O., Whalley, B. J., & Di Marzo, V. (2015). Cannabinoids in the treatment of neurological disorders. *Neurotherapeutics, 12*(4), 689–691. doi:10.1007/s13311-015-0388-0

Diamond, B. J., & Bailey, M. R. (2013). *Ginkgo biloba*: Indications, mechanisms, and safety. *Psychiatric Clinics of North America, 36*(1), 73–83. doi:10.1016/j.psc.2012.12.006

Dworkin, R. H., O'Connor, A. B., Audette, J., Baron, R., Gourlay, G. K., Haanpaa, M. L., . . . Wells, C. D. (2010). Recommendations for the pharmacological management of neuropathic pain: An overview and literature update. *Mayo Clinic Proceedings, 85*(Suppl. 3), S3–S14. doi:10.4065/mcp.2009.0649

Emet, M., Ozcan, H., Ozel, L., Yayla, M., Halici, Z., & Hacimuftuoglu, A. (2016). A review of melatonin, its receptors and drugs. *The Eurasian Journal of Medicine*, 48(2), 135–141. doi:10.5152/eurasianjmed.2015.0267

Ferguson, L. R. (2014). Nutrigenetics and Crohn's disease. In L. R. Ferguson (Ed.), *Nutrigenomics and nutrigenetics in functional foods and personalized nutrition* (pp. 153–168). Boca Raton, FL: CRC Press.

Fernandes de Abreu, D. A., Eyles, D., & Feron, F. (2009). Vitamin D, a neuro-immunomodulator: Implications for neurodegenerative and autoimmune diseases. *Psychoneuroendocrinology*, 34 (Suppl. 1), S265–S277. doi:10.1016/j.psyneuen.2009.05.023

Fernstrom, J. D., & Fernstrom, M. H. (2007). Tyrosine, phenylalanine, and catecholamine synthesis and function in the brain. *The Journal of Nutrition*, 137(6 Suppl. 1), 1539S–1547S; discussion 1548S. doi:10.1093/jn/137.6.1539S

Fintelmann, V., & Gruenwald, J. (2007). Efficacy and tolerability of a Rhodiola rosea extract in adults with physical and cognitive deficiencies. *Advances in Therapy*, 24(4), 929–939. doi:10.1007/BF02849986

Fleischhacker, M., Schulz, S., Johrens, K., von Lilienfeld-Toal, M., Held, T., Fietze, E., . . . Ruhnke, M. (2012). Diagnosis of chronic disseminated candidosis from liver biopsies by a novel PCR in patients with haematological malignancies. *Clinical Microbiology and Infection*, 18(10), 1010–1016. doi:10.1111/j.1469-0691.2011.03713.x

Gauthier, S., & Schlaefke, S. (2014). Efficacy and tolerability of Ginkgo biloba extract EGb 761® in dementia: A systematic review and meta-analysis of randomized placebo-controlled trials. *Clinical Interventions in Aging*, 9, 2065–2077. doi:10.2147/cia.s72728

Ghorayeb, I., Gamas, A., Mazurie, Z., & Mayo, W. (2017). Attention-deficit hyperactivity and obsessive-compulsive symptoms in adult patients with primary restless legs syndrome: Different phenotypes of the same disease? *Behavioral Sleep Medicine*, 17(3), 246–253. doi:10.1080/15402002.2017.1326919

Grant, J. E., Chamberlain, S. R., Redden, S. A., Leppink, E. W., Odlaug, B. L., & Kim, S. (2016). N-acetylcysteine in the treatment of excoriation disorder: A randomized clinical trial. *JAMA Psychiatry*, 73(5), 490–496. doi:10.1001/jamapsychiatry.2016.0060

Grober, U., Kisters, K., & Schmidt, J. (2013). Neuroenhancement with vitamin B12-underestimated neurological significance. *Nutrients*, 5(12), 5031–5045. doi:10.3390/nu5125031

Hariri, M., & Azadbakht, L. (2015). Magnesium, iron, and zinc supplementation for the treatment of attention deficit hyperactivity disorder: A systematic review on the recent literature. *International Journal of Preventive Medicine*, 6, 83. doi:10.4103/2008-7802.164313

Hashiguchi, M., Ohta, Y., Shimizu, M., Maruyama, J., & Mochizuki, M. (2015). Meta-analysis of the efficacy and safety of Ginkgo biloba extract for the treatment of dementia. *Journal of Pharmaceutical Health Care and Sciences*, 1, 14. doi:10.1186/s40780-015-0014-7

Henderson, L., Yue, Q. Y., Bergquist, C., Gerden, B., & Arlett, P. (2002). St John's wort (Hypericum perforatum): Drug interactions and clinical outcomes. *British Journal of Clinical Pharmacology*, 54(4), 349–356. doi:10.1046/j.1365-2125.2002.01683.x

Hendriks, T., de Jong, J., & Cramer, H. (2017). The effects of yoga on positive mental health among healthy adults: A systematic review and meta-analysis. *The Journal of Alternative and Complementary Medicine*, 23(7), 505–517. doi:10.1089/acm.2016.0334

Hennessey, J. V., Garber, J. R., Woeber, K. A., Cobin, R., & Klein, I. (2016). American Association of Clinical Endocrinologists and American College of Endocrinology position statement on thyroid dysfunction case finding. *Endocrine Practice*, 22(2), 262–270. doi:10.4158/ep151038.ps

Hurt, E. A., Arnold, L. E., & Lofthouse, N. (2011). Dietary and nutritional treatments for attention-deficit/hyperactivity disorder: Current research support and recommendations for practitioners. *Current Psychiatry Reports*, 13(5), 323–332. doi:10.1007/s11920-011-0217-z

Jahnke, R., Larkey, L., Rogers, C., Etnier, J., & Lin, F. (2010). A comprehensive review of health benefits of qigong and tai chi. *American Journal of Health Promotion*, 24(6), e1–e25. doi:10.4278/ajhp.081013-LIT-248

Johnson, M. T., McCammon, C. A., Mullins, M. E., & Halcomb, S. E. (2011). Evaluation of a simplified N-acetylcysteine dosing regimen for the treatment of acetaminophen toxicity. *Annals of Pharmacotherapy*, 45(6), 713–720. doi:10.1345/aph.1P613

Jones, D. S., Bland, J. S., & Quinn, S. (2010). What is functional medicine? In D. S. Jones & S. Quinn (Eds.), *Textbook of functional medicine* (pp. 5–14). Federal Way, WA: Institute for Functional Medicine. Original work published 2005.

Kakuda, T. (2011). Neuroprotective effects of theanine and its preventive effects on cognitive dysfunction. *Pharmacological Research, 64*(2), 162–168. doi:10.1016/j.phrs.2011.03.010

Kali, A. (2016). Psychobiotics: An emerging probiotic in psychiatric practice. *Biomedical Journal, 39*(3), 223–224. doi:10.1016/j.bj.2015.11.004

Kalueff, A. V., & Tuohimaa, P. (2007). Neurosteroid hormone vitamin D and its utility in clinical nutrition. *Current Opinion in Clinical Nutrition & Metabolic Care, 10*(1), 12–19. doi:10.1097/MCO.0b013e328010ca18

Kaplan, B. J., Crawford, S. G., Field, C. J., & Simpson, J. S. (2007). Vitamins, minerals, and mood. *Psychological Bulletin, 133*(5), 747–760. doi:10.1037/0033-2909.133.5.747

Khalsa, M. K., Greiner-Ferris, J. M., Hofmann, S. G., & Khalsa, S. B. (2015). Yoga-enhanced cognitive behavioural therapy (Y-CBT) for anxiety management: A pilot study. *Clinical Psychology & Psychotherapy, 22*(4), 364–371. doi:10.1002/cpp.1902

Kilpinen-Loisa, P., Nenonen, H., Pihko, H., & Makitie, O. (2007). High-dose vitamin D supplementation in children with cerebral palsy or neuromuscular disorder. *Neuropediatrics, 38*(4), 167–172. doi:10.1055/s-2007-990266

Krisanaprakornkit, T., Sriraj, W., Piyavhatkul, N., & Laopaiboon, M. (2006). Meditation therapy for anxiety disorders. *Cochrane Database of Systematic Reviews,* (1), CD004998. doi:10.1002/14651858.CD004998.pub2

Lakhan, S. E., & Vieira, K. F. (2008). Nutritional therapies for mental disorders. *Nutrition Journal, 7,* 2. doi:10.1186/1475-2891-7-2

Lauche, R., Wayne, P. M., Dobos, G., & Cramer, H. (2016). Prevalence, patterns, and predictors of t'ai chi and qigong use in the United States: Results of a nationally representative survey. *Journal of Alternative and Complementary Medicine, 22*(4), 336–342. doi:10.1089/acm.2015.0356

Linde, K., Berner, M. M., & Kriston, L. (2008). St John's wort for major depression. *The Cochrane Database of Systematic Reviews* (4), CD000448. doi:10.1002/14651858.CD000448.pub3

Liska, D. (2010). Functional medicine is science-based. In D. S. Jones & S. Quinn (Eds.), *Textbook of functional medicine* (pp. 49–54). Federal Way, WA: Institute of Functional Medicine. Original work published 2005.

Liu, J., Wan, G. B., Huang, M. S., Agyapong, G., Zou, T. L., Zhang, X. Y., . . . Kong, X. J. (2019). Probiotic therapy for treating behavioral and gastrointestinal symptoms in autism spectrum disorder: A systematic review of clinical trials. *Current Medical Science, 39*(2), 173–184. doi:10.1007/s11596-019-2016-4

Liu, L., & Zhu, G. (2018). Gut–brain axis and mood disorder. *Front Psychiatry, 9,* 223. doi:10.3389/fpsyt.2018.00223

Lombard, J. (2010). Clinical approaches to hormonal and neuroendocrine imbalances: Neurotransmitters: A functional medicine approach to neuropsychiatry. In D. S. Jones & S. Quinn (Eds.), *Textbook of functional medicine* (pp. 638–644). Federal Way, WA: Institute for Functional Medicine. Original work published 2005.

Lord, R., & Redmond, E. (2012). Vitamins. In R. S. Lord (Ed.), *Laboratory evaluations in functional medicine* (2nd ed., pp. 17–62). Duluth, GA: Genova Diagnostics.

Lukaczer, D. (2010). Clinical approaches to gastrointestinal balance: The "4R" program. In D. S. Jones & S. Quinn (Eds.), *Textbook of functional medicine* (pp. 462–479). Federal Way, WA: Institute for Functional Medicine. Original work published 2005.

Lumpkin, M. (2010). Clinical approaches to hormonal and neuroendocrine imbalances: The hypothalamus-pituitary-adrenal axis. In D. S. Jones & S. Quinn (Eds.), *Textbook of functional medicine* (pp. 610–618). Federal Way, WA: Institute for Functional Medicine. Original work published 2005.

Malamood, M., Roberts, A., Kataria, R., Parkman, H. P., & Schey, R. (2017). Mirtazapine for symptom control in refractory gastroparesis. *Drug Design, Development and Therapy, 11,* 1035–1041. doi:10.2147/dddt.S125743

Mao, J. J., Li, Q. S., Soeller, I., Xie, S. X., & Amsterdam, J. D. (2014). Rhodiola rosea therapy for major depressive disorder: A study protocol for a randomized, double-blind, placebo-controlled trial. *Journal of Clinical Trials, 4,* 170. doi:10.4172/2167-0870.1000170

Mao, J. J., Xie, S. X., Zee, J., Soeller, I., Li, Q. S., Rockwell, K., & Amsterdam, J. D. (2015). Rhodiola rosea versus sertraline for major depressive disorder: A randomized placebo-controlled trial. *Phytomedicine, 22*(3), 394–399. doi:10.1016/j.phymed.2015.01.010

Maroon, J., & Bost, J. (2018). Review of the neurological benefits of phytocannabinoids. *Surgical Neurology International, 9*, 91. doi:10.4103/sni.sni_45_18

Massoumi, L. (2016). Using natural supplements. *The Carlat Psychiatry Report, 14*(11& 12), 1–11.

McClure, E. A., Sonne, S. C., Winhusen, T., Carroll, K. M., Ghitza, U. E., McRae-Clark, A. L., . . . Gray, K. M. (2014). Achieving cannabis cessation—Evaluating N-acetylcysteine treatment (ACCENT): Design and implementation of a multi-site, randomized controlled study in the National Institute on Drug Abuse Clinical Trials Network. *Contemporary Clinical Trials, 39*(2), 211–223. doi:10.1016/j.cct.2014.08.011

McGrane, I. R., Leung, J. G., St Louis, E. K., & Boeve, B. F. (2015). Melatonin therapy for REM sleep behavior disorder: A critical review of evidence. *Sleep Medicine, 16*(1), 19–26. doi:10.1016/j.sleep.2014.09.011

Minich, D. (2016). *Nutrigenomics in clinical practice: Genes, food, and specialty diagnostics.* Retrieved from https://www.gdx.net/clinicians/medical-education/previous-webinars/nutrigenomics-in-clinical-practice

Mischoulon, D., & Freeman, M. P. (2013). Omega-3 fatty acids in psychiatry. *Psychiatric Clinics of North America, 36*(1), 15–23. doi:10.1016/j.psc.2012.12.002

Montiel-Castro, A. J., Gonzalez-Cervantes, R. M., Bravo-Ruiseco, G., & Pacheco-Lopez, G. (2013). The microbiota-gut-brain axis: Neurobehavioral correlates, health and sociality. *Frontiers in Integrative Neuroscience, 7*, 70. doi:10.3389/fnint.2013.00070

Moore, L. D., Le, T., & Fan, G. (2013). DNA methylation and its basic function. *Neuropsychopharmacology, 38*(1), 23–38. doi:10.1038/npp.2012.112

Morris, M. S., Jacques, P. F., Rosenberg, I. H., & Selhub, J. (2010). Circulating unmetabolized folic acid and 5-methyltetrahydrofolate in relation to anemia, macrocytosis, and cognitive test performance in American seniors. *The American Journal of Clinical Nutrition, 91*(6), 1733–1744. doi:10.3945/ajcn.2009.28671

Mullur, R., Liu, Y.-Y., & Brent, G. A. (2014). Thyroid hormone regulation of metabolism. *Physiological Reviews, 94*(2), 355–382. doi:10.1152/physrev.00030.2013

Muskin, P. R., Gerbarg, P. L., & Brown, R. P. (2013). Along roads less traveled: Complementary, alternative, and integrative treatments. *Psychiatric Clinics of North America, 36*(1), 13–15. doi:10.1016/j.psc.2013.01.009

National Institutes of Health. (2018). *Complementary, alternative, or integrative health: What's in a name?* Retrieved from https://nccih.nih.gov/health/integrative-health

Noone, P. G., Hamblett, N., Accurso, F., Aitken, M. L., Boyle, M., Dovey, M., . . . Ramsey, B. (2001). Safety of aerosolized INS 365 in patients with mild to moderate cystic fibrosis: Results of a phase I multi-center study. *Pediatric Pulmonology, 32*(2), 122–128. doi:10.1002/ppul.1098

Olsson, E. M., von Scheele, B., & Panossian, A. G. (2009). A randomised, double-blind, placebo-controlled, parallel-group study of the standardised extract shr-5 of the roots of Rhodiola rosea in the treatment of subjects with stress-related fatigue. *Planta Medica, 75*(2), 105–112. doi:10.1055/s-0028-1088346

Ortigoza-Escobar, J. D., Serrano, M., Molero, M., Oyarzabal, A., Rebollo, M., Muchart, J., . . . Perez-Duenas, B. (2014). Thiamine transporter-2 deficiency: Outcome and treatment monitoring. *Orphanet Journal of Rare Diseases, 9*, 92. doi:10.1186/1750-1172-9-92

Ortiz, J. G., Nieves-Natal, J., & Chavez, P. (1999). Effects of Valeriana officinalis extracts on [3H] flunitrazepam binding, synaptosomal [3H]GABA uptake, and hippocampal [3H]GABA release. *Neurochemical Research, 24*(11), 1373–1378. doi:10.1023/a:1022576405534

Panossian, A., & Wikman, G. (2010). Effects of adaptogens on the central nervous system and the molecular mechanisms associated with their stress-protective activity. *Pharmaceuticals (Basel), 3*(1), 188–224. doi:10.3390/ph3010188

Perica, M. M., & Delas, I. (2011). Essential fatty acids and psychiatric disorders. *Nutrition in Clinical Practice, 26*(4), 409–425. doi:10.1177/0884533611411306

Petroff, O. A. (2002). GABA and glutamate in the human brain. *Neuroscientist, 8*(6), 562–573. doi:10.1177/1073858402238515

Pizzorno, L., & Ferril, W. (2010). Clinical approaches to hormonal and neuroendocrine imbalances: Thyroid. In D. S. Jones & S. Quinn (Eds.), *Textbook of functional medicine* (pp. 644–667). Federal Way, WA: Institute for Functional Medicine. Original work published 2005.

Popper, C. W. (2014). Single-micronutrient and broad-spectrum micronutrient approaches for treating mood disorders in youth and adults. *Child and Adolescent Psychiatric Clinics, 23*(3), 591–672. doi:10.1016/j.chc.2014.04.001

Pratte, M. A., Nanavati, K. B., Young, V., & Morley, C. P. (2014). An alternative treatment for anxiety: A systematic review of human trial results reported for the Ayurvedic herb ashwagandha (Withania somnifera). *Journal of Alternative and Complementary Medicine, 20*(12), 901–908. doi:10.1089/acm.2014.0177

The Public Health and Welfare, 42 U.S.C. § 300gg–91(d)(16), 2018. Retrieved from https://www.law.cornell.edu/uscode/text/42/300gg-91

Rapin, J. R., & Wiernsperger, N. (2010). Possible links between intestinal permeablity and food processing: A potential therapeutic niche for glutamine. *Clinics (Sao Paolo), 65*(6), 635–643. doi:10.1590/S1807-59322010000600012

Raskin, M., Bali, L. R., & Peeke, H. V. (1980). Muscle biofeedback and transcendental meditation. A controlled evaluation of efficacy in the treatment of chronic anxiety. *Archives of General Psychiatry, 37*(1), 93–97. doi:10.1001/archpsyc.1980.01780140095011

Rohilla, S., Bhatt, D. C., & Gupta, A. (2018). Therapeutic potential of phytomedicines and novel polymeric strategies for significant management of candidiasis. *Current Pharmaceutical Design, 24*(16), 1748–1765. doi:10.2174/1381612824666180524102933

Rosenblat, J. D., & McIntyre, R. S. (2017). Bipolar disorder and immune dysfunction: Epidemiological findings, proposed pathophysiology and clinical implications. *Brain Sciences, 7*(11), 144. doi:10.3390/brainsci7110144

Sadock, B. J., Sadock, V. A., & Ruiz, P. (2015). *Kaplan & Sadock's synopsis of psychiatry: Behavioral sciences/clinical psychiatry* (11th ed.). Philadelphia, PA: Wolters Kluwer.

Sarris, J., Oliver, G., Camfield, D. A., Dean, O. M., Dowling, N., Smith, D. J., . . . Ng, C. H. (2015). N-Acetyl cysteine (NAC) in the treatment of obsessive-compulsive disorder: A 16-week, double-blind, randomised, placebo-controlled study. *CNS Drugs, 29*(9), 801–809. doi:10.1007/s40263-015-0272-9

Savage, K. M., Stough, C. K., Byrne, G. J., Scholey, A., Bousman, C., Murphy, J., . . . Sarris, J. (2015). Kava for the treatment of generalised anxiety disorder (K-GAD): Study protocol for a randomised controlled trial. *Trials, 16*, 493. doi:10.1186/s13063-015-0986-5

Schuwald, A. M., Noldner, M., Wilmes, T., Klugbauer, N., Leuner, K., & Muller, W. E. (2013). Lavender oil-potent anxiolytic properties via modulating voltage dependent calcium channels. *PLOS ONE, 8*(4), e59998. doi:10.1371/journal.pone.0059998

SNPedia. (2019). *rs1801133(T;T) homozygous form of the C677T allele for the MTHFR gene.* Bethesda, MD: National Center for Biotechnology Information. Retrieved from https://www.snpedia.com/index.php?title=Rs1801133(T;T)&oldid=1286608

Stafford, R. S. (2008). Regulating off-label drug use-rethinking the role of the FDA. *The New England Journal of Medicine, 358*(14), 1427–1429. doi:10.1056/NEJMp0802107

Stevens, J. E., Jones, K. L., Rayner, C. K., & Horowitz, M. (2013). Pathophysiology and pharmacotherapy of gastroparesis: Current and future perspectives. *Expert Opinion on Pharmacotherapy, 14*(9), 1171–1186. doi:10.1517/14656566.2013.795948

Strickland, K. C., Krupenko, N. I., & Krupenko, S. A. (2013). Molecular mechanisms underlying the potentially adverse effects of folate. *Clinical Chemistry and Laboratory Medicine: CCLM / FESCC, 51*(3), 607–616. doi:10.1515/cclm-2012-0561

Sult, T. (2010). Digestive, absorptive, and microbiological imbalances. In D. S. Jones & S. Quinn (Eds.), *Textbook of functional medicine* (pp. 327–338). Federal Way, WA: Institute for Functional Medicine. Original work published 2005.

Szabo, E. K., & MacCallum, D. M. (2011). The contribution of mouse models to our understanding of systemic candidiasis. *FEMS Microbiology Letters, 320*(1), 1–8. doi:10.1111/j.1574-6968.2011.02262.x

Teschke, R., Sarris, J., & Lebot, V. (2011). Kava hepatotoxicity solution: A six-point plan for new kava standardization. *Phytomedicine, 18*(2–3), 96–103. doi:10.1016/j.phymed.2010.10.002

Teschke, R., Sarris, J., & Lebot, V. (2013). Contaminant hepatotoxins as culprits for kava hepatotoxicity—Fact or fiction? *Phytotherapy Research, 27*(3), 472–474. doi:10.1002/ptr.4729

Unger, E. R., Lin, J. S., Brimmer, D. J., Lapp, C. W., Komaroff, A. L., Nath, A., . . . Iskander, J. (2016). CDC grand rounds: Chronic fatigue syndrome—Advancing research and clinical education. *MMWR Morbidity and Mortality Weekly Report, 65*(50–51), 1434–1438. doi:10.15585/mmwr.mm655051a4

U.S. Food and Drug Administration. (2016). *Dietary supplement alerts and safety information.* Retrieved from http://www.fda.gov/Food/RecallsOutbreaksEmergencies/SafetyAlertsAdvisories/default.htm

Ushiroyama, T., Ikeda, A., & Ueki, M. (2002). Effect of continuous combined therapy with vitamin K(2) and vitamin D(3) on bone mineral density and coagulofibrinolysis function in postmenopausal women. *Maturitas, 41*(3), 211–221.doi:10.1016/s0378-5122(01)00275-4

Vasquez, A. (2010). Clinical approaches to immune imbalance and inflammation: Inflammation and autoimmunity: A functional medicine approach. In D. S. Jones & S. Quinn (Eds.), *Textbook of functional medicine* (pp. 409–417). Federal Way, WA: Institute for Functional Medicine. Original work published 2005.

Vitetta, L., Bambling, M., & Alford, H. (2014). The gastrointestinal tract microbiome, probiotics, and mood. *Inflammopharmacology, 22*(6), 333–339. doi:10.1007/s10787-014-0216-x

Vonder Haar, C., Peterson, T. C., Martens, K. M., & Hoane, M. R. (2016). Vitamins and nutrients as primary treatments in experimental brain injury: Clinical implications for nutraceutical therapies. *Brain Research, 1640*(Pt. A), 114–129. doi:10.1016/j.brainres.2015.12.030

Wahls, T., Rubenstein, L., Hall, M., & Snetselaar, L. (2014). Assessment of dietary adequacy for important brain micronutrients in patients presenting to a traumatic brain injury clinic for evaluation. *Nutritional Neuroscience, 17*(6), 252–259. doi:10.1179/1476830513y.0000000088

Wang, Y., Huang, L., Zhang, L., Qu, Y., & Mu, D. (2017). Iron status in attention-deficit/hyperactivity disorder: A systematic review and meta-analysis. *PLOS ONE, 12*(1), e0169145. doi:10.1371/journal.pone.0169145

Wani, A. L., Bhat, S. A., & Ara, A. (2015). Omega-3 fatty acids and the treatment of depression: A review of scientific evidence. *Integrative Medicine Research, 4*(3), 132–141. doi:10.1016/j.imr.2015.07.003

Weil, P. (2012a). DNA organization, replication & repair. In B. D. Murray, D. A. Bender, K. M. Botham, P. J. Kennelly, V. W. Rodwell, & P. A. Weil (Eds.), *Harper's illustrated biochemistry* (29th ed., pp. 354–376). Philadelphia, PA: McGraw-Hill.

Weil, P. (2012b). Nucleic acid structure & function. In B. D. Murray, D. A. Bender, K. M. Botham, P. J. Kennelly, V. W. Rodwell, & P. A. Weil (Eds.), *Harper's illustrated biochemistry* (29th ed., pp. 343–354). Philadelphia, PA: McGraw-Hill.

Weil, P. (2012c). RNA synthesis, processing and modification. In B. D. Murray, D. A. Bender, K. M. Botham, P. J. Kennelly, V. W. Rodwell, & P. A. Weil (Eds.), *Harper's illlustrated biochemistry* (29th ed., pp. 377–394). Philadelphia, PA: McGraw-Hill.

Wittich, C. M., Burkle, C. M., & Lanier, W. L. (2012). Ten common questions (and their answers) about off-label drug use. *Mayo Clinic Proceedings, 87*(10), 982–990. doi:10.1016/j.mayocp.2012.04.017

Zhang, H.-F., Huang, L.-B., Zhong, Y.-B., Zhou, Q.-H., Wang, H.-L., Zheng, G.-Q., & Lin, Y. (2016). An overview of systematic reviews of Ginkgo biloba extracts for mild cognitive impairment and dementia. *Frontiers in Aging Neuroscience, 8*, 276. doi:10.3389/fnagi.2016.00276

Zhang, W.-F., Tan, Y.-L., Zhang, X.-Y., Chan, R. C., Wu, H.-R., & Zhou, D.-F. (2011). Extract of *Ginkgo biloba* treatment for tardive dyskinesia in schizophrenia: A randomized, double-blind, placebo-controlled trial. *The Journal of Clinical Psychiatry, 72*(5), 615–621. doi:10.4088/JCP.09m05125yel

IV

Psychotherapy With Special Populations

Stabilization for Trauma and Dissociation

Kathleen Wheeler

Trauma affects all dimensions of the person, dysregulating and disconnecting the person physiologically, emotionally, spiritually, cognitively, interpersonally, and socially. Trauma refers to an extremely stressful event or situation that is experienced as overwhelming to the individual and as a result, the experience/memory is stored dysfunctionally in the brain (Cozolino, 2017; Shapiro, 2018). Shapiro (2001) broadened the concept of trauma to include any adverse life experience that has a lasting effect on the self. These experiences may be small t traumas or big T traumas. The latter, big T trauma, coincides most closely with the *Diagnostic and Statistical Manual of Mental Disorders* (5th ed.; *DSM-5*; American Psychiatric Association [APA], 2013) Criterion A event for posttraumatic stress disorder (PTSD); that is, the person has experienced, witnessed, or was confronted with an event or events that involved actual or threatened death or serious injury, or a threat to the physical integrity of self or others. The small t traumas might include those events that are relatively common, such as a significant loss, illness, problems with relationships or work, bullying, neglect, and betrayal.

Wider recognition by the psychiatric establishment of the expanding conceptualization of traumatic experiences is reflected by a new *DSM-5* category of psychiatric diagnosis, trauma-related disorders (APA, 2013). Disorders in this category include acute stress disorder (ASD), PTSD, adjustment disorder, specified or unspecified trauma and stressor related disorder for those presentations that do not fully meet criteria for the previous three diagnoses, reactive attachment disorder (RAD), and disinhibited social engagement disorder, with the latter two exclusively for children.

Other diagnoses directly related to traumatic events include the *DSM-5* category of dissociative disorders (DDs), which include dissociative amnesia, depersonalization/derealization, and dissociative identity disorder (DID); and the *DSM-5* category somatic symptom and related disorder, which includes somatic symptom disorder, illness anxiety disorder, conversion disorder, and psychological factors affecting other medical conditions. Borderline personality disorder (BPD) is also thought to be caused by early relationship trauma and is discussed in Chapter 18. Other disorders not included in the *DSM-5* category of trauma-related disorders that are discussed in this chapter are disorders of extreme stress not otherwise specified (DESNOS) or complex trauma and psychosomatic disorders. However, the World Health Organization (WHO, 2018) announced a major change in the diagnostic classification of complex trauma that will go into effect in January 2022. The *International Classification of Diseases*, 11th revision (*ICD-11*) will for the first time include a diagnosis of Complex PTSD. This recognition is a major advance that acknowledges the existence and appropriate treatment that expands the diagnostic categories related to trauma.

This chapter further explicates the care of individuals who have suffered significant trauma and elaborates psychotherapeutic strategies for care using the treatment hierarchy framework presented in Chapters 1 and 2. Treatment of this population with a particular emphasis on stage 1 (stabilization) based on Porges's polyvagal theory (PVT) is discussed. Specific stabilization strategies are illustrated with clinical vignettes on how to work with those with complex trauma. Interventions are aimed toward safety, developing dual awareness through mindfulness, and managing physiological arousal. "When we consciously and deliberately engage in practices that produce physical calmness, we signal the limbic brain that we're safe at a physiological level" (Church, 2015, p. 49). These practices and strategies enhance and strengthen one's resilient zone (RZ) as described in Chapter 1.

SPECTRUM OF TRAUMATIC RESPONSE

The effects of adverse life experiences and traumatic events can be cumulative and significantly compromise functioning and lead to mental health problems, psychiatric disorders, and physical disorders. An individual's response and the long-term sequelae of trauma are highly individualistic and depend on the nature, chronicity, and severity of the traumatic events, the person's age, development stage, genetic vulnerability, prenatal factors, gender, past experiences, preexisting neural physiology, cognitive deficits, emotional maturity, coping skills, hardiness, relationships with others, intrafamilial involvement, sociocultural factors, and a host of other factors (Briere & Scott, 2013; Chu, 2011).

The spectrum of the traumatic stress response is illustrated in Figure 17.1. Traumatic stress disorders include several diagnoses that result from one or more traumatic events and often include symptoms of intrusive thoughts, avoidant behavior, and hyperarousal. These symptoms can be thought of as state-dependent memories that result from earlier experiences caused by a traumatic situation. These memories are stored differently from normal memories; are not integrated with other, more adaptive networks; and may be encoded as sensations and images in implicit memories rather than in verbal narrative and context. The traumatic memory is fragmented and not linked to other experience (neural networks) but lives on as a physical sensation, emotion, and/or image.

This unprocessed trauma leads to unexpected reexperiencing or intrusive thoughts related to the trauma, the numbing of awareness or avoidance of situations or circumstances that are associated with the trauma, and a persistent increase in physiological arousal. The patient may alternate between denial or numbing and experiencing intrusive thoughts or images. Figure 17.1 lists common numbing and intrusive symptoms. During denial states, increased activity such as work, sports, or sexual activities may take place, and to quell the intrusive states, substances such as alcohol may be used. Intrusive emotional states reenact the stressor, and through overgeneralization, situations that before the trauma were neutral are infused with anger, fear, and sadness. Chapter 2 explains the neurophysiology of these cycles. Although these symptoms might have been adaptive at the time of the trauma, their contribution to the present can create significant problems for the person in identity, interpersonal relationships, affect dysregulation, and cognitive distortions.

Acute Stress Disorder

ASD was a relatively new diagnosis in the *DSM-IV*, and the *DSM-5* has further honed this diagnosis to include nine out the following 14 symptoms that occur from 3 days to

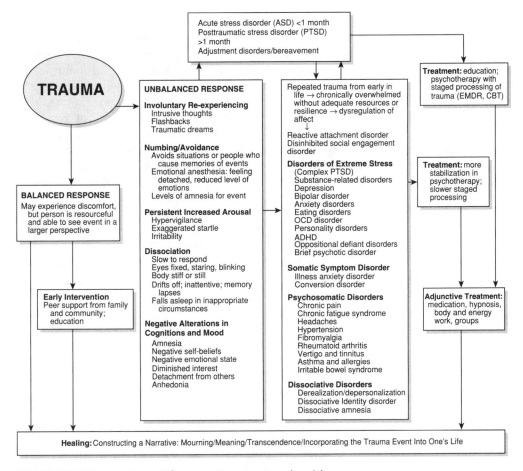

FIGURE 17.1 The spectrum of traumatic response algorithm.

ADHD, Attention deficit hyperactivity disorder; CBT, cognitive behavioral therapy; EMDR, eye movement desensitization and reprocessing; OCD, obsessive-compulsive disorder.

Source: Davis, K., & Weiss, L. (2004). *Traumatology: A workshop on traumatic stress disorders.* Hamden, CT: EMDR Humanitarian Assistance Programs.

1 month after a traumatic event. The essential features of ASD include a subjective sense of numbing; derealization (a sense of unreality related to the environment); inability to remember at least one important aspect of the event; intrusive distressing memories of the event; recurrent distressing dreams; feeling as if the event is recurring; intense prolonged distress or physiological reactivity; avoidance of thoughts or feelings about the event; sleep disturbances; hypervigilance; negative mood; exaggerated startle response; and agitation or restlessness. These symptoms develop after a traumatic event and last from 3 days to 1 month. If the symptoms persist after 4 weeks, the diagnosis changes to PTSD.

Posttraumatic Stress Disorder

The *DSM-5* describes PTSD as the result of having been exposed to, witnessing, or experiencing repeated or extreme exposure to aversive events; events occurring to a close relative or friend; or one or more of the following event(s): death or threatened serious injury, or actual or threatened sexual violence (APA, 2013). Intrusive thoughts, avoidance behaviors, negative thoughts and mood, and hyperarousal must be present for at least 1 month after the traumatic event. Duration of symptoms varies, with some individuals recovering in a few months and others who can remain symptomatic for 50 years. It is not uncommon for symptoms to exacerbate or reoccur in response to stressors or triggers of the original trauma. Intrusive states include nightmares and flashbacks, which are fragments of distressing recollections, along with the physical components of the trauma (i.e., smell, physical sensation, taste, emotion, sound, and visual image). Avoidance behaviors include feelings of detachment, not thinking about the event, staying away from places that remind the person of the event, not remembering part or all of the event, diminished participation in pleasurable activities, not feeling (i.e., psychic numbing), and believing that as a result of the event, the person will not have a normal life. Hyperarousal may manifest by bursts of anger, agitation, irritability, difficulty concentrating, hypervigilance, difficulty falling or staying asleep, and an exaggerated startle response.

The DSM 5 introduced a dissociative subtype for PTSD with symptoms of derealization and depersonalization. A recent study provides support that adverse childhood events (ACEs) and combined traumatic and non-traumatic stressors across the lifespan signficantly contribute to the development of PTSD symptoms (Frewin, Zhu, & Lanius, 2019).

Dissociative Disorders

In addition to the triad of hyperarousal, avoidance, and intrusive thoughts, one of the most disturbing symptoms for the patient is dissociation. People can experience dissociation from mild daydreaming and spacing out to depersonalization and derealization episodes to total unresponsiveness, although they are awake and responsive to their environment such as in dissociative amnesia and dissociative fugue. Severe episodes of dissociation occur in DDs and interfere with social or occupational functioning. DID, formerly called multiple personality disorder, is an extreme version of dissociation. Significant dissociative states are characterized by a disconnection of thoughts, emotions, sensations, and behaviors.

Dissociation indicates that neural networks are functioning independently and separately, that the networks are unintegrated, and that information processing has been disrupted. Dissociative states reflect discrete memory networks that have not been linked to other dimensions of consciousness. Dissociation is thought to be primarily a right-brain phenomenon (Schore, 2019). Those who suffer from severe dissociation are those who have suffered significant trauma. Putnam (1989) provides an excellent definition of dissociation from his seminal book on multiple personality disorders: "a normal process that is initially used defensively by an individual to handle traumatic experiences [that] evolves over time into a maladaptive or pathological process" (p. 9). Box 17.1 describes patient-reported signs of dissociation, and Box 17.2 lists the observable signs of dissociation that the clinician may notice.

Dissociation is also considered a primitive type of defense in that as anxiety rises, the person may dissociate without awareness that this is happening in an effort to avoid the perceived threat. Separation results in disturbances in memory, consciousness, self-identity, and perception. Dissociation reflects a disconnection of the flow of information in neural networks. This is consistent with the basic tenet of this book, that disconnected neural networks drive the symptoms that are considered psychopathological. Memories or information encoded in one state are not available to that person in another state. Neurophysiologically, the parasympathetic branch of the autonomic nervous system contributes to dissociation when the person experiences overwhelming

BOX 17.1 Patient-Reported Signs of Dissociation

- Things look different, tunnel vision, colors too vivid or washed out
- Things sound different, muffled or too loud, "tinny" or echoing
- Things seem to move in slow motion, or fast forward
- Emotions become flat, numb; no feelings
- Feeling out of touch with surroundings
- Feeling like an observer of their present circumstances
- Feeling like they are on autopilot
- People or the world does not seem real; or person feels like a stranger in familiar place
- Events seem like a dream
- It seems like one is watching things from outside the body
- Foggy feeling, clouding of alertness

BOX 17.2 Observable Signs of Dissociation

- Behavior that is an inappropriate response to stimuli, such as falling down after loud noise; disorientation
- Person is slow to respond
- Eyes fixed, staring into space, blinking rapidly without focusing, or staring downward
- Body becomes stiff or still
- Person drifts off, goes away, spaces out, blanks out, or loses track of what is happening; is inattentive and has memory lapses
- Person falls asleep in inappropriate circumstances

Source: Schiraldi, G. R. (2001). *The self-esteem workbook.* Oakland, CA: New Harbinger Publications..

stress (Porges, 2011). In this process, heart rate and blood pressure are reduced, and endogenous opioids are released (van der Kolk, 2014). This is a state of resignation or freeze in that the person cannot escape and the body responds by dissociating emotionally and mentally. This state may be associated with anhedonia, which is an inability to achieve or experience pleasure, and abulia, which is a state of profound apathy and inability to make decisions. Although dissociation is considered a dorsal vagal "shut down" response, dissociation can also occur when the person is behaviorally active (Rothschild, 2017).

This physiological state gets locked into the brain with all the attending sensations that occurred at the time of the event. This state-dependent dissociation results in fragmented memories disconnected from words and instead stored as images, sounds, smells, and body sensations. Later similar experiences triggered by internal or external stimuli may activate this material (Shapiro, 2018). For example, internal stimuli and the activation of a physiological state such as anxiety or pain may serve as a trigger along with external stimuli such as a sound or smell. The dissociated patient may cycle rapidly between arousal with hypervigilance and then numbing confusion, and it may be difficult to distinguish whether the person is aroused or numb. The trauma patient experiences repetitive episodes of sympathetic arousal that in turn reflexively trigger deep parasympathetic dissociation. The trauma patient lives in a state of involuntary and disruptive autonomic instability and cycling (van der Kolk, 2014). See Figure 17.2.

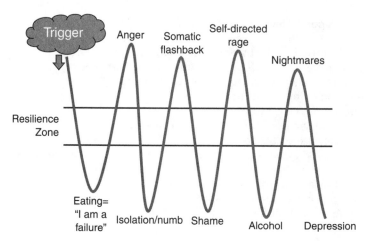

FIGURE 17.2 Autonomic cycles of disturbing emotions, behaviors and symptoms.

Dissociative states may include flashbacks that are disturbing to the patient which may occur automatically when the intensity of feeling becomes too strong and/or when triggers to the original trauma are encountered. Flashbacks reflect dissociated implicit capsules of memories (Howell, 2020). "Trauma interferes with the registration and consolidation of experience into narrative memory" (Howell, 2020, p. 32). Thus, the integrative function of memory consolidation fails and the memory is stored as somatic sensation, visual image, or sounds. Adults who experience trauma are not as likely to dissociate memories as children, because a child's brain does not have the associated neural networks needed to process the overwhelming affects that occur in trauma, particularly with repeated sexual trauma. In general, the younger the child when the trauma occurs and the more overwhelming the event(s), the more likely it is that the event will be dissociated (Schore, 2019). Research has found that children who are severely abused prior to adolescence have either partial or complete amnesia for the events (Waters, 2016). It is not only the negative events that are not remembered but the positive events too so that the person may not remember much about childhood at all. Dissociation is pathologic when it becomes the primary response to stress (Stien & Kendall, 2006) or becomes problematic to the person.

A dissociative disorder may develop after a significant adverse experience/trauma when the individual responded with a severe interruption of consciousness. Patients with DDs have intact reality testing; that is, although the person may have flashbacks or images, these are triggered by current events, relate to the past trauma, and are not delusions or hallucinations. Dissociation is involuntary and results in failure of the normal control over a person's mental processes and normal integration of conscious awareness (Steele, Boon, & van der Hart, 2017). Dimensions of a memory that should be linked are not and are fragmented. For example, a person may be aware of a sound or smell, but these sensations would not be linked to the actual event itself, leaving the person fearful and/or confused. In addition, the person may reenact, as well as reexperience, trauma without consciously knowing why.

Symptoms of dissociation may be either positive or negative. Positive symptoms refer to unwanted additions to mental activity such as flashbacks; negative symptoms refer to deficits such as memory problems or the inability to sense or control different parts of the body. It is thought that dissociation decreases the immediate subjective distress of the trauma and also continues to protect the individual from full awareness of the disturbing event. Dissociation actually reduces disturbing feelings and protects the person from full awareness of the trauma. This highlights the importance of attachments and relationships so the child can grow socially, intellectually, and cognitively. Factors that contribute to the development of DDs are early age of onset, severity of the trauma, the chronicity, and intrafamilial involvement (Waters, 2016). If abuse or neglect has occurred early in life, these memories become compartmentalized and often do not intrude into awareness until later in life when the person is in a stressful situation.

DDs include (a) depersonalization/derealization disorder, (b) dissociative amnesia/fugue, and (c) DID. Anyone may experience a transient or temporary depersonalization. In international studies, DDs have a 9% to 18% prevalence, and DID is present in 1% to 1.5% of the general population (Sar, 2011). Patients with this disorder usually seek treatment for another problem such as anxiety, substance use, or depression. Depersonalization is an extremely uncomfortable feeling of being an observer of one's own body or mental processes while derealization is a recurring feeling that one's surroundings are unreal or distant. The person may feel mechanical, dreamy, or detached from the body. Some people suffer episodes of these problems that come and go, while others have episodes that begin with stressors and eventually become constant. Dissociative amnesia is also fairly common with a prevalence of about 2% to 7% and may occur in any age group from children to adults. The amnesia is often related to trauma, and memory returns spontaneously after the individual is removed from the stressful situation (Blue Knot Foundation, 2019).

DID was formerly called multiple personality disorder, and a requirement for this diagnosis was the presence of alternate identities. Because switching from one personality to another happens infrequently, many people with this disorder are not properly diagnosed. DID may occur at any age but is diagnosed three to nine times more frequently in adult females than in adult males. There is usually a childhood history of severe physical or sexual abuse. Childhood physical, sexual, or emotional abuse and other traumatic life events are associated with adults experiencing dissociative symptoms. Patients with DID almost universally suffer from comorbid PTSD (Chu, 2011).

Comorbidity is common with DDs. Depression, panic attacks, eating disorders, PTSD, somatoform symptoms, eating disorders, obsessive–compulsive disorder (OCD), reactive attachment disorder (RAD), attention deficit disorder (ADD) with or without hyperactivity, personality disorders such as BPD, and substance-use disorders as well as sexual and sleep disorders commonly co-occur with all of the DDs (ISSTD, 2011). In addition, dissociative amnesia may be comorbid with conversion disorder or a personality disorder. Dissociative fugue, a type of dissociative amnesia, is associated with travel and may co-occur with PTSD. Depersonalization and derealization also occur in hypochondriasis, mood and anxiety disorders, OCD, and schizophrenia (Spiegel et al., 2011). Historically, the defense of repression was thought to underlie most psychiatric disturbances but more contemporary thinking posits that dissociation, one of the most primitive defenses, is key to understanding most psychiatric disturbances, including substance abuse, eating disorders, depression, panic anxiety, generalized anxiety, phobias, obsessive–compulsive anxiety and personality disorders, conversion disorders, brief psychotic disorders, as well as other psychiatric disorders (Howell, 2020; McWilliams, 2011).

Most clinicians view dissociation as on a continuum, with some dissociation considered a normal experience for most people. For example, we dissociate when we go to the movies, get lost in a good book, daydream, space out during a lecture, or drive from point A to point B without paying attention to how we got there. One study of the general population found that 25% of people report mild to severe episodes of dissociation

(Steinberg & Schnall, 2000). If trauma is severe or prolonged or occurs early in life, PTSD and DDs are likely to develop. It is curious that dissociation is considered rare in the United States when prevalence rates of DDs range from 2% to 10% occurrence at some time during a person's life (ISSTD, 2011). Steinberg and Schnall (2000) estimate that the 1-year prevalence rate for the general population is probably around 10%, which is the same as that for major depression and generalized anxiety disorder. A study of outpatients seeking psychotherapy found that 29% of the 84 subjects tested had a diagnosis of DD after being interviewed with a structured interview for DDs (Foote, Smolin, Kaplan, Legatt, & Lipschitz, 2006). Only 5% of these subjects had been diagnosed with a DD before the interview. DDs are often misdiagnosed and the person may have been treated in the mental health system for bipolar disorder, schizophrenia, schizoaffective disorder, BPD, panic attacks, eating disorders, somatoform symptoms, and major depressive disorder before being diagnosed correctly (McWilliams, 2011). As a result, the person with DID spends anywhere from 5 to 12 years in mental health treatment prior to being accurately diagnosed (Spiegel et al., 2011).

Disorders of Extreme Stress

If the trauma is particularly prolonged or severe, pervasive personality problems develop. This is usually what has been termed complex PTSD or DESNOS (Herman, 1992). Although neither of these are *DSM-5* diagnoses, the diagnostic classification of Complex PTSD will be added to the *ICD-11* in January 2022 (WHO, 2018). Herman, in her groundbreaking book "Trauma and Recovery", coined the term *complex post-traumatic syndrome* to refer to survivors of childhood abuse who may accumulate a number of diagnoses, including bipolar disorder, depression, anxiety disorders, substance abuse disorders, eating disorders, BPD, somatization disorder, and DDs, in their encounters with the mental health system. Stien and Kendall (2006) add attention deficit hyperactivity disorder (ADHD) and oppositional defiant disorder (ODD) to this list as diagnoses related to complex trauma for children. Some are considered secondary diagnoses, such as substance abuse, OCD, somatization disorder, and eating disorders, because these problems represent attempts by the traumatized person to cope with the effects of the trauma (Waters, 2016).

Brain and hormonal changes may occur as a result of early, prolonged trauma, and these changes contribute to long-term difficulties with memory, learning, and regulating impulses and emotions. Difficulties include problems with self-regulation and impulse control, including self-destructive activities; problems in information processing, particularly with dissociation; personal identity issues such as self-blame, shame, and being permanently damaged; somatization of external stress manifesting in the body as disease or physical disorders; problems in interpersonal relationships and being dysfunctionally attached to perpetrators (Howell, 2020). These individuals, referred to as the chronically disempowered by Chu (2011), are often survivors of childhood abuse and usually require long-term treatment extending over several years.

Somatic Symptoms and Related Disorders

Somatic complaints have been identified as one of the most clinically relevant symptoms linked to a childhood history of abuse, particularly sexual abuse (Briere & Scott, 2013). Trauma, dissociation, and physical symptoms are inexorably linked. Those with significant somatic symptoms that are not caused by a medical condition are diagnosed under the general heading of somatic symptom and related disorders and include the following diagnoses in the *DSM-5*: somatic symptom disorder, illness anxiety disorder, conversion disorder, psychological factors affecting other medical conditions, and factitious disorder. These individuals may have an excessive preoccupation with bodily dysfunction and manifest a variety of physical problems, such as neurological symptoms(especially headaches), gastrointestinal symptoms, and chronic pain that cannot be explained based on their medical condition. Conversion reactions include paralysis, anesthesia, blindness, deafness, and seizures (Briere & Scott, 2013). These disorders are characterized by a preoccupation with somatic problems and usually present in medical rather than mental health settings. Many cultures have somatization and dissociation syndromes. These are listed in the *DSM-5* Glossary of Cultural Concepts of Distress and include the following: Latin American cultures with *Nervios* and *Susto*, Cambodia with *Khyal cap*, Zimbabwe with *Kufungisisa*, Haiti with *Maladi moun*, China with *Shenjing shuairuo* and *Dhat*, and Japan with *Taijin kyofusho* (APA, 2013).

Psychosomatic Disorders

Psychosomatic disorders most likely overlap and are closely aligned with somatoform disorders but are not specifically delineated in the *DSM-5* because they are considered medical illnesses. Psychosomatic disorders include significant physiological changes in various tissues or organs in the body that are thought to be caused by childhood trauma or overwhelming stress. Psychosomatic disorders are induced by emotions and are mediated by the immune-peptide, autonomic-peptide, and neuroendocrine-peptide systems (Sarno, 2006). Sarno posits that these individuals are *repressors*; those who have a psychosomatic disorder subjectively do not experience painful and dangerous emotions and instead repress anger and anxiety. These emotions are thought to be too disturbing for the person if made conscious.

Psychosomatic medical illnesses are more commonly termed medically unexplained symptoms (MUS) and include tension myositis syndrome, which often manifests as back and neck pain; carpal tunnel syndrome; chronic fatigue syndrome; rheumatoid arthritis; fibromyalgia; allergies; asthma; psoriasis; eczema; acne; irritable bowel syndrome; tension and migraine headaches; vertigo and tinnitus; endocrine and autoimmune disorders; sleep-disordered breathing; and paroxysmal and essential hypertension. Additional disorders that may have a psychosomatic component are lupus erythematosus Graves disease, Hasimoto thyroiditis, Crohn disease, type 1 diabetes, multiple sclerosis, Sjögren syndrome, and reflex sympathetic dystrophy (Bergmann, 2019).

Scaer (2005) posits that the parasympathetic freeze response combined with autonomic dysregulation and abnormal cycling underlie psychosomatic disorders. He considers these to be the diseases and disorders of trauma. Although these diseases and disorders are sometimes associated with the presence of specific genes, he believes that they are primarily caused or triggered by early childhood and complex traumas that activate latent genetic tendencies. Because individuals with these disorders most often seek medical attention and usually do not seek psychotherapy and medical researchers are not particularly interested in psychology, there is no solid evidence base for psychotherapy as a first-line treatment. However, there is anecdotal and case study evidence for the efficacy of insight-oriented psychotherapy and eye movement desensitization and reprocessing (EMDR) therapy for some of these trauma-related medical problems. Scaer categorizes these disorders and diseases based on the predominant feature of their abnormal function (Scaer, 2005), as shown in Table 17.1.

TABLE 17.1 DISEASES AND DISORDERS OF TRAUMA	
Categories of Dysfunction	Diseases and Disorders
Diseases of abnormal autonomic regulation	Fibromyalgia, irritable bowel syndrome, chronic fatigue syndrome, gastroesophageal reflux disease, mitral valve prolapse or dysautonomia syndrome, multiple chemical sensitivities, migraine headache
Syndromes of procedural memory	Whiplash syndrome, cumulative trauma disorder, tics, phantom limb pain, chronic pain, premenstrual dysphoric syndrome, postpartum depression or psychosis
Diseases of somatic dissociation	Reflex sympathetic dystrophy, interstitial cystitis, chronic pelvic pain
Disorders of endocrine and immune system regulation	Hyperthyroidism, diabetes, rheumatoid arthritis, systemic lupus erythematosus, Sjögren syndrome, Graves disease, Hashimoto thyroiditis, multiple sclerosis
Disorders of cognition and sleep	Attention deficit disorder, sleep-disordered breathing, sleep apnea, narcolepsy, cataplexy, hypnagogic hallucination, sleep paralysis

Source: Scaer, R. (2005). *The trauma spectrum: Hidden wounds and human resiliency.* New York, NY: W. W. Norton.

STRUCTURAL DISSOCIATION THEORY

The theory of structural dissociation provides a cogent framework for working with those with dissociation (Steele, van der Hart, & Nijenhuis, 2005). Those with PTSD are thought to have one apparently normal part (ANP) and one emotional part (EP), termed primary dissociation; those with one ANP and more than one EP are said to have secondary dissociation, and these individuals are most likely diagnosed with BPD or DESNOS or dissociative disorders not otherwise specified (DDNOS); still others may have several ANPs and EPs and are diagnosed with DID, which is tertiary dissociation. See Figure 17.3. The EP holds the sadness and memories of the trauma while the ANP is phobic of the EP and is often unaware of the trauma. Defenses serve as a barrier between the ANP and the EP. The more parts there are, the more the fragmentation of the personality with the different parts experiencing themselves as younger than they really are. For example, the helpless little child EP who suffered abuse or neglect may take over the personality and leave the person feeling confused, afraid, and even ashamed as they are not sure what is happening. The person may hear an inner voice, an EP, who says: "You are worthless and should be dead" or "Shut up, you are stupid" even though nothing in reality seems to be wrong. They may even hear arguments going on in their head. Because of this, DID is often misdiagnosed as schizophrenia or another psychotic disorder instead of a DD. It is important to remember that all parts have a purpose or function with some parts "helpers" who by dissociating at the time of trauma allowed the person to escape and survive, whereas other parts may hold the anger and rage that were too threatening to experience at the time the trauma occurred. Treatment for those with significant DDs is focused toward increased communication and cooperation between parts with the ultimate goal of at least cooperation between the parts with integration the ideal.

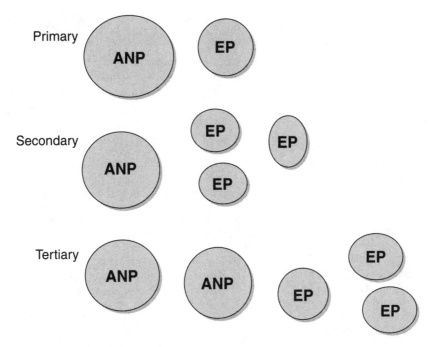

FIGURE 17.3 Structural dissociation: Primary, secondary, and tertiary dissociation.

ANP - Apparently Normal Part; EP = Emotional Part

Each part has its own responses, feelings, thoughts, perceptions, physical sensations, and behaviors to situations/people. These different parts may not be aware of each other with only one dominant personality operating depending on the situation and circumstance of the moment. For example, the person may be triggered by an outside event, such as a sound or situation, and the EP who holds the trauma will take over the personality. The EPs involve action defense systems that are ready to act and have been prevented from integration (Steele, van der Hart, & Nijenhuis, 2005). This is called switching. The day-to-day functioning is usually carried on by the ANP that avoids traumatic memories, that is phobic of the traumatic memory. Thus, the person may seem fine some of the time but cannot sustain this state due to outside environmental or even internal bodily events. Bodily sensations such as a rapidly beating heart and the sensation of anxiety can trigger an EP to be dominant. All parts are stuck in maladaptive states that maintain dissociation.

GOALS OF TREATMENT

Because many, if not most, outpatients and inpatients present with significant trauma histories, it is important that the advanced practice psychiatric nurse (APPN) learn to assess and treat this population. These patients come to treatment with a range of disturbing symptoms and present significant diagnostic and treatment challenges. The complexity of symptoms and multiple diagnoses confuse and challenge clinicians who care for this population. In general, the goals of treatment for PTSD can be applied to those who suffer from other trauma-related diagnoses. These are delineated in the American Psychiatric Association's practice guidelines for PTSD (APA, 2009) and include reducing the severity of symptoms, preventing or treating trauma-related

TABLE 17.2 ASSESSMENT/OUTCOME INSTRUMENTS FOR DISSOCIATION	
Instrument	**Purpose and How to Obtain**
Dissociative Experiences Scale (DES; Bernstein & Putnam, 1986) DES-Revised (Carlson & Putnam, 1993)	28 items; most often used self-report screening tool for dissociation (included in Chapter 3, Assessment and Diagnosis) Uses a Likert scale instead of percentages
Multidimensional Inventory of Dissociation (Dell, 2006)	Self-report with validity scales; available on the International Society for the Study of Trauma and Dissociation website (www.isst-d.org)
Multiscale Dissociation Inventory (Briere, 2002)	Available without cost from John Briere (www.johnbriere.com)
Somatoform Dissociation Questionnaire (SDQ-20 and SDQ-5; Nijenhuis, 2011)	Two forms, 20 items on a 5-point Likert scale pertaining to both negative (analgesia) and positive (pain) dissociative phenomena
Dissociative Disorders Interview Schedule (DDIS; Ross, 2013)	16 sections on this thorough diagnostic tool with no total score for the entire interview; available for free from www.rossinst.com/sample_forms.html
The Structured Clinical Interview for *DSM-IV* Dissociative Disorders – Revised (SCID-D; Steinberg, 1994)	Most widely used structured interview for dissociative disorders; evaluates the existence and severity of dissociative symptoms *Interviewer's Guide to the SCID-D* (Steinberg, 1994)

comorbid conditions that are present, improving adaptive functioning, restoring a psychological sense of safety and trust, protecting against relapse, and integrating the danger experienced into a constructive schema of risk, safety, prevention, and protection.

Because trauma aborts normal development and, consequently, interpersonal, professional, and educational opportunities are lost, assisting the person in restoring and promoting progress in the affected areas is important. Maturational social coping skills may be impaired, particularly for those who suffered trauma in childhood. McFarlane and van der Kolk (1996) observe that trauma causes the person to abandon hope because the person is unable to look beyond himself or herself to plan for the future. Clinical signs of recovery include being able to talk about the trauma without feeling upset or numb, functioning in daily life, feelings of being safe and confident, being in healthy relationships without feeling vulnerable, taking pleasure in life, having the ability to rely on self and others, experiencing minimal dissociation, managing emotions, feeling deserving, and being able to plan for the future.

Although these outcomes may seem daunting for patients who are chronically disempowered, they are achievable by following a progression of interventions that build on a strong foundation of safety and stabilization. Symptom outcome measures used for assessment can be used to track progress during treatment and to help determine whether the goals of treatment have been met. Tables 17.2 and 17.3 include dissociation and trauma assessment and outcome instruments.

Assessment

The assessment itself is therapeutic in that through the therapist's empathy, knowledge, and communication in the initial interview, the patient feels hopeful, and

TABLE 17.3 ASSESSMENT/OUTCOME INSTRUMENTS FOR TRAUMA	
Instrument	**Purpose and How to Obtain**
Impact of Event Scale-Revised (IES-R; Weiss & Marmar, 1997) PTSD Checklist for *DSM-5* (PCL-5; Weathers et al., 2013)	Most widely used self-report screening tool for single incident trauma; 22 items; included in Chapter 3, Assessment and Diagnosis 20 item self-report scale for screening for posttraumatic stress disorder (PTSD): www.ptsd.va.gov
Modified PTSD Symptom Scale: Self-Report Version (MPSS-SR; Falsetti, Resnick, Resick, & Kilpatrick, 1993)	Self-report 17-item checklist of PTSD symptoms; especially useful for patient with multiple traumas or when trauma history is unknown; does not key to a specific trauma Sherry Falsetti, PhD, Medical University of South Carolina, Crime Victims Research and Treatment Center, Medical University of North Carolina, 171 Ashley Ave., Charleston, SC 29425-0742
Trauma and Attachment Belief Scale (TABS; Pearlman, 2003)	Self-report scale that evaluates the needs and expectations of trauma survivors in relation to others; taps into underlying assumptions regarding relationships Western Psychological Services, 12031 Wilshire Blvd., Los Angeles, CA 90025-1251; telephone: 310-478-2061; fax: 310-478-7838; website: www.wpspublish.com
Primary Care PTSD Screen (PC-PTSD; Kimerling et al., 2006)	4-item screening tool for primary care and medical settings: www.mirecc.va.gov/docs/visn6/2_Primary_Care_PTSD_Screen.pdf
Short PTSD Rating Interview (SPRINT; Connor & Davidson, 2001)	8 items on a 5-point Likert scale measuring symptom severity and improvement since treatment; see Appendix 13.1 for tool
The structured interview for disorders of extreme stress (SIDES; Pelcovitz et al., 1997)	Clinician-administered 45-item tool that measures the symptom clusters of DESNOS: bvanderk@traumacenter.org HRI Trauma Center Research Dept. c/o Dr. J. Hopper 227 Babcock St. Brookline, MA 02116
The Clinician-Administered PTSD Scale (CAPS; Blake et al., 1995)	The most widely used clinician-administered structured interview for PTSD; assesses frequency and intensity of symptoms as well as effect on social and occupational functioning: www.ptsd.va.gov/professional/pages/assessments/assessment.asp Assessment Requests National Center for PTSD (116D) VA Medical Center 215 N. Main St. White River Junction, VT 05009

distress is diminished. Chapter 3 provides strategies that cultivate an assessment that is therapeutic. A thorough and accurate assessment includes selected appropriate assessment tools that help the APPN formulate a plan. Chapter 3 provides numerous instruments to use for screening and assessment. Chapter 24 provides a table of selected measures for outcome measurement. Assessment is ongoing throughout therapy as more is known about the patient and the therapist evaluates the effectiveness of interventions.

Given the ubiquity of trauma and the consequences of untreated trauma, all patients should be screened for trauma and dissociation; however, many professionals do not routinely do so, perhaps for a number of reasons. The clinician may be fearful of eliciting false memories by suggesting that trauma occurred or perhaps fearful of triggering pain and extreme emotional reactions, or the person may not remember whether the trauma did occur or the person may not reveal the trauma in the initial interview for fear of being emotionally overwhelmed and retraumatized or ashamed. Nonetheless, all patients should be screened for trauma and one way is to ask: "Have you ever suffered a situation or event as an adult or child that was highly disturbing and/or painful?" The use of common screening tools should be routine for all patients in your practice. These include the Dissociative Experiences Scale (DES) and the Adverse Childhood Experience (ACE) scale, both of which are included in Chapter 3, appendices.

Patients who score highly on the DES should be further evaluated by the Structured Clinical Interview for *DSM-IV* Dissociative Disorders (SCID-D) or the Dissociative Disorders Interview Schedule (DDIS). If a DD is present and you are not skilled in working with this population, it is best to either seek supervision from a therapist who is knowledgeable in this area or refer the patient to a clinician who is skilled in the treatment of these disorders because the patient may rapidly destabilize. Although the conventional wisdom is that these individuals need a prolonged period of stabilization before processing their trauma(s), a critical look at the research challenges this idea (De Jongh et al., 2016).

The Impact of Event Scale-Revised (IES-R) is the most widely used self-report screening tool for a specific trauma. The Short PTSD Rating Interview (SPRINT) is shorter and also screens for single incident traumatic symptoms. See Appendix 17.2 for the SPRINT and Appendix 3.4 for the IES. For patients with a high score on the IES and when significant trauma is suspected, more formal interview schedules are available and should be used. The Clinician-Administered PTSD Scale (CAPS) and the Structured Interview for Disorders of Extreme Stress (SIDES) are two such instruments, and each may require an hour or longer for completion. These interviews are especially useful if the trauma is in the past and the person is not currently distressed. The APPN should be careful not to reactivate trauma memories by encouraging the person to talk about the details of the trauma until stabilization is achieved.

Self-report measures include the Modified PTSD Symptom Scale: Self-Report Version (MPSS-SR) and the Trauma and Attachment Belief Scale (TABS). The former scale assesses all *DSM-5* criteria for PTSD for a single incident and the severity of the symptoms, whereas the latter does not key symptoms to any single traumatic event and measures disrupted cognitive schemas associated with complex trauma. The PTSD Checklist for *DSM-5* (PCL-5) is widely used as a screening tool for PTSD. All of the instruments discussed in this chapter have solid normative data, which means that they measure what they purport to measure and can be used and applied in various settings across situations for traumatized individuals.

Although all of these measures and the instruments in Tables 17.2 and 17.3 target specific symptoms and manifestations of dissociation and trauma, the effects of trauma are profound, pervasive, and wide ranging, and affect all dimensions of the person: emotional, intellectual, physical, relational, spiritual, vocational, environmental, and psychological. Holistic outcome measurements rather than symptom-specific instruments may more accurately reflect healing. Examples of measures reflecting holistic outcomes may include quality of life, self-efficacy, overall health status, connection to others (i.e., sense of belonging or social support), spiritual well-being, and resilience. These are listed in Chapter 24 and Table 24.2.

An important area of assessment is differentiating a thought disorder from a flashback if what appear to be psychotic symptoms are present. Flashbacks are trauma memories that come back as fragments: a sound, an image, a taste, an emotion, a scent, or a bodily sensation. Sometimes the flashback resembles a thought disorder. For example, one patient saw a naked woman on a bench. To determine whether this is trauma related, the APPN needs to know whether the content is about the trauma, is caused by a trigger, or is anxiety related and noninteractive. If the patient is observed talking or laughing to a person who is not there, he or she may be experiencing a hallucination rather than seeing an image related to a trauma. The patient knew that the naked woman was not real but said these images came to her at times, especially when she was tired or stressed. This is an important distinction between psychosis and flashbacks; if the person locates the image or object of interaction as coming from inside themselves, it is most likely a flashback and not considered a psychotic hallucination. By history, this patient had been sexually abused as a child in a cult, and the APPN concluded that the image was probably a flashback.

Sometimes, the patient with DID hears conversations going on in his or her head. The auditory hallucinations of 80% of DID patients are heard as emanating from inside the head, whereas for schizophrenic patients, 80% emanate from outside the person (Kluft, 1999). The voices for DID patients have a different quality from those of psychotic patients: the voices refer to a traumatic event; they are coherent; they often reflect an inner conversation among alternate personalities attempting to influence the identity; and they may be harsh and accusing but also may be comforting and helping (Kluft, 1999). In addition, the auditory halluncinations of DID are more like commentary, while in schizophrenia, they are more like one word or a command (Laddis & Dell, 2012). If the psychosis is transient and precipitated by a trigger or crisis, it most likely is not a thought disorder but is a flashback (Putnam, 1989). After the traumatic material is processed, the flashback will not be triggered again, in contrast to a hallucination, which is not affected by trauma processing. Visual hallucintations are also much more likely in DID and complex PTSD than in schizophrenia (Laddis & Dell, 2012).

Another particularly important area for assessment includes the presence of distorted cognitive schemas. Trauma affects patients' ideas about themselves and the world. This is especially true for adults who were traumatized as children and for children who have suffered interpersonal familial trauma. Because of basic cognitive immaturity and the normal egocentric viewpoint of children, the child who has been traumatized draws the conclusion that something is wrong with him or her. The child needs to preserve the idea that the caretaker is loving, because without an adult to care for the child, he or she would die, which is true for any immature mammal. The resulting negative schemas include self-blame, low self-esteem, trust and abandonment issues, need for control, difficulty setting boundaries, guilt, shame, helplessness, fear and yearning for dependency, and overall overestimation of danger in relationships and in the environment. These schemas persist into adulthood, embedded as a blueprint in the neural networks, and they are firmly entrenched in the person's way of thinking about himself or herself. Usually, these themes are readily apparent in sessions, but a more formalized assessment is provided by the TABS (see Table 17.3).

Constructing a Timeline

One method for assessing and organizing a trauma history is through constructing a timeline of the person's life. The APPN begins by explaining to the person that it is important to know both significant positive and negative events that have occurred in his or her life. The therapist draws a line on a piece of paper with the point at the beginning of the line, the person's birth date. The line is usually marked off in either 1-year or 5-year intervals to the present age depending on the age of the person.

Begin constructing the timeline by asking for factual information of events that occurred during the patient's early years such as siblings born, changes in schools or homes, early losses such as deaths of parents or grandparents, hospitalizations of self/parent, and so on. Some therapists begin with asking about important positive events/people that have made a significant impact on the person, and these are written above the line. The negative events that are elicited are stated below the line. It is important to structure this process in a way that will not require a great deal of detail about specific traumatic or disturbing events so that the person will not be triggered through the narrative. Once all positive and negative events are delineated on the timeline, the person is asked to rate each negative event on a 0 to 10 scale with 0 being no disturbance and 10 being the worst disturbance one can imagine. A timeline can be completed in one session for some people but often occurs over several sessions for those with more complex histories.

The timeline can also be used to clarify the person's psychiatric history and include times, dates, dosages of medications, symptoms, hospitalizations, and previous therapy or treatment. The advantage of collecting information in this way is that it creates a roadmap for treatment; is easy to explain to the patient; provides a quick visual for reference for the therapist and the patient as therapy progresses; helps the therapist assess positive memory networks and the presence of resources; promotes therapeutic rapport; and assists the person to form a narrative about his or her life experiences in a coherent way.

The pattern of events can also suggest the level of psychopathology. For example, if the person had many moves and changes in schools as a child, this may indicate family chaos and early developmental trauma. The timeline is dependent on the person's ability to remember and those who have suffered significant trauma may have a phobia of traumatic memory. Thus, if there are amnesic gaps in one's early years and there are no memories until age 20, this may indicate dissociation and significant trauma in one's childhood (Waters, 2016). It is of note that often all events, not just the abusive events, are forgotten. It is not until the trauma(s) are emotionally processed and remembered, that the person can remember positive events, too.

EVIDENCE-BASED INTERVENTIONS

There is consensus in the practice guidelines for PTSD that individual manualized trauma-focused psychotherapy, EMDR therapy, or CBT specifically prolonged exposure (PE) or cognitive processing therapy (CPT) are first-line interventions over pharmacological or other nonpharmacologic interventions (ISSTD, 2011; U.S. Department of Veterans Affairs, 2017; WHO, 2013), whereas other modalities are considered adjuncts to either of these approaches. A multidimensional meta-analysis revealed that most patients treated with CBT or EMDR therapy improve significantly (Bradley, Greene, Russ, Dutra, & Westen, 2005). However, further studies have found that exposure treatment for highly dissociative patients is not effective (Ebner-Priemer et al., 2009; Hagenaars, van Minnen, & Hoogduin, 2010). Box 17.3 provides resources for practice guidelines for trauma and dissociation.

BOX 17.3 Practice Guidelines for Trauma and Dissociation

Guidelines for the Evaluation and Treatment of Dissociative Symptoms in Children & Adolescents (International Society for the Study of Dissociation, 2004): www.isst-d.org/wp-content/uploads/2019/02/childguidelines-ISSTD-2003.pdf

Guidelines for Treating Dissociative Identity Disorder in Adults (International Society for the Study of Trauma and Dissociation [ISSTD], 2011): www.isstd.org/downloads/2011AdultTreatmentGuidelinesSummary.pdf

ISTSS PTSD Prevention and Treatment Guidelines for Complex PTSD (2018). Retrieved from https://istss.org/clinical-resources/treating-trauma/new-istss-prevention-and-treatment-guidelines

National Centre of Excellence for Complex Trauma: Practice Guidelines for Clinical Treatment of Complex Trauma (Blue Knot Foundation, 2019): www.blueknot.org.au/Portals/2/Practice%20Guidelines/BlueKnot_Practice_Guidelines_2019.pdf

Practice Guidelines for Identifying and Treating Complex Trauma-related Dissociation-May 2020: https://www.blueknot.org.au/Resources/Publications/Practice-Guidelines/Dissociation-Guidelines

VA/DoD Clinical Practice Guideline: Management of PTSD and Acute Stress Disorder (U.S. Department of Veterans Affairs, 2017): www.healthquality.va.gov/guidelines/MH/ptsd/VADoDPTSDCPGFinal012418.pdf

World Health Organization (WHO). Guidelines for the management of conditions specifically related to stress (WHO, 2013): apps.who.int/iris/bitstream/handle/10665/85119/9789241505406_eng.pdf;sequence=1

Practice guidelines for complex trauma and DID (Blue Knot Foundation, 2019; ISSTD, 2011) stress the importance of stabilization; the 2019 National Centre of Excellence developed by the Blue Knot Foundation in Australia noted that resilience and relationship trump technique. These guidelines confirm the centrality of managing physiological arousal and caution that talk therapies that emphasize "top-down" approaches or cognitive understanding limit one's ability to heal. That is, somatic approaches or a "bottom-up" nontraditional approach based on polyvagal theory (PVT) confirms the link between emotion and physiology and points to somatic stimulation as an emerging psychotherapeutic method for treating complex trauma (Blue Knot Foundation, 2019; Church, 2015). Please see Chapter 7 for EMDR therapy that includes a somatic phase in the protocol plus Chapter 11 for the Trauma Resilience Model that is a somatic therapy based on Peter Levine's (1997) somatic experiencing therapy. The National Centre of Excellence for Complex Trauma guidelines (Blue Knot Foundation, 2019) have been endorsed by numerous international practice guidelines such as the ISSTD, the Trauma and Dissociation Israel Organization, and the Clinic for Dissociative Studies in London in addition to numerous individuals who are trauma experts throughout the world.

Body and Energy Work

Although not evidence based, body and energy work are sometimes important adjuncts to trauma treatment. A number of trauma experts advocate using body therapies because trauma memories are stored in the brain and manifested in the body (Howell, 2020; Levine, 1997; Rothschild, 2017; Scaer, 2005; van der Kolk, 2014). van der Kolk (2003) reasons that because adults typically process information in a top-down manner from the cortex (thinking brain) to the amygdala (emotional brain), bottom-up therapy from the emotional brain to the thinking brain is important to access trauma memories in a more efficient way. Because psychotherapy is largely a left-brain cortex activity, body therapies are thought to be more likely to be effective and access areas involved where implicit memory is stored (amygdala). Also, body therapies enable ventral vagal modulation with attention to the body and breathing (Porges & Dana, 2018). This helps the person to become more comfortable with body sensations which previously may be experienced as threatening.

Body and energy work to bring the body back into conscious awareness may be needed if the person has somatic problems. Scaer (2005) says these individuals are parasympathetic dominant and suggests a number of body-based therapies for healing. These include somatic experiencing (SE), as described in Levine's book, *Walking the Tiger* (1997), and energy therapies, such as thought field therapy (TFT) and emotional freedom therapy (EFT), which use visual imagery, self-affirmations, and tapping on acupressure points. Movement therapies such as dance and other induced movement techniques, including touch, cranial sacral techniques, and gentle massage, may also be useful. Artistic endeavors such as sculpting, drawing, and painting can tap into right-brain states and may also be helpful. None of these methods are considered a sole evidence-based treatment for trauma. EMDR therapy is the only Level A evidence-based treatment that does have a somatic component.

The Trauma Resilience Model (TRM) has promising research and is primarily a somatic model of therapy. Please see Chapter 11. This model incorporates the resource building skills of the Community Resilience Model (CRM) with additional processing skills of pendulation, titration, and completion of the survival response. Foundational for stabilizing the nervous system is tracking, which means the person is able to sense what is happening inside his or her body (interoceptive awareness). Based on Porges's PVT, a form is included in Appendix 17.1 that helps the person to begin to notice nuances of internal sensations (tracking) and to link these to either immobilization or mobilization states of the nervous system. See Chapter 2 for further information about PVT and https://www.rhythmofregulation.com/resources/Beginner%27s%20Guide. pdf for A Beginner's Guide to Polyvagal Theory.

Cognitive Behavioral Strategies for Stabilization

There are many CBT strategies that are helpful for building in resources and stabilization (see Chapter 8). The APPN introduces, teaches, and practices with the patient in sessions. *Seeking Safety: A Treatment Manual for PTSD and Substance Abuse* by Najavits (2002), *The Anxiety and Phobia Workbook* by Bourne (2010), and *Coping With Trauma-Related Dissociation* (Boon, Steele, & van der Hart, 2011) are excellent resources for the APPN to use to assist the patient in developing these skills.

Stress inoculation therapy (SIT) is a type of CBT that emphasizes education, skill building, and application. SIT is also helpful in stabilization. SIT can be particularly helpful for those patients who have phobic avoidance due to trauma. For example, a patient may be fearful about leaving the house because of fear that an accident may occur. The APPN using SIT teaches the patient thought stopping, quieting, and guided self-dialogue and then assists the patient by following the steps outlined in Box 17.4.

BOX 17.4 Steps in Stress Inoculation

- Assess the probability of the feared event
- Use thought stopping and the quieting reflex
- Control self-criticism with guided self-dialogue
- Use role-playing and covert modeling
- Use self-reinforcement for skills

Cognitive processing, unlike emotional processing, can be safely done in the stabilization stage (Brand, 2001). Later in stage 2 (processing), more detailed and affective exploration can be done. Cognitive processing may be necessary to keep the person safe because trauma-induced beliefs contribute to safety problems. For example, many patients feel that they are bad and deserve to be punished for their abuse. Resolving or at least modifying the self-hatred and misattribution of blame underlying these beliefs is important before emotional processing, which may destabilize the person. Chapter 8 provides useful CBT strategies to modify this type of thinking, such as guided self-dialogue, thought stopping, cognitive restructuring, Socratic dialogue, labeling of distortions, questioning the evidence, reattribution, decatastrophizing, automatic thought record, and listing of advantages and disadvantages.

Another important adjunct to treatment is dialectical behavior therapy (DBT), which is discussed in Chapter 18. DBT was specifically developed for patients diagnosed with borderline personality disorder (BPD) and has great utility for all those who have difficulty with affect management. An important goal of DBT is to teach patients the skills needed for managing emotions, with mindfulness a key component of the treatment. DBT groups are offered in most major cities, and the therapist can refer a patient to a DBT group and/or use exercises with patients during individual sessions from *Skills Training Manual for Borderline Personality Disorder* by Linehan (1993b). A group provides the opportunity for the patient to gain valuable insights through support and feedback from others. In tandem with individual psychotherapy, group work is effective in developing affect management skills.

Group Therapy

Research on group treatment for PTSD is limited, but groups have been used for psychoeducation, cognitive therapy, psychodynamic therapy, supportive therapy, and exposure therapy (Ruzek, Young, & Walser, 2003). See Chapter 12. Group work is considered a useful adjunct to individual CBT or EMDR, and current findings do not support one type of group over another. Group therapy is thought to help the person cope with feelings of isolation, alienation, and anhedonia that are common for patients who have suffered significant trauma.

Debriefing

Debriefing involves talking about the trauma immediately after the event and is referred to as critical incident, stress debriefing, or some variation of these terms. Although debriefing is sometimes used, the APA practice guidelines do not support its efficacy (APA, 2009) and state that debriefing or single session techniques may increase symptoms and are ineffective for those with ASD and do not prevent PTSD. This may, in part, reflect the fact that subjects in these research studies did not choose whether to participate in the debriefing. Perhaps those who *choose* to participate would be more likely to benefit.

Miller-Karas (2015) reconceptualizes debriefing through a resilience lens and suggests that the following questions are helpful after a critical incident. This helps the person to stay in their resilient zone while answering questions about survival.

- Who helped you the most in the beginning?
- Can you remember the moment that help arrived?
- Can you remember the moment that you knew you were going to survive?
- Who else made it through?
- What gives you the strength to get through this now?
- When you have experienced other difficult times in your life, what or who helped you get through?
- Who is helping you the most now?
- What is helping you get through now?

Psychodynamic Psychotherapy

Research on psychodynamic psychotherapy for the treatment of trauma and dissociation is relatively sparse compared with that for CBT or EMDR therapy. Chapter 5, addresses methodological issues in psychodynamic research. The value of using psychodynamic psychotherapy for working with traumatized patients lies in the clinician's understanding of transference, countertransference, and resistance. Psychodynamic psychotherapy involves the activation of attachment relationships and interpersonal processes, but psychodynamic psychotherapy, unlike CBT, strives to deepen the person's understanding about how trauma has affected these processes. It may be particularly helpful to use psychodynamic approaches with patients who present with attachment and interpersonal difficulties with less specific memories of the trauma. As the interpersonal difficulties are connected with the trauma, the APPN may shift to more CBT strategies to build coping, distress tolerance, and functional skills. Through constructing a narrative, patients examine the meaning of the trauma experience in their lives. This can be enormously strengthening for the individual. Leichsenring and Steinert (2019) conclude in their comprehensive review of psychodynamic research that more randomized clinical trials are needed to describe outcomes among different populations of survivors.

A FRAMEWORK FOR TREATMENT

Given the complexity of responses to trauma, a framework for using psychotherapeutic interventions needs to address the bewildering symptoms and deficits that result, particularly when there has been severe and prolonged trauma. The treatment hierarchy outlined in Chapter 1 provides the framework for treatment (see Figure 1.8). This is a stage-oriented treatment model consistent with Porges's PVT and evidence-based models included in practice guidelines for trauma and dissociation (Blue Knot Foundation, 2019). Stage 1, safety and symptom stabilization, involves increasing external and internal resources, and stage 2 aims to process the painful memories so that the person can move toward enhancing future visioning. As trauma is processed, the person begins to expand his or her world from surviving the present to planning for the future. The final stage focuses on continued integration, rehabilitation, and personal growth. Educational, social, and vocational life skills may be needed that the person might have missed during aborted developmental periods when traumas occurred. This framework is based on the neuroscience underlying the adaptive information processing (AIP) model.

Beginning With Safety

To begin the healing process, decisions are made concerning where to target interventions based on a comprehensive assessment of the strengths and resources the person already has. Chapter 1 introduces PVT and the importance of neurophysiological equanimity for a felt sense of safety. Safety is always a priority in the stabilization stage, and crisis intervention may be needed. In general, the more urgent and basic the person's needs are on Maslow's hierarchy, the more directive the APPN's interventions. Physical safety and psychological stability must be ensured before discussing traumatic material. A Stabilization Checklist, included in Appendix 1.5, records indicators that should for the most part be accomplished in stage 1 before moving to stage 2 processing.

This checklist is intended to serve as a guide; thus, not every indicator must be met, but good clinical judgment based on these parameters is essential.

In stage 1 (stabilization), the therapist most often does not seek insight to accomplish therapeutic gains. Confrontation with family or others who deny the trauma is not encouraged. The therapist assists the patient in naming the problem, reframing asking for help as a sign of courage, and helping the person restore control. The APPN focus is on coping, distress tolerance, and stress management skills that build the patient's resources and self-efficacy while providing a safe structure for the therapeutic frame. As the work of stabilization continues, the therapeutic relationship is strengthened, and trust is developed.

In general, the patient's resources and the traumas experienced need to be balanced; that is, the greater the level of trauma, more resources may be needed to manage the deleterious effect of trauma on functioning. However, the number of traumas and trauma history do not necessarily dictate the number of resources needed. The person may have a significant history of trauma and many cumulative negative experiences, but this may be offset by the quality and quantity of his or her positive experiences and relationships. Positive experiences are essential so that the person can manage the state changes that are essential in trauma processing (Shapiro, 2018). van der Kolk (2006) agrees and says: "it is important to explore previous experiences of safety and competency and to activate memories of what it feels like to experience pleasure, enjoyment, focus, power and effectiveness, before activating trauma-related sensations and emotions" (p. 289). This speaks to the importance of increasing resources so that adaptive positive networks are present. Some patients may need positive experiences created particularly if they are resource impoverished and have an early history of neglect and trauma.

External resources are enhanced through case management techniques and supportive psychotherapy. Case management requires an active approach on the part of the therapist because the patient may need to be connected to nurturing and caring people and appropriate community resources such as rehabilitation or crisis center, child protection agency, a substance abuse or eating disorder program, or residential, partial hospital, or inpatient treatment. The APPN encourages the person to maintain functioning at work, home, or school and to cultivate and maintain supportive relationships. An excellent resource for case management is *Seeking Safety: A Treatment Manual for PTSD and Substance Abuse* by Najavits (2002). See Appendix 1.4 for a Treatment and Case Management Form. Crucial to case management is the ability of the therapist to set limits, to assess regressive and adaptive shifts in ego functioning, and to recognize conflict to help the person assuage anxiety without emphasizing interpretation.

Of particular concern is providing safety and protecting the person from self-harm. Affect dysregulation is cited as the most frequent reason for self-harm and self-mutilation, and patients often report that self-mutilation is an attempt to self-soothe (Blue Knot Foundation, 2019). The National Comorbidity Study found that PTSD was associated with a sixfold increase in the likelihood of an initial suicide attempt (Kessler, Borges, & Walters, 1999). This is higher than that for any other anxiety disorder. Numerous studies have found that childhood abuse is strongly associated with self-injury (Stien & Kendall, 2006; Waters, 2016). Self-injury may take the form of eating disorders, cutting, unsafe sexual practices, driving recklessly, alcohol or substance abuse, violent relationships, and parasuicidal behaviors. These behaviors are thought to be an attempt to self-regulate in that opioids are released.

Chapters 3 and 4 describe assessment for suicide and self-harm. Safety issues must be addressed directly and a plan established if necessary. As Chu (2011) observes, many survivors of childhood abuse are *addicted to crisis* and feel most alive when out of control.

These are sometimes the patients who want to rush into recovering memories before a foundation of safety is established. Such a strategy is doomed to failure as the person cycles through periods of intense emotions that alternate with numbing. Self-care and symptom control are foundational to the work of recovering memories and processing.

An important caveat regarding safety is that if the therapist primarily focuses on self-harm behaviors in the treatment, this may reinforce these behaviors. It is far better to provide minimal attention to self-harm behaviors and focus more on consequences and remediation so that the person is not rewarded with increased attention and therapist concern by being out of control. Identification of triggers for self-harm behaviors and education about other opioid-enhancing activities, such as exercise and self-soothing strategies, are essential to avert these cycles of self-harm. Linehan's (1993b) *Skills Training Manual for Borderline Personality Disorder* describes treatment strategies effective for working with parasuicidal behaviors. Please see Chapter 18.

Because comorbid disorders are prevalent, particularly in chronic PTSD, treatment interventions must be prioritized. What does the person need first to function and be safe? For example, many traumatized women suffer from panic attacks that are quite debilitating, and treatment initially may need to focus on how to manage these episodes. Helpful strategies may include psychoeducation, medication, making connections between symptoms and catastrophic self-statements, monitoring the attacks, rating the level of the anxiety, and developing coping strategies for when they occur. Coping strategies include abdominal breathing, muscle relaxation, distraction, and coping statements to counter negative self-talk.

For men who have suffered trauma, the priority may be anger management if aggression and violence are in the foreground initially. Anger management strategies may be necessary to ensure the safety of the patient and others. These methods may include psychoeducation, writing, drawing, painting, making a collage, cost–benefit analysis of anger, self-reflection and awareness of triggers, putting anger into words, distraction and self-soothing strategies, taking a time-out, enhancing the ability to communicate, channeling anger, exercise or physical work, relaxation strategies, and thought-stopping strategies (Boon et al., 2011).

There has been some controversy regarding whether to treat comorbid disorders such as alcohol abuse with PTSD simultaneously or separately. Current thinking provides an integrative model so that treatment focuses on both disorders. Without integrating stabilization strategies, exposure of the person to traumatic memories may intensify the need to use substances and trigger relapse. Self-medication with substances then may increase the person's risk to future trauma exposure. Because of the interdependent relationship between substance abuse and trauma, addressing out-of-control behaviors is a prerequisite for trauma treatment. This may entail a longer period of stabilization and eventually processing in small increments so that affect regulation is ensured. In any case, a first goal of treatment for those abusing substances is to reduce the abuse. For alcohol abuse, a 12-step program is usually part of the recommended treatment. See Chapter 19 for psychotherapeutic approaches for addictions.

Safety in the Therapeutic Relationship

The importance of safety in the therapeutic relationship cannot be overemphasized. The therapeutic alliance cultivates a healing environment for emotional safety and allows the patient to continue therapy and benefit from treatment. This relationship also fosters the patient's capacity toward building a healthy support system. Chapters 3 and 4 provide strategies for building a therapeutic alliance. Early implicit memories are activated in therapy and counterconditioning occurs; that is, the patient experiences fear-diminishing emotional states in the context of the therapist's positive regard, compassion, and caring attention (Briere & Scott, 2013; Chu, 2011). However, traumatized patients may have particular difficulty forming a therapeutic alliance, and trust issues are often fraught with anxiety. Often, these patients have been betrayed by those who were trusted and flee into isolation when faced with painful and overwhelming feelings that occur during therapy.

The term *traumatic transference* has been coined and refers to the particular transference constellations that form for those who have suffered childhood abuse (ISSTD, 2011). Therapy may begin to erode dissociative barriers and defenses, leading to greater intrusion of traumatic memories, and the person may fear loss of control due to increased awareness of disturbing emotions and cognitions. Thus, there may be fear and vulnerability that abuse and/or manipulation may occur as in childhood. The APPN who works with these individuals must be prepared to be the object of the person's anger and suspicion and he or she may even begin to feel as the patient feels: abused, enmeshed, helpless, and violated.

Even experienced therapists often seek supervision when working with those with complex trauma because transference and countertransference issues may be quite intense. Those who have suffered childhood abuse often have had chaotic relationships with caretakers who were supposed to love and protect them, and being close to others represents a threat, not a comfort. The therapeutic relationship offers a corrective emotional experience through collaborative support and connection. However, Chu (2011) cautions that therapy with those who have been significantly traumatized is not just about taking care of patients and that these individuals cannot be loved into health. Maintaining firm boundaries, setting limits, and explaining the inherent difficulties the person may encounter with trust are essential to promote a safe environment.

Patients with current trauma might have had previous complex traumas from the past that have shaped personality and are entangled with the present. They may need attention and longer-term intervention with cognitive behavior, psychodynamic, and interpersonal psychotherapies. Horowitz (2003) says these patients have themes that revolve around excessive fear of future victimization, enduring and irrational shame over vulnerability or incompetence, unusually intense anger and impulses for revenge, extreme sensitivity to guilt, and low thresholds for despair with an expectation of being abandoned. These themes may have reverberated in the person's life before the trauma, and through the work in resolving the present symptoms, the person may gain personal strengths and reduce prior personality conflicts.

The person's ability to tolerate painful affects and his or her strengths, resources, and coping skills are additional areas important to evaluate when targeting interventions. A primary goal of the stabilization stage is to attain self-regulation of internal states of arousal. What coping skills have worked for the person in the past? Often, the coping skills the person used as a child included dissociation, and although this was effective at the time for the child, it interferes significantly with adult functioning. What helps the person to relieve anxiety? After assessing current coping skills, new skills may need to be taught (see Appendix 1.2). Internal resources often need to be increased before processing. Internal resources are less tangible than external resources and include the person's ability to manage positive and negative emotions (i.e., affect regulation), symptom control, a sense of inner strength (i.e., ego strength), and a belief in himself or herself. Affect management skills can be learned, practiced and, over time, lead to internalization of self-soothing capacities.

MINDFULNESS

Because those who have suffered significant trauma have decreased activation of the prefrontal cortex under stress, strategies such as mindfulness that activate this area are extremely important to enhance control over emotions. See Chapter 11 for the neuroscience of mindfulness. Mindfulness underlies all stabilization and is an important skill to teach patients needing internal resources. Mindfulness is described as internal and having external awareness in abundance while dissociation is the deficiency of internal and external awarenss or as Forner (2017) states: "One is a basic function that is designed to know; the other is a brain function that is designed to not know" (p. xv). Mindfulness allows patients to become fully aware of their experiences and enables them to respond, rather than just react, to experiences. Jon Kabat-Zinn is credited with popularizing mindfulness and developing evidence-based protocols for use with chronic illness (Kabat-Zinn & Kabat-Zinn, 1990). Both DBT and TRM incorporate mindfulness and teach the importance of staying grounded in the moment and acceptance of oneself without judgment.

Although research supports the efficacy of mindfulness for a wide range of mental health problems numerous methodological considerations have been raised regarding the extant mindfulness research. These include the lack of clarity of the definition of mindfulness; the lack of specific terminology in the self-report questionnaires, and the inconsistency of clinical applications (van Dam et al., 2017). Despite this, mindfulness has been widely integrated and used in most psychotherapeutic approaches. An excellent resource for guided meditations that can be incorporated into sessions is *Guided Meditations, Explorations, and Healings* by Stephen Levine (1991). This book includes the loving kindness meditation and specific readings for addiction, pain, overwhelming emotional states, and grief. After using these techniques in sessions, the patient can begin to practice between sessions as a way to cultivate mindfulness at home.

It is helpful if the APPN learns and practices mindfulness first prior to teaching to patients. The teaching is then anchored in real experience, and it helps to protect the APPN from the secondary trauma that can occur from working with traumatized patients and bearing witness to violence or trauma. Professional training is available through workshops, conferences, and certification programs. Information about these workshops can be found through an Internet search on mindfulness-based professional stress-reduction training programs. An excellent free mindfulness certificate course is available for 8 weeks based on Kabat Zinn's Mindfulness-Based Stress Reduction program. Table 17.4 lists mindfulness resources and tapes.

Some patients have difficulty understanding the concept of mindfulness and may relate better to the terms *focusing* or *noticing*. Focusing on the breath may be a helpful starting point for some patients. Slow, deep breathing with exhalation twice as long as inhalation facilitates the parasympathetic nervous system and prevents further dissociation. The APPN has most likely taught patients in the hospital to deep breathe with abdominal muscles. This is similar and combined with instructions to notice the breath while staying in the moment and asking patients to place their hands on the abdomen; if done correctly, the hands will rise as breath is inhaled. It is most effective if the APPN does this with the person to illustrate the technique. This should be practiced for 10 minutes daily at a specific time during the day with no distractions. Breathing exercises assist the person in developing mindfulness, which aids in the identification of triggers and in modulating flashbacks. Progressive muscle relaxation may also be helpful and involves clenching and relaxing muscles from head to toe; this exercise is explained in Appendix 17.2. A caveat regarding progressive muscle relaxation is that it can lead to increased arousal and dissociation in a minority of patients. This may

TABLE 17.4 SELECTED MINDFULNESS RESOURCES

Resource	Description	Source
Educational Websites		
Palouse Mindfulness	8-week free online certification course based on Kabat-Zinn's Mindfulness-Based Stress Reduction program	palousemindfulness.com
Mindsight Institute	Daniel Siegel MD's educational organization that offers seminars, programs, and workshops on mindfulness	MindsightInstitute.com
Mindful Awareness Research Center (MARC)	UCLA research center devoted to identifying, evaluating, and disseminating mindfulness practices	www.uclahealth.org/marc
Books		
Mindfulness-Based Cognitive Therapy (MBCT)	The anxiety and stress solution deck: 55 CBT and mindfulness tips	Woods, Rockman, & Collins (2019)
Thoughts without a thinker: Psychotherapy from a Buddhist perspective	An expert account of the wedding of Buddhism & psychology	Epstein (2013)
Beginning Meditation Books		
	Wherever you go, there you are: mindfulness meditation in everyday life	Kabat-Zinn (2005)
	Complete introduction to "insight" meditation with bestselling author	*Meditation for Beginners by Jack Kornfield:* https://jackkornfield.com
	Real-world mindfulness for beginners: Navigate daily life one practice at a time	Salgado (2016)
Tapes		
Jon Kabat-Zinn Mindfulness for Beginners	Audiotape in enhanced digital book with five guided mindfulness meditations	Sounds True.com
Meditations for Everyday Mindfulness by Beryl Bender Birch	Award-winning audiotapes with guided imagery, 66-minute evidence-based practice of deep relaxation and meditation	Order from 1-888-NOW RELAX

be because in the person's brain a hypervigilant state has essentially served to keep the person safe so that relaxation triggers a physiological state of intense anxiety about being not safe. See at the end of Box 17.6 how to practice and teach deep breathing strategies to avert physiological arousal.

Mindfulness is helpful for patients in developing dual awareness. Dual awareness means being able to maintain awareness of more than one experience at a time, allowing the person to maintain a sense of the present here and now while experiencing sensations from the past then and there. Modulation through dual awareness is essential so that the person can control the level of hyperarousal and not be overwhelmed. Dual awareness activates the frontal lobes, which mediates arousal of the limbic system. This mechanism is compromised in those who have been severely traumatized in that internal sensations are associated with past events and reality is evaluated based on this restricted information (Siegel, 2010). The past becomes the present, and the person feels as if the event is happening now, with all the attendant hyperarousal that may be retraumatizing. See Box 17.5 for strategies that help to develop dual awareness.

Another useful strategy in developing dual awareness is rating the level of disturbance. In the session, the patient is asked to think of a mildly disturbing event and to rate his or her subjective unit of disturbance (SUD) on a scale of 0 to 10, with 10 being the worst they can imagine feeling and 0 being equal to no disturbance. After the rating is obtained, the therapist does deep breathing or progressive muscle relaxation exercises, or both, with the patient and asks him or her to turn the number lower, repeating this sequence several times. After the patient feels confident in the session, transferring this skill to home can be suggested as a homework exercise.

BOX 17.5 Dual Awareness Strategies

Ask the patient to remember a recent mildly distressing event, something where he or she was slightly anxious or embarrassed.

- What do you notice in your body?
- What happens in your muscles?
- What happens in your gut?
- How does your breathing change?
- Does your heart rate increase or decrease?
- Do you become warmer or colder?
- Is there any change in temperature?
- Is it uniform or variable in different parts of your body?

Then bring your awareness back into this room you are in now. Notice the color of the walls, the texture of the rug.

- What is the temperature of this room?
- What do you smell here?
- Does your breathing change as your focus of awareness changes?

Now try to keep awareness of your present surroundings while you remember that slightly distressing event.

- Is it possible for you to maintain awareness of where you are physically as you remember that event?
- End the exercise with your awareness focused on your current surroundings.

Source: Rothschild, B. (2000). *The body remembers: The psychopathology of trauma and trauma treatment* (p. 131). New York, NY: W. W. Norton.

MANAGING PHYSIOLOGICAL AROUSAL

For significantly traumatized patients, especially those with attachment trauma or severe and prolonged trauma, affect dysregulation is chronic, and deficits in arousal are present in the sympathetic nervous system (i.e., hyperarousal) and the parasympathetic nervous system (i.e., dissociation and underarousal). The underdeveloped cortex is unable to modulate and inhibit lower parts of the brain. These physiological changes occur in the brain and result in an autonomic signature in the body (Schore, 2019). Physiological arousal in general can trigger trauma-related memories, and conversely, trauma-related memories can precipitate generalized physiological arousal. It is thought that flashbacks and nightmares cause repeated release of stress hormones, which further entrenches the strength of the memory (van der Kolk, 2014).

The person may fluctuate rapidly between hyperarousal and hypoarousal with both the patient and the clinician confused about whether the person is in their resilient zone (window of tolerance) as depicted in Figure 1.3. There may be a very narrow resilient zone (RZ) so that the challenge for the APPN is to help the person widen their zone through relationship, safety, mindfulness, dual awareness, creating or strengthening resources, safe/calm place, and stress management exercises. See Chapter 11 for the Community Resilience Model (CRM) skills specifically developed to enhance the RZ. Decreasing emotional arousal is critical so that the person can manage triggers and reduce symptoms. If the person's level of disturbance is reported as greater than a 7 on the SUD scale, the person may not have access to their frontal lobes at that moment. At these times, anxiety and arousal are hyperattenuated, and the person may have difficulty assuaging anxiety and calming himself or herself.

A safe/calm place exercise is useful in decreasing autonomic arousal and is included in Appendix 1.7. The safe/calm place exercise can be practiced in the session with the patient and practiced as homework during the following week. Some patients may have difficulty with this exercise, and this response can be diagnostic in that there may not be anywhere that the person feels is or has been experienced as safe. Sometimes, attempting to relax may stimulate hyperarousal, which is counterproductive to the process. Explaining to patients that the safe/calm place can be an imagined place or a place they find relaxing or comfortable rather than safe may be helpful in accessing a calming image. Another way to use the safe/calm place is to ask for an image of a person with whom they feel safe and take the patient through the process of accessing somatic sensations related to being in the presence of someone connected with positive memories. This safe person can be an imagined person or a celebrity. One patient developed an Oprah image next to her as her safe person. It is helpful to close each session with the person's safe/calm place or person exercise. With regular practice, the safe/calm place lowers arousal levels, decreases biological reactivity, provides self-soothing, facilitates processing, and assists patients in leaving the session safely and calmly.

Stress management and affect-regulation strategies enhance internal resources so that arousal levels can be decreased. Often, those who have been significantly traumatized are alexithymic and cannot express their internal states. Expressive therapies such as art and movement may be safe ways for those who have difficulty in this area. Chapter 2 provides strategies for how to work with patients who have alexithymia. An important point about resource building is that nothing works for everyone all the time and that some things work better than others for certain patients. Understanding what works for this person at this time is essential, coupled with collaboration, trial and error, practice, and patience. The APPN helps the person develop a repertoire of skills that are readily available. The Weekly Plan for Increasing Resources from Chapter 1 is included in Appendix 1.2, and it is a helpful starting point for stress management so that resources can be identified that can reduce hyperarousal and enhance the person's sense of mastery. The patient may already be doing some of these techniques, and the APPN should review with the patient which strategies are already in place and then assist the person to choose an activity to focus on and practice the following week.

It is important for the APPN to provide a holding environment through the relationship with the person because it may be a bit daunting to see what is supposed to be done in the Weekly Plan for Increasing Resources when the patient is already feeling overwhelmed. Explain to the patient that the list represents a menu of all suggested strategies and that the focus will be on the one per week that will be most helpful at this time. Some items are more appropriate than others, depending on the person's problems, current resources, and preference and on the therapist's level of knowledge and skill in teaching selected techniques. For some patients, it may be preferable to use the blank Weekly Goal Worksheet in Appendix 1.3 and fill in a few activities because the person may be overwhelmed by the use of such a comprehensive list. In any case, the plan can then be revisited later as different strategies may be added that may be more appropriate as therapy progresses.

Box 17.6 describes selected strategies that facilitate the creation of new resources and strengthening of existing resources for a more robust RZ. Many of these are included in the Weekly Plan for Increasing Resources. Soothing activities might include smoothing on warm body lotion, taking a shower or bath, taking a long walk, looking at a tank full of fish swimming, looking at the sky, mindfully eating something delicious, gardening, and massaging feet or scalp. Deep breathing, progressive muscle relaxation, meditation, mindfulness, and yoga can also decrease arousal. Practicing these skills and helping the person access audiotapes, CDs, DVDs, videotapes, and books to be used to reinforce resources are important adjuncts to treatment. The patient can keep a daily log of the practice to track progress on the Weekly Plan for Increasing Resources or the Weekly Goal Worksheet. These strategies help to regulate the autonomic nervous system as do other strategies based on PVT that are included in Table 17.5.

BOX 17.6 Creating Resources

- Actual positive memories
- Circle of strength; see Appendix 7.2 (Chapter 7)
- Internalize a helper (real or pretend)
- Safe/calm place; see Appendix 1.7 (Chapter 1)
- Awareness of triggers; see Appendix 17.1
- Rating negative feelings on a 1 to 10 scale
- Soothing activities
- Basic self-care
- Yoga
- Progressive muscle relaxation; see Appendix 17.2
- Guided imagery
- Container; Appendix 1.8 (Chapter 1)
- Distancing/dual awareness
- Grounding; see Appendix 11.1
- Cognitive restructuring; see Table 8.5 (Chapter 8)
- Meditation/mindfulness
- Community Resilience Model Skills; see Appendix 11.1 (Chapter 11)
- Deep breathing*

---

*First introduce equal inhalation and exhalation as a deep inhalation may trigger a sympathetic response; then a longer, slower exhalation. Sighing is a parasympathetic response.

TABLE 17.5 STRATEGIES TO REGULATE THE AUTONOMIC NERVOUS SYSTEM		
Movement	**Sound**	**Touch**
Changing posture	Music	Tapping
Rocking chair	Prosody (soothing tone of voice)	Weighted blanket
Therapy ball	Conversation	Shawl
Soothing gestures	Hum or sing	Butterfly hug
Exercise	Chanting/praying	Massage
Dancing	Drumming	Grounding

Managing Flashbacks

Because flashbacks and dissociative periods cannot be reliably predicted, various strategies for when they occur can be helpful. These include identifying the phenomenon as a flashback or dissociative period and grounding techniques. *Grounding* means bringing the person's level of awareness to the immediate therapeutic environment by noticing things in the present (Miller-Karas, 2015): rubbing the upholstery on a chair, making sure the room is properly lighted, good eye contact, counting beads, stomping one's feet, touching an object such as a ring or watch that has been designated a safe object, deep breathing, playing with pets, exercising, taking a shower, holding an ice cube, walking outside, or supportive self-talk. An example of supportive self-talk may be repeatedly saying: "This is old stuff. I am scared right now. My feelings come and go. I am safe now. That was then. This is now. Take a deep breath, exhale long, and slow down."

After dual awareness and grounding skills are in place, further mindfulness strategies can be taught by asking patients to notice what happens during those times when they dissociate or have flashbacks. What happened before? What were they feeling physically and emotionally? What is the last thing they remember? How did they know they were dissociating? What were they trying to avoid? What else could they do? These types of questions assist the person in the development of nonjudgmental observation and enhanced awareness so that environmental triggers can be replaced with more adaptive ways of responding. As one patient reported after practicing mindfulness over a few months: "I'm onto myself now."

When working with the patient, consideration should be given to where the person is in the change process to aim interventions toward behavioral change. Chapter 9 explains the stages of change and appropriate interventions for each stage. If imagery is used that can be helpful in moving toward the contemplation phase of change, the person may experience dramatic relief through experiencing and expressing feelings about loss and change. However, the APPN should help the person modulate the intensity of the experience by naming the experience, rating the level of disturbance (0–10 scale) but not encourage detailed remembering of the trauma. After the patient has moved into the contemplation stage, the therapist helps the person to focus on the discrepancy between now and the way the person would like things to be. This can be accomplished through exploring questions. "How would you like things to be different in the future?" "What's keeping you from doing things you want to do?" "How does your current behavior fit into your future goals?"

SLEEP HYGIENE AND MEDICATION

Hyperarousal often compromises sleep and is discussed in Chapter 2. The nightmares that occur for the traumatized person may reflect the brain's unsuccessful attempt to integrate traumatic material into procedural memory networks (Shapiro, 2018). Because sleep disturbances are common for those who have suffered significant trauma and because they compromise daily functioning, good sleep hygiene, behavioral interventions, and medication may be indicated once other interventions proved to be ineffective. Sleep hygiene recommendations include exercising regularly; avoiding napping, nicotine, caffeine, alcohol, and heavy meals 4 to 6 hours before bedtime; maintaining a quiet, cool bedroom and a regular bedtime; using the bed for sleep or sex only; engaging in relaxing activities, and avoiding TV, computer and all screen time before bedtime. Behavioral strategies include progressive muscle relaxation exercises (see Appendix 17.3), paradoxical interventions (see Chapter 4) biofeedback, and CBT strategies (see Chapter 8).

Recommended medications for insomnia due to PTSD include nonbenzodiazepines such as eszopiclone (Lunesta) as well as risperidone and olanzapine as adjunct therapy for treating PTSD-related insomnia and nightmares (Lipinska, Baldwin, & Thomas, 2016). If the patient is already on an antidepressant, an antipsychotic, or mood stabilizer, switching from twice a day dosing to bedtime dosing may be helpful. If nightmares are present, prazosin (Minipress) should be considered. Melatonin and melatonin receptor agonists are sometimes helpful. It is important for the APPN to differentiate whether the insomnia is sleep avoidance rather than true insomnia. Medication may exacerbate sleep avoidance, or the patient may not take the medication. If the patient describes true fatigue and drowsiness when he or she goes to bed but becomes agitated or cognitively active, self-soothing and environmental safety strategies may be more effective than sedative hypnotics.

In addition to the affect management and coping skills discussed earlier, medication may be needed to decrease hyperarousal. However, antidepressants should not be offered as a first-line treatment in adults for PTSD and should only be considered if trauma-focused CBT or EMDR therapy have failed or are not available or if there is concurrent moderate . . . severe depression (U.S. Department of Veterans Affairs, 2017; WHO, 2013). Only paroxetine (Paxil), sertraline (Zoloft), and fluoxetine (Prozac) as well as the serotonin-norepinephrine reuptake Inhibitor (SNRI) venlafaxine are recommended by the U.S. Department of Veterans Affairs (2017) as adjunctive treatment if psychotherapy is not available. These medications ameliorate the symptoms of reexperiencing, avoidance or numbing, and hyperarousal, and are sometimes used to treat the comorbid disorders of depression, social phobia, OCD, and panic disorder that frequently occur with trauma. Naltrexone has been demonstrated to reduce dissociative symptoms and flashbacks in a few studies (Sutar & Sahu, 2019). These authors conclude that Paroxetine and Naloxone are the only medications where randomized clinical trials have found modest evidence for controlling depersonalizaiton and dissociative symptoms that are comorbid with PTSD and borderline personality disorder. Selected monoamine oxidase inhibitors (MAOIs) and tricyclic antidepressants (TCAs) have also been found to be effective, but because of the potential side effects and lethality in overdose, they have not been used as much.

Clonazepam (Klonopin) sometimes is used, but benzodiazepines are highly addictive and may interfere with the processing of trauma in psychotherapy. Research has not demonstrated benefit with clonazepam for those with PTSD (U.S. Department of Veterans Affairs, 2017). However, clonazepam is less likely to contribute to dependency than other benzodiazepines because it is a long-acting drug (half-life of 18 to 50 hours). Clonazepam is often used in the initial trial of a selective serotonin reuptake inhibitor

(SSRI) if needed to ameliorate anxiety until reaching the full effects of the drug. When clonazepam is used, the APPN should inform the patient of the intended use while waiting for the SSRI to take effect and to take the clonazepam daily, not just as needed. If taken only on an as-needed basis, clonazepam becomes an operant conditioning factor, which contributes to a sense of powerlessness and dependency.

Because of the metabolic side effects of typical and even some atypical antipsychotics, these medications should not be used unless tolerance to benzodiazepines has developed. Risperidone (Risperdal) or olanzapine (Zyprexa) in low doses is recommended if the person is having panic attacks or is having difficulty functioning due to anxiety. A number of concerns when prescribing for trauma survivors have been identified, which include problems with compliance, increased anxiety, interference with memory processing, substance abuse, distrust of authority, and fear of overmedication (Briere & Scott, 2013). It should also be kept in mind that research has found that medications do not cure PTSD. One study found that at 5-month follow-up after treatment, 60% of those on medication and 58% of those who received placebo still had PTSD while only 20% of those who received psychotherapy still had PTSD (Shalev et al., 2012). Given that medications have side effects and are only slightly more effective than placebo, caution should be used before prescribing. Initial doses of medication can increase anxiety at the beginning of treatment and panic attacks can occur. In addition, because the person may have memory problems, distractibility, arousal, dissociation, and trust issues, and may rely on their hypervigilance to keep them safe, compliance issues are common.

Recommendations for prescribers and therapists that may help to ameliorate compliance issues include:

- A follow-up appointment within a week of starting a new medication
- Cultivating trust to counter the patient's reluctance to take medications
- Titrate dose slowly to decrease side effects
- Educate thoroughly regarding side effects so that there are no surprises
- Consideration of abuse potential
- Document informed consent for medication
- Assuage concerns about overmedication because the patient may fear that he or she may be less responsive to danger if on medication (Briere & Scott, 2013)

Medication is an adjunct to treatment and does nothing to assuage the guilt, grief, and interpersonal difficulties that trauma patients suffer, but it is helpful in providing symptom relief and may discourage the person from leaving treatment prematurely and increase compliance. Medication does not directly promote new learning or processing, but if the person's anxiety level is decreased with medication, he or she may be more amenable to learning. Symptom reduction is enhanced and lasts longer with psychotherapy than with psychopharmacological interventions alone (van der Kolk et al., 2007). In a seminal review of the research for psychotherapy and psychopharmacology, the amount of symptom reduction from psychotherapy was considerably larger than that found for pharmacological interventions (Friedman et al., 2011). In addition, it is important to keep in mind that once the trauma is processed, sleep often improves.

FRASER TABLE TECHNIQUE

When working with those with DDs, it is important to be able to work with different alters or ego states; that is, different EPs of the personality. This can be accomplished through an ego state technique called the Fraser table technique, which is a useful adjunct to psychotherapy (Fraser, 1991). Even if the person does not have distinct alters, the use of this technique can be very helpful for those with complex trauma. Because this technique can seem strange, a solid therapeutic alliance is a prerequisite for its use. Originally used with hypnotic induction, it can be used as an imagery exercise without any formal induction. However, Fraser offers two caveats with the use of the table technique. First, the therapist should be knowledgeable about DDs or in supervision with someone who is, and second, there needs to be a plan for follow-up, as once it is used it can open up dissociative barriers that may be destabilizing without the proper resources in place.

There are at least six steps in this technique, depending on the person and the extent of the dissociation. Step 1 involves educating the person about the technique and normalizing the idea that we all have different states of ourselves that we are unaware of most of the time. For example, we may be one way at work, another way with a friend, or another way in our role as mom. All our different ages and states are still within us and this imagery exercise is a way to deepen our knowledge of these states. Step 2 involves an imagery using a safe/calm place to access relaxation in preparation for the table imagery. See Appendix 1.7 for the safe/calm place exercise. Step 3 involves leading the person through the table imagery to access the table; step 4 involves identifying those who come to the table with a full description of each; step 5 is communicating with the different states with various strategies delineated about how to accomplish this.

Communicating and working with the different states may involve using both stabilization and processing strategies for each state depending on the needs of that particular state. For example, one young woman who had significant attachment trauma identified a young part who was 4 years old who was sad and scared. This part needed resources to enhance attachment and subsequently attachment imagery exercises were used in many sessions that were very helpful in repairing attachment trauma (Steele, 2007). Therapists have developed a number of creative ways to use this technique. April Steele has imagery scripts available that can be accessed online for repairing attachment trauma at april-steele.ca/apr/imaginal-nurturing.

The final step is the fusion or integration of the different parts. The latter may not be necessary for those who do not have DID. It may be sufficient to develop an awareness of the different states and build in resources for those states that need stabilization and/or remediation.

PSYCHOEDUCATION

Psychoeducation is a key component to be integrated throughout all stages. It involves helping the person to understand that many current difficulties he or she is experiencing are adaptive responses to overwhelming events. The APPN may need to repeat intermittently throughout therapy that the person is not bad or crazy and that he or she is not responsible for what happened. In the case of childhood abuse, the patient's emotional denial of the reality of the abuse maintains a bond with the idealized caretaker and has most likely been an organizing force in the person's life (i.e., "I was hurt because I was bad"). This idea may be so entrenched that even when patients seemingly agree or intellectually know that they are not responsible, guilt and shame remain pervasive. These patients' faulty assumptions about themselves and others have permeated and colored all aspects of their lives. Intense attachment to the abuser protects the illusion of the child as safe. To acknowledge the reality would be admitting to an even greater horror, which is too anxiety provoking to face, that the people who were supposed to love and protect them did not. Recognizing that their parent(s) are selfish, cruel, and/or insane would mean abandonment and annihilation. The child achieves a measure of control and power through denial because if the child believes that he or she is being mistreated because he or she is bad, then the idealized parent is preserved and it is the child's fault, which allows the child the illusion of control.

Education about trauma and how the fear response develops and information about sympathetic nervous system arousal, depressive symptoms, panic, and an overview of trauma treatment are relevant according to the person's ability to understand and take in this information. This can be framed simply through a discussion about the RZ available at www.traumaresourceinstitute.com/ichill-app/ichill-app-1. Also, stress management techniques and specific strategies to use as resources are important areas to cover. Other important psychoeducational dimensions of trauma, which should be discussed, include reframing symptoms of flashbacks; avoidance, activated memories, and emotional numbing; prevalence of trauma; and safety plans, if necessary. Box 17.7 provides websites that offer educational material on trauma for patients and therapists.

Education about the psychotherapeutic process continues throughout all stages of treatment. Consciously experienced anxiety often occurs before or during symptom amelioration. It is important to explain to the patient that as positive changes occur, they may be followed temporarily by increased sadness, anger, or anxiety because change, even a positive change, may be experienced as a loss. The APPN keeps this in mind because the person may appear to be doing worse after significant gains. It is essential for the overall plan to be kept in mind with the therapeutic aims and gains in the foreground and to convey hope so that progress can continue.

The following example illustrates the use of education during the initial stage of treatment of a patient with DID. Dr. K, a 48-year-old university professor, came to treatment because she was becoming increasingly anxious about her partner, whom she suspected was having an affair. Dr. K described her memory as like "Swiss cheese" and said that she wanted to make sense of things and find out who she was. During the first several months of therapy, the sessions were fragmented and confusing, with the patient reporting strange sensations and images that came to her at seemingly random times. For example, she reported that when riding in a limousine to the airport, she became

BOX 17.7 Educational Information for Patients and Therapists

David Baldwin's Trauma Information Pages: www.trauma-pages.com/support.php

Ellen Lacter's website, End Ritual Abuse: endritualabuse.org

International Society for the Study of Trauma and Dissociation: www.isst-d.org

International Society for the Study of Trauma and Dissociation resources for special interest group on ritual abuse: endritualabuse.org/are-victims-responsible

International Society for Traumatic Stress Studies: www.istss.org/resources/index.htm

Justice Resource Institute (JRI), The Trauma Center: www.traumacenter.org

The National Child Traumatic Stress Network: www.nctsn.org

National Institute of Mental Health: www.nimh.nih.gov/health/topics/coping-with-traumatic-events/index.shtml

Sidran Traumatic Stress Institute (posttraumatic stress disorder, dissociative disorders, co-occurring addiction, self-injury, suicidality): www.sidran.org

Trauma Resource Institute: www.traumaresourceinstitute.com

U.S. Dept of Justice, Office on Violence Against Women (OVW): www.justice.gov/ovw

sexually aroused for no apparent reason and began to masturbate. In another instance, she recounted seeing dark figures in her bedroom at night. On questioning, Dr. K knew these images were not real but said she often had images come to her. She had been in therapy previously and remembered then that she had been sexually abused by her grandparents when she was a child. The therapist explained to Dr. K that her brain was trying to make sense of what had happened to her in the past and process those events. By not remembering, she had been able to distance herself from what had happened at the time of the trauma, and this was adaptive for her, allowing her to survive. She had functioned well, earning her doctorate, working as an academic, having friends, and creating a life for herself. These images and sensations were most likely flashbacks that may signal that she is ready to deal with the trauma that previously was completely dissociated. In other words, a flashback is an attempt by the brain to process what happened, but it is not quite successful. It is only a fragment of the memory and disconnected from other dimensions (i.e., memory networks) and the context of the original experience. These images and sensations are triggered by present circumstances and sensations.

The APPN then asked Dr. K to notice when she had strange images or sensations that did not seem to fit the situation and explained that together in sessions, the trigger for these events would be examined. She subsequently linked the sexual arousal in the limousine to being in the back seat of the car when she was driven by her grandfather to a place where she was sexually abused. Many patients are disturbed by linking sexual arousal with the abuse because the patient then assumes culpability for the sexual abuse. The therapist explained to Dr. K that sexual arousal naturally occurs when the genitals are touched and that this does not mean that it was her fault but only a normal physiological reaction to stimulation. The APPN reiterated: "Together we will deepen our understanding of how the trauma from your past affects you now. You are safe here." This was immensely reassuring to Dr. K, who thought she was "crazy." This illustrates how educating the patient about trauma in light of the person's experiences advances the therapeutic relationship and is integral to trauma treatment. See www.youtube.com/watch?v=L-q-tSHo9Ho

CASE EXAMPLE

Ms. H, an attractive, petite, 42-year-old full-time housewife came to psychotherapy initially for severe bulimia, vomiting as many as 40 times each day for the past year. She had previously been diagnosed with PTSD, anorexia nervosa, DDNOS, dependent personality disorder, panic anxiety, major depressive disorder, and polysubstance dependence. In the past, Ms. H self-medicated with alcohol, Vicodin, Xanax, and OxyContin. The Vicodin and OxyContin were taken to relieve her long-standing severe back pain. She was hospitalized twice for polysubstance abuse, and medications taken after hospitalization included Paxil (60 mg each day) and Depakote (250 mg twice daily). Ms. H was physically and emotionally abused as a child by a sadistic father and a neglectful, narcissistic mother. At intake, in addition to the bulimia, she reported depressive symptoms, trouble concentrating, anxiety, and periods of depersonalization and feeling dizzy and confused. She forgot periods of time; for example, she found herself in the grocery store and could not remember how she got there. This occurred particularly when she was stressed and anxious. She denied self-harm and suicide ideation. She had been married for 22 years and reported long-standing marital difficulties.

The history of childhood trauma and her tumultuous psychiatric history indicated that a long period of stabilization most likely would be needed. The APPN explained to Ms. H about her RZ and how it would be helpful to learn some strategies so she could stay regulated and in her RZ. The APPN worked with Ms. H once a week initially and, after several months, began twice-weekly psychotherapy, which continued over the next 5 years. Within

6 months of beginning treatment, her bulimia subsided. Much of the content of beginning sessions focused on building in resources and later on the abuse she suffered from her husband, which was ongoing and included emotional, sexual, and physical abuse. Ms. H initially appeared frightened and confused, especially when asked about her feelings. The therapist supported and validated Ms. H and told her that she was being abused as she vacillated between thinking that she deserved such punishment to feeling anger at her husband. She had idealized her husband, and as she began to see him more realistically, she also began to see herself in a different light, and her self-esteem increased. She began to assert herself more, and her marital relationship further deteriorated because her abusive husband was enraged that he was losing control of her. Plans for her safety were made, and 2 years after starting therapy, she filed for divorce and moved out of their house. This represented a significant turning point because stabilization was not possible previously as long as she was not safe. Her medication was changed to 20 mg of Prozac, and she found a full-time job shortly after the divorce. Over the course of treatment, various stabilization strategies were gradually integrated, which helped to widen her RZ so she could stay regulated. These included safe/calm place, container, circle of strength, rating negative feelings, basic self-care, yoga, progressive muscle relaxation, journaling, grounding, cognitive restructuring, walking, and deep breathing, in addition to other soothing activities. All were new to Ms. H; she had never practiced any of these before therapy.

Through mindfulness, Ms. H learned to manage her dissociative symptoms, and these periods decreased dramatically as she was able to stay in the present, understand the triggers, and talk about some of her traumatic experiences. Her back pain all but disappeared as she became aware that the triggers for these episodes were linked to feelings of anger. Her identification of her feelings in the present, the ability to experience these feelings, and understanding the meaning of her symptoms were crucial to her development of affect-regulation skills. Along with the deepening of her identity apart from her husband, her sense of humor and keen intelligence emerged. Some of her early childhood trauma was processed with EMDR therapy, but much of the work in psychotherapy focused on increasing resources, psychoeducation, and support, with the therapist bearing witness to her struggle and courage. Her healing reflected the return and expansion of her full consciousness through the integration of adaptive memory networks with dissociated neural networks. This was accomplished by creating positive experiences through the therapeutic relationship, learning and practicing specific resources, and weaving a narrative that connected her old and new memory experiences into a coherent tapestry reflecting a stronger, more resilient sense of self.

POST-MASTER'S TRAUMA TRAINING AND CERTIFICATION REQUIREMENTS

The APPN who wishes to attain competency treating traumatized patients should pursue additional training and ongoing supervision. Working with dissociative patients requires a high level of clinical expertise to do so successfully. The International Society for the Study of Dissociation (ISSD) offers post-master's training in the treatment of DDs but not certification. The program consists of nine monthly or biweekly sessions of 2.5 hours, which are held in many major cities listed on the website (www.issd.org). The sessions are designed to focus on readings and clinical situations. A distance-learning module is also available, along with advanced coursework.

In addition, integrative trauma psychotherapy programs are offered in large cities in the United States. An Integrative Trauma Psychotherapy Certificate Program is offered at Fairfield University and includes Basic Training in EMDR and the Trauma Resilience Model (TRM), a somatic therapy described in Chapter 11. See fairfield.edu/resiliencetraining.

CONCLUDING COMMENTS

Stabilization and safety are always the first order of business for any psychotherapy. This ensures that the processing needed to integrate the dissociated memory networks will not destabilize the patient. Enhancing resources ensures that positive adaptive memory networks exist for the eventual linking of dysfunctional material so that integration can occur. Strategies for stabilization are basic tools that all APPNs need to know to work with patients who present for psychotherapy. These skills build on the stress management techniques that registered nurses are familiar with. This foundation is deepened by understanding how and when to tailor specific stabilization strategies. Competency in stage 1 (stabilization) reflects the beginning-level skills needed for APPN practice.

There is a wide spectrum of trauma responses, and stabilization is needed before processing trauma. The limiting diagnosis of PTSD does not capture the complexity of traumatic experiences and their sequelae. Neurophysiological research demonstrates the importance of even subtle negative life events on the developing brain when a state of helplessness occurs (see Chapter 2). The physiological changes that occur and the perpetuation of those changes over time are determined by the meaning of life events in relation to past trauma (Shapiro, 2018). The learned associated responses embedded in memory networks are modified in the safety of the therapeutic relationship. Managing arousal and altering procedural memories begin the work of healing trauma.

The patients of severe childhood trauma are chronically disenfranchised and re-create betrayal and abandonment scenarios wherever they go, especially in the psychotherapeutic relationship as early attachment schemas are reactivated. Most complex child-onset trauma requires painstaking work as resources are increased and a narrative is woven about the nuances of the meaning of the events as the trauma is processed. Individuals who are survivors of childhood abuse present treatment challenges and the complexity and severity of symptoms can seem insurmountable to even the most experienced psychotherapist. However, healing occurs in this relationship with patience, caring, and skill. Novice APPN psychotherapists who continue to train and obtain supervision to develop skill in trauma treatment will be richly rewarded in their work. The APPN's presence bears witness with empathic resonance, creating the atmosphere needed for the most vulnerable of patients to be whole again. Those of us who work with this population marvel at the remarkable capacity for endurance, compassion, depth of character, and resilience of the human spirit. The honor of assisting in the growth of another person changes the patient and the therapist. In the healing journey with another, we heal ourselves.

DISCUSSION QUESTIONS

1. Discuss the spectrum of trauma-related diagnoses with respect to specific symptoms that overlap. Pick one trauma-related DSM diagnosis and identify what might be some, and differential diagnoses.
2. Identify goals of treatment for trauma.
3. What happens physiologically during dissociation, and what would you observe in the patient who dissociated during a session?
4. Fill out the DES, which is included in Chapter 3 on yourself and score it. Keep track with a log of all the times you notice yourself dissociating over the course of the next week.
5. How would you know whether a person was stabilized and ready to go on to processing?

6. Discuss why a person who has been traumatized as a child most likely has pervasive feelings of guilt.
7. Develop a comprehensive plan of all the potential issues and strategies that you need to teach a patient who has flashbacks.
8. Explain why mindfulness underlies all stabilization, why you should develop this skill, and how you plan to do so.
9. Practice the progressive muscle relaxation exercise and the safe/calm place exercise in Appendices 13.2 and 1.7 with a friend or family member. Ask for feedback so that you can improve.

REFERENCES

American Psychiatric Association. (2009). *Practice guidelines for the treatment of patients with acute stress disorder (ASD) and posttraumatic stress disorder (PTSD)*. Retrieved from https://psychiatryonline.org/pb/assets/raw/sitewide/practice_guidelines/guidelines/acutestressdisorderptsd.pdf

American Psychiatric Association. (2013). *Diagnostic and statistical manual of mental disorders* (5th ed.). Arlington, VA: American Psychiatric Publishing.

Bergmann, U. (2019). *Neurobiological foundations for EMDR practice* (2nd ed.). New York, NY: Springer Publishing Company.

Bernstein, C., & Putnam, F. W. (1986). Development, reliability, and validity of a dissociative scale. *Journal of Nervous and Mental Disease, 174*, 727–735. doi:10.1097/00005053-198612000-00004

Blake, D., Weathers, F. W., Nagy, L. M., Kaloupek, D. G., Gusman, F. D., Charney, D. S., & Keane, T. M. (1995). The development of a clinician-administered PTSD scale. *Journal of Traumatic Stress, 8*, 75–90. doi:10.1007/BF02105408

Blue Knot Foundation. (2019). *Practice guidelines for clinical treatment of complex trauma*. Retrieved from https://www.blueknot.org.au/Resources/Publications/Practice-Guidelines/Practice-Guidelines-2019

Boon, S., Steele, K., & van der Hart, O. (2011). *Coping with trauma-related dissociation*. New York, NY: W. W. Norton.

Bourne, E. J. (2010). *The anxiety and phobia workbook* (5th ed.). Oakland, CA: New Harbinger Publications.

Bradley, R., Greene, J., Russ, E., Dutra, L., & Westen, D. (2005). A multidimensional meta-analysis of psychotherapy for PTSD. *American Journal of Psychiatry, 162*, 214–227. doi:10.1176/appi.ajp.162.2.214

Brand, B. (2001). Establishing safety with patients with dissociative identity disorder. *Journal of Trauma & Dissociation, 2*(4), 133–155. doi:10.1300/J229v02n04_07

Briere, J. (2002). *Multiscale dissociation inventory*. Odessa, FL: Psychological Assessment Resources.

Briere, J., & Scott, C. (2013). *Principles of trauma therapy: A guide to symptoms, evaluation, and treatment* (2nd ed.). Thousand Oaks, CA: Sage.

Carlson, W.B., & Putnam, F.W. (1993). An update on the dissociative experiences scale. *Dissociation, 6*, 16-27.

Chu, J. A. (2011). *Rebuilding shattered lives: The responsible treatment of complex post-traumatic and dissociative disorders* (2nd ed.). New York, NY: John Wiley.

Church, D. (2015). *Psychological trauma: Healing its roots in brain, body, and mind*. Fulton, CA: Energy Psychology Press.

Cloitre, M., Courtois, C. A., Ford, J. D., Green, B. L., Alexander, P., Briere, J., . . . Van der Hart, O. (2012). *The ISTSS expert consensus treatment guidelines for complex PTSD in adults*. Retrieved from https://www.istss.org/ISTSS_Main/media/Documents/ISTSS-Expert-Concesnsus-Guidelines-for-Complex-PTSD-Updated-060315.pdf

Connor, K., & Davidson, J. (2001). SPRINT: A brief global assessment of post-traumatic stress disorder. *International Clinical Psychopharmacology, 16*, 279–284. doi:10.1097/00004850-200109000-00005

Cozolino, L. (2017). *The neuroscience of psychotherapy: Healing the social brain* (3rd ed.). New York, NY: W. W. Norton.

Davis, K., & Weiss, L. (2004). *Traumatology: A workshop on traumatic stress disorders*. Hamden, CT: EMDR Humanitarian Assistance Programs.

De Jongh, A., Resick, P., Zoellner, L., van Minnen, A., Lee, C. W., Monson, C., . . . Bicanic, I. (2016). Critical commentary on the ISTSS expert consensus treatment guidelines for complex PTSD in adults. *Journal of Anxiety and Depression, 33*, 359–369. doi:10.1002/da.22469

Dell, P. F. (2006). The multidimensional inventory of dissociation (MID): A comprehensive measure of pathological dissociation. *Journal of Trauma & Dissociation, 7*, 77–106. doi:10.1300/J229v07n02_06

Dworkin, M. (2005). *EMDR and the relational imperative*. New York, NY: Routledge.

Ebner-Priemer, U. W., Mauchnik, J., Kleindienst, N., Schmahl, C., Peper, M., Rosenthal, M. Z., & Bohus, M. (2009). Emotional learning during dissociative states in borderline personality disorder. *Journal of Psychiatry & Neuroscience, 34*, 214–222. Retrieved from http://jpn.ca/vol34-issue3/34-3-214

Epstein, M. (2013). Thoughts without a thinker: Psychotherapy from a Buddhist perspective. New York: Basic Books.

Falsetti, S. A., Resnick, H. S., Resick, P. A., & Kilpatrick, D. (1993). The modified PTSD symptom scale: A brief self-report measure of PTSD. *The Behavioral Therapist, 16*, 161–162.

Foote, B., Smolin, Y., Kaplan, M., Legatt, M., & Lipschitz, D. (2006). Prevalence of dissociative disorders in psychiatric outpatients. *American Journal of Psychiatry, 163*, 623–629. doi:10.1176/appi.ajp.163.4.623

Forner, C. (2017). *Dissociation, mindfulness and creative meditations*. New York, NY: Routledge.

Fraser, G. (1991). The dissociative table technique: A strategy for working with ego states in dissociative disorders and ego state therapy. *Dissociation, 4*(8), 205–213.

Frewem, P., Zhu, J., & Lanius, R. (2019). Lifetime traumatic stressors an adverse childhood experiences uniquely predict concurrent pTSD, complex PTSD, and dissociative subtype of PTSD symptoms whereas recent adult non-traumatic stressors do not: Results from an online survey study. *European Journal of Psychothraumatology, 10*. doi:10.1080/20008198.2019.1606625

Friedman, M. J., Resick, P. A., Bryant, R. A., Strain, J., Horowitz, M., & Spiegel, D. (2011). Classification of trauma and stressor-related disorders in *DSM-5*. *Depression and Anxiety, 28*(9), 737–749. doi:10.1002/da.20845

Hagenaars, M. A., van Minnen, A., & Hoogduin, K. A. (2010). The impact of dissociation and depression on the efficacy of prolonged exposure treatment for PTSD. *Behaviour Research and Therapy, 48*, 19–27. doi:10.1016/j.brat.2009.09.001

Heller, M. C. (2012). *Body psychotherapy: History, concepts, methods*. New York, NY: W. W. Norton.

Herman, J. (1992). *Trauma and recovery*. New York, NY: Basic Books.

Horowitz, M. J. (2003). *Treatment of stress response syndromes*. Washington, DC: American Psychiatric Publishing.

Howell, E. (2020). *Trauma and dissociation informed psychotherapy: Relational healing and the therapeutic connection*. New York, NY: W. W. Norton.

International Society for the Study of Dissociation. (2004). *Guidelines for the evaluation and treatment of dissociative symptoms in children and adolescents*. Retrieved from https://www.isst-d.org/wp-content/uploads/2019/02/childguidelines-ISSTD-2003.pdf

International Society for the Study of Trauma and Dissociation. (2011). Guidelines for treating dissociative identity disorder in adults. Third revision. *Journal of Trauma & Dissociation, 12*, 115–187. doi:10.1080/15299732.2011.537247

Kabat-Zinn, J. (2005). Wherever you go, there you are. New York: Hachette Books.

Kabat-Zinn, J., & Kabat-Zinn, J. (1990). *Full catastrophe living: Using the wisdom of your body and mind to face stress, pain and illness*. New York, NY: Dell Publishing.

Kessler, R. C., Borges, G., & Walters, E. E. (1999). Prevalence of and risk factors for lifetime suicide attempts in the National Comorbidity Survey. *Archives of General Psychiatry, 56*, 617–626.

Kimerling, R., Ouimette, P., Prins, A., Nisco, P., Lawler, C., Cronkite, R., & Moos, R. H. (2006). Brief report: Utility of a short screening scale for DSM-IV PTSD in primary care. *Journal General Internal Medicine, 21*(1), 65–67. doi:10.1111/j.1525-1497.2005.00292.x

Kluft, R. P. (1999). Current issues in dissociative identity disorder. *Journal of Practical Psychiatry and Behavioral Health, 5*, 3–19. Retrieved from https://journals.lww.com/practicalpsychiatry/Abstract/1999/01000/Current_Issues_in_Dissociative_Identity_Disorder.1.aspx

Laddis, A., & Dell, P. F. (2012). Dissociation and psychosis in dissociative identity disorder and schizophrenia. *Journal of Trauma & Dissociation, 13*(4), 397–413. doi:10.1080/15299732.2012.664967

Leichsenring, F., & Steinert, C. (2019). The efficacy of psychodynamic psychotherapy: An up-to-date review. In D. Kealy & J. S. Ogrodniczuk (Eds.), *Contemporary psychodynamic psychotherapy* (pp. 49–70). London, UK: Elsevier.

Levine, P. (1997). *Walking the tiger*. Berkley, CA: North Atlantic Books.

Levine, S. (1991). *Guided meditations, explorations, and healings*. New York, NY: Random House.

Linehan, M. M. (1993b). *Skills training manual for borderline personality disorder*. New York, NY: Guilford Press.

Lipinska, G., Baldwin, D. S., & Thomas, K. G. (2016). Pharmacology for sleep disturbance in PTSD. *Human Psychopharmacology: Clinical and Experimental, 31*, 156–163. doi:10.1002/hup.2522

McFarlane, A., & van der Kolk, B. (1996). Conclusions and future directions. In B. van der Kolk, A. D. McFarlane, & L. Weisaeth (Eds.), *Traumatic stress: The effects of overwhelming experience on mind, body, and society* (pp. 559–575). New York, NY: Guilford Press.

McWilliams, N. (2011). *Psychoanalytic diagnosis*. New York, NY: Guilford Press.

Najavits, L. M. (2002). *Seeking safety: A treatment manual for PTSD and substance abuse*. New York, NY: Guilford Press.

Nijenhuis, E. R. S. (2011). *Somatoform Dissociation questionnaire (SDQ-5 and SDQ-20)*. Retrieved from http://www.enijenhuis.nl/sdq

Pape, W., & Woller, W. (2015). Low dose naltrexone in the treatment of dissociative symptoms. *Nervenarzt, 86*(3), 346–351. doi:10.1007/s00115-014-4015-9

Pearlman, L. (2003). *Trauma and attachment belief scale*. Los Angeles, CA: Western Psychological Services.

Pelcovitz, D., van der Kolk, B., Roth, S., Mandel, F., Kaplan, S., & Resick, P. (1997). Development of a criteria set and a structured interview for disorder of extreme stress (SIDES). *Journal of Traumatic Stress, 10*, 3–16. doi:10.1023/a:1024800212070

Porges, S. W. (2011). *The polyvagal theory*. New York, NY: W. W. Norton.

Porges, S. W., & Dana, D. (2018). *Clinical applications of the Polyvagal theory: The emergence of Polyvagal-informed therapies*. New York, NY: W. W. Norton.

Putnam, F. W. (1989). *The diagnosis and treatment of multiple personality disorder*. New York, NY: Guilford Press.

Ross, C. (2013). *Dissociative disorders interview schedule*. Retrieved from https://www.rossinst.com/ddis

Rothschild, B. (2000). *The body remembers: The psychopathology of trauma and trauma treatment* (p. 131). New York, NY: W. W. Norton.

Rothschild, B. (2017). *The body remembers: Revolutionizing trauma treatment* (Vol. 2). New York, NY: W. W. Norton.

Ruzek, J., Young, B., & Walser, R. (2003). Group treatment of posttraumatic stress disorder and other trauma-related problems. *Primary Psychiatry, 10*(8), 53–57.

Salgado, B. (2016). *Real world mindfulness for beginners*. Berkley, Ca: Sonoma Press.

Sar, V. (2011). Epidemiology of dissociative disorders: An overview. *Epidemiology Research International, 2011*, 1–8. doi:10.1155/2011/404538

Sarno, J. E. (2006). *The divided mind: The epidemic of mind body disorders*. New York, NY: Harper Collins.

Scaer, R. (2005). *The trauma spectrum: Hidden wounds and human resiliency*. New York, NY: W. W. Norton.

Schiraldi, G. R. (2001). *The self-esteem workbook*. Oakland, CA: New Harbinger Publications.

Schore, A. (2019). *The development of the unconscious mind*. New York, NY: W. W. Norton.

Shalev, A. Y., Ankri, Y. L., Israeli-Shalev, Y., Peleg, T., Adessky, R. S., & Freedman, S. A. (2012). Prevention of posttraumatic stress disorder by early treatment: Results from the Jerusalem trauma outreach and prevention study. *Archives of General Psychiatry, 69*, 166–176. doi:10.1001/archgenpsychiatry.2011.127

Shapiro, F. (2001). *Eye movement desensitization and reprocessing (EMDR)*. New York: Basic Books.

Shapiro, F. (2018). *Eye movement desensitization and reprocessing (EMDR)* (3rd ed.). New York, NY: Guilford Press.

Siegel, D. (2010). *Mindsight: The new science of personal transformation*. New York, NY: Bantam Books.

Spiegel, D., Loewenstein, R., Lewis-Fernandez, R., Sar, V., Simeon, D., Vermetten, E., . . . Dell, P. (2011). Dissociative disorders in DSM-5. *Depression and Anxiety, 28*, 824–852. doi:10.1002/da.20874

Steele, A. (2007). *Developing a secure self: An attachment-based approach to adult psychotherapy*. Gabriola, BC, Canada: Author. Retrieved from www.april-steele.ca

Steele, K. (2012). *Coping with trauma-related dissociation: Skills training for patients and therapists*. New York, NY: W. W. Norton.

Steele, K., Boon, S., & van der Hart, O. (2017). *Treating trauma-related dissociation: A practical integrative approach*. New York, NY: W. W. Norton.

Steele, K., van der Hart, O., & Nijenhuis, E. (2005). Phase-oriented treatment of structural dissociation in complex traumatization: Overcoming trauma-related phobias. *Journal of Trauma & Dissociation, 6*(3), 11–53. doi:10.1300/J229v06n03_02

Steinberg, J. (1994). *Interviewer's guide to the structured clinical interview for DSM-IV dissociative disorders*. Washington, DC: American Psychiatric Publishing.

Steinberg, M., & Schnall, M. (2000). *The stranger in the mirror*. New York, NY: Cliff Street.

Stien, P., & Kendall, J. (2006). *Psychological trauma and the developing brain*. New York, NY: Hawthorne Press.

Sutar, R., & Sahu, S. (2019). Pharmacotherapy for dissociative disorders: A systematic review. *Psychiatry Research, 281*, 112529. doi:10.1016/j.psychres.2019.112529

U.S. Department of Veterans Affairs. (2017). *VA/DoD clinical practice guideline: Management of post-traumatic stress and acute stress disorder*. Washington, DC. Author. Retrieved from https://www.healthquality.va.gov/guidelines/MH/ptsd

Van Dam, N. T., van Vugt, M. K., Vago, D. R., Schmalzl, L., Saron, C. D., Olendzki, A., . . . Meyer, D. E. (2017). Mind the hype: A critical evaluation and prescriptive agenda for research on mindfulness and meditation. *Perspectives on Psychological Science, 13*(1), 36–61. doi:10.1177/1745691617709589

van der Kolk, B. (2003). Posttraumatic stress disorder and the nature of trauma. In M. Solomon & D. Siegel (Eds.), *Healing trauma*. New York, NY: W. W. Norton.

van der Kolk, B. (2006). Clinical implications of neuroscience research in PTSD. *Annals of New York Academy of Sciences, 1071*, 277–293. doi:10.1196/annals.1364.022

van der Kolk, B. (2014). *The body keeps the score: Brain, mind, and body in the healing of trauma*. New York, NY: Penguin Books.

van der Kolk, B., Spinazzola, J., Blaustein, M., Hopper, J., Hopper, E., Korn, D., & Simpson, W. (2007). A randomized clinical trial of EMDR, fluoxetine and pill placebo in the treatment of PTSD: Treatment effects and long-term maintenance. *Journal of Clinical Psychiatry, 68*, 37–46. doi:10.4088/jcp.v68n0105

Waters, F. S. (2016). *Healing the fractured child: Diagnosis and treatment of youth with dissociation*. New York, NY: Springer Publishing Company.

Weathers, F. W., Litz, B. T., Keane, T. M., Palmieri, P. A., Marx, B. P., & Schnurr, P. P. (2013). *The PTSD checklist for DSM-5 (PCL-5)*. Retrieved from https://www.ptsd.va.gov/professional/assessment/documents/PCL5_Standard_form.PDF

Weiss, D., & Marmar, C. (1997). The impact of event scale–Revised. In J. Wilson & T. Keane (Eds.), *Assessing psychological trauma and PTSD*. New York, NY: Guilford Press.

Woods, S.L., Rockman, P., & Collins, E. (2019). *Mindfulness-based cognitive therapy*. Oakland, Cal: Harbinger Pub, Inc.

World Health Organization. (2013). *WHO guidelines on conditions specifically related to stress*. Retrieved from http://www.who.int/mental_health/emergencies/stress_guidelines/en/index.html

World Health Organization. (2018, June 18). WHO releases new International Classification of Diseases (ICD 11) [Retrieved from http://www.who.int/news-room/detail/18-06-2018-who-releases-new-international-classification-of-diseases-(icd-11)

APPENDIX 17.1
Tracking Your Nervous System

Date	**I or M	Feeling/ Emotion	Body	*SUD (0–10)	Trigger

This form will help you learn how to track your nervous system. Please check in with how you are feeling at least once a day. Start with identifying whether you are in Immobilization or Mobilization (see list below). Then ask, What is the emotion I am feeling right now? Then ask, Where in my body do I feel that? Then, on a 0–10 scale, How disturbing is this feeling?

*SUD = Subjective Units of Disturbance, with 10 being the worst and 0 no disturbance

  **I = Immobilization (Dorsal Vagal)
Freeze
Shock/numb
Fatigue/no energy
Self-loathing
Memory problems
Shame/dissociation
Lack of appetite
Loneliness/disconnected
Depression
Shut down
**M = Mobilization (Sympathetic)
Fight/Flight
Heart pounding
Insomnia
Agitated
Anxiety/panic
Anger
Body tension
Shortness of breath
Irritability
Hyperactive
Hyperarousal

APPENDIX 17.2

ID#/Name: _____ Date: _____

Short PTSD Rating Interview (SPRINT)

Please identify the most distressing traumatic event: _____

	In the past week …	Not at all 0	A little bit 1	Moderately 2	Quite a lot 3	Very much 4
1	How much have you been bothered by unwanted memories, nightmares, or reminders of the event?					
2	How much effort have you made to avoid thinking or talking about the event, or doing things which remind you of what happened?					
3	To what extent have you lost enjoyment for things, kept your distance from people, or found it difficult to experience feelings?					
4	How much have you been bothered by poor sleep, poor concentration, jumpiness, irritability, or feeling watchful around you?					
5	How much have you been bothered by pain, aches, or tiredness?					

	In the past week …	Not at all 0	A little bit 1	Moderately 2	Quite a lot 3	Very much 4
6	How much would you get upset when stressful events or setbacks happen to you?					
7	How much have the above symptoms interfered with your ability to work or carry out daily activities?					
8	How much have the above symptoms interfered with your relationships with family or friends?					

Sum of 1 to 8 ☐

9	How much better do you feel since beginning treatment? (As a percentage) (%)					

0% ☐	10% ☐	20% ☐	30% ☐	40% ☐	50% ☐	60% ☐	70% ☐	80% ☐	90% ☐	100% ☐

10	How much have the above symptoms improved since starting treatment?

Worse 1	No change 2	Minimally 3	Much 4	Very much 5

APPENDIX 17.3

This exercise can be practiced with the patient during the session and it is often helpful if the APPN audiotapes a copy for the patient to listen to at home. If done properly, it may take 20 to 30 minutes. Begin with explaining that this is a relaxation exercise that will help to decrease physical tension and enhance the ability to identify where tension is stored in the body.

Progressive Muscle Relaxation

What you'll be doing is alternately tensing and relaxing specific groups of muscles. After tension, a muscle will be more relaxed than prior to the tensing. Concentrate on the feel of the muscles, specifically the contrast between tension and relaxation. In time, you will recognize tension in any specific muscle and be able to reduce that tension.

Don't tense muscles other than the specific group at each step. Breathe slowly and evenly and think only about the tension–relaxation contrast. Each tensing is for 10 seconds; each relaxing is for 10 or 15 seconds. Count "1,000 2,000 . . ." until you have a feel for the time span. Note that each step is really two steps—one cycle of tension–relaxation for each set of opposing muscles.

Please get in as comfortable a position as possible and take a deep breath; let it out slowly. Again a nice slow deep breath . . . take as deep a breath as possible—and then take a little more; let it out and breathe normally for 15 seconds. Let all the breath in your lungs out—and then a little more; inhale and breathe normally for 15 seconds.

> Begin with your muscles in your feet and your calves; tighten and pull your toes up while tensing each foot as tight as you can . . . hold that and just notice as you tense for 10 seconds . . . then relax your feet and next tense your calves . . . squeeze your calves as tight as you can . . . for 10 seconds 1...2...3...4...5...6...7...8...9...10... just notice and relax . . .

> Next tense your thigh muscles 1...2...3...4...5...6...7...8...9...10... hold … just notice then relax …

> Next tense the butt tightly and raise pelvis slightly off chair; relax. Dig buttocks into chair 1...2...3...4...5...6...7...8...9...10... just notice then relax…

> Pull in the stomach as far as possible … push out the stomach or tense it as if you were preparing for a punch in the gut ... 1...2...3...4...5...6...7...8...9...10... just notice then relax.

> Now tense your chest as tight as you can … 1...2...3...4...5...6...7...8...9...10 good, just tense then relax…

> Continue to breathe deeply as you pull your shoulders back ... 1...2...3...4...5...6...7...8...9...10... relax. Push the shoulders forward (hunch) 1...2...3...4...5...6...7...8...9...10 just notice and relax…

> Now flex your biceps 1...2...3...4...5...6...7...8...9...10 relax, take a deep breath … now tense your whole arm 1...2...3...4...5...6...7...8...9...10... and just notice as you relax … next flex squeeze your hands and fingers tight 1...2...3...4...5...6...7...8...9...10 and as you relax, take a deep breath.

(continued)

With the shoulders straight and relaxed, the head is turned slowly to the right, as far as you can; relax. Turn to the left; relax.

Dig your chin into your chest ...1...2...3...4...5...6...7...8...9...10... relax ... exhale nice deep breath…

Now your face, scrunch your face up as tight as you can 1...2...3...4...5...6...7...8...9...10... and as you relax take a deep breath letting all the air out.

Dig your tongue into the roof of your mouth ... 1...2...3...4...5...6...7...8...9...10 and relax. Dig it into the bottom of your mouth 1...2...3...4...5...6...7...8...9...10 and relax.

Open your eyes as wide as possible (furrow your brow) 1...2...3...4...5...6...7...8...9...10 and relax. Close your eyes tightly (squint) 1...2...3...4...5...6...7...8...9...10 relax.

Now just continue to breathe deeply and blow all the air out for a while.

These exercises will not eliminate tension, but when it arises, you will know it immediately, and you will be able to "tense–relax" it away or even simply wish it away.

Please note that an exercise program of any sort that stresses and stretches a full range of muscles can be used in this fashion if only you pay attention to the differences between tensions and relaxations of the muscles. Do the entire sequence once a day if you can, until you feel you are able to control your muscle tensions. This can also be combined with soothing music.

Dialectical Behavior Therapy for Complex Trauma

Barbara J. Limandri

Dialectical behavior therapy (DBT), first conceived by Marsha Linehan as a cognitive behavior based approach to treat those with chronic suicidal thoughts and diagnosed with borderline personality disorder, is highly relevant to treatment of those with complex trauma (Linehan, 1993a). Although not everyone with borderline personality disorder has comorbid posttraumatic stress disorder (PTSD), and not everyone with PTSD can be diagnosed with borderline personality disorder, there are important overlapping symptoms and neurophysiological correlates that they have in common. Some even believe that there is continuity in the two disorders that would be easier to accept clinically if there were not such a strong stigmatizing bias against borderline personality disorder diagnosis. Chu (2011) points out that the behavior and emotional response of one with borderline personality disorder can best be understood as reenactments of early abusive relationships, especially as one anticipates how others will behave. Key elements of borderline personality disorder related to PTSD include emotional reactivity and sensitivity (hyperarousal), history of invalidation (common in childhood abuse and sexual abuse), dissociation (intrusive symptoms and flashbacks), and affective instability (negative mood and thought changes). As noted in Chapter 16, the person with borderline personality disorder most likely fits the *Diagnostic and Statistical Manual of Mental Disorders*, Fourth Edition (DSM-IV) diagnosis of complex PTSD/disorder of extreme stress not otherwise specified (DESNOS).

This chapter discusses the use of DBT with particular focus on the utility and effectiveness in treating those with complex trauma histories. This includes an overview of DBT, including the research evidence to support DBT and its application to complex trauma, discussion of the interchange between trauma and borderline personality disorder, especially in relation to the consequences of trauma to the developing person, and the comorbidity of PTSD, personality disorder, depression, and substance use. The major focus of this chapter is evidence-based treatment approaches that are effective in treating complex trauma with emphasis on cognitive behavior, dialectical behavior, and exposure therapies that the APPN can use in thoughtful treatment planning. Separating these three psychotherapy approaches is artificial because they are contiguous, as will be evident later in this chapter. Although pharmacotherapy is an essential element of treatment, medications are adjunctive to psychotherapy and the reader is better served to consult more specific psychopharmacotherapy references. The APPN who wants to use DBT for treatment should seek a trained DBT therapist as a mentor and be trained in the model both at a basic level and eventually through an intensive training program. At the end of this chapter are resources for the APPN to consider in order to obtain appropriate training.

DIALECTICAL BEHAVIOR THERAPY

DBT may be described most simplistically as cognitive behavioral therapy (CBT) within a Zen Buddhist worldview. Dialectics refers to allowing the polarity of thesis (proposition or position) and antithesis (opposing perspective or position) to coexist and permitting a center position of synthesis, that is, instead of "this (thesis) or that (antithesis)" the truth is "this *and* that." The synthesis is a creative middle ground in which the conflict becomes a solution. The fundamental dialectic in DBT is that of change and acceptance. For example, the patient may profess that her life is one of misery and fear to such an extent that she can only see suicide as a solution. However, changing her behavior to step outside her comfort zone and experience new relationships or a different job further invites fear. The therapist's role is to guide the patient toward an alternative position (synthesis) of accepting her fear and pain as a motivating element to change her situation. The process of using dialectics in therapy is through "persuasive dialogue" (Linehan, 1993a) in which the therapist gradually invites the patient to new ways of viewing situations, thereby guiding the patient to develop more skills in achieving a greater quality of life. Frequently this is done through Socratic questioning that encourages the patient to analyze her thoughts, feelings, and behaviors in a nonjudgmental manner.

Basic to DBT are functions and modes of comprehensive treatment. The functions of treatment are (Dimeff, 2007):

1. Enhancing patients' capabilities
2. Motivating patients to use and expand their capabilities
3. Ensuring that patients can generalize their capabilities beyond the therapeutic relationship
4. Enhancing the therapist's skills and motivations
5. Structuring the environment for both the therapist and the patient to aid therapeutic progress

To achieve these functions, a DBT program has four essential elements:

1. Weekly individual therapy sessions for the patient of about 1 hour each
2. Weekly group skills training sessions for the patient of 2.5 hours each
3. Skills coaching via telephone or other electronic means as needed by the patient to manage in vivo situations
4. Team consultation to the therapist to maintain treatment fidelity and adherence

The research basis of DBT is based on faithful adherence to the functions and modes, even though this may not always be possible in different clinical situations and settings. When full fidelity is not possible, the clinician needs to be thoughtful about how best to adapt the treatment in keeping with the evidence and theory (Dimeff, 2007).

Assumptions About Patients and Treatment

There are some basic assumptions underlying DBT that were originally directed toward the patient with borderline personality disorder (Linehan, 1993a). These assumptions, however, apply more broadly to the patient who is struggling with emotional sensitivity, interpersonal crises, behavioral instability, and heightened vulnerability. When the APRN explains these assumptions to the patient and regularly revisits them both within the therapeutic relationship and in therapy consultation, treatment stays focused and authentic. Commonly in full DBT programs, the consultation team reviews these assumptions in part or as a whole each week. They include:

- Patients are doing the best they can at any given moment. Patients are more familiar with being invalidated and told they are not doing their best, are failing at whatever they are striving to do, or that they just are not trying.
- Patients want to improve. Even when patients are exasperating and stalling in their efforts, they keep their appointments, demonstrating their desire to improve.
- Patients need to do better, try harder, and be more motivated to change. This is a corollary to the first assumption. Getting better is work, hard work, and worth the effort. When the effort does not seem fruitful, the therapist needs to analyze with the patient what is interfering with therapy in a nonjudgmental, problem-solving manner.
- Patients may not have caused all of their problems, but they have to solve them anyway. This is especially true with the patient who has experienced trauma. What happened is in the past and the patient is struggling with behaviors that were adaptive at the time; however, those same behaviors may be holding the patient back now. Blaming the past maintains impotency in the patient, and the therapist provides the skills training and coaching for the patient to make the necessary changes for a worthwhile life.
- The lives of patients are unbearable as they are currently being lived. That is, the therapist must validate the patient's distress and accept that misery while also recognizing the only solution is to make a change.
- The patient must learn new behaviors in all relevant contexts. In the short term, hospitalization may seem the most appropriate way of handling suicidal ideation; however, to the chronically suicidal person hospitalization reinforces the status quo and abdicating the hard work of change. Instead, the therapist coaches the patient to practice skills that are more effective, albeit more difficult to use when distressed. Crisis is the peak of the learning moment and requires immense courage and effort for the therapist and patient to work together.
- Patient cannot fail in therapy. This is one of the most difficult assumptions for both the patient and the therapist. When patients stall in treatment, drop out of therapy, or even get worse, the therapy and therapist have failed. Of course, it is tempting to believe that the patient does not want to get better or does not have the capability to improve when patients do not get better. But such assumptions provide no direction for either the therapist or the patient. Instead the therapist needs to enhance the patient's engagement and commitment to treatment and reexamine the hypotheses of the treatment plan.
- Therapists treating the difficult patient need support. Consultation to the therapist is necessary in DBT to support the therapist and prevent burnout. The consultation group serves to treat the therapist by using the same skills that we ask the patient to use. In a weekly consultation group, the team prioritizes the needs of therapists, mindfully engages in discussing the effects of what we are doing, and advocates for each person to take care of self. When discussion shifts to clinical issues and case conferencing, it is the responsibility of each team member to address the avoidance of consultation to the therapist. When the therapist who is in solo practice tries to implement DBT without a consultation group, there is no sounding board for the therapist to find synthesis in one's work or to mediate over extension or burnout.

To practice within these assumptions, it helps for the APRN to consider the dialectics of the therapist, that is, the balancing skills and attitudes of providing treatment. Figure 18.1 illustrates the characteristics of the DBT therapist (Linehan, 1993a) in terms of the values of the therapist. To prevent passive acceptance of these characteristics, the authentic therapist needs to be confronting these balancing points constantly in providing care for the patient. Again the consultation to the therapist provides an opportunity to confront conflicts in self-beliefs and practices. At times the team member may need to

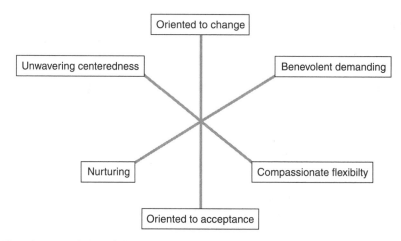

FIGURE 18.1 Characteristics of the DBT therapist.

Source: Adapted from Linehan, M. (1993a). *Cognitive-behavioral treatment of borderline personality disorder.* New York, NY: Guilford Press.

act as devil's advocate in challenging the therapist's therapeutic stance with a patient. Is the APRN seeing the patient as fragile, therefore, undermining the patient's capabilities? Is the APRN's unwavering centeredness preventing him or her from being compassionate toward the patient in finding a different solution to problematic behaviors? Sometimes the team may need to recommend the therapist take a break from therapy and ask a colleague to monitor the pager over the weekend or to fill in for the therapist in a skills group as the therapist takes the time to replenish personal reserves.

Principles of Practice

Within the DBT model the therapist orients the patient to some basic principles that guide the treatment. An important principle is that of giving the treatment time to work. DBT is designed to teach skills and encourage regularly practicing those skills to live life more fully. For patient who have had devastating experiences that have misshapen their lives, the least amount of time for DBT to be effective is 1 year. That includes at least 6 months of learning skills with necessary redundancy to practice them in different circumstances, then another 6 months of using the skills in daily living while analyzing how to improve on their effectiveness. Commonly the first 2 to 3 months of treatment may be stormy for the patient and therapist as the patient tests the limits of treatment and challenges the assumptions. After completing a full program many patients choose to continue additional peer group meetings to prepare them for living without therapy as a constant in their life. This group has a therapist who serves as a consultant to the group as needed. Not everyone chooses to participate in Accepting the Challenges of Exiting the System (ACES) and sometimes ACES is countertherapeutic in that it serves as a way for the patient to remain dependent on therapy or forestall venturing forth on her or his own. Some patients may terminate from DBT and seek continuing supportive psychotherapy.

There are some ground rules for ensuring the likelihood of success in treatment, the most basic of which is that the patient must attend the individual and group skills sessions consistently. If the patient misses more than three or four (depending on the ground rule the therapist/treatment team sets) consecutive sessions of any kind (individual therapy, group therapy, and pharmacological monitoring), treatment must end.

Usually this means a therapy hiatus of an established period in which the patient can reconsider his or her commitment to therapy. With such a rule stated in the beginning of therapy the patient has control over his or her commitment. When the patient misses two sessions in a row, the therapist sets a priority to examine the therapy-interfering behavior, identify vulnerability features, and arrive at some solutions to the problem. However, if the patient continues to miss the next session, it is essential that the therapist notify the patient of the unilateral termination and the conditions in which the patient is welcome to return to treatment, including a plan while on hiatus to improve commitment. To do otherwise would be reinforcing therapy-interfering behavior on the part of the patient and in turn would be therapy interfering on the part of the therapist. It is crucial to reinforce consistency in behavior in a clear and nonjudgmental manner. Frequently such nonjudgmental consistency was absent in early development, contributing to a sense of boundaryless relationships.

Another principle that the therapist discusses with the patient in the beginning of treatment as well as throughout therapy is that suicidal and self-harming behaviors are problems to be solved and are of the highest priority for treatment. Similarly, the patient must agree to reduce the behaviors as a goal for therapy and to work with the therapist before acting on self-harming urges. One of the most difficult agreements the therapist must make with the patient is that the patient can receive coaching on using skills to prevent self-harm but once the patient engages in target behavior and enters the ED or is admitted to the hospital, the therapist suspends direct consultation with the patient. At that point the inpatient staff takes over and may begin discharge planning with the therapist, but the therapist cannot talk with the patient until 24 hours after discharge from the facility. The underlying reasoning for such a rule is that hospitalization reinforces the patient's inability to care for self and use skills effectively. When that point is reached, DBT has failed. After discharge the patient likely returns to DBT and the focus must return to effective use of skills for safety and reengaging in treatment goals. The first order of resuming treatment is analyzing the behavioral events that led to target behavior.

The therapist also has some rules to follow that again are made explicitly clear in the orientation to therapy with the patient. First, the therapist agrees to make every reasonable effort to provide competent treatment for the patient. This means that the therapist is human and fallible. The patient may question the effectiveness of the therapist and has the responsibility to discuss this directly and nonjudgmentally with the therapist. In turn, the therapist works with the patient to clarify the treatment goals and strategies. The therapist also agrees to use consultation with the team to assure the patient of competent care, even though the patient may not see that consultation directly. The therapist may model use of skills at times, for example, if the therapist is feeling overly emotional within the session, he or she may say "let us both take a deep breath" and use mindfulness to balance emotional and rational mindedness. The patient sees the therapist being human and using skills to be more effective in the interpersonal situation.

Because frequently the patient seeking DBT has experienced poor boundary maintenance on the part of influential others, it is especially important for the therapist to make explicit the boundaries of the therapeutic relationship, including ethical conduct and separation of personal and professional roles. This does not mean maintaining a rigid and distant relationship with the patient, but rather assuring the patient that this is a professional relationship based on mutual respect and the desire for helping the patient. The patient needs to know that the therapist will maintain confidentiality within the limits of the law and ethical practice; however, there remains the duty to report a clear risk of harm to the patient or to vulnerable others. Reporting needs to occur in an as respectful and transparent way as possible to preserve the continuity of therapy. For the patient who has experienced childhood abuse, knowing the therapist has the role of protector and takes that role seriously is critically important in the validation process.

Stages of Treatment

The first stage of treatment is actually pretreatment. At this point, the patient and therapist negotiate the goals of therapy and arrive at a commitment to the treatment. The therapist may spend two or three sessions gathering information about the patient, his or her target behaviors, previous attempts to change behaviors, and what worked and did not work. This is also when the therapist makes explicit the assumptions and principles of therapy within the DBT model. Once the therapist and patient have committed to working together, the structure for the therapeutic relationship begins to take shape.

The focus of stage one in DBT is addressing life-threatening behaviors and therapy-interfering behaviors. Because the patient is simultaneously in individual therapy and group skills training, he or she is also learning to enhance his or her capabilities. This tends to be a stormy period as the patient adjusts to a class-type environment and expectations. For patients who have been in other types of therapy, this might feel awkward and strange, as they want quick fixes or answers to their personal problems. The focus is on behavioral control and management with emotions as a contextual element. Frequently the patient complains that the skills do not work, and the therapist needs to validate the patient's frustration while encouraging and reinforcing the use of skills. Diary cards are helpful for the patient to monitor his or her use of skills in association with behaviors and feelings. The emphasis is on practicing with the realization that results may take some time. Frequently the patient struggles with the homework of keeping a diary card as well as any assignments from the skills group, and instead wants to use therapy and group to talk about target behaviors. When the patient does not complete assignments or engages in target behaviors, the focus of treatment shifts to analyzing the behavior, the chain of events that led to the behavior, and the consequences of the behavior. This behavioral chain analysis becomes the staple of treatment in guiding the patient to become more mindful and use skills more effectively (see Figure 18.2).

Once the patient has progressed through the first phase of group skills training, he or she then can progress to addressing nontraumatizing emotional experiences. At this point therapy moves into stage two where he or she can regulate his or her emotions in such a way that he or she can think through them. He or she can bring together the dialectics of emotional mindedness and rational mindedness into wise mindedness, that is, a balanced experience of and response to emotions. It is only then that the patient can progress to working on trauma.

In stage three the patient integrates his or her skills, awareness of self, and interpersonal responsiveness to begin confronting the trauma he or she has experienced. This is when the therapist begins exposure therapy in which the patient gradually reexperiences elements of the trauma in small measured doses, using skills to regulate emotions and behavior. (See the discussion on exposure therapy later in this chapter.) As he or she can experience a memory without overwhelming distress, he or she gains a sense of mastery and self-efficacy. This is also when target behaviors may resurface, requiring the therapist to coach the patient in effectively using skills to manage urges

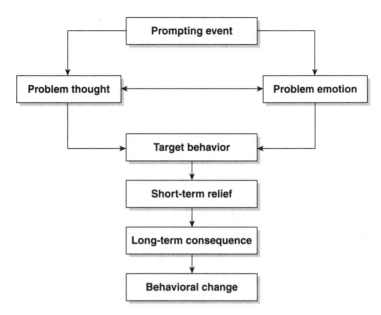

FIGURE 18.2 Behavioral chain analysis worksheet.

(e.g., self-harm behaviors and substance abuse). The therapist may also struggle with feelings of vicarious traumatization or victimizing the patient, and need consultation from other team members.

Finally, in stage four the patient shifts into a transcendent sense of self in which he or she focuses on self-efficacy, interdependence, and self-fulfillment. At this point the therapist prepares the patient to become his or her own therapist by decreasing the frequency and intensity of contact. The patient may become bored with therapy as a genuine response to self-responsibility. There may also be extinction bursts at this time (as well as earlier in treatment) when target behaviors and urges resurface but are quickly thwarted by the patient. The therapist's role here is to maintain calmness without overreacting to the patient's behavior, reassuring the patient that extinction bursts are reasonable and normal and serve more as a testing ground or dress rehearsal to letting go of therapy.

Although it appears that these stages are linear and progressive, the reality is more of a spiraling process. The analogy of the slinky toy traversing stairs is helpful here in that the coils of skills and successes can drive the patient in different directions, sometimes forward and sometimes backward. The overall movement is what counts and that there is progress in general.

DBT Skills Training

Skills training is the sine qua non of DBT because patients frequently lack the basic capabilities to manage their lives, thereby contributing to much of their misery. In fact, studies indicate that without the skills component, DBT is equally as effective as a variety of CBTs. The evidence supportive of full fidelity (including group skills training), however, demonstrates convincingly that DBT has positive and lasting outcomes, especially with those with borderline personality disorder but also with PTSD, substance abuse, eating disorders, and treatment-resistant depression (Andion, Ferrer, Matali, & Gancedo, 2012; Axelrod, Holtzman, & Sinha, 2011; Bloom, Woodward, Susmaras, & Pantalone, 2012; Ost, 2008; Safer, Robinson, & Jo, 2010).

Foundational to skills training is mindful meditation; therefore, these skills are taught in the orientation to group therapy in DBT and repeated at the beginning of each successive module in the 6-month therapy. There are two components to core mindfulness: the "what" skills (observing, describing, and participating) and the "how" skills (nonjudgmental stance, one minded in the moment, and effectiveness) that patients learn, then practice regularly, and include on their diary card (Linehan, 1993b). Although it seems to be a simplistic skill initially, many people (including therapists) struggle with mindfulness, and daily practice over time improves effectiveness and the utility of the other skills. Group sessions begin with mindfulness, team consultation incorporates mindfulness, and both therapists and patients remind each other of the need to stop and activate some brief mindfulness to regulate emotions and behavior. The actual practice of mindfulness can vary widely from quiet meditation to playful games that require full attention to the moment. In guiding the group in mindfulness, the leader provides some background for selecting the exercise and the reasoning for incorporating this activity at this time. Once everyone understands the activity and what to do, the leader signals at the beginning to first get into a comfortable, upright, and grounded position, then use deep breathing to relax, and finally begin the exercise. A Tibetan singing bowl or any kind of gentle cue may be used to signal each step.

Successive modules include sets of skills associated with each topic that help patients modulate their mood, behavior, and interpersonal relationships (Table 18.1).

TABLE 18.1 SKILLS MODULES IN DIALECTICAL BEHAVIOR THERAPY

Module	Common Exercises
Core mindfulness	Mindful abdominal breathing Focusing/observing Describing Wise mind Judgment diffusion
Distress tolerance	Radical acceptance Distract Relaxation Self-soothing
Emotional regulation	Recognizing emotions Reducing vulnerabilities Opposite action to emotion Problem-solving
Interpersonal effectiveness	Knowing what you want Making a request Passive vs. aggressive behavior Assertive listening Negotiating
Self-management	Realistic goal-setting Behavior analysis Contingency management Environmental control

Source: Adapted from McKay, M., Wood, J., & Brantley, J. (2007). *The dialectical behavior therapy skills workbook: Practical DBT exercises for learning mindfulness, interpersonal effectiveness, emotion regulation & distress tolerance.* Oakland, CA: New Harbinger Publications.

These include emotion regulation, interpersonal effectiveness, self-management, and distress tolerance skills. Each module requires about 4 weeks and follows carefully designed exercises and content from a skills manual (Linehan, 1993a; McKay, Wood, & Brantley, 2007). The manual ensures consistency and fidelity to the program, which is important for clinical practice and research to establish reliability and validity of the therapy. Each group session has a process to follow that can be adapted to different groups (e.g., teens, couples, and parents) to provide relevancy. Included in the group are review of content and reasoning, skill practice, homework assignments, and measurement of mastery when concluding a module. At the end of phase 1 that includes all the basic skill modules, the patient graduates to phase 2 that provides reinforcement of the skills and problem-solving effectiveness of skills in real life experiences. Phase 2 anchors skill effectiveness in the patient's life and prepares the patient to progress in more difficult therapy, especially when there is a trauma history. Some patients may elect to retake phase 1 or the therapist may recommend this. This is common for patients who experience a stormy orientation with resistance to full engagement or commitment to the program or other environmental barriers to mastery of skills. Finally, many patients elect to participate in a more advanced group after completing phases 1 and 2 and achieving their therapeutic goals in individual therapy. In the ACES group patients work together as peers to solidify their recovery and improve their functioning and quality of life. Those patients who progress through ACES show maintenance of positive outcomes including low use of emergency or hospital admissions, sustained employment or educational advancement, remission of self-injurious behaviors, and subjective satisfaction (Comtois, Kerbrat, Atkins, Harned, & Elwood, 2010).

Individual Therapy

Concurrent with group skills training, the full DBT model includes weekly individual 30- to 50-minute therapy sessions. Individual therapy follows a CBT approach that begins with several sessions of orientation to the therapy model and establishing the relationship and commitment to working together for the betterment of the patient. In the orientation, the patient and therapist arrive at a priority of behavioral targets with life-threatening behaviors as the highest priority, therapy interfering behaviors as the second highest priority, and quality of life-enhancing behaviors as the third priority area. This is also where the therapist introduces the patient to the diary card (see Exhibit 18.1 for a sample diary card) to monitor progress and give direction to each therapy session.

As the therapeutic relationship solidifies, the therapist progresses to basic treatment strategies including validation of the patient experience, problem-solving, and making changes (Linehan, 1993a). The therapist individualizes these strategies relative to the patient's needs and incorporates stylistic approaches to focus the patient in making the necessary changes in behavior to achieve therapeutic goals. More specific discussion of treatment strategies is beyond the scope of this chapter, and the reader would learn and enhance therapeutic abilities through specific training in DBT.

When a patient participates in target behavior, the therapist guides the patient in analyzing the events in a nonjudgmental and problem-solving way using the behavioral chain analysis. This begins with clearly identifying the problem behavior and describing the events that led to the behavior in a detailed and specific manner. Even though the patient may describe steps in the process in a general way, the therapist pushes for specificity and exquisite detail to identify antecedents and consequences of behavior and vulnerabilities that affect the process leading to the behavior. This detail is crucial for the patient to understand the various links in the chain of events and accompanying thoughts, feelings, and actions. The role of the therapist in this process is to be the naïve observer who is gathering data and seeking to understand every element of the

EXHIBIT 18.1

SAMPLE DIARY CARD FOR STANDARD DBT TREATMENT

Portland DBT Program: Standard Diary Card

Name:								Date Range:			How often did you fill out? __ Daily __ 2–3x __ Once

Day/ Date	Sad (0–5)	Guilt (0–5)	Anger (0–5)	Fear (0–5)	Happy (0–5)	SH U/A	SI U/A	Additional Target	Skills (0–5)	Notes

RATING SCALE FOR EMOTIONS AND URGES: 0 = none   1 = minimal   2 = mild   3 = moderate   4 = strong   5 = intense

USED SKILLS

0 = Didn't think about using
1 = Thought about using, but didn't want to use
2 = Thought about using, wanted to use, but didn't

3 = Used them but didn't help
4 = Used them, helped
5 = Didn't need them, but practiced

Urge to quit Individual (0–5)__
Urge to quit Group (0–5)__
Urge to quit Meds (0–5)__

revised 5.11.2009

FRONT

Instructions: Circle the days you worked on each skill.		How often did you use phone consult? __ daily __ 2–3x __ once __none							
Core Mindfulness	1. Wise mind: balance mind states	Mon	Tues	Wed	Thur	Fri	Sat	Sun
	2. Observe: just notice	Mon	Tues	Wed	Thur	Fri	Sat	Sun
	3. Describe: put words on	Mon	Tues	Wed	Thur	Fri	Sat	Sun
	4. Participate: enter into the experience	Mon	Tues	Wed	Thur	Fri	Sat	Sun
	5. Nonjudgmental stance	Mon	Tues	Wed	Thur	Fri	Sat	Sun
	6. One-mindfully: in the moment	Mon	Tues	Wed	Thur	Fri	Sat	Sun
	7. Effectiveness: focus on what works	Mon	Tues	Wed	Thur	Fri	Sat	Sun
Distress Tol.	8. Distract ACCEPTS	Mon	Tues	Wed	Thur	Fri	Sat	Sun
	9. Self-soothe with the senses	Mon	Tues	Wed	Thur	Fri	Sat	Sun
	10. IMPROVE the moment	Mon	Tues	Wed	Thur	Fri	Sat	Sun
	11. Pros and Cons	Mon	Tues	Wed	Thur	Fri	Sat	Sun
	12. Accepting reality (e.g. half-smile; breathing)	Mon	Tues	Wed	Thur	Fri	Sat	Sun
Emotion Reg.	13. Reduce vulnerability. PLEASE	Mon	Tues	Wed	Thur	Fri	Sat	Sun
	14. Challenge interpretation	Mon	Tues	Wed	Thur	Fri	Sat	Sun
	15. Build mastery	Mon	Tues	Wed	Thur	Fri	Sat	Sun
	16. Build postive experiences	Mon	Tues	Wed	Thur	Fri	Sat	Sun
	17. Opposite-to-emotion setion	Mon	Tues	Wed	Thur	Fri	Sat	Sun
Int Em.	18. Objective effectiveness: DEAR MAN	Mon	Tues	Wed	Thur	Fri	Sat	Sun
	19. Relationship effectiveness: GIVE	Mon	Tues	Wed	Thur	Fri	Sat	Sun
	20. Self-respect effectiveness: FAST	Mon	Tues	Wed	Thur	Fri	Sat	Sun
Prob Sol.	21. Check VITALS: motivate behavior	Mon	Tues	Wed	Thur	Fri	Sat	Sun
	22. Remove/add antecedent/consequence	Mon	Tues	Wed	Thur	Fri	Sat	Sun
	23. Exposure strategy	Mon	Tues	Wed	Thur	Fri	Sat	Sun

BACK

SH, self-harming behaviors; SI, suicidal ideas; U, urges; A, actions.

Source: University of Washington Behavioral Research and Therapy Clinics. (n.d.). *How to complete the diary card: instructions for therapists and patients.* Retrieved from https://depts.washington.edu/uwbrtc/wp-content/uploads/NIMH4-S-DBT-Diary-Cards-with-Instructions.pdf

behavioral chain for the purpose of guiding the patient to ascertain the function the behavior served. Figure 18.2 shows the basic form a behavioral chain analysis would take. It helps to draw the behavioral chain as it develops in the session on a whiteboard or tablet for the patient to see the process and learn how to use the behavioral chain independently. Figures 18.3 and 18.4 provide examples of behavioral chain analyses related to medication management and a nonpharmacological therapy issue. The last

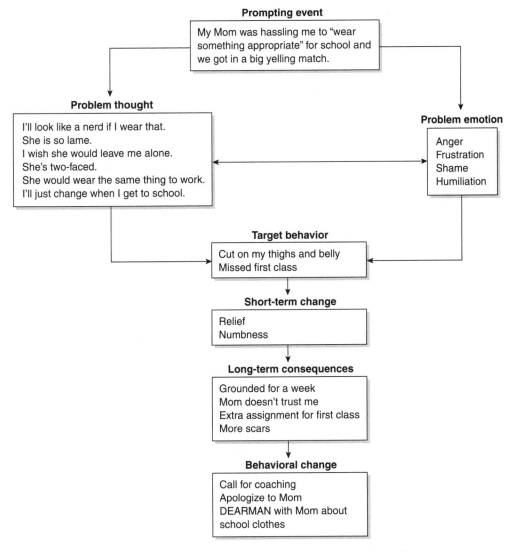

FIGURE 18.3 Sample behavioral chain analysis for teen conflict with mother.

step in the behavioral change involves the use of DEARMAN for the particular issue, which is an acronym for describe, express, assert, reinforce, be mindful, appear confident, and negotiate.

TRAUMA-FOCUSED THERAPY

When the patient is no longer engaging in life-threatening or therapy-interfering behaviors and has a strong trusting relationship with her or his therapist, the patient and therapist can begin to focus on the traumatic experience that brought the patient into therapy. Without the DBT skills and reinforcement of skills in everyday life it would likely be destabilizing to address trauma exposure, and may even contribute to worsening of the patient's condition. Inevitably traumatic experiences that have been held in abeyance begin to influence the person's thoughts, feelings, and behaviors. When done in an unmindful way they can wreak havoc on one's relationships and personal functioning. Most psychotherapeutic approaches recommend some kind of controlled

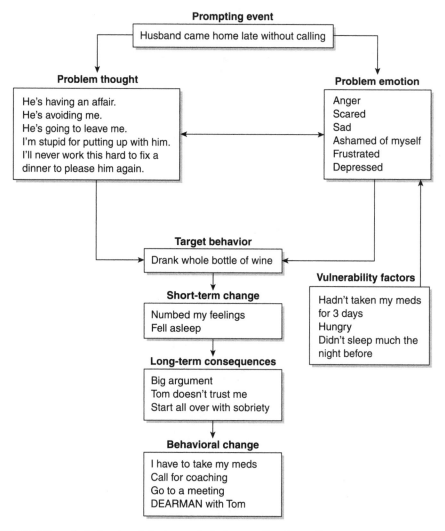

FIGURE 18.4 Sample behavioral chain analysis for medication adherence.

reexperiencing of the traumatic events to begin processing the memories in a more functional manner, thereby reducing symptoms. This may be through such similar strategies as abreaction, EMDR (eye movement desensitization and reprocessing therapy), or exposure therapy. All of these seem to produce results by connecting what currently seem like disconnected fragmented memories to neural circuits that allow cognitive processing and then storage in ordinary as opposed to fearful memory circuits. From a behavioral perspective, exposure therapy is a process of counterconditioning, that is, substituting an adaptive response for one that is nonadaptive. There are at least two basic types of exposure: imaginal exposure in which the patient experiences the stimulus in her or his imagination only, and in vivo exposure in which the patient experiences the actual stimulus in reality. In PTSD, in vivo exposure is limited to the people, places, and situations only and not the actual trauma, of course (Rauch, Foa, Furr, & Filip, 2004).

Preparing for Exposure

Prior to exposure work, the patient and the therapist need to do considerable preparatory work including what behaviors and emotions to target, the memory structures that are involved, the type of exposure to use, and the orientation of the patient to the process. This of course assumes the patient has sufficient stability and skills to begin the process. It is not uncommon to interrupt exposure work to restabilize the patient and provide some refresher skill development and scaffolding.

In identifying behavioral and emotional targets, it is helpful to consider a hierarchy and decide with the patient to address these from the least difficult to the most difficult (graduated exposure) or to begin with the big picture, that is, to rip off the Band-Aid (flooding). Then the patient and therapist discuss scheduling the exposure sessions, that is, scheduling sufficient time relative to the type of exposure that also allows debriefing and reconsolidation, possibly scheduling another therapy appointment for that week to simply debrief and review the diary card, dealing with how the patient will conduct the rest of the day, and addressing between-session symptom arousal. In orienting the patient, it may help to try a behavioral rehearsal for exposure, for example, choose a minor emotion such as embarrassment after a fall on the ice, and practice experiencing the emotions, then extinguishing them through repeated exposure, fully engaging in the emotion, using skills to manage the emotion, and preventing the behavioral response that usually accompanies the emotion (e.g., avoidance). This prepares the patient for the process of exposure and builds confidence in doing the exposure work. Because this is an unpleasant experience, it is essential that the patient understand and consent in a fully informed manner.

Conducting the Exposure

Begin by determining with the patient what situation elicits the unwanted emotional response and the discriminating conditions that influence the response (e.g., the patient may experience intense anxiety in small social gatherings among strangers but be comfortable in larger groups or with close friends). Then establish with the patient the intensity of the emotion before and after exposure, often using the subjective units of disturbance (SUD) scale that ranges from 0 to 100 with 0 being complete comfort and 100 being excruciating distress.

In graduated exposure, the targets for exposure are arranged in a hierarchy of initial SUD intensity and addressed from lower to higher intensity. The therapist then walks the patient through the stressful event from the very beginning while being attentive to the patient's emotional response and assisting the patient to tolerate the emotion while using skills to manage them, periodically asking the patient to rate the discomfort using the SUD scale. Repeat each situation until the SUD is much lower and the patient can tolerate reexperiencing with reasonable emotion and without negative behavioral responses. In traumatic events, it may be helpful to break the event into smaller units with lower SUDs and move gradually into more difficult elements. For example, a patient who was raped on her way home from work late at night spent several weeks imaging walking down the dark street, using mindfulness to observe and describe the cars parked along the street, the ambient sounds, the smells of early spring, and her rising sense of fear. When she was able to experience this without self-recrimination, her SUD rating dropped to 30 and she was ready to move on to the more frightening part of the experience. In this situation, the therapist combined imaginal and in vivo exposure in a progressive way.

Flooding exposure introduces cues with the highest SUD rating, and research indicates more sustaining long-term effectiveness than graduated exposure (Foa et al., 2005). It requires longer sessions and tends to be more distressing for the patient. The therapist approaches treatment the same as graduated exposure but focuses on the stimulus that the patient identifies as most distressing. The patient and therapist review the events repeatedly until the patient experiences a tolerable drop in SUDs. The treatment usually requires nine to 12 sessions and may include between-session CBT or DBT focused treatment, although research results indicate that additional cognitive treatments provide no additional benefits to the prolonged exposure (Foa et al., 2005). The patient may experience less between-session exacerbations of PTSD symptoms, however.

Following exposure treatment there usually is a period of stabilization and transition in therapy toward termination. Although some patients seek additional follow-up sessions, most show reduction in PTSD and depression symptoms to the extent that they return to work and ordinary social functioning. Much of the research has been done with women with acute and chronic PTSD and with veterans of both the Vietnam War and more recent wars. Less research has been done with women who have experienced military sexual assault alone or in conjunction with war trauma (Karlin et al., 2010; Nasasch et al., 2011; Powers, Halpern, Ferenschak, Gillihan, & Foa, 2010).

CASE EXAMPLE

Mr. M is a 68-year-old retired Marine who served for 13 months in combat posts in Vietnam during his service, and worked for a construction company as an electrician for 40 years. He has been married three times and has two adult sons and an adult daughter. His current wife was recently diagnosed with cervical cancer and Mr. M is struggling to maintain his 30 years of sobriety as he supports his wife during extensive surgery, radiation, and chemotherapy. His sponsor recommended he see a therapist for support. Although he was reluctant, he finally began to see a psychologist who saw him for three sessions, diagnosed chronic and complex PTSD; major depressive disorder, moderate and recurrent; and sustained remission but now threatened alcohol and cannabis dependency. The psychologist referred the patient for continued treatment with a DBT program due to the severity of PTSD and need for a wider treatment base, including group treatment and 24-hour availability for coaching.

In the assessment and orientation phase of treatment, Mr. M reported chronic insomnia characterized by frequent nightmares and sleep avoidance, delayed onset of sleep, frequent interruptions, and early awakening. He also has had several episodes of prolonged depression with suicidal thoughts and two serious attempts including hanging himself when he was 23 years old and within 6 months after discharge from the Marines. The patient's father came home from work early when he found Mr. M unconscious and hanging by his uniform belt in his bedroom closet. In another attempt a year later, Mr. M was drunk and tried to drown himself by walking into the ocean with rocks in his pockets; however, a bystander happened to notice Mr. M's activity while walking along the beach at 3 a.m. and called the police.

During the assessment, Mr. M endorsed symptoms of prolonged sadness and irritability, difficulty concentrating enough to even read the newspaper, frequent "spacing out" while at home when his wife was in the hospital or during waits during her treatments, poor appetite with 12-pound weight loss over the past month, intense self-demeaning statements and thoughts, self-blame for his wife's illness, and extreme leaden fatigue without motivation or interest in anything pleasurable. In the past, his four grandchildren usually made him happy but for the past 6 months even their presence seemed to annoy him. Additionally, Mr. M has strong cravings to drink alcohol, and the week before his first therapy appointment at the DBT program he found himself walking in an area of town where he knew he could buy drugs, even though he did not remember how he got there. He called his sponsor for a ride home.

Mr. M reported his early childhood history was marked by his parents divorcing when he was 3. He lived with his mother and older sister for 2 years but was eventually removed from the home when his mother attempted to kill both children and herself.

The father could not be located so both Mr. M and his sister were placed in a series of foster homes where both were physically and emotionally abused, and his sister was sexually abused in two separate homes. Eventually, Mr. M escaped foster care by participating in home robberies and drug possession and distribution and placed in juvenile detention until he was 18 years old.

He completed high school and joined the Marines early in the Vietnam War and was deployed within a year of enlistment. Most of his experience in Vietnam was in ground combat where he experienced the death and injuries of many of his friends to such an extent that he made a deliberate attempt to not form friendships, a pattern he maintained after returning to stateside.

During his year-long treatment he eventually described several particularly gruesome experiences in which he anticipated dying or severe injury. On only one occasion was he actually wounded in a firefight when he was hit with shrapnel from a bomb dropped on his quarters while he and his company were sleeping. Mr. M never described any of these experiences prior to this treatment, and he was particularly resistant to discuss them because he believed they were too long ago, irrelevant, and did not compare to the experience his wife was having with her cancer.

Initially the APPN focused on establishing a trusting relationship with Mr. M, which was quite challenging because he would frequently miss appointments, show up late, and not do his assigned homework. After 4 weeks he started in a phase 1 standard DBT treatment with all the other participants having substance abuse issues as well as trauma. Mr. M would fall asleep in the classes the first few weeks and the APPN individual therapist would conduct a behavioral chain analysis of this behavior as illustrated in Figure 18.5. His repair to the group was to discuss his homework first at the next three sessions and to bring a healthy snack for everyone to share. Eventually Mr. M became more consistent in his attendance and brought his diary card to sessions (see Exhibit 18.2 for sample).

In both group and individual therapy, Mr. M focused on the dialectic of his crisis-generating behaviors (e.g., fantasizing suicide/murder) and facing his inhibited grieving. It was critically important that he find a middle ground in living his life while allowing his feelings of grief both for his childhood and military experiences and his wife's illness. After 6 weeks of group therapy he was practicing his skills most days and was beginning to feel more confident of his ability to manage his emotions and behavior without internal or external upheaval or crisis-generating behavior. He continued to feel suicidal but frequency and intensity decreased significantly.

After 3 weeks of individual sessions the APPN recommended medications to target the sleep disturbance and depression. Initially Mr. M refused to consider medication because it was a sign of weakness and he was afraid of becoming addicted to the medications. The APPN spent considerable time explaining how medications work on the chemicals in his brain that were not effective, and finally Mr. M agreed to take prazosin (Minipress) 1 mg daily for his nightmares and this was titrated up to 5 mg at bedtime to get sustained relief of nighttime anxiety and improved dreaming. He later agreed to take citalopram (Celexa) 10 mg daily titrated up to 40 mg for his depression and anxiety; however, this was ineffective after 6 weeks and the APPN changed it to duloxetine 60 mg at which point, Mr. M began to feel more activated and motivated. He still had anxiety and agreed to a trial of lurasidone 20 mg, titrated up to 40 mg where he felt more activated, less anxious, and improved mood. After 3 months of therapy and medication he no longer felt suicidal and was making plans to visit the national parks in the United States with his wife in their recreational van.

After completing phase 1 and midway through phase 2 of DBT treatment both the therapist and patient began exploring Mr. M's anxiety related to his wife's illness and likely death. As he allowed his feelings to emerge he began having flashbacks of combat

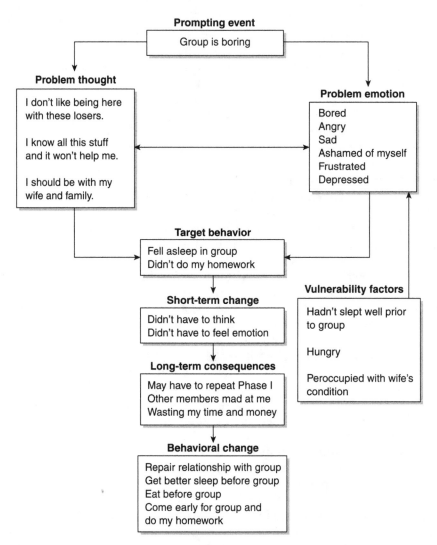

FIGURE 18.5 Behavioral chain analysis for Mr. M.

in Vietnam and feeling guilty that he was focusing on his problems instead of his wife. The therapist helped Mr. M consider the dialectics of accepting his wife's illness and self-compassion for his fears while also working to change his self-invalidating thoughts and angry outburst when he felt sadness. The therapist engaged Mr. M in practicing the skill of opposite action to emotion in which he would watch old comedies with his wife in the evenings following her treatments. He also began to face his emotional vulnerabilities and counteract his self-invalidation. At some point Mr. M began to feel real joy in his life along with the constant fear of his wife's eventual death. He spent more time with the family including his adult children and their children and took his wife for short trips to the beach.

The day after graduating from phase 2, Mr. M's wife suddenly died from a pulmonary embolus. Mr. M became rageful and help rejecting. Suicidal urges returned to such an extent that he began carrying his service revolver every day and would sit in his car and rehearse shooting himself. His daughter found him one day and yelled at him for being so selfish and self-absorbed. This shocked Mr. M and he gave his gun to his therapist. They scheduled twice-weekly appointments until he could get back into a

EXHIBIT 18.2

Mr. M's Early Diary Card

Portland DBT Program: Standard Diary Card

Name: SM								Date Range: 1/4 - 1/10			How often did you fill out? __ Daily ☒2–3x __ Once	

Day/ Date	Sad (0–5)	Guilt (0–5)	Anger (0–5)	Fear (0–5)	Happy (0–5)	SH U/A	SI U/A	Additional Target	Skills (0–5)	Notes
1/4	5	5	3	0	0	0 / 0	0 / 0		3+	
1/5	5	5	4	1	0	0 / 0	0 / 0		3+	
1/6	5	5	2	0	0	0 / 0	0 / 0		4	
1/10	4	4	3	0	0	0 / 0	0 / 0		4	

RATING SCALE FOR EMOTIONS AND URGES: 0 = none 1 = minimal 2 = mild 3 = moderate 4 = strong 5 = intense

USED SKILLS
0 = Didn't think about using
1 = Thought about using, but didn't want to use
2 = Thought about using, wanted to use, but didn't

3 = Used them but didn't help
4 = Used them, helped
5 = Didn't need them, but practiced

Urge to quit Individual (0–5) __
Urge to quit Group (0–5) 0
Urge to quit Meds (0–5) 0

revised 5.11.2009

FRONT

	Instructions: Circle the days you worked on each skill.					How often did you use phone consult? __ daily __ 2–3x __ once ☒ none		
Core Mindfulness	1. Wise mind: balance mind states	Mon	Tues	Wed	Thur	Fri	Sat	Sun
	2. Observe: just notice	(Mon)	(Tues)	(Wed)	(Thur)	(Fri)	(Sat)	(Sun)
	3. Describe: put words on	(Mon)	(Tues)	(Wed)	(Thur)	(Fri)	(Sat)	(Sun)
	4. Participate: enter into the experience	Mon	Tues	(Wed)	(Thur)	Fri	Sat	(Sun)
	5. Nonjudgmental stance	Mon	Tues	Wed	Thur	Fri	Sat	Sun
	6. One-mindfully: in the moment	(Mon)	(Tues)	Wed	Thur	Fri	Sat	Sun
	7. Effectiveness: focus on what works	Mon	Tues	Wed	Thur	(Fri)	(Sat)	(Sun)
Distress Tol.	8. Distract ACCEPTS	Mon	Tues	(Wed)	(Thur)	Fri	Sat	Sun
	9. Self-soothe with the senses	Mon	Tues	(Wed)	(Thur)	Fri	Sat	Sun
	10. IMPROVE the moment	Mon	Tues	(Wed)	(Thur)	Fri	Sat	Sun
	11. Pros and Cons	Mon	Tues	Wed	Thur	(Fri)	(Sat)	Sun
	12. Accepting reality (e.g. half-smile; breathing)	(Mon)	(Tues)	(Wed)	Thur	Fri	Sat	Sun
Emotion Reg.	13. Reduce vulnerability. PLEASE	Mon	Tues	Wed	Thur	Fri	Sat	Sun
	14. Challenge interpretation	Mon	Tues	Wed	Thur	Fri	Sat	Sun
	15. Build mastery	Mon	Tues	Wed	Thur	Fri	Sat	Sun
	16. Build postive experiences	Mon	Tues	Wed	Thur	Fri	Sat	Sun
	17. Opposite-to-emotion setion	Mon	Tues	Wed	Thur	Fri	Sat	Sun
Int Em.	18. Objective effectiveness: DEAR MAN	Mon	Tues	Wed	Thur	Fri	Sat	Sun
	19. Relationship effectiveness: GIVE	Mon	Tues	Wed	Thur	Fri	Sat	Sun
	20. Self-respect effectiveness: FAST	Mon	Tues	Wed	Thur	Fri	Sat	Sun
Prob Sol.	21. Check VITALS: motivate behavior	Mon	Tues	Wed	Thur	Fri	Sat	Sun
	22. Remove/add antecedent/consequence	Mon	Tues	Wed	Thur	Fri	Sat	Sun
	23. Exposure strategy	Mon	Tues	Wed	Thur	Fri	Sat	Sun

BACK

phase 2 group to focus on skills. He also attended a spouse bereavement group weekly and returned to daily Alcoholics Anonymous (AA) meetings. His daughter and one son joined him in family therapy at the DBT program and addressed issues of abandonment and invalidation. His daughter expressed her anger with Mr. M during her early years because he was so distant and "odd" and seemed "so together." Mr. M and his son began to address their respective apparent competence that prevented others from being able to be supportive or helpful.

Within 4 months of his wife's death, Mr. M began to connect his early childhood abuse with his military experiences. He recognized that joining the Marines was an attempt to get structure and stability but this backfired when he was sent to Vietnam where stability was impossible. His use of alcohol and marijuana was the only way he could cope. Returning to civilian life did not provide stability as he continued to numb his emotions with substances that eventually contributed to the demise of his significant relationships with his wives and his sister. He began the trauma program at DBT where the therapist first attempted gradual exposure. Mr. M was impatient with his progress, and the therapist and patient agreed that using flooding might be reasonable, given his effective use of skills and commitment to treatment. The Vietnam Veterans Association assisted him in gaining access to a virtual reality facility where the therapist and patient worked with his combat experiences. This was a difficult time for Mr. M, and his medications were adjusted several times to provide sufficient support in his recovery.

Eventually Mr. M stabilized behaviorally and emotionally. He reunited with his sister after decades of estrangement, and encouraged her to locate a DBT program in her state to address her traumatic events and the consequential life difficulties she continued to experience. Mr. M had continued in the ACES program to anchor his recovery in the reality of living his life outside of therapy. He jokes that he is the "poster child for DBT" because he was the worst patient ever initially and now is an avid spokesperson. He participates in online forums and maintains a DBT app on his cell phone to remind him of skills to use. Although he saw his treatment as tumultuous, Mr. M recognized how essential it was for him to learn new behaviors before he could tackle "Pandora's box."

POST-MASTER'S TRAINING

APPNs who would like to use DBT in their practice would be best served by taking a course through one of the certified training programs. Behavioral Tech, LLC, offers training through regional workshops and online. This organization, founded by Marsha Linehan, has a full staff of trainers who provide authorized certification in DBT and maintains a well-designed website (www.behavioraltech.org/training). Taking a beginner's course provides a complete orientation to DBT, in addition to reading the classic texts by Linehan (1993a, 1993b) noted in the references at the end of this chapter. Additionally, the book by Dimeff (2007) is an important book to read and use for reference when starting this practice approach. After completing a beginner's course, the APPN might locate a full DBT clinic to find a clinician as a mentor (www.dbtinformation.org/htm/clinics.html). Starting with skills training and using a skills manual or workbook such as those included in the references at the end of this chapter will help the APPN become more comfortable with the basics of DBT. Finally, it is important to eventually take an intensive workshop, usually a week long, that is offered around the country and builds confidence in practicing DBT. The Behavioral Tech, LLC, website provides an ongoing list of intensive workshops including those for independent practitioners. What is most important in using DBT with complex patients is to develop and maintain a consultative team of colleagues who use DBT not only in their practice but also in their lives. The consultation team provides support and reinforcement of skills needed in working with this vulnerable population.

CONCLUDING COMMENTS

Complex PTSD and borderline personality disorder have more in common both epidemiologically and diagnostically, and therefore have better outcome effectiveness when treated similarly. The most researched therapeutic approaches to produce effective and lasting improvement include prolonged exposure, CBT, and DBT (Foa et al., 2005; Harned, Korslund, Foa, & Linehan, 2012; Robertson, Humphreys, & Ray, 2004). These are treatments that the advanced practice psychiatric nurse can use with some additional training to provide quality effective treatment for patients. The evidence clearly establishes these treatments as the basis for the best clinical practice when properly used. In providing treatment for someone with complex PTSD, the therapist needs to be flexible and persistent in considering the most appropriate approach for this particular patient (Wagner, Rizvi, & Harned, 2007). The patient needs to trust the therapist's competence, skill, and sensitivity before engaging in this work.

With a fully functioning DBT model the therapist also receives the benefit of consultation from other team members when engaging in this difficult work with patients. The APPN who is trying to do this in a private practice would benefit from forming a consultation group of other clinicians using CBT and DBT to fortify his or her work and protect him or her from burnout and the added vulnerability of vicarious traumatization. Additionally, the discipline would benefit by APPNs conducting research and writing about clinical work in these situations to demonstrate the role of the advanced practice nursing in this area.

DISCUSSION QUESTIONS

1. How does mindfulness serve as a core skill in DBT and for the patient in therapy? How would the APPN guide the patient in adding mindfulness to the patient's daily practice?
2. What DBT skills would be essential for the chronically suicidal patient with complex PTSD? Why are these skills of higher priority than others?
3. How can the APPN incorporate DBT in a solo practice? What would be essential to maintain the clinician who uses DBT in solo practice? How would the APPN create the optimal environment to incorporate DBT in practice?
4. What would be the limitations of using DBT in solo practice? How would the APPN compensate for these limitations both for self and for the patient?
5. How are borderline personality disorder, complex PTSD, and bipolar disorder similar and different? What treatment strategies would the APPN consider in working with populations with these disorders? How might the practice be different with these disorders?
6. Consider a patient the student is currently working with or has strong recollections of working with in the past. How might DBT enhance the therapy with that patient? How might the APPN work with that patient now with knowledge about DBT?
7. What role does medication play in DBT? How would the APPN incorporate medication management and therapy with the patient in DBT? If providing only medication management, how would the APPN collaborate with the other providers? If conducting therapy with a DBT patient, how would the APPN decide whether to include medication management or refer to another provider for medication management?
8. What ethical issues arise in incorporating DBT in clinical practice? How does the APPN's values and beliefs affect incorporation of DBT in other forms of psychotherapy?

REFERENCES

Andion, O., Ferrer, M., Matali, J., & Gancedo, G. E. (2012). Effectiveness of combined individual and group dialectical behavior therapy compared to only individual dialectical behavior therapy: A preliminary study. *Psychotherapy, 49*(2), 241–250. doi:10.1037/a0027401

Axelrod, W. P., Holtzman, K., & Sinha, R. (2011). Emotion regulation and substance use frequency in women with substance dependence and borderline personality disorder receiving dialectical behavior therapy. *The American Journal of Drug and Alcohol Abuse, 37,* 37–42. doi:10.3109/00952990.2010.535582

Bloom, J., Woodward, E., Susmaras, T., & Pantalone, D. (2012). Use of dialectical behavior therapy in inpatient treatment of borderline personality disorder: A systematic review. *Psychiatric Services, 63,* 881–888. doi:10.1176/appi.ps.201100311

Chu, J. (2011). *Rebuilding shattered lives: Treating complex PTSD and dissociative disorders* (2nd ed.). Hoboken, NJ: John Wiley & Sons.

Comtois, K., Kerbrat, A., Atkins, D., Harned, M., & Elwood, L. (2010). Recovery from disability for individuals with borderline personality disorder: A feasiblity trial of DBT-ACES. *Psychiatric Services, 61*(11),1106–1111. doi:10.1176/ps.2010.61.11.1106

Dimeff, L. (Ed.). (2007). *Dialectical behavior therapy in clinical practice: Applications across disorders and settings.* New York, NY: Guilford Press.

Foa, E., Hembree, E., Cahill, S., Rauch, S., Riggs, D., Feny, N., & Yadin, E. (2005). Randomized trial of prolonged exposure for posttraumatic stress with and without cognitive restructuring: Outcome at academic and community clinics. *Journal of Consulting and Clinical Psychology, 73*(5), 953–964. doi:10.1037/0022-006X.73.5.953

Harned, M., Korslund, K., Foa, E., & Linehan, M. (2012). Treating PTSD in suicidal and self-injuring women with borderline personality disorder: Development and preliminary evaluation of a dialectical behavior therapy prolonged exposure protocol. *Behaviour Research and Therapy, 50,* 381–386. doi:10.1016/j.brat.2012.02.011

Karlin, B., Ruzek, J., Chard, K., Eftekhari, A., Monson, C. H., & Foa, E. (2010). Dissemination of evidence-based psychological treatments for posttraumatic stress disorder in the Veterans Health Administration. *Journal of Traumatic Stress, 23*(6), 663–672. doi:10.1002/jts.20588

Linehan, M. (1993a). *Cognitive-behavioral treatment of borderline personality disorder.* New York, NY: Guilford Press.

Linehan, M. (1993b). *Manual for treating borderline personality disorder.* New York, NY: Guilford Press.

McKay, M., Wood, J., & Brantley, J. (2007). *The dialectical behavior therapy skills workbook: Practical DBT exercises for learning mindfulness, interpersonal effectiveness, emotion regulation & distress tolerance.* Oakland, CA: New Harbinger Publications.

Nasasch, N., Foa, E., Huppert, J., Tzur, D., Fostick, L., Dinstein, Y., . . . Zohar, M. (2011). Prolonged exposure therapy for combat- and terror-related posttraumatic stress disorder: A randomized control comparison with treatment as usual. *The Journal of Clinical Psychiatry, 72,* 1174–1180. doi:10.4088/JCP.09m05682blu

Ost, L. G. (2008). Efficacy of the third wave of behavioral therapies: A systematic review and meta-analysis. *Behaviour Research and Therapy, 46,* 296–321. doi:10.1016/j.brat.2007.12.005

Powers, M., Halpern, J., Ferenschak, M., Gillihan, S., & Foa, E. (2010). A meta-analytic review of prolonged exposure for posttraumatic stress disorder. *Clinical Psychology Review, 30,* 635–641. doi:10.1016/j.cpr.2010.04.007

Rauch, S., Foa, E., Furr, J., & Filip, J. (2004). Imagery vividness and perceived anxious arousal in prolonged exposure treatment for PTSD. *Journal of Traumatic Stress, 17*(6), 461–465. doi:10.1007/s10960-004-5794-8

Robertson, M., Humphreys, L., & Ray, R. (2004). Psychological treatments for posttraumatic stress disorder: Recommendations for the clinician based on a review of the literature. *Journal of Psychiatric Practice, 10*(2), 106–118. doi:10.1097/00131746-200403000-00005

Safer, D., Robinson, A., & Jo, B. (2010). Outcome from a randomized controlled trial of group therapy for binge eating disorder: Comparing dialectical behavior therapy adapted for binge eating to an active comparison group therapy. *Behavior Therapy, 41*(1),106–120 doi:10.1016/j.beth.2009.01.006

Wagner, A., Rizvi, S., & Harned, M. (2007). Applications of dialectical behavior therapy to the treatment of complex trauma-related problems: When one case formulation does not fit all. *Journal of Traumatic Stress, 20*, 391–400. doi:10.1002/jts.20268.

Psychotherapeutic Approaches for Addictions and Related Disorders

Susie Adams

Coping with life stressors is an inevitable part of the human experience. Anxiety, depression, loss, neglect, illness, chronic pain, trauma, or other life stressors can result in dysregulation of the individual—physiologically, emotionally, cognitively, interpersonally, and spiritually. From infancy onward, biopsychosocial factors drive one's attempts to "self-soothe" or self-regulate feelings, thoughts, and emotions in response to the world around us. The use of mood altering substances and mood altering behaviors can be viewed as the individual's attempts to "self-soothe."

The cultural, social, and legal context frame the degree of acceptance of any given behavior or use of substances. Nicotine, caffeine, and alcohol are legally and socially accepted. The use of prescription anxiolytics, analgesics, opioids, sedatives, hypnotics, and stimulants is condoned when properly prescribed and used as directed to manage various conditions. Gambling, computer gaming, sexual intimacy, running marathons, Internet use, and shopping are socially acceptable behaviors. Although heroin and cocaine remain illicit substances, the legalization of marijuana for first medical use in over 17 states, and more recently legalization for recreational use in Colorado and Washington, are shifting the boundaries of what are considered illicit substances of abuse and addiction. It is the misuse, excessive use, dependence, and ultimately the inability to control one's use of mood-altering substances or mood-altering behaviors that are problematic.

Historically, addiction has been defined as the compulsive need for and use of a habit-forming substance (such as heroin, nicotine, or alcohol) characterized by tolerance and physiological symptoms of withdrawal and recognized to be physically, psychologically, or socially harmful (Merriam-Webster, 2020). There is growing recognition among researchers that a compulsive behavior can stimulate the same reward system in the brain that leads to pleasurable or "self-soothing" sensations similar to mood altering substances (Grant, Brewer, & Potenza, 2006). The individual becomes addicted to the behavior and the associated pleasurable feeling brought about by the particular behavior such as gambling, Internet pornography, exercise, or sexual behaviors. These compulsive behaviors are sometimes categorized as process addictions.

The purpose of this chapter is to present an integrated model of care supported by evidence-based psychotherapeutic interventions that facilitate lifelong recovery for individuals with substance and behavioral addictions. Pharmacological interventions for substance addictions, while well supported by research and clinical practice, are beyond the scope of this chapter. An overview of the prevalence, health risks, and the financial burden of addictive disorders provides a compelling context for addressing this global health problem. A discussion of *Diagnostic and Statistical Manual of Mental Disorders* (5th ed.; *DSM-5; American Psychiatric Association [APA], 2013*) criteria for addictions and related disorders provides a new context for understanding what was previously confined to substance use disorders (SUDs) in the *Diagnostic and Statistical Manual of Mental Disorders-Training Revision* (4th ed.; *DSM-IV-TR*; American Psychiatric Association, 2000). Definitions of key terms including addiction, SUDs, behavioral addiction, relapse, and recovery will be followed by a brief synopsis of causative factors (neurobiology, behavioral, and psychosocial factors). Principles of comprehensive treatment components will be presented followed by screening and assessment tools and a discussion of evidence-based psychotherapeutic interventions. The chapter concludes with a case study that demonstrates an integrated person-centered treatment approach.

OVERVIEW OF ADDICTIONS

Prevalence

The abuse of illicit and licit psychoactive substances is a serious U.S. and global public health problem. Table 19.1 and Table 19.2, respectively, provide a synopsis of the prevalence, health risks, and economic burden of addictions worldwide and in the United States. Despite regional differences, worldwide, alcohol causes greater harm to younger men (7.6% of deaths, 8.9% of disability-adjusted life years [DALYs] for men 15 to 49 years, 18.9% DALYs for men 50+ years) and greater harm to older women (4% of deaths, 2.3% of DALYs for women 15 to 49 years, 27.1% for women 50+ years), reflecting gender differences in quantity, frequency, and patterns of drinking (Global Burden of Disease [GBD] Alcohol Collaborators, 2018; United Nations Office of Drugs and Crime [UNODC], 2018; World Health Organization [WHO], 2012).

According to data from the U.S. National Survey on Drug Use and Health (NSDUH), the use of illicit and licit psychoactive substances has been on the rise between 2002 and 2018 across most age categories and for most substances (Substance Abuse and Mental Health Services Administration [SAMHSA], 2002, 2012, 2018). The steady rise in the amount of use, binge use, and heavy alcohol use from high school into the college years is significant. See Figure 19.1 for current alcohol use, binge drinking, and heavy drinking patterns by age group. Epidemiological studies indicate that delaying initial alcohol use until after the age of 14 years can significantly decrease lifetime risk of subsequent alcohol abuse and dependence (DeWitt, Adlaf, Offord, & Ogborne, 2000). Individuals who start to drink at age 11 or 12 years are nearly 10 times more likely to become alcohol dependent than those who started drinking later (ages 19 and older;) DeWitt et al., 2000). Other researchers have found that individuals who experienced two or more adverse childhood events also have a 1.37 times greater risk for lifetime alcohol dependence than individuals who had no adverse childhood events (Pilowsky, Keyes, & Hasin, 2009).

There are a number of "at-risk" populations within the United States where even higher prevalence of SUDs occurs. These include survivors of emotional, physical, and sexual abuse; people with physical, sensory, or cognitive disabilities; people who live with chronic pain; people with depression; people who are unemployed that have limited education and low socioeconomic status; and people with military combat service (Len et al., 2016; SAMHSA, 2012, 2018). Since the U.S. financial crisis in 2008, unemployment rates have soared along with concomitant home foreclosures, loss of healthcare coverage,

TABLE 19.1 WORLDWIDE PREVALENCE, HEALTH RISKS, AND ECONOMIC BURDEN OF ADDICTIONS

Use:[1,3]	
• Alcohol users	2.4 billion
• Daily tobacco smokers	1.1 billion
• Drug users	275 million
Alcohol Health-Related Risks & Disability:[1]	
• Seventh leading risk for death	
• Seventh leading risk for DALYs	
Alcohol Use Risk to Men vs. Risk to Women:[1,3]	
• Ages 15–49 yrs	8.9% of DALYs for men vs. 2.3% of DALYs for women
• Ages 50+ yrs	18.9% of DALYs for men vs. 27.1% of DALYs for women
• 7.6% of deaths for men	vs. 4.0% of deaths for women
Economic Burden:*[2]	
• Healthcare costs	1.3%–3.3%
• Public order/safety costs	6.4%–14.4%
• Criminal damages	0.3%–1.4%
• Drunk driving costs	1.0%–1.7%
• Workplace costs	2.7%–10.9%
• Total global cost estimates	$210–$665 billion

*Statistics only available on alcohol. Calculated as percent of Gross Domestic Product (GDP)

[1]Global Burden of Disease Alcohol Collaborators (2018)

[2]Institute of Alcohol Studies, UK (Baumberg, 2006)

[3]World Health Organization (2012)

DALYs = Disability-Adjusted Life Years

TABLE 19.2 U.S. PREVALENCE, HEALTH RISKS, AND ECONOMIC BURDEN OF ADDICTIONS

Use in Past Month (Age 12 Years and Older)[1]		
• Current illicit substance use	11.2%	30.5 million
• Current alcohol use	51.6%	140.6 million
• Binge drinking*	24.5%	66.6 million
• Heavy drinking**	6.1%	16.7 million
Past Month Misuse of Psychotherapeutic Prescription* (Age 12 Years and Older)[1]**		
• Psychotherapeutic prescription	2.2%	6.0 million
• Pain relievers	1.2%	3.2 million
• Stimulants	0.66%	1.8 million

(continued)

TABLE 19.2 U.S. PREVALENCE, HEALTH RISKS, AND ECONOMIC BURDEN OF ADDICTIONS (*CONTINUED*)		
• Tranquilizers	0.62%	1.7 million
• Sedatives	0.15%	0.4 million
Past Year Opioid Misuse**** (Age 12 Years and Older)[1]		
• Opioid misuse	4.2%	11.4 million
• Pain reliever misuse only	3.9%	10.5 million
• Heroin use only	0.3%	0.3 million
• Pain reliever misuse & heroin use	0.6%	0.6 million
Lifetime Prevalence[2]		
• Alcohol abuse	13.2%	
• Alcohol dependence	5.6%	
• Substance use disorder any kind	14.6%	
Medical Comorbidity Risks[3]		
• Drug abuse/dependence	1.5–2.6 × risk for	CHD
• Drug abuse/dependence	1.3–1.7 × risk for	HTN
• Drug abuse/dependence	1.4–1.7 × risk for	Arteriosclerosis
• Drug abuse/dependence	2.0–2.7 × risk for	Liver disease
• Drug abuse/dependence	1.3–2.0 × risk for	Arthritis
• Alcohol dependence	1.5 × risk for	CHD
• Alcohol dependence	1.8 × risk for	Liver disease
Estimated Economic Cost[4,5]		
• Alcohol	$249 billion/year	
• Tobacco	$300 billion/year	
• Illicit drugs	$193 billion/year	
• Prescription opioid misuse	$78.5 billion/year	
• Total	$820.5 billion/year	

*Since 2015 binge drinking is defined as four or more alcoholic beverages per occasion for women and five or more alcoholic beverages per occasion for men.

**Heavy drinking is defined as having five or more drinks a day with binge drinking during past month.

***The estimated numbers of past month misusers of different prescription psychotherapeutics are not mutually exclusive because people could have misused more than one type of prescription psychotherapeutic in past month.

****Opioid misuse is defined as heroin use or prescription pain reliever misuse.

[1]Substance Abuse and Mental Health Services Administration (2018).

[2]Kessler et al. (2005).

[3]Chou, Huang, Goldstein, & Grant (2013).

[4]Centers for Disease Control and Prevention (n.d.).

[5]National Institute on Drug Abuse (2017).

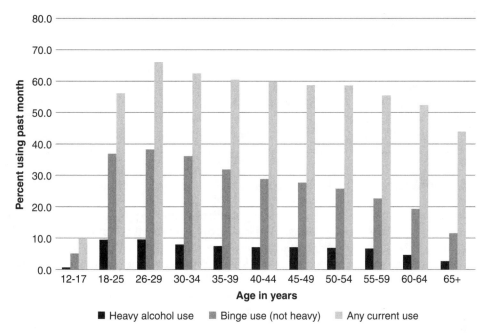

FIGURE 19.1 Current, binge, and heavy alcohol use among persons (age 12 years and older) by age group.

Source: Adapted from Substance Abuse and Mental Health Services Administration. (2018). *Key substance use and mental health indicators in the United States: Results from the 2017 National Survey on Drug Use and Health* (HHS Publication No. SMA 18-5068, NSDUH Series H-53). Rockville, MD: Center for Behavioral Health Statistics and Quality, Substance Abuse and Mental Health Services Administration. Retrieved from https://www.samhsa.gov/data/.

and economic insecurity. These socioeconomic stressors have historically been associated with increased risk for alcohol and substance use problems. News reports highlight the increasing rates of suicide, posttraumatic stress disorder (PTSD), traumatic brain injury, substance abuse, and domestic violence among returning military and veterans serving in over a decade of war in Iraq (Operation Iraqi Freedom [OIF]) and Afghanistan (Operation Enduring Freedom [OEF]). A recent Institute of Medicine (IOM) report on military personnel found that 20% engage in heavy drinking and 47% in binge drinking (Pittman, 2012).

Coexisting SUDs, psychiatric disorders, and medical disorders are linked to adverse or poorer treatment outcomes, decreased quality of life, marked disability, and higher healthcare utilization, including emergency and crisis services. Predictably, coexisting disorders destroy social and work relationships; correlate with increased intimate and family violence; and contribute to unstable housing, legal problems, and poverty, particularly when compared to having a single diagnosis (Prisciandaro et al., 2012).

The complexity of coexisting SUDs, as well as psychiatric and medical disorders, makes detection, accurate diagnoses, and formulation of appropriate treatment planning a challenge for both primary care providers and mental health specialists (Hasin & Kilcoyne, 2012). Failure to accurately diagnose these conditions is a barrier to timely access and specialized treatment for SUDs. These diagnostic challenges coupled with the stigma associated with SUDs are reflected in the disparity among the 20.7 million Americans (7.6% of the population) who reported alcohol and drug intake, indicating the need for specialized SUD treatment, and the 2.5 million (12.2% of the population) who actually received treatment in 2017 (SAMHSA, 2018).

Prevalence statistics and comorbidities can never aptly convey the emotional, physical, financial, and spiritual toll on the individuals and their families who struggle with addictive disorders. Substance abuse erodes the fabric of family life, meaningful relationships, and sows the genetic, psychosocial, and intergenerational seeds of addiction within the family. Although no single model has been identified for treating SUDs, three decades of research in this field provide increasing evidence of positive outcomes related to integrated treatment approaches that focus on principles of cognitive behavioral therapy (CBT), contingency management (CM), mindfulness, motivational interviewing (MI), and couple and family therapy along with pharmacotherapy. Early screening and detection of SUDs, assessing and encouraging motivation to change, and engagement in person-centered approaches that facilitate active participation in treatment planning and lifelong recovery are critical components of an integrated recovery model.

Addiction Concepts and Definitions

As previously mentioned, the concept of addiction has expanded to include both substance and behavior addictions. While sources such as the National Institute on Drug Abuse (NIDA) and the National Institute of Alcohol Abuse and Alcoholism (NIAAA) adhere to definitions focused solely on SUDs, the American Society of Addiction Medicine (ASAM) has broadened their definition of addiction to include substance use and other behaviors. Addiction is viewed as a chronic, progressive, yet treatable disease of the brain that involves the interaction of brain reward circuits, genetics, and environmental experiences. Compulsive substance use or other behaviors are pursued to self-soothe and/or prevent withdrawal symptoms despite harmful consequences (ASAM, 2019).

DSM-5

Although the *DSM-IV-TR* (APA, 2000) diagnostic criteria focused exclusively on drug or substance use and distinguished between disease categories of substance abuse and substance dependence, the *DSM-5*, released in May 2013 by the American Psychiatric Association, eliminates the distinction between abuse and dependence and broadens the diagnostic criteria to include "substance-related and addictive disorders" that includes the new category of "behavioral addictions." Pathological gambling is the only currently recognized behavioral addiction in the *DSM-5*, although this suggests that other behavioral disorders may be added in the future. Other behaviors such as sex, eating, shopping, and Internet use have the potential to become addictive and destructive. They were considered for inclusion in the *DSM-5*; however, these behaviors have been referenced within the appendix pending further research (Bickman, 2011; Curley, 2010; Markel, 2012).

The *DSM-5* criteria for addiction combines the 11 criteria previously used for abuse and dependence in the *DSM-IV-TR*, while eliminating the criterion of "substance-related legal problems" because this can no longer be uniformly applied across different states in the United States and internationally. The *DSM-5* lowers the diagnostic threshold, requiring that only two of the criteria be met to satisfy the diagnostic category of "substance use disorders," although there must be a maladaptive pattern of substance use or behavior that leads to clinically significant impairment or distress occurring at any time in the same 12-month period and two of the other diagnostic criteria from *DSM-IV-TR*:

- Failure to fulfill major role obligations at work, school, or home
- Recurrent substance use or behavior in situations in which it is physically hazardous
- Continued use or behavior despite having persistent recurrent social or interpersonal problems caused or exacerbated
- Tolerance

- Withdrawal
- Substance use in larger amounts or substance/behavior used over longer periods than intended
- Persistent desire or unsuccessful efforts to cut down or control use
- Great deal of time spent obtaining or pursuing
- Cravings or urges to engage in behavior or use substance
- Important social, occupational, or recreational activities are given up or reduced
- Behavior or substance use is continued despite knowledge of having a persistent or recurrent physical or psychological problem that interferes with functioning

The criteria of "tolerance" and "withdrawal" in the *DSM-IV-TR*, respectively, denotes increasing amounts of a substance needed to achieve the same desired effect and characteristic signs and symptoms when a particular drug/substance is discontinued. However, withdrawal symptoms can also be seen when medications such as beta-blockers or antidepressants are discontinued. Pharmacological withdrawal is a normal physiological response to the discontinuation of the medication and is not the same as addiction, which refers to the loss of control over the intense urges to take the drug even at the expense of adverse consequences (O'Brien, Volkow, & Li, 2006). There is considerable debate about unintended consequences that may ensue from lowering the diagnostic threshold for addictions, the implications for screening and access to treatment services, and the use of the term *addiction* versus the more neutral terms of *abuse* or *dependence* (Bickman, 2011; Curley, 2010; Markel, 2012).

Allen Frances, who chaired the *DSM-IV* task force and was a member of the *DSM-III-R* Task Force, voices his concern about collapsing the previously separate categories of substance abuse and substance dependence into one category of substance use disorders. Allen suggests that beyond increasing stigma, this collapsed label sends the wrong message to individuals who abuse substances that they are among the "addicted" (Frances, 2013). This message connotes that the substance already controls the individual's life; that it will be quite difficult to give up the substance; that this is biologically determined by genetic fate; and the addiction is beyond an individual's control, thereby diminishing personal responsibility for substance use and its consequences (Frances, 2013). Frances suggests that clinicians continue to use the ICD-10 codes implemented October 1, 2015, which continue to distinguish between substance abuse and substance dependence codes (APA, 2015; Frances, 2013).

Relapse

Relapse is the recurrence or return to substance use or addictive behaviors after periods of abstinence. Relapse is a persistent risk in addiction and can be triggered by exposure to the addictive/rewarding substances and behaviors, exposure to conditioned environmental cues, and by exposure to emotional stressors that trigger increased activity in the brain circuitry and the neurotransmitters involved. These three modes of relapse are supported by a body of neuroscience research: (a) drug or reward-triggered relapse, (b) cue-triggered relapse, and (c) stress-triggered relapse (ASAM, 2015).

It is important to recognize that relapse is not unique to addiction disorders; rather, it is characteristic of all chronic medical diseases. The relapse rate for drug addiction at 40% to 60% compares as well or better to the relapse rates for other chronic diseases when considering adherence to medication: type 1 diabetes at 30% to 50%, hypertension at 50% to 70%, and asthma at 50% to 70% (McLellan, Lewis, O'Brien, & Kleber, 2000). Relapse is not a treatment failure but an indicator that renewed and tailored intervention is needed.

Recovery

Although initial definitions of recovery applied to alcohol and drug problems, the most recent definition applies to recovery from mental disorders and SUDs and aptly applies to behavioral addictions as well:

> Recovery is a process of change through which individuals improve their health and wellness, live a self-directed life, and strive to reach their full potential. (SAMHSA, 2012)

According to behavioral health leaders including individuals in addiction recovery and mental health consumers, recovery is considered a lifelong process that encompasses four major dimensions:

1. **Health**—overcoming or managing one's disease(s) as well as living in a physically and emotionally healthy way.
2. **Home**—a stable and safe place to live.
3. **Purpose**—meaningful daily activities, such as a job, school, volunteerism, family care-taking, or creative endeavors, and independence, income, and resources to participate in society.
4. **Community**—relationships and social networks that provide support, friendship, love, and hope (SAMHSA, 2011a).

During the past decade, SAMHSA and the Center for Substance Abuse Treatment (CSAT) have convened summits and national conferences to develop and refine a consensus understanding of the recovery process (CSAT, 2009; Gaumond & Whitter, 2009; SAMHSA, 2011a; Sheedy & Whitter, 2009) informed by the Guiding Principles of Recovery (see Box 19.1).

Etiology

There are many pathways to addiction and multiple interacting factors that contribute to the etiology of both substance use and behavioral addictions. Although addiction is now recognized as a primary disease of the brain's neurocircuitry (Feltenstein & See, 2008; NIDA, 2010), genetic factors account for roughly half the likelihood that someone will develop an addiction (Prescott & Kendler, 1999; Schuckit et al., 2001). Environmental factors, culture, and an individual's personal resilience all interact with predisposing genetic vulnerabilities to further influence the likelihood and emergence of addictive behaviors or substance use. In addition to these factors and in contrast with the medical disease model, adaptive information processing (AIP) posits that addictions are disorders of memory, learning, and chronic affect dysregulation associated with maladaptive neuroplasticity (Shapiro, 2018). Many people experiment with alcohol and substance use in their teens and early 20s, with the majority using alcohol in moderation, typically in social settings, over the course of a lifetime. An estimated 15% to 20% of users adopt regular or frequent use of alcohol and/or drugs such as marijuana, cocaine, or other illicit drugs several times a week to cope with stress and mask or manipulate undesired feelings such as guilt or sadness. This second stage pattern of use has been recognized as "abuse" but did not meet the criteria for "dependence" in the *DSM-IV-TR*. An estimated 5% of substance users' progress to the third stage pattern of use, or "dependence," entails daily or nearly daily use, life centered on obtaining the alcohol or substance, using it, or recovering from its effects (withdrawal symptoms) to the detriment of family, work, school, and other social obligations despite increasing negative consequences. In this final stage of addiction, recognized as "dependence," the person's life and use of the alcohol or substance are entirely out of control. The cravings and urges are

BOX 19.1 Guiding Principles of Recovery

Recovery emerges from hope: The belief that recovery is real provides the essential and motivating message of a better future—that people can and do overcome the internal and external challenges, barriers, and obstacles that confront them.

Recovery is person driven: Self-determination and self-direction are the foundations for recovery as individuals define their own life goals and design their unique path(s).

Recovery occurs via many pathways: Individuals are unique with distinct needs, strengths, preferences, goals, culture, and backgrounds, including trauma experiences that affect and determine their pathway(s) to recovery. Abstinence is the safest approach for those with substance use disorders.

Recovery is holistic: Recovery encompasses an individual's whole life, including mind, body, spirit, and community. The array of services and supports available should be integrated and coordinated.

Recovery is supported by peers and allies: Mutual support and mutual aid groups, including the sharing of experiential knowledge and skills, as well as social learning, play an invaluable role in recovery.

Recovery is supported through relationship and social networks: An important factor in the recovery process is the presence and involvement of people who believe in the person's ability to recover; who offer hope, support, and encouragement; and who also suggest strategies and resources for change.

Recovery is culturally based and influenced: Culture and cultural background in all of its diverse representations including values, traditions, and beliefs are key to determining a person's journey and unique pathway to recovery.

Recovery is supported by addressing trauma: Services and supports should be trauma informed to foster safety (physical and emotional) and trust, as well as promote choice, empowerment, and collaboration.

Recovery involves individual, family, and community and responsibility: Individuals, families, and communities have strengths and resources that serve as a foundation for recovery.

Recovery is based on respect: Community, systems, and societal acceptance and appreciation for people affected by mental health and substance use problems—including protecting their rights and eliminating discrimination—are crucial in achieving recovery.

biologically and psychologically driven at this stage. The person has lost his or her sense of personal integrity and self-esteem. He or she will resort to any means to obtain the alcohol or drugs, including prostituting, pimping, selling drugs, selling his or her children for adoption, prostituting his or her children . . . anything to get the next fix. The personal despair, self-loathing, and sense that God (or a higher power) could never forgive him or her or love him or her as a human being is common. Thus, we have come to appreciate the bio-psycho-social-spiritual factors that contribute to the development of addictions.

For further detailed information about the new working recovery definition or the guiding principles of recovery, please see store.samhsa.gov/system/files/pep12-recdef.pdf

Neurobiology of the Reward System

During the last several decades, progress in neuroimaging studies has enabled scientists to examine the brains of individuals with SUD in real time and garner a better understanding and insight into neurobiological underpinnings of these complex disorders

(Goldstein & Volkow, 2011; Koob & Volkow, 2010). The basic neurobiological pathways of the reward system in the brain include projections from the ventral tegmental area (VTA), through the median forebrain (MFB), and terminate in the nucleus accumbens (NA) or the pleasure center of the brain, where there is a proliferation of dopamine (DA) neurons. The NA plays a central role in reward, fear, and aggression and is modulated by DA and other neurotransmitters, including norepinephrine (NE) and serotonin (5-HT). Together the NA, 5-HT, and DA modulate inhibitory behaviors (impulse control), learning, cognition, motivation, and the reward stimuli and play principal roles in the genesis of SUDs and behavioral addictions (Grant et al., 2006; Potenza, 2006). Most drugs of abuse and behavioral addictions flood the reward circuitry with DA, which appears to be the final common neurotransmitter in the reward pathway.

Chronic activation of the reward pathway by use of substances or behavioral additions has been linked to neuroadaptive effects occurring in the brain. Over time there is a generalized decrease in DA neurotransmission, induced by the intermittent increases in DA from substances or addictive behaviors. Chronic substance use and addictive behaviors also result in release of corticotropin releasing factor (CRF), implicated in activation of central stress pathways. Sensitization occurs when there is an increased response to the repeated administration of the substance or behavior and can be associated with increased "wanting" or "craving" after repeated intermittent use. This is followed by *counter adaptation* where the initial positive reward feelings are followed by the development of tolerance. Greater amounts of the substance or behaviors are required to achieve a diminishing level of positive rewards (Koob et al., 2004). Recent neurobiological findings support what previous addiction researchers had hypothesized, a "reward deficiency syndrome," where a hypodopaminergic state involving multiple genes and environmental stimuli puts individuals at high risk for multiple addictive, impulsive, and compulsive behaviors (Blum et al., 1996).

Memory consolidation is the process in which newly formed memories mediated by the hippocampus are pliable and subject to modification or updating by diverse processes including inhibition of new protein synthesis and gene expression and subject to subsequent reminders. Over time hippocampus-dependent memories are believed to become less pliable and resistant to updating new information to an established memory for relevance through consolidation, which is surmised to occur within 1 to 2 days, although these memories can be reactivated by subsequent reminders, such as triggers (Alberini, 2009). Reactivated memories are again pliable and restabilize through retrieval-dependent reconsolidation. Memory consolidation and reconsolidation are implicated in acute and chronic symptoms of addictive disorders and PTSD. Specifically, intense memories, such as a drug-related trauma, intensify NE hyperactivity, and stress hormones (e.g., CRF) are believed to play a role in the encoding and consolidation of these memories.

Of clinical importance is the role of memory consolidation in the treatment of addictive disorders and PTSD. Memories are dynamic and subject to updating with new information. *Memory reconsolidation* is believed to mediate memory updating as new memories to sustain their relevance. Evolving research indicates that the progressive benefit of reconsolidation is that newly formed and pliable memories of the drug-related or traumatic event may be modified through various therapies including CBT (e.g., Eye Movement Desensitization and Reprocessing [EMDR]), relapse prevention, and/or pharmacological interventions (e.g., receptor antagonists) that facilitate memory extinction (Koob, 2009; Lee, 2008, 2009; Soeter & Kindt, 2011).

Although the neurobiology of the reward system in the brain has been understood for decades, recent research has implicated a wider network of bidirectional brain circuitry involving the basal forebrain, frontal cortex, and midbrain structures with the reward circuitry that collectively mediate memory, motivation, impulse control, delayed gratification, cognitive appraisal of risks and rewards, selection of certain rewards, response to triggers or cues, altered judgment, and the dysfunctional pursuit of rewards seen in addiction (ASAM, 2015). There is mounting evidence that supports neurobiological, genetic, and phenomenological links between behavioral addictions (classified as impulse-control disorders in the *DSM-IV-TR*) and substance addictions (Blanco, Moreyra, Nunes, Saiz-Ruiz, & Ibanez, 2001; Grant & Potenza, 2005; Kalivas & Volkow, 2005; Potenza, 2006, 2008). Alcohol, marijuana, nicotine, other drugs, and compulsive behaviors such as pathological gambling act on the same reward circuitry in the brain. Under- standing the similar neurobiology of SUDs and behavioral disorders can inform clinical efforts of prevention and treatment.

TREATMENT APPROACHES

The overall goals of addiction treatment are to: (a) decrease the frequency and intensity of relapses, (b) sustain periods of remission, and (c) optimize the person's level of functioning during periods of remission (ASAM, 2015). Central to these three goals is the personal awareness that through the recovery process one can experience hope, even for those who initially may not perceive hope. In addition to the Guiding Principles of Recovery (Box 19.1), the NIDA synthesizes the latest evidence on addiction treatment in an ongoing effort to influence healthcare policy by informing the public, healthcare providers, and decision-making bodies on best practices (NIDA, 2012). Recognizing that addiction is a complex yet treatable disease that affects brain function and behavior, that no single treatment approach is appropriate for everyone (NIDA, 2012), and that treatment must be safe, effective, patient-centered, timely, efficient, accessible, and equitably available (Institute of Medicine [IOM], 2001), principles of effective treatment of addiction continue to be refined. Box 19.2, Principles of Effective Treatment for Addictions, and Figure 19.2, Components of Comprehensive Drug Abuse Treatment, summarize the latest knowledge, research, clinical practice, and evidence-based treatment approaches in the field of addiction. Although these documents predate the release of the *DSM-5* in 2013 and focus on drug addiction, the principles and components of comprehensive treatment largely apply to behavioral addictions as well.

Particularly relevant to the consideration of behavioral and psychotherapy approaches are the need to address the motivation to change, providing incentives for abstinence, building skills to resist behavioral or drug use, replacing behavioral or drug-using activities with constructive and rewarding activities, improving problem-solving skills, and facilitating better interpersonal relationships (NIDA, 2012). Participation in group therapy and other peer support programs such as 12-step programs during and following treatment helps maintain abstinence when that is the desired goal, particularly in substance use more so than behavioral addiction where the goal is to have a normal or healthy level of a given behavior, not complete abstinence.

Person-Centered Care

Substantial progress in the treatment of SUD alone or with concurring psychiatric disorders has occurred during the last 30 years. During this period, there has been a compilation of research and practice guidelines that indicates that the most effective treatment for SUD with and without concurrence with psychiatric disorders is one that is multidimensional and incorporates and addresses medical, psychosocial, and mental health issues. As a rule, these strategies are person centered and integrate individual assets, wishes, abilities, and personal choices that promote an understanding and awareness of the detrimental course of sustained drug use; mitigate drug use; facilitate a drug-free lifestyle; and attain an optimal level of functioning.

BOX 19.2 Principles of Effective Treatment for Addictions

1. Addiction is a complex but treatable disease that affects brain function and behavior.
2. No single treatment is appropriate for everyone.
3. Treatment needs to be readily available.
4. Effective treatment attends to the multiple needs of the individual, not just his or her drug abuse (or behavior).
5. Remaining in treatment for an adequate period of time is critical.
6. Behavioral therapies—including individual, family, or group counseling—are the most commonly used forms of drug abuse (and behavioral addiction) treatment.
7. Medications are an important element of treatment for many patients, especially when combined with counseling and other behavioral therapies.
8. An individual's treatment and services must be assessed continually and modified as necessary to ensure that it meets his or her changing needs.
9. Many drug-addicted individuals also have other mental disorders.
10. Medically assisted detoxification is only the first stage of (drug) addiction treatment and by itself does little to change long-term drug abuse.
11. Treatment does not need to be voluntary to be effective.
12. Drug use during treatment must be monitored continuously, as lapses during treatment do occur.
13. Treatment programs should test patients for the presence of HIV/AIDS, Hepatitis B and C, tuberculosis, and other infectious diseases, as well as provide targeted risk-reduction counseling, linking patients to treatment if necessary.

Source: National Institute on Drug Abuse. (2012). *Principles of drug addiction treatment: A research-based guide* (3rd ed.). Bethesda, MD: National Institute of Health, U.S. Department of Health and Human Services. Retrieved from http://www.drugabuse.gov/sites/default/files/podat_1.pdf

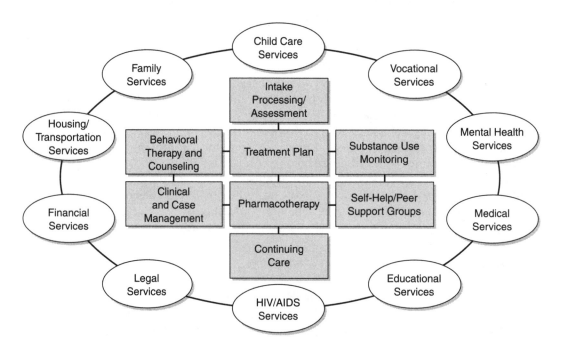

FIGURE 19.2 Components of comprehensive drug abuse treatment.

Source: Adapted from National Institute on Drug Abuse. (2012). *Principles of drug addiction treatment: A research-based guide* (3rd ed.). Bethesda, MD: National Institute of Health, U.S. Department of Health and Human Services. Retrieved from http://www.drugabuse.gov/sites/default/files/podat_1.pdf

CULTURE

Person-centric care encompasses various factors including degree of self-efficacy, culture and level of acculturation, ethnicity, preferred language, age, sexual orientation, socio-economic status, and spiritual and religious beliefs. Patients and families seeking SUD treatment must be assessed for individual uniqueness that comprises socioeconomic status, as well as personal strengths, needs, abilities, and choices. Secondly, assessing cultural influences necessary to facilitate community integration, support the role of family, and facilitate access to social support and natural resiliencies of various cultures provides a greater understanding of the person's experiences associated with SUD.

In a study involving the cause of alcohol and substance use in American Indian and Alaskan Native (AI/AN; Legha & Novins, 2012) communities, researchers emphasized the unique role culture has on treatment planning by underscoring the significance of community, family, and strong relationships with respect to cultural diversity and socio-economic challenges. In another study, researchers highlighted additional areas that enhance cultural competency, including cultural knowledge and skills; culturally sensitive attitude and appropriate behaviors; and community integration. They also stressed the importance of understanding family communication styles, perception of drug abuse and trauma, and culturally specific linguistics such as idioms, colloquial expressions, dialects, and nonverbal expressions (Rieckmann et al., 2012; Siegel, Haugland, Reid-Rose, & Hopper, 2011). Cultural, role delineation, and socioeconomic factors also have a significant impact on women with SUD and coexisting psychiatric conditions. Lastly, with changing societal demographics moving from a majority culture to a minority culture, it is imperative for psychiatric nurses to be mindful of their own culture, beliefs, and personal biases and their potential impact on how they evaluate symptoms, offer a diagnosis, and treat individuals seeking treatment for SUD.

WOMEN

Women seeking treatment often present with great social and psychological challenges, including psychiatric disorders and psychological distress, high rates of history of trauma and interpersonal violence, few vocational skills, and low income (Hunter, Robison, & Jason, 2012). Additional social challenges faced by women include child care, homelessness with minor children, pregnancy, and financial instability and transportation problems. Women seeking treatment for SUD are more likely than men to have experienced traumatic events and present with untreated PTSD. Due to the inordinate prevalence of PTSD in women with SUD, integrating trauma-focused treatment in substance abuse treatment programs is critical in decreasing symptoms during active treatment and community integration (Greenfield et al., 2011; Hien et al., 2009; Kulaga et al., 2009).

According to the CSAT (2009), women are more apt than men to continue treatment once it begins, particularly if treatment is supportive, collaborative with the provider, and includes on-site child care. Women are also more willing to participate in group therapy and seek professional mental health services than men. Positive treatment outcomes unique to women can be strengthened by the following:

- Valuing the significance of relationships
- Embracing unique psychobiological attributes and healthcare needs
- Understanding the importance of and influence of lifelong caregiver roles they assume
- Appreciating the meaning of societal roles and gender expectation across cultures, specifically about women who have SUD

- Accepting and using a trauma-competent perspective
- Integrating strengths into the evaluation, treatment, and symptom management
- Employing a strength-based treatment approach

Increasingly, as more women seek treatment for SUD and coexisting psychiatric disorders, psychiatric nurses are poised to evaluate potential barriers to treatment and utilize resources to develop gender-specific and trauma-focused approaches to ameliorate symptoms and facilitate an optimal level of functioning and integration into the community.

OLDER ADULTS (AGE 50 YEARS AND OLDER)

There is mounting evidence of an inordinate prevalence of older adults who will seek SUD treatment for prescription and illicit drugs in the upcoming decades. Of particular concern is the increased use of nonprescription opioids. Mental health and primary care providers contend that this dangerous disorder presents a challenge and requires early and routine screening to ensure accurate diagnosis and treatment. A major barrier to screening for SUD in older adults is that mental health providers are more likely to view these conditions as an afterthought rather than routine.

Age-related factors must also be considered when developing a person-centered treatment plan. Substance use disorders are predicted to rise significantly among older adults in the next 20 years. The prevalence of Americans over 50 years of age with an SUD is estimated to double from 2.8 million in 2002 to 5.7 million in 2020 (Han, Gfroerer, Colpe, Barker, & Colliver, 2011; SAMHSA, 2012).

Older adults differ from their younger counterparts in several areas that include unique features such as age- and drug-related cognitive function; physiological changes; and psychological, emotional, and socioeconomic factors. Clinical concerns associated with these changes include impact on learning or developing new coping skills to enhance relapse prevention, as well as heightened sensitivity to psychoactive drugs and interactions between them and medications used to treat coexisting psychiatric and medical conditions (Arndt, Clayton, & Schultz, 2011; Wu & Blazer, 2011). Outcomes studies also indicate that older adults are most likely to require lower doses of medications, such as methadone; have fewer legal problems; and remain in treatment longer than younger patients.

Treating older adults with an SUD and most likely a coexisting medical or psychiatric disorder requires expertise in age-related physiological and psychological changes and socioeconomic challenges. Unique age-related changes include diminished biological (e.g., slowed metabolism), cognitive, and neurobiological changes; disability along with reduced physical stamina; sensory deficits; financial constraints; few social support networks; and impaired driving and transportation issues. Due to a higher incidence of adverse effects of SUD in older adults, coexisting medical and psychiatric conditions require continuous monitoring and collaboration with primary care providers to minimize serious and adverse treatment outcomes. Treatment considerations for older adults include a candid and honest discussion about drug-related problems and treatment options.

Co-Occurring Disorders

Co-occurring disorders is a term used to describe the simultaneous occurrence of a substance use/abuse-related disorder and a nonsubstance-related mental health disorder based on *DSM* diagnostic categories (CSAT, 2006). Based on the National Survey on Drug Use and Health (2019), an estimated 47.6 million adults experienced mental illness in the past year, 19.3 million adults experienced an SUD, and, among those, 9.2 million adults had co-occurring disorders. Among the 9.2 million with co-occurring disorders, 51.4% received substance use treatment or mental health treatment, only an estimated 7% received treatment for both conditions, and 48.6% received no treatment at all (NSDUH, 2019). Although there is greater understanding for the need to treat both substance use and mental health disorders in an integrated approach rather than separately or sequentially, the limited access to care for integrated services results in fragmented and inadequate care for most people.

A classification system developed by the state program directors of mental health associations and alcohol and drug abuse programs provides a four-quadrant model to coordinate care for individuals with co-occurring disorders (see Figure 19.3 on co-occurring disorders by severity). As the severity of both disorders increases, the level of care, setting of care, and coordination of services intensify. In Quadrant I with low severity of both mental illness and alcohol/drug abuse, care is typically provided in primary healthcare settings with some consultation with specialized care providers. Patients in Quadrant II, having greater severity of mental illness and mild substance use issues, typically are seen through the mental health system of care. Those in Quadrant III, with greater severity of substance abuse problems and mild or moderate mental health problems, are typically seen in the substance abuse treatment system. Patients in Quadrant IV, with high severity of both addiction and mental illness problems, are typically seen in state psychiatric hospitals, jails, prisons, emergency rooms, or criminal justice systems on parole or probation. The greater the severity of the co-occurring disorders, the greater the need for integrated and trauma-informed services (CAST, 2006; SAMHSA, 2002).

Trauma-Informed Care

During the past 20 years, there has been increasing recognition of the impact of childhood abuse, childhood neglect, exposure to violence, and subsequent revictimization as adolescents and adults as risk factors and correlates for developing substance abuse and mental health disorders (Najt, Fusar-Poli, & Brambilla, 2011). There is an association

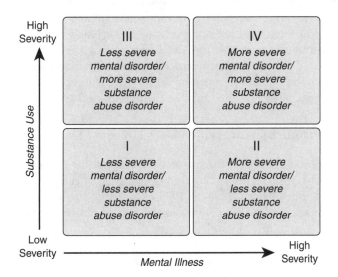

FIGURE 19.3 Level of severity quadrants for co-occurring substance use and mental disorders.

Source: Adapted from Center for Substance Abuse Treatment. (2005). *Substance abuse treatment for persons with co-occurring disorders* (Treatment Improvement Protocol [TIP] Series No. 42). DHHS Publication No. (SMA) 05-3922. Rockville, MD: Substance Abuse and Mental Health Services Administration. Retrieved from https://www.ncbi.nlm.nih.gov/books/NBK64197/.

that the younger the age of abuse/neglect/violence and the more prolonged the duration, the greater the likelihood of developing substance abuse and mental health disorders (Brems, Johnson, Neal, & Freemon, 2004; Dube et al., 2003).

Research indicates that women substance abusers have higher rates of comorbid PTSD than women in the general community and two to three times the incidence of comorbid PTSD than substance abusing men who are in treatment (Kessler et al., 2005; Kessler, Sonnega, Bromet, Hughes, & Nelson, 1995). Among women seeking substance abuse treatment, the rates of emotional, physical, and sexual abuse ranged from 55% to 9% (Adams et al., 2011; Najavits, Weiss, & Shaw, 1997). For these women, substance abuse became a means to dull the emotional pain of prior traumas or cope with ongoing trauma.

With the increased exposure to violence in combat zones during the wars in Iraq and Afghanistan, there has been a dramatic increase in rates of PTSD, substance abuse, and suicide among U.S. military servicemen and women and veterans (U.S. Department of Veterans Affairs [DVA], 2020). Three out of every four Vietnam combat veterans with PTSD had co-occurring SUDs. One in five veterans of the Iraq and Afghanistan wars has PTSD or depression. Although rates of co-occurring substance use have not been established, these veterans are at greater risk for experiencing SUDs due to combat exposure (Lan et al., 2016).

Regardless of whether the trauma is childhood abuse, domestic violence, combat exposure, natural disasters, or other forms of trauma, understanding the risk for using alcohol or drugs to "numb" the pain or "avoid" the bad memories, dreams, people, or places increases and thereby makes the PTSD symptoms worse. Clinicians need to learn evidence-based treatment approaches to simultaneously treat the underlying trauma and PTSD while addressing the alcohol and drug use. Addressing trauma-related symptoms early in treatment can increase the likelihood of recovery from SUDs because most individuals report using alcohol or drugs to manage PTSD symptoms such as flashbacks, sleep problems, nightmares, avoidance of trauma memories, and hypervigilance. A few studies suggest that using a selective serotonin reuptake inhibitor, such as sertraline, among those who have PTSD before the onset of the SUD results in a better treatment response (Brady et al., 2005; Labbate, Sonne, Randall, Anton, & Brady, 2004). A manualized CBT approach to increase coping skills for women with co-occurring PTSD and SUDs called "Seeking Safety" has demonstrated efficacy in treatment retention, reducing PTSD symptoms, and reducing relapse rates (Najavits, 2002). Other therapies such as Eye Movement Desensitization and Reprocessing therapy (EMDR), Dialectical Behavior Therapy (DBT), and mindfulness practice offer additional promising treatment approaches useful in addressing the underlying trauma, but empirical testing of their treatment efficacy for SUD needs to be further strengthened.

12-Step Peer Support Groups

The 12-step program is a set of guiding principles that outlines actions for recovery from addictions, compulsions, or other behavioral problems. These principles were initially proposed by Alcoholics Anonymous in 1939 as a method to recover from alcoholism and subsequently adapted as the foundation for other 12-step groups throughout the world. The guiding principles include:

- Admitting that one cannot control one's addiction or compulsion
- Recognizing a higher power that can give strength
- Examining past errors with the help of a sponsor (experienced member)
- Making amends for these errors
- Learning to live a new life with a new code of behavior
- Helping others who suffer from the same addictions or compulsions

Participation in 12-step groups during and after formal substance abuse treatment has been associated with positive outcomes among substance users. However, high attrition rates and low participation limit the effectiveness of 12-step groups. Common barriers to participation cited by patients are the religious aspect and emphasis on powerlessness. Clinicians cite convenience, scheduling issues, and finding the right "patient fit" for a particular 12-step group as barriers. Studies have found that the person's readiness to change, perceived need for help, and motivation are more critical factors in 12-step group participation (Laudet, 2003; Smith, Buxton, Bilal, & Seymour, 1993). Positive attitudes by clinicians about 12-step groups and their role in supporting recovery were associated with greater rates of referral, while resistance to the concepts of spirituality and powerlessness was associated with lower rates of referral by clinicians (Laudet & White, 2005).

Participation in 12-step groups can be viewed as a complementary treatment approach that helps the person to build a support network. Advanced practice psychiatric nurses (APPNs) who can address concerns about entering a new group, explain the concept of powerlessness and spirituality within the 12-step tradition, and use MI to contract for attendance at several different groups to find the right "fit" and encourage attendance, are more likely to successfully engage their patients in 12-step group participation as one aspect of their lifelong journey in recovery.

SCREENING AND ASSESSMENT

Recent results of the National Health Interview Survey revealed increasing use of alcohol with 51% of adults reporting regular alcohol use, 14% current infrequent drinkers, 6% former regular drinkers, 9% former infrequent drinkers, and only 20% abstainers (Schiller, Lucas, & Peregoy, 2012). These prevalence rates of drinking have increased since 2004 when 49% of adults in the United States were abstainers, 22% reported light or occasional drinking, and 29% reported "risky drinking" or individuals who regularly or occasionally exceed screening guidelines (U.S. Surgeon General, 2004). Rising alcohol-related emergency room visits and motor-vehicular deaths as well as rising prevalence of alcohol use in teens and adults have prompted ongoing efforts to train healthcare providers across disciplines to screen and assess patients for alcohol and drug use.

The Screening, Brief Intervention and Referral to Treatment, known as SBIRT, has been a public health approach supported by SAMHSA since early 2000 to train the healthcare workforce to deliver screening and early intervention for individuals with SUDs and those at risk for developing these disorders. SAMHSA has funded numerous and ongoing efforts to train current healthcare providers and integrate SBIRT skills into the education and curriculum of all health professionals as well as universal screening across healthcare settings. SBIRT is intended for widespread use in primary care centers, hospitals, emergency rooms, trauma centers, and other community settings for early interventions with at-risk substance users before more severe consequences occur. The SAMHSA SBIRT website (https://www.samhsa.gov/sbirt) provides information and resources on SBIRT grant funding, billing and coding, and training materials. The NIAAA has additional SBIRT resources and clinician guidelines for adults (NIAAA, 2005) and for youth (NIAAA, 2015). For individuals who screen positive for risky alcohol and drug use, healthcare providers can use an MI approach in ongoing brief periodic interactions to engage the patient in steps to reduce his or her risky alcohol use over time. For patients who meet criteria for more advanced alcohol use or dependence, clinicians are advised to refer those patients for specialized addiction treatment. Information on additional screening tools for age-specific and special populations such as pregnant women is provided in Table 19.3.

TABLE 19.3 SCREENING TOOLS FOR ALCOHOL AND DRUG USE

Screening Measure	Target Population	Groups Used With	Number of Items	Problem Screened	Cut-Off Score for Harmful Use	Time to Administer
CAGE*	Adults	Emergency departments (EDs), hospitals, primary care providers	4	Alcohol dependence	1 (range 0–4)	Less than 1 minute
CAGE-AID*	Adults	EDs, hospitals, primary care providers	4	Alcohol and drug dependence	1 (range 0–4)	Less than 1 minute
Alcohol Use Disorders Identification Test (AUDIT-C)*	Adults	Primary care providers, EDs, driving while intoxicated (DWI) offenders, workplace screening	10 (three subscales)	Harmful or hazardous alcohol use	8 (range 0–40)	3 to 5 minutes
CRAFFT[1]	Adolescents	EDs, hospitals, primary care providers, psychiatric settings	6	Alcohol and drug abuse	2 (0–6)	Less than 1 minute
Drug Abuse Screening Test (DAST-10)[2]	Adults Adapted for adolescents	Primary care providers, hospital, medical, and psychiatric settings	10	Drug abuse	Low: 1 to 2 Moderate: 3 to 5 Substantial: 6 to 10 (range 0–10)	1 to 2 minutes
TWEAK*	Pregnant women	OB/GYNs, midwives Labor and delivery settings	5	Alcohol abuse	2 (range 0–7)	Less than 2 minutes
UNCOPE*	Pregnant women	OB/GYNs, midwives, labor and delivery settings	6	Alcohol and drug abuse	2 (0–6)	Less than 1 minute

*Public domain.

[1] Copyright by Boston Children's Hospital; no cost, need approval of Center for Adolescent Substance Abuse Research (www.ceasar-boston.org).

[2] Copyright by Harvey Skinner, PhD; no cost, need approval through harvey.skinner@yorku.ca.

Clinicians who treat patients with SUDs or co-occurring disorders beyond the primary care setting understand the importance of establishing a therapeutic relationship; conducting a comprehensive biopsychosocial assessment including the risk for any urgent medical or psychiatric crisis; making differential diagnoses; and implementing and evaluating a person-centered, trauma-informed treatment plan. See Table 19.4 on biopsychosocial addiction assessment.

TABLE 19.4 BIOPSYCHOSOCIAL ADDICTION ASSESSMENT	
Chief Complaint	**Trauma History**

• Reason(s) for seeking treatment at this time: Priority is to assess level of patient safety (e.g., suicidality, homicidality)	• Trauma exposures
	  – Childhood abuse or neglect
	  – Rape or sexual assault
	  – Domestic violence
	  – Military/combat service
	  – Natural disasters
	• History of head injury; loss of consciousness; and/or seizures

History of Present Illness	**Substance Use History**
• Antecedent events • Pattern of presenting symptoms (depression, alcohol, drug use, and so on) • Current and recent stressors • Current coping skills/behaviors • Include patient and family's perception of alcohol or other drug consumption	• For each substance—identify type and details • Duration/frequency/last use • Blackouts • Withdrawal seizures • Drug-related psychosis • Legal, psychosocial, physical, interpersonal, and occupational consequences
Past Medical History	**General and Neurological Examination: (Germane to Treatment Setting and Situation)**
• Medical history/treatment and outcomes • Recent and past hospitalizations, surgeries • Include list of prior and any current medications, over-the-counter, herbal, or complementary treatments	• Appearance, height, weight, BMI • Current health status, last physical exam, allergies, dietary changes • Physical exam • Neurologic and mental status exam
Past Psychiatric History	**Lab Work**
• Psychiatric history/treatment and outcomes • Recent and past psychiatric or substance abuse hospitalizations, residential, or outpatient treatments • Include exposure to prescription opioids, psychotropic medications, side effects, treatment response	• Serum, breath, or urine for substance used as indicated • Chemistry profile, electrolytes, complete blood count • Hemoglobin, hematocrit • Liver, renal, and thyroid function tests • Comprehensive metabolic profile • Pregnancy test (women of child-bearing age) • HIV/AIDS, hepatitis C, tuberculosis • Toxicology screens (if indicated)

(continued)

TABLE 19.4 BIOPSYCHOSOCIAL ADDICTION ASSESSMENT (*CONTINUED*)	
Comprehensive Review of Systems	Other Tests
• Current and chronic health problems by system • Functional status • Nutritional status	• Electrocardiogram • CAGE, AUDIT-C, TWEAK, CRAFFT (appropriate to age, gender, setting)
Biological Family History	Differential Diagnoses
• Family medical history (two generations) • Family psychiatric and/or substance use history (two generations)	• *DSM-5* psychiatric and substance use disorders
Sociocultural History	Proposed Treatment Plan
• Family and social history • Work history/current employment • Legal history—active and past • Current support system • Marital status, children	• Based on safety needs, severity of medical, psychiatric, and substance use disorders
Development History (Especially for Children)	
• Pregnancy/delivery/in utero exposure to alcohol/drugs • Early developmental milestones • Social and interpersonal development	

AUDIT-C, Alcohol Use Disorders Identification Test-modified; BMI, body mass index; DSM-5, Diagnostic and Statistical Manual of Mental Disorders, 5th edition.

A mental status examination must be used initially as part of the assessment and continually throughout the treatment process to monitor symptom management and level of dangerousness to self and others. Evidence of acute psychiatric or SUD symptoms must be referred to the emergency department or services for further evaluation, detoxification, and psychiatric and medical stabilization. In the absence of active or acute symptoms of SUD and psychiatric conditions, an evaluation of the person's readiness and motivation to engage in treatment must be determined. Stressful life events, ineffective coping, or adaptive coping skills contribute to the chronic nature of SUDs. A critical concept of treatment is helping individuals understand that recovery is an ongoing process that requires a lifetime commitment. Recovery is not simply achieving sobriety or being drug free. Recovery establishes goals and supports steps to improve overall health, happiness, self-sufficiency, and a meaningful life without substances through education, employment, volunteerism, and developing a strong social network.

EVIDENCE-BASED PSYCHOTHERAPEUTIC INTERVENTIONS

During the past decade, the implementation of evidence-based practice (EBP) has permeated all healthcare systems including substance abuse treatment. Despite the promulgation of practice guidelines, protocols, and manualized psychosocial interventions such as the Treatment Improvement Protocol (TIP) series for addictions developed by

SAMHSA in the 1990s and 2000s, demonstration of improved treatment outcomes in the addiction field remains inconsistent across treatment settings and geographic areas. Some argue that a focus on specific evidence-based core skill sets that are broadly applicable and easily learned replaces the emphasis on manualized psychosocial interventions (Glasner-Edwards & Rawson, 2010). Critical goals of EBPs in addiction treatment involve (a) improving impulse control, (b) reducing craving, and (c) promoting an adaptive social environment (Glasner-Edwards & Rawson, 2010). Evidence-based skills that can best impact these three goals include (a) principles of CM, MI, and brief intervention skills training; (b) core cognitive behavioral coping skills and relapse prevention strategies; and (c) couple and family counseling techniques (Carroll & Rounsaville, 2006; Glasner-Edwards & Rawson, 2010).

Maintaining the Therapeutic Frame

Although the concept of the therapeutic frame originated from psychoanalytic therapy, it has been widely adopted by most psychotherapy schools including interpersonal, object relational, cognitive behavioral, and self-psychological theories (Cherry & Gold, 1989). The therapeutic frame consists of the conditions required to support a professional counseling relationship. Typically this includes setting and maintaining clear boundaries and role expectations to provide the patient with a secure, safe "holding" environment that facilitates personal growth and development (Modell, 1976). Conversely, the therapeutic frame also supports the clinician in maintaining a therapeutic stance of neutrality (nonjudgmental), anonymity (avoiding unnecessary self-disclosure), and nonintrusiveness, thereby keeping the focus on the person's thoughts, concerns, and needs. The "traditional" treatment frame consists of rules regarding:

- Making and keeping regular appointment times
- Enforcing established starting and ending times for each session
- Declining to disclose a home or cellular phone number or address
- Canceling sessions if the patient arrives under the influence of alcohol or psychoactive drugs
- Not having contact outside of therapy sessions
- Having no sexual contact or interactions that could reasonably be interpreted as sexual
- Terminating counseling if threats are made or acts of violence are committed against the counselor
- Allowing patients to explore thoughts and feelings without "acting out" thoughts/feelings of harm to self or others, or damaging property within a session
- Establishing and enforcing a clear policy in regard to payment

Exceptions to a particular rule may be supported by a particular treatment approach. For example, the use of telephone contact outside the therapy session may be appropriate within the context of DBT in managing suicidal feelings. Patients may feel abandoned if a telephone call is not returned, thereby damaging the therapeutic alliance (Center for Substance Abuse Treatment [CSAT], TIP #36, 2000).

Clinicians working in the addiction field must attend to issues of *transference, countertransference, secondary traumatization,* and *burnout.* Alcohol and drug counselors, as well as other mental health professionals, work with people who have often suffered abuse and neglect as children and revictimization as adolescents and adults. This is even more complex when the clinician may also be in recovery from SUDs and/or suffered abuse or neglect themselves. Clinicians must be mindful of their own feelings to avoid countertransference that can lead to negative judgments and rejection of certain patients or to "rescuing" helpless or defenseless patients. Finding the appropriate balance of providing support and distance to facilitate growth and recovery is an ongoing process. Supervision and consultation are useful strategies to provide the clinician with objective feedback and recognize or prevent boundary crossings or countertransference issues.

Patients with SUDs and especially those with a history of abuse are often mistrustful while at the same time seeking a trustworthy relationship. At times they may project intense feelings onto the clinician, which results in a "push-pull" dynamic. The person may test the clinician's limits, breach trust, act out, avoid engaging in meaningful counseling, or relapse. APPNs must be mindful of these dynamics and develop strategies to ensure effective care. Because child abuse and neglect represent the ultimate violation of trust, the *therapeutic frame* must be maintained with appropriate boundaries and limitations to provide a safe, trustworthy relationship and the opportunity to heal (CSAT, TIP #36, 2000).

By contrast, some patients may idealize the clinician as they experience perhaps the first relationship with a consistent trustworthy person who offers positive regard and validates their value and positive self-esteem. In those who have recently stopped abusing alcohol or drugs, tension may be reduced through obsessive romantic or sexual fantasies about the clinician. Patients who have used sex as their primary way of relating may misinterpret cues from the clinician and believe the clinician is sexually interested in them. The patient who is "in love" with his or her therapist/clinician poses a challenge and an opportunity for therapeutic growth. While the APPN must be alert to potential "romanticized" patient perceptions and avoid seduction, the situation presents the opportunity for the person to learn to examine the feelings, rather than act on them, and explore the underlying meaning. By maintaining the professional boundary of the patient–counselor relationship, the clinician can guide the patient to examine whether he or she is replacing substance use with romantic fantasies to reduce tension. The clinician may also guide the person to explore what he or she values about the therapeutic relationship—feelings of trust, safety, and positive regard—and how to seek this experience in nonsexual relationships with others who listen. This is potentially a "teachable moment" where the patient uses reflection to learn to better differentiate his or her own feelings (CSAT, Tip #36, 2000).

The ongoing daily stress of working with those who have experienced abuse, neglect, and violence can take a toll on clinicians. When repeatedly listening to disclosures of abuse, neglect, violence, and victimization, especially when perpetrated by parents or family members on their own children, the clinician may experience symptoms of trauma in the form of disturbing dreams, anxiety, irritability, withdrawal, and problems in interpersonal relationships. This phenomenon is recognized as secondary trauma. Untreated or ignored, this can progress to symptoms of PTSD and burnout. Clinicians experiencing these symptoms lose perspective and effectiveness in working with traumatized patients. The APPN may unintentionally minimize, negate, or fail to inquire about a person's abuse history, thereby unconsciously avoiding the distress raised by listening to disclosures of abuse or neglect. By contrast, the clinician may become overly focused on probing for histories of abuse or neglect, seeking detailed histories when the person may not be a survivor of abuse or may not feel safe or ready to disclose or have any memories of abuse. These clinicians are vulnerable to become overly involved with the desire to "rescue" the patient, and may direct anger at parents, mental health clinicians, former therapists, or child protective services (CPS) workers who had missed the abuse. When this loss of professional objectivity occurs, the relationship ceases to be therapeutic or beneficial to the patient (Briere & Scott, 2006).

Motivational Interviewing

Motivational interviewing (MI) was initially developed within the addiction field to motivate individuals to commit to healthy drug-free lifestyle change (Miller & Rollnik, 1991, 2002). See Chapter 9, for detailed discussion and applications of MI beyond the addiction field. The specific treatment goal of MI centers on identifying the opportunity to guide the individual in change talk and enhancing the motivation to change. This approach affords the APPN an opportunity to join and appreciate the person's experience that begins when treatment is started irrespective of the stage of change. Motivation to change is potentiated through the therapeutic alliance and specific communication strategies that direct the discussion. By encouraging the person to appraise problems linked to his or her addiction, the nurse can actively frame and use the individual's "own words" as a basis for adaptive change. Change talk reflects the motivation to change, the incentive to remain abstinent, and forecasts positive outcomes (Hallgren & Moyers, 2011; Miller, Moyers, Amrhein, & Rollnick, 2006).

MI also requires the APPN to avoid challenging the person's resistance and ambivalence and instead to "roll with the resistance," accepting that ambivalence and resistance to change are a natural part of change and growth. Eventually resistance to change diminishes, as the individual discovers personal options, accountability, and solutions to the current situation, while promoting autonomy and self-efficacy (Marlatt & Gordon, 1985). As the person becomes more confident through change talk and discovers healthy solutions to everyday problems, these sessions can be used to sustain motivation and support newly found self-esteem, hope, and self-efficacy. The most successful approaches for an SUD are likely to be those that encourage self-efficacy.

Contingency Management

CM is a behavioral reinforcement-based approach within the CBT model that employs positive or reward reinforcement that has proven efficacy in the treatment of SUD as evidenced by facilitating effective and adaptive behavioral changes based on four decades of research (Hser et al., 2011; Stitzer, Petry, & Peirce, 2010). Promising outcomes from these data consist of reduced substance use, increased group participation, and improved adherence to medication regimens (Schmitz, Lindsay, Stotts, Green, & Moeller, 2010).

Similar to CBT, CM is likely to be a part of an integrated treatment plan for SUD to reinforce homework completion and session participation to strengthen CBT through exposure to adaptive coping skills training by reinforcing abstinence and relapse prevention. Building coping skills enables the individual to sustain and maintain new behaviors primarily because they reinforce the brain's self-regulatory or impulsivity capacity. Typically, reinforcement involves provision of monetary-based reinforcers, such as vouchers for retail purchases for abstinence incentive (Hser et al., 2011). How one manages money is further influenced by culture and perception of money management and prudent use of one's money through impulse control (Hamilton & Potenza, 2012). Other forms of reinforcement may include treatment attendance, adherence to treatment goals, and medications.

Effectiveness of CM using reinforcement can be established using various reinforcers, such as monitoring drug screens and previously mentioned money-management tasks. Collecting and monitoring drug screens several times a week to identify brief episodes of abstinence reinforces adherence to pharmacological and psychotherapeutic interventions; reduces cravings and/or psychiatric symptoms; and promotes relapse prevention (Carroll et al., 2012). Positive reinforcement manifested by negative drug screens; adherence to treatment; reduced cravings; and absence of psychiatric symptoms expand with continuous lengths of abstinence. Positive reinforcement is also strengthened by incorporating additional psychotherapeutic interventions, such as MI, mindfulness and social skills training, and couples and family therapy, to target high-risk behavior associated with impulsive drug use and relapse.

Cognitive Behavioral Coping Skills and Relapse Prevention

Typically CM, MI, and CBT are integrated to help individuals increase coping skills and develop a relapse prevention plan by focusing on cognitive, behavioral, and lifestyle choices that might be changed or reinforced (Marlatt, 2006). One of the central components of this approach is identifying relapse triggers and developing a variety of coping strategies to successfully avoid or manage different triggers without reverting to substance use or addictive behavior patterns such as gambling.

Mindfulness is often part of an integrated plan of care utilizing other cognitive behavioral approaches. This approach necessitates awareness or mindfulness of triggers and high-risk situational cues and readiness to do something about it. Awareness and readiness enable the individuals to explore and develop an array of relapse prevention interventions, such as "stepping back" and appraising the trigger-related situation, which historically was deemed automatic, and using more adaptive coping behaviors to modulate triggers (Witkiewitz, Lustyk, & Bowen, 2013). Together, these proactive techniques reinforce adaptive coping behaviors and greater control over trigger-related situations, specifically physical and emotional responses. Similar to other cognitive behavioral techniques, mindfulness is most appropriate for individuals who have completed initial treatment, including symptom management of psychiatric conditions, and are clearly motivated to sustain treatment gains and formulate healthy lifestyles and recovery. See Chapter 8, for detailed discussion and applications of CBT beyond the addiction field.

Integrated Family Therapy

Quality family interactions and relationships and mental health of members are strongly correlated. Likewise, long-lasting committed relationships afford the most important form of social support for many individuals with an SUD. Conversely, distant, impaired, and dysfunctional family relationships typically result in divorce and separation and have a long-standing destructive impact on couples and families, as well as their children and communities, and overburden healthcare systems and resources. It is widely understood that abstinence and healthy communication and relationship functioning curtail societal costs, familial violence, and lifelong emotional and behavioral problems of children (O'Farrell & Clements, 2012; Rowe, 2012). Couples and family therapy is a necessary component of the integrated plan and a proven asset to helping individuals and their families and communities restore severed interpersonal relationships and improve social and occupational functioning related to SUD. Research findings consistently indicate couples and family therapy approaches among the most effective modalities in the treatment of adults with an SUD (Rowe, 2012).

Couples and family therapy offers venues for individuals and families to understand the impact of SUD within a social context and develop communication and social skills that restore trust, self-efficacy, and confidence and strengthen dysfunctional relationships associated with an SUD. These skills also help families and individuals appraise the role of high-risk situations and drug-induced triggers and develop coping techniques that restore healthy interactions and support relapse prevention. Specific communication and social skills training include assertiveness, anger and stress management, and active listening skills necessary to heal and repair family relationships through effective quality support and empathy. Furthermore, couples and family therapy plays key roles in moderating substance use; promoting higher levels of relationship satisfaction; improving child and marital functioning; reducing family and partner violence; sustaining sobriety; and facilitating community integration (CSAT, TIP #39, 2004).

Eye Movement Desensitization and Reprocessing Therapy

Research on using EMDR therapy for SUD includes case reports and one randomized controlled study (Abel & O'Brien, 2010; Bae & Kim, 2012, 2015; Brown et al., 2015; Cox & Howard, 2007; Hase, Schallmayer, & Sack, 2008; Henry, 1996; Marich, 2010). These studies show promising results but more research is needed. Several EMDR therapy protocols have been developed specifically to treat addictions, one of which is The Feeling-State Therapy (FST; Miller, 2010, 2011). Originally Jim Knipe (2019) conceptualized that addiction may arise as a defense against a traumatic disturbance. In order to keep disturbing feelings out of the person's awareness, a highly charged positive affect occurs as a result of using, which then reinforces the behavior of using. A "feeling state" comprises a feeling associated with a behavior that causes the urges and cravings associated with both substance and behavioral addictions. For example, Miller (2011) cites the example that a "feeling state" linked to compulsive shopping might be composed of the sensations and emotions of excitement and the anticipation of "getting what I want." The urge or craving is not the feeling that the person seeks but rather the drive for the positive feelings associated with the behavior linked with them. In this example, the urge to buy clothes was not the desired feeling, but it was the need to feel excitement and anticipation. If the therapist focused only on the craving or urge to shop, the therapist would miss the underlying need for excitement and anticipation and fail to break the feeling/behavior connection (Miller, 2011). In behavioral addictions, the goal is to enable the person to return to a normal system of functioning, not to totally abstain from the behavior. Shopping, eating, exercising, sexual intimacy, and even recreational gambling are normal behaviors. Once the "feeling-state" memory is processed, the individual automatically begins to use more appropriate ways to satisfy needs (Miller, 2011).

Behavioral and some substance addictions may also form as a response to a preexisting intense psychological need such that the use of the substance is associated with avoidance of undesirable emotional feelings such as dysphoria, depressed mood, and emptiness. Thus, the addiction is a solution to a problem. This is most easily illustrated by the urge or craving for substances such as alcohol, cocaine, or opioids when these substances are associated with the "feeling state" of "chilling out" on alcohol or opioids or "being productive" or having "great sex" on cocaine. The underlying drive may be avoidance of dysphoria or boredom by using alcohol or the need to feel alert, aware, and highly stimulated by using cocaine. Additionally, the physiological reaction to the drug also contributes the desired "feeling state" of euphoria. Thus, the compulsion to take the drug to achieve a euphoric state can and does occur even if there is not a preexisting psychological need the individual wishes to avoid. Because substance addictions can create intense experiences for the development of a "feeling state," the treatment goal is abstinence. It is also important to recognize that if you successfully eliminate a substance addiction through processing the positive feeling state, the underlying depression or anxiety disorder may emerge (Miller, 2011).

Individuals who struggle with addictions often have core beliefs that are shame-based, meaning they perceive themselves as "losers," "failures," and "hopeless." Shame drives a person to hide, withdraw, and avoid treatment. Guilt over actions taken while under the influence of substances or during compulsive, addictive behaviors is more event specific. The individual typically feels guilty that his or hertheir behavior may have been embarrassing or inappropriate while intoxicated or overspending while compulsively shopping, but the individual does not feel that he or she is inherently a "bad person" or a "loser." Guilt often motivates a person to seek treatment. A turning point for many people with addictions is when they feel guilty about their actions and want to repair interpersonal relationships and stop the destructive behavior patterns created by their addiction. Understanding the difference between guilt and shame and its impact on an individual's motivation or avoidance of treatment is critical to hope and the recovery process (Dearing, Stuewig, & Tangney, 2005).

Feeling-state addiction therapy (FSAT) combines the FST of behavioral and substance addiction (Miller, 2012) with a modification of EMDR (Shapiro, 2018). Guilt and shame are reactions to the behaviors caused by the "feeling state." In the Feeling-State Addiction Protocol (FSAP), the "feeling state" is the target for therapy. The theoretical basis of EMDR is the AIP Model that posits the innate information processing system of the brain is interrupted as a result of high arousal from events perceived as traumatic (Shapiro, 2018),. The memory of the event is encoded within an isolated neural network containing the heightened emotions, bodily sensations, and the associated cognitive appraisals at the time of the event. The memory node becomes fixed and isolated from linking the experience to more adaptive information, forming the basis for pathology. When the memory is triggered by current environmental stimuli, dysfunctional reactions and affects emerge. EMDR facilitates the adaptive reprocessing of such pathological memories (see Chapters 2, and 7, for further discussion of AIP and EMDR).

The primary modification of the EMDR protocol for FSAP is the identification of the specific positive FS (sensation + emotion + cognition) linked with the addictive behavior and its Positive Feeling Scale (PFS) level (0–10) and associated body sensations. Eye movement sets are then performed while the patient visualizes the addictive behavior until the PFS level drops to 0 or 1. Once the FS associated with the addictive behavior has been processed, the negative belief underlying the FS is determined, and the positive belief is chosen and installed using the standard EMDR protocol. See Box 19.3 on FSAP (Knipe, 2019; Miller, 2012).

Another widely used EMDR therapy protocol for addictions is the Desensitization of Triggers and Urge Reprocessing (DeTUR) Model (Popky, 2005). Popky uses bilateral eye movements or the bilateral stimulation component of EMDR to process the triggers, urges, and cravings associated with addiction using the Level of Urge (LOU) 0 to 10 scale. Popky's protocol includes the following steps: (a) building rapport; (b) performing a history, assessment, and diagnosis; (c) supporting resources; (d) accessing internal resource state; (e) setting a positive treatment goal; (f) ensuring an associated positive state; (g) identifying urge triggers; (h) desensitizing triggers; (i) installing positive state to each trigger; (j) testing and future check; (k) conducting closure and self-work; and (l) conducting follow-up sessions.

BOX 19.3 Feeling-State Addiction Protocol

1. Obtain history, frequency, and context of addictive behavior.
2. Evaluate the person for having the coping skills to manage feelings if he or she is no longer using the addictive behaviors to cope. If not, do resource development before continuing. Install future template if necessary.
3. Identify the specific aspect of the addictive behavior that has the most intensity associated with it. If the addiction is to a stimulant drug, then the rush/euphoria sensations are usually the first to be processed. However, if some other feeling is more intense, process that first. The starting memory may be the first time or the most recent—whatever is most potent.
4. Identify the specific positive feeling (sensation + emotion + cognition) linked with the addictive behavior and its Positive Feeling Score (PFS) level (0–10).
5. Locate and identify any physical sensations created by the positive feelings.
6. Have the patient visualize performing the addictive behavior—feeling the positive feeling combined with the physical sensations.
7. Eye movement sets are performed until the PFS level drops to 0 or 1.
8. Install future templates of how the person will live without having that feeling.
9. Between sessions, homework is given to evaluate the progress of therapy and to elicit any other feelings related to the addictive behavior.
10. In the next session, the addictive behavior is reevaluated for both the feeling identified in the last session as well as identifying other positive feelings associated with the behavior.
11. Steps 3 to 9 are performed again as necessary.
12. Once the FSs associated with the addictive behavior have been processed, the negative beliefs underlying the FSs are determined, and the desired positive beliefs are chosen.

Source: Miller, R. (2012). Treatment of behavioral addictions utilizing the feeling-state addiction protocol: A multiple baseline study. *Journal of EMDR Practice and Research, 6*(4), 159–169. doi:10.1891/1933-3196.6.4.159

CASE EXAMPLE

Ms. B, a thin, cachectic, 27-year-old woman entered residential treatment for co-occurring cocaine, marijuana, and alcohol addiction; substance-induced mood disorder; and chronic PTSD immediately following release from 30 months incarceration for prostitution and drug trafficking. She has lost custody of her 5-year-old daughter as a result of her incarceration. The biological father is unknown and her daughter has been in the custody of her aging parents since she was incarcerated. She relates a history of childhood neglect and physical abuse by her mother and stepfather, who were both reportedly alcoholics. The youngest of three girls, she denies sexual abuse until she dropped out of high school and left home at age 16 to live with her older boyfriend, age 24. He was emotionally, physically, and sexually abusive, and turned her onto alcohol, marijuana, cocaine, and opioids within their first year together. She began prostituting and selling drugs to get out of the abusive relationship, quickly finding herself victimized by johns and a series of pimps over the next 7 years. She was in and out of jail three to five times a year for prostituting until she ended up in the state prison for women for multiple violations and the drug-trafficking charge, a felony offense. She did engage in prison-based drug treatment which included 12-step groups, trauma-informed group therapy, and psychoeducation during the past 8 months, affiliated with the current residential treatment program for women with addictions in an urban setting. This was her first exposure to addiction and recovery services.

Ms. B entered residential treatment with trepidation, fearing she would be unable to adhere to the treatment program's expectations. An initial comprehensive intake evaluation was completed by a licensed addiction counselor, an educational and workforce evaluation by her case manager, a comprehensive mental health history and evaluation by the APPN, and she was assigned a "Big Sister" peer mentor in the 12-month residential program. The first month in the program provides all residents with an individual therapist for weekly counseling, a case manager for coaching and navigating program expectations, a daily series of trauma-informed group counseling based on the "Seeking Safety" program (Najavits, 2002), 12-step groups on-site twice weekly and off-site once weekly, and a weekly faith-based group with the option of a prayer-partner volunteer through local church affiliation. The second month focuses on job placement in a position that provides a living wage while continuing all of the program elements through evening programming on completion of the eight-session "Seeking Safety" group series. Within the context of this residential program, Ms. B engaged in all of the treatment components as she eventually pursued part-time and eventually full-time employment by the fourth month. Her APPN prescribed escitalopram 20 mg orally daily, which resolved her anxiety and improved her mood, energy, motivation, and sleep.

The case manager and APPN consistently used MI approaches. After a 6-month period of stabilization in the program and in weekly individual therapy with her APPN who was trained in EMDR, many of the traumatic memories of abuse by johns and pimps while prostituting were processed and the cravings and urges to use cocaine abated.

Individual Session Focused on Trigger and Urge to Use (Feeling State and DeTUR Protocols)

Ms. B has previously learned and used resources to stabilize her emotions both within and outside of sessions. In the prior session Ms. B processed the warm, dysphoric sensory feelings and thoughts associated with using opiates until the subjective unit of distress (SUDs) was zero on a 0 to 10 scale with 0 = no disturbance at all and 10 representing the worst disturbance.

APPN:	What would you like to focus on today?
Ms. B:	I'm struggling with thoughts of using marijuana again. . . (discouraged tone).
APPN:	Tell me more about what's happening.
Ms. B:	The kitchen staff at the restaurant where I wait tables all smoke weed. They keep offering me blunts . . . I know if I start using that jeopardizes getting custody of Angel (her 5-year-old daughter).
APPN:	What part of this situation has the most intensity?
	The desire to chill out? (*Urge*)
	Being around others who are smoking weed? (*Trigger*)
	The smell of weed? (*Trigger*)
	Something else?
Ms. B:	Probably the smell . . . even if I don't see them smoking, I can smell it on their clothes, their hair. . . .
APPN:	What are the positive thoughts and sensations you associate with the smell of weed?

Ms. B:	Hmmm. . . . I remember how relaxed I'd feel when smoking weed . . . nothing stressed me out or worried me . . . it would be nice not to feel the pressure of work, managing bills, court appearances to regain custody of Angel . . . I always feel the pressure. I have a warm, relaxed feeling when I smell weed.
APPN:	Would you like to process this trigger . . . the smell of weed . . . with bilateral eye movements as we have in the past?
Ms. B:	It's helped in the past . . . sure.
APPN:	On a scale of 0 to 10, with 0 being no sensation associated with the smell of weed and 10 being the most intense positive sensation associated with the smell of weed, where would you rate your level of sensation right now as you think of the smell of weed? (*Positive Feeling Score – PFS*)
Ms. B:	Probably a 7.
APPN:	I'd like you to visualize being with coworkers smoking weed and hold the smell of weed in your mind while your eyes follow the pencil I'm holding (*administer 30 to 40 repetitions of bilateral movements with APPN and patient seated almost side-by-side with chairs facing in opposite direction per the Feeling-State Addiction Protocols*) *Perform eye movement sets until the PFS score drops to 0 or 1.*)

An alternative approach focuses on decreasing the urge to use associated with the situational triggers to use.

APPN:	On a scale of 0 to 10 with 0 being no urge to use and 10 being the highest level of urge to use (LOU), where would you rate that level of urge to use when you think of coworkers inviting you to share a blunt?
Ms. B:	**Probably a 7.**
APPN:	I'd like you to visualize being with coworkers smoking weed and hold the smell of weed in your mind while your eyes follow the pencil I'm holding (*administer 30 to 40 repetitions of bilateral movements per the DeTUR protocol. Perform eye movement sets until the LOU score drops to 0 or 1.*)
APPN:	Now I'd like you to describe how you will respond to your coworkers when they invite you to share a blunt.
Ms. B:	Jay–you know I can't smoke weed. Please don't ask me anymore. You know the most important thing to me is getting Angel back. A relapse or a dirty urine isn't worth it.
APPN:	I'd like you to visualize this positive scenario at work as we do the bilateral eye movements. (*Perform 30 to 40 repetitions of bilateral movements. Repeat eye movement sets until the strength on a scale of 0 to 10 with 10 being the strongest positive affect is 8 to 10. This builds a future template of effective coping for the patient.*)

After desensitizing the urges with EMDR, Ms. B did not experience cravings or urges for alcohol or marijuana even at times when other residents relapsed and were either re-incarcerated or discharged from the program. Ms. B maintained clean urine drug screens throughout her year in residence, faithfully engaged in all aspects of the program, attended 12-step meetings, rarely missed an individual therapy session, mentored new program residents as a "Big Sister" during her final 6 months in residential treatment, and maintained employment with one of the large hotels, where she worked in the catering department.

On graduation from the 12-month residential treatment program, Ms. B transitioned to one of the program's apartment complexes dedicated to ongoing recovery. She was able to continue seeing her APPN monthly for ongoing medication management through the aftercare services. Treatment focused on reunification with her then 6-year-old daughter, referral to pro bono legal services to begin steps to regain custody of her daughter, and supportive therapy to manage daily work and life stressors without relapsing to drug or alcohol use. She received promotions at work over the next 2 years, enjoyed regular visitation with her daughter, and was engaged in therapy regarding issues of reconciliation with her aging parents. She was active in 12-step recovery groups and joined a church community where she was baptized. She attributes her recovery to the women and program staff who believed in her, her rekindled faith in God whom she thought had abandoned her long ago as a teenager, her unwavering desire to be a "good mom" to her daughter, her employer "who took a chance on a woman with a felony conviction," and the recovery community she relies on daily. Her future challenges will be the decision on whether or when to engage in a significant monogamous relationship. She anticipated ongoing work with her APPN as she embarks on that journey.

Ms. B's history of complex trauma alerted the APPN to provide a sufficient period of stabilization and a comprehensive multidisciplinary approach utilizing community resources, medication, MI, 12-step group work, and peer support. Processing Ms. B's traumas before she has sufficient resources would destabilize her and lead to a relapse as the barrier to the trauma is removed before the person can tolerate such disturbing emotion. The therapeutic alliance allowed Ms. B to remain in treatment, increase her resources, and process urges and her traumatic memories with EMDR therapy once she was stabilized with sufficient support and resources. Her motivation for treatment of reuniting with her daughter provided a strong motivation to continue her treatment. EMDR therapy is a powerful treatment and should only be used by those who have received Basic Training in EMDR from an EMDRIA Approved Trainer. Please see Chapter 7, for how to obtain training in EMDR therapy. Caution is also advised for those who do not know the intricacies of working with this complex population.

POST-MASTER'S ADDICTION NURSING TRAINING AND CERTIFICATION

Specialized certification as an addiction nurse is offered by the Addictions Nursing Certification Board (ANCB), an affiliate of the International Nurses Society on Addictions (IntNSA). The organization offers two levels of certification: Certified Addictions Registered Nurse (CARN) and Certified Addictions Registered Nurse–Advanced Practice (CARN-AP).

Eligibility for the CARN-AP requires:

- Current, full, unrestricted license as a registered nurse (RN) in the United States or Canada
- A master's degree or higher in nursing

- Documentation of a minimum of 500 hours of supervised, direct patient contact in advanced clinical practice working with individuals and families impacted by addictions/dual diagnoses. All 500 hours may be earned while in the master's program.
- Submission of master's program transcript verifying the hours of supervised clinical practice, or submission of verification form signed by supervisor/consultant of post-master's supervised direct patient contact, which together with hours of supervised contact in the master's program equals 500 or more hours.

Application and details for this program are available at www.intnsa.org/ancb/certification.

CONCLUDING COMMENTS

In conclusion, this chapter has provided an overview of the complexity of coexisting substance use, psychiatric, and medical disorders and underscores the importance for all healthcare providers to accurately screen, identify, provide, and/or link patients to appropriate, person-centered and integrated services. The APPN is uniquely prepared to provide diagnosis and treatment of psychiatric disorders and will find it increasingly important to refine skills in the diagnosis and treatment of substance use and behavioral addiction disorders, given the prevalence and co-occurring nature of these disorders.

DISCUSSION QUESTIONS

1. Discuss the potential impact of the *DSM-5* diagnostic criteria for addictions, which lowers the diagnostic threshold and includes both substance use and behavioral addictions.
2. What neurobiological pathways and neurotransmitters are implicated in both behavioral and substance use addictions?
3. Describe the goals of addiction treatment and the components of comprehensive addiction treatment.
4. Discuss the 10 guiding principles of recovery and how you would integrate these into the treatment of a crack-cocaine addicted pregnant woman who is entering residential treatment that will continue through 90 days postpartum including care of infant in residence.
5. What screening questions and measures would be most helpful in detecting behavioral and substance use addictions?
6. Describe motivational interviewing and how you would apply this approach to the individual described in the case study for this chapter.
7. Describe integrated family therapy and how you would apply this approach to the individual described in the case study for this chapter.
8. Describe the FSAP and how you would apply this approach to the individual described in the case study for this chapter.
9. Discuss the importance of maintaining the therapeutic frame and the role of boundaries in working with individuals with addictions.
10. Examine your own thoughts, feelings, and attitudes about individuals with substance use and behavioral addictions. How have addictions touched you, your family, or friends that may influence your ability to effectively work with individuals with addictive disorders?

REFERENCES

Abel, N. J., & O'Brien, J. M. (2010). EMDR treatment of comorbid PTSD and alcohol dependence: A case example. *Journal of EMDR Practice and Research, 4*(2), 50–59. doi:10.1891/1933-3196.4.2.50

Adams, S. M., Peden, A. R., Hall, L. A., Rayens, M. K., Staten, R. R., & Leukefeld, C. G. (2011). Predictors of retention of women offenders in a community-based residential substance abuse treatment program. *Journal of Addictions Nursing, 22*, 103–116. doi:10.3109/10884602.2011.585719

Alberini, C. M. (2009). Transcription factors in long-term memory and synaptic plasticity. *Physiological Reviews, 89*, 121–145. doi:10.1152/physrev.00017.2008

American Psychiatric Association. (2000). *Diagnostic and statistical manual of mental disorders* (4th ed., text rev.). Washington, DC: Author.

American Psychiatric Association. (2013). *Diagnostic and statistical manual of mental disorders* (5th ed.). Arlington, VA: American Psychiatric Publishing.

American Psychological Association. (2015). *Practice update: Substance use disorders and ICD-10 coding.* Retrieved from https://www.apaservices.org/practice/update/2015/09-10/substance-disorders

American Society of Addiction Medicine. (2015). *The ASAM national practice guideline for the use of medications in the treatment of addiction involving opioid use.* Retrieved from https://www.asam.org/docs/default-source/practice-support/guidelines-and-consensus-docs/asam-national-practice-guideline-supplement.pdf

American Society of Addiction Medicine. (2019). *Definition of addiction.* Retrieved from https://www.asam.org/quality-practice/definition-of-addiction

Arndt, S., Clayton, R., & Schultz, S. K. (2011). Trends in substance abuse treatment 1998–2008: Increasing older adult first-time admissions for illicit drugs. *American Journal of Geriatric Psychiatry, 19*, 704–711. doi:10.1097/JGP.0b013e31820d942b

Bae, H., & Kim, D. (2012). Desensitization of triggers and urge reprocessing for an adolescent with an Internet addiction disorder. *Journal of EMDR Practice and Research, 6*(2), 73–81. doi:10.1891/1933-3196.6.2.73

Bae, H., & Kim, D. (2015). Desensitization of triggers and urge reprocessing for pathological gambling: A case series. *Journal of Gambling Studies, 31*, 331–342. doi:10.1007/s10899-013-9422-5

Baumberg, B. (2006). The global economic burden of alcohol: A review and some suggestions. *Drug and Alcohol Review, 25*, 537–551. doi:10.1080/09595230600944479

Bickman, J. (2011). *Doctors spell out addiction for the next decade. The fix, addiction and recovery.* Retrieved from http://www.thefix.com/content/dvm-5-definition-addiction9110

Blanco, C., Moreyra, R., Nunes, E. V., Saiz-Ruiz, J., & Ibanez, A. (2001). Pathological gambling: Addiction or compulsion? *Seminars in Clinical Neuropsychiatry, 6*, 167–176. doi:10.1053/scnp.2001.22921

Blum, K., Sheridan, P. J., Wood, R. C., Braverman, E. R., Chen, T. J., Cull, J. G., . . . Comings, D. E. (1996). The D2 dopamine receptor gene as a determinant of reward deficiency syndrome. *Journal of the Royal Society of Medicine, 89*, 396–400. doi:10.1177/014107689608900711

Brady, K. T., Sonne, S., Anton, R. F., Randall, C. L., Back, S. E., & Simpson, K. (2005). Sertraline in the treatment of co-occurring alcohol dependence and posttraumatic stress disorder. *Alcoholism: Clinical and Experimental Research, 29*, 395–401. doi:10.1097/01.ALC.0000156129.98265.57

Brems, C., Johnson, M. E., Neal, D., & Freemon, M. (2004). Childhood abuse history and substance use among men and women receiving detoxification services. *American Journal of Drug and Alcohol Abuse, 30*, 799–821. doi:10.1081/ADA-200037546

Briere, J., & Scott, C. (2006). *Principles of trauma therapy: A guide to symptoms, evaluation and treatment.* Thousand Oaks, CA: Sage Publications.

Brown, S., Gilman, S. G., Goodman, E. G., Adler-Tapia, R., & Freng, S. (2015). Integrated trauma treatment in drug court: Combining EMDR and seeking safety. *Journal of EMDR Practice and Research, 9*(3), 123–136. doi:10.1891/1933-3196.9.3.123

Carroll, K. M., Nich, C., Lapaglia, D. M., Peters, E. N., Easton, C. J., & Petry, N. M. (2012). Combining cognitive behavioral therapy and contingency management to enhance their effects in treating cannabis dependence: Less can be more, more or less. *Addiction, 107,* 1650–1659. doi:10.1111/j.1360-0443.2012.03877.x

Carroll, K. M., & Rounsaville, B. J. (2006). Behavioral therapies: The glass would be half full if only we had a glass. In W. R. Miller & K. M. Carroll (Eds.), *Rethinking substance abuse: What science shows, and what we should do about it* (pp. 223–239). New York, NY: Guilford Press.

Centers for Disease Control and Prevention. (n.d.). *Excessive drinking is draining the U.S. economy.* Retrieved from https://www.cdc.gov/features/costsofdrinking/index.html

Center for Substance Abuse Treatment. (2000). *Substance abuse treatment for persons with child abuse and neglect issues* (Treatment Improvement Protocol [TIP] Series, No. 36, Chapter 4). Rockville, MD: Substance Abuse and Mental Health Services Administration. Retrieved from http://www.ncbi.nlm.nih.gov/books/NBK64902

Center for Substance Abuse Treatment. (2004). *Substance abuse treatment and family therapy.* (Treatment Improvement Protocol [TIP] Series, No. 39, Chapter 4). Rockville, MD: Substance Abuse and Mental Health Services Administration. Retrieved from http://www.ncbi.nlm. nih.gov/books/NBK64266

Center for Substance Abuse Treatment. (2005). *Substance abuse treatment for persons with co-occurring disorders* (Treatment Improvement Protocol [TIP] Series No. 42). DHHS Publication No. (SMA) 05-3922. Rockville, MD: Substance Abuse and Mental Health Services Administration. Retrieved from https://www.ncbi.nlm.nih.gov/books/NBK64197/

Center for Substance Abuse Treatment. (2006). *Definitions and terms relating to co-occurring disorders.* (COCE overview paper 1. DHHS Publication No. [SMA] 06–4163. Rockville, MD: Substance Abuse & Mental Health Services Administration. Retrieved from http:// store.samhsa.gov/shin/content//PHD1130/PHD1130.pdf

Center for Substance Abuse Treatment. (2009). *Substance abuse treatment: Addressing the specific needs of women.* (Treatment Improvement Protocol [TIP] Series, No. 51. HHS Publication No. [SMA] 09–4426). Rockville, MD: Substance Abuse and Mental Health Services Administration. Retrieved from http://kap.samhsa.gov/products/manualt/tips/pdf/ TIP51.pdf

Cherry, E. F., & Gold, S. M. (1989). The therapeutic frame revisited: A contemporary perspective. *Psychotherapy, 26*(2), 162–168. doi:10.1037/h0085415

Chou, S. P., Huang, B., Goldstein, R., & Grant, B. F. (2013). Temporal associations between physical illnesses and mental disorders—Results from the Wave 2 National Epidemiologic Survey on Alcohol and Related Conditions (NESARC). *Comprehensive Psychiatry.* Retrieved from doi:proxy.library.vanderbilt.edu/10.1016/j.comppsych.2012.12.020

Cox. R. P., & Howard, M. D. (2007). Utilization of EMDR in the treatment of sexual addiction: A case study. *Sexual Addiction and Compulsivity, 14*(1), 1–20. doi:10.1080/10720160601011299

Curley, B. (2010). *DSM-V* – Major changes to addictive diseases classifications. *Recovery Today* (online newsletter). Retrieved from https://www.naadac.org/assets/2416/naadacnews_ 2010_febmar.pdf

Dearing, R. L., Stuewig, J., & Tangney, J. P. (2005). On the importance of distinguishing shame from guilt: Relations to problematic alcohol and drug use. *Addictive Behaviors, 30,* 1392–1404. doi:10.1016/j.addbeh.2005.02.002

DeWitt, D. J., Adlaf, E. M., Offord, D. R., & Ogborne, A. C. (2000). Age at first alcohol use: A risk factor for the development of alcohol disorders. *American Journal of Psychiatry, 157,* 745–750. doi:10.1176/appi.ajp.157.5.745

Dube, S. R., Felitti, V. J., Dong, M., Chapman, D. P., Giles, W. H., & Anda, R. F. (2003). Childhood abuse, neglect and household dysfunction and the risk of illicit drug use: The Adverse Childhood Experiences Study. *Pediatrics, 111,* 564–572. doi:10.1542/peds.111.3.564

Feltenstein, M. W., & See, R. E. (2008). The neurocircuitry of addiction: An overview. *British Journal of Pharmacology, 154,* 261–274. doi:10.1038/bjp.2008.51

Frances, A. (2013). *Essentials of psychiatric diagnosis: Responding to the challenge of* DSM-5. New York, NY: Guilford Press.

Gaumond, P., & Whitter, M. (2009). *Access to Recovery (ATR) approaches to recovery-oriented systems of care: Three case studies* (HHS Publication No. [SMA] 09–4440). Rockville, MD: Center for

Substance Abuse Treatment, Substance Abuse and Mental Health Services Administration. Retrieved from https://www.samhsa.gov/sites/default/files/partnersforrecovery/docs/ATR_Approaches_to_ROSC.pdf

Glasner-Edwards, S., & Rawson, R. (2010). Evidence-based practices in addiction treatment: Review and recommendations for public policy. *Health Policy, 9*, 93–104. doi:10.1016/j.healthpol.2010.05.013

Global Burden of Disease Alcohol Collaborators. (2018). Alcohol use and burden for 195 countries and territories, 1990–2016: A systematic analysis for the Global Burden of Disease Study 2016. *The Lancet, 392*(10152), 1015–1035. doi:10.1016/S0140-6736(18)31310-2

Goldstein, R. Z., & Volkow, N. D. (2011). Dysfunction of the prefrontal cortex in addiction: Neuroimaging findings and clinical implications. *National Review of Neuroscience, 12*, 652–669. doi:10.1038/nrn3119

Grant, J. E., Brewer, J. A., & Potenza, M. N. (2006). The neurobiology of substance and behavioral addictions. *CNS Spectrums, 11*, 924–930. doi:10.1017/S109285290001511X

Grant, J. E., & Potenza, M. N. (2005). Pathological gambling and other behavioral addictions. In R. J. Frances, S. I. Miller, & A. H. Mack (Eds.), *Clinical textbook of addictive disorders* (3rd ed., pp. 303–320). New York, NY: Guilford Press.

Greenfield, S. F., Rosa, C., Putnins, S. I., Green, C. A., Brooks, A. J., Calysn, D. A., . . . Winhusen, T. (2011). Gender research in the National Institute on Drug Abuse National Treatment Clinical Trials Network: A summary of findings. *American Journal of Drug and Alcohol Abuse, 37*, 301–312. doi:10.3109/00952990.2011.596875

Hallgren, K. A., & Moyers, T. B. (2011). Does readiness to change predict in-session motivational language? Correspondence between two conceptualizations of client motivation. *Addiction, 106*, 1261–1269. doi:10.1111/j.1360-0443.2011.03421.x

Hamilton, K. R., & Potenza, M. N. (2012). Relations among delay discounting, addictions, and money mismanagement: Implications and future directions. *American Journal of Drug and Alcohol Abuse, 38*, 30–42. doi:10.3109/00952990.2011.643978

Han, B., Gfroerer, J. C., Colpe, L. J., Barker, P. R., & Colliver, J. D. (2011). Serious psychological distress and mental health service use among community-dwelling older U.S. adults. *Psychiatric Services, 62*, 291–298. doi:10.1176/ps.62.3.pss6203_0291

Hase, M., Schallmayer, S., & Sack, M. (2008). EMDR reprocessing of the addiction memory: Pretreatment, posttreatment, and 1-month follow-up. *Journal of EMDR Practice and Research, 2*(3), 170–179. doi:10.1891/1933-3196.2.3.170

Hasin, D., & Kilcoyne, B. (2012). Comorbidity of psychiatric and substance use disorders in the United States: Current issues and findings from the NESARC. *Current Opinions in Psychiatry, 25*, 165–171. doi:10.1097/YCO.0b013e3283523dcc

Henry, S. (1996). Pathological gambling: Etiological consideration and treatment efficacy of EMDR. *Journal of Gambling Studies, 12*(4), 395–405. doi:10.1007/BF01539184

Hien, D. A., Wells, E. A., Jiang, H., Suarez-Morales, L., Campbell, A. N., Cohen, L. R., ... Nunes, E. V. (2009). Multisite randomized trial of behavioral interventions for women with co-occurring PTSD and substance use disorders. *Journal of Consulting and Clinical Psychology, 77*, 607–619. doi:10.1037/a0016227

Hser, Y.-I., Li, J., Jiang, H., Zhang, R., Du, J., Zhang, C., . . . Zhao, M. (2011). Effects of a randomized contingency management intervention on opiate abstinence and retention in methadone maintenance treatment in China. *Addiction, 106*, 1801–1809. doi:10.1111/j.1360-0443.2011.03490.x

Hunter, B. A., Robison, E., & Jason, L. A. (2012). Characteristics of sexual assault and disclosure among women in substance abuse recovery homes. *Journal of Interpersonal Violence, 27*, 2627–2644. doi:10.1177/0886260512436389

Institute of Medicine, Committee on Quality of Health Care in America. (2001). *Crossing the quality chasm: A new health system for the 21st century*. Washington, DC: National Academies Press. doi:10.17226/10027

Kalivas, P. W., & Volkow, N. D. (2005). The neural basis of addiction: A pathology of motivation and choice. *American Journal of Psychiatry, 162*, 1403–1413. doi:10.1176/appi.ajp.162.8.1403

Kessler, R. C., Berglund, P., Demler, O., Jin, R., Merikangas, K. R., & Walters, E. E. (2005). Lifetime prevalence and age-of-onset distributions of *DSM-IV* disorders in the National

Comorbidity Survey Replication. *Archives of General Psychiatry, 62*, 593–602. doi:10.1001/archpsyc.62.6.593

Kessler, R. C., Sonnega, A., Bromet, E., Hughes, M., & Nelson, C. B. (1995). Posttraumatic stress disorder in the National Comorbidity Survey. *Archives of General Psychiatry, 52*, 1048–1060. doi:10.1001/archpsyc.1995.03950240066012

Knipe, J. (2019). Treating addictive disorders with adaptive information processing. In J. Knipe (Ed.), *EMDR toolbox: Theory and treatment of complex PTSD and dissociation* (2nd ed., pp. 125–156). New York, NY: Springer Publishing Company.

Koob, G. F. (2009). Dynamics of neuronal circuits in addiction: Reward, antireward, and emotional memory. *Pharmacopsychiatry, 42*, S32–S41. doi:10.1055/s-0029-1216356

Koob, G. F., Ahmed, S. H., Boutrel, B., Chen, S. A., Kenny, P. J., Markou, A., . . . Sanna, P. P. (2004). Neurobiological mechanisms in transition from drug use to drug dependence. *Neuroscience and Behavioral Reviews, 27*, 739–749. doi:10.1016/j.neubiorev.2003.11.007

Koob, G. F., & Volkow, N. D. (2010). Neurocircuitry of addiction. *Neuropsychopharmacology, 35*, 217–223. doi:10.1038/npp.2009.110

Kulaga, A., Kristman-Valente, A., Chu, M., Sage, R., Robinson, J. A., Liu, D., . . . Nunes, E. D. (2009). Multisite randomized trial of behavioral interventions for women with co-occurring PTSD and substance use disorders. *Journal of Consulting and Clinical Psychology, 77*, 607–619. doi:10.1037/a0016227

Labbate, L. A., Sonne, S. C., Randall, C. R., Anton, R. F., & Brady, K. T. (2004). Does comorbid anxiety or depression affect clinical outcomes in patients with post-traumatic stress disorder and alcohol use disorders? *Comprehensive Psychiatry, 45*, 304–310. doi:10.1016/j.comppsych .2004.03.015

Lan, C. W., Fiellin, D. A., Barry, D. T., Bryant, K. J., Gordon, A. J., Edelman, E. J., ... Marshall, B. D. L. (2016). The epidemiology of substance use disorders in US veterans: A systematic review and analysis of assessment methods. *American Journal of Addictions, 25*, 7–24. doi:10.1111/ajad.12319

Laudet, A. B. (2003). Attitudes and beliefs about 12-step groups among addiction treatment clients and clinicians: Toward identifying obstacles to participation. *Substance Use and Misuse, 38*, 2017–2047. doi:10.1081/JA-120025124

Laudet, A. B., & White, W. L. (2005). An exploratory investigation of the association between clinician's attitudes toward twelve-step groups and referral rates. *Alcohol Treatment Quarterly, 23*(1), 31–45. doi:10.1300/J020v23n01_04

Lee, J. L. (2008). Memory reconsolidation mediates the strengthening of memories by additional learning. *Nature and Neuroscience, 11*, 1264–1266. doi:10.1038/nn.2205

Lee, J. L. (2009). Reconsolidation: Maintaining memory relevance. *Trends in Neuroscience, 32*, 413–420. doi:10.1016/j.tins.2009.05.002

Legha, R. K., & Novins, D. (2012). The role of culture in substance abuse treatment programs for Indian and Alaska Native communities. *Psychiatric Services, 63*, 686–692. doi:10.1176/appi.ps .201100399

Marich, J. (2010). EMDR in addiction continuing care: A phenomenological study of women in recovery. *Psychology of Addictive Behaviors, 24*(3), 498–507. doi:10.1037/a0018574

Markel, H. (2012). The D.S.M. gets addiction right. *The New York Times*. New York, NY. Retrieved from http://www.nytimes.com/2012/06/06/opinion/the-dsm-gets-addiction-right.html?_r=0

Marlatt, G. A. (1997). *Cognitive-behavioral relapse prevention for addictions*. [DVD]. Washington, DC: American Psychological Association. Retrieved from https://www.apa.org/pubs/videos/4310746

Marlatt, G. A., & Gordon, J. R. (1985). *Relapse prevention: Maintenance strategies in the treatment of addictive behaviors*. New York, NY: Guilford Press.

McLellan, T. A., Lewis, D. C., O'Brien, C. P., & Kleber, H. D. (2000). Drug dependence, a chronic medical illness: Implications for treatment, insurance, and outcomes evaluation. *Journal of the American Medical Association, 284*, 1689–1695. doi:10.1001/jama.284.13.1689

Merriam-Webster. (2020). *Addiction*. Retrieved from https://www.merriam-webster.com/dictionary/addiction

Miller, R. (2010). The Feeling-State Theory of impulse-control disorders and the impulse-control disorder protocol. *Traumatology, 16*(3), 2–10. doi:10.1177/1534765610365912

Miller, R. (2016). *The Feeling-State Addiction Protocol (FSAP)*. Retrieved from http://www.imagetransformationtherapy.org/microsoft-word---the-fsap-4.pdf

Miller, R. (2012). Treatment of behavioral addictions utilizing the feeling-state addiction protocol: A multiple baseline study. *Journal of EMDR Practice and Research, 6*(4), 159–169. doi:10.1891/1933-3196.6.4.159

Miller, W. R., Moyers, T. B., Amrhein, P., & Rollnick, S. (2006). A consensus statement on defining change talk. *Motivational Interviewing Network of Trainers Bulletin, 13*(2), 6–7. Retrieved from https://motivationalinterviewing.org/sites/default/files/MINT13.2.pdf

Miller, W. R., & Rollnick, S. (1991). *Motivational interviewing: Preparing people for change.* New York, NY: Guilford Press.

Miller, W. R., & Rollnick, S. (2002). *Motivational interviewing: Preparing people for change* (2nd ed.). New York, NY: Guilford Press.

Modell, A. (1976). The holding environment and the therapeutic action of psychoanalysis. *Journal of the American Psychoanalytic Association, 24*, 285–308. doi:10.1177/000306517602400202

Najavits, L. M. (2002). *Seeking safety: Cognitive behavioral therapy for PTSD and substance abuse.* New York, NY: Guilford Press.

Najavits, L. M., Weiss, R. D., & Shaw, S. R. (1997). The link between substance abuse and posttraumatic stress disorder in women: A research review. *American Journal on Addictions, 6*(4), 273–283. doi:10.3109/10550499709005058

Najt, P., Fusar-Poli, P., & Brambilla, P. (2011). Co-occurring mental and substance abuse disorders: A review of the potential predictors and clinical outcomes. *Psychiatry Research, 186*, 159–164. doi:10.1016/j.psychres.2010.07.042

National Institute on Alcohol Abuse and Alcoholism. (2005). *Helping patients who drink too much: A clinician's guide. Updated 2005 edition.* National Institutes of Health, NIH Publication No. 07–3769. Retrieved from https://pubs.niaaa.nih.gov/publications/practitioner/cliniciansguide2005/guide.pdf

National Institute on Alcohol Abuse and Alcoholism. (2015). *Alcohol screening and brief intervention for youth: A practitioner's guide* (NIH Publication No. 11–7805). Retrieved from https://pubs.niaaa.nih.gov/publications/Practitioner/YouthGuide/YouthGuide.pdf

National Institute on Drug Abuse. (2010). *Drugs, brains, and behavior: The science of addiction.* Bethesda, MD: National Institute of Health Publication 10–5605: U.S. Department of Health and Human Services. Retrieved from http://www.drugabuse.gov/sites/default/files/sciofaddiction.pdf

National Institute on Drug Abuse. (2012). Principles of drug addiction treatment: A research-based guide (3rd ed.). Bethesda, MD: National Institute of Health, Publication 12–4180: U.S. Department of Health and Human Services. Retrieved from http://www.drugabuse.gov/sites/default/files/podat_1.pdf

National Institute on Drug Abuse. (2017). *Trends and statistics: The economic costs of substance abuse.* Retrieved from https://www.drugabuse.gov/related-topics/trends-statistics#supplemental-reeferences-for-economics-costs.

National Institute on Drug Abuse. (2018). *Drugs, brains, and behavior: The science of addiction.* U.S. Department of Health and Human Services, NIH Publication No. 18-DA-5605. Retrieved from https://www.drugabuse.gov/sites/default/files/soa.pdf

National Survey on Drug Use and Health. (2009). *Rates of co-occurring mental and substance use disorders.* Rockville, MD: Substance Abuse and Mental Health Services. Retrieved from http://www.samhsa.gov/co-occurring/topics/data/disorders.aspx#1

O'Brien, C. P., Volkow, N., & Li, T. K. (2006). What's in a word? Addiction versus dependence in *DSM-V.* (Editorial). *American Journal of Psychiatry, 163*, 764–765. doi:10.1176/ajp.2006.163.5.764

O'Farrell, T. J., & Clements, K. (2012). Review of outcome research on marital and family therapy in treatment for alcoholism. *Journal of Marital and Family Therapy, 38*, 122–144. doi:10.1111/j.1752-0606.2011.00242.x

Pilowsky, D. J., Keyes, K. M., & Hasin, D. S. (2009). Adverse childhood events and lifetime alcohol dependence. *American Journal of Public Health, 99*, 258–263. doi:10.2105/AJPH.2008.139006

Pittman, D. (2012). IOM: Military needs better care for addicts. *MedPage Today.* Retrieved from https://www.medpagetoday.com/publichealthpolicy/militarymedicine/34798

Popky, A. J. (2005). DeTUR, an urge reduction protocol for addictions and dysfunctional behavior. In F. Shapiro (Ed.), *EMDR solutions: Pathways to healing* (pp. 167–188). New York, NY: W. W. Norton.

Potenza, M. N. (2006). Should addictive disorders include non-substance-related conditions? *Addiction, 101*(1), 142–151. doi:10.1111/j.1360-0443.2006.01591.x

Potenza, M. N. (2008). The neurobiology of pathological gambling and drug addiction: An overview and new findings. *Philosophical Transactions of the Royal Society of Biological Sciences, 363*, 219–228. doi:10.1098/rstb.2008.0100

Prescott, C. A., & Kendler, K. S. (1999). Genetic and environmental contributions to alcohol abuse and dependence in a population-based sample of male twins. *American Journal of Psychiatry, 156*, 34–40. doi:10.1176/ajp.156.1.34

Prisciandaro, J. J., DeSantis, S. M., Chiuzan, C., Brown, D. G., Brady, K. T., & Tolliver, B. K. (2012). Impact of depressive symptoms on future alcohol use in patients with co-occurring bipolar disorder and alcohol dependence: A prospective analysis in an 8-week randomized controlled trial of acamprosate. *Alcohol, Clinical and Experimental Research, 36*, 490–496. doi:10.1111/j.1530-0277.2011.01645.x

Rieckmann, T., McCarty, D., Kovas, A., Spicer, P., Bray, J., Gilbert, S., . . . Mercer, J. (2012). American Indians with substance use disorders: Treatment needs and comorbid conditions. *American Journal of Drug and Alcohol Abuse, 38*, 498–504. doi:10.3109/00952990.2012.694530

Rowe, C. L. (2012). Family therapy for drug abuse: Review and updates 2003–2010. *Journal of Marital and Family Therapy, 38*, 59–81. doi:10.1111/j.1752-0606.2011.00280.x

Schiller, J. S., Lucas, J. W., & Peregoy, J. A. (2012). *Summary health statistics for U.S. adults: National Health Interview Survey, 2011. Vital Health Statistics, 10*(256). Hyattsville, MD: National Center for Health Statistics. Retrieved from http://www.cdc.gov/nchs/data/series/sr_10/sr10_256.pdf

Schmitz, J. M., Lindsay, J. A., Stotts, A. L., Green, C. E., & Moeller, F. G. (2010). Contingency management and levodopa-carbidopa for cocaine treatment: A comparison of three behavioral targets. *Experimental and Clinical Psychopharmacology, 18*, 238–244. doi:10.1037/a0019195

Schuckit, M. A., Edenberg, H. J., Kalmijn, J., Flury, L., Smith, T. L., Reich, T., . . . Foroud, T. (2001). A genome-wide search for genes that relate to a low level of response to alcohol. *Alcoholism: Clinical and Experimental Research, 25*, 323–329. doi:10.1111/j.1530-0277.2001.tb02217.x

Shapiro, F. (2018). *Eye Movement Desensitization and Reprocessing (EMDR): Basic principles, protocols, and procedures* (3rd ed.). New York, NY: Guilford Press.

Sheedy, C. K., & Whitter, M. (2009). *Guiding principles and elements of recovery-oriented systems of care: What do we know from the research?* (HHS Publication No. [SMA] 09–4439). Rockville, MD: Center for Substance Abuse Treatment, Substance Abuse and Mental Health Services Administration. Retrieved from https://www.samhsa.gov/sites/default/files/partnersforrecovery/docs/Guiding_Principles_Whitepaper.pdf

Siegel, C., Haugland, G., Reid-Rose, L., & Hopper, K. (2011). Components of cultural competence in three mental health programs. *Psychiatric Services, 2*, 626–631. doi:10.1176/ps.62.6.pss6206_0626

Smith, D. E., Buxton, M. E., Bilal, R., & Seymour, R. B. (1993). Cultural points of resistance to the 12-step recovery process. *Journal of Psychoactive Drugs, 25*(1), 97–108. doi:10.1080/02791072.1993.10472596

Soeter, M., & Kindt, M. (2011). Disrupting reconsolidation: Pharmacological and behavioral manipulations. *Learning & Memory, 18*, 357–366. doi:10.1101/lm.2148511

Stitzer, M. L., Petry, N. M., & Peirce, J. (2010). Motivational incentives research in the National Drug Abuse Treatment Clinical Trials Network. *Journal of Substance Abuse Treatment, 38*(1), S61–S69. doi:10.1016/j.jsat.2009.12.010

Substance Abuse and Mental Health Services Administration. (2002). *NASMHPD/NASADAD Joint Task Force Report to Congress on the prevention and treatment of co-occurring substance use disorders and mental disorders*. Rockville, MD. Retrieved from https://www.ncmhjj.com/wp-content/uploads/2014/10/Behavioral_Health-Primary_CoOccurringRTC.pdf

Substance Abuse and Mental Health Services Administration. (2011a). *SAMHSA announces a working definition of "recovery" from mental disorders and substance use disorders*. Retrieved from http://www.samhsa.gov/newsroom/advisories/1112223420.aspx

Substance Abuse and Mentral Health Services Administration. (2011b). *Substance use disorders in people with physical and sensory disabilities* (HHS Publication No. (SMA) 11–4648). In Brief, 6(1) Retrieved from https://store.samhsa.gov/sites/default/files/d7/priv/sma11-4648.

Substance Abuse and Mental Health Services Administration. (2012a). *Results from the 2011 National Survey on Drug Use and Health: Summary of national findings.* Retrieved from http://www.samhsa.gov/data/NSDUH/2k11Results/NSDUHresults2011.pdf

Substance Abuse and Mental Health Services Administration. (2012b). *SAMHSA's working definition of recovery.* Retrieved at https://store.samhsa.gov/product/SAMHSA-s-Working-Definition-of-Recovery/PEP12-RECDEF

Substance Abuse and Mental Health Services Administration. (2018). *Key substance use and mental health indicators in the United States: Results from the 2017 National Survey on Drug Use and Health* (HHS Publication No. SMA 18-5068, NSDUH Series H-53). Rockville, MD: Center for Behavioral Health Statistics and Quality, Substance Abuse and Mental Health Services Administration. Retrieved from https://www.samhsa.gov/data/

Substance Abuse and Mental Health Services Administration. (2019). *Key substance use and mental health indicators in the U.S.: Results from the 2018 National Survey on Drug Use and Health.* Retrieved from https://www.samhsa.gov/data/sites/default/files/cbhsq-reports/NSDUHNationalFindingsReport2018/NSDUHNationalFindingsReport2018.pdf

U.S. Department of Veterans Affairs. (n.d.). *PTSD and substance abuse in veterans.* Retrieved from https://www.ptsd.va.gov/professional/treat/cooccurring/tx_sud_va.asp

U.S. Surgeon General. (2004). *News release by U.S. Surgeon General Carmona: Face facts about drinking.* Retrieved from http://alcoholism.about.com/cs/support/a/blnih040407.htm

United Nations Office on Drugs and Crime. (2018). *World drug report 2018* (United Nations publication, Sales No. E.18.XI.9). Retrieved from https://www.unodc.org/wdr2018/prelaunch/WDR18_Booklet_1_EXSUM.pdf

Witkiewitz, K., Lustyk, M. K., & Bowen, S. (2013). Retraining the addicted brain: A review of hypothesized neurobiological mechanisms of mindfulness-based relapse prevention. *Psychology of Addictive Behaviors, 27*(2), 351–365. doi:10.1037/a0029258

World Health Organization. (2009). *Global health risks: Mortality and burden of disease attributable to selected major risks.* Retrieved from http://www.who.int/healthinfo/global_burden_disease/GlobalHealthRisks_report_full.pdf

Wu, L. T., & Blazer, D. G. (2011). Illicit and nonmedical drug use among older adults: A review. *Journal of Aging and Health, 23,* 481–504. doi:10.1177/0898264310386224

Psychotherapy With Children

Kathleen R. Delaney, Janiece DeSocio,
and Julie A. Carbray

In this chapter child psychotherapy is discussed in the context of the evolving science of evidence-based practices (EBPs). Viewing all intervention through a lens of supporting evidence is particularly important for child psychiatric nurses who hold a social commitment with families and children to provide effective treatment that promotes mental health and wellness. As described in the chapters on adult psychotherapy, psychiatric nursing interventions are always initiated in the context of the relationship. In the case of a child (unless specified, the term *child* is used to refer to treatment with both children and adolescents), that focus broadens to the relationship the APPN establishes with the family/parent/caregiver. The perspective of APPNs who treat children is also shaped by an orientation on prevention and promoting resiliency. Following a historical summary and exploration of underlying assumptions of child intervention, several basic principles of child psychotherapy will be described. Two therapeutic evidence-based psychotherapeutic approaches will be highlighted, then applied to select commonly occurring childhood disorders. As noted in Chapter 1, nurse psychotherapists are on a journey of novice to expert. To provide a sense of this growth, three cases are presented: one involving a novice nurse who uses a solution-focused common elements approach and two other cases detailing the approach of an expert psychiatric nurse who discusses her treatment plan for a child exhibiting complex behaviors indicative of comorbid serious emotional disorders.

HISTORICAL CONTEXT

What defines the field of child psychotherapy? For anyone over a certain age, a mention of child psychotherapy conjures up an image of play therapy and a dynamic, drive-theory orientation to a child's behavioral problems. Indeed, a history of child therapy would have most likely begun in the 1930s and early 1940s when the ideas of Anna Freud and Melanie Klein predominated (West & Evans, 1992). While psychodynamic and play-therapy techniques have continued refinement and broadened to include Jungian techniques (Chethik, 2000; Schaefer, 2003) and short-term models (Trowell et al., 2007), the dominance of the psychodynamic school has subsided (Ritvo et al., 1999).

Child psychodynamic practice has drawn consistent criticism for the lack of empirical data on its effectiveness (Barrnett, Docherty, & Frommelt, 1991; Remschmidt & Quashner, 2001; Ritvo, 2006), but recent reviews, particularly from the United Kingdom, indicate that psychodynamic approaches are effective for some children, particularly ones dealing with internalizing disorders, such as depression and anxiety (Midgley, O'Keeffe, French, & Kennedy, 2017). Today, psychodynamic therapy continues as an element of training in psychiatry (Kitts et al., 2019) and is recognized as a portal to concepts critical to the relationship, attunement, and narrative elements of treatment (Leonidaki, Lemma, & Hobbis, 2018; Myklebust & Bjørkly, 2019). The field is also supported by the American Academy of Child and Adolescent Psychiatry (AACAP), which has published a practice guideline on the implementation of psychodynamic therapy for children age 3 to 12 (Kernberg, Ritvo, Keable, & AACAP Committee on Quality Issues, 2012). In children and teens, there is also increasing interest in research that aimed to demonstrate its effectiveness with select populations (Abbass, Rabung, Leichsenring, Refseth, & Midgley, 2013).

Given that historical background, what propelled the current dominance of behavioral and cognitive-behavioral approaches in child psychotherapy? Hibbs (2001) proposed that a data-based, scientific approach to solving specific behavioral problems contributed to the ascendancy of child behavioral treatments in the 1960s and 1970s. Through the 1990s, the trend continued toward time-limited interventions aimed at producing symptom-specific outcomes and child psychotherapy was increasingly defined by techniques and their accompanying school of therapy (e.g., Interpersonal, Systemic, Cognitive-behavioral, and Family) (Roth & Fonagy, 1996). In their most recent policy statement on child psychotherapy, the AACAP endorsed the notion of psychotherapy as treatments residing in these established therapy schools (AACAP, 2014).

At the same time, a shift was occurring in how therapies were organized within these recognized psychotherapy schools; that is, they were increasingly classified by the major childhood disorders: anxiety, depression, attention deficit hyperactivity disorder (ADHD), and conduct disorders (Weisz, Hawley, & Doss, 2004). Organizing intervention by diagnosis was advanced by the work of the American Psychological Association Division 12 (1993), who created a scheme to rate the evidence supporting psychological interventions. In the child field, what followed were extensive treatment reviews for specific childhood disorders such as anxiety disorders, ADHD, and autism (Burns, 2003). This organizational scheme for rating evidence also lent itself to analysis of clinical trial research, which supplied the data for another emerging movement, defining EBPs (Hibbs & Jensen, 1996). What has emerged from this trend are sets of interventions for particular disorders and child psychotherapy being defined and organized by EBPs for both specific disorders (e.g., Wang et al., 2017) and a common elements approach of effective treatments that spans across disorders, for example, parent management training and problem-solving skills groups (Barth et al., 2012). Another emerging trend is a transdiagnostic approach where the treatment target is the underlying cognitive or emotional mechanism (such as emotional dysregulation) that is seen to drive mental health/behavioral symptoms across diagnostic categories, for example, mood and externalizing disorders (Aldao, Gee, De Los Reyes, & Seager, 2016).

APPN: TRAINING AND CERTIFICATION

Psychiatric nurses are key participants in the coordination of mental healthcare for children and bring a particular nursing orientation and expertise. The scope of practice for child psychiatric nurses sets down several areas of emphasis: the value of the relationship, a health focus, view of the child in relation to social systems, and the application of science to treatment, that is, both psychological interventions and the neurobiology of illness (American Nurses Association, 1985). Preparation for advanced practice psychiatric nurses (APPNs) occurs at the graduate level and includes training in multiple bodies of knowledge (medical science, neurobiology of psychiatric disorders, health systems, treatment methods, psychopharmacology, and relationship science). APPNs bring this distinct orientation into their work with children by the way they respond and view phenomena.

There are two groups of APPNs who are trained, certified, and licensed to provide child psychotherapy. The first are Child and Adolescent Clinical Specialists (C/A CSs), who, since the demarcation of their scope in 1985, have provided comprehensive psychiatric services to children and adolescents. At the start of the decade there were close to 990 certified C/A CSs, but through the early 2000s fewer C/A CSs sought ANCC certification, and thus there has been scant increase in this workforce over the past 15 years (Delaney & Vanderhoef, 2019). In 2001, when the PMH Nurse Practitioner (NP) exams were introduced, an adult and a family or life span PMH NP option were offered. The Family PMH NP is trained to deliver psychiatric services across the life span and function in a manner quite similar to the C/A CSs, although, as noted in a role differentiation study of the two groups, there was a greater emphasis on medication management among PMH NPs and therapy with C/A CSs (Weiss & Talley, 2009).

At the same time, the advanced practice registered nurse (APRN) consensus model was widely endorsed, which set the PMH specialty as a life-span population. As a result of an alignment of licensing, accreditation, certification, and education by 2015, only the PMH-NP (life span) certification exam was available for new APPNs (Delaney, 2017). However, the existing C/A CS workforce will continue to practice since, as with any specialty, once licensed, an APPN retains that state license and may renew certification by meeting the certifying body's certification practice requirements (see details at APNA, n.d.). The APRN consensus model delineates the positioning of a specialty practice level beyond the basic population/role license. In the near future, the PMH specialty must decide if creating specialty training would be the optimal path for addressing the mental health needs of particular child/adolescent populations, particularly those with complex serious emotional disorders (Delaney & Karnick, 2019).

UNDERLYING ASSUMPTIONS AND PRINCIPLES OF CHILD THERAPIES

Four underlying assumptions that differentiate child therapies from adult psychotherapy are developmental considerations, family inclusion, consideration of the interacting systems in a child's life, and the concept of resiliency. In the adult realm of mental health service delivery, the notion of recovery has become a prominent organizing principle of mental health treatment. In the child field, a parallel idea is the concept of resiliency. This principle is in direct contrast to the traditional approach to children, which was ground in a problem-based method. Resiliency as an overarching perspective moves the field to a strength-based approach that holds at its center a stance of therapeutic optimism (Meichenbaum, 2017).

Developmental Considerations The level of a child's development influences what he or she can understand and how he or she understands the world. For instance, depending on a child's developmental level, he or she may be unable to take another person's perspective into account and may explain an adult's action based on an egocentric view of the situation (Coburn, Bernstein, & Begeer, 2015). By about age 6, this egocentric thinking gives way to a more reasoned interpretation of another person's intention; thus an APPN should be aware of potential diagnostic issues when egocentric thinking is still apparent in a latency aged child (Begeer et al., 2016). As the APPN approaches a child's issues, he or she also considers the developmental norms that the child's behavior might or might not be violating. Are the parents'/teacher's expectations for sustained attention in line with what one might expect of a child of that age? Thus, understanding a child's developmental level of reasoning, perspective taking, language, and social emotional regulation facilitates treatment planning, therapies, and, at times, developmentally sensitive adaption of a particular method such as CBT (Kendall, 2016).

Just as in adult therapies where APPNs consider the notion of the neural integration that can be achieved via intervention, in the child world an overarching framework is the notion of how a child achieves self-regulation via integration of the thinking, emotional, memory, and motivational centers of the brain (Nigg, 2017). The field of developmental neuroscience has accelerated the view of children as striving to achieve integration largely on the heels of experience-dependent growth of critical areas of the brain (Siegel, 1999). This developmental view is particularly important when, after a thorough assessment, the APPN begins to piece together a formulation of the child's presentation with an eye on both the child's functioning and how the child/family has attempted to cope with the regulation issues they deal with, be it impulsivity or emotional dysregulation (Sloan et al., 2017; Southam-Gerow, 2013).

Developmental neuroscience also provides APPNs with a platform for combining the emerging neurobiology of illness/treatment with a service system organized around a family-centered approach. In one sense, neuroscience maps ways of helping children and adolescents engage in experiences that will help them reorganize, strengthen, and re-connect with developmental challenges (Dahlitz, 2015). Similar to the spiral of integration in Chapter 1, children engage in life, so they are making decisions that lead to behaviors that promote competence, which in turn increases esteem. To re-engage with social systems, children must respond to situations with appropriate control of their behaviors and emotions. This critical task is represented by the notion of self-regulation. Box 20.1 provides a brief summary and an example of how research informs efforts to understand childhood illness in the framework of neural integration and self- regulation.

Family Involvement A second underlying assumption of child psychotherapy is that clinicians operate from a norm of family involvement in treatment and treatment decisions. The idea of family involvement has an important history and critical place in child treatment (see Box 20.2). Family involvement begins when treatment is initiated, enlisting the parent's view of treatment needs and establishing goal congruence (a consensus about the goals of therapy and the means to accomplish those goals). This orientation, sometimes titled a family-centered systems of care approach or a patient-family-centered care approach (Conway et al., 2006), should be firmly integrated into all aspects of treatment planning. Focused efforts to involve families in care is also critical as the treatment proceeds since strengthening family's engagement has been demonstrated to improve outcomes and reduce treatment drop out (Warnick, Bearss, Weersing, Scahill, & Woolston, 2014). Evidence also supports that decreases in vulnerable youths' behavioral symptoms can be achieved via the development of family connections, school support, and strengthening community ties (Stoner, Leon, & Fuller, 2015).

A family-centered approach does not mean that the family is the focus of treatment. Family treatment is appropriate to improve family interactions, keep families engaged in services, or increase their knowledge about mental health. For some children, an individual approach with a family component may be the appropriate treatment combination, particularly if informed by evidence of parent-child interactions that reinforce a problematic behavioral pattern (Kendall, 2017). Children with conduct issues may require a multi-systematic approach where interventions are aimed at the various systems that interact with the child; in this instance, family involvement is a critical element to both setting goals and keeping them involved with the treatment (Henggeler, 2012).

Child's Systems Surround The third underlying assumption of child psychotherapy is consideration of the systems that promote a child's development, that is, family, school, peers, and community. Since interaction in these systems is a key to ongoing

BOX 20.1 Self-Regulation

At its most basic level, regulation is conceptualized as a developmental milestone of childhood whereupon the child controls behavior in the service of socially desirable conduct (Nigg, 2017). As a simple example, think of the 4-year-old who, as the preschool teacher puts down a plate of cookies, is told to wait for snack time to begin. What prevents that child's hand from snatching a treat? Neuroscientists would argue that the restraint arises from the development of inhibitory control and the integration of emotion with memory (e.g., what happened last time I snatched a cookie?). These processes help dampen the rush to reward so that the child can comply with the teacher's request and wait. It is within this almost simultaneous action and reaction of cognitive, emotional, and motor systems that individuals adjust to the demands of a particular situation. Neuroscience researchers illustrate how frontal lobe activities coordinate with limbic system structures to control attention and modulation of emotions, which in turn facilitates one's ability to respond appropriately to particular situations (Eisenberg & Spinrad, 2004).

Self-regulation depicts the pivotal developmental process of integrating emotion, reading the salience of a cue with a memory of past experience. As Nigg (2017) points out, there are many ways to approach self-regulation; that is, emotional regulation, executive functioning, or effortful control. While there are diverse ranges of constructs, it has important implications for how a child's behavioral issues are viewed and addressed. Indeed, the future of child psychotherapy may lie in how neuroscience informs the process of creating experiences such that the child strengthens neural pathways and develops adaptive ways of thinking, feeling, and behaving (e.g., Rothenberg, Weinstein, Dandes, & Jent, 2019). Self-regulation issues, particularly emotional regulation, are increasingly understood to cut across several dimensions of child psychopathology such as ADHD, PTSD, maltreatment, depression, and anxiety (Aldao et al., 2016; Anastopoulos et al., 2011; Tan et al., 2012).

Problems in the preschool child's self-regulation have also been tied to subsequent issues with aggression, social withdrawal, and conduct problems (Bell & Calkins, 2012). Since it may be one of the pivotal processes that drive several disorders, Nigg (2017) suggests it should be a component of any therapy program aimed at attention, self-awareness, or cognitive controls.

ADHD, attention deficit hyperactivity disorder; PTSD, posttraumatic stress disorder.

BOX 20.2 Key Events and Principles in Family Centered Care Approach

- **CASSP established** (Children and Adolescent Service System Program). The overarching goals of CASSP were to coordinate community services for children with serious emotional needs. CASSP principles also emphasized that parents should be empowered, treated as partners in care, and participate fully in treatment planning (Day & Roberts, 1991).
- **Systems of care (SOC) approach is defined.** These principles moved into a broader SOC approach to treatment (Stroul & Friedman, 1996) with the creation of agencies and funding that assured comprehensive community-based services would be available for families of children with serious emotional illness. Here the emphasis shifted to establishing networks for delivering individualized service plans embedded in comprehensive, culturally competent, coordinated service networks.
- **Comprehensive community SOC ideology is developed.** Via SOC grants, SOCs were developed that held parents as key players determining how services would be developed, delivered, managed, and evaluated to match the needs of the child. These SOC grants continue under the SAMHSA-supported Comprehensive Community Mental Health Services for Children Initiative. Recent data from CMHI programs has been combined with data from the National Survey of Children's Health to create a report on children's mental health and trauma (U.S. DHHS, 2018).

CMHI, Children's Mental Health Initiative; U.S. DHSS, U.S. Department of Health and Human Services; SAMHSA, Substance Abuse and Mental Health Services Administration.

development, a child's competence in these systems must also be facilitated. As articulated by parents, a *guiding principle* of child psychotherapy should be a focus on developing a package of services that contribute to a wide band of "real-world" outcomes (Lindsey et al., 2014). For instance, the goals of treatment should include a focus on improvements in critical areas of a child's life and the socioemotional skills they need to succeed in school and with peers (Gattis, 2014). We increasingly understand the role of family, socioeconomic status, and community supports in childhood developmental and behavioral disorders (Robinson et al., 2017). In line with a goal of supporting a child's strengths, reducing risk, and increasing protective factors, treatment should also extend to the development of a community support system that may serve as an important protective buffer (e.g., Crush, Arseneault, Jaffee, Danese, & Fisher, 2017: Lu & Xiao, 2019). Guidelines have not been formally written for this type of community systems approach but exemplars exist, particularly via school community collaborations (Lewallen, Hunt, Potts-Datema, Zaza, & Giles, 2015) as well as models for integrating EBPs into community services within the context of usual care at community-based practice settings (Vidal & Connell, 2019).

The idea of community-based systems of care has been supported by the Substance Abuse and Mental Health Services Administration's (SAMHSA) Children's Mental Health Initiative (CMHI). Since 1993 CMHI has funded over 300 demonstration and extension grants to states for creating systems of care that are more responsive to children with serious mental health conditions and their families (U.S. DHHS, 2018). All of the systems operate within four basic systems of care principles (family driven, youth driven, culturally and linguistically competent, and providing community-based services; Stroul, Goldman, Pires, & Manteuffel, 2012).

Resiliency In Chapter 1, healing was identified as an outcome of the psychotherapy process. Must child psychotherapy involve healing? Yes, but not healing in the cognitive sense where, as with adults, one comes to piece together a healing narrative. Rather, therapy should be healing such that children can regulate their behavior and emotions and thus stay positively connected with their school, family, and peers. It is regulation in the service of interacting and building the store of experiences that children/adolescents use to learn and practice how to plan, solve problems, build competence, and exercise agency. To accomplish these outcomes, therapy should be aimed at helping children build resilience. That may include addressing maladaptive behaviors, but equally important is constructing an environment and service system that builds on children's strengths and augments their vulnerabilities (Whitson, Bernard, & Kaufman, 2013).

Resiliency was initially conceptualized via a person-centered approach, isolating characteristics of children who were able to develop—and indeed thrive—in the face of significant adversity (Anthony, 1987). Increasingly, resiliency is viewed as a grounding conceptual framework for intervention programs that promote competency and minimize stress (Goldstein & Brooks, 2013). In line with this approach, interventions are not primarily focused on pathology but on strengths and promoting protective processes in families and systems that interface with the child (Masten & Barnes, 2018). A strength-based orientation moves beyond diagnosis-bound approaches to consider accommodations in the environment that will strengthen factors to help children and adolescents successfully deal with the challenges they may face.

A strength-based emphasis has been part of child psychiatric nursing since the first standards of practice written in 1985 (ANA, 1985). This orientation does not discount diagnosis but emphasizes that nurse psychotherapists combine symptom amelioration with building environments that allow for the mobilization of a positive developmental thrust, a potential long recognized as residing in children and re-set in an environment structured to support functioning (Emde, 1990). This orientation does not discount the need to intervene to help children regulate and/or alleviate distress.

Thus, any psychotherapist treating children must also know a range of interventions and what is efficacious for the treatment of a particular serious emotional disorder (e.g., Higa-McMillan, Francis, Rith-Najarian, & Chorpita, 2016). For instance, a child dealing with serious anxiety will need to learn regulation skills grounded in cognitive-behavioral techniques (Kendall, 2017). It would be an error in clinical reasoning not to initially consider these techniques given the substantial evidence supporting the use of behavioral, cognitive-behavioral, and, for some anxiety disorders, combined techniques (medication with CBT) to address anxiety issues.

Part of building resiliency might mean addressing the pivotal process that may be driving the disorder. For example, the treatment plan for a depressed adolescent may need to include interpersonal psychotherapy (IPT) when dysfunctional relationships are seen as central to the disorder (Markowitz & Weissman, 2012). Chapter 10 contains an excellent outline of the principles and basic techniques of IPT and a summary of the accommodations of the model in IPT protocols designed for adolescents. Alternately, therapy might be focused on affirming cognitive skills for a sexual and gender minority (SGM) youth who may experience disproportionate chronic stress, discrimination, and victimization associated his or her SGM identity (Craig & Austin, 2016). Either or both processes (interpersonal and cognitive) may be at play in adolescent depression and treatment should address the core issue. Combining evidence-based therapies (a traditional deficit approach) with a fundamental strength-based framework may seem like forging a meeting of opposites. What is essential is that the APPN weaves together targeted interventions within a plan for building systems that promotes a child/adolescent's competence. In doing so, the nurse aims to help the child get back on the developmental path of agency, choices, and eventually self-efficacy.

CURRENT EVIDENCE-BASED PRACTICES IN THE CHILD FIELD

Therapies and psychological approaches become evidence-based practices via clinical trials where defined groups of participants receive a standardized treatment. Members of this participant group have similar behaviors or presentations such that they meet select diagnostic criteria. Thus, a particular EBP often demonstrates efficacy for a particular diagnosis. The convention of linking EBPs to diagnosis is reinforced by publications such as practitioner reviews (Sayal, Prasad, Daley, Ford, & Coghill, 2018), research summaries of treatments for particular disorders (Daley et al., 2018), and texts describing specific EBPs in detail (Weisz & Kazdin, 2017).

Based on a review of the literature, it would seem that there was much to choose from when considering an EBP approach for children and adolescents. There are EBPs for particular child/adolescent serious emotional disorders (SEDs) that provide a clear roadmap to the psychosocial interventions that can be used to address specific aspects of a disorder, such as CBT techniques for adolescent depression (Spirito, Esposito-Smythers, Wolff, & Uhl, 2011). While the body of evidence-based child practices does not equal those amassed in the adult field, reviews and analysis of effective treatment modalities indicate the growing strength of the child specialty (Higa-McMillan et al., 2016). Organizing child interventions by EBPs and diagnosis envisions a future where the therapist will line up diagnosis and a suitable evidence-based intervention. This would seem a logical approach, but this convention is not without complications. Several issues of an EBP-based child psychotherapy therapy system are outlined in Box 20.3. With the advent

BOX 20.3 Issues of EBP and Child Psychosocial Treatment

There are several issues with building a child therapy system grounded in EBPs. One, it rests on the assumption that eventually there will be an EBP to match most of the child's SEDs. While significant strides have been made in developing a menu of evidence-based treatment for children (Weisz & Kazdin, 2017), the child specialty has not built a body of clinical–trial evidence to support psychosocial or combined treatment for every diagnostic category. Reviews of child-specific EBPs demonstrate progress in the treatment of adolescent depression, anxiety, and ADHD, but there is much work to be done, particularly in areas such as use of EBPs guided by diagnostic criteria with vulnerable populations (Klein, Damiani-Taraba, Koster, Campbell, & Scholz, 2015), children with bipolar disorder (Findling & Chang, 2018), or the transdiagnostic presentation of behaviors such as irritability (Brotman, Kircanski, & Leibenluft, 2017).

Even with the SEDs that have been the focus of significant research, there are issues with the way evidence reviews interpret and collect data, at times calling into question the conclusions of treatment that are considered evidence-based (Watson, Richels, Michalek, & Raymer, 2015). Over the last two decades in large scale studies and evidence reviews, medications have demonstrated effectiveness at addressing core ADHD symptoms (Cortese et al., 2018). Behavioral and psychosocial treatments are recommended as an adjunct to medication for ADHD (Cheung et al., 2018), and there is support for behavioral parent training, as well as some support for CBT approaches and classroom modifications (Gálvez-Lara et al., 2018). Yet debate continues on the effectiveness of a wider range for psychosocial treatments in ADHD (Fabiano, Schatz, Aloe, Chacko, & Chronis-Tuscano, 2015).

Another assumption of the evolving evidence-based system is that clinicians will proceed in a linear fashion from assessment to diagnosis to locating the appropriate EBP. However, diagnosis in the child and adolescent field comes with a host of considerations. Children's psychiatric diagnoses are not static; they can change over the years. The current popular taxonomies do not provide for a youth's presentation that might be a blend of behaviors, each akin to several disorders (Diler, 2018) or a combination of behaviors that do not fit into any existing diagnostic category. With children, comorbid disorders are common; 40% of affected youth report more than one class of mental health disorders (Merikangas et al., 2010).

Another issue is the assumption that EBPs, primarily designed and tested as child-centered approaches, will be what families want or need. Speaking for the voice of parents, Flynn (2005) noted families' issues with EBPs that continue into the present (Haine-Schlagel & Walsh, 2015); primarily there are too few, they are poorly translated into "real world practice", and they disregard the family's role in the treatment planning. As Flynn emphasized, children and adolescents must be treated in the context of their school lives, families, and communities. The outcomes families seek (improved school performance, competency, enhanced peer relationships) are not necessarily the direct outcomes of applying an EBP.

Finally, a therapy model organized solely around EBPs overlooks the reality that children and adolescents with SEDs have a variety of interconnected needs. Research demonstrates that youth with SED are likely to have a comorbid disorder, be severely impaired, and be experiencing problems in multiple areas of their lives (e.g., school, family) (Robinson et al., 2017). Within the youth SED population are cohorts of children with particular needs arising from maltreatment, being in foster care, or involvement in the Juvenile Justice system; for these children, specific EBPs are slowly emerging (Dorsey et al., 2017). Children with complex needs will require an approach that simultaneously addresses their multiple social needs as well as issues arising from their SED.[*]

ADHD, attention deficit hyperactivity disorder; CBT, cognitive behavioral therapy; EBP, evidence-based practice; SEDs, serious emotional disorders.

---

[*] It is beyond the scope of this chapter to review the issues with translation of EBPs with "usual" care in community settings (see Weisz, Krumholz, Santucci, Thomassin, & Ng, 2015).

of web-based searches and dashboard methods for organizing effective treatments, the hope is clinicians will achieve a comfort level with isolating the best available, most effective approach for a child's presentation (Weisz, 2015). Indeed, the logical result of this modular effort is moving the child field toward defining child psychotherapy by EBPs in line with a child's core issues, informed by diagnosis but not necessarily dictated by it (Weisz et al., 2015).

PSYCHOTHERAPY WITH CHILDREN: BASIC PRINCIPLES

Initial Contact, Assessment, Setting Shared Goals

There are numerous psychotherapy interventions for children, many of which fall within the major schools of therapy (e.g., cognitive-behavioral, psychodynamic, and supportive). The text has provided an excellent orientation to the underlying conceptual framework of these major schools, the drivers of change, and theoretically how particular methods achieve these aims. The basic structure of psychotherapy with children aligns with the principles forwarded for adults.

With children and families, as with adults, the APPN mindfully moves through the initial contact, aware that this first meeting sets the stage for the requisite therapeutic alliance. With children, one also considers that it is the parent, not the child or teen, that often initiates the treatment and thus for the youth there may be a mixture of both fear and resentment at this initial session. Thus, beginning with this first meeting, it is helpful to take a strength-based approach, for example, praise the teen for his or her efforts at maintaining control of some aspects of his or her life (Cepeda, 2010). All the principles of therapeutic communication also apply here, but the attending and listening are to both the family and the child. Cepeda (2010) also underscores the importance of picking up on the themes or the preoccupations of the child during the assessment process. For the beginning practitioner, several texts exist to guide this initial engagement process (Cepeda, 2010; Whitcomb, 2017).

Child Assessment

During initial meetings with a child and his or her family, the APPN conducts a thorough assessment. The basic elements are reviewed here since assessment drives treatment planning, which in turn drives the psychotherapeutic approach. However, the reader should refer to more extensive texts on child assessment for a comprehensive approach to the process (e.g., Mash & Barkley, 2010). In line with a family-focused, strength-based approach, the APPN does not conduct the assessment to place a label on the child, which might place constraints about how to think about the child and the family goals. Yet, while working within a strength-based framework, the APPN is aware that billing, service site treatment records, and, at times, communications with other providers will necessitate a diagnostic impression is recorded. Parents will also want to know within what category (mood, thought, behavior) the APPN places the focus of treatment.

The psychiatric assessment should be conducted in an organized fashion with particular categories of information explored, such as details of the current problem, strengths, functioning, psychiatric history, medical issues, and emotional/physical development. Given that 29% of psychiatric disorders that first appear in adolescents are associated with child adversities, screening for trauma circumstances is particularly important (McLaughlin et al., 2012).

The novice APPN might use the AACAP assessment practice parameter (King, 1997)[*] and incorporate specialized areas of assessment depending on the child's presentation. For instance, if a child/parent reports a significant history of anxiety, the APPN should consider the onset, duration, and intensity, along with the developmental considerations such as what would be considered normal childhood fears (Beesdo, Knappe, & Pine, 2009). A structured interview format appropriate to the child's presentation and specialized assessment tools might also be employed (Frick, Barry, & Kamphaus, 2010). Numerous rating scales exist for children; Lee (2012) provides a succinct summary of the gold standard tools and consideration for their use and interpretation.

Finally, the assessment process of children requires that the APPN develops a sense of the child's internal world. In his classic book, *The Clinical Interview of the Child*, Stanley Greenspan (Greenspan & Thorndike Greenspan, 2003) explains how one conducts an assessment of not just a child's problem behaviors but also how the child is organizing experiences and the developmental level of that organization. These key processes include the developmental level of the child's regulation and engagement, which is assessed by taking note of how the child attends to the interview and shares attention and focus. The second process involves how the child signals and communicates via gestures. The third has to do with the meaning system of the child and mental images or representations he or she creates, and the last involves how the child connects ideas and feelings and reflects on a global level. Taken together, these processes offer a vehicle for observing the often intangible aspects of children, that is, how they take in reality, how they take in you as an interviewer, how they signal needs, and how they manipulate ideas.

While the basic components of the assessment process in child treatment move in parallel with adults, there are several distinct features. As with adults, APPNs organize their assessment around guidelines that map out the essential content areas (Lempp, de Lange, Radeloff, & Bachmann, 2012). In an integrated approach, the assessment may also include a review of systems to rule out medical issues that may be present and impacting behavior (Johnson & Newland, 2012). The assessment also demands integrating data from multiple informants—parents, child, and school—as well as viewing the information through a developmental-systems lens (see Guerra, Williamson, & Lucas-Molina, 2012). Finally, the APPN considers presenting behaviors in terms of their setting, frequency, variability/consistency, and situational influences (Mash & Barkley, 2010). Considering the known issues of disparities in the treatment of racial and ethnic minority youth, the assessment incorporates ethnic and cultural contexts for both the child's behavior and the interpretation of the presenting problems, as well as the goals and expectations of the family (Alegria, Green, McLaughlin, & Loder, 2015). Rates of mood disorders, distress, and suicide ideations/attempts and completions are rising in adolescents (Twenge, Cooper, Joiner, Duffy, & Binau, 2019); thus, of course, the interview includes a careful suicide risk assessment.

Another important element of child psychotherapy involves goal setting with both the parent and child. Through careful listening, the APPN has come to understand the parent's perception of the core problem as well as how he or she has come to understand the behavior and what he or she believes the child needs to recover (Kelly & Coughlan, 2018).

For teens, collaboration is particularly important as often they are not the ones initiating treatment and fear the stigma they perceive accompanies a mental health diagnosis (Boyd, Butler, & Benton, 2018). Parents' beliefs, attitudes, and expectations about treatment and their sense of the effectiveness of the interventions are critical to their engagement with services (Becker, Boustani, Gellatly, & Chorpita, 2018). Among the reasons Horwitz and colleagues (2012) note for parents prematurely leaving treatment are issues around the cultural relevance of services, lack of consideration of family

---

[*]This guideline currently under revision by the AACAP.

preferences (particularly around medication), and seeing the treatment as irrelevant and/or ineffective. Thus, incorporating the family's ideas into treatment goals not only demonstrates respect but meeting the family's expectations increase the likelihood that parents/caregiver will stay with treatment (Horwitz et al., 2012).

Formulation

Following the assessment and discussion of shared goals, the APPN begins to build a formulation of the child's core issues, a synopsis of what the child and family are dealing with (Henderson & Martin, 2014). The formulation goes beyond diagnosis to explain the contexts of the child and family situation, what is unique about the child's presentation, and how the child/family is responding to situations, as well as their (and other informants') narratives of the events that shaped that interpretation. Constructing the formulation, the APPN might use a biopsychosocial framework such as the four P's model (predisposing, precipitating, perpetuating, and protective factors) or the Four Perspectives model, which includes consideration of disease, dimensions, behaviors, and life story (Henderson & Martin, 2014). With children, it is also important to include the developmental context and an understanding of why the child is struggling in particular areas of his or her life and what might be the processing/regulation/learning deficit underlying the behavior (McLaughlin, DeCross, Jovanovic, & Tottenham, 2019). The formulation should take into account the systems the child interacts with; his or her support network; and the cultural dimensions that impact on the particular SED, the way the adolescent views treatment, or a particular orientation to mental health (Alegria et al., 2015; DeFrino et al., 2016; Huang & Zane, 2016).

Treatment Planning

Treatment planning includes family goals, preferences, and beliefs, as well as the child's/adolescent's perspective on the problem and, for teens, their ideas on how best to address the issue (Boyd et al., 2018; Haine-Schlagel & Walsh, 2015). Given the issue, the APPN draws upon the evidence supporting a particular approach to formulate the treatment plan. Following an overview of general principles of child psychotherapy, I will discuss two methods of implementing evidence-based psychotherapy. The use of medications is indicated in combination with psychosocial interventions in several child and adolescent SEDs, such as pediatric bipolar disorder, and with moderate to severe levels of particular disorders (ADHD, OCD, and adolescent depression). A thorough treatment of this topic is beyond the scope of this chapter, so the reader is referred to the practice guidelines and most recent evidence on combined/pharmacological treatment strategies (e.g., Axelson, 2019; Cortese et al., 2018; Dobson, Bloch, & Strawn, 2019; Lawrence, Nangle, Schwartz-Mette, & Erdley, 2017; Wang et al., 2017).

General Principles of Child Psychotherapy

One way to approach child psychotherapy would be to discuss the major schools of therapy and exactly what a child version might entail. In many respects, the therapeutic mechanisms of CBT and interpersonal psychotherapy discussed in this text apply to work with children and teens. While the goals of CBT with children are in line with the general principles of the therapy school, there are important differences in their implementation with children and teens (Delaney & Hawkins-Walsh, 2012). For instance, the principles of cognitive therapy with children are similar, that is, sessions are problem focused, collaborative, and goal oriented (Friedberg & McClure, 2015). But as Friedberg and McClure (2015) point out, owing to the child's motivation for treatment and cognitive/verbal abilities, therapy tasks should be constructed in line with the child's developmental level and an orientation to the here and now. The actual use of CBT techniques with children and teens will also depend on the particular issues and their engagement with a particular CBT technique.

For the interested reader, Sharer (2012) provides excellent summaries of the major schools of therapy (e.g., psychodynamic, IPT, CBT) as well as multisystemic and Eye Movement Desensitization and Reprocessing (EMDR) therapy) in the context of child treatment and specific intervention techniques (e.g., behavioral parent training). For the APPN who decides to offer these therapies in his or her practice, Sharer also provides information about how one enrolls in specific training to become proficient at each particular type of therapy. Since the principles and core techniques of the CBT and IPT for children and teens are quite similar to their presentation in this text, I will spend the rest of the chapter discussing specific ways to implement these strategies within an evidence-based approach to psychotherapy for children.

While the discussion deals with various evidence-based approaches, intervention with children and families always includes consideration of the therapeutic alliance as it continues to be recognized as one of the core factors that create change in therapy (DeNadia et al., 2017). Of course, prioritizing the relationship in all encounters aligns well with a nursing framework (D'antonio, Beeber, Sills, & Naegle, 2014) and naturally combines with a planned use of evidence-based psychosocial interventions (Perraud et al., 2006). The relationship with the child draws upon similar APPN skills, such as use of interpersonal abilities (such as warmth and empathy) and attunement with the child's affect (Delaney, Shattell, & Johnson, 2017). Via this attunement, the APPN begins to form a bond with the child, and from that connection begins to collaborate on treatment planning (Karver, De Nadai, Monahan, & Shirk, 2019).

In child psychotherapy, the APPN also focuses on the alliance with the family, knowing that this will entail building trust and understanding the family's dilemma. Caring for a child with emotional difficulties creates stress, particularly in the years that families search for answers and they find none, or have problems accessing services or understanding exactly what the services offer (Clark, 2016; Mendenhall & Mount, 2011). Families must also deal with the stigma and blame that they sense from relatives and their community (Kaushik, Kostaki, & Kyriakopoulos, 2016). Building an alliance with families of traumatized children has been historically difficult and actively addressing barriers to treatment is critical to increasing engagement (Saxe et al., 2012).

EVIDENCE-BASED INTERVENTIONS

At the start of one's advanced practice career, an APPN may not have extensive or specialized training in a mode of therapy. As they begin to practice, APPNs will undoubtedly find they spend much time providing a full range of psychiatric services including diagnostic evaluations and medication management. Often it is within this framework that one provides the indicated psychotherapeutic or psychosocial interventions Chapter 21. As the novice APPN moves into a particular service sector, depending on the team and how they approach therapy, he or she might seek advanced therapy training in a particular modality such as IPT or psychodynamic. Perhaps the APPN finds that many of the children and teens in the practice are dealing with anxiety and thus finds it appropriate to acquire additional training in CBT (Kendall, 2017). For the beginner or novice APPN who finds that he or she is dealing with directing intervention for a wide variety of children, there are several methods for implementing evidence-based psychosocial therapies. An approach accessible for the novice APPN might incorporate a common elements/transdiagnostic approach. To begin, I discuss a manualized therapy approach so the reader understands the difference with this versus a common elements approach.

Treatment With Manualized Approach

In treatment planning, one way to address a child's issues is to utilize a specific method or manualized approach. For illustration, outlined here is the treatment approach for a child assessed with trauma issues. The treatment is being utilized with a 10-year-old boy who was brought to the mental health clinic with behaviors that began following a 6-month-long exposure to a domestic violence situation. The boy is assessed by the APPN, who determines that many of the presenting issues (poor sleep due to nightmares about the violence, irritability and refusal to talk about the domestic violence, minor aggression and restlessness) began following the domestic violence exposure. After gathering additional information and consultation with the boy's mother, the team agreed the evidence-based treatment of choice was trauma-focused cognitive behavioral therapy (TF-CBT) (Dorsey et al., 2017). TF-CBT is an empirically supported treatment model for children who have experienced some form of trauma. It aims at helping such children practice emotional expression, build emotion-event-cognition connection, and gradually process their abuse experience (Cohen, Deblinger, & Mannarino, 2018). TF-CBT is a components-based treatment where within a relationship-based approach parents and the child learn how to manage emotions, cope with stress, manage and process thoughts related to the trauma, and enhance feelings of safety. The acronym PRACTICE represents the components of TF-CBT.

The first component, psychoeducation, begins the process as the child and parent are taught about trauma response, what causes it, common responses (including PTSD symptoms), and how TF-CBT addresses these issues. Also included in this component is a review of the effective parenting skills that will be of use to the traumatized child, such as praise and positive attention. The R stands for relaxation and the skills taught to the child to deal with the physiologic response to the trauma. Affect modulation (A) provides skills such as affect identification and thought interruption to help children control thoughts attendant to anxious feelings. Enhancing safety (E) as well as cognitive coping (C) is critical and includes problem-solving to help the child both regulate negative thinking and recognize the relationship between thoughts, feelings, and behavior. In the final components, the child begins to construct the trauma narrative (T), which entails creating a narrative of the experience, correcting distortions about the experiences, and placing the trauma in the context of his whole life. Via graduated exposure to feared stimuli, the therapist leads the child through *in vivo* (I) mastery of trauma cues. Then in conjoint (C) parent–child sessions the child shares the trauma narrative with parents. Finally, the therapist and family work toward enhancing (E) the child's sense of future safety. In controlled studies, reviews of the method note children who completed the TF-CBT program had significantly reduced depression, anxiety, and PTSD symptoms (Dorsey et al., 2017).

The originators of TF-CBT demonstrate modifications of the method for children with complex trauma and reference single site studies where the method has been successfully used with these children (Cohen, Mannarino, Kliethermes, & Murray, 2012). Complex developmental trauma is defined by cumulative, poly victimization, which often results in greater impairment marked by problems in multiple developmental domains such as affect regulation, attachment, behavioral control, cognition, and self-concept (Cook et al., 2005). It should be noted that results from interventions specifically targeting these children have demonstrated positive outcomes but not clear superiority over treatment as usual, largely due to issues with the comparison groups (Dorsey et al., 2017). Thus, selection of treatment based on diagnosis for this highly vulnerable population should be approached with care and perhaps with consideration of a common elements or transdiagnostic approach.

Common Elements Approach

In some settings, TF-CBT may not be available, there might be a delay in the child entering treatment, or the child may present with a trauma history that has generated a host of regulation/behavioral issues. In this situation, an APPN might take a common elements approach in providing psychotherapeutic intervention for the child. Common elements refer to the individual treatment approaches such as affect regulation or psychoeducation that are component parts of many manualized treatments. The common elements approach has been in development for 15 years, and while the focus of the program drivers has evolved (Chorpita et al., 2017; McLeod et al., 2017; Weisz et al., 2012), the core idea of the common elements approach has remained consistent.

The program has its roots with the Child and Adolescent Health Division (CAMHD) of The Hawaii Department of Health where a team of practitioners mapped evidence-based interventions across child diagnoses and some 322 clinical trials to arrive at effective interventions for common childhood mental health problems such as aggression, withdrawn behaviors, and attention problems (Choripita & Daleiden, 2009). The investigators' goal was to conceptualize how the existing evidence on treatment, derived largely from controlled clinical trials, would be best implemented in real world practice where case managers usually select the services a child will receive. They posit that transportability of interventions would more likely occur when the common elements across diagnoses and the evidence of a particular strategy were isolated. For instance, a problem-solving approach might be contained in a package of CBT elements for adolescent depression (Curry & Meyer, 2018), but it is also a component for treatment of children with conduct issues and a wide variety of mental health issues (Nezu, Nezu, & Hays, 2019). The common elements approach views the evidence-based strategy in light of the actual intervention as well as the diagnostic categories where it fits best.

The distillation of methods and matching of models to the best fit of patient characteristics has continued (Chorpita, Daleiden et al., 2011; Lindsey et al., 2014) but has moved focus into how common elements might be used in what is called modular treatment, an approach that flexibly responds to the treatment setting, response to a treatment approach, and emerging issues (Chorpita et al., 2017). The common elements approach is now considered one method of a transdiagnostic approach, the use of a single protocol for an identified problem that cuts across diagnostic categories (see Marchette & Weisz, 2017, for a review of the transdiagnostic approach).

The originators of this method see it as a way to increase the use of evidence- based approaches in usual care as the unified/transdiagnostic protocols present straightforward tiered interventions to common issues. An example of a child-oriented transdiagnostic intervention is FIRST (Weisz, Bearman, Santucci, & Jensen-Doss, 2017). FIRST uses five core principles applicable to children dealing with anxiety, depression, and conduct issues; they are: techniques to self-calm, increasing motivation to make adaptive behavior more rewarding, repairing thoughts, problem-solving, and a technique called "trying the opposite." Early trials of FIRST report significant improvement on pre/post scores on multiple clinical measures including symptom checklists as well as reports on "top problems." These findings were derived from pre/post comparisons on standardized diagnoses and on standardized parent and youth symptom checklists, as well as trajectory of change analyses of weekly standardized problem reports by youth and caregivers. Interventions such as FIRST offer a useful and reasonable way to introduce evidence-based approaches into usual care since training can be brief and straightforward. Recently, Washington State reported significant gains from state-wide training throughout their public mental health system in a common elements approach to treating child/adolescent PTSD, anxiety, depression, and behavior problems (Dorsey, Berliner, Lyon, Pullmann, & Murray, 2016).

Common Elements Approach to Intervening With a Child With a Trauma History, ADHD Behaviors, and Aggressive Acting Out: Common Elements Approach

Children rarely present to specialty mental health services with just a single issue. Thus, while ADHD is a common childhood mental health issue, there is often co morbidity of externalizing and internalizing disorders. The problems with ADHD have long been viewed as a fundamental problem in regulation of attention, executive functions, and insufficient intrinsic motivation, leading to a high need for stimulation and levels of reinforcement to motivate performance (Hinshaw, 2018). Another area of increasing interest is the relationship between adverse childhood experiences (ACEs) and ADHD.

Using data from the National Survey of Children's Health, investigators found that a sample of 76,227 children with ADHD had higher levels of ACEs than the larger cohort, even after adjusting for socioeconomic status (Brown et al., 2017). Similar findings were reported for a large sample of children between 5 and 9 years old experiencing ACEs, who then demonstrated increased rates of ADHD at 9 years old (Jimenez, Wade, Schwartz-Soicher, Lin, & Reichman, 2017). These data raise the question of the overlap of ADHD and behaviors seen in exposure to traumatic events (difficultly concentrating, dysregulated affect, irritability, and hyperarousal) (Szymanski, Sapanski, & Conway, 2011). As these data build, clinicians should carefully consider a child's trauma history in their assessment of ADHD (Klein et al., 2015).

Understanding the complexity of the disorder, treatment approaches may target various difficulties the child is displaying in home and school. Consider the use of a common elements approach with a latency-aged youth with a history of trauma who carries a diagnosis of ADHD and anxiety. Despite stimulant medication, the child exhibits frequent angry outbursts, opposition, and aggression. To begin, the APPN would review the best available evidence for a behavioral, cognitive, or psychoeducational intervention to augment the medication and address these behavioral/regulation issues.

In treatment planning, the APPN realizes the family is unaware of the impact of trauma exposure and suggests that the child's angry outbursts suggest emotional regulation deficits. Considering the child's presentation, the parents' goals, and the availability of TF-CBT, the APPN might consider introducing strategies to address the child's immediate issues with dysregulation. In drawing sources together, the APPN realizes that children who have experienced trauma have multiple problems with regulation (cognitive/affective balance) (McLaughlin & Lambert, 2017) and manifest behaviors indicative of emotional regulation (ER) issues, for example, irritability, emotional flooding, or angry outbursts (Muller, Vascotto, Konanur, & Rosenkrantz, 2013). Also, given the common comorbidities with ADHD (including anxiety), psychosocial treatments are often indicated to address issues with emotional dysregulation or aggressive behaviors (Brotman et al., 2017; Rosen et al., 2019), even while the exact mechanisms of ER and the matching approach are still being honed (Chu, Chen, Mele, Temkin, & Xue, 2017). The following case example illustrates how a novice APPN and treatment team might use a common elements approach to address a child's outbursts that could be attributed to the ADHD, trauma history, or anxiety.

CASE EXAMPLE

A Common Elements Approach to Aggressive Outbursts

Jennifer, who is 10 years old, came to the hospital accompanied by her mother and father. They were seeking admission to a partial-hospitalization program for their daughter because of increasing aggression and emotional outbursts at home and school over the past several months. When frustrated, Jennifer lashed out at other children, particularly her brother. The APPN discussed with the family how the intake would proceed and explained that the first step was to hear the family's story about how they saw Jennifer's problems, as well as her strengths. Their stories depicted not just a child having problems with aggression but an unhappy child who seemed overwhelmed by her emotions. In addition, Jennifer's problems had created tremendous tension in the home.

The parents were frustrated with the services they had received in the past. Their daughter had been seen in the mental health system for several years. Jennifer was adopted at age 2 and the parents had a sense she experienced significant neglect in her early history. In reviewing her history, the APPN noted that Jennifer had been assigned a variety of diagnoses, most prominently ADHD, oppositional defiant disorder (ODD), and anxiety. Following a recent extensive diagnostic evaluation at the clinic, Jennifer was thought to be exhibiting behaviors consistent with ADHD and anxiety but was also displaying increasing aggression and emotional regulation issues, which might be tied to her trauma history. Jennifer was medically and neurologically clear. In the initial intake session, the APPN gathered ideas around the family's goals for treatment and what they considered to be a priority focus while building a relationship with the parents and Jennifer. This was accomplished by forming an empathic bridge with their disappointments with previous treatment and their sense of urgency to stop what they perceived to be a path of deteriorating behavior.

The APPN listened carefully, moving inside the family's narrative and how they pieced together events and assigned meaning to Jennifer's behavior and the school's response. Valuable information was attained in the initial interview about how the family framed the behaviors, what they believed treatment should accomplish, and what, in their own terms, improvement would look like. The APPN inquired about the child's strengths and competencies in order to capture an image of the child Jennifer can be at times, and a future vision of how she might increase those strengths. At the same time, Jennifer's behaviors during the intake were noted as well as her predominant affect and ability to contain strong emotions. After approximately 30 minutes with the parents and Jennifer, the APPN asked to see Jennifer alone. The APPN used conversation and expressive techniques to observe how she responded to some mild probing questions, the partial hospital setting, and the therapist's presence. During this phase of the interview, Jennifer said that she was somewhat confused by her outbursts and aggression. She could not describe the events that led up to a typical 'meltdown" but stated that she would like to get along better at home and at school. Thus, Jennifer and her parents exhibited motivation for change.

Following this immersion in the family narrative, clarification of their treatment goals, and the tentative exploration of how Jennifer experienced the world, the APPN worked with the family on selecting one area for change and eliciting their ideas on what might bring about this change. All agreed that they wanted the focus to be the aggressive behavior and emotional outbursts. The evidence-based CBT with good support was a family cognitive-behavioral psychoeducational intervention, drawing from components of the Coping Power program (Boxmeyer, Lochman, Kassing, Mitchell, & Romero, 2018). One aspect of Coping Power is to work with the child and family to increase emotional awareness and to identify triggers for anger arousal. The first step was teaching Jennifer and her family to recognize the signs of mounting tension/ frustration and then catching the escalation early. The severity of her outbursts was "scaled" with a target number for improvement. The parents and Jennifer drew a picture of what the future would look like when they had achieved the family goal. This session aimed at a family-centered, solution-oriented method for approaching one aspect of Jennifer's behavior.

The partial hospitalization program Jennifer attended, in a sense, mimicked a typical day at school and employed a similar strategy. During the time on the unit, staff carefully watched and patterned Jennifer's behavior. This close observation gave some clues to how Jennifer became frustrated; this was especially evident when events did not unfold as expected. As the staff and APPN talked with Jennifer, it was noted that Jennifer could identify basic feelings but did not have a large emotional vocabulary and could not connect her feelings to the events that triggered them. Observing the signs of mounting frustrations, the APPN and staff stepped in early and interrupted the behavior before it escalated. A plan was agreed on that Jennifer might "take space" and avoid any involved conversation during tense times. Once calm, role-playing was initiated to help Jennifer learn how one uses an emotional vocabulary to describe events.

These simple strategies, which were effective on the unit, were discussed with Jennifer's parents. Each evening, upon leaving the partial hospital program, the APPN discussed Jennifer's day with the parent who picked her up and planned on what they might work on at home. In the morning, the time at home was reviewed with the parents. The family and Jennifer began to regain their confidence that they could dampen down mounting escalation. They scaled her improvement in the positive zone. The family began to see the "old" Jennifer, an energetic, curious child. After 10 days in the partial program, both Jennifer and her family thought they were ready to transition to outpatient care. At that point the parents were provided several options. One, they decided to remain with the psychiatrist for medication management aimed at her ADHD. Two, they chose to continue working with the APPN, who continued to approach Jennifer's outbursts by working with the components of the Coping Power Program, moving now to perspective taking and anger management.

Expert Nursing Practice

As child/adolescent APPNs gain experience, their use of evidence-based practices expands. In a recent qualitative study, 15 expert child APPNs talked about their approach to treatment (Delaney & McInosh, in press). Each participant discussed the importance of relationships he or she formed with children and their families and also the "everydayness" of how they interacted. As explained by one APRN, "I'm trying to be more of a coach, a teacher, a model for them and what to do." Another APPN echoed a similar view, saying, "What's most effective in when we're trying to help the child in the family environment is that the parents actually feel better, and then they feel more confident, and then they're able to do what we're asking to do with the child, which is, often, something that doesn't come naturally in their parenting." The base for participants' practical, problem-focused approach varied.

The following two clinical examples are provided to illustrate the approach of expert nurses: one with a young girl teen presenting with an eating disorder and obsessive-compulsive behaviors, and another with a latency aged youth with bipolar disorder. The case examples illustrate how the APPNs built an approach based on the neurobiology of the disorder and combining components of EBPs to direct psychoeducation and family engagement, as well as provide strategies to address target behaviors.

CASE EXAMPLE

Expert Nursing Approach to a Child Exhibiting Comorbid Serious Emotional Disorders

10-Year-Old Alicia: A Psychiatric Mental Health Nurse Practitioner Approach to Treatment Planning

Janiece DeSocio, PhD, RN, PMHNP-BC

Alicia, age 10, was referred by her primary care provider (PCP) for a psychiatric evaluation due to a seven-pound weight loss, an increase in handwashing, and fears of germs over the past 2 months. Her symptoms began following an episode of the flu when she experienced several days of nausea, vomiting, and sore throat. Following her recovery, Alicia weighed 64 pounds and returned to school and swim team but continued to complain of stomachaches when she ingested even small amounts of food. Within the past month she has continued to complain of stomachaches with eating, resulting in further weight loss. Today she weighs 60 pounds at 4'6" tall with a BMI of 14.5. The most Alicia has ever weighed is 67 pounds at her last physical exam 6 months ago. After Alicia's recovery from the flu, her mother noticed Alicia was washing her hands multiple times a day to the point that her hands were always red and chapped. She is fretful and anxious, and has difficulty falling asleep. Last week the school called Alicia's parents to report that Alicia was refusing to use the girl's bathroom. She has been pulling her sleeves over her hands to avoid touching doorknobs and frequently wipes her desk with anti-bacterial gel. Her mother found several discarded school lunches in Alicia's room and, when confronted, Alicia acknowledged she does not eat or drink at school because she is afraid she will need to use the bathroom and it is full of germs.

Given this history, the PMHNP identifies several areas for further assessment and interprofessional collaboration. Administration of the Children's Yale-Brown Obsessive Compulsive Scale (CY-BOCS) reveals symptoms sufficient for a diagnosis of obsessive-compulsive disorder (OCD). Alicia's acute onset of symptoms after a sore throat warrants evaluation for Pediatric Acute-Onset Neuropsychiatric Syndrome/Pediatric Autoimmune Neuropsychiatric Disorder Associated With Streptococcus infection (PANS/PANDAS) (Toufexis et al., 2015). The PMHNP collaborates with Alicia's PCP, who agrees to follow up with laboratory tests (CBC, throat culture, anti-streptolysin O titer, and anti-DNase-B titer); if a strep infection is confirmed, the PCP will prescribe an antibiotic to treat the infection.

The PMHNP also notes that Alicia's weight loss and reduction of nutritional intake due to stomachaches and contamination fears increase her risk for medical destabilization (Lenton-Brym, Rodrigues, Johnson, Couturier, & Toulany, 2019). A referral is made to a pediatric eating disorder specialist for an evaluation. The eating disorder evaluation confirms a diagnosis of avoidant restrictive food intake disorder (ARFID) for Alicia and results in a recommendation for family-based eating disorder treatment for Alicia and her parents (Lock, La Via, & American Academy of Child and Adolescent Psychiatry Committee on Quality Issues, 2015).

A collaborative relationship develops between the PCP, eating disorder specialist, and the PMHNP who will follow Alicia for management of her continuing OCD symptoms. The PMHNP adapts her approach in consideration of the developmental tasks of industry versus inferiority in this school-age child (Guerra et al., 2012). The Practice Parameter for the Assessment and Treatment of Children and Adolescents with OCD (Lock et al., 2015) is a useful reference to share with Alicia's parents in discussing evidence-based treatment options. Additionally, the PMHNP cites research findings of the Pediatric OCD Treatment Study and others indicating combined cognitive behavioral therapy (CBT) and the SSRI, sertraline, are more effective than CBT or sertraline alone in treatment of childhood OCD (Grados, Torrico, Frederick, & Riley, 2016; Pediatric OCD

Treatment Study Team, 2004). Parental education also includes a discussion about managing Alicia's anxiety and avoiding proliferation of her compulsive rituals by calmly withdrawing attention and redirecting Alicia away from the performance of new compulsive routines (Storch, McGuire, & McKay, 2018). Additionally, the PMHNP offers to consult with Alicia's school to develop a school plan for responding to Alicia's needs and support her return to normal developmental functioning.

CASE EXAMPLE

Expert Nursing Approach to a Child Exhibiting Behaviors Consistent With Pediatric Bipolar Disorder

8-Year Old Thomas: A Psychiatric Mental Health Nurse Practitioner Approach to Treatment Planning, Medication Management, and Family Support
Julie A. Carbray PhD, PMHNP-BC, PMHCNS-BC, APN

Thomas is an 8-year-old cherubic, energetic, and loud Caucasian boy who presents with his parents to the outpatient clinic. His family is concerned about the level of mood dysregulation Thomas shows at home, where he is always irritable, demanding, and volatile, especially when things do not go as he desires. Thomas has an uncle with bipolar disorder and his parents note that sometimes they worry Thomas shares similar symptoms with his uncle. He does well at school, is proud of his grades, but his intense moods keep peers at a distance. Those who try to be his friend soon abandon him for less intense peers, despite his creative and witty personality. At home, his family feels they are always on eggshells, anticipating what they say or do might trigger him to explode. When he explodes, he throws shoes or toys, will hit whoever is in his way, and has run out of his home and into the street without paying attention to safety.

Although a more chronic concern, Thomas has never been a good sleeper. His parents look forward to when he is finally sleeping each night, but he seldom can sleep before 10 p.m. and awakens before the rest of the house each morning and starts his busy day while all are sleeping. Thomas shows intensity and struggled with mood regulation throughout the intake interview with themes of hopelessness, negative cognitions, and frustration fueling his angry responses to questions. Quietly, his parents shared that they have been worried that these symptoms will leave Thomas disabled as an adult, like his uncle, and they want to stop the course of these symptoms to prevent the same outcome. Developmentally, Thomas wants to show his parents that he is more independent. They have noticed he has begun to want more privacy, especially around talking about his symptoms.

Although Thomas understands what can trigger his anger, he feels frustrated with his inability to articulate what he needs when frustrated or to stop himself. After he has a rage, he is embarrassed, exhausted, and wants his family to not talk about it because he is better. However, the family does not recuperate as quickly. Thomas had been treated for ADHD previously, but his parents are concerned that his symptoms of mood dysregulation went beyond what they have read about ADHD symptoms. Given his symptoms, I gave his parents the Child Mania Rating Scale (Pavuluri et al., 2006) to further illicit any positive symptoms of mania. Thomas's parent responses to the rating scale indicated that his symptoms were likely to indicate mania, and I shared with them that their instincts were correct that his symptoms were beyond his previous ADHD diagnosis and that a pediatric bipolar disorder diagnosis seemed likely.

We discussed together the predominant challenges for Thomas, his irritability, mood dysregulation, and his struggle with self-soothing, especially when he does not get his way. I showed Thomas and his parents a picture of a brain and discussed with them how the emotional center of the brain (amygdala) seems to become so active that it shuts off the part of the brain that helps people solve problems and shift expectations (frontal cortex), allowing the emotions to take over and how medications and therapy have been designed specifically for children like Thomas to help them regulate better. I shared with Thomas and his family how chemicals in the body help the brain regulate those actions and that sometimes medications can help to better regulate the emotions so that a child can work with his or her family on better problem-solving and keeping his or her moods (both anger and hyperarousal) more manageable (Singh, Garrett, & Chang, 2015). We reviewed medications that had the most evidence for effectiveness with irritability, mania, and hyperarousal, and we discussed what benefits and potential risks were involved with these medication choices. After this review, Thomas and his family decided to start with preliminary lab work done to rule out thyroid illness, vitamin deficiencies, and lead poisoning, and get a baseline for kidney, liver, and metabolic function, and then to start risperidone, 0.25 mg in a bid to control his symptoms.

In addition, we talked about starting a family psychotherapy regimen that would help Thomas to track his moods, control his responses to a shift in his mood states or arousal, and would also help his parents to better understand techniques they could use to help Thomas when his brain circuits seemed "stuck." I told them about RAINBOW therapy, specifically designed for children with pediatric bipolar spectrum illnesses (Weinstein, West, & Pavuluri, 2013). The group also helps kids understand and regulate their moods and engage with their parents in solving problems due to their illness. As a start, Thomas and his family would begin to track his moods and together collect information about triggers for rage episodes as well as to see what helps to soothe Thomas when he begins to become angry. Most importantly I shared how research consistently demonstrates that early intervention, academic successes, a supportive family system, and treatments work and show great promise for Thomas and his family's recovery. I told the family I would be their coach along the way, and offered my confidence that together we could help Thomas gain better control over his symptoms and for their family to see hope and more peace in their everyday living—and that the disability of his uncle did not need to be in the future for Thomas.

CONCLUDING COMMENTS

Paradigms are slow to change. For 50 years the prevailing notion in child psychotherapy has led to an approach grounded in a deficit model, and often interventions based solely on the label assigned to the child. However, this traditional diagnosis-driven model has not adequately addressed the global burden of child mental health (Kazdin, 2019), particularly for vulnerable children with SEDs (Delaney, Burke, DeSocio, Greenberg, & Sharp, 2018). The need is great. Latest data inform that approximately one in every four or five U.S. children and adolescents meets criteria for a mental disorder with severe impairment across their lifetime (Merikangas et al., 2010), yet half of the 7.7 million children with a treatable mental health disorder do not receive needed treatment from a mental health professional (Whitney & Peterson, 2019). While the incidence of the most common mental health issues continues and in some cases expands, such as anxiety, depression, and externalizing disorders (ADHD and ODD), the understanding of these disorders and how their underlying constructs fit together continue to be modified by the emerging science (e.g., Hinshaw, 2018). Circumstances also change such as the increase in bullying and social media, which influence child mental health. Populations emerge. While developmental trauma has been in the literature for many years (Cook et al., 2005), the impact of ACEs on developmental processes and their link to psychopathology is increasingly clear (McLauglin et al., 2019).

As discussed here, approaches change as evidence moves into practice across new platforms. The change is a welcome one. The traditional methods of addressing child mental distress have not demonstrated appreciable growth in change curves over the last 40 years (Weisz, Kuppens, et al., 2017). It is time to reach toward a new frontier. Neuroscience might help get us there if children are approached with a family-centered framework with a view on building resources to promote resiliency. Of particular importance in the future will be the use of evidence-based approaches to promote mental health and early intervention into childhood mental distress (Baber et al., 2019). It is imperative that APPNs call upon all their relationship skills, as well as their knowledge of neuroscience and evidence-based therapies, to build a public health model of treatment that is strength based and family centered. Child mental health APPNs will be increasingly important clinicians in the mental health service delivery and it will be critical that they learn to integrate the vast amount of science that is emerging around child mental health and treatment and put that knowledge into practice.

DISCUSSION QUESTIONS

1. How might the traditional structure of mental health treatment and professional relationships block family participation in treatment decisions?
2. Discuss your experiences with accessing and using evidence-based therapies in child/adolescent treatment.
3. Name the quality and characteristics you would include when listing a child's strengths.
4. Discuss how you might build an environment around a child that would support competency and augment vulnerabilities.
5. What developmental issues of adolescence might pose difficulties in relationship building during psychotherapy?
6. How might you use the neurobiology material in this chapter in your approach to children/adolescents with serious emotional illness?
7. This chapter contained a case example of how to intervene using a common factors method. How does this differ from your notion of the process of child psychotherapy?

REFERENCES

Abbass, A. A., Rabung, S., Leichsenring, F., Refseth, J. S., & Midgley, N. (2013). Psychodynamic psychotherapy for children and adolescents: A meta-analysis of short-term psychodynamic models. *Journal of the American Academy of Child & Adolescent Psychiatry, 52*, 863–875. doi:10.1016/j.jaac.2013.05.014

Aldao, A., Gee, D. G., De Los Reyes, A., & Seager, I. (2016). Emotion regulation as a transdiagnostic factor in the development of internalizing and externalizing psychopathology: Current and future directions. *Development and Psychopathology, 28*, 927–946. doi:10.1017/S0954579416000638

Alegría, M., Green, J. G., McLaughlin, K. A., & Loder, S. (2015). *Disparities in child and adolescent mental health and mental health services in the US*. New York, NY: William T. Grant Foundation. Retrieved from http://wtgrantfoundation.org/library/uploads/2015/09/Disparities -in-Child-and-Adolescent-Mental-Health.pdf

American Academy of Child and Adolescent Psychiatry. (2014). *Psychotherapy as a core competency of child and adolescent psychiatrist*. Retrieved from https://www.aacap.org/ AACAP/Policy_Statements/2014/Psychotherapy_as_a_Core_Competence_of_Child_and_ Adolescent_Psychiatrist.aspx

American Nurses Association Council on Psychiatric and Mental Health Nursing. (1985). *Standards of child and adolescent psychiatric and mental health nursing practice* [Unpublished document]. Silver Spring, MD: Author.

American Psychiatric Nurses Association. (n.d.). *Consensus model for APRN regulation.* Retrieved from http://www.apna.org/i4a/pages/index.cfm?pageid=3745#sthash.O3dG0kLH.dpbs

American Psychological Association, Division 12. (1993). *Task force on promotion and dissemination of psychological procedures. A report adopted by the division 12 board.* Retrieved from http://www.div12.org/sites/default/files/InitialReportOfTheChamblessTaskForce.pdf

Anastopoulos, A. D., Smith, T. F., Garrett, M. E., Morrissey-Kane, E., Schatz, N. K., Sommer, J. L., . . . & Ashley-Koch, A. (2011). Self-regulation of emotion, functional impairment, and comorbidity among children with ADHD. *Journal of Attention Disorders, 15,* 583–592. doi:10.1177/1087054710370567

Anthony, E. J. (1987). Risk, vulnerability, and resilience: An overview. In E. J. Anthony & B. J. Cohler (Eds.), *The invulnerable child* (pp. 3–48). New York, NY: Guilford Press.

Axelson, D. (2019). *Pediatric bipolar disorder: Overview of choosing treatment.* In D. Brent (Ed.), *UpToDate.* Retrieved from https://www.uptodate.com/contents/pediatric-bipolar-disorder-overview-of-choosing-treatment

Baber, M., Gough, A., Jamieson, J., Milne, R., Pham, H., Walters, E., . . . & Ji, E. (2019). Reducing the risk of mental ill health: The importance of the early years of life. *Perspectives in Public Health, 139*(3), 126–127. doi:10.1177/1757913919839003

Barrnett, R. J., Docherty, J. P., & Frommelt, G. M. (1991). A review of child psychotherapy research since 1963. *Journal of the American Academy of Child & Adolescent Psychiatry, 30*(1), 1–14. doi:10.1097/00004583-199101000-00001

Barth, R. P., Lee, B. R., Lindsey, M. A., Collins, K. S., Strieder, F., & Sparks, J. A. (2012). Evidence-based practice at a crossroads: The timely emergence of common elements and common factors. *Research on Social Work Practice, 22,* 108–119. doi:10.1177/1049731511408440

Becker, K. D., Boustani, M., Gellatly, R., & Chorpita, B. F. (2018). Forty years of engagement research in children's mental health services: Multidimensional measurement and practice elements. *Journal of Clinical Child & Adolescent Psychology, 47*(1), 1–23. doi:10.1080/15374416.2017.1326121

Beesdo, K., Knappe, S., & Pine, D. S. (2009). Anxiety and anxiety disorders in children and adolescents: Developmental issues and implications for *DSM-V. Psychiatric Clinics, 32,* 483–524. doi:10.1016/j.psc.2009.06.002

Begeer, S., Bernstein, D. M., Aßfalg, A., Azdad, H., Glasbergen, T., Wierda, M., & Koot, H. M. (2016). Equal egocentric bias in school-aged children with and without autism spectrum disorders. *Journal of Experimental Child Psychology, 144,* 15–26. doi:10.1016/j.jecp.2015.10.018

Bell, M. A., & Calkins, S. D. (2012). Attentional control and emotion regulation in early development. In M. I. Posner (Ed.), *Cognitive neuroscience of attention* (2nd ed., pp. 322–330). New York, NY: Guilford Press.

Boxmeyer, C. L., Lochman, J. E., Kassing, F., Mitchell, Q. P., & Romero, D. (2018). Cognitive therapies: Anger management. In M. M. Martel (Ed.), *Developmental pathways to disruptive, impulse-control and conduct disorders* (pp. 239–262). New York, NY: Elsevier. doi:10.1016/B978-0-12-811323-3.00010-9

Boyd, R. C., Butler, L., & Benton, T. D. (2018). Understanding adolescents' experiences with depression and behavioral health treatment. *Journal of Behavioral Health Services & Research, 45,* 105–111. doi:10.1007/s11414-017-9558-7

Brotman, M. A., Kircanski, K., & Leibenluft, E. (2017). Irritability in children and adolescents. *Annual Review of Clinical Psychology, 13,* 317–341. doi:10.1146/annurev-clinpsy-032816-044941

Brown, N. M., Brown, S. N., Briggs, R. D., Germán, M., Belamarich, P. F., & Oyeku, S. O. (2017). Associations between adverse childhood experiences and ADHD diagnosis and severity. *Academic Pediatrics, 17*(4), 349–355. doi:10.1016/j.acap.2016.08.013

Burns, B. J. (2003). Children and evidence-based practice. *Psychiatric Clinics of North America, 26*(4), 955–970. doi:10.1016/S0193-953X(03)00071-6

Cepeda, C. (2010). *Clinical manual for the psychiatric interview of children and adolescents.* Arlington, VA: American Psychiatric Publishing.

Chethik, M. (2000). *Techniques of child therapy: Psychodynamic strategies* (2nd ed.). New York, NY: Guilford Press.

Cheung, A. H., Zuckerbrot, R. A., Jensen, P. S., Laraque, D., Stein, R. E., & GLAD-PC STEERING GROUP. (2018). Guidelines for adolescent depression in primary care (GLAD-PC): Part II. Treatment and ongoing management. *Pediatrics, 141,* e20174082. doi:10.1542/peds.2017-4082

Chorpita, B. F., & Daleiden, E. L. (2009). Mapping evidence-based treatments for children and adolescents: Application of the distillation and matching model to 615 treatments from 322 randomized trials. *Journal of Consulting and Clinical Psychology, 77*, 566–579. doi:10.1037/a0014565

Chorpita, B. F., Daleiden, E. L., Ebesutani, C., Young, J., Becker, K. D., Nakamura, B. J., . . . Starace, N. (2011). Evidence-based treatments for children and adolescents: An updated review of indicators of efficacy and effectiveness. *Clinical Psychology: Science and Practice, 18*, 154–172. doi:10.1111/j.1468-2850.2011.01247.x

Chorpita, B. F., Daleiden, E. L., Park, A. L., Ward, A. M., Levy, M. C., Cromley, T., . . . Krull, J. L. (2017). Child STEPs in California: A cluster randomized effectiveness trial comparing modular treatment with community implemented treatment for youth with anxiety, depression, conduct problems, or traumatic stress. *Journal of Consulting and Clinical Psychology, 85*, 13–25. doi:10.1037/ccp0000133

Chu, B. C., Chen, J., Mele, C., Temkin, A., & Xue, J. (2017). Transdiagnostic approaches to emotion regulation: Basic mechanisms and treatment research. In C. A. Essau, S. LeBlanc, & T. H. Ollendick (Eds.), *Emotion regulation and psychopathology in children and adolescents* (pp. 419–451). New York, NY: Oxford University Press.

Clark, J. (2016). *My child and me: A qualitative exploration of the experiences of parents who have had a child or children receive psychological therapy* (Doctoral dissertation). City, University of London, London, UK. Retrieved from https://openaccess.city.ac.uk/id/eprint/17026

Coburn, P. I., Bernstein, D. M., & Begeer, S. (2015). A new paper and pencil task reveals adult false belief reasoning bias. *Psychological Research, 79*, 739–749. doi:10.1007/s00426-014-0606-0

Cohen, J. A., Deblinger, E., & Mannarino, A. P. (2018). Trauma-focused cognitive behavioral therapy for children and families. *Psychotherapy Research, 28*, 47–57. doi:10.1080/10503307.2016.1208375

Cohen, J. A., Mannarino, A. P., Kliethermes, M., & Murray, L. A. (2012). Trauma-focused CBT for youth with complex trauma. *Child Abuse & Neglect, 36*, 528–541. doi:10.1016/j.chiabu.2012.03.007

Conway, J., Johnson, B., Edgman-Levitan, S., Schlucter, J., Ford, D., Sodomka, P., & Simmons, L. (2006). *Partnering with patients and families to design a patient- and family-centered health care system: A roadmap for the future. A work in progress* [Unpublished manuscript]. Boston, MA: Institute for Family-Centered Care and Institute for Healthcare Improvement. Retrieved from http://www.ihi.org/knowledge/Pages/Publications/PartneringwithPatientsandFamilies.aspx

Cook, A., Spinazzola, J., Ford, J., Lanktree, C., Blaustein, M., Cloitre, M., . . . van der Kolk, B. (2005). Complex trauma in children and adolescents. *Psychiatric Annals, 35*, 390–398. doi:10.3928/00485713-20050501-05

Cortese, S., Adamo, N., Del Giovane, C., Mohr-Jensen, C., Hayes, A. J., Carucci, S., . . . Hollis, C. (2018). Comparative efficacy and tolerability of medications for attention-deficit hyperactivity disorder in children, adolescents, and adults: A systematic review and network meta-analysis. *The Lancet Psychiatry, 5*(9), 727–738. doi:10.1016/S2215-0366(18)30269-4

Craig, S. L., & Austin, A. (2016). The AFFIRM open pilot feasibility study: A brief affirmative cognitive behavioral coping skills group intervention for sexual and gender minority youth. *Children and Youth Services Review, 64*, 136–144. doi:10.1016/j.childyouth.2016.02.022

Crush, E., Arseneault, L., Jaffee, S. R., Danese, A., & Fisher, H. L. (2017). Protective factors for psychotic symptoms among poly-victimized children. *Schizophrenia Bulletin, 44*(3), 691–700. doi:10.1093/schbul/sbx111

Curry, J. F., & Meyer, A. E. (2018). Treatment of depression. In P. Kendall (Ed.), *Cognitive therapy with children and adolescents: A casebook for clinical practice* (3rd ed., pp. 94–122). New York, NY: Guilford Press.

D'antonio, P., Beeber, L., Sills, G., & Naegle, M. (2014). The future in the past: Hildegard Peplau and interpersonal relations in nursing. *Nursing Inquiry, 21*, 311–317. doi:10.1111/nin.12056

Dahlitz, M. (2015). Neuropsychotherapy: Defining the emerging paradigm of neurobiologically informed psychotherapy. *International Journal of Neuropsychotherapy, 3*(1), 47–69. doi:10.12744/ijnpt.2015.0047-0069

Daley, D., Van Der Oord, S., Ferrin, M., Cortese, S., Danckaerts, M., Doepfner, M., . . . Banaschewski, T. (2018). Practitioner review: Current best practice in the use of parent training and other behavioural interventions in the treatment of children and adolescents with attention deficit hyperactivity disorder. *Journal of Child Psychology and Psychiatry, 59,* 932–947. doi:10.1111/jcpp.12825

Day, C., & Roberts, M. C. (1991). Activities of the child and adolescent service system. Program for improving mental health services for children and families. *Journal of Clinical Child Psychology, 20,* 340–350. doi:10.1207/s15374424jccp2004_2

DeFrino, D. T., Marko-Holguin, M., Cordel, S., Anker, L., Bansa, M., & Van Voorhees, B. (2016). "Why should I tell my business?": An emerging theory of coping and disclosure in teens. *Research and Theory for Nursing Practice, 30,* 124–142. doi:10.1891/1541-6577.30.2.124

Delaney, K. R. (2017). Psychiatric mental health advanced practice nursing workforce: Capacity to address mental health professional workforce shortages. *Psychiatric Services, 68,* 952–954. doi:10.1176/appi.ps.201600405

Delaney, K. R., Burke, P., DeSocio, J., Greenberg, C., & Sharp, D. (2018). Building mental health and caring for vulnerable children: Increasing prevention, access, and equity. *Nursing Outlook, 66,* 590–593. doi:10.1016/j.outlook.2018.10.004

Delaney, K. R., Drew, B. L., & Rushton, A. (2018). Report on the APNA national psychiatric mental health advanced practice registered nurse survey. *Journal of the American Psychiatric Nurses Association, 25,* 146–155. doi:10.1177/1078390318777873

Delaney, K. R., & Hawkins-Walsh, E. (2012). Cognitive and behavioral treatment with children. In E. Yearwood, G. Pearson, & J. Newland (Eds.), *Child & adolescent behavioral health: A source for advanced practice psychiatric and primary care practitioners in nursing* (pp. 313–331). Hoboken, NJ: Wiley-Blackwell. doi:10.1002/9781118704660.ch17

Delaney, K. R., & Karnik, N. S. (2019). Building a child mental health workforce for the 21st century: Closing the training gap. *Journal of Professional Nursing, 35*(2), 133–137. doi:10.1016/j.profnurs.2018.07.002

Delaney, K. R., & McIntosh, D. (in press). Exploring the thinking, reasoning and clinical approach of Expert Child Psychiatric Nurses. *Journal of Child and Adolescent Psychiatric Nursing.*

Delaney, K. R., Shattell, M., & Johnson, M. E. (2017). Capturing the interpersonal process of psychiatric nurses: A model for engagement. *Archives of Psychiatric Nursing, 31,* 634–640. doi:10.1016/j.apnu.2017.08.003

Delaney, K. R., & Vanderhoef, D. M. (2019). Psychiatric mental health advanced practice registered nurse workforce: Charting the future. *Journal of the American Psychiatric Nurses Association, 25,* 11–18. doi:10.1177/1078390318806571

De Nadai, A. S., Karver, M. S., Murphy, T. K., Cavitt, M. A., Alvaro, J. L., Bengtson, M., . . . Storch, E. A. (2017). Common factors in pediatric psychiatry: A review of essential and adjunctive mechanisms of treatment outcome. *Journal of Child and Adolescent Psychopharmacology, 27,* 10–18. doi:10.1089/cap.2015.0263

DeSocio, J. (2013). The neurobiology of risk and pre-emptive interventions for anorexia nervosa. *Journal of Child and Adolescent Psychiatric Nursing, 26,* 16–22. doi:10.1111/jcap.12018

Diler, R. S. (2018). Pediatric bipolar disorders and ADHD. In W. B. Daviss (Ed.), *Moodiness in ADHD* (pp. 111–127). New York, NY: Springer.

Dobson, E. T., Bloch, M. H., & Strawn, J. R. (2019). Efficacy and tolerability of pharmacotherapy for pediatric anxiety disorders: A network meta-analysis. *Journal of Clinical Psychiatry, 80*(1), 17r12064. doi:10.4088/JCP.17r12064

Dorsey, S., Berliner, L., Lyon, A. R., Pullmann, M. D., & Murray, L. K. (2016). A statewide common elements initiative for children's mental health. *Journal of Behavioral Health Services & Research, 43*(2), 246–261. doi:10.1007/s11414-014-9430-y

Dorsey, S., McLaughlin, K. A., Kerns, S. E., Harrison, J. P., Lambert, H. K., Briggs, E. C., . . . Amaya-Jackson, L. (2017). Evidence base update for psychosocial treatments for children and adolescents exposed to traumatic events. *Journal of Clinical Child & Adolescent Psychology, 46,* 303–330. doi:10.1080/15374416.2016.1220309

Eisenberg, N., & Spinrad, T. L. (2004). Emotion-related regulation: Sharpening the definition. *Child Development, 75,* 334–339. doi:10.1111/j.1467-8624.2004.00674.x

Emde, R. N. (1990). Mobilizing fundamental modes of development: Empathic availability and therapeutic action. *Journal of the American Psychoanalytical Association, 38,* 881–913. doi:10.1177/000306519003800402

Fabiano, G. A., Schatz, N. K., Aloe, A. M., Chacko, A., & Chronis-Tuscano, A. (2015). A systematic review of meta-analyses of psychosocial treatment for attention-deficit/hyperactivity disorder. *Clinical Child and Family Psychology Review, 18,* 77–97. doi:10.1007/s10567-015-0178-6

Findling, R. L., & Chang, K. D. (2018). Improving the diagnosis and treatment of pediatric bipolar disorder. *Journal of Clinical Psychiatry, 79*(2), 1–4. doi:10.4088/JCP.su17023ah3c

Flynn, L. M. (2005). Family perspectives on evidence-based practice. *Child and Adolescent Psychiatric Clinics, 14*(2), 217–224.

Frick, P. J., Barry, C. T., & Kamphaus, R. W. (2010). *Clinical assessment of child and adolescent personality and behavior.* New York, NY: Springer Science + Business Media.

Friedberg, R., & McClure, J. (2015). *Clinical practice of cognitive therapy with children and adolescents: The nuts and bolts* (2nd ed.). New York, NY: Guilford Press.

Gálvez-Lara, M., Corpas, J., Moreno, E., Venceslá, J. F., Sánchez-Raya, A., & Moriana, J. A. (2018). Psychological treatments for mental disorders in children and adolescents: A review of the evidence of leading international organizations. *Clinical Child and Family Psychology Review, 21,* 366–387. doi:10.1007/s10567-018-0257-6

Gattis, M. N. (2014). Are family communication and school belonging protective factors against depressive symptoms in homeless youth in Toronto? *Canadian Journal of Community Mental Health, 32,* 75–83. doi:10.7870/cjcmh-2013-034

Goldstein, S., & Brooks, R. B. (2013). Why study resilience. In S. Goldstein & R. B. Brooks (Eds.), *Handbook of resilience in children* (pp. 3–14). New York, NY: Springer.

Grados, M. A., Torrico, H., Frederick, J., & Riley, T. (2016). Pediatric obsessive-compulsive disorder: A psychopharmacology update. *Child & Adolescent Psychopharmacology News, 21*(1), 1–5, 8. doi:10.1521/capn.2016.21.1.1

Greenspan, S. I., & Thorndike Greenspan, N. (2003). *The clinical interview of the child* (3rd ed.). Arlington, VA: American Psychiatric Publishing.

Guerra, N. G., Williamson, A. A., & Lucas-Molina, B. (2012). Normal development: Infancy, childhood and adolescence. In J. M. Rey (Ed.), *IACAPAP e-textbook of child and adolescent mental health* (pp. 1–39). Geneva, Switzerland: International Association for Child and Adolescent Psychiatry and Allied Professions.

Haine-Schlagel, R., & Walsh, N. E. (2015). A review of parent participation engagement in child and family mental health treatment. *Clinical Child and Family Psychology Review, 18,* 133–150. doi:10.1007/s10567-015-0182-x

Henderson, S. W., & Martin, A. (2014). Case formulation and integration of information in child and adolescent mental health. In J. M. Rey (Ed.), *IACAPAP e-textbook of child and adolescent mental health* (pp. 1–20). Geneva, Switzerland: International Association for Child and Adolescent Psychiatry and Allied Professions.

Henggeler, S. W. (2012). Multisystemic therapy: Clinical foundations and research outcomes. *Psychosocial Interventions, 21,* 181–193. doi:10.5093/in2012a12

Hibbs, E. D. (2001). Evaluating empirically based psychotherapy research for children and adolescents. *European Child and Adolescent Psychiatry, 10,* 3–11. doi:10.1007/s007870170002

Hibbs, E. D., & Jensen, P. S. (Eds.). (1996). *Psychosocial treatments for child and adolescent disorders. Empirically based strategies for clinical practice.* Washington, DC: American Psychological Association. doi:10.1037/10196-000

Higa-McMillan, C. K., Francis, S. E., Rith-Najarian, L., & Chorpita, B. F. (2016). Evidence base update: 50 years of research on treatment for child and adolescent anxiety. *Journal of Clinical Child & Adolescent Psychology, 45,* 91–113. doi:10.1080/15374416.2015.1046177

Hinshaw, S. P. (2018). Attention deficit hyperactivity disorder (ADHD): Controversy, developmental mechanisms, and multiple levels of analysis. *Annual Review of Clinical Psychology, 14*(1), 291–316. doi:10.1146/annurev-clinpsy-050817-084917

Horwitz, S. M., Demeter, C., Hayden, M., Storfer-Isser, A., Frazier, T. W., Fristad, M. A., . . . & Findling, R. L. (2012). Parents' perceptions of benefit of children's mental health treatment and continued use of services. *Psychiatric Services, 63,* 793–801. doi:10.1176/appi.ps.201100460a

Huang, C. Y., & Zane, N. (2016). Cultural influences in mental health treatment. *Current Opinion in Psychology, 8,* 131–136. doi:10.1016/j.copsyc.2015.10.009

Jimenez, M. E., Wade Jr, R., Schwartz-Soicher, O., Lin, Y., & Reichman, N. E. (2017). Adverse childhood experiences and ADHD diagnosis at age 9 years in a national urban sample. *Academic Pediatrics, 17,* 356–361. doi:10.1016/j.acap.2016.12.009

Johnson, B. S., & Newland, J. A. (2012). Integration of physical and psychiatric assessment. In E. L. Yearwood, G. S Pearson, & J. A. Newland (Eds.), *Child and adolescent behavioral health. A resource for psychiatric and primary care practitioners in nursing* (pp. 57–88). Ames, Iowa: Wiley-Blackwell. doi:10.1002/9781118704660.ch4

Karver, M. S., De Nadai, A. S., Monahan, M., & Shirk, S. R. (2019). Alliance in child and adolescent psychotherapy. In J. C Norcross & M. J. Lambert (Eds.), *Psychotherapy relationships that work* (3rd ed., pp. 79–116). New York, NY: Oxford University Press.

Kaushik, A., Kostaki, E., & Kyriakopoulos, M. (2016). The stigma of mental illness in children and adolescents: A systematic review. *Psychiatry Research, 243,* 469–494. doi:10.1016/j .psychres.2016.04.042

Kazdin, A. E. (2019). Annual research review: Expanding mental health services through novel models of intervention delivery. *Journal of Child Psychology and Psychiatry, 60,* 455–472. doi:10.1111/jcpp.12937

Kelly, M., & Coughlan, B. (2018). A theory of youth mental health recovery from a parental perspective. *Child and Adolescent Mental Health, 24,* 161–169. doi:10.1111/ camh.12300

Kendall, P. C. (2016). *Child and adolescent therapy* (4th ed.). New York, NY: Guilford Press.

Kendall, P. C. (Ed.). (2017). *Cognitive therapy with children and adolescents: A casebook for clinical practice.* New York, NY: Guilford Press.

Kernberg, P., Ritvo, R., Keable, H., & American Academy of Child and Adolescent Psychiatry Committee on Quality Issues. (2012). Practice parameter for psychodynamic psychotherapy with children. *Journal of the American Academy of Child & Adolescent Psychiatry, 51,* 541–557. doi:10.1016/j.jaac.2012.02.015

King, R. A. (1997). Practice parameters for the psychiatric assessment of child and adolescents. *Journal of the American Academy of Child and Adolescent Psychiatry, 36*(10 Suppl.), 4S–20S. doi:10.1097/00004583-199710001-00002

Kitts, R. L., Isberg, R. S., Lee, P. C., Sharma, N., Goldman, V., & Hunt, J. (2019). Child psychotherapy training in the United States: A national survey of child and adolescent psychiatry fellowship program directors. *Academic Psychiatry, 43,* 23–27. doi:10.1007/ s40596-018-0998-z

Klein, B., Damiani-Taraba, G., Koster, A., Campbell, J., & Scholz, C. (2015). Diagnosing attention-deficit hyperactivity disorder (ADHD) in children involved with child protection services: Are current diagnostic guidelines acceptable for vulnerable populations? *Child: Care, Health and Development, 41*(2), 178–185. doi:10.1111/cch.12168

Lawrence, H. R., Nangle, D. W., Schwartz-Mette, R. A., & Erdley, C. A. (2017). Medication for child and adolescent depression: Questions, answers, clarifications, and caveats. *Practice Innovations, 2*(1), 39–53. doi:10.1037/pri0000042

Lee, P. H. (2012). The use of rating scales in diagnostic assessment of children. *The Carlat Child Psychiatry Report, 3*(3), 1–37. Retrieved from https://www.thecarlatreport.com/ the-carlat-child-psychiatry-report/use-rating-scales-diagnostic-assessment-children

Lempp, T. J., de Lange, D., Radeloff, D. M., & Bachmann, C. (2012). The clinical examination of children, adolescents and their families. In J. M. Rey (Ed.), *IACAPAP e-textbook of child and adolescent mental health* (pp. 1–25). Geneva, Switzerland: International Association for Child and Adolescent Psychiatry and Allied Professions.

Lenton-Brym, T., Rodrigues, A., Johnson, N., Couturier, J., & Toulany, A. (2019). A scoping review of the role of primary care providers and primary care-based interventions in the treatment of pediatric eating disorders. *Eating Disorders, 27,* 1–20. doi:10.1080/10640266.2018.1560853

Leonidaki, V., Lemma, A., & Hobbis, I. (2018). The active ingredients of dynamic interpersonal therapy (DIT): An exploration of clients' experiences. *Psychoanalytic Psychotherapy, 32*(2), 140–156. doi:10.1080/02668734.2017.1418761

Lewallen, T. C., Hunt, H., Potts-Datema, W., Zaza, S., & Giles, W. (2015). The whole school, whole community, whole child model: A new approach for improving educational attainment and healthy development for students. *Journal of School Health, 85*(11), 729–739. doi:10.1111/josh.12310

Lindsey, M. A., Brandt, N. E., Becker, K. D., Lee, B. R., Barth, R. P., Daleiden, E. L., & Chorpita, B. F. (2014). Identifying the common elements of treatment engagement interventions in children's mental health services. *Clinical Child and Family Psychology Review, 17*(3), 283–298. doi:10.1007/s10567-013-0163-x

Lock, J., La Via, M. C., & American Academy of Child and Adolescent Psychiatry Committee on Quality Issues. (2015). Practice parameter for the assessment and treatment of children and adolescents with eating disorders. *Journal of the American Academy of Child & Adolescent Psychiatry, 54*(5), 412–425. doi:10.1016/j.jaac.2015.01.018

Lu, W., & Xiao, Y. (2019). Adverse childhood experiences and adolescent mental disorders: Protective mechanisms of family functioning, social capital, and civic engagement. *Health Behavior Research, 2*(1), 3. doi:10.4148/2572-1836.1035

Marchette, L. K., & Weisz, J. R. (2017). Practitioner review: Empirical evolution of youth psychotherapy toward transdiagnostic approaches. *Journal of Child Psychology and Psychiatry, 58*(9), 970–984. doi:10.1111/jcpp.12747

Markowitz, J. C., & Weissman, M. M. (2012). Interpersonal psychotherapy: Past, present and future. *Clinical Psychology & Psychotherapy, 19*(2), 99–105. doi:10.1002/cpp.1774

Mash, E. J., & Barkley, R. A. (2010). *Assessment of childhood disorders* (4th ed.). New York, NY: Guilford Press.

Masten, A., & Barnes, A. (2018). Resilience in children: Developmental perspectives. *Children, 5*(7), 98. doi:10.3390/children5070098

McLaughlin, K. A., DeCross, S. N., Jovanovic, T., & Tottenham, N. (2019). Mechanisms linking childhood adversity with psychopathology: Learning as an intervention target. *Behaviour Research and Therapy, 118*, 101–109. doi: 10.1016/j.brat.2019.04.008

McLaughlin, K. A., Green, J. G., Gruber, M. J., Sampson, N. A., Zaslavsky, A. M., & Kessler, R. C. (2012). Childhood adversities and first onset of psychiatric disorders in a national sample of U.S. adolescents. *Archives of General Psychiatry, 69*(11), 1151–1160. doi:10.1001/archgenpsychiatry.2011.2277

McLaughlin, K. A., & Lambert, H. K. (2017). Child trauma exposure and psychopathology: Mechanisms of risk and resilience. *Current Opinion in Psychology, 14*, 29–34. doi:10.1016/j.copsyc.2016.10.004

McLeod, B. D., Sutherland, K. S., Martinez, R. G., Conroy, M. A., Snyder, P. A., & Southam-Gerow, M. A. (2017). Identifying common practice elements to improve social, emotional, and behavioral outcomes of young children in early childhood classrooms. *Prevention Science, 18*(2), 204–213. doi:10.1007/s11121-016-0703-y

Meichenbaum, D. (2017). Bolstering resilience. In D. Meichenbaum (Ed.), *The evolution of cognitive behavior therapy: A personal and professional journey* (pp. 172–117). New York, NY: Routledge.

Mendenhall, A. N., & Mount, K. (2011). Parents of children with mental illness: Exploring the caregiver experience and caregiver focused interventions. *Families in Society: The Journal of Contemporary Social Services, 92*, 183–190. doi:10.1606/1044-3894.4097

Merikangas, K. R., He, M. J. P., Burstein, M., Swanson, M. S. A., Avenevoli, S., Cui, M. L., . . . Swendsen, J. (2010). Lifetime prevalence of mental disorders in U.S. adolescents: Results from the National Comorbidity Study-Adolescent supplement (NCS-A). *Journal of the American Academy of Child and Adolescent Psychiatry, 49*, 980–989. doi:10.1016/j.jaac.2010.05.017

Midgley, N., O'Keeffe, S., French, L., & Kennedy, E. (2017). Psychodynamic psychotherapy for children and adolescents: An updated narrative review of the evidence base. *Journal of Child Psychotherapy, 43*(3), 307–329. doi:10.1080/0075417X.2017.1323945

Muller, R. T., Vascotto, N. A., Konanur, S., & Rosenkranz, S. (2013). Emotion regulation and psychopathology in a sample of maltreated children. *Journal of Child & Adolescent Trauma, 6*(1), 25–40. doi:10.1080/19361521.2013.737441

Myklebust, K. K., & Bjørkly, S. (2019). Development and reliability testing of the scale for the evaluation of staff-patient interactions in progress notes (SESPI): An assessment instrument of mental health nursing documentation. *Nursing Open, 6*(3), 790–798. doi:10.1002/nop2.254

Nezu, A. M., Nezu, C. M., & Hays, A. M. (2019). Emotion-centered problem-solving therapy. In K. S. Dobson & D. J. A. Dozois (Eds.), *Handbook of cognitive-behavioral therapies* (4th ed., pp. 171–180). New York, NY: Guilford Press.

Nigg, J. T. (2017). Annual research review: On the relations among self-regulation, self-control, executive functioning, effortful control, cognitive control, impulsivity, risk-taking, and inhibition for developmental psychopathology. *Journal of Child Psychology and Psychiatry, 58*(4), 361–383. doi:10.1111/jcpp.12675

Pavuluri, M. N., Henry, D. B., Devineni, B., Carbray, J. A., & Birmaher, B. (2006). Child Mania Rating Scale: Development, reliability, and validity. *Journal of the American Academy of Child & Adolescent Psychiatry, 45*(5), 550–560. doi:10.1097/01.chi.0000205700.40700.50

Pediatric OCD Treatment Study Team. (2004). Cognitive-behavior therapy, sertraline, and their combination for children and adolescents with obsessive-compulsive disorder. *Journal of the American Medical Association, 292*, 1969–1976. doi:10.1001/jama.292.16.1969

Perraud, S., Delaney, K. R., Carlson-Sabelli, L., Johnson, M. E., Shephard, R., & Paun, O. (2006). Advanced practice psychiatric mental health nursing, finding our core: The therapeutic relationship in the 21st century. *Perspectives in Psychiatric Care, 42*, 215–226. doi:10.1111/j.1744-6163.2006.00097.x

Remschmidt, H., & Quashner, K. (2001). Psychodynamic therapy. In H. Remschmidt (Ed.), *Psychotherapy with children and adolescents* (pp. 81–97). Cambridge, UK: Cambridge University Press.

Ritvo, R. (2006). Is there research to support psychodynamic psychotherapy, Part I. AACAP News, July/August, 200–201. Retrieved from https://www.yumpu.com/en/document/read/48086872/is-there-research-to-support-psychodynamic-psychotherapy

Ritvo, R., Al-mateen, C., Asherman, L., Beardslee, W., Hartman, L., & Lewis, O., . . . Szigethy, E. (1999). Report of the Psychotherapy Task Force of the American Academy of Child and Adolescent Psychiatry. *Journal of Psychotherapy Practice and Research, 8*, 93–102. Retrieved from https://www.ncbi.nlm.nih.gov/pmc/articles/PMC3330534

Robinson, L. R., Holbrook, J. R., Bitsko, R. H., Hartwig, S. A., Kaminski, J. W., Ghandour, R. M., . . . Boyle, C. A. (2017). Differences in health care, family, and community factors associated with mental, behavioral, and developmental disorders among children aged 2–8 years in rural and urban areas—United States, 2011–2012. *MMWR Surveillance Summaries, 66*(8), 1. doi:10.15585/mmwr.ss6608a1

Rosen, P. J., Leaberry, K. D., Slaughter, K., Fogleman, N. D., Walerius, D. M., Loren, R. E., & Epstein, J. N. (2019). Managing frustration for children (MFC) group intervention for ADHD: An open trial of a novel group intervention for deficient emotion regulation. *Cognitive and Behavioral Practice, 26*(3), 522–534. doi:10.1016/j.cbpra.2018.04.002

Roth, A., & Fonagy, P. (1996). *What works for whom? A critical review of psychotherapy research.* New York, NY: Guilford Press.

Rothenberg, W. A., Weinstein, A., Dandes, E. A., & Jent, J. F. (2019). Improving child emotion regulation: Effects of parent–child interaction-therapy and emotion socialization strategies. *Journal of Child and Family Studies, 28*(3), 720–731. doi:10.1007/s10826-018-1302-2

Saxe, G. N., Ellis, B. H., Fogler, J., & Navalta, C. P. (2012). Innovations in practice: Preliminary evidence for effective family engagement in treatment for child traumatic stress–trauma systems therapy approach to preventing dropout. *Child and Adolescent Mental Health, 17*, 58–61. doi:10.1111/j.1475-3588.2011.00626.x

Sayal, K., Prasad, V., Daley, D., Ford, T., & Coghill, D. (2018). ADHD in children and young people: Prevalence, care pathways, and service provision. *The Lancet Psychiatry, 5*(2), 175–186. doi:10.1016/S2215-0366(17)30167-0

Schaefer, C. E. (Ed.). (2003). *Foundations of play therapy.* Hoboken, NJ: Wiley.

Sharer, K. (2012). Individual and family therapies. In E. Yearwood, G. Pearson, & J. Newland (Eds.), *Child & adolescent behavioral health: A source for advanced practice psychiatric and primary care practitioners in nursing* (pp. 291–312). Hoboken, NJ: Wiley-Blackwell.

Siegel, D. J. (1999). *The developing mind: How relationships and the brain interact to shape who we are.* New York, NY: Guilford Press.

Singh, M. K., Garrett, A. S., & Chang, K. D. (2015). Using neuroimaging to evaluate and guide pharmacological and psychotherapeutic treatments for mood disorders in children. *CNS Spectrums, 20*(4), 359–368. doi:10.1017/S1092852914000819

Sloan, E., Hall, K., Moulding, R., Bryce, S., Mildred, H., & Staiger, P. K. (2017). Emotion regulation as a transdiagnostic treatment construct across anxiety, depression, substance, eating and borderline personality disorders: A systematic review. *Clinical Psychology Review, 57*, 141–163. doi:10.1016/j.cpr.2017.09.002

Southam-Gerow, M. A. (2013). *Emotion regulation in children and adolescents: A practitioner's guide.* New York, NY: Guilford Press.

Spirito, A., Esposito-Smythers, C., Wolff, J., & Uhl, K. (2011). Cognitive-behavioral therapy for adolescent depression and suicidality. *Child and Adolescent Psychiatric Clinics of North America, 20*(2), 191–204. doi:10.1016/j.chc.2011.01.012

Stoner, A. M., Leon, S. C., & Fuller, A. K. (2015). Predictors of reduction in symptoms of depression for children and adolescents in foster care. *Journal of Child and Family Studies, 24*(3), 784–797. doi:10.1007/s10826-013-9889-9

Storch, E. A., McGuire, J. F., & McKay, D. (Eds.). (2018). *The clinician's guide to cognitive-bheavioral therapy for childhood obsessive-compulsive disorder.* San Diego, CA: Academic Press. Retrieved from https://www.sciencedirect.com/book/9780128114278/the-clinicians-guide-to-cognitive-behavioral-therapy-for-childhood-obsessive-compulsive-disorder

Stroul, B. A., & Friedman, R. M. (1996). *A system of care for children and adolescents with severe emotional disturbances* (Revised Ed.). Washington, DC: National Technical Assistance Center for Child Mental Health, Georgetown University Child Development Center.

Stroul, B., Goldman, S., Pires, S., & Manteuffel, B. (2012). *Expanding systems of care: Improving the lives of children, youth and families.* Washington, DC: Georgetown University Center for Child and Human Development, National Technical Assistance Center for Children's Mental Health.

Szymanski, K., Sapanski, L., & Conway, F. (2011). Trauma and ADHD–association or diagnostic confusion? A clinical perspective. *Journal of Infant, Child, and Adolescent Psychotherapy, 10*(1), 51–59. doi:10.1080/15289168.2011.575704

Tan, P. Z., Forbes, E. E., Dahl, R. E., Ryan, N. D., Siegle, G. J., Ladouceur, C. D., & Silk, J. S. (2012). Emotional reactivity and regulation in anxious and nonanxious youth: A cell-phone ecological momentary assessment study. *Journal of Child Psychology and Psychiatry, 53,* 197–206. doi:10.1111/j.1469-7610.2011.02469.x

Toufexis, M. D., Hommer, R., Gerardi, D. M., Grant, P., Rothschild, L., D'Souza, P., . . . Murphy, T. K. (2015). Disordered eating and food restrictions in children with PANDAS/PANS. *Journal of Child and Adolescent Psychopharmacology, 25*(1), 48–56. doi:10.1089/cap.2014.0063

Trowell, J., Joffe, I., Campbell, J., Clemente, C., Almqvist, F., Soininen, M., . . . Tsiantis, J. (2007). Childhood depression: A place for psychotherapy. *European Child & Adolescent Psychiatry, 16,* 157–167. doi:10.1007/s00787-006-0584-x

Twenge, J. M., Cooper, A. B., Joiner, T. E., Duffy, M. E., & Binau, S. G. (2019). Age, period, and cohort trends in mood disorder indicators and suicide-related outcomes in a nationally representative dataset, 2005–2017. *Journal of Abnormal Psychology, 128*(3), 185–199. doi:10.1037/abn0000410

U.S. Department of Health and Human Services, Substance Abuse and Mental Health Services Administration. (2017). *The comprehensive community mental health services for children with serious emotional disturbances program, Report to Congress, 2016.* Retrieved from https://store.samhsa.gov/product/The-Comprehensive-Community-Mental-Health-Services-for-Children-with-Serious-Emotional-Disturbances/PEP18-CMHI2016

U.S. Department of Health and Human Services, Substance Abuse and Mental Health Services Administration. (2018). *Helping children and youth who have traumatic experiences.* Retrieved from https://www.samhsa.gov/sites/default/files/brief_report_natl_childrens_mh_awareness_day.pdf

Vidal, S., & Connell, C. M. (2019). Treatment effects of parent–child focused evidence-based programs on problem severity and functioning among children and adolescents with disruptive behavior. *Journal of Clinical Child & Adolescent Psychology, 48*(Supp. 1), S326–S336. doi:10.1080/15374416.2018.1469092

Wang, Z., Whiteside, S. P., Sim, L., Farah, W., Morrow, A. S., Alsawas, M., . . . Daraz, L. (2017). Comparative effectiveness and safety of cognitive behavioral therapy and pharmacotherapy for childhood anxiety disorders: A systematic review and meta-analysis. *JAMA Pediatrics, 171*(11), 1049–1056. doi:10.1001/jamapediatrics.2017.3036

Warnick, E. M., Bearss, K., Weersing, V. R., Scahill, L., & Woolston, J. (2014). Shifting the treatment model: Impact on engagement in outpatient therapy. *Administration and Policy in Mental Health, 41,* 93–103. doi:10.1007/s10488-012-0439-3

Watson, S. M. R., Richels, C., Michalek, A. P., & Raymer, A. (2015). Psychosocial treatments for ADHD: A systematic appraisal of the evidence. *Journal of Attention Disorders, 19*(1), 3–10. doi:10.1177/1087054712447857

Weinstein, S. M., West, A. E., & Pavuluri, M. (2013). Psychosocial intervention for pediatric bipolar disorder: Current and future directions. *Expert Review of Neurotherapeutics, 13*(7), 843–850. doi:10.1586/14737175.2013.811985

Weiss, S. J., & Talley, S. (2009). A comparison of the practices of psychiatric clinical nurse specialists and nurse practitioners who are certified to provide mental health care for children and adolescents. *Journal of the American Psychiatric Nurses Association, 15*(2), 111–119. doi:10.1177/1078390309333546

Weisz, J. R. (2015). Promoting youth self-regulation through psychotherapy redesigning treatments to fit complex youths in clinical care. In G. Oettingen & P. M. Gollwitzer (Eds.), *Self-regulation in adolescence* (pp. 311–332). Cambridge, UK: Cambridge University Press. doi:10.1017/CBO9781139565790.016

Weisz, J. R., Bearman, S. K., Santucci, L. C., & Jensen-Doss, A. (2017). Initial test of a principle-guided approach to transdiagnostic psychotherapy with children and adolescents. *Journal of Clinical Child & Adolescent Psychology, 46*(1), 44–58. doi:10.1080/15374416.2016.1163708

Weisz, J. R., Chorpita, B. F., Palinkas, L. A., Schoenwald, S. K., Miranda, J., Bearman, S. K., . . . Gibbons, R. D. (2012). Testing standard and modular designs for psychotherapy treating depression, anxiety, and conduct problems in youth: A randomized effectiveness trial. *Archives of General Psychiatry, 69*, 274–282. doi:10.1001/archgenpsychiatry.2011.147

Weisz, J. R., Hawley, K. M., & Doss, A. J. (2004). Empirically tested psychotherapies for youth internalizing and externalizing problems and disorders. *Child and Adolescent Psychiatric Clinics of North America, 13*, 729–815. doi:10.1016/j.chc.2004.05.006

Weisz, J. R., & Kazdin, A. D. (Eds.). (2017). *Evidence-based psychotherapies for children and adolescents* (3rd ed.). New York, NY: Guilford Press.

Weisz, J. R., Krumholz, L. S., Santucci, L., Thomassin, K., & Ng, M. Y. (2015). Shrinking the gap between research and practice: Tailoring and testing youth psychotherapies in clinical care contexts. *Annual Review of Clinical Psychology, 11*, 139–163. doi:10.1146/annurev-clinpsy-032814-112820

Weisz, J. R., Kuppens, S., Ng, M. Y., Eckshtain, D., Ugueto, A. M., Vaughn-Coaxum, R., . . . Weersing, V. R. (2017). What five decades of research tells us about the effects of youth psychological therapy: A multilevel meta-analysis and implications for science and practice. *American Psychologist, 72*(2), 79. doi:10.1037/a0040360

West, P., & Evans, C. L. S. (1992). The specialty of child and adolescent psychiatric nursing. In P. West & C. L. S. Evans (Eds.), *Psychiatric and mental health nursing with children and adolescents* (pp. 1–10). Gaithersburg, MD: Aspen Publications.

Whitcomb, S. A. (2017). *Behavioral, social, and emotional assessment of children and adolescents* (5th ed.). New York, NY: Routledge/Taylor & Francis Group.

Whitney, D. G., & Peterson, M. D. (2019). U.S. national and state-level prevalence of mental health disorders and disparities of mental health care use in children. *JAMA Pediatrics, 173*(4), 389-391. doi:10.1001/jamapediatrics.2018.5399

Whitson, M. L., Bernard, S., & Kaufman, J. S. (2013). The effects of cumulative risk and protection on problem behaviors for youth in an urban school-based system of care. *Community Mental Health Journal, 49*(5), 576–586. doi:10.1007/s10597-012-9535-9VA

Psychotherapeutic Approaches With Children and Adolescents

Pamela Lusk and
Anka Roberto

This chapter on psychotherapy approaches for children and adolescents comes at a time when children appear to be more vulnerable than ever. Perhaps an overarching concern is about safety, particularly with violence between community groups, school shootings, the emergence of infectious diseases that reach the level of pandemic, school shootings shattering generations-old assumptions that children can be safe in school; and at home, children are not safe with Internet access to predators and sexually explicit material. This heightened concern makes adults, parents, and teachers perhaps more attentive and protective than ever. Other factors that make children and adolescents appear to be more vulnerable, seemingly due to a variety of changes in child rearing and education. are identified in the list that follows:

- Focus on performance on tests rather than encouraging curiosity and learning because it is exciting and enjoyable
- Test performance as a measure of a child's success
- Discomfort with individual differences in learning and ability, so that those who "deviate" are not just different, they have "learning differences" that are regarded as "disabilities" and seem to overlap with emotional and behavioral disturbances
- Differences that may appropriately be viewed as developmental, transitional adjustments are nowadays often readily diagnosed, giving a lifelong "sentence." These include attention deficit hyperactivity disorder (ADHD), anxiety, depression, mood disorders, obsessive-compulsive disorder (OCD), and even schizophrenia
- Because of a diagnosis orientation, there is less recognition and promotion of resilience, less expectation of healing, and less focus on strengths and assets

   There are changes in family and community life which include:

- Family time together may be diluted with "electronics"
- Possible inconsistency in parts of the day that work better with routines, such as morning preparation and bedtime
- Children have had their social and school life disrupted (including school closures for health/safety)
- More exposure to violence on TV and video games
- In some neighborhoods violence between groups and racism with accompanying violence

Those who work with children have become acutely aware in the past few years of the need to provide trauma-informed care with the many children and adolescents who have experienced adverse childhood experiences (ACEs). In a 1998 study, "Relationship of Childhood Abuse and Household Dysfunction to Many of the Leading Causes of Death in Adults: The Adverse Childhood Experiences (ACE) Study (Felitti et al., 1998), findings suggest that the impact of adverse childhood experiences on adult health is strong and cumulative. ACEs contribute to increased mental health and medical problems and negatively affect the neurodevelopment of the growing child. The need to consider ACEs when assessing, evaluating, and planning treatment for children and adolescents is important in current clinical practice.

For advanced practice psychiatric nurses (APPNs) skilled in child and adolescent behavioral health, the challenges include sorting through what might be really serious and enduring, requiring a more intense treatment, and what is more likely reactive, and may require more focus on supporting resilience. This requires grounding in both developmental and family theory as aspects of the child's life. Being grounded in family means being able to sit with families, engage with them in describing what worries they have, and inviting them to participate in solutions. In traditional face to face meetings and when telepsychiatry is the format, the APPN strives to identify how the family functions as a supportive, healthy, holding context in which the children can grow. And if they are not, how can they be helped to do so? Being comfortably grounded in these two critical aspects of the child's experience and evolution makes it possible to assess what is amiss, if anything, and to proceed with some confidence in finding solutions. See Chapter 13, on family therapy.

While there is increasing exploration into the brain biology of development, and behavioral and emotional experience and expression, the more palpable evidence provided by APPN's observations and experiences with the child and child in interaction with critical people in his or her life best shapes the practitioners' hypotheses, formulations, and treatment plans. And, of course, these are all best refined in collaboration with child, family, and other involved and concerned people, such as teachers and pediatricians. It is important to remember that children live with other people, and a practice that includes these others in understanding and intervening is most likely to have lasting benefits. Daniel Seigel's model of the interplay between flow of energy in the brain, mind as an interpreter of experience, and interpersonal context invites us to pay attention to what we can see, with the recognition that the mind and the interpersonal context can change the brain (Seigel, 2001).

This chapter discusses the importance of developmental theory, principles in conducting therapy with children/adolescents, establishing a therapeutic relationship, involving the family, and application of specific psychotherapeutic approaches in working with children/adolescents. Two evidence-based child therapies, cognitive behavioral therapy (CBT) and eye movement desensitization and reprocessing (EMDR) therapy, are highlighted with case examples provided.

DEVELOPMENTAL THEORY

Being grounded in development means first recognizing that children are in motion, that they are developing, and the first big outcome of child development is to become a healthy adult–able to be a contributing member of a community. Keeping this motion toward the future in mind always requires that the clinician think not only of where the child is now, but where the child is going. Of what community(ies) will she or he be a member? And what contributions will he or she be making? Second, being grounded in development means being able to identify where a child is in the range of tasks from basic ego functions to developing language and communication, to increasing cognitive sophistication, and to socializing with increasing affection and empathy. And importantly, APPNs must always keep in mind the trajectory of development, helping to distinguish between moving along well, to apparent delays, to possible disabilities, but never becoming so focused on now that one ignores the fact that as all of us are on developmental journeys. Children and adolescents are moving more quickly and perceptibly toward their futures, and the future is to become a contributing member of a community.

Before the APPN receives training in specific psychotherapeutic approaches, there are foundational assumptions based on growth and development that are the basis of practice with children and adolescents. As children grow in years, their bodies grow, their brains develop, and they learn from their interactions with their environment. Science, including advanced neuroscience with new imaging capabilities and information regarding the plasticity of the developing brain, informs our understanding of neurodevelopment and the ways psychotherapeutic interventions change the brain. Theories of growth and development have long been a basis for how the child therapist assesses the individual child, considers his or her strengths and needs, forms a diagnostic impression, and develops a plan of treatment in collaboration with the child/adolescent and parent.

Communication with children and adolescents is developmentally based and usually visits are conducted in a child-friendly room/office. Strategies for engaging the child and/or teen in the therapeutic process and ways to involve parents in treatment are discussed later in this chapter. Because the child/adolescent's initial psychiatric interview/evaluation differs from the usual adult interview, a step-by-step template is provided in Appendix 21.1 to guide an initial diagnostic interview with a child or teen.

Though there have been different descriptive frameworks, using different language, as professionals have tried to describe the changes experienced and expected as children grow, there are two developmental frameworks, Erickson and Piaget, that are most helpful in guiding therapists in thinking about where children/adolescents are in their journeys. When seeing the child and parent for the comprehensive evaluation, the child psychotherapist compares how this child is mastering developmental tasks and moving forward through the stages relative to his or her chronological age based on these developmental frameworks.

Erikson's stages of psychosocial development, first published in his book, *Childhood and Society* (1950), provides descriptions that focus on the interactions between the developing child and the surrounding "society," for example, family, school, peer context, and later work context, and then also noting the child's response as well as others' response to the child. Thus, a child in school is assessing himself and his success in the context of the expectation of his schooling as well as comparing himself to his peers and the response of his family members to his progress. The name of this stage is industry (mastering the "Industry" of the society) versus inferiority (a sense of failure at mastering). Using this framework for assessing a child struggling in school helps to put together the child's ability, the family's support and encouragement, peers' response to the child, and the expectations of performance in school and emotional and behavioral difficulties the child might be experiencing. See Table 5.3 in Chapter 5, for Erikson's stages of development.

Piaget's stages of cognitive development give some further clarification to the readiness of a child to tackle both academic tasks as well as social interaction tasks. Piaget's framework explicates how one's thinking evolves. For example, the adolescent stage of propositional thinking allows the flexibility of thinking "what if?" and of predicting intellectually, a flexibility that is not as readily usable in the "preoperational" thinking of the stage of "concrete operations." Thus, an adolescent fully in the operational stage is able to do more complicated math, to make judgments about things to do with his or her peers and things not to do, and be able to present a persuasive case to her or his parents or teachers about something she or he would like them to consider. See Table 21.1 for Piaget's stages of cognitive development.

TABLE 21.1 PIAGET'S STAGES OF COGNITIVE DEVELOPMENT		
Typical Age Range	**Description of Stage**	**Developmental Phenomena**
Birth to nearly 2 years	Sensorimotor Experiencing the world through senses and actions (looking, hearing, touching, mouthing, and grasping)	• Object permanence • Stranger anxiety
About 2 to about 6 or 7 years	Preoperational Representing things with words and images; using intuitive rather than logical reasoning	• Pretend play • Egocentrism
About 7–11 years	Concrete operational Thinking logically about concrete events; grasping concrete analogies and performing arithmetical operations	• Conservation • Mathematical transformations
About 12 through adulthood	Formal operational Abstract reasoning	• Abstract logic • Potential for mature moral reasoning

Source: Piaget, J. (1936). *Origins of intelligence in the child.* London, England: Routledge & Kegan Paul.

The APPNs' knowledge of normal growth and development through ages/stages informs the assessment of that child/adolescent's current level of functioning at home, at school, and in social situations. When seeing the child and parent for the comprehensive evaluation, the child psychotherapist compares how this child is mastering developmental tasks and moving forward through the stages of development relative to his or her chronological age. Since progression through predictable stages of growth and development is our overarching assumption, then it follows every child/adolescent has the potential to grow and develop, as well as master new skills, accomplish goals, and contribute to others. This can be communicated with confidence to parents and the young person. The message, "I hear your struggles and concerns now. We can work together, using the evidence-based interventions that have been effective with other children/ adolescents with similar concerns, and with your strengths and efforts, we expect positive outcomes" (Lusk & Melnyk, 2011b, p. 298). The APPN instills hope and outlines positive expectations from the initial consultation visit.

PRINCIPLES OF CHILD PSYCHOTHERAPY

The Setting

Settings where APPNs specialize in psychiatric/mental healthcare of children and adolescents include inpatient or partial hospitalization units, outpatient mental health organizations, private practice, and integrated pediatric and primary care practices.

APPNs conduct initial evaluations with children/teens, diagnose psychiatric disorders, develop and maintain a therapeutic relationship, plan treatment in collaboration with the family, and manage psychiatric/mental health disorders over time. The role requires knowledge and skills in delivering psychotherapeutic interventions as well as psycho-pharmacology. A good understanding of psychotherapy with children and adolescents is important for all APPNs.

Utilizing a developmental approach to child/adolescent work, the office/therapy room is adapted to be appealing to the child and relaxing and interesting for the adolescent. It is helpful to keep the desk or a table and chairs for the traditional face-to-face interview with parents and adolescents if they prefer to interact that way. The table or desk also can be used for art projects or activities with the therapist. Some place colorful and interesting toys in easy reach, and the child is encouraged to play with the toys as he or she wishes, while others prefer a more structured situation where toys are available at the appropriate time. For example, in the first meeting with a child and family, and often at the beginning of following psychotherapy sessions, it is useful to have the child sit with the family and talk about what is happening. In the first meeting with the child, the APPN asks the child why the child's parents brought him or her in today, and what follows is a conversation between the child and parents (and sometimes siblings) about what is going on, what are the problems, what works well, and so forth. In later sessions, the opening should be a review of accomplishments or difficulties, or how the child did with the various things that had been suggested/prescribed. Children usually know how to talk, and their family members can help them express themselves.

Toys and play bring another element of discovery to the sessions. When families are involved, as we believe they should be, they can be invited to watch the child at play and ask questions about what is happening in the play, and they can also be invited to join the child in play. Therapists differ in how wide a variety of toys or other materials they might find useful in their offices. For some, drawing materials may be enough. For others, a variety of puppets or a sand tray may expand the opportunities for the child's expression and "work." For children with dissociative states, there is a whole range of special materials that can facilitate discovery and integration. An excellent resource for working with children with dissociation is the book *Healing the Fractured Child: Diagnosis and Treatment of Youth With Dissociation* by Frances Waters (2016). However, working with dissociation is a specialty that requires a high degree of skill and details will not be covered in this chapter. When the therapist conveys an interest in the child and his or her play, she or he may also include the parents as they watch the child and inquire about what is happening. Often if siblings are present, they, too, may be involved in play, and the relationship to materials is enriched by the relationships between the children, their affection, sharing, fighting, competition, and so on. All can be observed, and some can be modified, by a parent or the therapist suggesting a way to share or resolve a fight.

Adolescents may want to draw on paper, with an Etch a Sketch, or fidget with other items in the office as they talk. With younger children, toys kept in the office are chosen to facilitate communication through play. The younger child doesn't communicate with words like an older child/teen or adult; rather, he or she uses play to express thoughts/strengths/fears/joys/struggles. These children often talk as they play, but it may be to the doll or animal toy, or as a running narrative as they play. Unless there is a therapeutic reason to limit play materials in a session, the child can move around the room freely and choose how to play with the toys. In every office, it is helpful for the APPN to have a basket or box of toys/art supplies/books available even if his or her practice is "across the life span," and he or she sees primarily adults. Basic props can be used by any child who is there for assessment or treatment, as well as by children attending visits with their parents. See Box 21.1 for suggested toys for a therapeutic playroom.

BOX 21.1 Toys for a Therapeutic Playroom

Doll house with furniture and a toilet
Baby doll, box or bed, and bottles
Family of small dolls with mother, father, and children
Family groups of animals also with parents, young animals
Dolls with ethnic features (Asian, White, Black, etc.); Lego makes a set of "Children of the World," which includes all skin tones
Set of blocks or Legos
Play-Doh or clay
Puppets (including a puppet with teeth)
Paper and pencil, crayons, washable markers
Sand in trays
Table games and other structured games, checkers, cards
Action figures–helpers, police figure or car, firefighter, medical person
Soft balls (swoosh or nerf)
Books
Toy phones
An animal toy or puppet with big teeth, which can be used to express aggression
Etch a Sketch

Establishing a Therapeutic Relationship

Young people communicate differently, especially at different developmental stages. Many will not have mastered talking as their primary way of communicating, and even those children and teens who are excellent conversationalists might not have the experience or vocabulary to identify and describe emotional states. Toys and props, such as those previously listed, allow for many ways of communicating. Props/toys also allow for the child/teen to draw or fidget with his or her hands to help manage anxiety as he or she talks. The therapist who conveys openness, patience, a nonjudgmental approach, and a natural curiosity about why people do what they do and who takes the time to listen will be most successful in establishing a therapeutic connection with children and adolescents (Wissow, 2015).

The therapist is knowledgeable about play and is skillful at using play in the therapeutic situation. Children's play therapy tends to fall into the following categories: physical activities, solo imaginary play games with rules, creative projects, and imaginary play with the therapist as participant (Kernberg, Litvo, & Keable, 2012, p. 551). When working with a very young child who is communicating through play, the therapist's role is to remain present with the child, follow his or her play, and make timely observations about the child's actions. The therapist remains curious about the child's inner world expressed through play. For example, a small child might have the sister doll aggressively kick the brother doll. The therapist can calmly state: "The sister really kicked the brother" and then wait for elaboration from the child. The child will form the story; the therapist follows and facilitates the child's continued expression.

Sometimes new therapists are hesitant to provide positive comments in interactions with the child, fearing they might imply judgment–"If you did this, you are good," or "If you did that, you are a bad person." There is a distinction between judging a person to be good or bad and commenting on a behavior or thought or feeling. As an example, a young child who lines all the play figures up by color might elicit a reinforcing positive comment by the therapist such as, "Look, you put them all in a line.

The line starts with the yellows and goes all the way up to the reds and then greens." This is an honest observation of what the child has just done and, therefore, a reinforcing statement, not a judgment on whether the child is good. The statement reflects the child's play. The therapist can then add a comment or question, to further encourage the child's creative play. "They are all in a straight line. I wonder why they are all in a line?" Because children line up at preschool, the child may respond, "Oh they are going outside to wait for the mommies to pick them up"; or "The teacher told them to"; or "They like to be with their color and make a rainbow line"; or the child may shrug and move on to another activity.

Children, as they become comfortable in the playroom and develop a trusting relationship (therapeutic relationship) with the APPN, will re-enact the same play scenarios over and over. This repetition is expected. That is how young children use play to work out their feelings/fears/worries. The therapist continues to calmly follow the play and, after a time, the scenario as set up by the child will change. For instance, the child who acted out the sister doll kicking the brother doll with great energy may enter the playroom each session, go to the playhouse, and in the play have the sister doll kick the brother doll aggressively. Then, after repeating this scene over and over and over, the sister doll might get ready to kick the brother doll, and the mother doll will come into the room. The child will script the rest of the story, but the therapist notes the play has changed. There is movement to resolve that issue. The therapist remains a calm, sounding board, supporting the active, energetic play the child chooses. In the therapy room the child can have a doll being aggressive without the play being stopped as "not nice." The child can express emotions freely, with the supportive therapist reflecting and predictably keeping the playroom a safe place to express feelings/fears/anger. Generally, a calm soft tone of voice is comforting to the child.

As children get older in years and spend more time at school and with other children and adults, they develop a command of language and an increased ability to express themselves verbally. They still enjoy play and will use the toys in the office/playroom, sometimes competitively with the therapist, to work out their feelings/fears/worries. They are still learning the words to express emotions and describe their difficulties. The therapist can assist the school-age child while playing, in putting words to emotions and learning problem-solving skills. With the school-age child, self-regulation is often a focus of therapy. Self-regulation can be addressed and practiced in most all the therapeutic play activities with the therapist positively reinforcing the child's ability to express normal emotions such as anger, fear, and jealousy while remaining in control.

The school-age child, with his or her developmental tasks of industry versus inferiority, will often initiate games, and often competitive games, with the therapist. An ability to genuinely enjoy each child with his or her interests, strengths, and views of the world is a most valued trait in child therapists. The goal for each session is to prepare yourself to be aware and to "listen" for themes in the child's communication, verbal and nonverbal, as expressed through play or art, or activities with the therapist, and provide therapeutic responses. The therapist who is dependable and remains present, calm, and open to that child's world expressed in play or with words facilitates the establishment of a strong therapeutic relationship.

When interviewing adolescents, it is best to follow their lead. If they choose to sit chair to chair, or at the table to converse, the therapist can follow that. If they choose to build with Legos or draw with an Etch a Sketch as they talk, go along with that. Teens can create incredible structures/diagrams, and so on, with the same props/toys younger children use simply. They demonstrate their strengths and abilities, which can be leveraged in the therapy. A recent study of adolescents ages 14 to 19 in focus groups identified "what adolescents need from psychotherapists in change process" (Lavik, Veseth, Frøysa, Binder, & Moltu, 2018). From the words of the adolescent participants: (a) if the teen is facing a scary situation, attend to the adolescent's starting point; (b) be warm, invested, and emotionally engaged; (c) offer live company and presence as a real human being; (d) have integrity as an adult and a professional; (e) know the world of a teenager and get into his or her stories; and (f) have mutuality as a virtue and treat the adolescent as an equal.

Some specific strategies for working with adolescents versus adults include the therapist assuming a more active role in setting the agenda (with the teen's input) for the sessions and providing interesting, developmentally based content such as evidence-based adolescent treatment manuals. In working with the adolescent, it is also good to allow for plenty of time for them to finish their thought and initiate conversation, but it is not helpful to allow for so much silence between interactions that their anxiety rises to uncomfortable levels. Remaining attuned to the teen's nonverbal communication can let the therapist know that the teen's anxiety is increasing. For instance, in response to a question such as, "What are some of your positive qualities?" there may be a long pause, and the teen may become flushed, fidget, and appear nearly panicked with wide eyes and fearful facial expression. The therapist then is cued to break the silence and move on to another line of conversation or provide prompts or possible responses to the question such as, "I remember a very positive thing from what your mom said when she was in the office with us. Your mom told me that the family dog is your responsibility and you *always* feed him in the mornings and walk him every evening even when you are tired from basketball practice. She said she can always count on you." Providing this example can prompt the teen to think of more positive qualities. It also demonstrates that the therapist is interested, is listening, and recognizes the teen's individual strengths.

Another therapeutic strategy when working with adolescents is maintaining a predictable beginning, middle, and end of each session. Providing structure and having goal-focused content prepared for the session is a comfort for the adolescent. Adolescents generally want to know reasons for the content chosen for sessions, and their questions are very fresh and perceptive. When the therapist explains the theoretical framework of the therapy, and why the sessions are formatted as they are (at the adolescent's level of comprehension), then the teen is much more likely to follow through with treatment (Beck, 2011). As the therapist and adolescent get to know each other, a therapeutic alliance develops. Adolescents are generally open and honest and will provide feedback when asked about how the therapy is going. This mutual feedback as part of the therapy models positive interpersonal communication and strengthens the therapeutic relationship.

Involving the Family in Psychotherapy

APPNs should invite the parent/s to share behavioral information privately with the clinician before the child enters the room or by phone before the session. This can be helpful to shift to a positive approach so the child does not feel discouraged and criticized (Wesselmann et al., 2014). Parents provide the information for the history of the chief complaint, history of prior treatment, and the medical and developmental history. The therapist establishes a collaborative alliance with the parent/s through which they participate as partners in the treatment. After the problem is discussed and the child is seen with the parent present, it is helpful to spend time with the parent and child together to observe their interaction. A focus on the child's strengths enhances a positive self-view through questions such as: "What characteristics do you enjoy about your child/teen?" What are your favorite early memories of your child/teen?" "What activities do you most enjoy about your child/teen?" (Wesselmann, Schweitzer, & Armstrong, 2014). It is also ideal, if the child is old enough and willing, for the APPN to spend some time alone with the child to allow him or her to express any fears related to his or her safety and speak confidentially about any concerns. Risk assessment is part of the interview as is a clear discussion of confidentiality. As the evaluation is completed, the therapist, teen, and parent collaboratively identify a treatment plan. Evidence-based care includes (a) the best evidence from research literature about treatment modalities with best outcomes, (b) the parents'/teen's values and preferences for treatment, and (c) the therapist's training and comfort in delivering the recommended evidence-based therapy (Lusk & Melnyk, 2011a).

Resources for treatment, time, finances, and available transportation are also important considerations in establishing a treatment plan. Ideally, the parent, teen, and therapist all agree with the treatment plan. When working with parents and teens, occasionally parent/teen conflict occurs. The best approach for the therapist is to maintain the stance: the therapist, teen, and parents all are on the same team in treatment. All are on the team battling depression or anxiety (the identified presenting problem). If the parent/teen/child conflict is the most pressing concern, a referral for family therapy is considered.

It can be very helpful when parents attend the sessions because the child/teen and parent can develop a shared language and understanding of the therapy process. This strengthens the parent/child relationship. If the youth, parent, and therapist collaboratively decide the teen or other youth should be seen individually, the therapist will check in with the parent regularly to discuss progress, to discuss new goals, and to be available for parents' comments and concerns. It is a team approach to work toward positive outcomes and any modeling and facilitation of an improved parent–child relationship is very valuable.

The Initial Psychiatric Evaluation

A template for an initial psychiatric evaluation with a child/adolescent in Appendix 21.1 is scripted to be used just as it is written for new child therapists and for experienced child/adolescent clinicians. The template can help assure that no important questions are inadvertently omitted. The evaluation begins with a direct question about why the child or adolescent is meeting with a mental health specialist now. It is important to get that response in the child/teen's own words. The parents can also provide their input, but the child/teen's understanding of his or her "need for help" with regards to seeing a specialist in child/adolescent mental health is very valuable for framing the therapeutic work to follow.

After establishing the presenting problem, the template follows a strength-based format. This initial evaluation template has proved to be acceptable to children, teens and parents and comprehensive enough to allow for an initial treatment plan to be identified at the end of the evaluation. It generally can be completed in a 1-hour visit.

Screening instruments are often used in primary care or psychiatric practices and can be reviewed before beginning the psychiatric evaluation. See Table 21.2.

TABLE 21.2   SCREENING TOOLS FOR CHILDREN AND ADOLESCENTS

Assessment Tool	Brief Description	Availability/Source
Open Access Screening Instruments		
ACE	CYW Adverse Childhood Experiences Questionnaire (ACE-Q) CYW ACE-Q Versions 1. CYW Adverse Childhood Experiences Questionnaire for Children (CYW ACE-Q Child) 17-item instrument completed by the parent/caregiver for children age 0 to 12 2. CYW Adverse Childhood Experiences Questionnaire for Adolescents (CYW ACE-Q Teen) 19-item instrument completed by the parent/caregiver for youth age 13 to 19 3. CYW Adverse Childhood Experiences Questionnaire for Adolescents: Self-Report (CYW ACE-Q Teen SR) 19-item instrument completed by youth age 13 to 19	Burke Harris, N. and Renschler, T. (version 7/2015). Center for Youth Wellness ACE Questionnaire (CYW ACE-Q Child, Teen, Teen SR). Center for Youth Wellness. San Francisco, CA. centerforyouthwellness. org/aceq-pdf
A-DES	The A-DES is a version of the Dissociative Experiences Scale developed specifically for use with *adolescents*. The approximate age range for this version is 10–21 years.	www.emdrworks.org/ Downloads/a-des.pdf
CDC	The Child Dissociative Checklist (CDC) Version 3 is designed to be used as a clinical screening tool for the identification of dissociative pathology in children. This is a checklist of 20 symptoms that are rated as very true, somewhat true, or not true.	www.icctc.org/ August2013/PMM%20 Handouts/Child%20 Dissociative%20 Checklist.pdf
CRAFFT	The CRAFFT is a behavioral health screening tool for use with children under the age of 21 and is recommended by the American Academy of Pediatrics' Committee on Substance Abuse for use with adolescents. It consists of a series of six questions developed to screen adolescents for high risk alcohol and other drug use disorders.	www.ceasarboston.org/ CRAFFT

(continued)

TABLE 21.2 SCREENING TOOLS FOR CHILDREN AND ADOLESCENTS (*CONTINUED*)		
Assessment Tool	**Brief Description**	**Availability/Source**
GAD 7	GAD 7 is a screening tool most commonly used in primary care ages 13–17 years. Validated as a diagnostic tool and severity assessment scale, GAD 7 is a 3-point Likert-type self-report questionnaire with seven items. Scores >10 have good diagnostic sensitivity and specificity for generalized anxiety disorder. Higher scores correlate with more functional impairment.	www.phqscreeners.com/ images/sites/g/files/ g10060481/f/201412/ GAD-7_English.pdf
PHQ 9 – Modified for Teens	The Patient Health Questionnaire is a depression scale. PhQ9 for Depression Adolescent version – same 9 questions as PhQ9 but scoring is modified. Modified with permission from the PHQ (Spitzer, Williams, & Kroenke, 1999) by J. Johnson (Johnson, 2002)	www.aacap.org/App_ Themes/AACAP/docs/ member_resources/ toolbox_for_clinical_ practice_and_ outcomes/symptoms/ GLAD-PC_PHQ-9.pdf
PSC	The Pediatric Symptom Checklist is a psychosocial screen designed to facilitate the recognition of cognitive, emotional, and behavioral problems so that appropriate interventions can be initiated as early as possible. Included here are two versions, the parent completed version (PSC) and the youth self-report (Y-PSC). The Y-PSC can be administered to adolescents ages 11 and up.	www.brightfutures.org/ mentalhealth/pdf/ professionals/ped_ sympton_chklst.pdf (Bimaher et al., 1997; Monga et al., 2000).
SCARED	For younger children and adolescents, the SCARED (Screen for Child Anxiety Related Disorders) is used (ages 8–17 years). The SCARED has a Child Version and Parent 17	sspediatricassociates.com/ Forms-and-Policies/ Forms/Behavioral,- Mental-Health- Assessment-Forms/ SCARED-form-Parent- and-Child-version.aspx

PSYCHOTHERAPY APPROACHES

The current emphasis of evidence-based interventions organized by problem areas in the Evidence-Based Child and Adolescent Psychosocial Interventions chart represents over 900 randomized trials of psychosocial treatments for youth and can be accessed online at the American Academy of Pediatrics website at the link that follows:

www.aap.org/en-us/Documents/CRPsychosocialInterventions.pdf

Many of the psychotherapy modalities discussed at length in earlier chapters of this book, such as psychodynamic therapy (Chapter 5), interpersonal therapy (Chapter 10), cognitive behavioral therapy (Chapter 8), Eye Movement Desensitization and Reprocessing therapy (Chapter 7), and motivational interviewing (Chapter 9), have adaptations that are used very successfully with children and teens. The theoretical frameworks remain the same; however, the delivery is developmentally appropriate for the age/stage of the child or adolescent. In this section, the application of the theory for child/teen therapy is discussed. Parent management training (PMT) and problem-solving skills therapy (PSST) are evidence-based approaches for disruptive behaviors and are also included here.

Psychodynamic Psychotherapy

Psychodynamic psychotherapy has continued to be a primary modality of psychotherapy for younger children to facilitate the child's expression of emotions and experiences through art, free play, sand trays, movement, and other nonverbal mediums. Because it is difficult to conduct randomized controlled trials with young children in play therapy (since the very nature of the therapy is that it is nondirective and the therapist "follows" the child as he or she initiates the play), there is a paucity of research studies to support play therapy as an evidence-based therapy. Play, however, provides a way for the child to communicate with the therapist and is the vehicle for resolution of emotional distress.

The framework of psychodynamic psychotherapy seeks to be predictable–same time, same place. It progresses through three stages: the opening phase, the middle phase, and the termination phase. The psychodynamic approach is especially helpful in complex cases because it addresses the underlying dynamics of the problem. From the 2012 Practice Parameter of the Academy of Child and Adolescent Psychiatry (Practice Parameters are now called "Clinical Practice Guidelines"), "The practice of psychodynamic psychotherapy (ages 3–12) provides an essential, developmental perspective on normality and pathology, applicable to the individual child and his family facilitating optimal development and adaptive resilience vis-à-vis stressors and trauma" (Kernberg et al., 2012, p. 541).

Psychodynamic psychotherapy is useful with internalizing disorders, mild to moderate externalizing disorders, developmental difficulties, and maladaptive responses to life events (Kernberg et al., 2012). Internalizing disorders refer to behaviors that result from negativity that is focused inward and are associated with "quiet" temperaments. For example, the child may become depressed and blame herself or himself when there is conflict in the home. Externalizing disorders refer to behavior that may include oppositional behaviors such as temper tantrums, substance use, and conduct disorders. Externalizing disorders are most associated with children who have more difficulty controlling reactive impulses, have lower ability to self-regulate, and have a higher need for intensity pleasure, low task persistence, and lower need for closeness. Children with the externalizing "loud" disorders typically do better with behavioral therapy approaches (Yearwood, Pearson, & Newland, 2012, pp. 31, 32).

Psychodynamic therapy emphasizes "following the child" in deciding what will be done in each session. The course of therapy, thus, is very open-ended. The length of therapy is based on the child's progress. The role of the therapist is to be empathetic, predictable, nonjudgmental, and dependable. Children often play and replay scenarios through the family dolls, expressive art supplies, or role-playing with the therapist. The therapist follows as the child works through his or her concerns and the play scenarios begin to change and resolve. Patterns in play reveal the child's inner conflicts, developmental difficulties, and maladaptive relational patterns (Kernberg et al., 2012, p. 544). The therapist seeks to help the child understand his or her feelings and conflicts in developmentally appropriate terms, and then the child and therapist can think together about behaviors the child can do for himself or herself or enlist parents or caregivers to relieve the child's distress and move forward through healthy mastery of developmental tasks. The process of repetition and elaboration is the "working through" phase.

When the child's progress indicates it is time to terminate therapy, some regression can be anticipated. The therapist at the termination phase addresses gains made during therapy, as well as issues of dependency and separation, and addresses issues of loss and separation activated in the parents with the close of therapy. For the teen, more expressive therapy may be indicated, which is discussed in Chapter 5.

Interpersonal Psychotherapy With Adolescents

Interpersonal psychotherapy (IPT) is based on the theory of Harry Stack Sullivan, who emphasized interpersonal relationships and social experiences in shaping personality. Interpersonal psychotherapy is directive with the focus on the relationship between the patient and therapist. IPT-A (adolescent) is evidence-based therapy for adolescent depression and is included with CBT by the United States Preventive Services Task Force recommendations for treatment of adolescents who are depressed. IPT-A was developed to treat major depressive disorder in short-term therapy of about 12 to 16 sessions. It is a manualized therapy with a specific manual for adolescent depression (Mufson et al., 2004). There is also an adolescent skills-based model IPT-AST that has been particularly helpful in school settings, thus returning adolescents to school, work, and other activities quickly (Yearwood et al., 2012).

The therapist role is collaborative and warm but adheres strictly to the treatment manual. Because it is interpersonally based, termination of the short-term therapy is discussed at every visit. Sessions are usually for an hour weekly. The focus of the working phase of therapy is on problems in current relationships in the patient's life, including role transitions, grief, interpersonal disputes, and interpersonal deficits. Teens are encouraged to identify solutions to problems on their own as much as possible. Teens learn to initiate their own changes, and this learning accounts for improvements that continue for months after treatment. See Chapter 10.

Motivational Interviewing

Motivational interviewing (MI) is an evidence-based approach used as a brief mental health intervention for adolescents at risk for problem substance use. The Substance Abuse and Mental Health Services Administration (SAMHSA; 2017) endorses the SBIRT model (Screening, Brief Intervention, Referral, Treatment; https://www.sbirttraining .com/training) in primary care and other healthcare settings where adolescents are seen. SBIRT ensures that health professionals are screening all adolescents for risk of substance use. It is important to follow a positive screening with a brief intervention such as MI (https://www.zurinstitute.com/course/motivational-interviewing/). MI is a collaborative, person-centered communication process designed to help individuals resolve ambivalence and plan for change. For adolescents, MI helps build motivation for behavior change. Brief MI interventions consisting of one or two sessions targeted toward increasing a teen's motivation to decrease substance use have produced good outcomes in several studies (Davis, Houk, Rowell, Benson, & Smith, 2016). The therapist utilizes a non-confrontational, Socratic questioning approach to increase awareness of benefits and consequences related to substance use, engages the adolescent into treatment, and increases motivation for change (Weisz & Kazdin, 2017). For adolescents who place a high value on making their own decisions, this approach is particularly effective. MI respects the autonomy and ability of the adolescent to consider all aspects of behaviors and come to his or her own conclusion about any changes in behavior that will facilitate his or her best outcomes. Teens appreciate not being told what is best for them by a healthcare professional. They respond well to the respectful, collaborative interaction. See Chapter 9 for a thorough discussion of MI.

Parent Management Training

The Parent Management Training Oregon (PMTO) model is designed to treat or prevent antisocial behavior problems in children and adolescents. It was developed at the Oregon Social Learning Center (OSLC). This training is based on social learning, social interaction, and behavioral theories (Yearwood et al., 2012). Over 25 studies have demonstrated the efficacy of the model. PMTO can be delivered in single family or group sessions. Family sessions usually run 60 minutes and continue for 25 to 30 sessions. Group treatment is usually 14 sessions for 90 minutes each. Treatment sessions are structured and include homework. Children may be included in the sessions, according to therapist/family preference. Behaviors are broken down into manageable steps, using positive reinforcement to teach children socially appropriate behaviors and to teach parents skills such as limit setting, problem-solving skills, and positive involvement with other parents. Parents are taught to emphasize positive reinforcement and not use harsh, coercive discipline. Examples of appropriate discipline methods include using time-outs and extra chores in response to behavioral issues such as lying or stealing. This approach has strong evidence to support it with disruptive behavior disorders and delinquency.

Training information can be obtained from the OSLC website at https://www .parentmanagementtraininginstitute.com/professional-training.html. Implementation Scientists International, Inc. was developed at OSLC to provide training in PMTO. There is an emphasis on fidelity to the core dimensions of the program.

Problem-Solving Skills Training

For children and adolescents with disruptive behaviors, Parent Management Training is the best evidence-based approach; however, there are instances where the parents aren't available, and the child/teen is seen individually (Weisz & Kazdin, 2017). Problem-Solving Skills Training (PSST) is effective for individual work. PSST focuses on cognitive processes including identifying alternative solutions to interpersonal problems, identifying the means to making friends, and identifying the consequences of one's actions. Difficulties with these processes are associated with disruptive behaviors (Yearwood et al., 2012). PSST consists of weekly 30- to 50-minute sessions with the child, and the core program is 12 sessions. Central to the treatment is using these problem-solving steps: (a) What am I supposed to do? (b) I need to figure out what to DO, (c) What will HAPPEN? (d) I need to make a choice, and (e) I need to find out how I did. Early sessions use simple tasks and games to teach the problem-solving steps and to practice not responding impulsively. The therapist prompts the child/teen verbally and nonverbally to guide the actions and provide a lot of praise as well as give specific feedback for performance. The therapist also models appropriate ways of performing. Children begin sessions with tokens that can be exchanged for prizes after the session. During the session, the child can lose chips for not using the steps. The therapist uses social reinforcement and extinction to shape behaviors. Studies have shown that "PMT and PSST alone or in combination produce reliable and significant reductions in oppositional, aggressive, and antisocial behavior, and increases in prosocial behavior among children" (Weisz & Kazdin, 2017, p. 153). There is a session-by-session guide but no published treatment manual yet. The website is yaleparentingcenter.yale.edu/store.

Cognitive Behavioral Therapy

Cognitive behavioral therapy (CBT) is the most recommended psychotherapy for children older than 8 years old, and adolescents. The theory and development of CBT is presented in Chapter 8. CBT is a brief, time-limited psychotherapy that focuses on cognitive restructuring, behavioral activation (increasing pleasurable activities), and problem-solving. CBT has been adapted to be developmentally appropriate for children with their concrete cognition and for adolescents who, as they enter puberty, start thinking abstractly. The 2018 updated *Guidelines for Adolescent Depression in Primary Care: Treatment and Ongoing Management* reaffirms that CBT has been shown to be effective in treating adolescents with major depressive disorder in tertiary care as well as in community settings (Cheung et al., 2018). See Table 21.3 for research on CBT with children and adolescents.

In CBT sessions, young people identify their strengths and goals and map out the path with steps to work toward their goals. Parents are invited to participate in the sessions as their child learns the CBT model of cognitive restructuring–explained as "catch it, check it, change it." The child/teen practices and learns to quickly catch negative or not very accurate thoughts ("I always mess up. I am a loser"), then challenge that thought ("Is it true? Is it always true all the time? Or is there an alternative, more realistic explanation?"). Then the child is asked to change the "dysfunctional," not accurate thought to a positive, more accurate thought. For behavioral activation, the child/teen identifies activities that he or she enjoys and makes a plan to spend more time with those activities. Parents can help schedule bike riding time or time for teens to throw a ball to their dog and reinforce the importance of pleasurable activities. Problem-solving is taught throughout the CBT program, both in identifying their own problematic thoughts and solving ways to modify those, as well as learning how to solve problems with peers and tough situations at school and at home. Children and teens seem to enjoy the feeling of accomplishment when they figure out their own thoughts that are not accurate, and they identify the strategy that works best for them to deal with problematic triggers and thoughts. CBT is time limited, usually 4 to 14 sessions (Beck, 2011). Manuals are colorful, clear, concise, and interesting. CBT for children and adolescents is often conducted using treatment manuals. Commonly used manuals are included in Table 21.4.

In choosing a manual for CBT for the child, the APPN utilizes the Piaget stages of cognitive development when choosing the CBT treatment manual for the patient. For children 7 to 11 years who think concretely, the COPE (Creating Opportunities for Personal Empowerment) for Children manual is used. The content and examples in the child manual are colorful and include colorful activities appropriate for the child who thinks concretely. The COPE teen manual (for youth that have reached the Piaget stage of formal operations) has skill building activities and case examples at a higher level. The teen patient is challenged to use abstract thinking to "solve" the situations in the case study. In practice, the APPN will get a sense of the stage of thinking of the child/teen through talking with him or her in the initial assessment. Asking the child/teen to interpret a proverb provides information for the therapist re: if the child/teen thinks abstractly and the teen manual will be appropriate for him or her. For those pre-teens or teens where developmental level/intellectual ability is not clearly in the "formal operations" stage, the therapist can share both the child and teen CBT manual with the patient and parent and ask which manual will be best.

TABLE 21.3   CBT RESEARCH: SELECTED RANDOMIZED CLINICAL TRIALS AND META-ANALYSES

Author	Study	Results
Meta-Analyses/Systematic Reviews		
Weersing, Jeffreys, Do, Schwartz, and Bolano (2017)	Evidence base update of psychosocial treatments for child and adolescent depression. Review of 42 RCTs 2008–2014	Evidence for child treatments are notably weaker than for adolescent interventions. CBT for depressed children is possibly efficacious. For depressed adolescents both CBT and interpersonal psychotherapy are well established interventions with evidence of efficacy in multiple trials by independent investigative teams.
Higa-McMillan, Francis, Najarian, and Chorpita (2016)	Evidence base update: 50 years of research on treatment for child and adolescent anxiety. 111 treatment studies examined. 1967– mid 2013	This review "suggests substantial support for CBT as an appropriate and first line treatment for youth with anxiety disorders." There are other treatment approaches that were probably efficacious.
Williams, O'Connor, Eder, and Whitlock (2009)	Systematic Evidence Review for the U.S. Preventive Services Task Force (USPSTF). Recommendation for screening for Adolescent Depression in Primary Care	Ten fair- or good-quality RCTs evaluated short-term efficacy of psychotherapy among 757 children or adolescents aged 9–18 years. Most psychotherapy trials demonstrated an improvement in depression symptoms based on proportion achieving remission, change in mean depression score, or improved global functioning. USPSTF recommended screening with follow up and cognitive behavioral therapy or interpersonal therapy available.
Watanabe, Hunot, Omori, Churchill, and Furukawa (2007)	Systematic Review: Psychotherapy for depression among children and adolescents. 27 studies included in meta-analysis	At post treatment, psychotherapy was superior to usual care, and wait list CBT and IPT were effective therapies for treatment of adolescent and child depression. 6 months post treatment the superiority was not significant. No adverse effects were reported in any of the studies.

(continued)

TABLE 21.3 CBT RESEARCH: SELECTED RANDOMIZED CLINICAL TRIALS AND META-ANALYSES (*CONTINUED*)		
Author	**Study**	**Results**
Zhou et al. (2019)	Meta-analysis published in JAMA Psychiatry–Comparison of types and acceptability of psychotherapies for acute anxiety disorders of children and adolescents.	101 unique trials included. Group CBT was significantly more effective than the other psychotherapies; for acceptability, CBT bibliotherapy had more discontinuations, in terms of quality of life, and functional improvement CBT (delivered in different ways) was significantly beneficial compared to placebo and wait list conditions.
Reynolds, Wilson, Austin, and Hooper (2012)	Meta-analysis of 55 RCTs. Effects of psychotherapy for anxiety in children and adolescents	Psychotherapy for specific disorders had larger effects than generic therapy. Effect size for CBT interventions was higher. Individual therapy had larger effects than group therapy. Studies need effective follow up and cost effectiveness analysis.
Yang et al. (2017)	Systematic Review and Meta-Analysis: Efficacy and acceptability of CBT for depression in children less than 13 years old	Most studies are re: depression in adolescents, so a study of depression in children is a great contribution to the literature. At posttreatment CBT was significantly more effective than control conditions in decreasing depressive symptoms and permission of depression. CBT had no more discontinuations than control. Still there are small size ($n = 9$) of trials.

(continued)

TABLE 21.3 CBT RESEARCH: SELECTED RANDOMIZED CLINICAL TRIALS AND META-ANALYSES (CONTINUED)

Author	Study	Results
Randomized Clinical Trials		
Kennard et al. (2009)	TADS (2004–2007) Treatment of Adolescent Study multisite RCT comparing four conditions: (1) CBT 15 session (2) fluoxetine (3) combination CBT/ fluoxetine (4) pill placebo. N = 439	Combination superior to other conditions which were ns 12-week response: 43% vs. 61% vs. 71% vs. 35% 12-week remission: 16% vs. 23% vs. 37 % vs. 17% At 18 weeks CBT outcomes were comparable to fluoxetine
Rohde, Waldron, Turner, Brody, and Jorgensen (2014)	RCT comparing three conditions (1) CWD-A coping with depression-adolescent 12 session CBT then FFT (functional family therapy) vs. (2) FFT then CWD-A, vs. (3) coordinated CWD-A + FFT	Post treatment depression: 45% CWD-A/FFT vs. 44% FFT.CWD-A vs. 52% coordinated Tx. 60% depression remission across conditions by 1 yr. follow up. CWD-A is a manualized CBT program that has been studied since 1990. Developed by Lewinsohn & Clarke
Rohde, Clarke, Mace, Jorgensen, and Seeley (2004)	RCT two conditions (1) CWD-A (adolescents only) vs. (2) life skills/tutoring (matched on duration & modality) N = 93	Post treatment MDD recovery: 39% vs. 19% (sig. difference) MDD recovery rates at 1-month follow up 63% vs. 63%
Clarke et al. (2005)	Two conditions: (1) individual CWD-A CBT (5–9) sessions, + usual care SSRI vs. (2) Usual care SSRI	Remission 6 wk. follow up: 57% vs. 43% Remission 12 wk. follow up: 77% vs. 72% Remission 53 wk. follow up: 89% vs. 94% (all ns)

(continued)

TABLE 21.3   CBT RESEARCH: SELECTED RANDOMIZED CLINICAL TRIALS AND META-ANALYSES (*CONTINUED*)

Author	Study	Results
Walkup et al. (2008)	Child-Adolescent Anxiety Multi-Modal Study CAMS. Compared Kendall's Coping Cat CBT for youth, sertraline SSRI, COMBINATION, and pill placebo. 488 children ages 7–17 yrs.	Results: 80% of youth who receive COMB were found to be improved or very much improved. Both CBT 60% and medication 55% were also significantly better than placebo (24%), Coping Cat is a manualized CBT program, which is the gold standard in CBT for anxiety in children studies. The majority (>80%) of acute responders maintained positive response at both weeks 24 and 36. Consistent with acute outcomes, COMB maintained advantage over CBT and SRT.
Dickerson et al. (2018)	Important RCT cost-effectiveness of CBT for depressed youth declining antidepressants in pediatrics	Assessment of a brief CBT program for depressed adolescents in primary care. vs. treatment as usual over 12 months. Random assignment of 212 youth. Costs calculated per QALY. Brief primary care CBT is cost-effective – becomes more dominant over TAU over time as revealed by a statistically significant cost offset at end of 2 yr. follow up.
Melnyk et al. (2013)	RCT – COPE CBT program delivered in classrooms of culturally diverse high school students. $N = 779$ students, vs. attention control in the same high schools. Delivered by teachers in 9th grade health class	Results measured post intervention and 6 and 12 months post intervention. The students with significantly elevated depression scores pre-intervention had the most robust improvement in depression. There were also improvements in health (decreased BMI, better school attendance).

TABLE 21.4 SELECTED CBT MANUALS FOR CHILDREN / ADOLESCENTS		
CBT Manuals	**Authors**	**Description**
"Coping Cat"	Kendall & Hedtke (2006)	CBT manual for children with anxiety
"CWD-A"	Lewisohn, Clarke, Hops, and Andrews (1990)	CBT manual: Coping with depression/adolescence
"COPE for Teens"	Melnyk (2003a)	CBT manual for teens' anxiety/depression
"COPE Child"	Melnyk (2003)	CBT manual for children's anxiety/depression

CBT, cognitive behavioral therapy; COPE, Creating Opportunies for Personal Empowerment.

In CBT, following the Beck model, sessions have this consistent structure (Beck, 2011).

- Check in–Bridge from previous session
- Setting the agenda
- Homework/action plan review
- Work on problems
- Summary
- Feedback (both ways)
- Assign action plan/ homework

CBT manuals typically follow this CBT session structure. The agenda is set for each session in manuals for children and adolescents. The child/adolescent CBT session will begin with a "check in" with the young person as he or she arrives for the session. This "check in" allows for risk assessment as well as monitoring symptoms, progress, and current concerns in his or her life. Next, the therapist asks the child/adolescent what he or she has written in the last session's homework pages. CBT manuals include homework pages, now called "action plans," for each session so the skills learned in the session with the therapist can be applied to the child's or teen's home, school, and social life during the week. Homework pages with drawings or matching activities are generally used with the children; however, the adolescent pages look more like a traditional workbook with some questions and some illustrations. The questions ask how the skills from last week's session with the therapist were helpful in specific situations during the teen's week. After the check in and review of the homework "action plan," the therapist reads the content from the child or teen manual.

The core CBT theme that is reinforced in every session is: How you think (cognition) affects how you feel and how you behave. This is generally represented as a Thinking, Feeling, Behaving Triangle (Melnyk, 2003a). See Figure 21.1. The Thinking, Feeling, Behaving Triangle is reviewed each session. The sessions use this framework to discuss content on self-concept, dealing with emotions (self-regulation), problem-solving, thoughts, feelings, and actions associated with anxiety and depression and strategies for coping with emotions in healthy ways. Several evidence-based coping strategies are taught such as: self-talk, guided imagery, staying in the moment, thought stopping, deep breathing, exercise, and seeking out someone to talk with.

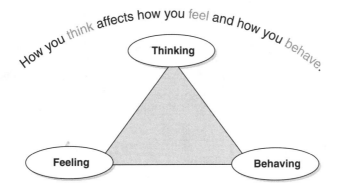

FIGURE 21.1 Cognitive behavioral therapy theme

Source: Used with permission from Melnyk, B. M. (2003a). Creating Opportunities for Personal Empowerment (COPE) manual for teens. Retrieved from https://www. cope2thrive.org

This is an explanation of the Thinking, Feeling, Behaving Triangle using a child example:

Two children are walking down the sidewalk—Mary and Tony. They look down and see an anthill with a lot of ants crawling in circles and lines. Mary <u>thinks</u> (her cognition), "I think ants are such interesting insects." She <u>feels</u> excited to see all the ants and the anthill. She <u>bends down</u> and moves to observe the ants closely (behavior). Tony, on the other hand, sees the moving ants and <u>thinks</u>, "Oh no, I have heard if an ant bites you, you could swell up and die. I might die." With that cognition, or <u>thought</u>, Toby <u>feels</u> fear, and Toby is breathing fast as he <u>runs away</u> (behavior). The two children had very different thoughts about the "trigger"—the anthill with busy ants. Their thoughts affected their feelings and then how they acted (behavior).

The therapeutic alliance is central to CBT. In CBT, the APPN takes an active role, checking in at the beginning of the session, reviewing and assigning homework, eliciting feedback from the child/teen, and presenting the actual session content with fidelity to the manual, but also with enough flexibility that the examples the child or teen provides can be explored individually. This has been termed "fidelity with flexibility" (Beidas & Kendall, 2014, p. 233). The APPN summarizes the session and reviews the action plan for putting the skills learned into practice in the next week. The APPN establishes a therapeutic alliance with the child/teen and his or her parent and works collaboratively with the young person, as the child/teen becomes a detective, figuring out his or her own thoughts, feelings, and behaviors and identifies coping strategies that work well for him or her. The child/teen becomes an active participant in this present-oriented psychotherapy. The APPN also keeps the intervention, examples, and homework developmentally appropriate. For example, with younger children, before they can start the program, they use flashcards to learn what is a thought (usually a sentence, I am looking forward to that class), a feeling (sad, mad, happy), and what is a behavior (kicking the bike, running away, dancing for joy).

Parents and children/ adolescents are taught to be their own therapists. As they finish the CBT program, they review what they have learned and plan for situations that might come up in the future that will trigger negative, not so accurate thoughts, strong feelings, or behaviors that aren't helpful, and they review the coping strategies that they have been practicing so that coping skills they learned are strong and available when they face challenges.

Training Opportunities for CBT with Children

The Beck Institute offers 3-day basic CBT workshops at the Beck Training Institute as well as online trainings in CBT. The CBT for Children and Adolescents 3-day workshop is available at the Beck Institute in Philadelphia, Pennsylvania. Its website is beckinstitute .org/get-training/. When ordering the Kendall Coping Cat Manual, there is an accompanying therapist manual. For the COPE manuals, there is an online training available at cope2thrive.com.

CBT CASE STUDY

Chris is a 13-year-old eighth grader who was referred to the APPN by his pediatrician for assessment of possible attention deficit disorder (ADD). Chris's medical record indicates he is having difficulties at home and at school. Chris came to the initial evaluation accompanied by his mother. He is average height and weight, dressed neatly in jeans and t-shirt. He was wearing a baseball cap and looked down, averting direct eye contact. He chose the chair next to the wall and leaned against the wall throughout the visit. His mood was predominantly sad, with an irritable tone to his voice. He always responded when he was asked a question. His responses were always appropriate to the question, but minimal, usually only two or three words. He shrugged when asked why he was referred to the APPN and said, "Ask her" as he pointed to his mother. Mom reports he is constantly aggravating his three older sisters. She added, "He can't walk into a room with them without slamming their laptop closed, tapping them on the shoulder, or scattering their papers." His difficulty at school was described as "a change in behavior," which was a concern for his main teacher. The teacher called Chris's parents to tell them Chris has been avoiding his friends and spending most of his time alone during school breaks outside on the grass field. He is not concentrating on his schoolwork and his usual good grades have dropped.

Chris said "Yes," he feels terrible most of the time. He endorsed irritability and depression. He denied any thoughts of self-harm or suicide. He and his mom relate comfortably. He was very respectful with her and if he responded to a question at the same time she did, he would, say, "Sorry mom" and wait for her to speak. We agreed to have the Vanderbilt questionnaires filled out to r/o ADD. Chris has no history of ADD. He has always made good grades and focused well at school and at home. He had not been paying attention as well lately at school, and has "poor concentration" according to the teacher.

On Chris's return visit to the clinic, the Vanderbilt questionnaires returned by Chris's parents and his teacher were reviewed. He did not score positively for ADD or ADHD; rather, his anxiety and depression scores were elevated. We discussed a treatment plan. His mother was very interested in Chris getting into counseling and added that it is "awful for her and her husband to see Chris feel so bad." He is "not himself." The parents have been to the school where they were told about bullying going on in the Jr. High, with one boy in particular identified as the leader of a group of eighth grade students who yell loud insults to individuals at recess. Chris's mother says Chris is asking more and more to stay home from school. He seemed depressed and anxious. As the issues at school are discussed, Chris mostly shrugs, is not very verbal, but appears sad, almost tearful and shakes his head yes, he is depressed. He adds he always feels terrible and does not want to go to school and be exposed to that popular kid (the bully). Chris said he doesn't care whether he comes for counseling or not, but his mom interjects that she wants him to feel better, and says she will schedule the sessions and bring him on Fridays when he doesn't have school. He nodded and softly said OK.

We reviewed the CBT manual we would be using because Chris is 13 and cognitive development can vary between preteens and early teens. Chris and his mom reviewed both the child CBT manual and the teen CBT manual and they chose the teen manual. Chris has reached the developmental level of formal operations according to the Piaget Cognitive Stages of Development Model (Piaget, 1936). In the initial psychiatric evaluation with the APPN, Chris was able to interpret a proverb abstractly. This confirms he has entered the formal operational stage of development. Chris, in this developmental stage, which is consistent with his chronological age, is able to think abstractly, logically test hypotheses, and use more mature moral reasoning (Piaget, 1936). See Table 21.1.

Chris's CBT sessions were set up for weekly Friday appointments. For the CBT program used by the APPN, COPE, the visits are 30 minutes (Lusk & Melnyk, 2011b). Brief visits are appreciated by teens and their parents. Each session in the manual can be covered easily in 30 minutes and the homework/action plan serves to "extend the session" as the content is reviewed during the week. Chris came accompanied by his mother for his sessions and continued his minimal but appropriate responses the first couple of sessions. He always wore a baseball cap pulled down over his eyes, so eye contact was minimal. It was clear that he was listening to the session content by his responses to the questions about the examples in the manual. As he continued the sessions, he did the homework pages, with his mom's urging, and he began warming up and started arguing with the therapist about statements and questions in the COPE lessons (indicative of his abstract thinking and developing moral reasoning abilities). He was very bright, and very good at presenting arguments for his point of view. He was interested in the COPE session content and liked to offer his opinion of the examples. As he developed an alliance with the therapist, he became more forthcoming with his thoughts and feelings, and he explained his thought about his experience at school, "What you (therapist, mom) have to understand is, I am a loser. Yes, J. teases me on the playground, but bullies want kids like me to know I am a loser. Popular kids like J. always have lots of friends around them, losers like me don't have many friends." Chris's negative <u>thought</u> (cognition) "I am a loser" was held by him as the Truth. He described <u>feeling</u> depressed, discouraged, hopeless, and resigned to his loser status. He dreaded going to the school playground. His <u>behavior</u> had become avoidant. He was isolating himself from his friends and asking every day to stay home from school.

The Socratic questioning used in CBT was presented as "Suppose I (therapist) am a Superior Court Judge. What is your evidence that you are a loser?" This CBT approach was very effective with this bright, argumentative 13-year-old. He found it interesting to challenge his own negative thoughts. He agreed with his mother that he has real strengths and abilities. He has always maintained good grades, has always been incredibly good at math, and was the computer whiz at school and especially at home. He was often thanked by his parents and sisters for problem-solving computer issues. He likes spending time building things with his dad and his goal is to work with his dad and then take over the family business. When asked to list the evidence that he is a loser, he had a hard time providing the proof. He identified: He has not grown up a loser and isn't a loser at home. He is not a loser at academics. He is not a loser as far as athletic ability. He has played the usual team sports at the school. He isn't a loser in the classroom, the teacher respects him (his mother concurred). He isn't a loser with his three good friends that have been together since kindergarten and share the same interests in computer games. He does believe that popular kids like J. always have about 10 friends with them on the playground and he has only a few friends, so that is less than J. and J. is louder.

Chris became increasingly active in the COPE sessions, and by the time he finished the seven sessions he had some coping strategies for dealing with his discomfort and stress at school. In fact, he became more assertive with peers at school. As far as cognitive restructuring, he re-examined his belief/thought that he is a "loser" and came to the conclusion he in fact is *not* a loser at all in most of his life. Instead, he identified his strengths at school: He is intelligent, he is very good at debate, and he is very talented with building and with computers. Chris became able to sort out what was accurate about the bully's comments and what was just name-calling (cognitive restructuring). He became more aware of the bully's routine communication, that of name-calling, and realized he wasn't the only recipient of the mean remarks. His friends were also being called names and they could stick together through the stressful times on the playground. For behavioral activation, he returned to his time on the school field, walking and talking with his friends during school breaks. He also tried, with his parents' encouragement, to spend more time in the workshop with his dad. They enjoyed building things out of wood for the home. Problem-solving was Chris's area of strength and he thoroughly enjoyed all the problem-solving situations in the CBT manual. He would always take the problem to a higher level, and then work through the possible solutions and choose the best one. He also was able to sort out the solutions to his "bully" problem and strategize a way to solve his misery at school. As he completed the seven CBT sessions from the COPE manual, Chris's mood clearly lifted. His vitality returned. He had stopped begging to stay home from school and his sisters and mom thought it was OK if he was in the room with them. His mother attended all the sessions with him, as she was also really interested in learning the CBT approach. His dad came for one of the sessions to meet the therapist and experience a session. Both parents were genuinely impressed with Chris's ability to come up with his own strategy for changing his situation and they told him so. Chris basked in the praise and it was clear he was proud of himself. Post CBT depression and anxiety questionnaires indicated he was no longer seriously depressed. Chris was seen yearly for the next 4 years, just to check in with the therapist when he was at the clinic for his yearly visit with the pediatrician. At the most recent visit, he was happy to see the therapist. He reports he is a high school junior but is taking some college courses. He is still very talented at working with computers and describes himself as "an IT guy"; he helps family, friends, and teachers at school when there are computer problems. In the visit, his mother thought back to his COPE, CBT sessions. She asked, "Chris, are there bullies at your school now?" He thought for awhile, looked puzzled, and said, "No, I don't think so." He doesn't remember much about the specific CBT content from the sessions, but remembers the Thinking, Feeling, Behaving Triangle diagram that was in every session. He can still give an example of how his thoughts affect his feelings and his behavior.

As Chris moved through the seven COPE CBT sessions, he was able to explore and evaluate his self "identity." Chris began to move from Erikson's stage of "school age" self-evaluation based on how well one performs" tasks "in comparison to peers (e.g., when Chris first came for evaluation and stated he was a "loser" based on his school yard performance), to Erikson's stage of development—more focused on "identity." In the CBT sessions, Chris explored his individual strengths, abilities, and goals for his life. As he explored his contributions to his family, at school and with friends, he began to identify a possible future adult role, what Erikson refers to as "occupational identity" (e.g., When he described himself, at his yearly check-in when he was finishing his last year of high school, he stated: "I am an IT guy," and told of his IT responsibilities and specialty knowledge).

Eye Movement Desensitization and Reprocessing Therapy

As APPNs embark to work with the patients within the general population, it is important to know that Eye Movement Desensitization and Reprocessing (EMDR) therapy has been proven to be effective in treating children and adolescents with mental health disorders including PTSD, depression, anxiety, and phobias (Shapiro, 2018). The use of EMDR therapy with children is a successful approach to help children overcome trauma symptoms from a variety of causes including medical conditions and adverse childhood events in children (Barron, Bourgaize, Lempertz, Swinden, & Darker-Smith, 2019). EMDR therapy helps distressing memories to lose their tenacity and impact on the limbic system, which ultimately affects one's somatic and cognitive sense of self and safety (Adler-Tapia & Settle, 2017; Shapiro, 2018). The basics of applying EMDR therapy as a therapeutic approach with children allows for children to become experts in their own trauma and for the APPN to help children reprocess traumatizing experiences in an adaptive way to decrease PTSD and anxiety-related symptoms (Adler-Tapia & Settle, 2017). See Table 21.5 for selected EMDR research with children and adolescents.

When working with a child, it is evident that one's fight and flight reaction to adversity startles the young mind, leading to a disruption in executive functioning, blocking thoughts and affecting emotional reactions to perceived benign situations (Greenwald, 1999). This often manifests as problems in focusing and academic struggles as well as emotional dysregulation, which many times mimics symptoms of ADHD. Attachment theory (Bowlby, 1988) says that healing the traumatized child will allow for stability in the mind-body connection, allowing for interpersonal connection to take place. This, in turn, allows for trusting relationships with others to be possible and healthy adult–child

TABLE 21.5   EMDR RANDOMIZED CLINICAL TRIALS WITH CHILDREN AND ADOLESCENTS

Author	Study	Results
Ahmad, Larsson, and Sundelin-Wahlsten (2007)	EMDR for 33 children (ages 6–16) diagnosed with PTSD and with various traumatic experiences. EMDR for 8 weekly sessions.	Posttraumatic Stress Symptom Scale for Children: Treatment group demonstrated decreased PTSD-related symptoms compared with waitlist control.
Brown et al. (2017)	Meta-analysis of 36 RCTs. Reviewed therapies for children after disasters	CBT, EMDR, KIDnet, and classroom-based interventions are effective and demonstrated significant reductions in PTSD with large effect sizes in pre-post comparisons.
Chemtob, Nakashima, and Carlson (2002)	ABA design brief therapy with EMDR	Substantial sustained improvement in PTSD symptoms compared with waitlist control.
Chen et al. (2018)	Reviewed six RCTs for PTSD in children and adults with complex trauma	EMDR-reduced PTSD symptoms, depression, and/or anxiety post tx and at follow-up compared with CBT, individual/group therapy, and fluoxetine.

(continued)

TABLE 21.5   EMDR RANDOMIZED CLINICAL TRIALS WITH CHILDREN AND ADOLESCENTS (*CONTINUED*)

Author	Study	Results
de Roos et al. (2017)	Explored efficacy of EMDR and CBT writing therapy on PTSD as a result of single trauma	Large effect size for both CBT and EMDR; large remission rates for PTSD and comorbid problems in children and adolescents; both tx were well tolerated as compared to waitlist controls; post after 6 wks and follow-ups at 3 & 6 months after only six sessions.
de Roos et al. (2009)	EMDR vs. CBT (fireworks explosion)	Substantial sustained improvement in PTSD symptoms and EMDR; fewer sessions required
Diehle, Opmeer, Boer, Mannarino, and Lindauer (2015)	48 (8–18 yr. old) Treated with TF-CBT or EMDR	Clinician-administered PTSD scale for children and adolescents (CAPS-CA); difference in reduction was small and not statistically significant. Significant effect for time for EMDR vs. TF-CBT. Both EMDR and TF-CBT were effective with reducing PTSD in children.
Farkas, Cyr, Lebeau, and Lemay (2010)	40 adolescents with conduct problems (all under youth protective services due to maltreatment)	Diagnostic Interview Schedule for Children (DISC) and Trauma Symptom Checklist for Children (TSCC). Significantly greater decreases in PTSD symptoms post-test and at 3-month follow up. Significantly greater decreases in depression and anxiety scores post-test in those who received EMDR compared to those who received routine care.

(*continued*)

TABLE 21.5 EMDR RANDOMIZED CLINICAL TRIALS WITH CHILDREN AND ADOLESCENTS (*CONTINUED*)		
Author	**Study**	**Results**
Jaberghaderi, Greenwald, Rubin, Zand, and Dolatabadim (2004)	CBT vs. EMDR with sexually abused Iranian girls ages 12–13.	Child Report of Posttraumatic Symptoms and Parent Report of Post-traumatic Symptoms (PROPS) showed decrease in symptoms post-treatment. A decrease in PTSD symptoms for both treatments: EMDR had fewer sessions. No statistical significance due to lack of statistical power; however, EMDR showed greater treatment efficacy in a shorter period of time compared to CBT. 6.1 (mean) sessions as opposed to 11.6 (mean) sessions.
Khan et al. (2018)	Meta-analysis comparing 14 RCTs	Found that EMDR is better than CBT in reducing posttraumatic symptoms and anxiety; however, four studies found no difference at 3-month follow-up; there was no difference in reducing depression.
Kemp, Drummond, and McDermott (2010)	27 children and adolescents who experienced a single motor vehicle accident, waitlist control (EMDR tx for 6 weeks every 7–10 days)	PTSD diagnostic criteria and Child Posttraumatic Stress-Reaction Index; Child Postraumatic Stress Reaction (parent) and Impact of Event Scale (IES). PTSD was reduced dramatically (25% positive DSM criteria) in EMDR vs. control (100% positive DSM criteria). PTSD decreased over time and sustained at 12 months.

(*continued*)

TABLE 21.5 EMDR RANDOMIZED CLINICAL TRIALS WITH CHILDREN AND ADOLESCENTS (*CONTINUED*)

Author	Study	Results
Moreno-Alcázar et al. (2017)	Meta-analysis of 8 EMDR efficacy for children with PTSD sx.	EMDR was superior to waitlist control and showed comparable efficacy to CBT in reducing posttraumatic and anxiety symptoms; depression symptoms were reduced but were not statistically significant.
Soberman, Greenwald, and Rule (2002)	29 male adolescents with conduct disorder with complex trauma in RCT or day treatment standard care vs. standard plus 3 sessions of EMDR.	Impact of Event Scale (IES), Child Report of Posttraumatic Symptoms and Parent Report of Posttraumatic Symptoms (PROPS). EMDR group had greater decreases in PROPS scores post-test, and a trend for greater decreases in IES scores at 2-month follow-up.
Wanders, Serra, and de Jongh (2008)	EMDR vs. CBT for behavioral problems	EMDR produced larger changes in target behaviors. Increase in self-esteem scores (significant increases). Significant decreases in behavioral problems as reported by parents.

CBT, cognitive behavioral therapy; DSM, Diagnostic and Statistical Manual of Mental Disorders; EMDR, eye movement desensitization and reprocessing; PTSD, posttraumatic stress disorder; RCTs, randomized control trials; sx, symptoms; TF-CBT, trauma-focused cognitive behavioral therapy; tx, treatment.

relationships to develop. Children are dependent on their environment and the people in it for emotional stability. Depending on the age of the child, it may be essential for a successful EMDR therapy child session to include parental figures or caregivers in sessions to ensure safety and promote nurturing. Safety is a foundational need in order to be successful in growth and development. As the APPN works with children, establishing a safe environment is imperative.

A friendly, open space allows for the child to explore his or her surroundings with age-appropriate toys and objects that can allow for engagement of the therapeutic relationship. Essential to the beginning stages of EMDR therapy, the therapist helps the child to establish a safe place/space in a play space that allows for exploration of other feelings or emotions that may be difficult to manage. The steps to conducting a successful and therapeutic EMDR therapy session with a child differs from child to child. No two children are alike, and it is important for the APPN to be flexible in his or her approach in accessing memories, reprocessing them, and ensuring a return to a stable place at the conclusion of each session. Ensuring that the APPN uses the framework of the eight phases of EMDR therapy with the child is essential. Children seem to reprocess traumatic life events faster and more fluidly than adults if the therapeutic environment is stable enough to ensure safety and healthy attachments are present (Adler-Tapia & Settle, 2017). See Table 7.4 in Chapter 7, for the eight phases of EMDR. The following are some adaptations of the phases for children:

Phase 1: History Taking/Case Conceptualization/Treatment Planning Phase: This phase involves a few steps to ensure the emotional safety of the child; this, in turn, allows for the APPN and child to establish rapport. This is a time of exploration in a neutral safe environment for the child through drawing, play, or talking/playing games. Essential in Phase 1 is the assessment of dissociation through parent interviews and observation of the child during play sessions. See emdrtherapyvolusia.com/wp-content/uploads/2016/12/Child_Dissociative_Checklist_Packet-1.pdf for the Child Dissociative Checklist (CDC) assessment and scoring for dissociation. This may take several sessions with and without the parent to allow for symptoms to present themselves in a therapeutic space. The APPN may also need to collaborate with school or daycare staff to assess for dissociation or self-harm or harm to others. Targets that are usually the disturbing event are identified for processing during this phase.

Phase 2: Preparation Phase: During this phase the APPN gathers informed consent for the child and family and educates the family and child on the use of EMDR therapy. Resource identification also takes place during this phase: The APPN assesses whether there are consistent care providers as well as whether there are healthy attachments present for the child and the identification of safe people and safe places for the child. The APPN also allows for exploration of resources for the child to allow for stabilization throughout treatment; for example, teaching meditation techniques, breathing exercises (see Chapter 8), calming exercises, and allowing for the imaging or drawing of a safe place/fun place or creating a safe container that holds negative thoughts and feelings about oneself. Children also need to be able to identify their feeling states during the assessment phase. This can happen by using emoji faces/expressions or exploring different cartoon characters/pictures of other children in discussing feeling states. As the APPN teaches and learns from the child what his or her "happy, sad, mad, confused, or fearful" states look and feel like in their bodies, the therapeutic relationship begins to develop. This is an important preparation phase of EMDR therapy for children and allows for the child to get in touch with how he or she feels and where he or she feels these feelings. As the APPN is educating the child and the child is educating the APPN, the parent or caregiver in the room is observing with the hopes that he or she will become more aware of what these feeling states look like in his or her child; that is, a child who shares that when his or her "belly hurts" he or she feels worried and scared or a child who states he or she feels "mixed up in the head" when he or she is confused and sad. Examples of accounts when he or she feels these things provides an opportunity to actively engage the parent or caregiver and helps outside the therapy session for healthy communication to take place at home.

Facilitating the creation of a happy/fun/calm place. Explore with the child what a happy/fun/calm place feels and looks like. This is a resource that the APPN will use throughout the EMDR therapy session. Creating a happy/fun/calm experience can take place in a sand tray as the child uses miniatures to create a world that feels happy/fun/calm or on paper as the child draws a happy/fun/calm place with colored pencils, crayons, or markers. Many children display creations that look very much like their home or school environments with safe people or animals that represent their calm place or a favorite vacation experience. Once a calm place is identified, the child is taught bilateral stimulation to tap in the resource. This helps stabilization to take place after reprocessing of traumatic or stressful events.

Creating a container. The APPN then engages the child in creating a container that will allow for containment of disturbing thoughts/feelings or memories that have come up in the reprocessing session. Many children build Lego-like structures, draw their container in three dimensions, or decorate a box/Tupperware bin to allow for the feelings and thoughts to stay in the office. An essential piece in developing the container is to allow the child to understand how to access the container, if needed, from home. Many times, imagining teleporting their thoughts or feelings to the office into the container is helpful. Some children benefit from taking a smaller container home with them and returning their container to the office each week to "dump" their negative feelings, thoughts, or beliefs into their "bigger "container. Sometimes a child will ask for help from his or her parents in writing down his or her thoughts on a sticky note to return to the office weekly.

The final portion of the preparatory phase for the child with EMDR therapy is the exploration of bilateral stimulation with the child via differing techniques, that is, following a finger puppet from left to right; watching a paintbrush safely touch the tops of hands from left to right; child holding buzzies in hands, in shoes, or on ears that make a buzzing sensation from left to right; or even using drumsticks from left to right with the APPN. The APPN teaches the child about bilateral stimulation and shows the child the stop sign to use if he or she becomes uncomfortable and wants to stop.

Phase 3: Assessment Phase: This begins by deciding what to work on (target). Many children use many different play vehicles, objects, dolls, and figurines to re-create the "bad thing that happened" in their play. The APPN helps each child to identify the disturbing event or expression of his or her "not so good" feelings with the image, negative cognition (NC), positive cognition (PC), validity of cognition (VoC), emotions, subjective units of disturbances scale (SUDS), and body sensations. Using a sand tray, drawing a picture, or using play figures to express the unpleasant feelings or event allows the child to express the NC. The APPN then asks the child what he or she would like to believe about himself or herself when thinking of the event to establish a PC and then ask how true that statement or the VoC feels to him or her now when he or she thinks of the event on a 1 to 7 scale, with 1 not at all and 7 very true. For example: "I am safe" when the child thinks of the bad thing that happened not feeling very true might be a 2. After asking the child about what feelings he or she has, the APPN measures the level of disturbance on a scale of 0 to 10 to establish the SUDS. One way to illustrate this is to show the child that his or her arms opened wide is a 10 and hands closed together is a 0. After this, the APPN asks the child where in his or her body the child feels the disturbance, that is, belly, head, heart, hands, or feet.

Phase 4: Desensitization Phase: Reprocessing begins here with the APPN using bilateral stimulation (BLS) in whichever form is most comfortable to the child. It is important to allow for the parent or caregiver to be close to the child. Sometimes the child sits in the parents' lap or beside them, which ensures that the child is safe and not alone (if helpful for the child, which should be established in the assessment phase). Bilateral stimulation continues until the SUDS goes down to a 0, taking breaks in between sets (approximately 20 bilateral movements) to allow for deep breathing and letting go of the emotion. The APPN notes the child's facial expressions; physical manifestations such as agitation, tears, or anger; and bodily sensations (if verbalized), and assures the child he or she is safe in the room, if necessary. If the child displays any signs of distress such as aggressive behavior toward the clinician, parent, or self, or if the child uses the stop signal, the APPN helps the child to re-establish safety and grounding with the parent figure or caregiver with a hug (if that feels safe for the child); the use of a transitional object such as a blanket, stuffed animal, and so on; swaying left and right; swinging in a swing or a hammock; or cuddling in a bean bag chair of some sort. This sense of safety and containment is helpful to allow for a womb-like experience to be felt by the child. This may also warrant returning to the child's happy/fun/calm place for stabilization with the parent and APPN for a brief period. As reprocessing continues, the child will learn to work through the negative emotion with ease and feel relief from symptoms of anxiety and distress. The child is now asked if anything in the sand tray or the picture needs to change. If so, the child can do so at this point. Remember that each child is different; one may work through reprocessing without the need to stabilize in between; in contrast, another child may need to go back and forth from the disturbing event to his or her happy/fun/calm place. This continues until the SUDS reaches a zero or no disturbance. When the SUDS is a zero, the Desensitization Phase is completed and therapy moves to the next phase.

Phase 5: Installation Phase: The Installation Phase begins when the APPN asks the child to bring the original target back up and asks if the original PC still makes sense or if there is one that fits better now. If it still makes sense, the same PC is used; if not, a new one can be chosen. The child can be assisted by showing cards with pictures of various PCs from an EMDR thought kit for kids (Gomez, 2009). When the new PC is chosen and the validity of cognition (VoC) is less than a 7; the APPN then uses BLS to strengthen the VoC to a 7.

Phase 6: Body Scan: At this point, the APPN asks the child to go back to the original target that he or she worked on via play/drawing or talk and has the child pick his or her PC. With a magnifying glass or a special detector, the child is asked to scan his or her body to look or feel for any "funny/weird" feelings that don't feel good to the child. If something is detected by the child, the APPN can use BLS while the child is focusing on the disturbance. This continues until the child notices a clear body scan with no disturbance.

Phase 7: Closure Phase: This phase can come about during the completion of a single incomplete session or during the completion of a particular target. The use of a container and calm place is helpful during this phase in between sessions or at the completion of the target in the process of EMDR therapy.

Containing negative thoughts, feelings, or memories. At the end of each reprocessing session, children need to be able to contain their emotions, memories, or negative thoughts. The APPN should instruct the child to "pour" bad feelings into his or her constructed containers. Sometimes this is done literally, such as children bowing their heads into a Lego structure as the APPN opens the top block, allowing for a safe opening to be able to be closed when they are done "emptying" their thoughts, or blowing their thoughts out through their mouths. Children should leave the therapeutic space with some level of relief. Engaging with their happy/fun/ calm place with slow BLS is key. Two to three sets of slow BLS can assist with this. The APPN engages the child and parent in a rhythmic swing or rocking motion to allow for engaging the child in calming/soothing his or her body. A hammock or a swing that can move from left to right is a great resource, or allowing the parent to hold the child and rock him or her from left to right slowly (if the child allows for such act to take place) is another great alternative.

Phase 8: Re-evaluation Phase: At the following session, the APPN spends time communicating with the parent/caregiver about any changes in behavior in between sessions, asking about eating and sleeping patterns. The APPN should also assess, by parent report, the child's adjustment/presentation in his or her home and school environment with other children/adults and/or pets. The child should also be asked if there are any feelings or thoughts that came up in between sessions. Some children will return their smaller container to empty or give the APPN pieces of paper that they and their parents wrote on that need to go into their containers. The APPN can re-assess the child by having him or her recreate the happy/fun/calm place in half of the sand tray/picture as well as his or her feeling state or negative feelings/disturbing event in the other half of the sand tray/picture. The APPN may note that the sand tray or picture changes dramatically, informing progress or regression. Each phase 3 to 8 should continue as the goal for each disturbing event is to decrease the SUD level to a 0 and increase the VOC to 7. At the end of EMDR therapy, parents/caregivers have observed and been active participants in their child's therapy session. This ensures that the parent/s have gained skills in assisting the child to calm his or her body and mind. Empowering parents with these tools is key to a successful re-integration in the home and school environment. APPNs should also collaborate with school staff such as teachers, counselors, paraprofessional staff, and primary care providers (if necessary) to allow for the child's holistic health to be a priority throughout therapy.

EMDR CASE STUDY

Session 1 (Phase 1): B is an 8-year-old male who resides at home with his mother, father, sister, and dog in a suburban town. B comes to the office with anxiety, phobia, loss of appetite, weight loss, and panic when he is in school. B is in the second grade. B verbalizes each morning to his mother that he "will die at school," resists getting on the bus each morning, and many times needs parental supervision to acclimate to the school environment at the beginning of the school day. B is overly consumed with fears of dying due to allergies, bee stings, and natural disasters. His home environment is conflictual with his parents arguing and threats of divorce have been overheard by B. He resides in a town in which a school shooting took place when he was in preschool. His parents report that B is unaware of the school shooting for "he hasn't asked or talked about it at home." The APPN noted that B was 4 years old at the time of the school shooting and at the onset of marital discord. Research indicates that the impact of trauma on the brain makes an imprint during precise developmental milestones (Adler-Tapia & Settle, 2017). This informed the APPN that B's cognitive development was in the preoperational phase where pretend play allows for accessing memories, thoughts, feelings, and belief systems. Thus, the approach for starting sand tray therapy with B was thought to be appropriate. According to Erikson's theory of development, B was navigating industry versus inferiority, and in his case fear and anxiety were overriding his ability to engage in his school environment to gain knowledge and develop new skills (Erikson, 1950).

B's anxiety symptoms started 6 months ago and have now necessitated intervention because the school counselor reported that B cannot tolerate being in the classroom without being disruptive to the school environment. Before B's first appointment, his APPN assessed the school environment by counselor report and Mom and Dad report. The counselor stated there is some marital discord, no friendship issues, and B has never asked about the school shooting nor has he watched any news media on the event because his parents are careful not to expose him to the news.

Session 2 (with child and parents; Phases 2 and 3): B presented to the office fidgety; he was hypervigilant as evidenced by looking behind his shoulder frequently and making eye contact with his mom and dad for reassurance. B explored the office space, playing with Legos and looking through the APPN's miniature collection. B was assisted to create a happy/fun/calm place in the sand tray. He created a recent trip to Florida with his family placing an airplane in the sand tray as well as trees and seashells. B and this APPN spent some time talking about the positive emotions of the calm place and getting to know all the things that B likes to do. He mentioned that he used to like soccer and baseball, but that he gets nervous on the field now. B was encouraged to create a container out of Legos that became a 4 × 4 box with no doors or windows and tightly closed in a pyramid fashion at the top, leaving no openings. B was instructed to think of all his mixed-up thoughts and put them in the container as the APPN opened the top of the pyramid structure. B leaned his head over and made a rushing water sound and emptied his mixed-up thoughts into the container. B was then asked if he liked a certain smell from an essential oil collection. B selected cinnamon, and as he focused on his fun/happy/calm place, he was taught the butterfly hug (an EMDR self-soothing technique) as he inhaled the smell of cinnamon. B took deep breaths while holding his cupped hands in front of his face like he was drinking an invisible bowl of soup. He inhaled the bowl of soup and then blew the soup, cooling it off slowly, focusing on belly breathing. B was then given a stack of sticky notes and a zip lock bag to take home, and he and his parents were instructed to write down the things that happen through the week that make him have mixed-up thoughts. B asked if he could take a little treasure chest home with him to put his worries in so he could bring them back to the office next week. The session then ended as he skipped out of the room.

Session 3: (Phases 3 to 7): B returned to the next session exclaiming how excited he was to bring his mixed-up feelings back to the office. B gave the APPN his smaller treasure box and he put them in his pyramid container. The APPN then continued the assessment phase. B was asked to share what home was like on one side of the sand tray and on the other side what school was like. B created the home environment by placing a play cell phone (mom) in the middle of the sand, a boy figure (self) with two guard robot men next to the boy, a little girl (sister) playing in a corner of the sand with My Little Pony figures, and a man figure (dad) in a separate corner up on a hill by himself laying down sleeping. All figures in the home environment were separated in different corners of the sand. When B was asked to share what school was like with the APPN, B placed a little boy (self) in the middle of the sand with snakes all around him, three little snakes (his teacher, the principal, and his school therapist), and one large snake (not designated by B as any particular person) draped across the sand tray. B was introduced to a BLS handheld tapping (buzzing) device and orientated to how it worked. B was excited to use the buzzies with one in each sock and stated they "feel good buzzing in my feet." B was asked to label the emotion in both sides of the sand tray. B stated "lonely" in his home environment, and "nervous" in the school environment. B was then asked what he believed about himself when he feels nervous; for example, "if he was wearing a T shirt that said something about himself when he felt nervous, what would it say?" B stated that, "It would say I am not safe." B was then asked how he would like to think about himself. He stated: "I am safe," which he rated as a 2/7 VOC. B was then asked to rate how much that bothered him from 0 to 10. B stated that he felt it big with his arms wide open as a 10 and that the feeling lived in his belly. B verbalized who each object stood for on each side of the sand tray without being asked. He then placed the buzzies in his sneakers as he focused his attention on his school environment with the buzzing left, then right (BLS). In between each set, B was asked to take a deep breath and let go of the feeling as well as rate the thought of feeling unsafe from 0 to 10. After 10 to 12 sets of BLS, B rated his level of unsafe to be a 0 and proceeded to remove the snakes from the school side of the sand tray, leaving only the boy by himself in the sand tray. B then moved onto playing with a truck in the office. B's focus was then redirected to his happy/fun/calm place with three to four slow sets of BLS. At the end of the session, the APPN removed the top Lego of the container to allow for B to let the negative thoughts, images, and feelings in the container. He walked outside to the hammock and his mom was asked to swing him in the hammock slowly as he closed his eyes and imagined his happy/fun/calm place. He left again with his treasure chest and holding his mom's hand.

Session 4: (Phases 3 to 7): Continuation of reprocessing: B arrived at the next session with the treasure chest as he emptied it into the bigger Lego container in the office, all by himself this time. B and the APPN discussed the week and how things were at school. B informed his APPN that he is afraid when he is on the playground at school. B stated that he again "was unsafe" and it was a big 10 feeling in his belly. The APPN asked B to use the sand tray to show the playground. B placed a boy in the middle of the sand tray with 10 to 12 army figures all around the boy with guns facing him. He then placed the big snake (the same one he used during the last session) in the middle of the sand tray. He asked for the buzzies to put in his sneakers again. The APPN handed the buzzies to him, letting him know that he can use the stop word like they had talked about in the last session if he wanted to stop. B continued to play in the sand tray, this time moving the figures around, taking a two-headed dragon and blowing all the army men out of the sand tray and throwing the snake out of the sand tray. He continued by replacing the army men with a few other boy-like figures in the sand. He then stated, "I'm done." The APPN asked him how big the unsafe was now. He stated, "It's all gone now." The session ended with a body scan and B swinging in the hammock, asking his mom to swing with him in the hammock. They swung for 15 minutes together.

Subsequent sessions (Phases 3 to 8): These continued through the reprocessing of the "unsafe" NC at school for two more sessions. Within 1 month, B was able to tolerate being in the classroom without event and started riding the bus to school with his peers. His parents were counseled on having a talk with him about the school shooting. Upon disclosure, he stated to the parents that he had known for months and was waiting for them to tell him about it. This conversation and sand tray EMDR therapy allowed B's anxiety symptoms to decrease, which helped him to re-socialize and play soccer and baseball again. These family conversations allowed B to reintegrate into a developmentally competent industrious school-aged boy, learning new skills and becoming social again, regaining Erikson's development stage of industry. B spent his summer at a local summer camp with no panic episodes.

RESOURCES FOR WORKING WITH CHILDREN

Technology advances are augmenting our practice and education. Telepsychiatry is an ever-expanding practice opportunity for APPNs and has dramatically increased access to mental healthcare for families who don't have accessible services in their communities. Therapists are practicing via the Internet in real time sessions with patients. See Chapter 4, on tele mental health. Virtual reality via goggles can provide exposure therapy in the office with virtual reality simulations, and adolescents can practice problem-solving skills with virtual school or peer situations. Therapeutic games can provide mastery experiences that are very engaging for children and adolescents. Applications or apps provide a way for children to record and measure healthy behaviors and/or chart moods. See Table 21.6.

Therapists are receiving training with avatars, virtual patients who respond to the therapist's questions and comments and provide a safe learning environment for acquiring new psychotherapy skills.

TABLE 21.6 APPS FOR CHILDREN		
Application Name	**Description**	**Usability/Cost**
MoodKit	-Exportable mood charts with 7- and 30-day views -Unlimited mood ratings and notes per day -Over 200 mood improvement activities -Includes a thought checker -Good for teens	-Easy to use -$4.99
Headspace: Mindfulness App	-Guided meditation -Good for teens.	-Easy to use -$12.99/month
Stop, Breathe, and Think Kids	40+ missions to develop the superpowers of quiet, focus, and a more peaceful sleep.	-Easy to use -Free
Breathe2Relax	-Stress reduction and stress management tool provides info on toxic stressors -Engages diaphragmatic breathing -Log level of stress -Good for teens	-Easy to use -Free
Optimism	-Mood charting app -Captures triggers that induce stress -Wellness planning -Good for teens	-Easy to use -Free
Calm Kids	-Mindfulness/Meditation through story telling/music/sound -Daily tracker -Age categories: teaching children meditative practices (all ages)	-Easy to use –$20.00
Finger Driver	-Left right (bilateral) games to allow for finger to drive a car on screen to initiate calming reflex. Ages 4+	-Easy to use- Free
CBT Tools for Youth	Allows children ages 4+ to label feelings, find level of the emotion, locate feeling in body, recognize tools to use to decrease negative emotions, and perform a guided muscle relaxation exercise within app.	-Easy to use- $2.99 a year
Binaural Beats	Ages 12+ Anxiety Stress/Relief app	-Easy to use- Free

Other resources for advanced practice psychiatric nurses who specialize with children include:

- *Journal of Child and Adolescent Psychiatric Nursing*
- American Psychiatric Nurses' Association—Child and Adolescent Council
- See Table 21.7 for resources for therapists and families

TABLE 21.7 RESOURCES FOR THERAPISTS AND FAMILIES	
Therapist Resources:	
American Academy of Child and Adolescent Psychiatry	www.aacap.org
American Academy of Pediatrics/ Mental Health Initiatives	www.aap.org/mentalhealth
Evidence-Based Child and Adolescent Psychosocial Interventions	www.aap.org/enus/Documents/ CRPsychosocialInterventions.pdf
State Statutes Child Abuse & Neglect	www.childwelfare.gov/topics/systemwide/ laws-policies/state
Best Children's Books About Mental Health	childmind.org/article/best-childrens-books-about-mental-health
Resources for Families:	
Facts for Families	www.aacap.org/aacap/families_and_youth/ facts_for_families/fff-guide/FFF-Guide-Home.aspx
Center for Disease Control and Prevention/ Children's Mental Health	www.cdc.gov/childrensmentalhealth/index. html
Reach Institute: Evidence-based mental health information for families	www.thereachinstitute.org
Attachment and Trauma Center of Nebraska: Free resources and free parent class for parents raising children with a history of trauma	www.atcnebraska.com

POST-MASTERS TRAINING FOR CBT & EMDR THERAPY

APPNs who love working with children and adolescents can have a challenging and rewarding career as a nurse psychotherapist. Graduates leave psychiatric mental health nurse practitioner (PMHNP) programs with beginning competencies in psychotherapy. Study, consultation, further training, and experience with different schools of psychotherapy and with different age groups allow students to "try on" the role of psychotherapist and see which therapeutic approach and which population resonates with them. As a licensed mental health provider, you will have many educational workshops available so you can develop expertise. Ongoing supervision with a master child therapist is essential for expert practice.

CBT Training

Beck Institute for CBT Training - CBT for Children & Adolescents, now also online. In order to achieve certification as a trauma-focused cognitive behavioral theraoy (TF-CBT) therapist, one must be a licensed mental health practitioner; participate in a live TF-CBT 2-day training; participate in 12 consultation sessions by an approved

TF-CBT consultant; complete three TF-CBT cases with measurable outcomes; and pass a TF-CBT knowledge-based exam. The criteria are available at tfcbt.org/TF-CBT-certification-criteria/

EMDR Therapy Training

Therapists start by participating in an Eye Movement Desensitization and Reprocessing International Organization (EMDRIA) approved basic training that is 50 hours, which includes 20 hours of didactic, 20 hours of practice and 10 hours of consultation. See Chapter 7. Some EMDRIA approved basic trainings focus on teaching therapists to work with developmentally grounded EMDR therapy focused on children (Adler-Tapia & Settle, 2017). There is also EMDR therapy advanced training to work with children available after basic training and certification in EMDR is completed. Additional training in EMDR therapy for working with children is available from:

- Ana Gomez, LPC: Online and in person intensives on EMDR with children as well as sand tray therapy with EMDR www.anagomez.org
- Robbie Adler-Tapia, PhD: Offers basic training and advanced training approved by the EMDRIA Institute with in-person training and remote clinical supervision https://www.drrobbie.org/trainings-workhops

CONCLUDING COMMENTS

Child/Adolescent specialists are on the forefront of some exciting trends in psychiatric/mental health practice. "There is accumulating evidence that some behavior problems can be prevented. Effective strategies include supporting parents' mental health, reducing exposure to stresses, helping parents learn to both read and help modulate infant's emotions, and helping parents learn ways to stimulate and have positive interactions with their infants and young children" (Adam & Foy, 2015, p. 203). Another prevention opportunity is the incorporation of psychoeducation into school health curriculums so that all children and teens receive instruction in mental health resources, coping strategies, and problem-solving knowledge and disemination about to build resilience. This is beginning to happen in response to school tragedies and the impact of ACEs on mental and physical health.

Integration of behavioral health into primary care/pediatric settings provides new practice opportunities for APPNs. Screening of all children for depression is recommended by the United States Preventive Services Task Force (USPSTF) and American Academy of Pediatrics. APPNs also advocate for routine screening for anxiety, substance use risk, and adverse childhood experiences in all health settings for children and adolescents. Early intervention is key to improving the trajectory of psychiatric disorders that begin in childhood and adolescence. Also, teaching and providing brief evidence-based interventions such as MI for young people at risk of substance use and other risky behaviors is essential.

In working with children and adolescents with common age-related adjustment struggles, those who have trauma and stressor-related disorders, and other psychiatric disorders that generally present in childhood, the nurse therapist can facilitate optimal growth and mastery. From what we know from neuroscience, change is always possible with children and teens, and the young person's ongoing growth and development is on the side of learning and positive outcomes as they work with the APPN in therapy. With so much potential for positive change, child and adolescent psychiatric/mental health nursing is an exciting and rewarding practice specialty for APPNs.

DISCUSSION QUESTIONS

1. Discuss your experiences with using evidence-based therapies in child/adolescent treatment.
2. Compare/contrast the development of a therapeutic relationship with adolescents versus adults.
3. Describe how the APPN can partner with parents in psychotherapy with adolescents/children.
4. Review the "Evidence-Based Child and Adolescent Psychosocial Interventions" chart at www.aap.org/en-us/Documents/CRPsychosocialInterventions.pdf
   What surprised you? What did you assume was an evidence-based intervention that has little evidence to support it?
5. Discuss the pros and cons of using therapy treatment manuals with children/adolescents.
6. Discuss the role of the therapist with the child who has experienced significant trauma.
7. How does the APPN conduct an initial interview with a child/adolescent differently than the initial psychiatric evaluation with an adult?
8. Describe how the APPN can integrate psychotherapy and pharmacotherapy in an outpatient practice.

REFERENCES

Adam, H., & Foy, J. (Eds). (2015). *Signs and symptoms in pediatrics*. Itasca, IL: American Academy of Pediatrics.

Adler-Tapia, R. (2012). *Child psychotherapy: Integrating developmental theory into clinical practice*. New York, NY: Springer Publishing Company.

Adler-Tapia, R., & Settle, C. (2017). *EMDR and the art of psychotherapy with children: Infants to adolescents* (2nd ed.). New York, NY: Springer Publishing Company.

Ahmad, A., Larsson, B., & Sundelin-Wahlsten, V. (2007). EMDR treatment for children with PTSD: Results of a randomized controlled trial. *Nordic Journal of Psychiatry, 61*(5), 349–354. doi:10.1080/08039480701643464

Barron, I. G., Bourgaize, C., Lempertz, D., Swinden, C. L., & Darker-Smith, S. (2019). Eye Movement Desensitization Reprocessing for children and adolescents with posttraumatic stress disorder: A systematic narrative review. *Journal of EMDR Practice and Research, 13*(4), 270–283. doi:10.1891/1933-3196.13.4.270

Beck, J. (2011). *Cognitive behavior therapy: Basics and beyond*. New York, NY: Guilford Press.

Beidas, R., & Kendall, P. (2014). *Dissemination and implementation of evidence-based practices in child and adolescent mental health*. New York, NY: Oxford University Press.

Bowlby, J. (1988). *A secure base*. New York, NY: Basic Books.

Brown, R. C., Witt, A., Fegert, J. M., Keller, F., Rassenhofer, M., & Plener, P. L. (2017). Psychosocial interventions for children and adolescents after man-made and natural disasters: A meta-analysis and systematic review. *Psychological Medicine, 47*, 1893–1905. doi:10.1017/S0033291717000496

Chemtob, C., Nakashima, J., & Carlson, J. (2002). Brief treatment for elementary school children with disaster related posttraumatic stress disorder: A field study. *Journal of Clinical Psychology, 58*(1), 99–112. doi:10.1002/jclp.1131

Chen, R., Gillespie, A., Zhao, Y., Xi, Y., Ren, Y., & McLean, L. (2018). The efficacy of Eye Movement Desensitization and Reprocessing in children and adults who have experienced complex childhood trauma: A systematic review of randomized controlled trials. *Frontiers in Psychology, 9*(534), 1–11. doi:10.3389/fpsyg.2018.00534

Cheung, A., Zuckerbrot, R., Jensen, P., Laraque, D., Stein, R., & GLAD-PC Steering Group. (2018). Guidelines for adolescent depression in primary care (GLAD-PC): Part II. Treatment and ongoing management. *Pediatrics, 141(3)*, e20174082. doi:10.1542/peds.2017-4082

Clarke, G., Debar, L., Lynch, F., Powell, J., Gale, J., O'Connor, E., . . . Hertert, S. (2005). An randomized effectiveness trial of brief cognitive–behavioral therapy for depressed adolescents receiving antidepressant medication. *Journal of the American Academy of Child & Adolescent Psychiatry, 44(9)*, 888–898. doi:10.1016/S0890-8567(09)62194-8

Davis, J., Houk, J., Rowell, L., Benson, J., & Smith, D. (2016). Brief motivational interviewing and normative feedback for adolescents: Change language and alcohol use outcomes. *Journal of Substance Abuse Treatment, 65*, 66–73. doi:10.1016/j.jsat.2015.10.004

de Roos, C., van der Oord, S., Zijlstra, B., Lucassen, S., Perrin, S., Emmelkamp, P., & de Jongh, A. (2017). Comparison of Eye Movement Desensitization and Reprocessing therapy, cognitive behavioral writing therapy, and wait-list in pediatric posttraumatic stress disorder following single-incident trauma: A multicenter randomized clinical trial. *Journal of Child Psychology and Psychiatry, 58(11)*, 1219–1228. doi:10.1111/jcpp.12768

Dickerson, J. F., Lynch, F. L., Leo, M. C., DeBar, L. L., Pearson, J., & Clarke, G. N. (2018). Cost-effectiveness of cognitive behavioral therapy for depressed youth declining antidepressants. *Pediatrics, 141(2)*, e20171969. doi:10.1542/peds.2017-1969

Diehle, J., Opmeer, B., Boer, F., Mannarino, A., & Lindauer, R. (2015). Trauma focused cognitive behavioral therapy or Eye Movement Desensitization and Reprocessing: What works in children with posttraumatic stress symptoms? A randomized control trial. *European Child & Adolescent Psychiatry, 24(2)*, 227–236. doi:10.1007/s00787-014-0572-5

Erikson, E. (1950). *Childhood and society*. New York, NY: W. W. Norton.

Evidence-Based Child and Adolescent Psychosocial Interventions. (2018). Satellite Beach, FL: PracticeWise. Retrieved from https://www.aap.org/en-us/Documents/CRPsychosocialInterventions.pdf

Farkas, L., Cyr, M., Lebeau, T. M., & Lemay, J. (2010). Effectiveness of MASTR EMDR therapy for traumatized adolescents. *Journal of Child & Adolescent Trauma, 3*, 125–142. doi:10.1080/19361521003761325

Felitti, V., Anda, R., Nordenberg, D., Williamson, D., Spitz, A., Edwards, V., & Marks, J. (1998). Relationship of childhood abuse and household dysfunction to many of the leading causes of death in adults. The adverse childhood experiences (ACE) study. *American Journal of Preventative Medicine, 14(4)*, 245–248. doi:10.1016/S0749-3797(98)00017-8

Gomez, A. M. (2009). *The thoughts kit for kids*. Ana Gomez Products. ISBN: 978-0-9795274-1-8. Retrieved from https://www.anagomez.org/product/the-thoughts-kit-for-kids/

Greenwald, R. (1999). *Eye Movement Desensitization and Reprocessing (EMDR) in child and adolescent psychotherapy*. New Jersey, NJ: Book-mart Press.

Higa-McMillan, C., Francis, S., Najarian, L., & Chorpita, B. (2016). Evidence-base update: 50 years of research on treatment for child and adolescent anxiety. *Journal of Clinical Child & Adolescent Psychology, 45(2)*, 91–113. doi:10.1080/15374416.2015.1046177

Jaberghaderi, N., Greenwald, R., Rubin, A., Zand, S. O., & Dolatabadim, S. (2004). A comparison of CBT and EMDR for sexually-abused Iranian girls. *Clinical Psychology and Psychotherapy, 11*, 358–368. doi:10.1002/cpp.395

Kemp, M., Drummond, P., & McDermott, B. (2010). A wait-list controlled pilot study of Eye Movement Desensitization and Reprocessing (EMDR) for children with post-traumatic stress disorder (PTSD) symptoms from motor vehicle accidents. *Clinical Child Psychology and Psychiatry, 15(1)*, 5–25. doi:10.1177/1359104509339086

Kendall, P. C., & Hedtke, K. (2006). *Coping cat workbook* (2nd ed.). Ardmore, PA: Workbook Publishing.

Kennard, B. D., Silva, S. G., Toney, S., Rohde, P., Hughes, J. L., Vitiello, B., . . . March, J. (2009). Remission and recovery in the Treatment for Adolescents with Depression Study (TADS): Acute and long-term outcomes. *Journal of the American Academy of Child & Adolescent Psychiatry, 48(2)*, 186–195. doi:10.1097/CHI.0b013e31819176f9

Kernberg, P., Litvo, R., & Keable, H. (2012). Practice parameter for psychodynamic psychotherapy with children. *Journal of the American Academy of Child & Adolescent Psychiatry, 51(5)*, 541–557. doi:10.1016/j.jaac.2012.02.015

Khan, A. M., Dar, S., Ahmed, R., Bachu, R., Adnan, M., & Kotapati, V. P. (2018). Cognitive behavioral therapy versus Eye Movement Desensitization and Reprocessing in patients with post-traumatic stress disorder: Systematic review and meta-analysis of randomized clinical trials. *Cureus, 10*(9), e3250. doi:10.7759/cureus.3250

Lavik, K., Veseth, M., Frøysa, H., Binder, P., & Moltu, C. (2018). 'Nobody else can lead your life': What adolescents need from psychotherapists in change processes. *Counselling and Psychotherapy Research, 18*(3), 262–273. doi:10.1002/capr.12166

Lewisohn, P. M., Clarke, G. N., Hops, H., & Andrews, J. (1990). Cognitive-behavioral treatment for depressed adolescents. *Behavior Therapy, 21*, 385–401. doi:10.1016/S0005 -7894(05)80353-3

Lusk, P., & Melnyk, B. M. (2011a). COPE for the treatment of depressed adolescents. Lessons learned from implementing an evidence-based practice change. *Journal of the American Psychiatric Nurses Association, 17*(4), 297–309. doi:10.1177/1078390311416117

Lusk, P., & Melnyk, B. M. (2011b). The brief cognitive-behavioral COPE intervention for depressed adolescents: Outcomes and feasibility of delivery in 30-minute outpatient visits. *Journal of the American Psychiatric Nurses Association, 17*(3), 226–236. doi:10.1177/ 1078390311404067

Melnyk, B. M. (2003a). *Creating Opportunities for Personal Empowerment (COPE) manual for teens.* Retrieved from https://www.cope2thrive.org

Melnyk, B. M. (2003b). *Creating opportunities for personal empowerment COPE.* Retrieved from www.cope2thrive.com

Melnyk, B. M., Kelly, S., Jacobson, D., Belyea, M., Shaibi, G., Small, L., . . . Marsiglia, F. F. (2013). The COPE healthy lifestyles TEEN randomized controlled trial with culturally diverse high school adolescents: Baseline characteristics and methods. *Conteporary Clinical Trials, 36*(1), 41–53. doi:10.1016/j.cct.2013.05.013

Moreno-Alcázar, A., Treen, D., Valiente-Gómez, A., Sio-Eroles, A., Pérez, V., Amann, B. L., & Radua, J. (2017). Efficacy of Eye Movement Desensitization and Reprocessing in children and adolescent with post- traumatic stress disorder: A meta-analysis of randomized controlled trials. *Frontiers in Psychology, 8*, 1750. doi:10.3389/fpsyg.2017.01750

Mufson, L., Dorta, K., Wickramarantne, P., Nomura, Y., Olfson, M., & Weissman, M. (2004). A randomized effectiveness trial of interpersonal psychotherapy for depressed adolescents. *Archives of General Psychiatry, 61*, 577–584. doi:10.1001/archpsyc.61.6.577

Piaget, J. (1936). *Origins of intelligence in the child.* London: Routledge & Kegan Paul.

Reynolds, S., Wilson, C., Austin, J., & Hooper, L. (2012). Effects of psychotherapy for anxiety in children and adolescents: A meta-analytic review. *Clinical Psychology Review, 32*(4), 251–262. doi:10.1016/j.cpr.2012.01.005

Rohde, P., Clarke, G. N., Mace, D. E., Jorgensen, J. S., & Seeley, J. R. (2004). An efficacy/ effectiveness study of cognitive–behavioral treatment for adolescents with comorbid major depression and conduct disorder. *Journal of the American Academy of Child & Adolescent Psychiatry, 43*(6), 660–668. doi:10.1097/01.chi.0000121067.29744.41

Rohde, P., Waldron, H. B., Turner, C. W., Brody, J., & Jorgensen, J. (2014). Sequenced versus coordinated treatment for adolescents with comorbid depressive and substance use disorders. *Journal of Consulting and Clinical Psychology, 82*(2), 342–348. doi:10.1037/a0035808

Seigel, D. (2001). Toward an interpersonal neurobiology of the developing mind: Attachment relationships, "mindsight," and neural integration. *Infant Mental Health Journal, 22*(1–2), 67–94. doi:10.1002/1097-0355(200101/04)22:1<67::AID-IMHJ3>3.0.CO;2-G

Shapiro, F. (2018). *Eye Movement Desensitization and Reprocessing: Basic principles, protocols, and procedures* (3rd ed.). New York, NY: Guilford Press

Soberman, G., Greenwald, R., & Rule, D. (2002). A controlled study of Eye Movement Desensitization and Reprocessing (EMDR) for boys with conduct problems. *Journal of Aggression, Maltreatment and Trauma, 6*(1), 217–236. doi:10.1300/J146v06n01_11

Substance Abuse Medical Health and Services Administration. (2017). *Integrating screening, brief intervention, and referral treatment into primary care.* Retrieved from https://www.samhsa.gov/ sbirt/about

Walkup, J. T., Albano, A. M., Piacentini, J., Birmaher, B., Compton, S. C., Sherril, J. T., . . . Kendall, P. C. (2008). Cognitive behavioral therapy, sertraline, or a combination in childhood anxiety. *New England Journal of Medicine, 359*(26), 2753–2766. doi:10.1056/NEJMoa0804633

Wanders, F., Serra, M., & de Jongh, A. (2008). EMDR versus CBT for children with self-esteem and behavioral problems: A randomized controlled trial. *Journal of EMDR Practice and Research, 2*(3), 180–189. doi:10.1891/1933-3196.2.3.180

Watanabe, N., Hunot, V., Omori, I. M., Churchill, R., & Furukawa, T. A. (2007). Psychotherapy for depression among children and adolescents: A systematic review. *Acta Psychiatrica Scandinavica, 116*(2), 84–95. doi:10.1111/j.1600-0447.2007.01018.x

Waters, F. S. (2016). *Healing the fractured child: Diagnosis and treatment of youth with dissociation.* New York, NY: Springer Publishing Company.

Weersing, V., Jeffreys, M., Do, M., Schwartz, K., & Bolano, C (2017). Evidence-base update of psychosocial treatments for child and adolescent depression. *Journal of Clinical Child & Adolescent Psychology, 46*(1), 11–43. doi:10.1080/15374416.2016.1220310

Weisz, J., & Kazdin, A. (2017). *Evidence-based psychotherapies for children and adolescents* (3rd ed.). New York, NY: Guilford Press.

Wesselmann, D., Schweitzer, C., & Armstrong, S. (2014). *Integrative parenting: Strategies for raising children affected by attachment trauma.* New York, NY: W. W. Norton.

Williams, S. B., O'Connor, E. A., Eder, M., & Whitlock, E. P. (2009). Screening for child and adolescent depression in primary care settings: A systematic evidence review for the US Preventive Services Task Force. *Pediatrics, 123*(4), e716–e735. doi:10.1542/peds.2008-2415

Wissow, L. (2015). Disruptive behavior and aggression. In H. Adam & J. Foy (Eds), *Signs and symptoms in pediatrics* (pp. 203–214). Elk Grove Village, IL: American Academy of Pediatrics.

Yang, L., Zhou, X., Zhou, C., Zhang, Y., Pu, J., Liu, L., . . . Xie, P. (2017). Efficacy and acceptability of cognitive behavioral therapy for depression in children: A systematic review and meta-analysis. *Academic Pediatrics, 17*(1), 9–16. doi:10.1016/j.acap.2016.08.002

Yearwood, E., Pearson, G., & Newland, J. (2012). *Child and adolescent behavioral health: A resource for advanced practice psychiatric and primary care practitioners in nursing.* Ames, IA: Wiley-Blackwell.

Zhou, X., Zhang, Y., Furukawa, T. A., Cuijpers, P., Pu, J., Weisz, J. R., . . . Xie, P. (2019). Different types and acceptability of psychotherapies for acute anxiety disorders in children and adolescents: A network meta-analysis. *JAMA Psychiatry, 76*(1), 41–50. doi:10.1001/jamapsychiatry.2018.3070

APPENDIX 21.1
Child / Adolescent Initial Psychiatric Evaluation Template

Initial Child/Adolescent Psychiatric Interview/Evaluation

Patient Initials: Date:
Age:
Sex:
Preferred Pronoun:
Year in School:
Screening Tools/Scores:
Identifying Information/Reason for Visit: in child/teen's own words
   Accompanied by:
Additional information–reason for visit in parent's (or other adult's) own words:
   When did the problem/situation begin?
   When was this "behavior/mood" identified as a concern?
    Difficulty/Changes in Functioning:
    At School:
    At Home:
    Socially:
    Child's Favorite Activities:
   Is the child still enjoying these activities?
    Strengths of Child/Teen: (What does that child do well or love to learn about?)
    Jobs/Volunteer Activities:
    Names of Friends? (In their words)
    Goals/Dreams—What do they see themselves doing in the future?
   When they have a decision to make, or a problem to discuss, who do you talk to?
    Main Supports:
    Three Wishes (Pretend you meet someone magical, and he or she can grant you three wishes)
    What would your three wishes be?
    Current Living Situation: (Who lives with you?)

Do you feel safe where you live? Have you ever been mistreated? Parent: or another adult–Do you feel safe?
Have there been adverse childhood experiences (trauma, violence, legal issues) that the child has been exposed to?
   General Healthy Habits—Exercise, Appetite (diet), Sleep:
   (Religious beliefs, cultural practices/traditions, dietary observances. pets. community supports):
   Contributions: Ways they help others, family, friends, volunteer work:

History of Presenting Problem:

At what age was the child's first referral for evaluation/counseling?
   Individual education plan at school?
   Previous counseling?
   When?
   Child's response:
   Any medications prescribed along with the counseling?
   Response to medication? Any adverse effects?
   Past Psychiatric Hospitalizations?
   When:
   Reason for Admission:
   Past Drug or Alcohol Treatment:
   Inpatient:
   Outpatient, Intensive:
   12 Step Programs:
   All Current Medications (medical & mental health):
   Allergies to medications:

Health History:

Birth/Developmental History:
   Head Injuries/Concussions:
   Seizures:
   Other:

Family & Social History:

<u>Family History</u> (medical and psychiatric):

Depression:

Anxiety:

Bipolar Disorder:

Schizophrenia:

<u>Social History:</u>

Recent Changes in Family or Living Situation:

Sexual History: heterosexual, homosexual, bisexual, questioning:

Substance use: ETOH, RX drugs not prescribed, drugs of abuse, MJ

Eating Disorders:

<u>Mental Status Exam:</u>

Appearance: (Appears stated age? Outstanding characteristics?)

Mood:

Mood Instability:

Affect:

Behavior:

Speech:

Attention:

Intellect, Judgment, Reasoning:

Self-perception is realistic

Perceptual distortions:

Subjective: Hallucinations?

Impulse Control:

Thoughts: Abstract thinking? Concrete thinking?

Grandiose?

Pervasively Negative, Hopeless?

Times when you feel hopeless?

Thoughts of wanting to not be around, to be dead?

Past thoughts of hurting self?

Past self-injurious behavior?

Thoughts of wishing you weren't around, wanting to be dead?

Thoughts of killing yourself?

When did you last have suicidal thoughts? How would you do it?

Is that method available to you? Guns? Pills?

What did you think about that stopped you from acting on these thoughts?

Protective Factors:

Thoughts of hurting someone else.

Identified target? Method?

Is that method available? Guns in the home? Available? Other weapons?

Can child/teen keep himself or herself safe? (Can refrain from harmful action)?

Safety plan: Contact numbers (MY3 app)

What is the Family's Crisis Plan?

Diagnostic Impression:

Plan:

22

Psychotherapy With Older Adults

Georgia L. Stevens, Merrie J. Kaas, and Kristin Linda Hjartardottir

The demographics of aging and mental health service use as well as the continuing workforce shortage documented by the Institute of Medicine (IOM; 2008) should encourage nurses to seize the opportunity to create new models of mental healthcare for the growing population of older adults. Older adults comprised 15.6% of the United States population in 2017. This percentage will increase to 21.6% by 2040 with the greatest growth among the oldest old, those who are 85 years of age or older (Administration for Community Living, 2019). The population of older adults in this country is becoming increasingly diverse as minorities become emerging majorities, and there are multiple cohorts among older adults (Kropf & Cummings, 2017; Wazwaz, 2015). These shifts in aging demographics provide us with the opportunity to continue to rethink our concept of aging from inevitable decline to what is possible with optimal aging (Depp & Jeste, 2010). Furthermore, the changing demographics impact our conceptual models of mental health and highlight new areas for mental healthcare.

Although mental illness is not a normal part of aging, at least 20% of older adults have one or more mental health or substance use conditions (Eden, Maslow, Le, & Blazer, 2012; World Health Organization [WHO], 2017). Mental disorders include those that emerge in later life such as dementia and geriatric depression, as well as serious mental illness (SMI) that has been experienced over a lifetime. People with SMI are living longer into late adulthood, have more chronic conditions, and require fewer needed resources (Kropf & Cummings, 2017). Aging baby boomers are at greater risk for mental disorders as well as changing rates and types of substance use disorders than the two older cohorts of elders, thereby increasing the need for behavioral health and substance abuse specialty services in both primary care and psychiatric care settings. The 1999 Surgeon General's groundbreaking report on mental health stressing the growing prevalence of psychiatric disorders among the elderly and the need for evidence-based services has been borne out (U.S. Department of Health and Human Services [USDHHS], 1999). Unfortunately, mental health policy and treatment of older adults have lagged to the extent that they remain critically underserved (Boyd & Stevens, 2018; Friedman, Williams, Kidder, & Furst, 2018).

There have been significant changes in academic and research interests in aging and the elderly in the past few decades. New scientific findings and hypotheses have addressed illness and the concepts of health promotion and preventive medicine to move studies beyond what aging *is* to what *is possible* with aging. Understanding *potential* in relation to aging is profound, because doing so can enable older people to access latent skills and talents in later life and will challenge younger age groups to think in a different way about what is possible in their later years (Jeste & Depp, 2010; Kropf & Cummings, 2017). A focus on potential can also challenge mental health professionals to address factors that impact the mental health and well-being of older adults as well as reduce psychiatric symptoms.

The MacArthur Study of Successful Aging demonstrated that positive mental attitude and participation in social activities, including regularly scheduled activities, appear to exert a protective factor similar to exercise on mental and cognitive functioning and successful aging. In fact, combining social engagement and exercise seems to give extra protection against cognitive and physical decline. These positive effects were also found among those with chronic conditions, thus encouraging the adoption of a healthy lifestyle (Rowe & Kahn, 1998). Since this study, we have in fact seen the positive impact of lifestyle management, social support, cognitive engagement, self-care enhancement, spiritual support, and community services in mental health promotion among older adults (Boyd & Stevens, 2018; Jeste, Savla, Thompson, & Depp, 2013; Turk, Elci, Resick, & Kalarchian, 2016). Nurses are ideally suited to provide such interventions for mental health promotion for older adults with late onset as well as chronic mental illness.

This chapter provides the advanced practice psychiatric nurse (APPN) with the foundation for conducting psychotherapy with the older adult to enhance mental health and reduce psychiatric symptoms. The first section of this chapter addresses the underlying assumptions and principles for psychotherapy with older adults including life context and care considerations. The next section covers common presentations, diagnostic considerations, and goals in selecting therapy approaches for late-life psychiatric disorders. These sections are followed by general guidelines for psychotherapy with older adults, the evidence base for specific therapy modalities, and implementation strategies for cognitive behavioral therapy (CBT), mindfulness, interpersonal psychotherapy (IPT), reminiscence therapy (RT), and life review therapy (LRT) with older adults. This is followed by a case illustrating the use of LRT. The final section of the chapter addresses the role of the APPN as well as certification and education for APPNs who wish to attain further education in the care of this population.

Advanced practice nurses who work with older adults should be proficient at assessing the status of their patients' cognitive, affective, functional, physical, and behavioral function as well as their family dynamics. They must also be knowledgeable about the effects of psychotropic medications on elderly people and the factors that increase older adults' risk for drug toxicity such as age, polypharmacy, adherence, and comorbidity. Specialized advanced practice geropsychiatric nurses are challenged to integrate multiple psychotherapeutic modalities with knowledge of the normal aging process, physiologic disorders, and sociocultural influences when working with older adults and their families.

UNDERLYING ASSUMPTIONS AND PRINCIPLES

Effective psychotherapy with older adults relies on an understanding of individual, family, collective, and systemic issues, which together provide basic principles for psychotherapy with older adults. The next section summarizes basic considerations and principles that underlie the conduct of psychotherapy with older adults.

Developmental Considerations in Late Adulthood

Although late adulthood development has not been as well delineated as other stages, Erik Erikson described the developmental task of "integrity versus despair," which his wife extended to a ninth stage of gerotranscendence. Gerotranscendence emphasizes ongoing growth over decrements (Erikson & Erikson, 1997; Jewell, 2014).

The transition from young-old (ages 65 to 74 years) to middle-old (ages 75 to 84 years) to old-old (ages 85 years and older) is more than a series of birthdays; it is a gradual biopsychosocial developmental process that may be viewed as both positive and negative. Relationships with family and friends change in both positive and negative ways. From a positive perspective, the later years allow time for personal growth and development that were impossible when work and family responsibilities were priorities. Retirement requires finding new meaning in life. Travel, friendships, and engaging in neglected hobbies can enhance quality of life and improve well-being. However, such freedom may not be possible with limitations in health, resources, social support, and individual perceptions of aging (Boyd & Stevens, 2018). Psychotherapy interventions need to be tailored to the individual needs of elders at different stages of late adulthood. Interventions that address these developmental transitions can strengthen quality of life, well-being, and resilience.

Strengths, Resilience, and Wisdom

While there are positive and negative outcomes as we age, our understanding of successful aging has evolved as we have learned more from research. A view of inevitable decline was derived from past cross-sectional studies of a point in time, while more recent longitudinal and qualitative studies have yielded a more optimistic picture of aging with less cognitive and physical decline and more wisdom as major contributors to successful aging (Vaillant, 2007). Older adults have described a balance between self-acceptance and self-contentedness along with engagement and continuing self-growth in later life.

Positive mental aging is greater than the absence of impairment; it involves older adults' resilience in recovery, a sense of personal control and empowerment, and decisional control. These factors support emotional stability and well-being.

Wisdom has been associated with successful aging and conceptualized as social decision-making, emotional regulation or balance, and tolerance accrued from life experience. Age may be a source of strength from a lifetime of experience, associated wisdom, flexibility, and more mature coping strategies from which the elder and APPN can share a sense of optimism (Blood & Guthrie, 2018; Jeste et al., 2013,). Psychotherapy interventions to support successful aging might include information to support informed decision-making, strengthening coping strategies, and promoting meaningful activities, social engagement, and social support (Blood & Guthrie, 2018).

Functional Status

Functional status refers to a person's capacity to manage activities of daily living independently. Functional dependency generally increases with advancing age, with mental and physical health problems contributing significantly to frailty and functional decline. Race, ethnicity, gender, and poverty contribute to considerable variability in health status (Kropf & Cummings, 2017). Comorbidity of medical and mental health problems is actually the norm rather than unusual. Strategies to address these limitations can be part of psychotherapy with older adults and their caregivers to decrease excess disability.

Chronic health problems are prevalent in late adulthood, with 80% having at least one and 68.4% having at least two chronic conditions (National Council on Aging, n.d.). The prevalence of chronic conditions contribute to somatic and mental comorbidites, as well as polypharmacy, both of which can have significant negative consequences including reduced functional capacity (McGrath, Hajjir, Kumar, Hwang, & Salzman, 2017). Although chronic illness need not determine an older adult's sense of strength and value, living with chronic illness can be a topic of psychotherapy as the APPN addresses comorbidity, health management strategies, doctor visits, and medication management.

Mobility is critical to a person's perception of being healthy. Exercise should be encouraged for its beneficial effect on mobility and for its impact on emotions, depression, and sense of well-being (Saxon, Etten, & Perkins, 2015; Turk et al., 2016). Personal independence and self-mastery in everyday life are significantly impacted by visual and auditory losses. Given that visual and auditory changes impact functional capacity and lifestyle, one's capacity for adaptation and compensation is crucial. Such losses can be accommodated in psychotherapy by using large-print materials, ensuring that personal assistive devices are working properly at each session, clearly articulating, and audio-taping sessions for later review and learning at home.

The impact of cognitive issues on psychotherapy with older adults is extremely important because research has revealed that cognitive deficits are an integral component of all late-life psychiatric disorders and that they significantly impact functional capacity and disability. Multiple studies have revealed that cognitive impairment does not respond to treatment for other disorders, such as depression, and therefore requires simultaneous treatment (Twamley & Harvey, 2006). Cognitive principles suggest targeting cognitive symptoms and taking functional deficits into account when doing psychotherapy using accommodations such as conducting shorter sessions, using memory aids and mnemonic devices, summarizing previous sessions, and taking notes.

Cohort Issues and Changes

Late adulthood is comprised of three birth cohorts: baby boomers, 65 to 74 years of age; survivors of World War II, 75 to 84 years of age; and survivors of the Great Depression, aged 85 and older (Kropf & Cummings, 2017). Among the most important considerations for the APPN conducting psychotherapy with older adults is an understanding of the diversity that comes from individual variation and from cohort effects, or the impact of having been socialized with certain personality dimensions, abilities, beliefs, attitudes, and experiences, for example, the stigma of mental illness is different in the current cohorts of more senior elders from the cohort of baby boomers. Such stigma of mental illness has contributed to psychiatric symptoms being expressed with physical symptoms, less discussion of emotions, and a preference for primary care rather than specialized mental health. Models that involve collaboration of psychiatric-mental health clinical nurse specialists (PMHCNS) in primary care settings have been well received and yield positive outcomes.

The social cultural context of the boomers' coming of age involved the Vietnam War, Watergate, and the civil rights movement, followed by gender and sexual orientation empowerment and immersion in digital technology (Knight & Pachana, 2015). There is an opportunity to build on the principles of the recovery movement with more person-centered, collaborative approaches toward improving their health and wellness, living a self-directed life, and striving to reach their full potential The baby boomer cohort is leading the way in the empowerment and education of older adults, their families, providers, and the public to overcome the barriers imposed by stigma. Outreach and peer support groups will likely have a bigger role in treatment.

Social Support and Family Issues

By late adulthood, there have been a number of structural and role changes in families that will require the development of specialized services to address their needs. Women outnumber men in all racial and ethnic groups, such that widowhood is a normative role and women are more likely to live in poverty (Arias, 2014). Childrearing responsibilities are less prevalent as adult children are involved with their own families, although older adults may still be caring for their adult children with disabilities, as well as the 10% of grandchildren being raised by grandparents (Ellis & Simmons, 2014; Kropf & Cummings, 2017). The two million lesbian, gay, bisexual, and transgender (LGBT) adults aged 50 and older is expected to double by 2030 (Fredriksen-Goldsen et al., 2011). Aging lesbian, gay, bisexual, and transgender older adults face a multitude of challenges in housing, healthcare, and long-term care because of bias and discrimination.

Most older adults value their capacity to live independently at home, although they may be supported and cared for by family and friends. Social support is critical to successful aging. It is important to understand the older adult's relationship and social engagement histories and preferences in order to promote effective social networks and coping. This must include an understanding of the changes and losses of significant relationships in order to be able to decrease potential isolation and strengthen a sense of well-being and a trusted and safe social network.

When the impact of functional decline necessitates a higher level of support, older adults rely primarily on the help of family caregivers, especially adult daughters. The birth cohort of baby boomers has fewer younger family members available for caregiving than prior birth cohorts. Contemporary LBGT older adults are less likely to have children or other family members to rely on, and "family of choice" may not be granted the same legal authority to make healthcare decisions. Family support may be rewarding while also being quite stressful with substantial costs in labor and money for the caregivers themselves. When older adults become more dependent on family caregiving, it is imperative that we provide effective family caregiver support to address the mental, emotional, physical, and financial stresses that caregivers face as an older adult's health deteriorates. Individual, family, and group therapy interventions can be tailored to the individualized caregiver needs. Although existing scientific evidence and clinical experience have largely evolved from a treatment model of therapeutic interventions for caregivers of those with dementia, they also address the treatment needs of those caring for elders with chronic and late-onset mental and physical disorders. Therapy goals may include caregiver education, specific problem-solving skills, resource acquisition, long-range planning, emotional support, respite, and the reduction of caregiver burden (National Alliance on Caregiving, 2009; Redfoot, Feinberg, & Houser, 2013).

Societal Issues

Ageism, racism, and poverty contribute to the health disparities among older adults of different cultures. In addition, ageism and bias have contributed to a historically pessimistic perspective on the effectiveness of psychotherapy with the elderly. Stigma is a collective and cohort issue. As more accurate information about aging has evolved, clinical psychotherapy practice and research have developed over the past two decades. This research is yielding an evidence base to support specific therapy approaches for psychiatric disorders in late adulthood and specific information about adapting psychotherapy approaches for older adults. There is a great need for more qualified, specially trained APPNs to provide mental healthcare, including psychotherapy, to older adults.

Existing funding streams and service delivery models need to be adapted to meet the need for long-term, community-based treatment, housing, and support for older adults from all cultures. Organizational barriers such as therapy time, transportation, and available providers and interpreters may not match the needs of the current cohorts of older adults. Our fragmented healthcare system contributes to the vulnerability of older adults with late-life psychiatric disorders that are complicated by significant physical comorbidity issues. APPNs, certified in psychiatric-mental health or gerontology, can make a significant contribution to the elder mental health crisis.

Life Context and Care Considerations

The life preferences and issues of older adults provide the context for care considerations. Contrary to popular beliefs, a small percentage of older adults live in nursing homes; 3.1% of those over 65% and 9% of those over 85 years of age (ACL, 2018). Most older adults prefer to live in their own homes, and this trend is expected to increase. There are gender differences in household arrangements with more men than women living with a spouse (72% vs. 48%) and more women than men living alone (34% vs. 20%; ACL, 2018). These solo housing arrangements point to potential care issues of loss, isolation, and vulnerability. Supportive community models have the potential to strengthen engagement, social relations, and healthy functioning (Kropf & Cummings, 2017). As health issues accumulate, vulnerability and dependency may require a move to long-term care settings of assisted living facilities (ALF) or nursing homes for short-term or long-term care. Residential moves are major transitions that require a focus on knowing the resident's history and preferences to support maximal integration, engagement, and comfort in the new environment.

Nurses providing psychiatric care for older adults may work in a wide variety of settings. In the community, these may include inpatient and emergency psychiatric services; outpatient mental health clinics, substance abuse treatment centers, and primary care; and adult day care, senior centers, peer support clubhouses, meal sites, and home care. In residential facilities, these settings may include continuing care communities, ALFs, and long-term care facilities.

In addition, given some of the emerging demographic and societal issues, psychiatric nurses will be practicing in nontraditional ways and settings such as school systems to address the needs of custodial grandparents (Ellis & Simmons, 2014). Given the recognition of the specialized needs of the aging LGBT community, mental healthcare must also be adapted to meet their needs in a culturally sensitive way. Prisoners are aging in place and comprise 28% of all who are incarcerated, requiring geropsychiatric expertise in correctional facilities (Kim & Peterson, 2014). The doubling of the number of homeless older adults between 2010 and 2050 requires understanding their needs and the integration of mental health and medical healthcare in nontraditional settings. APPNs need to be prepared to provide mental health and illness treatment in a variety of community, institutional, and nontraditional settings if we are to meet older adults where they are in their life circumstances.

PSYCHIATRIC DISORDERS IN OLDER ADULTS

This section provides an overview of significant late-life psychiatric disorders, changes in symptoms, and assessment strategies. Websites for resources and practice guidelines are included in Box 22.1. Challenges assessing psychiatric symptoms in the elderly include the masking of symptoms by comorbid disorders and medications, difficulty in obtaining an accurate mental health history, age-related variations in symptom presentation, and denial of symptoms. Assessment tools frequently used in geriatric psychiatry are included in Table 22.1.

BOX 22.1 Websites for Geriatric Mental Health Resources and Practice Guidelines

www.POGOe.org: Portal of Geriatric Online Education (CornellCARES.com): Geriatrics psychosocial patient handouts

giaging.org/issues/mental-health-and-aging: Grantmakers in Aging: Resources on mental health disorders and treatment including psychotherapies and evidence-based programs

https://www.alz.org/alzheimers-dementia/what-is-alzheimers

www.geronurse-online.org

psychiatryonline.org/pb/assets/raw/sitewide/practice_guidelines/guidelines/alzheimer-watch.pdf: *Practice guideline for the treatment of patients with Alzheimer's disease and other dementias of late life*

www.aagponline.org: American Association for Geriatric Psychiatry provides information and resources about geriatric mental health practice

www.nimh.nih.gov/health/topics/older-adults-and-mental-health/index.shtml#part_153484

http://reminiscenceandlifereview.org/: International Institute for Reminiscence and Life Review

www.integration.samhsa.gov/integrated-care-models/older-adults

www.thebcat.com

TABLE 22.1 ASSESSMENT TOOLS IN GERIATRIC PSYCHIATRY	
Geriatric Depression Scale (GDS)*	Widely used as a screening tool for depression (see Appendix 3.6; Yesavage et al., 1983).
The Montgomery–Åsberg Depression Rating Scale[†]	Can be used to measure symptom severity over time and the impact of psychotherapy (Montgomery & Åsberg, 1979).
Cornell Scale for Depression in Dementia[†]	The most widely used diagnostic scale for depression in dementia (Alexopoulos, Abrams, Young, & Shamoian, 1998).
Mood Disorder Questionnaire (MDQ)[‡]	Screens also for bipolar disorder (Hirschfeld et al., 2000).
Young Mania Rating Scale (YMRS)[§]	Screens for bipolar disorder (see Appendix 3.8; Young, Biggs, Ziegler, & Meyer, 1978).
The Clinical Anxiety Scale (CAS)*	Six-item scale derived from the (Hamilton Anxiety Rating Scale), excluding items that overlap with depression. Used as a screening tool and to measure severity over time (Westhuis & Thyer, 1989).
The Penn State Worry Questionnaire (PSWQ)*	16-item inventory that is reliable with older adults and used to measure pathological worry—central symptom of generalized anxiety disorder. Eight-item version is also available. Can be used to measure impact of psychotherapy (Hopko et al., 2003).

(continued)

TABLE 22.1 ASSESSMENT TOOLS IN GERIATRIC PSYCHIATRY (*CONTINUED*)	
Brief Psychiatric Rating Scale (BPRS)* [†]	Used for psychosis evaluation (Overall & Gorham, 1988).
Abnormal Involuntary Movement Scale (AIMS)*	Used for the evaluation of medication side effects of antipsychotic medications (Guy, 1976).
Mini-Mental State Examination (MMSE)[†]	Considered the gold standard for evaluation of dementia but is no longer a public domain (Folstein, Folstein, & McHugh, 1975).
The Saint Louis University Mental Status (SLUMS)[†]	Superior than MMSE in detecting mild neurocognitive disorder (Tariq, Tumosa, Chibnall, Perry, & Morley, 2006).
The Montreal Cognitive Assessment tool (MOCA)[†]	Another brief screening tool for detection of mild cognitive impairment (Nasreddine et al., 2005).
Mini-Cog[†]	Clock drawing test combined with a three-item recall test for dementia screen (Borson, Scanlan, Brush, Vitaliano, & Dokmak, 2000).
Neuropsychiatric Inventory (NPI)[†]	Comprehensive assessment of psychopathology in dementia as reported by caregiver (Cummings et al., 1994).
Behavioral Pathologic Rating Scale for Alzheimer's Disease (BEHAVE-AD)[‡]	Used for assessment of behavioral problems in dementia (Reisberg, Borenstein, Salob, Ferris, & Franssen, 1987).
The Brief Biosocial Gambling Screen (BBGS)*	Used as a quick three-question screening survey (Gebauer, LaBrie, & Shaffer, 2010).

*Self-report.

[†]Observer rated.

[‡]Self-report or observer rated.

[§]Self-report and observer rated.

Depression

Depression, including subsyndromal depression, and other mood disorders are common among the elderly but are not a natural aspect of aging. Prevalence rates of depression for older adults tend to be lower than for younger adults. Older adults living in long-term care facilities, however, have higher rates of depression than those who live in the community (Seitz, Purandare, & Conn, 2010). Although rates of remission are comparable between adults and older adults, poorer outcomes may be impacted by chronicity, external locus of control, and comorbid somatic illnesses, factors that are frequently experienced by older adults (Licht-Strunk et al., 2007). The Depression and Bipolar Support Alliance has indicated that mood disorders are under-recognized, inadequately treated, and underserviced in older adults. Under-recognition is a particular problem in primary care, the healthcare setting most often used by older adults. Worsening of depression symptoms leads to a decrease in cognitive function, functional impairment, poorer well-being, and increased risk of death for older adults. Thus, appropriate diagnosis and timely treatment, especially in primary care settings, are critical in the care of older adults (Kuchibhatla, Fillenbaum, Hybels, & Blazer, 2012).

Symptoms of depression in older adults often include an emphasis on physical ailments (e.g., aches, pains, and gastrointestinal problems), as well as changes in sleep, appetite, and use of pain medication. Older adults with depression often complain of cognitive problems such as memory problems or executive dysfunction mimicking symptoms of dementia, thus requiring special attention for diagnostic purposes. Psychologically, older adults with depression are more likely to express an exaggerated sense of helplessness, apathy, and emptiness or loneliness, rather than other emotions such as sadness, and often seem more agitated than younger adults with depression. As individuals get older they tend to under-report symptoms of depression, warning that depression might be further underestimated in the oldest of old (Hegeman, de Waal, Comijs, Kok, & van der Mast, 2015); Husain et al., 2005).

Bipolar Disorder

For a long time, there was paucity in research on bipolar disorder among older adults. As the demographics have changed, research has increased in the last decade (Sajatovic & Chen, 2011). About 5% to 19% of older adults presenting to psychiatric clinics have bipolar disorder. Psychopathology for those with longstanding illness can be severe with a high prevalence of cognitive dysfunction, incomplete treatment responses, relapses, and high mortality (Young, 2005). Compared to younger adults, the clinical presentation for older adults includes more depressed mood, poor sleep, low appetite, disturbance in activity level, and cognitive impairment (Nivoli et al., 2014). Bipolar mania in late life usually is milder than in younger patients; can present as mixed, dysphoric, or agitated states; and has a higher probability of irritability (Young, 2005). Primary bipolar disorder may be early onset (i.e., recurring in later years) or late onset (first episode at age greater than 50 years). Older adults with late-onset bipolar disorder are more likely to have bipolar II, may not have a family history of bipolar disorder, but have higher rates of neurological and medical comorbidity, as well as a higher vulnerability to relapse (García-López, Ezquiaga, De Dios, & Agud, 2017; Trinh & Forester, 2007).

Longitudinal assessment is especially important because depression is more prevalent than mania; depression often precedes mania; mania presents with paranoia, agitation, and delusions; and symptoms overlap with other psychotic and cognitive disorders (Sajatovic et al., 2005). Given the higher rates of alcohol abuse and suicide among older adults with bipolar disorder, it is important to screen for both. Alcohol use, treatment non-adherence, sleep quality, and cognitive failure have been found to be predictors of suicidal ideations (O'Rourke, Heisel, Canham, & Sixsmith, 2017). There are significant diagnostic challenges associated with bipolar disorder in older adults and include patient under-reporting, vague or nonclassic symptoms, comorbid health conditions, and the fact that depressive and manic symptoms can be induced by somatic conditions and medications.

Anxiety Disorders

It is estimated that the prevalence of anxiety disorders among older adults is between 7% and 14.2% and that it is more prevalent than depression. Those estimates include all *Diagnostic and Statistical Manual of Mental Disorders (DSM-5)* diagnoses of anxiety disorders (Reynolds, Pietrzak, El-Gabalawy, Mackenzie, Sareen, 2015; Wolitzky-Taylor, Castriotta, Lenze, Stanley, & Craske, 2010). However, the prevalence of anxiety symptoms not meeting the threshold of an anxiety disorder is estimated to be even higher. More age-appropriate diagnostic measures are needed to understand anxiety symptoms and subsyndromal presentation, prevalence, and appropriate treatment. This is especially important because anxiety not only negatively impacts current functioning and life but increases risk for other problems including depression and cognitive dysfunction (Lenze & Wetherell, 2011; Sami & Nilforooshan, 2015; Tung Fung, Wa Lee, Chun Lee, & Wa Lam, 2018).

Some anxiety disorders are more likely to occur during late adulthood. These include generalized anxiety disorder (GAD), agoraphobia, anxious depression, and anxiety associated with medical illnesses. Although treatable, these later occurring anxiety disorders may be difficult because of greater severity and higher mortality, yielding poorer outcomes (Sami & Nilforooshan, 2015; van Hout et al., 2004). Obsessive–compulsive disorder and panic disorder with or without agorapbia usually have much earlier onset and tend to be more severe and disabling. There are several risk factors for geriatric anxiety, including gender (female), single for any reason versus married, poor physical health, low socioeconomic status, high-stress life events, depression, and physical limitations in daily activities (Wolitzky-Taylor et al., 2010).

Somatic symptoms, such as dyspnea, dizziness, chest pain, irritable bowel, heartburn, tremors, initial insomnia, and hypochondriasis, are predominant in older adults experiencing anxiety disorders. Anxiety disorders may also be expressed as irritability, nervousness, trouble concentrating, worry, and fear. It may be difficult to determine whether the symptoms reflect anxiety or an underlying physical cause, such as endocrine imbalance, pulmonary disease, delirium or dementia, or medication side effects or interactions (Subramanyam, Kedare, Singh, & Pinto, 2018).

Posttraumatic Stress Disorder

Recently, more research has been done on posttraumatic stress disorder (PTSD) prevalence and impact on older adults. The incidence of PTSD in older adults is between 4.5% and 5.5% (Pietrzak, Goldstein, Southwick, & Grant, 2012). PTSD impacts psychosocial functioning negatively, and exposure to trauma early in life can cause more severe symptoms late in life, as well as impacting coping abilities (Ogle, Rubin, & Siegler, 2013). As with many psychiatric disorders, older adults with PTSD tend to have more cognitive problems later in life when compared to younger adults, or those without exposure to trauma (Schuitevoerder et al., 2013). Most PTSD research in older adults has examined individuals who are Holocaust survivors or who were prisoners of war during World War II. In these populations, symptoms of PTSD tend to be chronic, causing more social, emotional, and physical health problems in later years (Chopra et al., 2014; Ogle, Rubin, Berntsen, & Siegler, 2013). In one study, spouses of those who had suffered traumatic experiences and PTSD in World War II also had PTSD symptoms (Bramsen, van der Ploeg, & Twisk, 2002). This study speaks to the potential life-long impact of war and early trauma experiences on the whole family and the importance of family work and a systems approach for treatment if one partner has suffered significant trauma. Newer studies are looking at different sources of trauma for older adults such as weather disasters, severe medical diagnosis, and falls, and the impact on potential PTSD. Further research will be needed to evaluate the impact of different traumatic life experiences on older adults, as well as identifying protective factors for late life PTSD.

Schizophrenia

Older adults with early-onset schizophrenia have lived with a debilitating chronic disorder most of their lives. The course of the disorder in later years is relatively stable, with some changes in symptom intensity: positive symptoms become less prominent, whereas negative symptoms persist. Hospitalizations become less frequent for mental illness symptoms, but there is an increase in hospitalizations due to medical comorbities.

Severity of movement disorders in older patients as side effects from medications is greater than in younger patients, and they are more likely to have cardiovascular disease, COPD, and hypothyroidism as a result of the mental illness and the antipsychotics used to treat its symptoms. Cognitive decline is similar in older adults with schizophrenia regardless of age, age of onset, or illness duration, but much greater when compared with older adults who do not have the illness (Hendrie et al., 2014; Lowenstein, Czaja, Bowie, & Harvey, 2012). Depressive symptoms are common in older adults with chronic schizophrenia and are linked to physical, social, and financial distress, not unlike older adults without schizophrenia. On a positive note, older adults with schizophrenia have improved social functioning and lower rates of substance abuse (Jeste & Maglione, 2013).

Late-onset schizophrenia occurs after the age of 45 years and accounts for 20% to 25% of older adults with schizophrenia. It differs from early-onset schizophrenia in that it is more common in women, is mostly a paranoid subtype, and has less severe symptoms, including less severe negative symptoms, less impairment in learning and abstraction or cognitive flexibility, and less affective blunting or personality deterioration, thereby requiring lower doses of antipsychotics (Rabins & Lavrisha, 2003). Up to 20% of older adults with schizophrenia may maintain remission, and age does not negatively impact remission rate (Barak & Swartz, 2012; Jeste & Twamley, 2003).

Psychiatric assessment should address the full range of schizophrenia symptoms, including presence and severity of psychosis and psychotic-related symptoms, positive and negative symptoms, depression, cognitive changes associated with the negative symptoms, and neurocognitive impairment. Given the widespread use of older antipsychotic medication in this cohort with an increased prevalence of tardive dyskinesia, it is important to assess for involuntary movement side effects and the potential for decreased independence in the activities of daily living.

Dementia

Dementia symptoms may occur as a result of a number of disorders and underlying causes. Alzheimer's disease (AD), with 4.5 million victims, accounts for 50% to 60% of the dementias; vascular or multi-infarct disease for up to 20%; and diffuse Lewy body disease for 5% to 20% of dementia disorders, with more overlap than previously thought. In each case, the classic symptoms of dementia (i.e., cognitive impairments along with a number of functional, behavioral, and psychological deficits) are present. Increasing attention has been paid in recent years to mild cognitive impairment (MCI), which may or may not progress to dementia. Studies suggest that baseline depression with MCI is associated with increased risk of dementia, particularly vascular dementia (Richard et al., 2013; Rosenberg et al., 2013). Furthermore apathy without other symptoms of depression has been associated with progression from MCI to AD (Richard et al., 2012). Diagnostic challenges include distinguishing between depression, dementia, and delirium, all common in older adults, often with overlapping symptoms. Accurate history and assessment of mood, memory, and attention span is important. As with other psychiatric illnesses, special attention should be made to ensure that underlying medical conditions or chemical imbalances are evaluated.

Neuropsychiatric symptoms, such as apathy, depression, anxiety, and sleep-wake cycle reversal, as well as agitation, delusions, disinhibition, and hallucinations, are common in patients with dementia (van der Linde et al., 2016; Zhao et al., 2016). These emotional and behavioral disturbances are a significant cause of stress in the older adult and caregiver and require appropriate intervention (Rabins & Pearlson, 2009). Given the prevalence and significance of concurrent depression and anxiety, the APPN should include early diagnosis and treatment of these conditions (Richard et al., 2013; Tampi et al., 2011).

Substance Abuse and Gambling

Rates of substance use and addiction for older adults has increased significantly with the baby boomer generation. This generation is bringing changes in attitudes both toward alcohol use as well as recreational use of illicit substances and prescription medications. Changes in diagnosis of substance use disorder, as defined by the *DSM-5*, moves away from defining degrees of using to more focus on patterns of using and functional impairment. For older adults, adaptation for screening and diagnosis might be needed due to age-related functional changes and fewer role obligations, cognitive impairment, small amounts causing more impairment, and lack of insight in terms of connection between negative outcomes and substance use.

Alcohol use among older adults has steadily increased. According to the National Epidemiologic Survey on Alcohol and Related Conditions in 2013, alcohol use disorder was estimated to be present for 5.1% men and 2.4% women older than 65 years old. Rates of binge drinking in the year prior were 21.5% for men and 9.1% for women (Substance Abuse and Mental Health Services Administration [SAMHSA], 2014). Due to the increased sensitivity for alcohol, and increased morbitidy and mortality rates, the guidelines for alcohol use in older adults who are otherwise healthy and not on medications have been lowered to no more than three drinks on a given day and no more than seven drinks in a week (National Institute on Alcohol Abuse and Alcoholism [NIAAA], n.d.).

Marijuana and other cannabis use has steadily increased in the community, and with legal changes and increased uses for medicinal purposes this trend is expected to continue. Almost 3% of individuals older than 65 years reported marijuana use in the last 12 months on the National Survey on Drug Use and Health in 2015 (Han & Palamar, 2018). There are not many studies available on the risks of marijuana for older adults but some studies have linked marijuana use with cardiovascular problems, negative drug interactions with prescription medications, and both short- and long-term negative effects on cognitive functioning (Lloyd & Striley, 2018). Also, older adults who use marijuana have higher prevalence for alcohol use disorder, nicotine dependence, stimulant use, and misuse of prescription medications.

Older adults are commonly prescribed medications and it is estimated that at least 25% of older adults are prescribed controlled substances with potential for abuse or misuse. As with younger adults, opioid prescriptions have multiplied in the last decade; however, there are few studies about the misuse of opioids in older adults. The limited research suggests that misuse tends to be higher for older adults than for younger adults with more serious consequences (West, Severtson, Green, & Dart, 2015).

Gambling

Gambling disorders among older adults are becoming a significant problem. The prevalence of lifetime gambling disorder in older adults ranged from 0.01% to 10.6% across 25 studies in a 2014 systematic review of gambling in older adults. Older adults with a gambling disorder were more likely to be men, single/divorced or separated, and people who gamble to ameliorate depression and increase socialization (Subramaniam et al., 2015). Concerns about problem gambling in older adults include the loss of financial stability given fixed incomes; lower levels of socialization and higher levels of loneliness, albeit older adults may go to casinos and bingo parlors to be with other people; and increased physical/medical conditions such as COPD and diabetes (van der Maas et al., 2017). Clearly the rising rates of gambling disorders in all populations make the explicit screening for geriatric gambling a necessary addition to any addiction disorder evaluation. See Table 22.1 for a quick three-question gambling screening tool.

Suicide Risk, Assessment, and Intervention

Suicide is a tragic event for the individual and family at any age. Recent statistics show that suicide rates in the United States have increased by 27% from 1999 to 2016 and are now the tenth leading cause for overall death. The National Institute of Mental Health (NIMH) reports that older adults die by suicide proportionately more than younger age groups. Older men, both White and Black over 65 years of age, have the highest suicide rates of all gender, race, and age groups (National Institute of Mental Health [NIMH], 2019). The baby boomer cohort appears to have a higher rate of suicide at any given age than subsequent cohorts, giving rise to increasing concern about suicide as these adults age (Conwell, Van Orden, & Caine, 2011). Suicide risk factors are multifaceted and include social isolation and poor social support, depression, prevalent anxiety, loss of a loved one, physical illness(es) and/or uncontrollable pain, impaired functioning, and insomnia (Almeida et al., 2012; Conwell, 2014; Lapierre et al., 2012). These contributing factors need to be routinely assessed when working with older adults. For the APPN, forming a therapeutic alliance with the older adult is vital because some reports suggest older adults are less likely to report suicidal ideations to medical and mental health providers (Conwell & Thompson, 2008). Relief of symptoms, working with complex grief, and helping older adults to find meaning in life and maintain social connections are important goals in therapy with suicidal individuals.

Even though there is high lethality associated with suicidal behaviors in older adults, research about suicide prevention is rare (Okolie, Dennis, Thomas, & John, 2017). Large multicenter studies utilizing collaborative care strategies, problem-solving and interpersonal psychotherapies, and provider education aimed at reducing suicidal ideation and depression have shown lower suicide rates in older adults. PROSPECT (Prevention of Suicide in Primary Care Elderly: Collaborative Trial; Alexopoulos et al., 2009; Bruce et al., 2004), IMPACT (Improved Mood Promoting Access to Collaborative Care Treatment; Unützer et al., 2006), and DEPS-GP (Depression and Early Prevention of Suicide in General Practice; Almeida et al., 2012) have shown early and lasting effects of reducing suicidal behavior. Use of specific psychotherapies such as problem-solving therapy (PST; Gustavson et al., 2016) and problem adaptation therapy (PATH; Kiosses et al., 2015) have also shown reductions in suicidal ideation older adults more than supportive therapy.

GENERAL GUIDELINES FOR PSYCHOTHERAPY WITH OLDER ADULTS

The following section provides an overview of general considerations and guidelines for providing psychotherapy to older adults. Websites for resources and practice guidelines are included in Box 22.1. Challenges identifying appropriate therapy approaches lie, in part, with the difficulties in assessing psychiatric symptoms in the elderly, which include the masking of symptoms by comorbid disorders and medications, difficulty in obtaining an accurate mental health history, age-related variations in symptom presentation, and denial of symptoms. Assessment tools frequently used in geriatric psychiatry are included in Table 22.1.

Before the discussion of specific therapies and their application with older adults, it is important to consider general issues related to conducting psychotherapy with older adults as noted in the literature by clinicians and researchers (Areán, 2004; Knight &

Pachana, 2015; Knight & Poon, 2008; Sullivan, Zeff, & Zweig, 2018). One psychotherapy issue concerns the development of the therapeutic alliance between the clinician and the older adult. The cohort of older adults who are now in their 70s, 80s, 90s, or older, have had few experiences with the process of psychotherapy. But Dakin and Areán (2013) report when older adults do need mental healthcare, the most common causes for seeking depression treatment were interpersonal relationships, challenges due to cognitive changes and health conditions, finances, housing, and grief/loss issues.

Knight (2004) describes points to discuss when teaching older adults about psychotherapy. He suggests the following ideas be discussed early in the therapy process: normalizing the therapy process as assistance with problems in living; setting goals and priorities for therapy and teaching older adults how to set realistic goals for themselves; explaining how the therapy process works to improve symptoms; describing the conduct of therapy sessions, including the responsibilities of the patient and APPN; the length, number, and cost of therapy sessions, as well as the projected outcome of the therapy; and talking about the confidentiality of the information that is discussed in therapy. This list is useful to discuss with all patients, but repeated discussions and written materials about these topics may be most helpful when working with older adults.

Comorbidity

Older adults have a number of medical, psychological, and social issues to manage and a thorough assessment of the presenting problems must be done to be clear about the mental health issues and what concerns need to be addressed medically. APPNs who work with older adults must know about the particular issues related to the elderly and aging. For example, they need to know about the psychological effects of medications commonly taken by older adults to understand whether the presenting symptoms are psychologically or medicinally driven.

In a recent review of psychotherapies developed for older adults with chronic and acute medical conditions and cognitive impairments, cognitive-behavioral and problem-solving therapies were found to be effective, but more research is needed to identify effective psychotherapies with older adults who have coexisting medical conditions (Raue, McGovern, Kiosses, & Sirey, 2017).

Another important but often overlooked issue related to comorbidity is the impact of the current and long-standing early traumatic experiences of the older adult. There is less research on trauma and PTSD in older adults than younger and middle-aged adults, and it is likely older adults and healthcare professionals may under-recognize these conditions, leading to more cognitive and health problems (Cook, McCarthy, & Thorp, 2017; Lohr et al., 2015). The experience of cumulative and early childhood trauma for the older adult is unfortunately all too common. Even if the person has been highly functional throughout life, current and ongoing losses may trigger implicit memory and previous abuse that has been dormant for decades. Trauma is sometimes overlooked in the older adult because it may be difficult for the APPN to imagine the older person as a vulnerable little girl who was raped by her father 70 years ago. The person's life might have been spent in an effort to deal with the anxiety and the long-term sequelae of the abuse. Assessment of current and past trauma is an essential first step toward helping the older adult manage the effects of the trauma in light of other aging issues.

Another overlooked comorbidity is complicated grief. Grief is a process that is impacted by the individual's feelings about the loss and the ability to use new coping skills to find meaningful ways of managing the realities of the loss. Complicated grief is a syndrome that occurs in about 10% of older bereaved adults (Perng & Renz, 2018; Zisook & Shear, 2009). As a result of the inability of the older adult to accept the loss and move beyond the acute grief response, some older adults experience prolonged grief, which becomes a major focus of their lives. Risk factors for complicated grief include difficult early relationships marked by separation anxiety, history of mood disorders, and experience with multiple and/or concurrent important losses including relationships, health, home, income, pets, and the lack of social support. Complicated grief may be an early signal of depression or complicate an existing mood disorder. Recognition of complicated grief as a serious response to multiple significant losses can be the first step in appropriate targeted grief psychotherapy treatment (Perng & Renz, 2018).

Collaboration

Because many older adults have multiple chronic illnesses, APPNs must be able to recognize common red flags that may signal a medical problem and have available medical resources for referral and collaboration. The APPN must recognize the limits of his or her expertise in assessment and seek referrals to a specialist when needed. In some instances, the presenting problem in an older adult is a physical or memory problem that needs a referral to a medical practitioner. In other cases, the problem is a social one, such as isolation, and requires a referral to social services. Too often, psychological problems coexist with medical and social problems, which make coordination of care a very important component of the APPN's role. When a decision is made to initiate psychotherapy, a choice of therapy is based on the scientific evidence, patient and clinician values and abilities, projected treatment outcomes, and financial concerns. Researchers and practitioners have suggested an integration of psychotherapies in primary care settings and other non-mental health settings such as community centers, homeless shelters, and prisons to achieve more successful and long-lasting medical and emotional outcomes with older adults (Bruce et al., 2004; Unützer et al., 2006).

Working with older adults means collaborating with a multimember team, which includes the patient, the family, and the healthcare organization. Many older adults live with chronic illnesses that are being treated by a variety of healthcare providers who may have a stake in the outcome of psychotherapy. Families request that their parent, grandparent, or sibling be seen by an APPN and consequently are interested in the process and outcome of the therapy. Institutions such as nursing homes and assisted-living facilities also request psychotherapy for an older resident and expect communication about the problem, treatment, and follow-up. In the process of providing psychotherapy services, collaboration with families, institutions, and other healthcare providers is essential to obtain the information needed to conduct a thorough assessment, validate patient information provided in therapy, teach families and staff to work with a particular older adult, and document outcomes of treatment over time. This is especially true when the older adult has impaired cognitive or physical abilities.

Transference and Countertransference

After therapy begins, issues of transference and countertransference may occur between any clinician and patient, but there are likely to be different issues when the patient is older. Because of the variety of lived experiences of the older adult, the origin of transference can come from many stages of life and from any family setting. There are many life experiences from which relationship distortions can occur. Knight (2004) and others describe situations in which the patient may respond to the APPN as a child, grandchild, parent, spouse, sibling, erotic object, or social authority figure. Unfortunately, there is little guidance from the literature for the clinician to understand, explicate, and use this transference process effectively with older patients to resolve problems in living. However, the first step is that the APPN recognizes his or her own feelings toward the patient in addition to recognizing the patient's feelings. Exploring one's own feelings as well as the patient's feelings are essential strategies for good psychotherapy.

Countertransference issues affect the APPN's perception of the older patient. Most psychotherapy programs do not offer substantial training to students about how to work with the elderly. However, when faced with a therapy situation with an older adult, projections of past relationships with older adults can significantly impact the APPN's ability to establish and maintain a therapeutic alliance. Unresolved issues with parents, personal fears about aging and death, and experiences with caretaking responsibilities of parents or grandparents may distort images of the older patients APPNs serve. Learning about these types of transference and countertransference issues is extremely important to work effectively with older adults. Ongoing clinical supervision is essential for working through these challenges during the psychotherapy process. See Chapter 4, for a further discussion of transference and countertransference.

Termination

Another psychotherapy issue that may be different with older adults is that of termination. Termination of psychotherapy should occur by a mutual decision between the APPN and the patient based on the therapy goals attained. However, terminating psychotherapy can be very difficult for the APPN and an older adult patient because of fears that the older patient will have no one else with whom to share personal thoughts and feelings. Granted, these feelings can originate because of transference and countertransference issues or the APPN's personal sense of importance, but it is exactly for these reasons that it may be easier to cross the professional boundary from APPN to friend with older adults. To mitigate the potential for inappropriate boundary crossing, it is essential to discuss the criteria for termination from therapy and the importance of endings early in the therapy process; to identify potential options for replacing the social and emotional intimacy of therapy as therapy draws to an end; and to examine at the end of therapy what was learned by both the patient and the APPN as a result of the psychotherapy process to foster a sense of reciprocity, sharing, and completion (Sullivan, Zeff, & Zweig, 2018).

Practical Issues

Practical issues such as physical arrangement of the therapy office to accommodate diminished sight and hearing are issues to be addressed when working with older adults. Environmental noise should be kept to a minimum, and the APPN and older patient need to be seated facing each other to facilitate communication. Accommodations may also have to be made for assistive devices such as walkers and wheelchairs when entering the building and office. Chairs may need to be situated so that older adults have access to something firm and stable to help them rise after sitting through a long therapy session. Therapy sessions may need to be shortened. Bathrooms need to be available and easily accessible, even with ambulatory assistive devices. Patient information materials should be written in at least a 14-point font and easily available. It is also useful to call and remind the patient about the therapy session 1 or 2 days in advance until the sessions become routine.

Complementary and Alternative Medicine Therapies and Older Adults

Complementary medicine refers to use of complementary and alternative medicine (CAM) *together with* conventional medicine, such as using meditation practices in addition to medications to help reduce anxiety. Most use of CAM by Americans is complementary. Alternative medicine refers to the use of CAM *in place of* conventional medicine, such as using dietary supplements or traditional Chinese medicine for the depressive effects of seasonal affective disorder or depression. Integrative medicine combines treatments from conventional medicine and CAM for which there is some high-quality evidence of safety and effectiveness (American Association for Retired Persons and National Center for Complementary and Alternative Medicine [AARP & NCCAM], 2007).

Increasingly, middle-aged and older adults are using CAM therapies for the management of health and mental health concerns. In a 2007 study by the American Association of Retired Persons (AARP) and the National Center for Complementary and Alternative Medicine (NCCAM), 63% of survey respondents who were 50 to 65 years of age and older reported having used one or more CAM therapies. The two most common types of CAM therapies were bodywork (e.g., massage and chiropractic manipulation) and herbal products or dietary supplements for the use of treating specific conditions and for overall wellness (AARP & NCCAM, 2007). An earlier study found similar results from older adult survey respondents aged 66 to 100 years who reported using CAM therapies such as chiropractic, herbal medicines, massage, and acupuncture for pain relief, improved quality of life, and maintenance of health and fitness (Williamson, Fletcher, & Dawson, 2003). But findings from a more recent analysis of the national Collaborative Psychiatric Epidemiology Survey (Groden, Woodward, Chatters, & Taylor, 2017) to distinguish CAM use between pre-boomers (born prior to 1945) and boomers (born between 1946 and 1964) showed that 23% of older adults used CAM interventions. Pre-boomers used more prayer and spiritual practices than boomers, boomers used a variety of CAM approaches for mental health care, and boomers sought out mental healthcare for mental disorders.

So why should information about CAM therapies be part of this chapter? This is because CAM therapies can be used in conjunction with psychotherapy to provide effective, evidence-based treatments to older adults with psychiatric disorders who request them. See Chapter 16, on integrating CAM into psychotherapy. APPNs need to understand that many of their patients may already be using CAM therapies and will continue using them as part of the treatment for psychiatric disorders; therefore, we need to ask patients about any CAM therapy use. APPNs can develop their own competencies and licensure to provide various CAM therapies directly to their patients in conjunction with psychotherapy, such as energy or bodywork therapies. APPNs can also include prayer and other spiritual practices in mental healthcare as appropriate and important to the patient. APPNs should develop a network of relationships with professional CAM providers to whom patients can be referred. Future graduate programs in psychiatric and geriatric nursing will need to teach students to assess patients for CAM use and teach about the use of effective CAM therapies for maximizing the health and well-being of older adults and for the treatment of mood and cognitive symptoms of various psychiatric disorders.

EVIDENCE-BASED RESEARCH AND PSYCHOTHERAPY

At one time, psychotherapy for the treatment of psychiatric disorders in late life was not enthusiastically endorsed by the mental health community. This perspective has changed in the past 20 years, largely because of clinical trials demonstrating that mood disorders, especially depression, can be treated successfully in older adults when psychotherapies are adapted to meet the physical and cognitive requirements of older adults.

Recent studies suggest that older community-living adults may benefit from psychotherapy just as younger adults and they prefer psychotherapy over medications (Gum et al., 2006). Yet, they may not receive psychotherapy services as often as younger adults. Challenges to accessibility of psychotherapy include the lack of psychotherapy options for depression and anxiety disorders in primary care, difficulties reaching homebound and rural elders, and limited professional mental health workforce with expertise working with older adults (Nurit, Dana, & Yuval, 2016; Raue et al., 2017).

Although some of the issues about the use of psychotherapy with older adults are similar to those of any age, there are differences that need to be considered before commencing therapy. A number of psychotherapies have been reported in the literature to be used successfully with older adults, especially those with depression. In a review of 40 years of research about psychotherapies for adult depression, Cuijpers (2017) reports that all therapies (cognitive behavioral, interpersonal, problem-solving, supportive, behavioral activation, and short-term psychodynamic) are effective with older adults without significant differences among them in the reduction of depression symptoms. Psychotherapies have been adapted more recently for older adults with cognitive impairment, such as Problem-Solving Therapy for Executive Dysfunction (PST-ED), Problem Adaptation Therapy (PATH), Cognitive Behavioral Therapy for Mild Dementia (CBT-MD), Interpersonal Therapy for Mild Cognitive Impairment (IPT-CT), and, for older adults with medical illnesses, for example, Personalized Adherence Intervention for Depression (PID-C) and Ecosystem-Focused Therapy (EFT) for post-stroke depression (McGovern et al., 2014). Dialectical Behavior Therapy (DBT) has been shown to be effective in reducing depressive symptoms and suicidality in older adults with coexisting personality disorders (Lynch & Cheavers, 2007). Mindfulness-based interventions are also being studied for their impact on the health and mental health of older adults with the best evidence for decreasing depression, anxiety, and stress (Geiger et al., 2016). Emerging research findings suggest mindfulness interventions may be beneficial to reduce the negative symptoms of adult psychosis, but no studies have been done with older adults (Aust & Bradshaw, 2017). Most often, these approaches have been used for individual therapy with older adults, although the literature does report the effectiveness of group and family therapy (Cuijpers, 2017; Tavares & Barbosa, 2018). Scientific evidence supports the use of psychotherapy with older adults alone, with medications, and with complementary and alternative therapies (Table 22.2). This section reviews the evidence for using three of the most common psychotherapies with older adults and discusses the modifications needed to assist elders to be successful in using these psychotherapies.

Cognitive Behavioral Therapy

The most extensively studied of the psychotherapies with older adults is CBT. Over 500 clinical trials have compared CBT with other therapies, medications, or usual care for the treatment of adult depression over the last 40 years (Cuijpers, 2017). Results of systematic reviews and meta-analyses of psychosocial treatments for depression and anxiety in the older adults, including CBT, indicate that CBT can be effective in the treatment of depression and anxiety, albeit with some age-specific modifications, that are described in Table 22.3 (Cuijpers, 2017; Hall, Kellett, Berrios, Bains, & Scott, 2016; Shah, Scogin, & Floyd, 2012).

TABLE 22.2 TREATMENT OPTIONS FOR COMMON PSYCHIATRIC DISORDERS IN OLDER ADULTS			
Goals of Therapy	**Foci/Themes of Therapy**	**Evidence-Based Psychotherapy Modalities**	**Evidence-Based CAM Modalities***
Depression			
Healthcare management adherence to healthcare regimen, relapse recognition and prevention, symptom reduction to remission, suicide prevention	Isolation, grief, caretaker's burden, finding meaning in life, balancing resources, how to improve quality of life	CBT, IPT, PST, reminiscence therapy, DBT, group and family therapy	St. John's wort, SAMe, exercise, bright light exposure, mindfulness-based interventions
Anxiety			
Symptom reduction to remission, adherence to healthcare regimen, reduction in inappropriate use of primary care, relapse prevention	Specific worries of older adults such as about death, health, and becoming dependent, concrete suggestions for managing acute anxiety	Behavioral therapy, relaxation training, biofeedback, CBT, IPT, psychoeducation	Kava, yoga, MBSR, guided imagery, biofeedback, rosemary and lavender essential oils, music therapy
Schizophrenia			
Healthcare management, enhancing quality of life, optimizing adherence with medications, preventing relapse	Skills for daily living, maintaining meaningful relationships, health status, substance use, coping skills	Psychoeducation, psychosocial skills training, CBT, family therapy	Mindfulness-based therapies show promise in adults with psychosis

(continued)

TABLE 22.2   TREATMENT OPTIONS FOR COMMON PSYCHIATRIC DISORDERS IN OLDER ADULTS (*CONTINUED*)

Goals of Therapy	Foci/Themes of Therapy	Evidence-Based Psychotherapy Modalities	Evidence-Based CAM Modalities*
Bipolar Disorder			
Healthcare management, enhancing quality of life, optimizing adherence with medications, achieving remission, suicide prevention	Skills for daily living, maintaining meaningful relationships, health status, substance use, coping skills	Psychoeducation, psychosocial skills training, CBT, family therapy	No CAM therapies have been substantiated for treatment of cyclic mood changes in older adults
Dementia			
Acceptance of changing mental status; maintaining meaningful relationships, health; optimizing life activities within changing cognitive status	Coping skills for daily living, depression prevention, and/or management	Psychoeducation, psychosocial skills training, CBT-MD, IPT-CI, PATH, family therapy	Ginkgo biloba, B vitamins, Snoezelen sensory stimulation, music therapy

*Lake, J. (2007). *Textbook of integrative mental health care*. New York, NY: Thieme Medical Publishers.

CAM, complementary and alternative medicine; CBT, cognitive behavioral therapy; CBT-MD, cognitive behavioral therapy for mild dementia; DBT, dialectical behavior therapy; IPT, interpersonal therapy; IPT-CI, interpersonal psychotherapy for mild cognitive impairment; MBSR, mindfulness-based stress reduction; PATH, problem adaptive therapy; PST, problem-solving therapy; SAMe, S-adenosyl-L-methionine.

TABLE 22.3   MODIFICATION OF CBT FOR OLDER ADULTS

CBT Issue	CBT Modifications
Difficulty in increasing pleasant events due to social isolation and physical limitations	Adapt the pleasant event list to activities that are realistic. Ask patient to identify only 5–10 pleasant events. Consider appropriate nonphysical pleasant events. Remind patient of events to engage in.
Multiple physical, social, and cognitive problems identified each week	Set agenda each week. Set priorities for work and skill building each week.

(*continued*)

TABLE 22.3 MODIFICATION OF CBT FOR OLDER ADULTS (*CONTINUED*)	
CBT Issue	**CBT Modifications**
	Refocus on abilities as well as disabilities. Use "faces" chart to identify feelings.
Confuses thoughts and feelings Worries about writing things down because of hand tremors or embarrassment about ability to express thoughts and feelings	Adapt worksheets to provide adequate space; consider lined paper for guide to writing. Ask patient to use audiotape or voice mail as option to writing or use keyboard and computer. Reassure patient that writing is a memory and learning tool; penmanship is not evaluated. Encourage patient to use a writing prosthesis.
Forgets to complete weekly activity schedules and dysfunctional thought records	Ask patient to use audiotape recorder or voice mail. Develop reminders (calendar, voice mail, friend, or family) for patient.

CBT, cognitive behavioral therapy.

CBT has been used with older adults as a treatment for physical illnesses such as tinnitus (Andersson, Porsaeus, Wiklund, Kaldo, & Larsen, 2005), chronic insomnia (Brewster, Riegel, & Gehrman, 2018; Haynes, Talbert, Fox, & Close, 2018), and chronic pain (Reid, Otis, Barry, & Kerns, 2003), and to promote improving self-care and function in people with heart failure (Freedland et al., 2015) and Parkinson's disease (Calleo et al., 2015). CBT has been combined with other therapies, such as social skills training, to manage the symptoms of schizophrenia in older persons (Granholm, Holden, Link, McQuaid, & Jeste, 2013). CBT has also been delivered successfully by telephone to rural older adults with depression and anxiety (Brenes, Danhauer, Lyles, Anderson, & Miller, 2016).

Because CBT has been explained in Chapter 8, this discussion focuses on the use of CBT with older adults and the modifications that may be needed for this population. Although many older adults do not require significant modifications of CBT to be successful in learning and applying the CBT tools in their lives, some common CBT issues and suggested modifications are summarized in Table 22.3. Other resources can provide explicit descriptions of using CBT techniques with older adults (Gallagher & Thompson, 1981; Granholm, Auslander, Gottlieb, McQuaid, & McClure, 2006). Although CBT has been provided to older adults in individual and group modalities, this review focuses on individual CBT.

CBT generally consists of 16 to 20 sessions, divided into three phases: introductory or early phase, working or middle phase, and termination or late phase (Areán, 2004). These phases usually do not change when working with older adults, although each phase may be extended. The focus of the initial phase (i.e., approximately sessions 1 through 3) of CBT is to socialize the patient to psychotherapy and CBT and build the therapeutic alliance. This is also the time to begin to identify goals of therapy and any barriers that may impact working toward or achieving these goals (e.g., family support, transportation, and physical limitations). After the older patient is comfortable with the CBT model and begins to ask questions about how the therapy works, it is time to move into the middle phase of CBT.

During the middle phase of CBT (i.e., approximately sessions 4 through 16), the focus is on building behavioral skills to increase pleasant activities, cognitive skills to challenge negative thinking, and social skills to improve problem-solving communication.

The weekly activity schedule and the automatic thought diary may need to be modified so that the older person is able to use these tools easily. Because most older persons are not used to identifying their feelings and thoughts and writing them down and then challenging their way of thinking, learning to use the CBT tools during this phase may take longer than in younger adults. Completing homework can be a problem because of vision and writing barriers. Reading and homework assignments may seem too much like school to be acceptable to some older adults, and others seem to appreciate the structured, educational approach of CBT. Using motivational interviewing techniques may be helpful in overcoming reluctance to doing the homework. Sometimes it may be more efficient to do the homework during the therapy session.

The later phase (i.e., approximately sessions 16 through 20) addresses termination and relapse prevention. Movement into this phase is dictated by goal attainment and the resolution of major complaints and symptoms. Skill building during these last sessions aims to consolidate learning by reinforcing the behavioral and cognitive skills learned, identifying expected "rough spots" when maintaining treatment outcomes, and developing a guide for surviving those difficult times. During this last phase of CBT, the APPN may find it helpful, with the patient's consent, to teach family members and healthcare staff ways to support the patient in maintaining therapeutic gains and prevent relapse.

In summary, CBT has been shown to be an effective intervention for a variety of physical and mental conditions affecting older adults, but the most common use of CBT has been to treat depression and anxiety disorders. CBT has been provided effectively in face-to face-sessions with older individuals and in groups, and delivered using telephone CBT. Assisted Internet-delivered CBT has also been studied to meet the needs of rural populations with depressed older adults (Titov et al., 2015) and older adults with knee arthritis (O'Moore et al., 2017).

A number of manuals have been developed to assist the clinician to adapt and conduct CBT with older adults. Many older adults do not require extensive modifications to the structured CBT approach, but when modifications are required, they usually focus on improving physical and memory capabilities to engage successfully in CBT. A thorough description of the use of CBT in the elderly is provided in *Cognitive Behavioral Therapy With Older People* (Laidlaw, Thompson, Gallagher-Thompson, & Dick-Siskin, 2003), in *Treating Late Life Depression: A Cognitive-Behavioral Therapy Approach* (Gallagher-Thompson & Thompson, 2009), and by Mark Floyd in *Making Evidence-Based Psychological Treatments Work With Older Adults* (Shah et al., 2012).

Interpersonal Psychotherapy

Interpersonal therapy (IPT), like CBT, has been studied for its effectiveness in reducing depression and anxiety in older adults. IPT gained attention as a therapeutic intervention in the 1970s' work by Gerald Klerman and Myrna Weissman and has been shown in clinical trials to be an effective intervention for depression compared with antidepressants. Unfortunately, the early clinical trials (DiMascio et al., 1979; Elkin et al., 1989) did not include a significant elderly population and did not identify age-specific outcomes. For the last 20 years, IPT has been used in a number of populations, with and without modifications to the original IPT manual, and is an empirically validated psychotherapy for depression (Cuijpers, 2017; Weissman, Markowitz, & Klerman, 2000). See Chapter 10, for IPT. The discussion that follows applies to using IPT with older adults.

Sholomskas et al. (1983) published an article that argued IPT could be used with older adults. Since then, there have been randomized clinical trials of IPT for the treatment of acute depression and for maintenance therapy for prolonging relapse and preventing

TABLE 22.4 MODIFICATION OF INTERPERSONAL PSYCHOTHERAPY FOR OLDER ADULTS	
IPT Issues	**IPT Modifications**
Initial Sessions	
Many problems are presented by patient, and there is too much life history to cover. Patient does not understand he or she has depression. Patient wants the therapist to "cure" depression.	Link presenting problems to one or two focus areas, and have patient prioritize these. Quantify depression with standardized scales; use these scales to educate the patient and family or support system about depression. Take an active role to structure therapy sessions using the IPT manual. Give the patient permission to temporarily take on the sick role so that energy can be focused on getting healthier rather than external demands.
Intermediate Sessions	
Patient is reluctant to talk about conflictual, negative feelings. Patient does not understand he or she has depression. Patient has difficulty staying focused on problem areas. Patient is reluctant to identify changes needed in his or her behavior. Patient wants to include family and other support in sessions.	Educate the patient about basic communication principles and identification of feelings. Quantify depression with standardized scales; use these scales to educate the patient and family or support system about depression. Address the patient's difficulty staying focused on the topic; look for patterns of distraction, and correlate feelings with distraction. Take an active role in therapy, but do not provide advice about therapy dilemmas presented by the patient; encourage the patient to state what can be done about the problem. Include joint meetings if appropriate, and IPT issues can be addressed.
Termination Sessions	
Patient experiences ongoing physical problems or stressors and wants to continue IPT.	Every few sessions, remind the patient of the number of sessions left. Remind the patient about the contract, and address sadness due to loss or change in the interpersonal relationship.

IPT, interpersonal therapy.

recurrence of major depression in older adults (Miller et al., 2001, 2003; van Schaik et al., 2007). Most of the available research studies have evaluated IPT in combination with psychopharmacology for the treatment of depression in adults, including some older adults in the study population (Mackin & Areán, 2005). Significant addition to the literature about IPT for older adults is *Interpersonal Psychotherapy for Depressed Older Adults,* written by Hinrichsen and Clougherty (2006); *Clinician's Guide to Interpersonal Psychotherapy in Late Life* by Miller (2009), and the "Interpersonal Psychotherapy for the Treatment of Late-Life Depression" chapter by Hinrichsen and Iselin (2014). These author clinicians review the information available on IPT and discuss the specific strategies for using IPT in older adults and the modifications needed for older adults with mood disorders and with cognitive impairments. The most recent IPT manual (Hinrichsen & Iselin, 2014) includes a review of the research, a user-friendly description for conducting IPT, clinical case summaries, and fidelity scales.

IPT can be an important vehicle for reflection and resolution of roles and relationships. Gerontologists have long discussed the changing roles and relationships of older adults as they traverse the landscape of old age (Rosow, 1967). Many publications have focused on the loss of social roles, the transition from one role to another (e.g., in retirement and widowhood), and the resulting sense of isolation and grief experienced by some older adults. Well-known theorists such as Erikson (1982) and Levinson (1986) have identified the importance of interpersonal relationships in maintaining stable physical and emotional health across life's stages. During transition from one life stage to another, adults often reflect on what is important and what needs to be changed. In adult development and aging, social relationships are often the focal point of these reflections. With older adults, IPT can be the vehicle for this reflection and resolution.

Clinician authors who have used IPT with depressed older adults suggest that there are few modifications needed when translating IPT for use with an older population (Areán, 2004; Hinrichsen & Clougherty, 2006; Hinrichsen & Iselin, 2014; Miller, 2009). Their perspective is that the structure of IPT provides a workable therapy framework to focus on bereavement, role transitions, and role conflict. Table 22.4 describes the modifications of IPT for older adults. The modifications commonly identified are those needed to support the physical and cognitive capabilities of older adults.

Reasons for choosing IPT over CBT include the comfort of the APPN with the type of therapy and whether the older patient is able and willing to address a specific here-and-now problem within a brief period. If the older adult presents with concerns focused on loss, grief, interpersonal conflicts, or role transitions; is cognitively intact; and is mildly to moderately depressed without a clear personality disorder, IPT appears to be a good choice for therapy. If the older adult presents with moderate or chronic or partially remitted depression or with MCI and expresses concerns about a negative life event and perceives himself or herself as helpless, CBT may be the better choice for therapy, especially the adapted CBT for mild dementia, CBT-MD.

Hinrichsen and Clougherty (2006) suggest that the modifications needed when applying IPT to older adults are those that clinicians need to make. They suggest that novice APPNs with little experience working with older adults may have less success with IPT than with other therapies because of conflicting attitudes and values about the responsiveness of older adults to therapy. Clinicians may have difficulty maintaining the structure of IPT when older adults lose focus and become reflective and tangential during sessions. They may become overwhelmed with the multitude of problems and have difficulty prioritizing problems appropriate for IPT. When this occurs, APPNs may not present a clear plan for treatment and then have difficulty moving through the phases of IPT in a timely fashion. Sometimes, APPNs may choose to extend the contract for IPT past the 16 weeks of treatment, which may reinforce dependency in the clinician/patient interpersonal relationship.

Mindfulness-Based Interventions

Older depressed adults often do not get treatment or delay getting treatment for their depression because they do not want to take medications or options for getting psychotherapy are limited by access and/or cost. Becoming more common with older adults, mindfulness-based interventions combining meditation, guided imagery, and relaxation aim to improve psychological well-being. Mindfulness-Based Stress Reduction (MBSR) programs are based on the work of Jon Kabat-Zinn (1990) and initially designed to address stress management. MBSR is now used to treat a variety of mental health and physical health conditions in many different populations. The usual 8-week MBSR program includes eight weekly 2.5-hour sessions and a 6-hour silent retreat on a different day during week 6. Participants are expected to engage in homework activities during the week which include body scans, relaxation and meditation exercises, yoga, and journaling, and discussions during the classes. The purpose of MBSR is to learn to be present in the moment non-judgmentally.

Although few in number currently, studies that have reported using MBSR for older adult subjects have shown the effectiveness of mindful-based interventions on disabilities related to physical health problems such as pain, arthritis, and cognitive impairment (Geiger et al., 2016). Some authors have suggested possible modifications such as 90-minute sessions, simplified yoga exercises, shortened or eliminated all-day retreat, shortened sitting meditations, fewer days of homework, and repetition of materials (Geiger et al., 2016). ELDERSHINE, an adapted MBSR program for older adults (Szanton, Wenzel, Connolly, & Piferi, 2011), is designed to promote positive mental and physical health. ELDERSHINE modifications include shorter meditation periods, shorter 90-minute 8-weekly sessions, seated rather than walking meditations, and no all day retreat. Large type weekly handouts are used instead of workbooks. This adapted program is one of the first developed specifically for older adults.

Reminiscence and Life Review

Reminiscence therapy (RT) and life review therapy (LRT) are approaches that focus on reflecting on life, the aging process, and on constructing a sense of self-continuity. Both approaches can be less challenging for the patient to use because they use remote memory processes to integrate a lifetime of successes and challenges rather than working memory, which might be less available to some older adults. To clarify these therapies, we offer a brief theoretical overview, differentiate these two concepts, and summarize the evidence using them with older adults.

The common roots of reminiscence and life review are found in the seminal article by Robert Butler (1963), a geropsychiatrist, who described the "looking back" process he observed in his patients and observed the therapeutic value of reflecting on the there and then, rather than as an escape from the here and now. Butler distinguished life review from reminiscence by saying that life review is a type of reminiscence. In 1974, Lewis and Butler described LRT as an effective method with older adults to assist them during developmental transitions. About the same time, Erikson (1982) described more fully the last developmental stage in late adulthood: ego integrity versus despair. Applying the concepts of RT and LRT in clinical practice was emphasized during the 1970s and 1980s because these concepts provided positive outcomes to what had been assumed to be old-age forgetfulness and escape from the realities of old age. New roles and goals were described for older adults.

Since that time, many study authors have struggled with distinguishing reminiscence and life review from each other and from other types of autobiographical reflections. Table 22.5 differentiates reminiscence from life review. This ambiguity has limited empirical study of their effectiveness in research and clinical practice. Burnside and Haight (1992) provide a conceptual analysis of reminiscence and life review therapies. In their analysis, *reminiscence* is defined as "a process of recalling long-forgotten experiences, events which are memorable to the person" (p. 856). *Life review* is defined as "a retrospective survey or existence, a critical study of a life, or a second look at one's life" (p. 856). Both processes depend on memory recall, but reminiscence is thought to reconstruct life events from memory (Staudinger, 2001) and life review as deconstructing life events into a more positive life narrative (Molinari, 1999).

TABLE 22.5 DISTINGUISHING REMINISCENCE AND LIFE REVIEW		
Criteria	**Reminiscence**	**Life Review**
Attributes	Verbal interaction between two or more people who are eliciting memories Involves "flash bulb" recall and spontaneous interaction or theme-focused group discussion No evaluation of life; focus is on pleasurable memories Focused on past events or experiences, not current events	Done between a therapeutic listener and reviewer on 1:1 basis Recall process covers entire life span, usually chronologically Recall must contain an evaluative or analytical component to prepare for the future Recall past or recent events and experiences
Recalled events Time frame goals	Both happy and sad times No specific time allotted Decreased isolation Increased socialization, connectedness, and friendships Increased self-esteem Increased life satisfaction	Both happy and sad times Usually takes 4 to 6 weeks Integrity Increased self-esteem Decreased depression Increased life satisfaction Peace
Patient characteristics	Cognitively intact and mild to moderately impaired older adults Able to focus on self and others in the group May be difficult in group setting to reminisce if patient has many traumatic events or is guarded	Cognitively intact to mildly impaired Self-focused Usually experiencing a life event trigger

At the risk of oversimplifying the distinctions between reminiscence and life review, Table 22.5 is provided so that the APPN can begin to understand the difference and choose the most appropriate intervention for the situation. These distinctions are drawn from a number of resources, including Molinari (1999), Burnside and Haight (1992), Haight and Burnside (1993), Staudinger (2001), and Knight (2004). Webster, Bohlmeijer, and Westerhof (2010) characterized reminiscence into three types: simple and unstructured, structured life review or reminiscence, and LRT. Simple or unstructured reminiscence is telling the story of life events focusing on positive events to enhance well-being. This type of reminiscence can be provided using non-professional providers such as support groups and memorists. Structured life review or reminiscence is more than just story-telling. It takes a more graded process proceeding through specific life timelines with the goal of reframing these events and integrating them into a more positive self-view. LRT is generally used with depressed and/or anxious individuals with the goal of changing one's view of himself or herself and correcting emotional responses to life events (Bhar, 2014). The goal of LRT is to replace negative beliefs about self and the past with more positive beliefs. Structured reminiscence and LRT should be provided by mental health professionals with psychotherapy training so that when remembering and talking about past events precipitates unexpected negative responses, appropriate professional interventions can be initiated. For example, Dick, a 78-year-old veteran, started talking about his Korean war experiences during a medication management session with Tony, a PMHNP working in the outpatient psychiatric department at the Veterans Medical Center. Instead of focusing on current symptoms, Tony asked questions that allowed Dick time to reflect on his memories about a particular skirmish in which Dick was wounded and accidentally shot another U.S. soldier. This brought up intense feelings of guilt and sadness for Dick. Tony understood that Dick needed to sort through his feelings about this past event and spent more time with him and then scheduled ongoing weekly psychotherapy appointments rather than medication management sessions. Differentiating these types of reminiscence interventions could be useful in developing protocols for different mental health problems for older adult populations (Bhar, 2014).

The focus on practical, clinical application of reminiscence and life review rather than on empirical study of its efficacy has led to conclusions by some geropsychiatric clinicians that these therapies are not useful for treating psychiatric illnesses but are reserved as more global psychosocial interventions for healthier older adults. Authors' recent systematic reviews of research related to life review and reminiscence suggest that LRT and RT can be effective in early treatment of depression with older adults who experience loss of meaning in life (Bohlmeijer, Roemer, Cuijpers, & Smit, 2007; Francis & Kumar, 2013; Hsieh & Wang, 2003; Shah et al., 2012) but also report a lack of consistent findings about the efficacy of both therapies due to different outcomes and outcome measurements, small and varied samples, ambiguous and diverse intervention protocols, and methodological flaws. Results from randomized controlled trials (Korte, Bohlmeijer, Cappeliez, Smit, & Westerhof, 2012; Pot et al., 2010) provide some evidence for the positive effects of reminiscence and life review for the treatment of depressive symptoms in older adults. Further study will help to clarify for whom these therapies are appropriate, when to provide these therapies, and how to use these therapies to alleviate psychiatric symptoms (Shah et al., 2012; Webster et al., 2010).

There is no standard structure or method of life review and reminiscence. Knight (2004) suggests using a timeline to guide the life review, such as reviewing life events over each decade. Another approach is to review various domains of life such as family of origin, educational experiences, military experiences, sexual development, and religious or spiritual history. Dutch researchers (Pot et al., 2010) developed a structured life review course, "Looking for Meaning," that improved coping skill and decreased depressive symptoms and anxiety. Each of the twelve 2-hour sessions centered on a topic and included sensory recall exercises, creative activities, and discussions. Approaching life review with an overall structure in mind facilitates discovering gaps in recall of significant events, which can open the door to discussions of positive and negative emotional issues that can be evaluated in light of the person's self-concept.

Haight and Olson (1989) offer sample questions that can be asked to direct life review following Haight's Life Review and Experiencing Form (Haight, Coleman, & Lord, 1995). They also suggest structuring the life review around developmental stages of life, such as childhood (What was your childhood like? What were your parents like?), adolescence (Who were important people for you? Do you remember feeling alone?), adulthood (Do/did you enjoy your work? How were you appreciated for your work?), and older age (What have been some of the disappointments in your life? What are the happiest moments in your life? What would you do differently?). Burnside and Haight (1992) suggest using pictures, books, autobiographical writing or journaling, audio-taping or videotaping, and letter writing to elicit memories. They also suggest asking questions to encourage a self-examination and exploration of how patients might have changed things if they had the opportunity.

In summary, reminiscence and life review therapies are useful techniques for helping older adults recall life events and, in the process of talking about their lives, come to an understanding of who they are as whole persons. The empirical evidence for the effectiveness of reminiscence and life review therapies is growing and these therapies have been reported to improve self-esteem, increase socialization, and decrease depressive symptoms (Francis & Kumar, 2013). Authors agree that the less structured approaches may prove to be a vital option for older adults in normal developmental transitions or experiencing dramatic life events, and the more structured LRT is more appropriate for the treatment of significant depressive symptoms.

Reminiscence and life review therapies are not manualized therapies consistently used by therapists. Although some personal historians and autobiographers in the private sector have developed their own products and processes for assisting persons to write their personal memoirs, these contracted personal memoirs are not done for the primary purpose of developing a coherent sense of self or reducing depressive symptoms. Biennial conferences of the International Institute of Reminiscence and Life Review demonstrate the variety of applications of reminiscence and life review therapies for different populations. See Appendix 22.1 for Haight's Life Review and Experiencing Form.

CASE EXAMPLE

This case study reflects the life review process familiar to the author, using the timeline approach rather than the event approach, and was agreeable to the patient.

Violet wheeled herself into the APPN's office and told her that she was 98 years old, soon to be 99, and wanted to get ready for her 100th birthday in just over a year. When the APPN asked Violet what she meant by "getting ready," she replied she wanted to clear up some things in her life to feel good about what she had accomplished. The APPN asked her where they should begin, and she replied, "At the beginning, as far back as I can remember." That was the start of a long but interesting journey with Violet as she sorted through her life on her way to being a centenarian.

Violet was living in a nursing home on a senior housing campus that included a primary geriatric clinic. Violet was referred by one of the geriatricians because she requested "someone to talk to about things." Little did he know how much talking she had to do! Violet was in a wheelchair because she was no longer able to walk independently because of peripheral vascular disease, which caused her leg tremors and pain.

At the first meeting, the APPN discussed with Violet her time frame for sorting things out. She planned to come for about 6 months and was able to come to therapy about every 2 weeks. A timeline was developed from her birth to current age, and then 100 was added at the end of the timeline, which was drawn on large paper sheets taped together and put on the office wall. The timeline was marked off in decades, much like a ruler, and notes on the paper were written during the therapy sessions. Because Violet could not remember much of her life before 3 years of age, the beginning of the timeline was information she remembered from family stories. The focus of each session was on a particular time in Violet's life. Structured questions centered on her family, work, decisions she had made, challenges she experienced, and what she had learned from the experiences during that time. She reminisced about the happy times and the sad times. Sometimes, Violet brought family pictures or letters to talk about. When there were gaps in her memory, another decade became the focus, with a return later to fill in the gaps.

When the APPN asked Violet how she had decided to do this life review, she replied that she wanted to know who she was and wanted to tell people about her life at the

100th birthday party she was planning. Her life was charted through her 98th year, and she noted this life review on her life chart. When the review of her 90s was completed, Violet thanked the APPN and invited her to the upcoming 100th birthday party. The value of the relationship for both Violet and the APPN was discussed. The APPN did attend her 100th birthday party, and the life review chart was on the wall for all to see.

The patient's goal of "clearing things up" was met during LRT as Violet became clearer about what the significant events were in her life, when these events happened, and how her emotional response impacted her self-identity and later relationships with her husband and children. The collaborative goal was met because Violet was able to emotionally disengage from past mistakes and negative experiences and to find some comfort in her sense of self at 100 years.

ROLE AND EDUCATIONAL RESOURCES FOR THE ADVANCED PRACTICE NURSE IN GEROPSYCHIATRIC NURSING

Due to the demographic imperative of the aging population, there is increasing awareness of the complex needs of older adults and the need for more nurses to help meet those needs in diverse settings. Unfortunately, gerontological nursing and especially geropsychiatric nursing (GPN) do not attract the nurses needed for an adequate workforce. As noted in a guest editorial in the *Journal of Gerontological Nursing*, this is reflected in the numbers of nurses holding national certification in gerontological nursing as both generalists and advanced practice nurses (APN; Melillo, 2017). There are 2.9 million RNs in the United States (USDHHS, 2014). The American Nurses Credentialing Center (ANCC) reports that in 2018 only 15% of the ANCC certified NPs and 13.6% of the ANCC certified clinical nurse specialists (CNS) had a gerontological focus (ANCC, 2019). Currently, there is no geropsychiatric advanced practice nursing certification available.

APPNs provide specialized psychiatric care to persons of all ages, including complex psychiatric diagnostic assessments and psychotropic medication prescribing and management, and are required to achieve competency in psychotherapy. APPNs (CNS and nurse practitioners [NP]) practice independently and collaboratively to manage the psychiatric care of older adults in settings such as inpatient and emergency psychiatric services, outpatient mental health clinics, psychiatric home care, long-term care facilities, and substance abuse treatment centers. Although APPNs can assess for common medical conditions often comorbid with psychiatric conditions, they do not generally diagnose and manage complex medical conditions of older adults. Generally, the medication prescribing practice of an APPN is focused on psychotropic medications and drugs to manage the side effects of these medications.

Some advanced practice nurses have expertise in both gerontologic and psychiatric nursing, and although fewer in number, they practice in settings where the elderly receive medical and psychiatric care and have been shown to be effective catalysts for improved clinical outcomes (Kaas & Beattie, 2006). The subspecialty of gerontologic mental health nursing was developed in the 1970s. Core content for this specialty was identified in the 1980s by Beverly Baldwin, but few specialized GPN programs have been developed (Morris & Mentes, 2006). Although the dearth of gerontological and geropsychiatric nurses is discouraging, there are a number of gerontological nurses, professional associations, and organizations who have and are continuing to develop the resources, knowledge, and skills to address the core competencies needed in GPN (Melillo, 2017).

The American Academy of Nursing's GPN Collaborative developed a definition of GPN to stimulate discussion about the preparation of nurses to work with older adults who have mental health concerns..

BOX 22.2 GPN Resources

1. *The GPN Collaborative*: Core competency enhancements in GPN at all levels of nursing education. The enhancements can be accessed under Teaching Tools at the Portal of Geriatric Online Education (www.pogoe.org).
2. *The GPN Initiative* (GPNI): Partnership of the National Hartford Center of Gerontological Nursing Excellence (NHCGNE), Hartford Institute for Geriatric Nursing, and AACN. Continuing education modules on mental health and aging can be accessed at (consultgeri.org/education-training/e-learning-resources/ geropsychiatric-nursing-initiative-modules).
3. *The Gerontological Advanced Practice Nurses Association (GAPNA)*: Web-based toolkit and consensus statement of 12 proficiencies for APN gerontological specialists. These can be accessed at www.pogoe.org.
4. *The University of Iowa's College of Nursing*: Evidence-Based Practice Guidelines addressing the needs of older adults in long-term care settings, half of these address geropsychiatric and mental health nursing. These can be accessed at (http://www .uiowacsomaygeroresources.com/)
5. *The Portal of Geriatrics Online Education (POGOe)*: Collection of expert-contributed geriatrics educational and assessment materials for educators and learners. These can be accessed under Educational Materials at www.pogoe.org.

GPN, geropsychiatric nursing.

[GPN] practice includes holistic support for and care of older adults and their families as they anticipate and/or experience developmental and cognitive challenges, mental health concerns and psychiatric/substance misuse disorders across a variety of health and mental health care settings. GPN practice is based on expert knowledge of normal age-related changes and common psychiatric, cognitive and co-morbid medical disorders in later life. Promotion of mental health and treatment of psychiatric/substance misuse and cognitive disorders emphasize strengths and potentials; integrate biopsychosocial, functional, and spiritual, cultural, economic and environmental factors, and address stressors that affect mental health of older adults and their families. (Beck, Buckwalter, & Evans, 2012, "Geropsychiatric Nursing Definition").

See Box 22.2 for GPN resources. Within this box you will find resources, their sources, and online access information (Butcher, 2016; Harrison, 2016; Melillo, 2017; National Hartford Center of Gerontological Nursing Excellence [NHCGNE], 2016).

CONCLUDING COMMENTS

Some psychotherapies have been shown to be effective with older adults with few modifications from the original theoretical or practice frameworks. When modifications are necessary, they are individualized to address the physical and cognitive impairments of an older adult. The scientific evidence shows us that longer sessions or extended treatment of individual therapy may positively impact the outcomes of therapy, yet increased age and the severity of psychiatric and medical illnesses may limit the type of therapies used with older adults. There is less information about how to use psychotherapies with older adults with coexisting substance use and medical illness, and how to use any particular psychotherapy with specific ethnic/cultural populations of older adults.

The literature regarding specific psychotherapy interventions for psychiatric disorders in late life is growing with nurses making significant contributions to the body of knowledge. This is encouraging because it is important for APPNs to look to the future and develop the evidence for the use of psychotherapies that promote mental health and effective coping. Our understanding of how to adapt these therapies to older adults may provide the basis of targeted health promotion psychotherapy, which can address the needs of the youngest birth cohort of older adults for whom psychiatric disorders and psychotherapy carry less stigma and for whom health promotion is more frequently perceived to be a personal responsibility.

DISCUSSION QUESTIONS

1. Discuss education and certification issues for APPNs working with geropsychiatric patients.
2. Describe how individual, collective, and system issues influence psychotherapy with older adults.
3. Describe general characteristics, assessment tools, treatment goals, and psychotherapy considerations for the following late-life psychiatric disorders: mood disorders, anxiety, schizophrenia, and dementia.
4. Discuss general modifications for the effective conduct of psychotherapy with older adults.
5. Discuss the evidence base and implementation strategies with older adults for each of the following psychotherapies: CBT, IPT, psychodynamic psychotherapy, and LRT.
6. Discuss the evidence and significance of family caregiver therapy.
7. Describe innovative diagnostic and strategic uses of psychotherapy with older adults.
8. Describe factors contributing to the impending geriatric mental health crisis.
9. Discuss contributions that APPNs can make to geriatric mental health promotion and treatment.

REFERENCES

Administration for Community Living. (2019). *2018 profile of older Americans*. Retrieved from https://acl.gov/sites/default/files/Aging%20and%20Disability%20in%20America/2018Old erAmericansProfile.pdf

Almeida, O. P., Pirkis, J., Kerse, N., Sim, M., Flicker, L., Snowdon, J., . . . Pfaff, J. J. (2012). A randomized control trial to reduce the prevalence of depression and self-harm behaviour in older primary care patients. *Annuals of Family Medicine, 10*(4), 347–356. doi:10.1370/afm.1368

Alexopoulos, G. S., Abrams, R. C., Young, R. C., & Shamoian, C. A. (1998). Cornell scale for depression in dementia. *Biological Psychiatry, 23*, 271–284. doi:10.1016/0006-3223(88)90038-8

Alexopoulos, G. S., Reynolds, C. F., III, Bruce, M. L., Katz, I. R., Raue, P. J., Mulsant, B. H., . . . Ten Have, T. (2009). Reducing suicidal ideation and depression in older primary care patients: 24-month outcomes of the PROSPECT study. *American Journal of Psychiatry, 166*(8), 882–890. doi:10.1176/appi.ajp.2009.08121779

American Association of Retired Persons and National Center for Complementary and Alternative Medicine. (2007). *Complementary and alternative medicine: What people 50 and older are using and discussing with their physicians*. Retrieved from https://www.aarp.org/health/alternative-medicine/info-2007/cam_2007.html

American Nurses Credentialing Center. (2019). *2018 ANCC certification data*. Retrieved from https://www.nursingworld.org/~499e5e/globalassets/docs/ancc/2017-certification-data-for-website.pdf

Andersson, G., Porsaeus, D., Wiklund, M., Kaldo, V., & Larsen, H. C. (2005). Treatment of tinnitus in the elderly: A controlled trial of cognitive behavior therapy. *International Journal of Audiology, 44*(11), 671–675. doi:10.1080/14992020500266720

Areán, P. A. (2004). Psychosocial treatments for depression in the elderly. *Primary Psychiatry, 11*(5), 48–53. Retrieved from http://primarypsychiatry.com/psychosocial-treatments-for-depression-in-the-elderly/

Arias, E. (2014). United States life tables, 2009. *National Vital Statistics Reports, 62*(7), 1–63. Retrieved from http://www.cdc.gov/nchs/data/nvsr/nvsr62/nvsr62_07.pdf

Aust, J., & Bradshaw, T. (2017). Mindfulness interventions for psychosis: A systematic review of the literature. *Journal of Psychiatric and Mental Health Nursing, 24*(1), 69–83. doi:10.1111/jpm.12357

Barak, Y., & Swartz, M. (2012). Remission amongst elderly schizophrenia patients. *European Psychiatry, 27*(1), 62–64. doi:10.1016/j.eurpsy.2010.12.012

Beck, C., Buckwalter, K., & Evans, L. (2012). *Geropsychiatric nursing competency enhancements: Geropsychiatric nursing definition.* Retrieved from https://pogoe.org/sites/default/files/Definition_Geropsych_Nursing.pdf

Bhar, S. (2014). Reminiscence therapy: A review. In N. Pachana & K. Laidlaw (Eds.), *Oxford handbook of clinical geropsychology* (pp. 675–690). Oxford, UK: Oxford University Press.

Blood, I., & Guthrie, L. (2018). *Supporting older people using attachment-informed and strengths-based approaches.* Philadelphia, PA: Jessica Kingsley Publishers.

Bohlmeijer, E., Roemer, M., Cuijpers, P., & Smit, F. (2007). The effects of reminiscence on psychological well-being in older adults: A meta-analysis. *Aging & Mental Health, 11*(3), 291–300. doi:10.1080/13607860600963547

Borson, S., Scanlan, J., Brush, M., Vitaliano, P., & Dokmak, A. (2000). The Mini-Cog: A cognitive "vital signs" measure for dementia screening in multi-lingual elderly. *International Journal of Geriatric Psychiatry, 15*, 1021–1027. doi:10.1002/1099-1166(200011)15:11<1021::AID-GPS234>3.0.CO;2-6

Boyd, M. A., & Stevens, G. (2018). Mental health promotion for older adults. In M. A. Boyd (Ed.), *Psychiatric nursing: Contemporary practice* (6th ed., pp. 254–266). Philadelphia, PA: Wolters Kluwer.

Bramsen, I., van der Ploeg, H. M., & Twisk, J. W. R. (2002). Secondary traumatization in Dutch couples of World War II survivors. *Journal of Consulting & Clinical Psychology, 70*(1), 241–245. doi:10.1037/0022-006X.70.1.241

Brenes, G. A., Danhauer, S. C., Lyles, M. F., Anderson, A., & Miller, M. E. (2016). Effects of telephone-delivered cognitive-behavioral therapy and nondirective supportive therapy on sleep, health-related quality of life, and disability. *American Journal of Geriatric Psychiatry, 24*(10), 846–854. doi:10.1016/j.jagp.2016.04.002

Brewster, G. S., Riegel, B., & Gehrman, P. R. (2018). Insomnia in the older adult. *Sleep Medicine Clinics, 13*, 13–19. doi:10.1016/j.jsmc.2017.09.002

Bruce, M. L., Ten Have, T. R., Reynolds, C. F., III, Katz, I. I., Schulberg, H. C., Mulsant, B. H., . . . Alexopoulos, G. S. (2004). Reducing suicidal ideation and depressive symptoms in depressed older primary care patients: A randomized controlled trial. *Journal of the American Medical Association, 291*(9), 1081–1091. doi:10.1001/jama.291.9.1081

Burnside, I., & Haight, B. K. (1992). Reminiscence and life review: Analysing each concept. *Journal of Advanced Nursing, 17*, 855–862. doi:10.1111/j.1365-2648.1992.tb02008.x

Butcher, H. K. (2016). Development and use of gerontological evidence-based practice guidelines. *Journal of Gerontological Nursing, 42*(7), 25–32. doi:10.3928/00989134-20160613-02

Butler, R. (1963). The life review: An interpretation of reminiscence in the aged. *Psychiatry, 26*, 65–76. doi:10.1080/00332747.1963.11023339

Calleo, J. S., Amspoker, A. B., Sarwar, A. I., Kunik, M. E., Jankovic, J., Marsh, L., . . . Stanley, M. A. (2015). A pilot study of a cognitive-behavioral treatment for anxiety and depression in patients with Parkinson disease. *Journal of Geriatric Psychiatry and Neurology, 28*(3), 210–217. doi:10.1177/0891988715588831

Chopra, M. P., Zhang, H., Pless Kaiser, A., Moye, J. A., Llorente, M. D., Oslin, D. W., & Spiro, A., III. (2014). PTSD is a chronic, fluctuating disorder affecting the mental quality of life in older adults. *American Journal of Geriatric Psychiatry, 22*(1), 86–97. doi:10.1016/j.jagp.2013.01.064

Conwell, Y., & Thompson, C. (2008). Suicidal behavior in elders. *Psychiatric Clinics of North America, 31*(2), 333–356. doi:10.1016/j.psc.2008.01.004

Conwell, Y., Van Orden, K., & Caine, E. D. (2011). Suicide in older adults. *Psychiatric Clinics of North America, 34*(2), 451–468. doi:10.1016/j.psc.2011.02.002

Conwell, Y. (2014). Suicide Later in Life: Challenges and Priorities for Prevention. American Journal of Preventive Medicine, 47(3), S244-S250. doi:10.1016/j.amepre.2014.05.040

Cook, J. M., McCarthy, E., & Thorp, S. R. (2017). Older adults with PTSD: Brief state of research and evidence-based psychotherapy case illustration. *American Journal of Geriatric Psychiatry, 25*, 522–530. doi:10.1016/j.jagp.2016.12.016

Cuijpers, P. (2017). Four decades of outcome research on psychotherapies for adult depression: An overview of a series of meta-analyses. *Canadian Psychology, 58*(1), 7–19. doi:10.1037/cap0000096

Cummings, J., Mega, M., Gray, K., Rosenberg-Thompson, S., Carusi, A., & Gornbein, J. (1994). The Neuropsychiatric Inventory: Comprehensive assessment of psychopathology in dementia. *Neurology, 44*(12), 2308. doi:10.1212/WNL.44.12.2308

Dakin, E. K., & Areán, P. (2013). Patient perspectives on the benefits of psychotherapy for late-life depression. *American Journal of Geriatric Psychiatry, 21*, 155–163. doi:10.1016/j.jagp.2012.10.016

Depp, C. A., & Jeste, D. V. (2010). Phenotypes of successful aging: Historical overview. In C. A. Depp & D. V. Jeste (Eds.), *Successful cognitive and emotional aging* (pp. 1–16). Washington, DC: American Psychiatric Publishing.

DiMascio, A., Weissman, M. M., Prusoff, P. A., Neu, C., Zwilling, M., & Klerman, G. L. (1979). Differential symptom reduction by drugs and psychotherapy in acute depression. *Archives of General Psychiatry, 36*, 1450–1456. doi:10.1001/archpsyc.1979.01780130068008

Eden, J., Maslow, K., Le, M., & Blazer, D. (Eds.). (2012). *The mental health and substance use workforce for older adults: In whose hands?* Washington, DC: National Academies Press.

Elkin, I., Shea, M. T., Watkins, J. T., Imber, S. D., Sotsky, S. M., Collins, J. F., . . . Parloff, M. B. (1989). National Institute of Mental Health Treatment of Depression collaborative research program: General effectiveness of treatments. *Archives of General Psychiatry, 46*, 971–982. doi:10.1001/archpsyc.1989.01810110013002

Ellis, R. R., & Simmons, T. (2014). *Coresident grandparents and their grandchildren: 2012.* Retrieved from https://www.census.gov/content/dam/Census/library/publications/2014/demo/p20-576.pdf

Erikson, E. (1982). *The life cycle completed.* New York, NY: W. W. Norton.

Erikson, E. H., & Erikson, J. M. (1997). *The lifecycle completed (Extended version).* New York, NY: W. W. Norton.

Folstein, M., Folstein, S. E., & McHugh, P. R. (1975). "Mini-mental state": A practical method for grading the cognitive state of patients for the clinician. *Journal of Psychiatric Research, 12*(3), 189–198. doi:10.1016/0022-3956(75)90026-6

Francis, J. L., & Kumar, A. (2013). Psychological treatment of late-life depression. *Psychiatric Clinics of North America, 36*, 561–575. doi:10.1016/j.psc.2013.08.005

Fredriksen-Goldsen, K. I., Kim, H.-J., Emlet, C. A., Muraco, A., Erosheva, E. A., Hoy-Ellis, C. P., . . . Petry, H. (2011). *The aging and health report: Disparities and resilience among lesbian, gay, bisexual, and transgender older adults.* Retrieved from https://www.lgbtagingcenter.org/resources/pdfs/LGBT%20Aging%20and%20Health%20Report_final.pdf

Freedland, K. E., Carney, R. M., Rich, M. W., Steinmeyer, B. C., & Rubin, E. H. (2015). Cognitive behavior therapy for depression and self-care in heart failure patients: A randomized clinical trial. *JAMA Internal Medicine, 175*(11), 1773–1782. doi:10.1001/jamainternmed.2015.5220

Friedman, M. B., Nestadt, P. S., Furst, L., & Williams, K. A. (2018). Meeting the mental health challenges of the elder boom. In S. J. Rosenberg & J. Rosenberg (Eds.), *Community mental health: Challenges for the 21st century* (3rd ed., pp. 133–158). New York, NY: Routledge/Taylor & Francis Group.

Gallagher, D., & Thompson, L. (1981). *Depression in the elderly: A behavioral treatment manual.* Los Angeles: University of Southern California Press.

Gallagher-Thompson, D., & Thompson, L. (2009). *Treating late life depression: A Cognitive Behavioral Approach.* New York, NY: Oxford University Press.

García-López, A., Ezquiaga, E., De Dios, C., & Agud, J. L. (2017). Depressive symptoms in early- and late-onset older bipolar patients compared with younger ones. *International Journal of Geriatric Psychiatry*, 32(2), 201–207. doi:10.1002/gps.4465

Gebauer, L., LaBrie, R., & Shaffer, H. J. (2010). Optimizing *DSM-IV-TR* classification accuracy: A brief biosocial screen for detecting current gambling disorders among gamblers in the general household population. *Canadian Journal of Psychiatry*, 55(2), 82–90. doi:10.1177/070674371005500204

Geiger, P. J., Boggero, I. A., Brake, C. A., Caldera, C. A., Combs, H. L., Peters, J. R., & Baer, R. A. (2016). Mindfulness-based interventions for older adults: A review of the effects on physical and emotional well-being. *Mindfulness*, 7(2), 296–307. doi:10.1007/s12671-015-0444-1

Granholm, E., Auslander, L., Gottlieb, J., McQuaid, J., & McClure, F. (2006). Therapeutic factors contributing to change in cognitive-behavioral group therapy for older persons with schizophrenia. *Journal of Contemporary Psychotherapy*, 36(1), 31. doi:10.1007/s10879-005-9004-7

Granholm, E., Holden, J., Link, P. C., McQuaid, J. R., & Jeste, D. V. (2013). Randomized controlled trial of cognitive behavioral social skills training for older consumers with schizophrenia: Defeatist performance attitudes and functional outcome. *American Journal of Geriatric Psychiatry*, 21(3), 251–262. doi:10.1016/j.jagp.2012.10.014

Groden, S. R., Woodward, A. T., Chatters, L. M., & Taylor, R. J. (2017). Use of complementary and alternative medicine among older adults: Differences between baby boomers and pre-boomers. *American Journal of Geriatric Psychiatry*, 25(12), 1393–1401. doi:10.1016/j.jagp.2017.08.001

Gum, A. M., Areán, P. A., Hunkler, E., Tang, L., Katon, W., Hitchcock, P., . . . Unützer, J. (2006). Depression treatment preferences in older primary care patients. *The Gerontologist*, 46(1), 14–22. doi:10.1093/geront/46.1.14

Gustavson, K. A., Alexopoulous, G. S., Niu, G. C., Mcculloch, C., Meade, T., & Areán, P. A. (2016). Problem-solving therapy reduces suicidal ideation in depressed older adults with executive dysfunction. *American Journal of Geriatric Psychiatry*, 24(1), 11–17. doi:10.1016/j.jagp.2015.07.010

Guy, W. (1976). *ECDEU assessment manual for psychopharmacology* (Rev. ed.). Rockville, MD: U.S. Department of Health, Education, and Welfare.

Haight, B., & Burnside, I. (1993). Reminiscence and life review: Explaining the differences. *Archives of Psychiatric Nursing*, 7(2), 91–98. doi:10.1016/S0883-9417(09)90007-3

Haight, B., Coleman, P., & Lord, K. (1995). The linchpins of a successful life review: Structure, evaluation and individuality. In B. K. Haight & J. D. Webster (Eds.), *The art and science of reminiscence: Theory, research, methods, and applications* (p. 179–192). Washington, DC: Taylor & Francis.

Haight, B., & Olson, M. (1989). Teaching home health aides the use of life review. *Journal of Nursing Staff Development*, 5(1), 11–16. PMID: 2921615

Hall, J., Kellett, S., Berrios, R., Bains, M. K., & Scott, S. (2016). Efficacy of cognitive behavioral therapy for generalized anxiety disorder in older adults: Systematic review, meta-analysis, and meta-regression. *American Journal of Geriatric Psychiatry*, 24, 1063–1073. doi:10.1016/j.jagp.2016.06.006

Han, B. H., & Palamar, J. J. (2018). Marijuana use by middle-aged and older adults in the United States, 2015–2016. *Drug and Alcohol Dependence*, 191, 374–381. doi:10.1016/j.drugalcdep.2018.07.006

Harrison, B. E. (2016). GAPNA toolkit available online. *Geriatric Nursing*, 37, 321. doi:10.1016/j.gerinurse.2016.06.008

Haynes, J., Talbert, M., Fox, S., & Close, E. (2018). Cognitive behavioral therapy in the treatment of insomnia. *Southern Medical Journal*, 111(2), 75–80. doi:10.14423/SMJ.0000000000000769

Hegeman, J. M., de Waal, M. W., Comijs, H. C., Kok, R. M., & van der Mast, R. C. (2015). Depression in later life: A more somatic presentation? *Journal of Affective Disorders*, 170, 196–202. doi:10.1016/j.jad.2014.08.032

Hendrie, H. C., Tu, W., Tabbey, R., Purnell, C. E., Ambuehl, R. J., & Callahan, C. M. (2014). Health outcomes and cost of care among older adults with schizophrenia: A 10-year study using medical records across the continuum of care. *American Journal of Geriatric Psychiatry*, 22(5), 427–436. doi:10.1016/j.jagp.2012.10.025

Hinrichsen, G. A., & Clougherty, K. (2006). *Interpersonal psychotherapy for depressed older adults.* Washington, DC: American Psychological Association.

Hinrichsen, G. A., & Iselin, M. G. (2014). Interpersonal psychotherapy for the treatment of late-life depression. In N. Pachana & K. Laidlaw (Eds), *Oxford handbook of clinical geropsychology* (pp. 622–636). Oxford, UK: Oxford University Press.

Hirschfeld, R., Williams, J. B. W., Spitzer, R. L., Calabrese, J. R., Flynn, L., Keck, P. E. Jr., . . . Zajecka, J. (2000). Development and validation of a screening instrument for bipolar spectrum disorder: The Mood Disorder Questionnaire. *American Journal of Psychiatry, 157,* 1873–1875. doi:10.1176/appi.ajp.157.11.1873

Hopko, D. R., Reas, D. L., Beck, J. G., Stanley, M. A., Wetherell, J. L,, Novy, D., & Averill, P. M. (2003). Assessing worry in older adults: Confirmatory factor analysis of the Penn State Worry Questionnaire and psychometric properties of an abbreviated model. *Psychological Assessment, 15,* 173–183. doi:10.1037/1040-3590.15.2.173

Hsieh, H.-F., & Wang, J.-J. (2003). Effect of reminiscence therapy on depression in older adults: A systematic review. *International Journal of Nursing Studies, 40,* 335–345. doi:10.1016/S0020-7489(02)00101-3

Husain, M., Rush, A. J., Sackeim, H. A., Wisniewski, S. R., McClintock, S. M., Craven, N., . . . Hauger, R. (2005). Age-related characteristics of depression: A preliminary STAR*D report. *American Journal of Geriatric Psychiatry, 13*(10), 852–860. doi:10.1097/00019442-200510000-00004

Institute of Medicine. (2008). *Retooling for an aging America: Building the health care workforce.* Washington, DC: National Academies Press. Retrieved from https://www.ncbi.nlm.nih.gov/books/NBK215401

Jeste, D. V., & Depp, C. A. (2010). Positive mental aging. *American Journal of Geriatric Psychiatry, 18*(1), 1–3. doi:10.1097/JGP.0b013e3181c3ef09

Jeste, D. V., & Maglione, J. E. (2013). Treating older adults with schizophrenia: Challenges and opportunities. *Schizophrenia Bulletin, 39*(5), 966–968. doi:10.1093/schbul/sbt043

Jeste, D. V., Savla, G. N., Thompson, W. K., & Depp, C. A. (2013). Association between older age and more successful aging: Critical role of resilience and depression. *American Journal of Psychiatry, 170,* 188. doi:10.1176/appi.ajp.2012.12030386

Jeste, D. V., & Twamley, E. (2003). Understanding and managing psychosis in late life. *Psychiatric Times, 20*(3), 19. Retrieved from https://www.psychiatrictimes.com/schizophrenia/understanding-and-managing-psychosis-late-life

Jewell, A. J. (2014). Tornstam's notion of gerotranscendence: Re-examining and questioning the theory. *Journal of Aging Studies, 30,* 112–120. doi:10.1016/j.jaging.2014.04.003

Kaas, M., & Beattie, E. (2006). Geropsychiatric nursing practice in the United States: Present trends and future directions. *Journal of the American Psychiatric Nurses Association, 12*(3), 142–155. doi:10.1177/1078390306292161

Kabat-Zinn, J. (1990). *Full catastrophic living. Using the wisdom of your body and mind to face stress, pain, and illness.* New York, NY: Bnmtam Dell.

Kim, K., & Peterson, B. (2014). *Aging behind bars: Trends and implications of graying prisoners in the federal prison system.* Washington, DC: Urban Institure. Retrieved from https://www.urban.org/sites/default/files/publication/33801/413222-Aging-Behind-Bars-Trends-and-Implications-of-Graying-Prisoners-in-the-Federal-Prison-System.PDF

Kiosses, D. N., Rosenberg, P. B., McGovern, A., Fonzetti, P., Zaydens, H., & Alexopoulos, G. S. (2015). Depression and suicidal ideation during two psychosocial treatments in older adults with major depression and dementia. *Journal of Alzheimer's Disease, 48,* 453–462. doi:10.3233/JAD-150200

Knight, B. (2004). *Psychotherapy with older adults* (3rd ed.). Thousand Oaks, CA: Sage.

Knight, B. G., & Pachana, N. A. (2015). *Psychological assessment and therapy with older adults.* New York, NY: Oxford University Press.

Knight, B. G., & Poon, C. Y. (2008). Contextual adult life span theory for adapting psychotherapy with older adults. *Journal of Rational-Emotive & Cognitive-Behavior Therapy, 26*(4), 232. doi:10.1007/s10942-008-0084-7

Korte, J., Bohlmeijer, E. T., Cappeliez, P., Smit, F., & Westerhof, G. J. (2012). Life review therapy for older adults with moderate depressive symptomology: A pragmatic randomized controlled trial. *Psychological Medicine, 42*(6), 1163–1173. doi:10.1017/S0033291711002042

Kropf, N., & Cummings, S. (2017). *Evidence-based treatment with older adults: Theory, practice, and research (Evidence-based practices series)*. New York, NY: Oxford University Press.

Kuchibhatla, M. N., Fillenbaum, G. G., Hybels, C. F., & Blazer, D. G. (2012). Trajectory classes of depressive symptoms in a community sample of older adults. *Acta Psychiatrica Scandinavica, 125*(6), 492–501. doi:10.1111/j.1600-0447.2011.01801.x

Laidlaw, K., Thompson, L. W., Gallagher-Thompson, D., & Dick-Siskin, L. (2003). *Cognitive behaviour therapy with older people*. West Sussex, UK: John Wiley & Sons.

Lake, J. (2007). *Textbook of integrative mental health care*. New York, NY: Thieme Medical Publishers.

Lapierre, S., Boyer, R., Desjardins, S., Dubé, M., Lorrain, D., Préville, M., & Brassard, J. (2012). Daily hassles, physical illness, and sleep problems in older adults with wishes to die. *International Psychogeriatrics, 24*(2), 243–252. doi:10.1017/S1041610211001591

Lenze, E. J., & Wetherell, J. L. (2011). Anxiety disorders: New developments in old age. *American Journal of Geriatric Psychiatry, 19*(4), 301–304. doi:10.1097/JGP.0b013e31820db34f

Levinson, D. J. (1986). A conception of adult development. *American Psychologist, 41*, 3–13. doi:10.1037/0003-066X.41.1.3

Lewis, M. I., & Butler, R. N. (1974). Life review therapy: Putting memories to work in individual and group psychotherapy. *Geriatrics, 29*, 165–173. PMID: 4417455

Licht-Strunk, E., van der Windt, D. A., van Marwijk, H. W., de Haan, M., & Beekman, A. T. (2007). The prognosis of depression in older patients in general practice and the community. A systematic review. *Family Practice, 24*(2), 168–180. doi:10.1093/fampra/cml071

Lloyd, S. L., & Striley, C. W. (2018). Marijuana use among adults 50 years or older in the 21st century. *Geronotology and Geriatric Medicine*. Advance online publication. doi:10.1177/2333721418781668

Lohr, J. B., Palmer, B. W., Eidt, C. A., Aailaboyina, S., Mausbach, B. T., Wolkowitz, O. M., . . . Jeste, D. V. (2015). Is post-traumatic stress disorder associated with premature senescence? A review of the literature. *American Journal of Geriatric Psychiatry, 23*(7), 709–725. doi:10.1016/j.jagp.2015.04.001

Lowenstein, D. A., Czaja, S. J., Bowie, C. R., & Harvey, P. D. (2012). Age-associated differences in cognitive performance in older patients with schizophrenia: A comparison with healthy older adults. *American Journal of Geriatric Psychiatry, 20*(1), 29–40. doi:10.1097/JGP.0b013e31823bc08c

Lynch, T. R., & Cheavens, J. S. (2007). Dialectical behavior therapy for depression with comorbid personality disorder: An extension of standard dialectical behavior therapy with a special emphasis on the treatment of older adults. In L. A. Dimeff & K. Koerner (Eds), *Dialectical behavior therapy in clinical practice. Applications across disorders and settings* (pp. 264–297). New York, NY: Guilford Press.

Mackin, R., & Areán, P. (2005). Evidence-based psychotherapeutic interventions for geriatric depression. *Psychiatric Clinics of North America, 28*(4), 805–820. doi:10.1016/j.psc.2005.09.009

McGovern, A., Kiosses, D., Raue, P., Wilkins, V., & Alexopoulos, G. (2014). Psychotherapies for late-life depression. Psychiatric Annals, 44(3), 147-152. doi:10.3928/00485713-20140306-07

McGrath, K., Hajjar, E. D. R., Kumar, C., Hwang, C., & Salzman, B. (2017). Deprescribing: A simple method for reducing polypharmacy. *Journal Family Practice, 66*, 436–445. Retrieved from https://mdedge-files-live.s3.us-east-2.amazonaws.com/files/s3fs-public/Document/June-2017/JFP06607436.PDF

Melillo, K. D. (2017). Geropsychiatric nursing: What's in your toolkit? [Guest editorial]. *Journal of Gerontological Nursing, 43*(1), 3–6. doi:10.3928/00989134-20161215-01

Miller, M. D. (2009). *Clinician's guide to interpersonal psychotherapy in late life*. New York, NY: Oxford University Press.

Miller, M. D., Cornes, C., Frank, E., Ehrenpreis, L., Silberman, R., Schlernitzauer, M. A., . . . Reynolds, C. F., III (2001). Interpersonal psychotherapy for late-life depression: Past, present, and future. *Journal of Psychotherapy Practice Research, 10*(4), 231–238. Retrieved from https://www.ncbi.nlm.nih.gov/pmc/articles/PMC3330668

Miller, M. D., Frank, E., Cornes, C., Houck, P., & Reynolds, C. F., III. (2003). The value of maintenance interpersonal psychotherapy (IPT) in older adults with different IPT foci. *American Journal of Geriatric Psychiatry, 11*(1), 97–102. doi:10.1097/00019442-200301000-00013

Molinari, V. (1999). Using reminiscence and life review as natural therapeutic strategies in group therapy. In M. Duffy (Ed.), *Handbook of counseling and psychotherapy with older adults* p. 154–165. New York, NY: John Wiley & Sons.

Montgomery, S., & Åsberg, M. (1979). A new depression scale designed to be sensitive to change. *British Journal of Psychiatry, 134*, 382–389. doi:10.1192/bjp.134.4.382

Morris, D., & Mentes, J. (2006). Geropsychiatric nursing education: Challenge and opportunity. *Journal of the American Psychiatric Nurses Association, 12*(2), 105–115. doi:10.1177/1078390306292154

Nasreddine, Z. S., Phillips, N. A., Bédirian, N. A., Charbonneau, S., Whitehead, V., Collin, I., . . . Chertkow, H. (2005). The Montreal Cognitive Assessment, MoCA: A brief screening tool for mild cognitive impairment. *Journal of the American Geriatrics Society, 53*(4), 695–699. doi:10.1111/j.1532-5415.2005.53221.x

National Alliance on Caregiving. (2009). *Caregiving in the U.S. 2009.* Retrieved from https://www.caregiving.org/wp-content/uploads/2020/05/Caregiving_in_the_US_2009_full_report.pdf

National Council on Aging. (n.d.). *Chronic disease self-managment fact.* Retrieved from https://www.ncoa.org/news/resources-for-reporters/get-the-facts/chronic-disease-facts

National Hartford Center of Gerontological Nursing Excellence. (2016, July/August). Opportunities, resources, and tools. *New Directions Newsletter.*

National Institute of Mental Health. (2019). *Suicide.* Retrieved from https://www.nimh.nih.gov/health/statistics/suicide.shtml

National Institute on Alcohol Abuse and Alcoholism. (n.d.). *Older adults.* Retrieved from https://www.niaaa.nih.gov/alcohol-health/special-populations-co-occurring-disorders/older-adults

Nivoli, A. M., Murru, A., Pacchiarotti, I., Valenti, M., Rosa, A. R., Hidalgo, D., . . . Colom, F. (2014). Bipolar disorder in the elderly: A cohort study comparing older and younger patients. *Acta Psychiatica Scandinavica, 130*(5), 364–373. doi:10.1111/acps.12272

Nurit, G. Y., Dana, P., & Yuval, P. (2016). Predictors of psychotherapy use among community-dwelling older adults with depressive symptoms. *Clinical Gerontologist, 39*(2), 127–138. doi:10.1080/07317115.2015.1124957

Ogle, C. M., Rubin, D. C., Berntsen, D., & Siegler, I. C. (2013). The frequency and impact of exposure to potentially traumatic events over the life course. *Clinical Psychological Science, 1*(4), 426–434. doi:10.1177/2167702613485076

Ogle, C. M., Rubin, D. C., & Siegler, I. C. (2013). The impact of the developmental timing of trauma exposure on PTSD symptoms and psychosocial functioning among older adults. *Developmental Psychology, 49*(11), 2191–2200. doi:10.1037/a0031985

Okolie, C., Dennis, M., Thomas, E. S., & John, A. (2017). A systematic review of interventions to prevent suicidal behaviors and reduce suicidal ideation in older people. *International Psychogeriatrics, 29*(11), 1801–1824. doi:10.1017/S1041610217001430

O'Moore, K. A., Newby, J. M., Andrews, G., Hunter, D. J., Bennell, K., Smith, J., & Williams, A. D. (2017). Internet cognitive-behavioral therapy for depression in older adults with knee osteoarthritis: A randomized controlled trial. *Arthritis Care Research, 70*(1), 61–70. doi:10.1002/acr.23257

Overall, J., & Gorham, D. (1988). The Brief Psychiatric Rating Scale (BPRS): Recent developments in ascertainment and scaling. *Psychopharmacology Bulletin, 24*, 97–99.

Perng, A., & Renz, S. (2018). Identifying and treating complicated grief in older adults. *Journal for Nurse Practitioners, 14*(4), 289–295. doi:10.1016/j.nurpra.2017.12.001

Pietrzak, R. H., Goldstein, R. B., Southwick, S. M., & Grant, B. F. (2012). Psychiatric comorbidity

Pot, A. M., Bohlmeijer, E. T., Onrust, S., Melenhorst, A.-S., Verbeek, M., & De Vries, W. (2010). The impact of life review on depression in older adults: A randomized controlled trial. *International Psychogeriatrics, 22*(4), 572–581. doi:10.1017/S104161020999175X

Rabins, P., & Lavrisha, M. (2003). Long-term follow-up and phenomenologic differences distinguish among late-onset schizophrenia, late-life depression, and progressive dementia. *American Journal of Geriatric Psychiatry, 11*(6), 589–594. doi:10.1097/00019442-200311000-00002

Rabins, P., & Pearlson, G. (2009). Treating dementia: Progress and promise. *American Journal of Geriatric Psychiatry, 17*(9), 723–725. doi:10.1097/JGP.0b013e3181b1222f

Raue, P. J., McGovern, A. R., Kiosses, D. N., & Sirey, J. A. (2017). Advances in psychotherapy for depressed older adults. *Current Psychiatry Reports, 19*, 57. doi:10.1007/s11920-017-0812-8

Redfoot, D., Feinberg, L., & Houser, A. (2013, August). *The aging of the baby boom and the growing care gap: A look at future declines in the availability of family caregivers.* Retrieved from https://www.aarp.org/content/dam/aarp/research/public_policy_institute/ltc/2013/baby-boom-and-the-growing-care-gap-in-brief-AARP-ppi-ltc.pdf

Reid, M., Otis, J., Barry, L., & Kerns, R. (2003). Cognitive-behavioral therapy for chronic low back pain in older persons: A preliminary study. *Pain Medicine, 4*(3), 223–230. doi:10.1046/j.1526-4637.2003.03030.x

Reisberg, B., Borenstein, J., Salob, S. P., Ferris, S. H., & Franssen, E. (1987). Behavioral symptoms in Alzheimer's disease: Phenomenology and treatment. *Journal of Clinical Psychiatry, 48*, 9. PMID: 3553166

Reynolds, K., Pietrzak, R. H., El-Gabalawy, R., Mackenzie, C. S., & Sareen, J. (2015). Prevalence of psychiatric disorders in U.S. older adults: Findings from a nationally representative survey. *World Psychiatry, 14*(1), 74–81. doi:10.1002/wps.20193

Richard, E., Reitz, C., Honig, L. H., Schupf, N., Tang, M. X., Manly, J. J., . . . Luchsinger, J. A. (2013). Late- life depression, mild cognitive impairment, and dementia. *JAMA Neurology, 70*(3), 383–389. doi:10.1001/jamaneurol.2013.603

Richard, E., Schmand, B., Eikelenboom, P., Yang, S. C., Ligthart, S. A., van Charante, E. P., & van Gool, W. A. (2012). Symptoms of apathy are associated with progression from mild cognitive impairment to Alzheimer's disease in non-depressed subjects. *Dementia and Geriatric Cognitive Disorders, 33*(2–3), 204–209. doi:10.1159/000338239

Rosenberg, P. B., Mielke, M. M., Appleby, B. S., Oh, E. S., Geda, Y. E., & Lyketsos, C. G. (2013). The association of neuropsychiatric symptoms in MCI with incident dementia and Alzheimer disease. *American Journal of Geriatric Psychiatry, 21*(7), 685–695. doi:10.1016/j.jagp.2013.01.006

Rosow, I. (1967). *Social integration of the aged.* New York, NY: Free Press.

Rowe, J. W., & Kahn, R. L. (1998). *Successful aging.* New York, NY: Random House.

Sajatovic, M., & Chen, P. (2011). Geriatric bipolar disorder. *Psychiatric Clinics of North America, 34*(2), 319–333. doi:10.1016/j.psc.2011.02.007

Sajatovic, M., Gyulai, L., Calabrese, J. R., Thompson, T. R., Wilson, B. G., White, R., & Evonjuk, G. (2005). Maintenance treatment outcomes in older patients with bipolar I disorder. *American Journal of Geriatric Psychiatry, 13*(4), 305–311. doi:10.1097/00019442-200504000-00006

Sami, M. B., & Nilforooshan, R. (2015). The natural course of anxiety disorders in the elderly: A systematic review of longitudinal trials. *International Psychogeriatrics, 27*(Special Issue 7), 1061–1069. doi:10.1017/S1041610214001847

Saxon, S. V., Etten, M. J., & Perkins, E. A. (2015). *Physical change and aging* (6th ed.). New York, NY: Springer Publishing Company.

Schuitevoerder, S., Rosen, J. W., Twanley, E. W., Ayers, C. R., Sones, H., Lohr, J. B., . . . Thorp, S. R. (2013). A meta-analysis of cognitive functioning in older adults with PTSD. *Journal of Anxiety Disorders, 27*(6), 550–558. doi:10.1016/j.janxdis.2013.01.001

Seitz, D., Purandare, N., & Conn, D. (2010). Prevalence of psychiatric disorders among older adults in long-term care homes: A systematic review. *International Psychogeriatrics, 22*(7), 1025–1039. doi:10.1017/S1041610210000608

Shah, A., Scogin, F., & Floyd, M. (2012). Evidence-based psychological treatment for geriatric depression. In F. Scogin & A. Shah (Eds.), *Making evidence-based psychological treatment work with older adults* 87–130. https://doi.org/10.1037/13753-004. Washington, DC: American Psychological Association.

Sholomskas, A., Chevron, E. S., Prusoff, B. A., & Berry, C. (1983). Short-term interpersonal therapy (IPT) with the depressed elderly: Case reports and discussion. *American Journal of Psychotherapy, 37*(4), 552–566. doi:10.1176/appi.psychotherapy.1983.37.4.552

Staudinger, U. (2001). Life reflection: A social–cognitive analysis of life review. *Review of General Psychology, 5*(2), 148–160. doi:10.1037/1089-2680.5.2.148

Subramanian, M., Wang, P., Soh, P., Vaingankar, J. A., Chong, S. A., Browning, C. J., & Thomas, S. A. (2015). Prevalence and determinants of gambling disorder among older adults: A systematic review. *Addictive Behaviors, 41*, 199–209. doi:10.1016/j.addbeh.2014.10.007

Subramanyam, A.A., Kedare, J., Singh, O.P., & Pinto, C. (2018). Clinical practice guidelines for geriatric anxiety disorders. Indian Journal of Psychiatry, 60(Suppl 3): S371-382.

Substance Abuse and Mental Health Services Administration. (2014). *Results from the 2013 National Survey on Drug Use and Health: Summary of national findings* (HHS Publication No. [SMA] 14-4863). Rockville, MD: Author. Retrieved from https://www.samhsa.gov/data/sites/default/files/NSDUHresultsPDFWHTML2013/Web/NSDUHresults2013.pdf

Sullivan, D. J., Zeff, P., & Zweig, R. A. (2018). Psychotherapy termination practices with older adults: Impact of patient and therapist characteristics. *Clinical Gerontologist, 41*(5), 399–411. doi:10.1080/07317115.2018.1437101

Szanton, S. L., Wenzel, J., Connolly, A. B., & Piferi, R. L. (2011). Examining mindfulness-based stress reduction: Perceptions from minority older adults residing in a low-income housing facility. *BMC Complementary and Alternative Medicine, 11*, 44. doi:10.1186/1472-6882-11-44

Tampi, R. R., Williamson, D., Mittal, V., McEnerney, N., Thomas, J., . . . Cash, M. (2011). Behavioral and psychological symptoms of dementia: Part II-Treatment. *Clinical Geriatrics, 19*(6), 31. Retrieved from https://www.consultant360.com/articles/behavioral-and-psychological-symptoms-dementia-part-ii-treatment

Tariq, S. H, Tumosa, N., Chibnall, J. T., Perry M. H. III., & Morley, J. E. (2006). Comparison of the Saint Louis University mental status examination and the Mini-Mental State Examination for detecting dementia and mild neurocognitive disorder–A pilot study. *American Journal of Geriatric Psychiatry, 14*(11), 900–910. doi:10.1097/01.JGP.0000221510.33817.86

Tavares, L. R., & Barbosa, M. R. (2018). Efficacy of group psychotherapy for geriatric depression: A systematic review. *Archives of Gerontology and Geriatrics, 78*, 71–80. doi:10.1016/j.archger.2018.06.001

Titov, N., Dear, B. F., Ali, S., Zou, J. B., Lorian, C. N., Johnston, L., . . . Fogliati, V. J. (2015). Clinical and cost-effectiveness of therapist-guided internet-delivered cognitive behavior therapy for older adults with symptoms of depression: A randomized controlled trial. *Behavioral Therapy, 46*(2), 193–205. doi:10.1016/j.beth.2014.09.008

Trinh, N., & Forester, B. (2007). Bipolar disorder in the elderly: Differential diagnosis and treatment. *Psychiatric Times, 24*(14), 38. Retrieved from https://www.psychiatrictimes.com/addiction/bipolar-disorder-elderly-differential-diagnosis-and-treatment

Tung Fung, A. W., Wa Lee, J. S., Chun Lee, A. T., & Wa Lam, L. C. (2018). Anxiety symptoms predicted decline in episodic memory in cognitively healthy older adults: A 3-year prospective study. *International Journal of Geriatric Psychiatry, 33*(5), 748–754. doi:10.1002/gps.4850

Turk, M. T., Elci, O. U., Resick, L. K., & Kalarchian, M. A. (2016). Wise choices: Nutrition and exercise for older adults: A community-based health promotion intervention. *Family & Community Health, 39*(4), 263–272. doi:10.1097/FCH.0000000000000116

Twamley, E., & Harvey, P. (2006). The importance of cognition in the conceptualization of both dementia and severe mental illness in older people. *American Journal of Geriatric Psychiatry, 14*(5), 387–390. doi:10.1097/01.JGP.0000220883.94784.aa

Unützer, J., Tang, L., Oishi, S., Katon, W., Williams, J. W., Jr., Hunkeler, E., . . . Langston, C. (2006). Reducing suicidal ideation in depressed older primary care patients. *Journal of the American Geriatrics Society, 54*(10), 1550–1556. doi:10.1111/j.1532-5415.2006.00882.x

U.S. Department of Health and Human Services. (1999). Older adults and mental health. In H. H. Goldman, P. Rye, & P. Sirovatka (Eds.), *Mental health: A report of the Surgeon General—Older adults and mental health* (pp. 331–402). Rockville, MD: Author Retrieved from https://www.hsdl.org/?view&did=730796

U.S. Department of Health and Human Services. (2014). *The future of the nursing workforce: National- and state-level projections, 2012–2025.* Retrieved from http://bhw.hrsa.gov/sites/default/files/bhw/nchwa/projections/nursingprojections.pdf

Vaillant, G. E. (2007). Aging well. *American Journal of Geriatric Psychiatry*, *15*(3), 181–183. doi:10.1097/JGP.0b013e31803190e0

van der Linde, R. M., Dening, T., Stephan, B. C., Prina, A. M., Evans, E., & Brayne, C. (2016). Longitudinal course of behavioural and psychological symptoms of dementia: Systematic review. *The British Journal of Psychiatry*, *209*(5), 366–377. doi:10.1192/bjp.bp.114.148403

van der Maas, M., Mann, R. E., McCready, J., Matheson, F. I., Turner, N. E., Hamilton, H. A., . . . Ialomiteanu, A. (2017). Problem gambling in a sample of older adult casino gamblers: Associations with gambling participation and motivations. *Journal of Geriatric Psychiatry and Neurology*, *30*(1), 3–10. doi:10.1177/0891988716673468

van Hout, H., Beekman, A. T., de Beurs, E., Comijs, H., van Marwijk, H., de Haan, M., . . . Deeg, D. J. (2004). Anxiety and the risk of death in older men and women. *British Journal of Psychiatry*, *185*, 399–404. doi:10.1192/bjp.185.5.399

van Schaik, D. J. F., van Marwijk, H. W. J., Beekman, A. T. F., de Haan, M., & van Dyck, R. (2007). Interpersonal psychotherapy (IPT) for late-life depression in general practice: Uptake and satisfaction by patients, therapists, and physicians. *BMC Family Practice*, *8*, 52. doi:10.1186/1471-2296-8-52

Wazwaz, N. (2015, July 6). It's official: The US is becoming a minority-majority nation. *US News*. Retrieved from https://www.usnews.com/news/articles/2015/07/06/its-official-the-us-is-becoming-a-minority-majority-nation

Webster, J. D., Bohlmeijer, E. T., & Westerhof, G. J. (2010). Mapping the future of reminiscence: A conceptual guide for research and practice. *Research on Aging*, *32*, 527–564. doi:10.1177/0164027510364122

Weissman, M., Markowitz, J., & Klerman, G. (2000). *Comprehensive guide to interpersonal psychotherapy*. New York, NY: Basic Books.

West, N. A., Severtson, S. G., Green, J. L., & Dart, R. C. (2015). Trends in abuse and misuse of prescription opioids among older adults. *Drug and Alcohol Dependence*, *149*(1), 117–121. doi:10.1016/j.drugalcdep.2015.01.027

Westhuis, D., & Thyer, B. (1989). Development and validation of the Clinical Anxiety Scale: A rapid assessment instrument for empirical practice. *Educational and Psychological Measurement*, *49*(1), 153–163. doi:10.1177/0013164489491016

Williamson, A. T., Fletcher, P. C., & Dawson, K. A. (2003). Complementary and alternative medicine: Use in an older population. *Journal of Gerontological Nursing*, *29*(5), 20–28. doi:10.3928/0098-9134-20030501-06

Wolitzky-Taylor, K. B., Castriotta, N., Lenze, E. J., Stanley, M. A., & Craske, M. G. (2010). Anxiety disorders in older adults: A comprehensive review. *Depression and Anxiety*, *27*, 190–211. doi:10.1002/da.20653

World Health Organization. (2017). *Mental health of older adults*. Retrieved from https://www.who.int/news-room/fact-sheets/detail/mental-health-of-older-adults

Yesavage, J. A., Brink, T. L., Rose, T. L., Lum, O., Huang, V., Adey, M., & Leirer, V. O. (1983). Development and validation of a geriatric depression screening scale: A preliminary report. *Journal of PsychiatricResearch*, *17*, 37–49. doi: 10.1016/0022-3956(82)90033-4

Young, R. (2005). Bipolar disorder in older persons: Perspectives and new findings. *American Journal of Geriatric Psychiatry*, *13*(4), 265–267. doi:10.1097/00019442-200504000-00001

Young, R., Biggs, J. T., Ziegler, V. E., & Meyer, D. A. (1978). A rating scale for mania: Reliability, validity and sensitivity. *British Journal of Psychiatry*, *133*, 429–435. doi:10.1192/bjp.133.5.429

Zhao, Q.-F., Tan, L., Wang, H.-F., Jiang, T., Tan, M.-S., Tan, L., . . . Yu, J.-T. (2016). The prevalence of neuropsychiatric symptoms in Alzheimer's disease: Systematic review and meta-analysis. *Journal of Affective Disorders*, *190*, 264–271. doi:10.1016/j.jad.2015.09.069

Zisook, S., & Shear, K. (2009). Grief and bereavement: What psychiatrists need to know. *World Psychiatry*, *8*(2), 67–74. doi:10.1002/j.2051-5545.2009.tb00217.x

APPENDIX 22.1
Haight's Life Review and Experiencing Form

Childhood

1. What is the very first thing you can remember in your life? Go as far back as you can.
2. What other things can you remember about when you were very young?
3. What was life like for you as a child?
4. What were your parents like? What were their weaknesses, strengths?
5. Did you have any brothers or sisters? Tell me what each was like?
6. Did someone close to you die when you were growing up?
7. Did someone important to you go away?
8. Do you ever remember being very sick?
9. Do you remember having an accident?
10. Do you remember being in a very dangerous situation?
11. Was there anything that was important to you that was lost or destroyed?
12. Was church a large part of your life?
13. Did you enjoy being a boy/girl?

Adolescence

1. When you think about yourself and your life as a teenager, what is the first thing you can remember about that time?
2. What other things stand out in your memory about being a teenager?
3. Who were the important people for you? Tell me about them. Parents, brothers, sisters, friends, teachers, those you were especially close to, those you admired, those you wanted to be like.
4. Did you attend church and youth groups?
5. Did you go to school? What was the meaning for you?
6. Did you work during these years?
7. Tell me of any hardships you experienced at this time.
8. Do you remember feeling that there wasn't enough food or necessities of life as a child or adolescent?
9. Do you remember feeling left alone, abandoned, not having enough love or care as a child or adolescent?
10. What were the pleasant things about your adolescence?
11. What was the most unpleasant thing about your adolescence?
12. All things considered, would you say you were happy or unhappy as a teenager?
13. Do you remember your first attraction to another person?
14. How did you feel about sexual activities and your own sexual identity?

(continued)

Family and Home

1. How did your parents get along?
2. How did other people in your home get along?
3. What was the atmosphere in your home?
4. Were you punished as a child? For what? Who did the punishing? Who was "boss"?
5. When you wanted something from your parents, how did you go about getting it?
6. What kind of person did your parents like the most? The least?
7. Who were you closest to in your family?
8. Who in your family were you most like? In what way?

Adulthood

1. What place did religion play in your life?
2. Now I'd like to talk to you about your life as an adult, starting when you were in your 20s up to today. Tell me of the most important events that happened in your adulthood.
3. What was life like for you in your 20s and 30s?
4. What kind of person were you? What did you enjoy?
5. Tell me about your work. Did you enjoy your work? Did you earn an adequate living? Did you work hard during those years? Were you appreciated?
6. Did you form significant relationships with other people?
7. Did you marry?
      (yes) What kind of person was your spouse?
      (no) Why not?
8. Do you think marriages get better or worse over time? Were you married more than once?
9. On the whole, would you say you had a happy or unhappy marriage?
10. Was sexual intimacy important to you?
11. What were some of the main difficulties you encountered during your adult and older years?
      a. Did someone close to you die? Go away?
      b. Were you ever sick? Have an accident?
      c. Did you move often? Change jobs?
      d. Did you ever feel alone? Abandoned?
      e. Did you ever feel need?

Summary

1. On the whole, what kind of life do you think you've had?
2. If everything were to be the same, would you like to live your life over again?
3. If you were going to live your life over again, what would you change? Leave unchanged?

(continued)

4. We've been talking about your life for quite some time now. Let's discuss your overall feelings and ideas about your life. What would you say the main satisfactions in your life have been? Try for three. Why were they satisfying?

5. Everyone has had disappointments. What have been the main disappointments in your life?

6. What was the hardest thing you had to face in your life? Please describe it.

7. What was the happiest period of your life? What about it made it the happiest period? Why is your life less happy now?

8. What was the unhappiest period of your life? Why is your life happier now?

9. What was the proudest moment in your life?

10. If you could stay the same age all your life, what age would you choose and why?

11. How do you think you've made out in life? Better or worse than what you hoped for?

12. Let's talk a little about you as you are now. What are the best things about the age you are now?

13. What are the worst things about being the age you are now?

14. What are the most important things to you in your life today?

15. What do you hope will happen to you as you grow older?

16. What do you fear will happen to you as you grow older?

17. Have you enjoyed participating in this review of your life?

Source: Haight,, B. K., Coleman, P., & Lord, K. (1985). The Linchpins of a successful life review: Structure, evaluation, and individuality. In B. K. Haight & J. D. Webser (Eds.), *The art and science of reminiscing. Theory, research, methods, and applications* (pp. 179–191). Washington, DC: Taylor & Francis.

V

Termination and Reimbursement

23

Reimbursement and Documentation

Mary D. Moller

The ability to be sufficiently reimbursed for all types of clinical services is critical for the psychiatric mental health advanced practice psychiatric nurse (APPN). Reimbursement is currently based on the valuation of current procedural terminology (CPT) codes. In January 2013 the way reimbursement had occurred for psychiatric services over the previous 40 years came to an abrupt halt. Previously, psychiatric services were primarily billed using psychiatric specialty billing codes. Recognizing that psychiatry is a complex branch of medicine, medical evaluation and management (E/M) codes (99xxx) were at last identified as the base codes for psychiatric services and the psychotherapy codes (908xx) were identified as procedure codes to be used as add-on codes.

Documentation requirements were also revised. For those accustomed to the narrative or SOAP format, progress notes were changed to represent the standard format of chief complaint, history of present illness, review of systems, past psychiatric history, mental status exam, diagnostic formulation, and treatment plan. The purpose of this chapter is to clarify the who, what, why, when, and where of how to use the current psychiatry billing codes and required documentation.

UNDERSTANDING CPT CODES

The first CPT manual was developed in 1966 in order to standardize the language used by various medical professionals to accurately describe the medical, surgical, and diagnostic services provided in an encounter for Medicare and other insurance companies. CPT codes are devised, maintained, owned, copyrighted, revised, retired, and published annually by the American Medical Association (AMA, 2020). These codes are used to identify accepted medical procedures and services provided by licensed medical providers including advanced practice registered nurses (APRNs). The CPT manual (AMA, 2020) is available from the AMA website and other retail vendors. All advanced practice psychiatric nurses (APPNs) are encouraged to purchase this book. CPT codes are continually updated to reflect changes in levels of complexity, practice management costs, and changes in the overall nature of clinical work as medical and surgical advances occur.

Every 5 years, the Centers for Medicare and Medicaid (CMS) requires that all codes are reviewed, revised, and/or eliminated. A two-part process, each involving a separate committee, occurs for each new/revised code. A CMS representative sits on both committees. First, the CPT editorial panel evaluates and votes on the rationale and language of the code. Each code is then assigned a reimbursement value based on a very complex process that takes into account the variables of practice expense, provider work, and malpractice costs. This process is overseen by a committee referred to as the *resource-based relative value scale update committee* (RUC) which was specifically formed in 1992 to offer recommendations on the valuation of CPT codes to the CMS. By 2002 after an evolving process, all aspects of medical reimbursement were resource based. Please see how rates are calculated at the CMS.gov website (www.cms.gov/apps/physician-fee-schedule/overview.aspx). This information is also published annually in the Federal Register. Private insurance companies are permitted to reimburse at rates higher than the CMS minimums. There are also regional differences around the country that are available on the CMS website.

Timeline and Process of the 2012 Review of Psychiatry Codes

The RUC, composed of 21 members from medical specialty associations, had not formally revalued the 24 existing major CMS code categories for psychotherapy services since 1998. In 2008, the professional societies began the mandatory review process of requesting a revaluation when it was recognized that the existing psychotherapy codes used by psychiatrists and APRNs were valued lower than the E/M codes used by all other physicians and APRNs. An additional concern was that the psychotherapy codes did not adequately differentiate the difference in the work performed by a psychiatrist or APPN from that provided by a psychologist, social worker, or licensed counselor.

The detailed process of code review and revaluation is subject to strict scrutiny and numerous checks and balances. The group recommending code changes must present "compelling evidence" to increase the value of a code. The evidence is based on changes in technology or the typical patient, flawed methodology of the current values, relativity analysis between the values, and actual time spent with patients related to various codes. Finally, there must be budget neutrality, meaning an increased relative value unit (RVU) for one service will lead to a decrease in the final payment for all other services (AMA, 2020). Ultimately, it was determined that psychiatrists, psychiatric APRNs, and prescribing clinical psychologists would use the standard E/M codes and selected codes from the annually updated CPT codebook published by the American Medical Association (Dewan et al., 2018).

Advantages of Coding With E/M Language

The use of the nontimed 99xxx E/M codes allows the provider to create an itemized bill of the services delivered. The bundled 908xx codes did not account for an inability the intensity of the service provided resulting in a lack of understanding and an ability to communicate the complexity involved in delivering psychiatric care. Evaluation and management codes refer to just that—the work that goes into both the evaluation of the patient and management of the diagnoses. These codes also have the added benefit of allowing the provider to bill based on the time spent in counseling and coordination of care (CCC) if greater than 50% of the encounter is spent in these kinds of discussions. The selection of the nontimed code is determined by the level of medical decision-making (MDM), which takes into account the complexity of treatment risk, number of problems/diagnoses, and amount of collateral information required to provide care. An invaluable guide, the *Evaluation and Management Services Guide* is published through the Medicare Learning Network and updated regularly. The current guide was published in January 2020. This comprehensive resource is embedded with active web links that will assist you (DHHS, 2020).

Most outpatient medical encounters are coded with a basic E/M code plus an add-on code or two. For example, if you go to your provider for a primary care visit and any kind of lab work, x-ray, or procedure is done, those services are billed with add-on codes. With the 2013 revision, *psychotherapy codes* became *add-on codes* as psychotherapy is one of psychiatry's major procedures. See Table 23.1 for psychotherapy CPT codes. An additional add-on code is *interactive complexity,* which refers to any kind of communication difficulty such as working with irate family members or patients who have lost control, hearing impairments, cognitive and intellectual disabilities, or the need for language translation, as well as work with children. A complex visit can now be fully documented and reimbursed for all the work that is required in a given patient encounter/session including therapy and management of complex family and/or patient interactions. There are also codes to bill for visits that extend beyond the scheduled time.

Nurse Psychotherapists

Nurse psychotherapists can still bill for stand-alone psychotherapy using the psychiatry specialty codes, but if the encounter involves discussing medications and/or diagnosis, and requires CCC with the prescriber, the APRN should bill using an E/M base code with a psychotherapy add-on procedure code. All APRNs need to remember that complex physiological and psychopharmacological content is part of our education and training and is reflected in our assessment, diagnosis, and treatment. Reimbursement is typically greater for an E/M code with a psychotherapy add-on than a stand-alone psychotherapy code. The documentation needs to reflect both of these billing codes. An example of this type of progress note is provided later in this chapter. As a reminder, psychotherapy *process* notes represent a unique Health Insurance Portability and Accountability Act (HIPAA) protected form of chart note. In circumstances where psychodynamic psychotherapy is being conducted, separate process notes can be maintained and are uniquely protected (Focht, Rodriguez, & Fuchs, 2017; Gutheil, 1980).

The Codes that Did Not Change

The psychotherapy codes that did not change include: psychoanalysis (90845); family psychotherapy without the patient present (90846) and conjoint with the patient present (90847); multifamily group psychotherapy (90849); and group psychotherapy (90853). In addition, the psychotherapy procedural codes that did not change include narcosynthesis (90865); therapeutic repetitive transcranial magnetic stimulation (90867), subsequent (90868) and subsequent w/motor threshold redetermination (90869); and electroconvulsive therapy (90870). These codes did not change because the complexity of the work that is involved with those codes had been adequately captured in the original valuation process.

Codes that Were Eliminated

The two codes that were eliminated include were group psychotherapy (90857) and pharmacologic management (90862). This caused a ripple effect throughout the profession as 90862 was the most commonly billed code used throughout psychiatry. However, this code had been very problematic as it was a nontimed code that frequently had high reimbursement. Yet, sometimes it had low reimbursement and providers were finding themselves trying to see more patients in order to receive adequate compensation for the work that was being done. A vestige of this code remains as an add-on code (+90863) and is to be used by prescribing psychologists with stand-alone psychotherapy services.

Codes that Were Added

The previous code for a new patient without interactive complexity was 90801, and with interactive complexity was 90802. These codes have been eliminated. A new patient evaluation without any medical evaluation and management is now coded as a 90791 and is most commonly used by nonprescribing psychologists, therapists, and social workers. There is a code for a new patient evaluation that includes medical services (90792). Psychiatrists and APPNs should use the new patient E/M codes (99203-5); however, it is appropriate to use 90792 when there is medical evaluation beyond the mental status exam and there is prescribing of medications and ordering or discussion of laboratory or other diagnostic tests. This code can also be used for an existing patient seen in a medical practice that is referred for an initial psychiatric evaluation. However, this code cannot be used on the same day with another E/M or psychotherapy code. This code can be billed annually, which has a great advantage for providing ongoing comprehensive psychiatric diagnostic and treatment re-evaluation as it typically reimburses more than an extended office visit or the most comprehensive outpatient visit for an ongoing patient.

New timed stand-alone codes, for the provision of psychotherapy only, were developed and include 30 minutes (90832), 45 minutes (90834), and 60 minutes (90837). They were simplified and include time spent with the family. These codes can be used by the APRN when there are no E/M services provided; however, these codes were primarily meant for use by psychologists, social workers, and licensed counselors. When a psychiatrist or APPN provides therapy within a standard E/M encounter, the new add-on psychotherapy codes should be used. Psychotherapy with E/M services is based on time: +90833 is to be used when the psychotherapy delivered is from 23 to 37 minutes; +90836 is used when the range is between 37 and 52 minutes; and +90838 is used if the encounter extends beyond 52 minutes.

New codes were added for crisis intervention; 90839 was to be used for initial contact and +90840 was used as an add-on to capture subsequent crisis intervention, which can be added on in 30-minute increments. The caveat with these codes is that CMS has not yet sanctioned a value for reimbursement. Currently, the crisis intervention codes are reimbursed depending on the protocol set forth by individual insurance carriers (carrier priced). CMS will be asking for these carrier-priced codes to be surveyed at a later date as well as several of the new codes after they have been used for a sufficient time period. See Table 23.2 for old and new CPT codes.

DOCUMENTATION REQUIREMENTS FOR THE PSYCHIATRIC RECORD, PSYCHOTHERAPY ONLY AND PSYCHOTHERAPY ADD-ON CODES

Many providers wonder about the minimum requirement for psychiatric documentation. As HIPAA requirements continue to unfold, the American Psychiatric Association (APA) developed a position statement on the minimum necessary guidelines for disclosure to third-party payers for psychiatric treatment (APA, 2007). There are three categories described: outpatient treatment that has been preauthorized, outpatient requiring preauthorization, and inpatient hospitalization. Specific guidance includes the documention of risk assessment, the disclosure of only a minimum of content in order to justify the billing code, and the protection of personal health information at all costs. The provider also needs to document the risk/benefits of various treatment options, record pertinent and significant changes, and provide evidence of adhering to best practices and standards of care (Focht, Rodriguez, & Fuchs, 2017).

Recent Medicare audits of psychotherapy notes neccessitate the inclusion of specific content. It will be important to include narrative comments related to target symptoms; goals of therapy; method of monitoring outcomes; frequency of treatment; clinical records to support relevant medical history; results of diagnostic tests or procedures; prognosis or progress to date; and estimated duration of treatment. The types of psychotherapy recognized by CMS include psychodynamic, behavioral, and ego supportive. It is suggested to create a template that you can modify with changes that have occurred since the last session. Medicare requirements for psychotherapy session documentation are included in Box 23.1.

BOX 23.1 Medicare Requirements for Psychotherapy Sessions

- Target symptoms
- Goals of therapy
- Method of monitoring outcomes
- Frequency of treatment
- Clinical records to support relevant medical history
- Results of diagnostic tests or procedures
- Prognosis or progress to date
- Estimated duration of treatment

TABLE 23.1 REVISED PSYCHOTHERAPY CODES

2019 Procedure	2019 Billing Code
Diagnostic interview	90791 (no medical) 90792 (with medical) (report with interactive complexity add-on [+90785] when appropriate)
Individual psychotherapy, 20–30 min	90832—Psychotherapy, 30 (16–37) min (report with interactive complexity add-on [+90785] when appropriate)
Individual psychotherapy, 45–50 min	90834—Psychotherapy, 45 (38–52) min (report with interactive complexity add-on [+90785] when appropriate)
Individual psychotherapy, 75–80 min	90837—Psychotherapy, 60 (53+) min (report with interactive complexity add-on [+90785] when appropriate)
Individual psychotherapy with E/M, 20–30 min	+90833—Psychotherapy, 30 (16–37) min, use only add-on code to selected E/M code (report with interactive complexity add-on [+90785] when appropriate)
Individual psychotherapy with E/M, 45–50 min	Use only as add-on code to selected E/M code +90836—Psychotherapy, 45 (38–52) min (report with interactive complexity add-on [+90785] when appropriate)

(continued)

TABLE 23.1 REVISED PSYCHOTHERAPY CODES (*CONTINUED*)	
2019 Procedure	**2019 Billing Code**
Individual psychotherapy with E/M, 75–80 min	Use only as add-on code to selected E/M code +90838—Psychotherapy, 60 (53+) min (report with interactive complexity add-on [+90785] when appropriate)
Group psychotherapy	90853, group psychotherapy (reported with interactive complexity add-on [+90785] when appropriate) *CPT, current procedural terminology; E/M, evaluation and management.*

Source: Adapted from American Psychiatric Association. (n.d.). *CPT primer for psychiatrists.* Retrieved from https://www. psychiatry.org/File%20Library/Psychiatrists/Practice/Practice-Management/Coding-Reimbursement-Medicare-Medicaid/Coding-Reimbursement/cpt-primer-for-psychiatrists.pdf

THE BASICS OF AN E/M CODE

The ins and outs of using E/M codes are thoroughly outlined in the Medicare Learning Network publication entitled *Evaluation and Management Services Guide* (DHHS, 2020). This guide is freely available to the public and all APPNs are encouraged to download this publication, which is referenced at the end of this chapter.

Understanding the Five Digits of an E/M Code

The specific 5-digit E/M code is selected based on the type of patient, location of service, and level of service. The first two digits, 99, indicate that it is an E/M code. The third and fourth digits identify the type of patient and location of service. The fifth digit indicates the level of service, which is determined by the complexity of history, physical exam, and MDM. The level of service is different in the outpatient and inpatient settings. In the outpatient setting, the fifth digit is on a range of 1 to 5, while the inpatient range is 1 to 3. In an office or other outpatient settings, a fifth digit of 1 or 2 is a problem-focused encounter involving straightforward MDM of minimal complexity. It should be noted that a level 1 does not require a licensed provider and is typically reserved for encounters where a patient is coming to an office to receive medical assistant type services. A fifth digit identified with a 3 indicates an expanded problem-focused encounter involving MDM of low complexity. A fifth digit identified with a 4 indicates a detailed encounter involving MDM of moderate complexity. Lastly, a fifth digit identified with a 5 indicates a comprehensive encounter involving MDM of high complexity. In the initial or subsequent hospitalization for the same problem, a 1 is straightforward, a 2 is moderate, and a 3 indicates high complexity. Table 23.2 depicts the standard CPT (outpatient, new patient, and established patient) facility codes and RVU designation for 2019.

Assigning the Five Digits

A *new patient* is one who has not received services from the provider or a provider in the same specialty or subspecialty in a medical group in the past 3 years. An *established patient* is one who has been seen by the provider or a provider in the same specialty

TABLE 23.2 COMMONLY USED CPT CODES			
Office/Outpatient Visit New CPT	**Office/Outpatient Visit Established CPT**	**Office/Outpatient Consultation CPT**	**Initial Hospital Care CPT**
99201	99211	99241	99221
99202	99212	99242	99222
99203	99213	99243	99223
99204	99214	99244	
99205	99215	99245	

CPT, current procedural terminology

or subspecialty in the medical group within the past 3 years. Even if the APPN is on call for the practice and has not personally seen the patient, the patient is considered an established patient for E/M purposes. If the APPN is in a primary care setting and is referred an existing clinic patient who is new to the psychiatry/behavioral health service, the documentation would be for a new patient. The location of service is designated as hospital inpatient, office or other outpatient, nursing facility, or emergency department. A new patient seen in an office or other outpatient setting that is highly complex would be identified by the E/M code of 99205. When this patient returns as an established patient who remains complex, the E/M code changes to 99215. A new patient who is highly complex and seen in a hospital-type setting would be identified by the E/M code of 99223. If this patient is seen in a subsequent hospitalization setting, the code would change to 99233. The add-on codes of psychotherapy (+90833) and/or interactive complexity (+90785) can be added to any encounter but must be properly documented. If the diagnostic interview extends beyond 60 minutes, or if regular encounters extend beyond the schedule time, the billing codes 99354 (use for each additional 60 minutes) and 99355 (use for each additional 30 minutes) can be billed.

The complexity level designated by the fifth digit of an E/M code for an outpatient is determined by three specific components: (a) history including the history of the present illness, past family and social history, and review of systems; (b) physical examination, which in psychiatry is designated as single system (psychiatric) and includes mental status exam and cognitive function; and (c) the MDM, which includes number of diagnoses, complexity of records to review, collaboration with other members of the team, and complexity of the treatment regimen. Each component has a specific label that indicates the amount and type of information required (Table 23.3). A new vocabulary has been created with specific guidelines as to how to determine the MDM, and ultimately the level of service for a given encounter. These terms will be described in detail for each of the major levels of service used to code and bill an outpatient encounter.

UNDERSTANDING THE MAJOR ELEMENTS OF AN E/M CODE

There are three broad elements in an E/M visit: history, physical exam, and MDM. Of these elements, the history is the most familiar to psychiatric providers. The physical exam and MDM are less well known, and APPNs may feel uncomfortable with the terminology. One reason why psychiatry has been reluctant to embrace E/M codes is because of the concept of a physical exam. However, in 1997, CMS changed the documentation

TABLE 23.3	LANGUAGE ASSOCIATED WITH E/M CODES						
History HPI	History PFSH	History ROS	# Diagnoses # Data	Risk	Medical Decision-Making	Level of Service
Brief	Pertinent	Problem pertinent	Minimal	Minimal	Straightforward	Problem focused (PF)
Extended	Complete	Extended	Limited	Low	Low complexity	Expanded problem focused (EPF)
		Complete	Multiple	Moderate	Moderate complexity	Detailed (DET)
			Extensive	High	High complexity	Comprehensive (COMP)

HPI, history of present illness; PFSH, past, family, and social history; ROS, review of systems

Source: U.S. Department of Health and Human Services. (2020). Evaluation and management services guide. Retrieved from https://www.cms.gov/Outreach-and-Education/Medicare-Learning-Network-MLN/MLNProducts/MLN-Publications-Items/CMS1243514.html

requirements and created 11 single-system specialty exams of which psychiatry was included: cardiovascular; ears, nose, mouth, and throat; eyes; genitourinary (female); genitourinary (male); hematologic, lymphatic, and immunologic; musculoskeletal; neurological; psychiatric; respiratory; and skin. In a level 5 complex patient, the psychiatric specialty exam (physical exam) only requires that the constitutional, psychiatric, and musculoskeletal systems be included. Each of these systems has specific bullet points that must be included and is described in a later section. As mentioned earlier, the MDM component comprises three sections: the number of diagnoses or management options; the amount and/or complexity of data to be reviewed; and the risk of significant complications, morbidity, and/or mortality. In order to objectify each of these MDM components for audit purposes, specific criteria in the form of points were developed and approved by CMS in the early 1990s by the Marshfield Clinic (over 600 multispecialty providers in 32 clinics throughout Wisconsin). It is to be noted that CPT itself does not require the Marshfield criteria, but CMS does. In order to be at the top of the documentation bar, it is suggested to include them in every encounter. Each of these three broad elements will now be reviewed.

History

Obtaining the history is no different in psychiatry than in any other branch of medicine. However, the verbiage that is used for medical symptoms has been adapted. Elements of the history include the chief complaint (CC) or, better stated, reason for encounter; history of present illness (HPI); review of systems (ROS); and the past, family, and social history (PFSH). The specified elements for each level of service are summarized in Table 23.4.

CHIEF COMPLAINT (REASON FOR ENCOUNTER)

The CC should be documented in the patient's exact words with quotation marks. An example is "I feel like life isn't worth living at all anymore. This has been going on for about a month," and encompass the problem and the duration.

TABLE 23.4 CPT REQUIREMENTS: HISTORY			
Level of Service	HPI	PFSH	ROS
Problem focused 99202/99212	Brief: one to three elements or one to two chronic conditions	N/A	N/A
Expanded problem focused 99203/99213	Brief: one to three elements or one to two chronic conditions	N/A	Problem pertinent: 1 system
Detailed 99204/99214	Extended: one to three elements or one to two chronic conditions	Pertinent 1 element*	Extended: 2–9 systems

(continued)

TABLE 23.4 CPT REQUIREMENTS: HISTORY (*CONTINUED*)			
Level of Service	HPI	PFSH	ROS
Comprehensive 99205/99215	Extended: four elements or three chronic conditions	Complete 3 elements**	Complete: 10–14 systems *CPT, current procedural terminology; HPI, history of present illness; PFSH, past family, and social history; ROS, review of systems.*

Source: U.S. Department of Health and Human Services. (2020). Evaluation and management services guide. Retrieved from https://www.cms.gov/Outreach-and-Education/Medicare-Learning-Network-MLN/MLNProducts/MLN-Publications-Items/CMS1243514.html

*No PFSH required for subsequent hospital visits. **Only two elements required for established patient.

HISTORY OF PRESENT ILLNESS

The HPI is a very familiar element to APPNs as it encompasses a portion of what used to go into the subjective section of a traditional narrative progress note documenting subjective and objective patient data, assignment and diagnosis, and plan (SOAP). What is different are the names of the elements that comprise the HPI. There are eight elements used to qualify and quantify the HPI: location (emotion and behavior are types of location in psychiatry), quality (description of symptom, i.e., sadness), severity, duration, timing, context, modifying factors, and associated signs/symptoms. The following is an example of all eight elements in a typical patient description of HPI:

> The patient reports ongoing (timing) emotional (location) problems of moderate (severity) anger (symptom) starting with the discovery of spousal marital affair (context) 2 weeks ago (duration), and now does not want to live in the same house (modifying factors) and associated with disrupted sleep and loss of appetite (associated signs/symptoms).

There are two major levels of HPI. The first is referred to as *brief* and consists of one to three elements or the status of one to two chronic or inactive conditions. Brief HPI is required for problem-focused (99212) and *expanded* problem-focused encounters (99213). The second level of HPI is referred to as extended and consists of four or more elements or the status of three or more chronic or inactive conditions. Extended HPI is required for detailed (99214) and comprehensive (99215) encounters (see Table 19.4).

REVIEW OF SYSTEMS

The ROS is exactly what it says. There are 14 systems that could potentially be reviewed: constitutional (vital signs and general appearance including nutritional status and fever); eyes; cardiovascular; neurological; genitourinary; ears, nose, throat, and mouth; gastrointestinal; integumentary (skin and/or breast); musculoskeletal; psychiatric; respiratory; hematologic/lymphatic; endocrine; and allergic/immune. The ROS is only a very brief comment related to the system being reviewed. There is no requirement for ROS for a problem-focused (99202, 99212) encounter.

There are three levels of ROS: problem pertinent (1 system), extended (2–9 systems), and complete (10–14). An expanded problem-focused encounter (99203, 99213) requires only the problem-pertinent system to be reviewed. A detailed encounter (99204, 99214) requires two to nine systems and typically comprises psychiatric and constitutional, although the system to be reviewed could be related to a reported side effect. A comprehensive encounter (99205, 99215) requires all 10 to 14 systems to be reviewed. The documentation of complete ROS must include individual systems and may include positive or pertinent negative responses, and the following statement in addition is permissible: "All other systems reviewed and are negative." In the absence of such a notation, at least 10 systems must be individually documented (see Table 23.5).

PAST, FAMILY, AND SOCIAL HISTORY

The elements of PFSH are also very familiar to psychiatric providers as this component similarly includes information that was contained in the objective section of a traditional SOAP note. *Past history* for a new patient includes current medications, illnesses and injuries, operations and hospitalizations, allergies, treatments, dietary status, and age-appropriate immunizations. Past history for an established patient would include any update since the last encounter/session.

Family history for a new patient includes medical events in the patient's family related to CC, HPI, PFSH, and ROS. Other elements of family history include hereditary or high-risk diseases, as well as health status or cause of death of parents, siblings, and children. Family history for an established patient would include any updates since the last encounter/session.

The final element of PFSH is the *social history*. Social history for a new patient includes: marital status; living arrangements; occupational history; use of drugs, alcohol, and tobacco; extent of education, sexual history, and current employment. Social history for an established patient would include any updates since the last encounter/session.

There are also two levels of PFSH: *pertinent* and *complete*. Pertinent is one item from one of the three areas and is required only for a detailed (99214) encounter. Complete is

TABLE 23.5 CPT PHYSICAL EXAM REQUIREMENTS FOR PSYCHIATRY	
Level	**Elements of Examination**
Problem focused 99202, 99212	One to five bulleted elements from psychiatric exam
Expanded problem focused 99203, 99213	At least six bulleted elements from psychiatric exam
Detailed 99204, 99214	At least nine bulleted elements from psychiatric exam
Comprehensive 99205, 99215	All bulleted elements from psychiatric exam Three of seven components of vital signs and general appearance (two bullets) from constitutional One bullet element from unshaded border from musculoskeletal *CPT, current procedural terminology.*

Source: U.S. Department of Health and Human Services. (2020). Evaluation and management services guide. Retrieved from https://www.cms.gov/Outreach-and-Education/Medicare-Learning-Network-MLN/MLNProducts/MLN-Publications-Items/CMS1243514.html

three out of three areas for a new patient and two out of three areas for an established patient and is required only for comprehensive (99215) encounters. PFSH is not required for problem-focused or expanded problem-focused encounters or in subsequent inpatient visits (see Table 23.4).

PHYSICAL EXAM

As mentioned earlier, the physical exam was an intimidating requirement for psychiatric providers, but with the 1997 CMS changes to include a single-system specialty there are now 11 possible systems: cardiovascular; ears, nose, mouth, and throat; eyes; genitourinary (female); genitourinary (male); hematologic, lymphatic, and immunologic; musculoskeletal; neurological; psychiatric; respiratory; and skin. There are some differences from the traditional mental status exam in how CMS defines the elements of the *psychiatric single system*.

Psychiatric Single-System/Specialty Exam—CMS Guidelines

The CMS Handbook lists all requirements for each of the single-system exams in alphabetical order. Each system has bulleted areas and shaded areas that must be included. The reader is encouraged to go now to the website and look at the psychiatric single-system exam requirements (pp. 76–77) in order to more clearly understand these requirements (https://www.cms.gov/Outreach-and-Education/Medicare-Learning-Network-MLN/MLNProducts/MLN-Publications-Items/CMS1243514.html). The psychiatric single-system exam consists of 11 bullets that are divided into two sections: descriptive statements and a complete mental status including cognitive exam. The groupings of symptoms include general, neurologic, psychiatric, and mental status/cognitive (see Boxes 23.3 and 23.4).

A problem-focused exam (99202, 99212) requires one to five bulleted areas. An expanded problem-focused exam (99203, 99213) requires at least six bulleted areas. A detailed exam (99204, 99214) requires at least nine bulleted areas.

The comprehensive exam (99205, 99215) requires all 11 bullets from the psychiatric single system plus a different set of bullets and elements from the constitutional (shaded border) and musculoskeletal (unshaded border). The 1997 CMS guidelines include detailed instructions for completion and documentation of the comprehensive physical exam. Each of the 11 major single systems has individual guidelines regarding which elements from each of the 11 major single systems are required for a comprehensive single-system exam.

BOX 23.2 Descriptive Statements

- Description of speech including: rate; volume; articulation; coherence; and spontaneity with notation of abnormalities (e.g., perseveration, paucity of language)
- Description of thought processes including: rate of thoughts; content of thoughts (e.g., logical vs. illogical, tangential); abstract reasoning; and computation
- Description of associations (e.g., loose, tangential, circumstantial, intact)
- Description of abnormal or psychotic thoughts including: hallucinations; delusions; preoccupation with violence; homicidal or suicidal ideation; and obsessions
- Description of the patient's judgment (e.g., concerning everyday activities and social situations) and insight (e.g., concerning psychiatric condition)

Source: U.S. Department of Health and Human Services. (2020). Evaluation and management services guide. *Retrieved from https://www.cms.gov/Outreach-and-Education/Medicare-Learning-Network-MLN/MLNProducts/MLN-Publications-Items/CMS1243514.html*

BOX 23.3 Complete Mental Status Exam Including Cognitive Function

- Orientation to time, place, and person
- Recent and remote memory
- Attention span and concentration
- Language (e.g., naming objects, repeating phrases)
- Fund of knowledge (e.g., awareness of current events, past history, vocabulary)
- Mood and affect (e.g., depression, anxiety, agitation, hypomania, lability)

Source: U.S. Department of Health and Human Services. (2020). Evaluation and management services guide. *Retrieved from https://www.cms.gov/Outreach-and-Education/Medicare-Learning-Network-MLN/MLNProducts/MLN-Publications-Items/CMS1243514.html*

The requirements are identified by shaded and unshaded sections. The psychiatric exam requires all elements in the shaded border from the constitutional exam and all elements in the shaded border from the psychiatric exam as well as one element from the two in the unshaded border of the musculoskeletal exam. Nothing from the other single-system exams is required for a comprehensive psychiatric single-system exam.

The constitutional system (shaded border) consists of two bullets that cover eight major areas:

- Measurement of any three of the seven vital signs: BP__ sitting or standing, BP__ supine, P__, R__, T__, Ht__, Wt__
- General appearance which includes grooming, deformities, nutrition, and development

The musculoskeletal system (unshaded border) consists of two bullets that cover a broad area:

- Assessment of muscle strength and tone (e.g., flaccid, cog wheel, and spastic), with notation of any atrophy and abnormal movements (e.g., motor tics, tremors, and vermiform tongue movements), or
- Examination of gait and station

Table 23.5 summarizes the required elements of the physical exam for psychiatry.

MEDICAL DECISION MAKING

The MDM in psychiatry is based on the nature of the presenting problem and is comprised of three components: the number of diagnoses, the amount of data to be reviewed, and risk of mortality/morbidity. In a typical medical visit, the Medical Decision is what drives everything else in the encounter including the history, psychiatric specialty exam, and intensity of the service delivered. In a psychiatric visit much of content of the session is driven by presemting symptoms, the ROS, and the PFSH so the MDM is determined at the end of the session. Psychiatric providers have always done this intuitively but now are being asked to make explicit what has been implicit in how an encounter is conducted. Medical decision making is a sort of "thinking out loud" for the record and often "transposes into the key of psychiatry" (R. Burd, personal communication, November 3, 2013). The three components have distinct guidelines and are summarized in Tables 23.6 and 23.7. Appendix 23.1 includes an example of an Evaluation and Management Established Patient Office Progress Note created as a worksheet that incorporates the major elements of MDM.

No. of Diagnoses or Management Options	Points	Amount and Complexity of Data	Points	Risk Factors of Presenting Problems
Self-limiting	1	Review and/or order lab data	1	One self-limited or minor problem (e.g., dysthymia well managed) Management options include minimal risk
Established problem to examining provider—stable or improved	1	Review and/or order radiology tests	1	Two or more self-limited or minor problems One stable chronic illness Acute uncomplicated illness Management options include low risk such as OTC medications
Established problem to examining provider—worsening	2	Review and/or order tests in the medical section of CPT	1	One or more chronic illnesses with mild exacerbation, progression, or side effects Two or more stable chronic illnesses Undiagnosed new problem with uncertain prognosis Acute illness with systemic symptoms Management options include any prescription medication—this elevates risk to moderate
New problem to examining provider—no additional workup or diagnostic procedures ordered (Max 2)	3	Discussion of test results with performing provider	1	One or more chronic illnesses with severe exacerbation, progression, or side effects Acute or chronic illnesses that pose a threat to life or bodily function Management options are elevated to extensive risk because the pharmacological prescription requires intensive management

No. of Diagnoses or Management Options	Points	Amount and Complexity of Data	Points	Risk Factors of Presenting Problems
New problem to examining provider—additional workup planned		Review and summarization of old records and/or obtaining history from someone other than the patient Review and summarization of old records and/or obtaining history from someone other than the patient and/or discussion of case with another provider Independent visualization of image tracing, or specimen itself (not simply review report)	1 2 2	
Minimal	Less than 1	Minimal	Less than 1	Minimal
Limited	2	Limited	2	Low
Multiple	3	Multiple	3	Moderate
Extensive	4	Extensive	4	Extensive

CPT, current procedural terminology; OTC, over-the-counter; MDM, medical decision making.

Source: U.S. Department of Health and Human Services. (2020). Evaluation and management services guide. Retrieved from the Medicare learning network: https://www.cms.gov/Outreach-and-Education/Medicare-Learning-Network-MLN/MLNProducts/MLN-Publications-Items/CMS1243514.html

TABLE 23.7	DETERMINATION OF LEVEL OF MDM		
Designated Level of MDM	No. of Diagnoses or Management Options	Amount and/ or Complexity of Data to be Reviewed	Risk of Complications and/or Morbidity/ Mortality
Straight forward 99202–99212	Minimal (0–1 problem points)	Minimal or none (0–1 data points)	Minimal
Low complexity 99203–99213	Limited (2 problem points)	Limited (2 data points)	Low
Moderate complexity 99204–99214	Multiple (3 problem points)	Multiple (3 data points)	Moderate
High complexity 99205–99215	High complexity (4 problem points)	Extensive (4 data points)	Extensive

MDM, medical decision making

Source: Department of Health and Human Services. (2020). Evaluation and management services guide. Retrieved from the Medicare learning network: https://www.cms.gov/Outreach-and-Education/Medicare-Learning-Network-MLN/MLNProducts/MLN-Publications-Items/CMS1243514.html

The Number of Diagnoses or Management Options

The MDM component of establishing the number of diagnoses and management options can be determined by using the Marshfield problem point chart developed for CMS audit purposes. This component is based on the number and types of problems, the complexity of establishing a diagnosis, and the potential clinical management decisions. These are influenced by undiagnosed problems, the number and type of tests that need to be ordered, the need to seek advice from others, and problems worsening or failing to respond to the existing treatment plan.

The Marshfield scoring of this component is as follows. A self-limiting problem with minimal management options is scored with 1 point. An established problem that is stable or improved and also has minimal management options is also scored with 1 point. An established problem that is worsening is scored with 2 points. This level typically requires prescription medications, which elevate the level of complexity. A new problem that requires no additional workup or diagnostic procedures ordered is scored with 3 points. There is a maximum of two new problems that can be scored in one encounter. Lastly, a new problem that requires additional workup is scored with 4 points. These last two options typically require complex pharmacological management and/or procedures such as TMS or ECT. The management options are scored according to the following algorithm: minimal = less than 1; limited = 2; multiple = 3; and extensive = 4.

The Amount and Complexity of Data

The amount and complexity of data are also based on a data point chart for audit purposes because the basic language is ambiguous. This component is based on the types of diagnostic tests, the need to obtain records, and the need to obtain history from other sources. This information is influenced by unexpected findings, independent interpretation of images and specimens and diagnostic tests, and the need to discuss test results with the provider performing the test.

The scoring of this section is as follows. The need to review and/or order lab data, review and/or order radiology tests, review and/or order tests in the medical section of the CPT manual, discussion of test results with the performing provider, and a review and summarization of old records and/or obtaining history from someone other than the patient are each scored with 1 point. The review and summarization of old records and/or obtaining history from someone other than the patient and/or discussion of case with another provider and the need for independent visualization of image tracing, or specimen itself and not simply reviewing the report are each scored with a 2. This component is scored according to the following algorithm: minimal or none = 0 to 1; limited = 2; multiple = 3; and extensive = 4.

Risk Factors of Presenting Problems

This MDM component is based on the risk involved in the presenting problem, diagnostic procedures, and management options. This information is influenced by several factors including: comorbidities, underlying conditions, and risk factors; uncertain prognosis, exacerbations, and/or complications; decision to order prescription drugs and/or the need for intravenous (IV) medications; and a decision to perform invasive tests, procedures, or major surgery. The scoring for this section is different from the first two MDM elements. One self-limited or minor problem, such as mild anxiety, that does not require medication and minimal therapy is rated as minimal risk. Two or more self-limited or minor problems, one stable chronic illness, or an acute uncomplicated illness that can be treated with brief therapy and/or over-the-counter medications are rated as low risk. Two or more chronic illnesses with mild exacerbation, progression, or side effects; two or more stable chronic illnesses; undiagnosed new problem with uncertain prognosis; or an acute illness with systemic symptoms are rated as moderate risk. Lastly, one or more chronic illnesses with severe exacerbation, progression, or side effects; or acute or chronic illnesses that pose a threat to life or bodily function and require medications involving intensive management and monitoring are rated as high risk.

SELECTING THE LEVEL OF MEDICAL DECISION-MAKING

The selection of the appropriate level of MDM in the office or other outpatient settings is determined by the highest two out of three ratings in the three overall elements (presenting problem, diagnostic procedures, and management options). For example, let us calculate the MDM for a patient who has persistent depressive disorder and is responding to standard dose selective serotonin reuptake inhibitor (SSRI) treatment with a side effect of sexual dysfunction and brief, solution-focused therapy provided by another therapist who has mailed you a copy of rating scales and asked you to review progress to determine whether therapy needs to be continued. You have taken the history and conducted the psychiatric exam based on the nature of the presenting problem and you have also been asked to provide a report to the insurance company. Under the diagnoses or management options, there is one established problem that is stable or improving (1 point) for a score of 1. Under the amount and complexity of data, you will review the rating scale scores (1 point) and obtain history from the therapist (1 point), and you will summarize the records and provide documentation to the insurance company (2 points) for a score of 4. Under the risk section, there is the need for prescription psychotropic medications that require monitoring of side effects, elevating the risk to moderate. The highest two out of three yields a score of extensive for the amount and complexity of data and moderate risk for an MDM score of moderate complexity. This would result in a level 4 service, or a 99214.

Documentation of MDM should include: assessment; impression; diagnosis, status of established diagnosis, differential diagnosis, probable diagnoses, and rule-outs for potential diagnoses; initiation/changes in treatment; and referrals, request, and advice from other providers. Additional MDM documentation includes type of tests, review and findings of tests, relevant findings from records, discussion of test results, direct visualization of images, comorbidities/underlying conditions, and the type of surgical or invasive procedure. See Table 23.6 for tabulation of MDM elements.

COUNSELING AND COORDINATION OF CARE

The purpose of the CPT coding process is to capture the work required to deliver a level of service and is not time dependent. Depending on the complexity of the patient, a level 5 service could occur in less than 30 minutes. However, in some situations the bulk of the work may occur in delivering what is referred to as counseling and CCC. If this type of care comprises over 50% of the encounter, then time becomes the controlling factor in designating the level of service. See Box 23.3 for examples of CCC discussions.

In the outpatient setting, care is required to be delivered face to face and must be documented as such. Additional documentation requirements include the length of time of the encounter and of the time spent in CCC. Many payors require documentation of encounter start and end times. The presence of family members present for the encounter must also be documented. The time designations for counseling/CCC are: 99212 = 10 minutes; 99213 = 15 minutes; 99214 = 25 minutes; and 99215 = 40 minutes.

Table 23.8 summarizes all that has been presented related to documenting E/M codes for a new or established patient in an office or other outpatient settings.

Case Example

Following are case examples of patient scenarios depicting typical outpatient psychiatric encounters and how they should be documented using E/M codes. The goal of the chart note is to demonstrate how ill the patient is, document the care given, and provide documentation for the itemized bill submitted for reimbursement.

BOX 23.3 Examples of CCC Discussions

- Diagnostic results
- Impressions related to the diagnosis
- Recommended diagnostic studies
- Prognosis
- Risks and benefits of management options
- Instructions for management and/or follow-up
- Importance of compliance with chosen management options
- Risk factor reduction
- Patient and family education

CCC, counseling and coordination of care.
Source: U.S. Department of Health and Human Services. (2020). Evaluation and management services guide. Retrieved from https://www.cms.gov/Outreach-and-Education/Medicare-Learning-Network-MLN/MLNProducts/MLN-Publications-Items/CMS1243514.html

TABLE 23.8   ALL REQUIRED EVALUATION AND MANAGEMENT ELEMENTS

New/Established Office or Other Outpatient Services

	99202/99212 Problem focused	99203/99213 Expanded problem focused	99204/99214 Detailed	99205/99215 Comprehensive
History				
CC	Required	Required	Required	Required
HPI	One to three elements	One to three elements	Greater than four elements	Greater than four elements
ROS	One system	One system	Two to nine systems	10 to 14 systems
PFSH	N/A	N/A	1/3 elements	2/3 elements (3/3 new patient)
Physical Exam				
1997	One to five bullets from psychiatric exam	At least six bullets from psychiatric exam	At least nine bullets from psychiatric exam	All bullets from constitutional and psychiatric, one from musculoskeletal
Medical Complexity Decision-Making				
	Straightforward	Low complexity	Moderate complexity	High complexity
Counseling/Coordination of Care				
Face to face	10 min	15 min	25 min	40 min

Source: U.S. Department of Health and Human Services. (2020). Evaluation and management services guide. Retrieved from https://www.cms.gov/Outreach-and-Education/Medicare-Learning-Network-MLN/MLNProducts/MLN-Publications-Items/CMS1243514.html

99212—ESTABLISHED PATIENT

Case

Thirty-year-old female with a history of depression who is stable on an SSRI for the past 4 months and reports no depressive symptoms. She comes for a prescription renewal. There are no treatment changes, no side effects, and her medication is prescribed at the same dose.

Presenting Problem

Patient is stable and requesting a 3-month medication refill.

History

For a 99212, there is no ROS or PFSH required. The HPI requires one to three elements or one to two chronic conditions.

Physical Exam

Only one to five bulleted points from the psychiatric single-system exam are required.

Medical Decision-Making

This patient has 1 problem point under diagnoses and management options for her stable diagnosis. Reviewing her record from 4 months ago results in 1 data point. Her risk is low due to being stabilized on an SSRI with no side effects. This averages to a straightforward level of MDM which translates to a problem-focused 99212.

99212—PROGRESS NOTE

CC/Reason for Encounter

"I'm here to get my citalopram renewed, everything is going well."

HPI

A 40-year-old married, African American female, comes to office for follow-up visit for treatment of depression that is stable with no exacerbations, no side effects.

PE

Speech: normal rate and tone. Mood: "I'm feeling good." Affect: broad, congruent, animated. Presentation: good hygiene and grooming. No S/I. Sleeping well.

Impression

Patient is stable and responding to SSRI. Diagnosis: *DSM-5* 300.4 Persistent depressive disorder, in remission. *ICD-10* F34.1 —improved on citalopram.

Plan

Continue same medication dose, wrote script for citalopram 20 mg #30 2 refills. Patient to notify office if there is a change in level of remission. Return visit in 3 months.

99213—ESTABLISHED PATIENT

Case

Office visit for a 32-year-old single Hispanic female with major depression, moderate, without psychotic features who is stable 6 months on an SSRI and who wants to decrease her current dosage due to sexual dysfunction.

History

An expanded problem-focused encounter requires a brief HPI consisting of one to three elements or one to two chronic conditions, PFSH is not required, and the ROS is problem pertinent for one system.

Physical Exam

At least six bulleted points from the psychiatric single-system exam are required.

Medical Decision-Making

This patient has 1 problem point under diagnoses and management options for an established problem that is stable. She has 3 problem points for a new problem that may require additional workup. Reviewing her record from 6 months ago results in 1 data point. Her risk is moderate due to being on an SSRI and having a side effect. This averages to a low level of MDM which translates to an expanded problem-focused 99213.

99213—PROGRESS NOTE

CC/Reason for Encounter

A 32-year-old married Hispanic female reports, "My depression is okay, but my sex drive is zero. I think it's from my medication."

HPI

The patient reports ongoing (timing) decreased libido (location) creating moderate (severity) frustration (quality) that has been going on for the last 6 weeks (duration). Now that her depression is better, she wants an active sex life (context). Her husband is supportive and not pressuring her (modifying factors). (*Although only one to three elements are required, seven are captured as she describes the HPI which often happens with psychiatric E/M documentation.*)

ROS

Psychiatric—no symptoms of depression or anxiety. Genitourinary—reports decreased libido.

PE

Psychiatric: Appearance: appropriately dressed, verbal, and cooperative; speech: normal rate and tone; mood: euthymic; affect: full and appropriate; thought process: logical, associations intact, no suicidal or homicidal ideation.

Problem

Depression responding to treatment but patient presents with a new problem of sexual side effects.

Diagnostic Impression

DSM: 296.32 *ICD-10*: F33.1 Major depression, moderate without psychotic features responding to SSRI.

Plan

Decrease fluoxetine from 40 to 20 mg. Called pharmacy with change. Return visit in 1 month.

99214—ESTABLISHED PATIENT

Case

Office visit for a 52-year-old married man, with a 16-year history of bipolar disorder responding to lithium carbonate and brief insight-oriented psychotherapy. Patient reports tremors and some diarrhea. Psychoeducation and prescription provided. Ordered laboratory tests.

History

A detailed encounter requires an extended HPI that includes 4/8 elements or greater than three chronic conditions. This level of encounter requires a pertinent level of PFSH which is one element. An extended ROS of two to nine systems is required.

Physical Exam

A 99214 detailed encounter requires nine bulleted items from the psychiatric single-system exam.

Medical Decision-Making

This patient has 4 points under diagnoses and management options for a new problem that requires additional workup. There are 2 points under amount and complexity of data for the need to order lab data and review of old records and labs. He is on lithium which has a moderate risk for side effects and requires monitoring. The highest two out of three rates the MDM at the moderate complexity level. The appropriate level of service is 99214.

PROGRESS NOTE

CC/Reason for Encounter

A 52-year-old single White male. Scheduled visit for treatment of bipolar disorder, stable on lithium for 16 months. Complains of tremors and diarrhea.

HPI

The patient reports increased tremors and diarrhea (location) creating moderate difficulty (severity) with fine motor tasks and fear of not being around a bathroom (associated signs and symptoms) that has been going on for the last 3 weeks (duration). This has happened since having the "bad GI flu" (context). He has decreased his salt and fluid intake but continued his lithium (modifying factors). He is also feeling dizzy.

PFSH

He is concerned he won't be able to work.

ROS

(Required only two systems)

Psychiatric: reports no change in mood, thinking, speech; continued taking lithium· while he had the flu.
Constitutional: reports changes in diet after experiencing fever, nausea, vomiting, and diarrhea for 4 days. No blood in vomitus or diarrhea.
GI: reports ongoing diarrhea and cramping after getting over the flu.
Musculoskeletal: complains of tremors and weakness on getting up too fast.

PE

(Nine elements)

Psychiatric: Appearance: appropriately dressed, verbal, and cooperative; speech: clear with no slurring or increased rate; thought process: normal; associations: normal; thought content: normal with no grandiosity; judgment: adequate; mood: euthymic; affect: broad, congruent, and animated; orientation: fully oriented; memory: intact.
Constitutional: BP = 168/110, P = 92 RSR, R = 18, unlabored, T = 99, weight = 224 (increase of 10#), well groomed with good hygiene.
Musculoskeletal: normal strength, fine tremors observable in both extremities that have never occurred before, gait normal, balance normal.

Impression

Diagnosis: *DSM-5* 296.46 *ICD-10* (F31.7) Bipolar I disorder, currently in remission. Mild lithium toxicity related to continuing lithium while experiencing vomiting and diarrhea, possible dehydration.

Plan

Continue lithium, psychoeducation, and supportive psychotherapy. Called lab and ordered stat lithium level, comprehensive metabolic panel, renal function, thyroid function. Reviewed diet and instructed to return to normal diet and increase water intake back to normal 2 liters/day. Reviewed effects of lithium during dehydration. Call patient with lab results. Return visit in 2 weeks to recheck vitals.

99215—ESTABLISHED PATIENT

Case

Office visit for a 32-year-old male with a 12-year history of schizophrenia, type 2 diabetes, hypertension, opioid dependence on medication-assisted treatment, and PTSD who has been seen bimonthly and has difficulty with adherence to oral antipsychotic medication, statin, antihypertensive, and antidiabetic medications. He lives in a group home and has a case manager. He is brought in by his parents. Patient reports a new kind of auditory hallucinations and increased paranoia. He is unkempt and withdrawn.

History

A comprehensive encounter requires an extended HPI that includes 4/8 elements or greater than three chronic conditions. This level of encounter requires a complete level of PFSH which is two elements. A complete ROS of 10 to 14 systems is required.

Physical Exam

A 99215 comprehensive encounter requires all bullets in constitutional and psychiatric shaded boxes and one bullet from the musculoskeletal unshaded box.

Medical Decision-Making

This patient has 4 points under diagnoses and management options for a new problem that requires additional workup. There are 3 points under amount and complexity of data for the need to order lab data (1); review of old records and labs, obtain history from someone other than the patient; and conduct discussion with a case manager (2). He is on medications that require monitoring and has one or more chronic illnesses with severe exacerbation (high risk). The highest two out of three rates the MDM at the high complexity level. The appropriate level of service is 99215.

PROGRESS NOTE

CC/Reason for Encounter

A 32-year-old single White male. Scheduled visit for treatment of schizophrenia. "I'm hearing these really weird and scary voices. I've never heard voices like this before, I feel like I need to blow my ears off my head because they are telling me I would be better off dead. I'm afraid to answer the telephone because I hear them from the phone wires and can't tell who I'm talking to."

HPI

The patient reports a new symptom, increased auditory hallucinations (location), creating severe difficulty (severity) because of persecutory nature (quality) that has been going on for the last 3 weeks (duration). He has never heard these kinds of voices before (context). This has happened since increasing marijuana intake to three times daily (timing and modifying factors). Dealing with the voices is causing him to feel lethargic (associated signs and symptoms).

PFSH

He has moved into a new group home that is known to have drug dealers in the vicinity. He has increased marijuana use. He may be using other drugs as well. His family insisted he come in for an appointment and brought him to the appointment.

ROS

(Required 10 systems) Psychiatric: anxious, paranoid; appearance: disheveled and unkempt, strong body odor, fingers stained yellow from smoking; constitutional: hasn't eaten in 2 days; sleep: disrupted; nutrition: gaining weight; respiratory: he is developing a smoker's cough. All other systems reviewed and are negative.

PE

(All bullets in constitutional and psychiatric and one bullet in musculoskeletal)

> **Constitutional:** BP = 140/98, P = 90 RSR, R = 20; weight = 235—gain of 10 pounds. Appearance: unkempt, bizarre, unable to maintain eye contact, reluctant to engage in conversation, frequently turns head, and mumbles to unseen voices.
> **Psychiatric:** Attitude: guarded; speech: soft, slowed, mumbles, incoherent; mood: agitated; affect: restricted, incongruent; thought process: illogical, paranoid, loose associations; thought content: persecutory auditory hallucination, ideas of

reference, paranoid ideation, delusions; orientation: self, place; memory: impaired for both recent and remote; judgment and insight: poor; attention and concentration: impaired; language: named 1/3 items after 3 minutes; fund of knowledge: poor, doesn't know president.

Musculoskeletal: Gait—shuffles; station: slightly off balance.

Problem/Diagnostic Impression

DSM-5: 295.9 *ICD-10* (F20. 0 Schizophrenia, paranoid type, in exacerbation related to substance use and medication nonadherence). In addition to delusions and negative symptoms, now has new-onset auditory hallucinations and is unable to care for self (corroborated by family). Smoking increasing. Comorbid medical conditions are exacerbating.

Plan

Switch oral olanzapine to long-acting aripiprazole following standard titration and switch methodology to hopefully reverse metabolic syndrome that may be related to olanzapine; order drug screen and comprehensive metabolic panel (CMP), lipid profile, hemoglobin A1C, methylfolate, vitamin D. Consult with internist regarding metabolic status and other medications. Temporarily move home with family to monitor substance use and assist with medication administration and activities of daily living (ADLs). Contact Acceptance and Commitment Therapy (ACT) team, refer family to National Alliance on Mental Illness, discuss group home situation with case manager prior to going back to this group home. Return visit in 1 week; may need hospitalization if unable to stabilize.

99215—ESTABLISHED PATIENT SEEN FOR COUNSELING AND COORDINATION OF CARE

Counseling and CCC is based on time, individuals present during the encounter, and the fact that over 50% of the encounter is spent discussing one or more of the following: diagnostic results; impressions related to the diagnosis; recommended diagnostic studies; prognosis; risks and benefits of management options; instructions for management and/or follow-up; importance of compliance with chosen management options; risk factor reduction; and patient and family education. There are no specific documentation requirements for history, physical exam, and MDM in a CCC encounter. Using the patient with schizophrenia described in the previous case, his follow-up appointment the next week is now described using language specific to CCC.

PROGRESS NOTE: COUNSELING AND COORDINATION OF CARE

Session Started

2:00 p.m.

Session Ended

2:45 p.m.

Persons Present

Patient, mother, father, case manager

Narrative Note

The entire appointment was spent in counseling and CCC. The first 10 minutes was spent discussing the diagnosis of schizophrenia and the differences between positive and negative symptoms. Misconceptions were clarified. The next 15 minutes was spent discussing the risks/benefits of switching to a long-acting injectable medication and the rationale for doing so. The patient was in agreement by the end of this section of the encounter, and an informed consent was signed. Ten minutes was spent coordinating the medical care with the case manager who would be present with the patient in the visit to the internist. The case manager was instructed in helping the patient check his blood sugars and to assuring that reliable test strips were used. Instructions about diet, smoking, and metabolic syndrome were provided. The last 10 minutes of the session was spent in explaining how to switch from oral olanzapine to long-acting injectable aripiprazole and the need to first take oral aripiprazole. We will have weekly CCC sessions during the medication switch.

CONCLUDING COMMENTS

The goal of this chapter is to inform the APPN on the ins and outs of using evaluation and management CPT. Added suggestions and clinical pearls include the following. For new patient intakes, you will probably be reimbursed more for a 99205 than a 90792, as the latter code does not take MDM into consideration. However, this is dependent on the carrier and if the patient is already in your practice. You are allowed one 90792 each calendar year. Always remember to use the code that best describes the care given. Medication follow-up encounters should never be coded less than a 99214 unless it is a very simple patient. Do not hesitate to use the CCC option for standard encounters that you know ahead of time will be spent discussing the components of CCC. However, be cognizant that CCC and psychotherapy are not the same. Avoid billing a 99212 or a 99202 because these codes are for 10 minutes of low complexity, which is probably not something the APPN would regularly do such as giving samples or taking vital signs. Remember to use the interactive complexity add-on code when encounters become heated or the family gets involved, but you probably will not be reimbursed very much. Remember to use the psychotherapy add-on codes, even though they do not reimburse that much when you are engaging in specific psychotherapy modalities. If the content is more CCC, use that to your advantage as a 99215 will likely reimburse more than a 99213 with a 90833 add-on. Seriously consider how much education is done in a typical encounter, particularly when explaining labs and drug interactions and neurobiology to the patient and family. Do not be afraid to use 99215, even though it may trigger an audit. Don't worry about a session running long and not getting reimbursed because you can bill a 99354 for an additional hour and a 99355 for each additional half-hour.

Please be aware that in 2018, CMS attempted to collapse the five levels of outpatient codes into just two codes under the premise that it would reduce documentation time. This unleashed a strong backlash from all medical specialities, not just psychiatry. The code change was delayed to 2021, but the following changes were approved that affect psychiatric billing: www.cms.gov/Outreach-and-Education/Medicare-Learning-Network-MLN/MLNProducts/MLN-Publications-Items/CMS1243514.html

- For established patient office/outpatient visits, when relevant information is already contained in the medical record, practitioners may choose to focus their documentation on what has changed since the last visit, or on pertinent items that have not changed, and need not re-record the defined list of required elements if there is evidence that the practitioner reviewed the previous information and updated it as needed.

- For new and established patients for visits, practitioners need not re-enter in the medical record information on the patient's chief complaint and history that has already been entered by ancillary staff or the beneficiary. The practitioner may simply indicate in the medical record that he or she reviewed and verified this information.

A helpful documentation guide is available through one of the Medicare carriers (Celerian Group Systems [CGS], 2020). Once the auditors see your excellent documentation you will probably be spared future audits. Lastly, the more you use the codes and adjust your documentation, the easier it will become. Please view the helpful web pages listed in this text and download the materials. It will take some study, but you may actually find you like the new way of doing business as it definitely does a better job of capturing the outstanding and comprehensive work of the APPN.

DISCUSSION QUESTIONS

1. After reading the Knopf 3-page article the AMA document titled "CPT® and RBRVS 2019 Annual Symposium" (AMA, 2018), what are your thoughts about the process that led to the conclusion of changing the major focus of psychiatric billing, coding, and documentation to that of the E/M codes? Do you agree? Why or why not?
2. Think of one of your past patient and family encounters in which members were shouting and not listening to you or each other and it took you 2 hours to de-escalate and salvage the situation. Were you reimbursed adequately for that amount of work? Or did you just "write it off" to one of those days when you knew you were not going to get reimbursed nearly enough to compensate for the time?
3. Even though you are primarily a psychotherapist, you are still an APRN and as such you are aware of the interrelatedness of the body and mind. Have you had psychotherapy sessions derail into discussion of medications in which you spent the majority of the session clarifying perceptions? Were you able to be reimbursed for that psychoeducation using a psychotherapy code? How did you document that as a psychotherapy session?
4. In your discussions with colleagues about the use of E/M codes, what have been some of the common themes? Are you better able to understand the rationale for coding after reading this chapter?
5. What could be some of the advantages to using E/M language in communicating with medical colleagues?
6. Can you identify the similarities between SOAP language and the language of HPI, PFSH, and ROS?
7. In thinking about an insurance audit of a 99215 chart note, what is your greatest fear related to your current method of documentation?

ACKNOWLEDGMENT

A special thank you to Ronald Burd, MD, for his thoughtful review and editorial comments to this chapter.

REFERENCES

American Medical Association. (2018). *CPT® and RBRVS 2019 annual symposium*. Retrieved from https://commerce.ama-assn.org/store/catalog/productDetail.jsp?product_id=prod2900018&sku_id=sku2920048&navAction=push

American Medical Association. (2020). *CPT® 2019 professional edition*. Chicago, IL: American Medical Association Publishing.

American Psychiatric Association. (2007). *Position statement on minimum necessary guidelines for third-party payers for psychiatric treatment*. Retreived from https://www.psychiatry.org/File%20Library/About-APA/Organization-Documents-Policies/Policies/Position-2007-Minimum-Necessary-Guidelines.pdf

Celerian Group Systems. (2020). CPT code 99215 office or other outpatient visit for established patient: Fact sheet. Retrieved from https://cgsmedicare.com/partb/mr/PDF/99215.pdf

Centers for Medicare and Medicaid Services. (n.d.). *Physician fee schedule search*. Retrieved from http://www.cms.gov/apps/physician-fee-schedule

Dewan, N. A., Burd, R. M., Anderson, A. A., Carlson, E. S., Harris, G. G., Jaffe, E. M., . . . Yowell, R. K. (2018). Understanding coding and payment for psychiatrists' services: How we got here and where we're going. *Focus, 16*(4), 407–414. doi:10.1176/appi.focus.20180002

Focht, A., Rodriguez, G. J., & Fuchs, B. (2017). Clinical documentation: What to include in the psychiatric record. In A. B. Simon, A. S. New, & W. K. Goodman (Eds.), *Mount Sinai expert guides: Psychiatry* (pp. 52–56). Hoboken, NJ: Wiley Blackwell.

Gutheil, T. (1980). Paranoia and progress notes: A guide to forensically informed psychiatric recordkeeping. *Hospital and Community Psychiatry, 31*, 479–482. doi:10.1176/ps.31.7.479

Knopf, A. (2013). Code with care: CPT code changes abound for 2013: Major billing code revision brings more billing options—And a steep learning curve. *Behavioral Healthcare, 33*(1), 12.

U.S. Department of Health and Human Services. (2020). *Evaluation and management services guide*. Retrieved from https://www.cms.gov/Outreach-and-Education/Medicare-Learning-Network-MLN/MLNProducts/MLN-Publications-Items/CMS1243514.html

APPENDIX 23.1
Evaluation and Management Established Patient Office Progress Note

Patient Name: _____

Date of Service: _____

Provider Name: _____

Time In: _____ a.m./p.m.   Time Out: _____ a.m./p.m.

Total Time Spent (minutes): _____

Level of Service: 99212 _____ 99213 _____ 99214 _____ 99215 _____

Counseling/Coordination > 50% of time (explain) _____

_____

_____

_____

TABULATION OF MEDICAL DECISION-MAKING ELEMENTS—HIGHEST TWO OUT OF THREE FOR OVERALL MDM

No. of Diagnoses or Management Options	Points	Amount and Complexity of Data	Points	Risk Factors of Presenting Problems	Number of Management Options
Self-limiting	1	Review and/or order lab data	1	• One self-limited or minor problem (e.g., dysthymia well-managed)	Rest; minimal risk
Established problem to examining provider—stable or improved	1	Review and/or order radiology tests	1	• Two or more self-limited or minor problems • One stable chronic illness • Acute uncomplicated illness	OTC meds; low risk

(continued)

TABULATION OF MEDICAL DECISION-MAKING ELEMENTS—HIGHEST TWO OUT OF THREE FOR OVERALL MDM (CONTINUED)

No. of Diagnoses or Management Options	Points	Amount and Complexity of Data	Points	Risk Factors of Presenting Problems	Number of Management Options
Established problem to examining provider—worsening	2	Review and/or order tests in the medical section of CPT	1	• One or more chronic illnesses with mild exacerbation, progression, or side effects • Two or more stable chronic illnesses • Undiagnosed new problem with uncertain prognosis • Acute illness with systemic symptoms	Prescription RX; moderate risk
New problem to examining provider—no additional workup or diagnostic procedures ordered (Max 2)	3	Discussion of test results with performing provider	1	• One or more chronic illnesses with severe exacerbation, progression, or side effects • Acute or chronic illnesses that pose a threat to life or bodily function	RX requiring intensive management; high risk

(continued)

No. of Diagnoses or Management Options	Points	Amount and Complexity of Data	Points	Risk Factors of Presenting Problems	Number of Management Options
New problem to examining provider—additional workup planned	4	Review and summarization of old records and/or obtaining history from someone other than the patient Review and summarization of old records and/or obtaining history from someone other than the patient and/or discussion of case with another provider Independent visualization of image tracing, or specimen itself (not simply review report)	1 2 2		
Straightforward	<1	Straightforward	<1	Straightforward	Minimal
Low complexity	2	Low complexity	2	Low complexity	Low
Moderate complexity	3	Moderate complexity	3	Moderate complexity	Moderate
High complexity	4	High complexity	4	High complexity	High
Notes:					

(continued)

HPI Location, quality, severity, duration, timing, context, modifying factors, associated signs and symptoms **OR** status of three or more chronic diseases.

Elements Documented: 99212-Problem Focused = 1–3
99214-Detailed = 4 Or >3 Chronic Conditions

99213-Expanded Problem Focused = 1–3
99215 Comprehensive = 4 HPI Or >3 Chronic Conditions

ROS	NL	NOTE
Const	☐	☐
Musculo	☐	☐
Psych	☐	☐
CV	☐	☐
Resp	☐	☐
GI	☐	☐
Skin/breasts	☐	☐
Neuro	☐	☐
Genitourinary	☐	☐
ENT/mouth	☐	☐
Endocrine	☐	☐

(continued)

Hem/lymph	☐	☐
Allerg/immun	☐	☐
Eyes	☐	☐

99212-Problem focused = None
99214-Detailed = 2–9 Systems

99213-Expanded Problem Focused = 1 System
99215-Comprehensive =>10 Systems

PFSH	No Chng	See Note
Past	☐	☐
Family	☐	☐
Social	☐	☐

99212-Problem Focused = None
99214-Detailed = At Least 1 Item From 1 Category

Exam–Single System 2 Bullets	NL	See Note
• 3 out of 7 Constitutional	☐	☐
Blood Pressure:		
Pulse:		

99213-Expanded Problem Focused = None
99215-Comprehensive Specifics of at Least Two Items

Exam–Single System 2 Bullets	NL	See Note
Musculoskeletal		
• Gait and station	☐	☐
• Muscle strength or tone, atrophy, abnormal movements (e.g., flaccid, cog wheel)	☐	☐

(continued)

Temperature:				
Respiration:				
Height:			Note:	
Weight:				
• **General appearance of patient**	☐	☐		
(e.g., development, nutrition, body habits, deformities)				

☐ Well Groomed ☐ Disheveled ☐ Bizarre ☐ Inappropriate

Notes:

Psychiatric Single System Exam—11 Bullets

Attitude: ☐ Cooperative ☐ Guarded ☐ Suspicious ☐ Uncooperative

• Speech: ☐ Normal ☐ Delayed ☐ Excessive ☐ Pressured ☐ Articulation clear ☐ Soft ☐ Loud ☐ Perseverating ☐ Spontaneous ☐ Paucity

• Thought Process: ☐ Intact ☐ Circumstantial ☐ LOA ☐ Flight of ideas ☐ Illogical ☐ Logical/Coherent ☐ Abstract reasoning ☐ Computations

• Associations: ☐ Tangential ☐ Loose ☐ Intact ☐ Tangential ☐ Tangential

• Thought Content: ☐ Delusions ☐ Phobias ☐ Poverty of Content ☐ Obsessions ☐ Compulsions ☐ Paranoid ideation ☐ Ideas of reference ☐ Preoccupation with violence ☐ Homicidal ideation ☐ Suicidal ideation

(continued)

- Judgment: □ Intact □ Impaired: □ Minimal □ Moderate □ Severe
- Insight: □ Intact □ Impaired: □ Minimal □ Moderate □ Severe

Complete Mental Status Examination Including

- Orientation: □ Fully orientated □ Disorientated: □ Time □ Person □ Place
- Memory: Recent = □ Intact □ Impaired: □ Minimal □ Moderate □ Severe Remote = □ Intact □ Impaired: □ Minimal □ Moderate □ Severe
- Attention span and concentration
- Language (naming objects, repeating phrases)
- Fund of knowledge (awareness of current events, past history, vocabulary)
- Mood: □ Euthymic □ Depressed □ Anxious □ Euphoric □ Agitation affect: □ Appropriate □ Labile □ Blunted □ Flat □ Expansive □ Constricted

Level of Exam	Content and Documentation Requirements
99212-Problem Focused	One to five elements identified by a bullet
99213-Expanded Problem Focused	At least six elements identified by a bullet
99214-Detailed	At least nine elements identified by a bullet
99215-Comprehensive	Perform ALL elements identified by a bullet; document every element in psychiatric and constitutional exam and at least one element in musculoskeletal

(continued)

DESCRIPTION OF SESSION (must include effects of meds, modifications, psychosocial issues, and HPI, if applicable):

Service Provided: ☐ Individual ☐ Family/Couple ☐ Group

Treatment Implemented: ☐ Cognitive behavioral ☐ Supportive ☐ Psychoeducation ☐ Insight oriented ☐ Pharmacological ☐ Lab work ordered, Rationale:

Does AIMS test need to be completed? : ☐ Yes _____ ☐ No _____ ☐ N/A _____

Substance Abuse:

Records/Progress Notes Reviewed/Collateral Contacts:

Medications (Dosage, S/E): _____

ASSESSMENT (response to treatment)

REMINDERS: Is the medication sheet updated after each visit? ☐ Yes ☐ No

If you prescribed medication, did the patient sign an informed consent? ☐ Yes ☐ No Does patient/family understand the treatment plan? ☐ Yes ☐ No

Was patient referred for preventive/ancillary services? ☐ Yes ☐ No

Diagnosis Imp _____ / _____ / _____

MDM Plan, Estimated Discharge Date, and Next Appointment:

Signature: _____ Date of Signature: _____

(continued)

Sample of non-checklist progress note

DATE: TIME IN: TIME OUT: OTHERS PRESENT:

REASON FOR ENCOUNTER _____ is a 27-year-old female who presents today with the following chief complaint.

CPT code: _____

CC:

HPI:

ROS: No headache, no diarrhea, no nausea, no constipation, no dysuria, no chest pain, no SOB. All other systems are negative.

CURRENT MEDICATIONS:

ALLERGIES:

PFSH:

EXAM:

<u>Constitutional</u>: VS: BP: P: R: Weight: (Document assessment/discussion of weight, nutrition, exercise, sleep

Psych: xx presents on time in calm and pleasant manner. *Appearance:* Hygiene and grooming are xx and appropriate for the season. Eyes are clear and bright. *Attitude:* cooperative. Able to initiate and maintain normal eye contact. Patient sits in a relaxed manner during the session. *Speech:* Able to initiate and maintain normal conversation; clear with no slurring. Speech has normal rate, rhythm, pitch, volume, and intensity *Thought process and associations:* absence of tangentiality, circumstantiality, loose associations, flight of ideas, and illogical speech. Abstraction and registration are present. *Thought content/Perceptual functioning:* There is no evidence of grandiosity, paranoia, delusions, ideas of reference, derailed speech, or internal stimuli . *Judgment/insight* realizes there is a problem and is actively seeking treatment. *Mood:* described as xx . There is no suicidal or homicidal ideation or intent. *Affect:* xxx broad, congruent, able to demonstrate full range of emotion.

Depression Self-rating: 0–10

Anxiety Self-rating: 0–10

(continued)

Any other formal rating scales administered during the session.

MEDICAL DECISION-MAKING:

(Fxx.xx) (primary encounter diagnosis-*ICD-10*) (List all diagnoses including comment and plan for each)

Comment:

Plan:

DIAGNOSTIC RESULTS REVIEWED: (Labs, x-ray, records from other providers)

<u>Lab Ordered:</u>

<u>Prescriptions Written:</u>

<u>Therapeutic Modality Implemented Today:</u> medication management, psychoeducation, supportive therapy.

<u>Return to Office:</u>

Estimated Completion of Treatment:

<u>Patient Education and Instructions:</u>

I have discussed the nature of the condition(s) and the reason I am recommending the treatment listed in the previous text. I have discussed with the patient the usual and FDA-approved uses of the prescribed medications, the research supporting use in this application, the reasons for recommending this medication for this patient, the potential risks and benefits of the medication, alternative treatments (including no treatment) and the attendant risks and benefits, and the consequences of not taking the medication. I have explained potential side effects, drug interactions, how to start or stop treatment, and how to deal with missed doses. The patient has provided consent for this treatment plan.

This information is privileged and confidential, for recipient only. It is not to be released without the written consent of the patient. A general authorization for release of medical or other information is NOT sufficient for this purpose.

_____ APRN

Signature

Termination and Outcome Evaluation

Kathleen Wheeler
and Danielle M. Conklin

This last chapter presents a general overview of termination: when to terminate, how to handle the patient who terminates prematurely, under what circumstances the therapist initiates termination, and ethical issues related to termination. The termination issues discussed in this chapter are germane to all psychotherapy approaches. In addition, practice guidelines and outcome evaluation in psychotherapy are discussed. Evidence-based practice guidelines are essential in order to make conscientious clinical decisions about patients so that appropriate goals can be set, which when met will then determine when to terminate psychotherapy. Outcome measurement helps to ensure that goals are met for an effective and ethical practice. These outcomes may reflect various levels of measurement. The chapter ends with a case example illustrating termination and the use of practice guidelines and outcome measures in time-limited psychodynamic psychotherapy.

WHEN TO TERMINATE

In contrast to the literature on the therapeutic alliance and other phases of the psycho-therapeutic relationship, there is little literature and almost no empirical evidence about the best way for therapists to deal with termination. Competency in the last phase of psychotherapy reflects the therapist's ability to assess the patient's readiness for termination and to manage termination issues within the context of the approach utilized in the treatment. Termination is an essential phase of the therapeutic relationship and there should be a plan in place by the therapist in order to process relevant issues that arise as the end to the relationship nears.

Binder (2004) reviews the few studies that have been conducted on termination and the duration of therapy, and arrives at these tentative conclusions: (a) limiting the duration of therapy may influence the rate of change; (b) acute symptoms exhibit more rapid change than characterological problems; and (c) more time in therapy leads to more change. However, there are no longitudinal studies, proving that longer-term psycho-therapy results in better outcomes than shorter-term psychotherapies.

Hopefully, the goals that have been set at the outset of therapy have been success-fully met. Research suggests that at least 11 to 13 sessions of evidence-based therapy are needed for 50% to 60% of patients to have good outcomes (Lambert, 2007). Unfortunately, this often is not the case. Patients frequently drop out of treatment without a plan for termination, especially in community mental health centers. Approximately 50% of patients drop out of therapy by session 3, while 35% end therapy after the first session (Barrett et al., 2008). There are many reasons for termination, including:

1. Mutually agreed on based on achievement of goals
2. Preplanned based on number of sessions
3. Forced termination because therapist graduates or changes clinical assignment
4. Forced termination because the patient moves
5. Forced termination because patient cannot afford fee or insurance will not pay
6. Patient terminates because he or she feels not helped
7. Therapist refers patient elsewhere because therapist feels there is no value in continuing
8. Setting ends the treatment for any reason (Gabbard, 2017)

An extensive review of the literature on termination revealed six strategies that reduce premature termination (Swift, Greenberg, Whipple, & Kominiak, 2012). These are: (a) providing education about the duration and pattern of change because studies have shown that most patients expect to attend five sessions or less; (b) providing role induction such as instructing the patient that he or she will be doing most of the talking; (c) incorporating patient preferences such as type of therapy, directive or manualized, versus less directive, homework or no homework; (d) strengthening early hope, which can be done by expressing confidence in the patient and his or her ability to have a successful therapy outcome and commending the person for seeking therapy; (e) fostering the therapeutic alliance; and (f) assessing and discussing treatment progress, which can be done through outcome measurement and sharing the results with the patient.

Termination optimally occurs when coping and functioning have improved, symptoms are reduced, and the goals of treatment are met. The achievement of goals depends on the collaborative goals set with the patient at the outset of treatment as well as the type of approach or model utilized. For example, supportive psychodynamic psychotherapy criteria for termination would include the strengthening of the ego, reversal of regression, and symptom improvement. In contrast, historically, more expressive psychoanalytic psychotherapy criteria for termination would involve the resolution of the transference neurosis, an acceptance of the futility of perfectionist strivings and childhood fantasies, a reduction in the intensity of core conflicts, and the development of a self-analytic capacity (Wolitzky, 2011). Self-analytic capacity means that the person has learned to be reflective and become his or her own therapist. This would occur after patterns of defenses emerge again and again and are observed and interpreted until the patient accepts the therapist's interpretations in the working through process (Gabbard, 2017). A more contemporary view is that relationships change for the better. This illustrates that new neural networks involving a different kind of relationship are developed.

The advanced practice psychiatric nurse (APPN) can usually detect that this has been achieved by what the patient says and does. Often, for example, the person may say: "I thought about what you would say when I was in that situation" or "I had a whole conversation in my head with you before I talked to him." These kinds of statements reflect the patient's internalization of the therapist's reflective function. Sometimes nothing is said but the person's functioning has greatly improved, and it is obvious to the therapist from what the person says about how he or she has handled various situations that a newfound ability to self-reflect and/or self-soothe is operating.

For cognitive behavioral therapy (CBT), termination begins in the first session and the expected duration is usually discussed at that time when issues and goals for treatment are clarified. The therapist usually sets a specific number of sessions, a predetermined date to end, or informs the patient that the treatment will not go longer than a few weeks or months without specifying an exact date (Binder, 2004). The idea is for the therapist and patient to keep a problem focus and momentum moving forward. Dienes, Torres-Harding, Reinecke, Freeman, and Sauer (2011) recommend setting parameters for treatment at the outset because studies have found no correlation between duration of therapy and effectiveness. Improvement after 12 to 15 sessions has been found to be minimal so it is the first 3 to 4 months in which most of the positive changes occur. It is a generally accepted practice in CBT to remind the person, from time to time throughout the treatment, of when termination will occur so that the person has an opportunity to discuss how he or she feels about ending and can prepare for it.

The goals of treatment in CBT involve changes in maladaptive thinking and behaviors toward more positive adaptive thinking and behavior and more effective coping skills. The last session reviews the goals and skills the person has developed as well as discussing how to prevent a relapse. Cognitive and behavioral factors that are unique for the person that brought them into treatment and that were ameliorated, such as perfectionism, negative thinking, lack of assertiveness, and so on, are highlighted with new strategies that were learned and consolidated. Usually termination for CBT is gradual with the person coming to sessions every other week, then every month, every 3 months, and then every 6 months so that modifications or changes can be addressed in order to ensure success.

In interpersonal psychotherapy (IPT), major goals of treatment relate to the resolution of interpersonal problems in the here and now. To that end, alternative strategies for interpersonal relationships are identified, new relational patterns are practiced, and old ways of relating are grieved. Once the patient is successfully implementing the new ways of being, goals of therapy are met. Termination begins as early as the middle phase of treatment and is embedded in the work of that phase, working with the sadness about the loss of the relationship with the therapist as well as issues of relapse prevention. As with CBT, there are a finite number of sessions delineated (16), and this provides incentive for the person to do the work within circumscribed parameters of the treatment. The therapy does not really end at the last session in that the work continues with the person working independently. For termination strategies suggested for successful outcomes for IPT and for CBT, see Chapters 8 and 10 respectively.

In Eye Movement Desensitization and Reprocessing (EMDR) therapy, therapy is ended when the collaboratively identified targets representing the adverse life experience or trauma are reprocessed and the subjective units of disturbance (SUD) scale is 0 and the validity of cognition (VOC) is 7. The EMDR therapist reevaluates the target of the previous reprocessing by asking the patient to bring the incident to mind after each reprocessing session. When a past event has been completely processed and there is no disturbance in the body, the person is guided to present triggers and then develops a future template. A future template is a mental imagery or video of how the person wants to be with respect to the trauma or adverse life experience going forward. At the final session, all the targets that have been identified for treatment will be reviewed in order to determine if each is resolved. There may be follow-up appointments as the person evaluates if there are any disturbances, new distortions, or psychoeducation needed (Shapiro, 2018). If outcome/assessment measures were given at the beginning of therapy, the patient will be asked to take these again and these results are shared with the person.

HOW TO TERMINATE

Historically, psychodynamic psychotherapists thought that termination represented a crisis that needed to be worked through as earlier losses or separations are revived and inevitable. For example, if a patient suffered abandonment issues, then this would get enacted and exacerbated in the transference just prior to termination. Termination has been likened to the rapprochement crisis as delineated by Mahler, Pine, and Bergman (2000). That is, the patient's core conflict centers on the need to be autonomous and self-reliant while at the same time to be dependent. These opposing forces are always in the background of the therapeutic process and as such must be understood in order for a successful termination to occur (Quintar, 2001).

The idea that separation anxiety about termination occurs has largely changed as psychotherapy is briefer and therapy is viewed now more from a primary care perspective, that is, that patients feel they can come in and out of psychotherapy and use it as a resource much as one would any healthcare provider (Gabbard, 2017). In fact, an intermittent psychotherapy model has evolved that treats termination as an interruption of services rather than an end-point. Proponents of this model posit that complications inherent in termination, such as exacerbation of symptoms and transference issues, are avoided if termination is reframed as an interruption of services (Cummings, 2001).

In intermittent psychotherapy, the word *termination* is not used; rather, therapy is only *interrupted*. It may be resumed in several months or several decades depending on the patient. The person is encouraged to write to the therapist about how he or she is doing after interrupting treatment and the therapist responds to all communications warmly. If the person is doing well, the therapist responds by offering positive comments on the person's problem-solving skills. On the other hand, if the person is having difficulties, the therapist asks the patient whether it is time to come in for a session. Foundational to this process is the therapeutic contract, homework, and resiliency. In this model, the patient is required to complete assigned homework as part of the therapeutic contract and failure to do so results in sending the person home or even termination of treatment. Although seemingly a severe punishment for such a transgression, the author points out that if enforced, there is rarely the forfeiture of a second session.

From a psychodynamic viewpoint, all requests from the patient to terminate should be explored. Often the patient's desire to end treatment is thought to reflect resistance. Gabbard (2017) states that underlying motives should always be explored with these questions in mind: Is the patient anxious and afraid and running from something? Is the patient angry at the therapist? Is the patient enacting a flight into health? Is the patient discouraged about the therapy, and feeling judged by the therapist? If the goals of treatment have not been met, it is likely that anxiety is underlying the wish to terminate. The person may not be aware of any underlying reason other than the stated: "I am fine now." For example, one patient who had been in treatment for depression and had difficulty in sustaining long-term relationships came only for several sessions and then unexpectedly announced that this would be her last session because she was feeling much better. The therapist was quite surprised and taken aback, as in the previous session the patient had talked about how sad she had felt as a little girl about her mother's absence in her life due to her alcoholism. This issue of loss seemed to permeate all relationships and situations, and the therapist had been moved by the previous session. The therapist gently explored whether the patient felt that her goal of being able to sustain a long-term relationship and trust someone was already met. As the session unfolded, the therapist wondered aloud whether her desire to leave now was based on some of the sad feelings she had expressed during the last session. Tearfully, the patient realized that she was fleeing as she was beginning to feel vulnerable in therapy.

Once expressed, she was able to stay and continue to work in ongoing psychotherapy. The inability to tolerate intense emotions speaks to the importance of the therapist assisting the person in affect management strategies and titrating the amount of arousal during treatment. Patients may be well-served to flee treatment if their defenses are fragile and they are not assisted with controlling overwhelming states of anxiety, rage, depression, and guilt. See Chapter 17, for stabilization and affect management strategies.

For those patients who are unable to tolerate success, treatment may be terminated by the patient as soon as the person begins to improve, leaving a perplexed therapist wondering what happened. These individuals may mistake early gains in well-being as recovery and see little benefit from continuing. This issue can be triaged through their history of self-defeating behavior because times of happiness and success trigger feelings of vulnerability. The therapist can point out to the patient that this may happen in therapy too and stress the importance of discussing ending treatment when the patient wants to leave treatment. Underlying this may be a great deal of guilt and masochism as the person may unconsciously feel that he or she does not deserve to be happy or successful. Dynamic interpretations about this issue can be helpful throughout the treatment and the vigilant therapist keeps this in mind as the person improves.

Perhaps the devaluing patient is the most difficult to work with as the person insists that the therapy was not worth the time and did not help and the therapist most likely feels demoralized. Often these individuals do not keep their last appointment. Of course, they may be accurate in their assessment, but it is important for the therapist to keep in mind that these feelings may be anxiety-driven and unconsciously the person may need to minimize the loss by not acknowledging the importance of the relationship. Underlying the devaluation may be deep feelings of inadequacy and worthlessness with the person perceiving the therapist as critical and uncaring. Maintaining an empathic, exploring stance without defensiveness in the face of a barrage of devaluation is extremely difficult. Sometimes the best that can be hoped for in such situations is providing the patient a new type of relationship experience through the therapist's benign presence. The overall goal then is that the person will be more likely to seek help at some point in the future.

If the APPN knows that the person has a history of anger, it may be helpful to include the family in treatment, especially initially (Stevenson, 2000). The therapist can then prepare the patient and family member for the likelihood of anger at the therapist and premature treatment at the beginning of treatment. In this way, Stevenson posits that the anger will seem like a "normal" part of the therapy and a healthy triangulation with the family, therapist, and patient will be established at the outset. In addition, these patients are often not self-referred and may be less than willing participants in therapy. Stevenson also suggests reframing anger as a problem for the patient's physical health in order to normalize anger and motivate the person for treatment.

For patients who are aggressive, termination can be seen as the ultimate rupture in the therapeutic alliance. Relational psychodynamic theorists posit that these patients are counterdependent and that termination provides a rich opportunity to rework conflicts of dependency versus autonomy. Safran and Muran (2000) say that when patients are aggressive and counterdependent in therapy, the therapist's work involves ultimately working toward an exploration of the dependency that is being defended against. In contrast, when patients are more dependent and deferential, the therapist's job is to help the person access the angry feelings that are being defended against. This gives the person the opportunity to learn that the therapist can survive his or her aggression. The therapist empathizes with and validates feelings of anger that emerge during termination, such as feelings of disappointment and resentment at not getting what the person wanted from therapy.

Gabbard (2017) points out that termination involves mourning by both the therapist and the patient. This is thought to be especially true for those who have been significantly traumatized in that the loss of termination relates to the loss components of the traumatic event (Horowitz, 2002). The person has emerged from the trauma having lost a sense of personal invulnerability. The loss of the therapeutic relationship and acceptance of the idea provide a context for mourning other past major losses. The patient realizes that ultimately no one can take care of him or her and love him or her unconditionally. The therapist also mourns the loss of the relationship with the patient. In addition, the therapist must reconcile with the limitations of what the therapy has accomplished. Novice APPNs sometimes have unrealistic expectations about what therapy can accomplish. Both parties may harbor unconscious fantasies about being healed and healing and must come to terms about the limitations of what one person can do for another.

However, if the goals of therapy have been met, typically the patient does not have much to say about termination when asked other than expressing appreciation and some sadness about terminating. No matter which psychotherapy approach the therapist is using, once a termination date has been set, whether a month, 6 weeks, or several months hence, the patient's feelings about termination should be explored intermittently in the time left. Even if the patient initiates termination, the therapist's agreement to terminate may be experienced as a rejection and abandonment.

Toward the end of treatment, the patient may have an exacerbation of symptoms that brought the person into therapy in the first place or a decrease in functioning. For this reason, it may be important for the therapist to inform the patient that this commonly occurs beforehand. The APPN should be aware and watchful for recidivism so that the person can be encouraged to express his or her feelings of sadness, abandonment, and loss rather than acting them out. Important work can be accomplished during termination, particularly for those patients with significant issues revolving around loss and dependency. These painful feelings are associated with earlier memories of loss and/or abandonment and related neural networks are often triggered by the present loss of relationship. This is important to point out to the patient; however, the therapist needs to explore this issue with sensitivity so that the treatment does not end on a bad note with the person feeling battered by repeated interpretations that only serve to further entrench the patient's position that there is no connection. Leaving therapy feeling misunderstood can feel better to the patient than the pain of separation and loss but this is not the ideal way to terminate. A useful analogy to keep in mind is the nearly universal experience of most adolescents in senior year of high school who turn their parents into ogres and become so obnoxious that all parties concerned are glad when they finally leave home. This helps to assuage sadness about leaving but is a less than ideal way to terminate a therapeutic relationship.

In addition to understanding the patient's unconscious issues related to termination, the therapist needs to be aware of his or her own issues. It is a good time for the therapist to reflect on whether his or her goals are congruent with what the patient wants. The therapist's goals may be too ambitious for the person and wanting the person to function at a higher level may not be appropriate at this time for this person. The APPN may be busy rescuing the person who does not share the same values or aspirations. In addition, the therapist may have his or her own abandonment issues and feel comfortable and rewarded from working with the patient and find termination difficult. These issues affect both the therapist and the patient. For the therapist, unresolved personal conflicts may predispose the therapist to use the therapeutic relationship to satisfy his or her own social and emotional needs. On the other hand, patients who have been difficult to work with may engender a sense of relief when they terminate. In that case, the therapist may neglect to adequately explore their wish to stop. Thus, it is important for the APPN to self-reflect and examine his or her own feelings about the patient's termination to ensure that the patient's best interests are in the foreground of the therapeutic process.

As noted previously, there are various models for whether to taper sessions or schedule follow-up sessions depending on the therapist's orientation, the goals, and the needs of the patient. Most psychoanalytic psychotherapies do not taper off sessions but some contemporary relational psychodynamic-oriented therapists do feel that it is useful in order for patients to see how they manage on their own (Gabbard, 2017). Other therapists schedule an appointment for a month or two after the last session as a follow-up session. A review of the treatment and how the person has changed may be conducted in the last session. Scheduled periodic phone calls may also be helpful for the therapist to monitor how the person is able to handle stresses outside of therapy. Some patients find regular ongoing support after therapy crucial in keeping on an even keel, and checking in periodically helps the person to maintain functioning at a high level. This may be especially important for the patient who has suffered severe and/or complex trauma.

Kluft (1999) suggests that for these patients, follow-up sessions may need to be held every few months indefinitely. It is prudent to ask the patient what would be good for him or her if you suspect that ongoing support is needed. However, it is important not to convey to the person that you expect that he or she will have problems in the future. One patient who had been severely depressed and came intensively over a period of 2 years achieved much higher functioning than he ever dreamed possible and continued to schedule appointments over the next several years every few months to "touch base." The focus of these sessions reflected his eagerness to share with the therapist his successes, and the therapist shared his pleasure but she also further explored how he did not believe that these changes belonged to him and were long-lasting. As his confidence grew in his newfound ability to deal with his life, he was able to lengthen the time between sessions further and further. Some patients may never wean themselves completely from therapy. Gabbard (2017) calls these individuals "therapeutic lifers" and suggests that consultation be sought to be sure about whether this arrangement is beneficial for the patient.

An important point about termination is that the door should always be left open for the patient to return. Hopefully, if the experience was a positive one, the person will be able to use therapy as a resource and feel comfortable about seeking help in the future. However, if the patient is being transferred to another therapist, it may not be appropriate to "leave the door open" for the person to return to you as this can cultivate splitting. In these situations, when the person is being transferred to another colleague, particularly if it is in a clinic setting, it may be helpful to introduce the patient to the new therapist and/or have the new therapist come to a few sessions pre-termination to ensure a smooth transition (Gabbard, 2017).

Reviewing the patient's file prior to termination in order to identify issues and important themes highlighted during treatment is helpful so that the APPN can organize his or her own thinking about the progress that has been made during the therapy process. In addition to the APPN's reflections, it is important to ask the patient what was and was not helpful in the treatment. Reflecting and reminiscing with the patient and outlining the ways that the person is functioning better are important in the sessions leading up to the last session or at the very least in the last session. This discussion should emphasize that these accomplishments are a consequence of changing maladaptive thinking patterns and/or insight gained and/or better ways of handling situations and/or increased ability to manage emotions, and so on. In examining the changes that have occurred, the therapist can reinforce education about how to maintain the gains made during times of stress and explore patient expectations about accessing resources in the future. Hopefully, educating the person has been part of the therapy all along but reinforcing again is essential during termination.

WHEN THE THERAPIST INITIATES TERMINATION

Occasionally, the therapist initiates termination because the patient is noncompliant, refuses to pay, is not benefiting from therapy, or needs other treatment not in the therapist's expertise. All these situations would probably benefit from consulting with a colleague prior to ending the treatment in order to clarify countertransference and ethical issues and plan how best to proceed. Chapter 4, discusses how to handle missed sessions and how and when to terminate when the person does not come to scheduled appointments. A termination letter that states one's concerns, the reasons for recommending continued treatment, and the referral should be sent to the patient with a copy of the letter kept in the patient's file. See Appendix 4.6 for a sample termination letter. However, if in the opinion of the APPN the person needs further care, it is incumbent on the therapist to make sure that the patient is not in crisis and then refer the person to a specific therapist as well as follow up on the appointment. This is important not only to protect the patient's well-being but also the APPN's legal liability.

Ethical issues may arise, particularly when managed care has denied authorization. For example, one patient with a panic anxiety disorder began to have fewer panic attacks so that he could drive to work, which he previously was unable to do. After the six authorized sessions, the APPN submitted the required outpatient treatment report (OTR) for further sessions and was denied. The therapist was alarmed and felt strongly that the progress that had been made would be jeopardized without further solidification and support for the gains made. If the therapist believes that the person's safety will be compromised by termination, it is incumbent on the therapist to ensure that treatment continues either at a lower cost by offering a sliding scale fee or payment plan, or referring the patient to a lower cost clinic and assist in treatment transition. It is important to not terminate abruptly because of an unpaid bill without first attempting to work things out and giving the person suitable warning.

Although the American Nurses Association (ANA) Code of Ethics (2015) does not specifically address abandonment of the patient, it clearly states: "The nurse's primary commitment is . . . the patient." However, the American Psychological Association Ethics Code (2017) does specifically address abandonment, and this should be followed by APPNs who are working with patients in psychotherapy. The American Psychological Association Code of Ethics requires that arrangements must be made for the patient's ongoing treatment, if needed, despite employment and/or contractual agreements. Courts have ruled that if health professionals terminate treatment because of managed care's failure to authorize sessions, the health professional is liable for harm as a result of abandonment (*Wickline vs. State of California*, 1986). The standard of care must be followed even if the managed care company denies payment or authorization to the provider. Managed care companies protect themselves from liability because of loopholes in the Employees Retirement Insurance Security Act (ERISA). The licensed health professional is responsible for the patient's care until treatment is ended by the patient or until treatment is no longer necessary. The APPN must refer the patient to a specific therapist and ensure that an appointment is set up, and must be especially careful if the person is in crisis. These efforts need to be carefully documented including consultations with colleagues, decisions made and rationale, and patient follow-through. Along the same lines, a therapist must neither propose nor agree to see a seriously ill patient infrequently. An important point to consider is if emotional or physical harm occurs to the patient as a result of failure of the therapist to meet a standard of care, the therapist is legally liable.

On the other hand, a mental health professional can also be sued for continuing to work with a patient when the treatment is not working. Again, the key here is, was the standard of care followed? And was there damage to the patient? One such case involved a patient who was in psychodynamic psychotherapy and was hospitalized for major depressive disorder (*Osheroff v. Chestnut Lodge*, 1985). Eventually the patient, who was a physician himself, was given antidepressants by another psychiatrist and he rapidly improved. The patient sued the hospital and psychiatrists who did not treat him with antidepressants. The case was settled out of court. However, APPNs who practice psychotherapy must follow practice guidelines and standards of care developed by other mental health professionals for psychotherapy and psychopharmacotherapy. APPNs are beginning to be more visible on some consensus panels that develop these guidelines.

PRACTICE GUIDELINES

Practice guidelines are official statements that summarize research findings and present the appropriate management for specific problems. It is important for the APPN to be familiar with those that are relevant for practice and incorporate the suggestions as appropriate. The guidelines are recommendations only and the APPN should tailor the guidelines to each individual patient's needs. Practice guidelines are intended to be flexible while standards of care should be followed for all cases. Although practice guidelines are foundational to improving healthcare, they are not in themselves legally binding, they do not replace clinical judgment, and they are not in and of themselves standards of care. Standards of care are determined based on *all* clinical data available for an individual case and subject to change as knowledge advances. The ultimate judgment regarding care for a specific patient should always be based on the patient and family's circumstances as well as available resources. The APPN should be knowledgeable about the practice guideline for the specific diagnosis treated and document if there is a deviation in care from the suggested guideline and why.

Relevant practice guidelines have been identified in this book for the specific topics discussed as appropriate. In addition to those developed by professional associations, academic centers, and government agencies, managed care organizations have also developed their own. Many practice guidelines are available on the web. These evidence-based guidelines are based on systematic reviews of randomized controlled studies. Reviews are based on electronic searches of databases such as Medline, PsychLit, the Cochrane Library, and meta-analysis, as well as hand-searching journals. Once the literature is reviewed, consensus opinion of an expert panel is sought regarding the appropriateness, safety, and efficacy of treatment options (Parry, 2000). The quality of the evidence is usually stated for each recommendation. The American Psychiatric Association and the American Academy of Child & Adolescent Psychiatry (AACAP) have developed a number of practice guidelines for psychiatric disorders, and these are available at www.psychiatry.org/psychiatrists/practice/clinical-practice-guidelines and www.aacap.org/AACAP/Resources_for_Primary_Care/Practice_Parameters_and_Resource_Centers/Practice_Parameters.aspx, respectively. The National Guideline Clearing House provides the ability to access and compare practice guidelines at the following website: www.guideline.gov/browse/by-topic.aspx

Because controlled clinical trials require strict inclusion criteria and few confounding variables, rarely does clinical practice reflect these stringent requirements. Most subjects with more than one diagnosis are excluded from the study and those who qualify and are asked to participate are not representative of the majority of patients (Insel, 2013). In addition, clinicians rarely adhere to one specific method but tailor the therapy to meet the individual's needs and integrate various methods and models to achieve efficacy. Psychotherapy approaches that utilize structured techniques and protocols lend themselves better to experimental design criteria. Therefore, approaches such as CBT and EMDR therapy have been studied more than less structured approaches such as psychodynamic psychotherapy. Psychodynamic interventions such as free association and dynamic interpretations are harder to quantify. However, this does not mean that less structured psychotherapy approaches are not effective, only that efficacy has not been established. See Chapter 5, for discussion of some of the inherent validity problems of evidence-based research in clinical practice.

Practice guidelines are based on the person's diagnosis. As Chapter 3, noted the, *Diagnostic and Statistical Manual of Mental Disorders (DSM)* diagnoses are highly variable and reflect only a snapshot in time. Many voice concern about diagnostic inflation with the new *DSM-5* diagnoses of binge eating disorder, bereavement, disruptive mood dysregulation for children with temper tantrums, somatic symptom disorder for those worried about a medical illness, mild neurocognitive disorder for those who are forgetful in old age, and an expanded attention deficit disorder for adults (Frances, 2013). In addition to the stigma of pathologizing normal responses to life situations, there is a danger of overtreating patients with medication. Despite a petition from an independent scientific review that more than 50 mental health associations endorsed, the American Psychiatric Association refused to discuss or be transparent in the process of developing the *DSM-5*.

The National Institute of Mental Health recognized the limitations of the *DSM-5* and research based on these diagnostic categories and symptom amelioration. A new system for decisions about research funding will incorporate genetics, imaging, cognitive science, and other levels of information instead of relying on *DSM* diagnostic categories. Although the *DSM* is reliable, that is, consistent with clinicians agreeing that certain symptoms constitute a specific label for a patient, it does not have validity in that the clusters of symptoms are not based on any objective measure. Without validity, reliability is not sufficient to base treatment decisions. With such a dramatic change in funding criteria, there may be important implications for future practice guidelines because practice guidelines are based largely on large federally funded randomized clinical trials, which in the past were based on a specific diagnostic category.

In addition to a *DSM* diagnosis, many other factors should be considered when deciding which psychotherapy treatment approach and interventions to use with the patient. These include clinical presentation, severity of symptoms, progression, coexisting conditions, gender, genetic or biologic variations, susceptibility to complications, and allergies to medications (Latov, 2005). In addition, the developmental history, defenses, pattern of relating, behavioral analysis, placebo response, coping skills, patient preference, compliance, intelligence, personality, and support system vary from person to person. It is not possible for practice guidelines to address all the nuances of clinical practice and it is important that guidelines do not override clinical judgment and common sense. Of course, the therapist's personality and training, therapeutic relationship with the patient, and the treatment setting are also important considerations in deciding what approach and interventions to use. In fact, given the research on therapist effectiveness, patient outcome, and the therapeutic alliance, Binder (2004) suggests that psychotherapy outcome studies should focus on empirically supported psychotherapists, not empirically supported treatments.

Yet, despite the complexity of clinical problems and inherent difficulties with evidence-based research in clinical practice, psychotherapy practice guidelines remain important in that empirical data for effective practice promotes accountability and positive outcomes. What is curious is that although studies have found that guidelines increase a research-based practice and improve patient outcomes, often clinical practice does not reflect that the person will receive the intervention(s) that are evidence based. For example, Sanderson (2002) points out that only a small percentage (15%–38%) of patients who have panic and phobic disorders receive the evidence-based psychotherapy interventions of exposure and cognitive restructuring, which are recommended by numerous practice guidelines. This gap between evidence-based treatments and real-world practice may be due to clinicians' inadequate training in these modalities or ignorance about practice guidelines.

OUTCOME EVALUATION

Outcome evaluation has become a critical issue in healthcare for everyone. The Institute of Medicine's (IOM; 2001) *Crossing the Quality Chasm* report emphasizes that healthcare should be safe, accessible, timely, equitable, efficient, cost effective, patient-centered, and *evidence-based,* based on *latest scientific evidence* coupled with the provider's clinical judgment, and informed by the patient's preferences. The $787 billion economic stimulus bill provided substantial amounts of money for the federal government to compare the effectiveness of different treatments for the same illness, and researchers received $1.1 billion to compare interventions for treating specific conditions (Pear, 2009).

The move toward evidence-based care began in earnest in 2010 with the initiation of health reform policy in order to lower costs and improve outcomes (National Research Council, 2011). Inpatient medical settings adopted quality indicators that include such markers as 30-day readmission, discharge planning, and follow-up in the community for specific diagnoses. For example, if a patient has been discharged from an inpatient setting with a diagnosis of congestive heart failure (CHF) and is readmitted within the next 30 days, the hospital will not get paid for the readmission inpatient hospitalization costs because research shows that if proper discharge instructions are given regarding diet, medication, and follow-up, the person would not suffer CHF again so soon after discharge. Although linking outcomes of treatment and quality indicators to reimbursement for outpatient behavioral healthcare have been slower to develop, there are already 300 process measures for assessment and improvement of mental health and substance abuse. See www.cqaimh.org/quality.html for examples of screening and assessment quality measures for behavioral health.

Starting in 2013, quality measures were mandated by the Centers for Medicare and Medicaid Services (CMS) including financial penalties for therapists who were noncompliant with the Physician Quality Reporting System (PQRS). With the passage of the Medicare Access and CHIP Reauthorization Act (MACRA) in 2015, the PQRS program was sunsetted and replaced by the Quality Payment Program (QPP) in January 2017. The QPP includes the Merit-Based Incentive Payment System (MIPS) and the Alternative Payment Model (APM), which requires direct reporting of at least six quality indicators from a mental behavioral health set of over 25 individual measures. Participating clinicians providing high value and quality care are rewarded with payment increases whereas clinicians who are not meeting performance standards are penalized with reduced payment for services. This is a beginning step toward linking reimbursement to the "best" mental health treatments available.

The best treatments are those that are evidence-based; in the future, those that are not considered evidence-based may not be reimbursed. Outcome effectiveness is predicted to be part of an organized care delivery system (Bobbitt, Cate, Beardsley, Azocar, & McCulloch, 2012). APPNs must document outcomes of psychiatric care to satisfy employers, consumers, insurers, policy makers, the general public, and themselves. Accountability and quality are hallmarks of professional nursing practice and are based on measurement of outcomes. Clinical rating scales and outcome measures should be essential to APPN practice. Outcomes can include clinical, functional, satisfaction, and financial indicators.

An outcome measure should have demonstrated validity and reliability as well as sensitivity to clinically important changes over time. The AACAP has developed a toolbox of resources that includes outcomes scales and other downloadable instruments for use in clinical practice available at www.aacap.org/AACAP/Member_Resources/AACAP_Toolbox_for_Clinical_Practice_and_Outcomes/Home.aspx. Appropriate symptom scales such as the clinical rating scales included in Table 3.6 in Chapter 3, have good normative data as do the measures in Tables 17.2 and 17.3 in Chapter 17. Medication targets discrete symptoms such as anxiety and so on; thus, symptom outcome measures reflect specific decreases in these parameters and are most appropriate when measuring outcome indicators of psychopharmacology. Appendix 24.1 includes a table of common outcome measures used in psychotherapy research and practice.

Psychotherapy, on the other hand, facilitates more holistic outcomes and affects all dimensions of the person: emotional, intellectual, physical, relational, spiritual, vocational, and psychological. The holistic model presented in Chapter 1, is embedded in relationships with others with a change in one dimension of the person affecting all other dimensions. Healing is "an emergent process . . . bringing together aspects of one's self and the body, mind, emotion, spirit, and environment at deeper levels of inner knowing, leading to an integration and balance" (Mariano, 2015, p. 59). Thus, although symptom measures are one parameter of change for psychotherapy treatment, global holistic outcomes reflecting relationships and overall health may be more accurate indicators of healing. Examples of measures reflecting holistic outcomes might include hope, resilience, connection to others, relationships with others, quality of life, overall health status, and spiritual well-being. Many of these instruments have been developed by nurse researchers. Selected holistic outcome measures are included in Table 24.1.

Another way to think about meeting the goals of psychotherapy and outcome measurement is according to how immediate to the patient's experience the outcome measure is (see Figure 24.1). The level of measurement reflects the degree of abstraction of the construct. The collaborative goal(s) of psychotherapy are reflected in outcome measures that are concrete, patient-centered, and quantifiable. Hopefully, if these are met, all levels of measurement reflect positive outcomes as significant change would reverberate toward the larger global measurement of holistic outcomes that are more abstract. For example, a patient came to treatment with panic disorder and was disturbed by the intensity and frequency of these episodes she was experiencing each day. The immediate collaborative goal set with the patient was to decrease the number of panic episodes per day, so the first step was to establish a baseline measure of how many times she was currently experiencing panic throughout the day. The APPN set an appropriate goal collaboratively with the patient to decrease that number by a certain date and initiated interventions to decrease the baseline number. Accomplishing this then decreased the patient's overall anxiety and depression that were measured with appropriate instruments measuring these respective clinical indicators. The psychotherapy approach employed to accomplish this was Eye Movement Desensitization and Reprocessing (EMDR) therapy, so a measure reflecting outcomes for this model was the subjective units of disturbance (SUDs) for each episode targeted with EMDR. These measures then were validated and reflected in the holistic outcome measurement of the construct of resilience. It is up to the clinician to decide which level of measurement to assess. Obviously, the more levels assessed, the more certain the APPN can be that significant change and healing have occurred. This type of outcome measurement strategy is called multimodal measurement.

Another consideration in choosing a measure for treatment effectiveness is who is reporting on the improvement. There is a growing focus on the value of patient-reported

TABLE 24.1	SELECTED HOLISTIC OUTCOME MEASURES	
Outcome	**Instrument**	**Type of Tool and How to Obtain**
Hope	Herth Hope Scale (Herth, 1992)	12-item self-report on a 1–4 Likert scale Contact kaye.herth@mnsu.edu
Resilience	Brief Resilient Coping Scale (Sinclair & Wallston, 2004)	4-item self-report rated on a 1–5 Likert scale Contact: vaughn.sinclair@Vanderbilt.Edu for tool
Connection to others	Sense of Belonging Instrument (Hagerty & Patusky, 1995)	18-item self-report questionnaire, respondents rate their sense of connection to others on a 1–4 Likert scale Contact: bmkh@umich.edu for tool
Relationships with others	Interpersonal Relationship Inventory (IPRI; Tilden, Nelson, & May, 1990)	30-item self-report on a 1–5 Likert scale that asks the respondent how he or she feels about personal relationships Contact: vtilden@unmc.edu for tool
Quality of life	Quality of Life Scale (Flanagan, 1982)	See Chapter 3, Assessment and Diagnosis
Spiritual well-being	WHO Spirituality, Religiousness and Personal Beliefs (SRPS; WHO, 2002)	See Chapter 3, Assessment and Diagnosis

WHO, World Health Organization.

outcomes, that is, patient self-report measures. A baseline outcome measure should be obtained on assessment and measurement should again be done at termination and also at several points during the treatment in order to monitor progress. Although very few clinicians routinely monitor outcomes during the course of treatment, the data can be quite useful not only for research purposes but also when therapy is stagnating. This can alert the APPN so that interventions and treatment can be reevaluated and modified. In addition, measuring outcomes intermittently, comparing the patient's own scores with each other at different points in time, is considered a rigorous time-series research design and sidesteps the validity issues inherent when comparing patients who have the same diagnosis with each other. Documenting patient outcomes using a time-series design would make an excellent empirically valid case study for publication. The following case example illustrates termination and the use of practice guidelines and outcome measures.

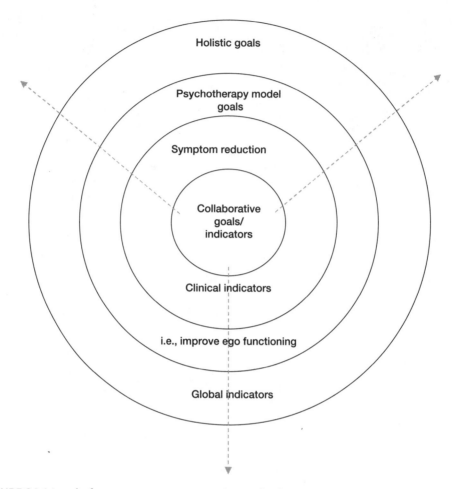

FIGURE 24.1 Level of outcome measurement in psychotherapy.

CASE EXAMPLE

Ms. K, a 60-year-old divorced, home health aide, presented for outpatient psychother-apy a week after discharge from a 5-day inpatient stay at the local psychiatric hospital after her ex-husband moved in with another woman. Ms. K had subsequently recurrent suicidal thoughts and voluntarily admitted herself. She was started on fluoxetine 30 mg and participated in group therapy but remained depressed after discharge.

In her initial session with the therapist, Ms. K scored 40 on the Beck Depression Inventory (BDI), indicating severe depression and described sadness, loss of interest in pleasurable activities, guilt, loss of energy, tearfulness, hopelessness, fatigue, loss of appetite, middle of the night insomnia, a 10-pound weight loss, and concentration prob-lems over the past month. The patient's identified complaint at the time of intake was, "I am helpless, hopeless and will never have a good life." She denied memory problems, substance abuse, delusions, or present suicidal ideation. Her depression, lack of social supports, hopelessness, and no spouse were risk factors for suicide. However, she did not have an organized plan to hurt herself and her voluntary hospitalization for previ-ous suicidal ideation as well as current denial of suicidal thoughts indicated that the risk for self-harm was present but not high. The APPN knew that risk might increase as she began to feel better and that Ms. K should continue to be closely monitored.

There was no history of mania, hypomania, or illicit drug use. Two prior episodes of depression were reported. The first episode was 10 years previously when she suffered an automobile accident that fractured her left arm and lacerated her face after she was thrown face first through the passenger side of a non-safety-plate windshield. She was diagnosed with major depressive disorder after this event and treated with fluoxetine for a year. Eight years after this accident, she was diagnosed with breast cancer and underwent a mastectomy followed by a course of chemotherapy and radiation. She was treated at that time with CBT for 16 sessions and venlafaxine for 2 years with a partial response.

Ms. K had a history of early traumatic relationships. She reported that her early childhood was marked by emotional and physical abuse from her rageful, alcoholic father and emotional neglect by her mother. Although she had amnesia for much of her childhood, one of her few early memories was of her father demeaning her and calling her "stupid" when she made a mistake. Her mother too was berated by her father and Ms. K felt her mother was afraid to intercede on her daughter's behalf. Her father insisted that she adhere to a strict regimen throughout her childhood; when she did not comply, he was angry and punishing. For example, she recalled that when she was learning to tie her shoes around the age of 4, her father slapped her across the face each time she did not correctly remember the proper sequence of steps to accomplish this task. She was expected to take care of her two younger sisters at an early age and was not allowed to play with other children. At the age of 10, her parents divorced, leaving her with her depressed, emotionally unavailable mother and her two sisters. Her mother remarried a year later and her stepfather frequently beat her while her mother did nothing about it. The continuing emotional and physical abuse interfered with her ability in school. She finally left home at age 17 and lived at a convent where she took classes to become a home health aide. At age 20, she met her ex-husband whom she married several months later.

She reported that her marriage of 30 years was not happy and that she was physically and emotionally abused by her husband, who was an alcoholic with frequent angry outbursts. On several occasions, he had punched and slapped her. Her husband had divorced her 10 years previously, leaving her without alimony or financial security. In fact, he financially exploited her by coming to her for money whenever he ran out. She had no children and expressed great regret at never being able to conceive but believed that she did not deserve children anyway. Her parents were both deceased at the time of intake and her relationship with her two sisters was distant and passive. Ms. K had been able to work full-time as a home health aide until her recent hospitalization and lived alone. She stated that she was hardworking and conscientious and liked helping others. Her work was a significant area of gratification for her.

Ms. K had recently had a physical exam at her nurse practitioner's office with complete blood count (CBC) with differential and chemistry profile all within normal limits. After a comprehensive psychiatric assessment and history, a diagnosis of major depressive disorder, recurrent, severe without psychotic features was made. In addition, her chronic dysphoria and poor self-esteem warranted an additional diagnosis of persistent depressive disorder (dysthymia). Medical diagnoses included obesity, type 2 diabetes, and hypertension. Medications included IC lisinopril–HCTZ 10/12.5, Toprol XL 100 mg, and Actoplus Met 15/500 mg. A Global Assessment of Functioning (GAF) score was 45/60 at intake. A treatment plan was developed using the practice treatment guidelines from the American Psychiatric Association (2010).

Practice guidelines suggest that frequent monitoring to assess suicidality and response to psychopharmacology is important in the acute phase of treatment. CBT and IPT are identified as the psychotherapeutic approaches that have the best documented efficacy. In addition, the guidelines state that if CBT was used before with some success yet did not result in longer-term change, a combination of psychodynamic and CBT approaches should be utilized. Ms. K's stated goal for therapy was first and foremost "to sleep better" and second to "be less lonely." Collaborative goals were set to sleep 6 hours a night within a month and to develop two new friends within 3 months. Sessions were scheduled for once a week for the next 40 weeks.

The acute phase of treatment aims to eliminate the symptoms and restore psychosocial functioning. Although Ms. K acknowledged that her depression was significant, she was passive and subdued in sessions and resisted attempts to discuss her feelings, focusing instead on her physical symptoms of fatigue, insomnia, and anorexia. She was not enthusiastic about the antidepressant medication, saying that she had tried it in the past and it was not particularly helpful. Trazodone 50 mg was prescribed at night for sleep. Given her tumultuous early relationship history, it was felt that stabilization was needed with supportive psychodynamic psychotherapy and cognitive behavioral education strategies designed to increase her resources so she could more easily stay in her resilient zone. Therapeutic communication techniques for stabilization as outlined in Table 4.1 based on the treatment hierarchy for this book were used. Patient outcome measures chosen to monitor progress were the Beck Depression Inventory (BDI) and the Sense of Belonging Instrument (SBI) because of their ease of administration, adequate normative data, appropriateness to goals of treatment, and the ability to provide both symptom-specific as well as a more holistic outcome measure. The SBI addressed the latter and would reflect the patient's stated outcome "to be less lonely." At the beginning of her second session, she scored 58 on the SBI, indicating a low sense of belonging. This was explained to Ms. K as important so that the APPN could monitor her functioning and improvement as therapy progressed.

Integrated treatment with the APPN both prescribing and conducting the psychotherapy was thought to be the most effective model to ensure coordination of care. Also, given her proclivity to focus on her physical symptoms and difficulty with emotional expression, it was felt that integrated rather than split treatment might help to provide a model for uniting her emotions with her physical symptoms. In this way, splitting and resistance to emotional exploration might be ameliorated. In light of her negative comments about her medication and her difficulty with identifying and expressing her feelings, the APPN did not increase her fluoxetine and joined with her initially in discussing her physical symptoms as the focus of treatment. Further testing with the Toronto Alexithymia Scale (TAS) indicated significant difficulties in identifying and describing feelings with an overall score of 62, with 51 or more significant for alexithymia. This is common for those who have suffered early trauma. It is therefore important that the APPN provide an emotional vocabulary through empathically linking the patient's feelings to events and her somatic symptoms.

As treatment evolved, the APPN felt that by Ms. K giving voice to her life narrative, she might be able to remember childhood events and integrate her dysfunctional memories into more adaptive memory networks. In doing so, the implicit beliefs that claimed responsibility for her own neglect and abuse could change by deepening her understanding of her family of origin and her ex-husband's psychopathology. One of the most powerful experiences in therapy, particularly for someone who has been disempowered and disrespected, is to be carefully listened to and taken seriously by another person. Ms. K's fear of dependency and abandonment issues were great and, as such, the APPN attended to the relationship and used countertransferential feelings as a source of data and a barometer for how the work was progressing. At times, there was significant deadness in the sessions with Ms. K filling the hour with her litany of somatic complaints and the APPN struggling to maintain a sense of emotional engagement, wishing that the sessions would end. The APPN noted these times gently to

Ms. K and explored her underlying feelings contributing to this way of communicating. Ms. K was able to articulate that she protected herself from caring too much about coming to therapy.

After 16 sessions, outcome indicators showed a significant decrease in symptoms on the BDI with a score of 26, indicating moderate depression as the patient entered the continuation phase of treatment. As her depression abated, her self-esteem increased and she was able to go back to work. She began to take increasing responsibility for her role in creating her loneliness and the unhealthy ways of getting her dependency needs met though passivity and withdrawing. Given the recurrent and chronic nature of Ms. K's depression and the improvement noted with combined psychotherapy and medication, ongoing psychodynamic psychotherapy was continued on a one time a week basis. At the 30th session, the APPN reviewed with Ms. K the number of sessions that were left and explored her feelings about the upcoming termination.

APPN:	We have 10 more sessions left.
Ms. K:	Okay, well, how can we speed this up? I don't think that this has helped that much.
APPN:	How frustrating to feel the lack of progress here and so little time left. Can you tell me more how you are feeling?
Ms. K:	Well, I am not blaming you but I need more direction and more from you.
APPN:	Tell me more about what you need from me.
Ms. K:	I don't know. I know you tried to do your best.
APPN:	How does that feel for you to tell me that?
Ms. K:	Scary, like you won't like me now and won't want to see me anymore.
APPN:	That I will abandon you by not caring if you say what you need?
Ms. K:	Well, I guess. It seems that this has brought out so much sadness that instead of feeling better, I just want to avoid the loneliness and pain. I guess I just shut down and am scared when I think about therapy ending.

In this session, Ms. K linked her withdrawing (defense) to her pain (anxiety) and this is an important step in understanding how she creates her own loneliness (response). Her ability to self-reflect had markedly improved. Over the next several months, she continued to deepen her emotional awareness about how the termination of therapy revived earlier pain of significant abandonment experiences relating to her childhood. At the 40th session, the BDI and the SBI were administered with scores of 20 and 40, respectively, indicating significant improvement on both indicators. Her GAF was 70/60. Ms. K continued to come every 4 to 6 weeks for medication management and psychotherapy over the next 6 months. Given the severity of her initial depression and the long-term nature of her chronic dysthymia, she remained on 30 mg of fluoxetine and returned every 3 months for ongoing support in the maintenance phase of treatment. This is consistent with the American Psychiatric Association's practice guideline recommendations for the maintenance phase of treatment.

Ms. K's therapy was unremarkable in the sense that there are many stories like hers in mental health clinics for those who have been ravaged by trauma. Yet what is remarkable is that it is the Ms. Ks who most need and benefit from the APPN's expertise, time, and caring. When a patient is psychologically savvy and engaging to work with, it is interesting and easy to invest the psychic energy needed to affect positive changes. Ms. K found relief in knowing that someone was willing to listen to her about her physical complaints and this led to discussing and linking her somatic symptoms to her emotional issues in a safe, supportive environment. Understanding the connection between conditioned somatic and emotional responses to internal and external sources allowed Ms. K to enhance self-regulatory skills. This understanding coupled with her experiencing emotions in an empathic relationship with the APPN facilitated integration of neural connections and healing. Careful attention was paid to pacing each session to what Ms. K could handle so that she would not be overwhelmed. She initially believed that her problems were all her own fault and that she did not deserve to get any better. Although demoralized and "resistant," she gradually began to look forward to her sessions and never missed once after the first month of treatment.

CONCLUDING COMMENTS

In addition to using measuring instruments and framing the goals of therapy according to the overall model of therapy used, it is incumbent on the therapist to check throughout therapy and at termination whether the specific collaborative goal(s) the patient and therapist identified are being met. For example, the problem of social isolation for Ms. K was addressed by the collaborative goal, "to feel less lonely." Thus, the specific outcome identified was to develop two new friends within 3 months. Her other problem of insomnia was addressed by the goal "to sleep better" and was measured by setting a specific date 1 month hence, by which she would be able to sleep 6 hours a night. Both goals were met and were clearly measurable, patient-centered, and easily quantified. Because APPNs are used to developing nursing care plans, identification of collaborative specific outcomes for psychotherapy is usually easily accomplished. An excellent adjunct to assist in developing specific goals, objectives, and interventions for psychotherapy treatment is *The Complete Psychotherapy Treatment Planner* (Jongsma, Peterson, & Bruce, 2014).

Integrating outcome measures into your clinical practice is prudent not only to determine whether collaborative goals are being met but also to meet the growing mandate for linking reimbursement to quality indicators. In addition, administering selected instruments at intake and throughout treatment allows the APPN to monitor the treatment process. Tracking the process of therapy can provide valuable information related to dynamics and determinants that help us to understand the process of therapeutic change. Which intervention is most effective for what problem for which population at which time in treatment? Not only does this assist with practice decisions for individual patients, but these data can also be disseminated to colleagues through reporting a single case or through a case series (a collection of cases with a similar problem or presentation). The case study has traditionally been the primary means of inquiry, teaching, and learning in psychotherapy.

DISCUSSION QUESTIONS

1. What tools do you believe would be appropriate outcome measures for psychodynamic, cognitive behavior, and interpersonal psychotherapy approaches? Review the instruments included in this book and identify specific tools reflecting indicators theoretically consistent for each model.

2. A patient says that he or she will be stopping psychotherapy after the current session. You do not believe this is in the person's best interests. Discuss how you would handle this.

3. Compare and contrast several practice guidelines available for a specific diagnosis. Identify any discrepancies. How would you go about choosing the best one for use for a patient you are seeing for outpatient psychotherapy?

4. You have a patient who has not paid you in several months but says that he or she will. Discuss how you would deal with this situation and how you would decide whether to terminate.

5. Review the ANA Code of Ethics. Do you believe that it adequately addresses issues related to the APPN conducting psychotherapy? If yes, state how it does so; if not, discuss how it does not and whether you feel it should.

6. Discuss the importance of outcome measurement for APPNs conducting psychotherapy.

7. Review the literature and identify three or four other specific outcome measures not listed in this chapter that you think would be good holistic indicators of improvement in psychotherapy. Provide the instrument's name, the concept measured, type of tool, why it would be an appropriate holistic measure, normative data (reliability and validity), and how to obtain it.

8. What psychotherapy approaches "fit" the best with how you like to work? How do you plan to continue to expand the ways you work with patients?

REFERENCES

Alden, L., Wiggins, J., & Pincus, A. (1990). Construction of circumplex scales for the inventory of interpersonal problems. *Journal of Personality Assessment, 55*, 521–536. doi:10.1080/00223891.1990.9674088

American Nurses Association. (2015). *Code of ethics for nurses*. Washington, DC: American Nurses Publishing. Retrieved from https://www.princetonhcs.org/-/media/princeton/documentrepository/documentrepository/nurses/code-of-ethics.pdf

American Psychiatric Association. (2010). *Practice guidelines for the treatment of psychiatric disorders* (3rd ed.). Arlington, VA: Author.

American Psychological Association. (2017). *Ethical principles of psychologists and code of conduct*. Retrieved from http://www.apa.org/ethics/code/index.aspx

Barrett, M. S., Chua, W.-J., Crits-Christoph, P., Gibbons, M. B., Casiano, D., & Thompson, D. (2008). Early withdrawal from mental health treatment: Implications for psychotherapy practice. *Psychotherapy, 45*(2), 247–267. doi:10.1037/0033-3204.45.2.247

Beck, A., Steer, R., & Garbin, M. (1988). Psychometric properties of the Beck Depression Inventory: Twenty-five years of evaluation. *Clinical Psychology Review, 8*(1), 77–100. doi:10.1016/0272-7358(88)90050-5

Bernstein, E., & Putnam, F. (1986). Development, reliability, & validity of a dissociation scale. *Journal of Nervous and Mental Disease, 174*, 727–735. doi:10.1097/00005053-198612000-00004

Binder, J. L. (2004). *Key competencies in brief dynamic psychotherapy*. New York, NY: Guilford Press.

Bobbitt, B. L., Cate, R. A., Beardsley, S. D., Azocar, F., & McCulloch, J. (2012). Quality improvement and outcomes in the future of professional psychology: Opportunities and challenges. *Professional Psychology: Research & Practice, 43*(6), 551–559. doi:10.1037/a0028899

Bovin, M. J., Marx, B. P., Weathers, F. W., Gallagher, M. W., Rodriguez, P., Schnurr, P. P., & Keane, T. M. (2016). Psychometric properties of the PTSD checklist for diagnostic and statistical manual of mental disorders–fifth edition (PCL-5) in veterans. *Psychological Assessment, 28*(11), 1379–1391. doi:10.1037/pas0000254

Cummings, N. (2001). Interruption, not termination: The model from focused, intermittent psychotherapy throughout the life cycle. *Journal of Psychotherapy in Independent Practice, 2*(3), 3–17. doi:10.1300/J288v02n03_02

Derogatis, L. R. (2004). SCL-90-R, Brief symptom inventory, and matching clinical rating scales. In M. E. Maruish (Ed.), *The use of psychological testing for treatment planning and outcomes assessment* (3rd ed., Vol. 3, pp. 1 -42). Mahwah, NJ: Erlbaum.

Dienes, K., Torres-Harding, S., Reinecke, M., Freeman, A., & Sauer, A. (2011). Cognitive therapy. In A. Gurman & S. Messer (Eds.), *Essential psychotherapies* (3rd ed., pp. 143–183). New York, NY: Guilford Press.

Flanagan, J. C. (1982). Measurement of quality of life: Current state of the art. *Archives of Physical Medicine and Rehabilitation, 63,* 56–59.

Frances, A. (2013). The new crisis of confidence in psychiatric diagnosis. *Annals of Internal Medicine, 159*(3), 221–222. doi:10.7326/0003-4819-159-3-201308060-00655

Gabbard, G. O. (2017). *Long-term psychodynamic psychotherapy: A basic text* (3rd ed.). Washington, DC: American Psychiatric Publishing.

Hagerty, B., & Patusky, K. (1995). Developing a measure of sense of belonging. *Nursing Research, 44*(1), 9–13. doi:10.1097/00006199-199501000-00003

Herth, K. (1992). Abbreviated instrument to measure hope: Development and psychometric evaluation. *Journal of Advanced Nursing, 17*(10), 1251–1259. doi:10.1111/j.1365-2648.1992 .tb01843.x

Horowitz, M. J. (2002). *Treatment of stress response syndromes.* Washington, DC: American Psychiatric Publishing.

Horowitz, M. J., Wilner, N. J., & Alvarez, W. (1979). Impact of events scale: A measure of subjective stress. *Psychosomatic Medicine, 41,* 209–218. doi:10.1097/00006842-197905000-00004

Insel, T. (2013). *Transforming diagnosis* [Blog post]. Retrieved from https://www.nimh.nih.gov/ about/directors/thomas-insel/blog/2013/transforming-diagnosis.shtml

Institute of Medicine. (2001). *Crossing the quality chasm: A new health system for the 21st century.* Washington, DC: National Academies Press.

Jongsma, A. E., Peterson, M., & Bruce, T. (Eds.). (2014). *The complete adult psychotherapy treatment planner* (5th ed.). Hoboken, NJ: Wiley.

Keane, T., Fairbank, J., Caddell, J., Zimering, R., Taylor, K., & Mora, C. (1989). Clinical evaluation of a measure to assess combat exposure. *Psychological Assessment, 1,* 53–55. doi:10.1037/1040-3590.1.1.53

Kellner, R. (1986). The Brief Depression Rating Scale. In N. Sartorius & T. Bain (Eds.), *Assessment of depression* (pp. 179–183). Berlin, Germany: Springer-Verlag. doi:10.1007/978-3-642-70486-4_17

Kluft, R. P. (1999). Current issues in dissociative identity disorder. *Journal of Pyschiatric Practice, 5,* 3–19. doi:10.1097/00131746-199901000-00001

Lambert, M. J. (2007). Presidential address: What we have learned from a decade of research aimed at improving psychotherapy outcome in routine care. *Psychotherapy Research, 17,* 1–14. doi:10.1080/10503300601032506

Larsen, D., Attkisson, C., Hargreaves, W., & Nguyen, T. (1979). Assessment of client/patient satisfaction: Development of a general scale. *Evaluation & Program Planning, 2,* 197–207. doi:10.1016/0149-7189(79)90094-6

Latov, N. (2005). Evidence-based guidelines: Not recommended. *Journal of American Physicians and Surgeons, 10*(1), 18–19.

Lorig, K., Stewart, A., Ritter, P., González, V., Laurent, D., & Lynch, J. (1996). *Outcome measures for health education and other health care interventions* (pp. 24–25). Thousand Oaks CA: Sage.

Mahler, M., Pine, F., & Bergman, A. (2000). *The psychological birth of the human infant symbiosis and individuation.* New York, NY: Basic Books.

Mariano, C. (2015). Holistic nursing: Scope and standards of practice. In B. Dossey, L. Keegan, C. Barrere, M. Blaszko Helming, D. Shields, & K. Avino (Eds.), *Holistic nursing: A handbook for practice* (7th ed., pp. 53–76). Burlington, MA: Jones& Bartlett.

National Research Council. (2011). *Report to Congress: National strategy for quality improvement in health care.* Retrieved from https://www.cms.gov/CCIIO/Resources/ Forms-Reports-and-Other-Resources/quality03212011a#es

Osheroff v. Chestnut Lodge (490 A2d 720, 722 Md App 1985). In R. Simon (Ed.), *Clinical psychiatry and the law.* Washington, DC: American Psychiatric Pub. 495.

Parry, G. (2000). Developing treatment choice guidelines in psychotherapy. *Journal of Mental Health, 9*(3), 273–281. doi:10.1080/jmh.9.3.273.281

Pear, R. (2009, February 15). U.S. to compare medical treatments. *The New York Times*. Retrieved from https://www.nytimes.com/2009/02/16/health/policy/16health.html

Quintar, B. (2001). Termination phase. *Journal of Psychotherapy in Independent Practice*, 2(3), 43–59. doi:10.1300/J288v02n03_04

Radloff, L. S. (1977). The CES-D scale: A self-report depression scale for research in the general population. *Applied Psychological Measurement 1*, 385–401. doi:10.1177/014662167700100306

Safran, J. D., & Muran, J. C. (2000). *Negotiating the therapeutic alliance*. New York, NY: Guilford Press.

Sanderson, W. (2002). *Why we need evidence-based psychotherapy practice guidelines*. Retrieved from http://www.medscape.com/viewarticle/445080

Shapiro, F. (2018). *Eye movement desensitization and reprocessing (EMDR)* (3rd ed.). New York, NY: Guilford Press.

Sinclair, V. G., & Wallston, K. (2004). The development and psychometric evaluation of the brief resilient coping scale. *Assessment*, 11(1), 94–101. doi:10.1177/1073191103258144

Spielberger, C. D. (1983). *State-Trait Anxiety Inventory for Adults™ manual*. Palo Alto, CA: Mind Garden.

Staats, S., & Partlo, C. (1992). A brief report on hope in peace & war, and in good times & in bad. *Social Indicators Research*, 24, 229–243. doi:10.1007/BF01077897

Stevenson, V. (2000). Premature treatment by angry patients with combat-related post-traumatic stress disorder. *Military Medicine*, 165(5), 422–424. doi:10.1093/milmed/165.5.422

Swift, J., Greenberg, R. P., Whipple, J. L., & Kominiak, N. (2012). Practice recommendations for reducing premature termination in therapy. *Professional Psychology: Research & Practice*, 43(4), 379–387. doi:10.1037/a0028291

Tilden, V., Nelson, C., & May, B. (1990). The IPR inventory: Development and psychometric characteristics. *Nursing Research*, 39(6), 337–343. doi:10.1097/00006199-199011000-00004

Trajkovic, G., Starcevic, V., Latas, M., Lestarevic, M., Ille, T., Bukumiric, Z., & Marinkovic, K. (2011). Reliability of the Hamilton rating scale for depression: A meta-analysis over a period of 49 years. *Psychiatry Research*, 189(1), 1–9.

Ware, J., Kosinski, M., & Keller, S. (1994). *SF-36 physical & mental health summary scales: A user's manual*. Boston, MA: Medical Outcomes Trust.

Wickline v. State of California (183 Cal App 3d 1175, 228 Cal Prtr 661; Cal Ct App 1986). In L. E. Lifson & R. I. Simon (Eds.), *The mental health practitioner and the law: A comprehensive handbook*. Cambridge, MA: Harvard University Press.

Wolitzky, D. (2011). Contemporary Freudian psychoanalytic psychotherapy. In A. Gurman & S. Messer (Eds.), *Essential psychotherapies* (3rd ed., pp. 33–71). New York, NY: Guilford Press.

World Health Organization. (2002). *WHOQOL-SRPB field-test instrument*. Retrieved from http://www.who.int/mental_health/media/en/622.pdf

Yesavage, J., Brink, T., Rose, T., Lum, O., Huang, V., Adey, M. & Leirer, V. (1983). Development and validation of a geriatric depression screening scale: A preliminary report. *Journal of Psychiatric Research*, 17, 37–49. doi:10.1016/0022-3956(82)90033-4

APPENDIX 24.1

Selected Instruments for Psychotherapy Outcome Measurement

The table that follows is a selected list of instruments that may be used in psychotherapy research. This is not a comprehensive list but does include many instruments that have been used in EMDR research. Sources of other instruments include journals and publishing houses, as well as the following publications:

American Psychiatric Association. (2000). *Handbook of psychiatric measures*. Washington DC: APA.

Antony, M., Orsillo, S., & Roemer, L. (Eds.). (2001). *Practitioner's guide to empirically based measures of anxiety*. New York, NY: Kluwer Academic/Plenum.

Conoley, J. D., & Impara, J. C. (Eds.).. (1995). *The twelfth mental measurements yearbook*. Lincoln: University of Nebraska Press.

Fischer, J., & Corcoran, K. (2007). *Measures for clinical practice & research* (Vol. 1 & 2). New York, NY: Oxford University Press.

Self-Management Resource Center. (2020). *Research and evaluation tools*. Retrieved from https://www.selfmanagementresource. com/resources/evaluation-tools/

Tool	Description	Reliability/Validity	Reference	Available
Beck Depression Inventory (BDI-II)	21-item self-report measure of depressive symptoms	Content, construct, and factorial validity; reliability 0.86–0.93	Beck, Steer, and Garbin (1988)	Purchase from: PearsonAssessments.com
Brief Depression Rating Scale (BDRS)	8-item therapist-rated observation measure of depressive symptoms	Concurrent validity 0.83; reliability 0.91–0.94	Kellner (1986)	Dr. Robert Kellner Department of Psychiatry University of Mexico 2400 Tucker, NE, NM 87131

(continued)

Tool	Description	Reliability/Validity	Reference	Available
Brief Resilience Coping Scale (BRCS)	4-item self-report scale on a 5-point Likert scale measuring perception of resilient coping	Construct and criterion validity; new tool with minimal reliability 0.7	Sinclair and Wallston (2004)	In public domain, but contact Vaughn Sinclair, PhD, Professor of Nursing Vanderbilt University vaughn.sinclair@vanderbilt.edu
Patient Satisfaction Questionnaire	18-item 4-point Likert scale to measure patient satisfaction with treatment	Good concurrent validity; reliability 0.86–0.94	Larsen, Attkisson, Hargreaves, and Nguyen (1979)	Dr. C. Attkisson, Professor of Medical Psychology Department of Psychiatry Box 33-C University of California, San Francisco San Francisco, CA 94143
Combat Exposure Scale	7-item measure of wartime stressors experienced by combatants	Good discriminate validity; reliability 0.85–0.97	Keane et al. (1989)	In public domain https://www.ptsd.va.gov/professional/assessment/documents/CES.pdf
Depression Scale (CES-D)	20-item Likert self-report scale screening test for depression	Validity construct based on DSM-IV; reliability 0.85 internal consistency	Radloff (1977)	In public domain

(continued)

Tool	Description	Reliability/Validity	Reference	Available
Dissociative Experiences Scale (DES)	28-item self-report to measure dissociation	Construct validity; reliability 0.79–0.86	Bernstein and Putnam (1986)	In public domain
Geriatric Depression Scale (GDS)	30 yes/no items self-report to rate depression in the elderly	Concurrent validity 0.83; reliability 0.94	Yesavage et al. (1983)	In public domain
Hamilton Rating Scale for Depression (HAM-D)	Clinician-rated 17-item checklist of depressive symptoms	Internal consistency, inter-relater reliability; test-retest reliability 0.65–0.98	Trajkovic et al. (2011)	In public domain
Visits to Providers	4 items asking numerical information about frequency of healthcare visits/use over the past 6 months	Test-retest reliability 0.76–0.97	Lorig et al. (1996)	In public domain
Health Survey Short Forms (SF-36 & SF-12)	2 self-report forms, one 36 items and the other 12 items, that measure perceived physical and mental health	Excellent concurrent, construct, and discriminate validity; reliability 0.76–0.93 with longer form higher	Ware, Kosinski, and Keller (1994)	Optum Optum.com

(continued)

Tool	Description	Reliability/Validity	Reference	Available
Hope Index	16-item self-report measure of hope	Construct and discriminative validity; reliability 0.78–0.85	Staats and Partlo (1992)	In public domain Dr. Staats staats1@osu.edu
Impact of Events Scale (IES)	15-item self-report Likert scale assessing current subjective distress related to a specific event	Good criterion, content, and construct validity; reliability 0.79–0.92	Horowitz, Wilner, and Alvarez (1979)	In public domain Daniel Weiss, PhD Department of Psychiatry University of California - San Francisco PO Box 0984-F San Francisco, CA 94143-0984 Phone: (415) 476-7557
Inventory of Interpersonal Problems (IIP)	32-item self-report Likert scale assessing interpersonal problems	Validity for longer version 127 items adequate; convergent validity with longer scale 0.90; reliability 0.88–0.89	Alden, Wiggins, and Pincus (1990)	Purchase from: Mind Garden https://www.mindgarden.com/113-inventory-of-interpersonal-problems
Interpersonal Relationship Inventory (IPRI)	30-item self-report 5-point Likert scale that asks respondents how they feel about personal relationships	Content and construct validity; reliability >0.80	Tilden et al. (1990)	Contact vtilden@unmc.edu

(continued)

Tool	Description	Reliability/Validity	Reference	Available
PTSD Checklist (PCL-5)	17-item self-report Likert scale assessing symptoms of PTSD. There is a civilian, military, and specific version with the latter focusing on a particular event	Convergent and concurrent validity; test-retest reliability 0.84	Bovin et al. (2016)	In public domain https://www.ptsd.va.gov/professional/assessment/adult-sr/ptsd-checklist.asp
Sense of Belonging Instrument	18-item self-report questionnaire with respondents rating sense of connection to others on a Likert scale	Content and construct validity; reliability test-retest 0.88	Hagerty and Patusky (1995)	Contact bmkh@umich.edu
Symptom Checklist-90-Revised (SLC-90-R)	90-item single-page self-report Likert screening tool designed to measure symptoms of psychopathology	Convergent validity 0.89 with MMPI; internal consistency reliability 0.89	Derogatis (2004)	Purchase from: PearsonAssessments.com
State-Trait Anxiety Inventory (STAI)	20-item self-report with a 4-point Likert scale; 2 forms with STAI-1 for state anxiety and STAI-2 for trait anxiety	Good convergent validity; reliability	Spielberger (1983)	Purchase from: Mind Garden https://www.mindgarden.com/145-state-trait-anxiety-inventory-for-adults

Afterword

This book is a how-to compendium of evidence-based approaches. The novice advanced practice psychiatric nurse (APPN) may feel a bit overwhelmed after reading this book and wonder where and how to begin to integrate these approaches into practice. Keep in mind that all the authors of the chapters in this book were also all beginners at one time. The contributing authors have generously shared their considerable clinical knowledge and expertise to provide a how-to for each respective approach and/or population for both novice and experienced APPNs. Expert clinicians continue seeking individual and group supervision, ongoing education, and further certification throughout their professional career. An ethical, compassionate practice requires no less.

The work of psychotherapy requires lifelong learning and ongoing education and supervision in order to practice competently and effectively. To ensure lifelong education, mandating a minimum of 25 contact hours of psychotherapy for the psychiatric mental health nurse practitioner (PMHNP) recertification in addition to the current requirement of 25 contact hours of pharmacotherapeutics is one possible cogent solution. This would highlight how essential psychotherapy is for APPN practice as well as encourage PMHNP graduate curricula to place greater emphasis on psychotherapy skills and content. In order for this to occur, our professional associations must endorse and propose such a mandate to the American Nurses Credentialing Center (ANCC). This speaks to the importance of joining our professional organizations that support psychiatric nursing, the American Psychiatric Nurses Association, the International Society of Psychiatric Nursing, and the National Organization of Nurse Practitioner Faculty. It is imperative and crucial for the growth, credibility, and viability of the psychotherapy role to our profession to raise a collective voice endorsing ongoing education.

It is curious that there seems to be concern by some nursing editors and authors that nurses do not have their own body of research demonstrating the effectiveness of psychotherapy. There is abundant research demonstrating the efficacy and cost-effectiveness of the psychotherapy approaches included in this book. The research is not discipline specific; that is, the focus is not on who is delivering the intervention but the particular intervention(s) and the specific problem/diagnosis that is treated. Nurse-delivered psychotherapy research is not essential to support the practice of nurses as psychotherapists any more than nurse-delivered pharmacotherapy research is necessary in order to prescribe. If a particular intervention or medication is effective, it will be effective if properly delivered no matter which discipline is delivering the treatment. Building our own evidence base for psychotherapeutic approaches that already have solid outcome data is redundant and reflects our own anxiety and insecurity about the APPN psychotherapy role. There are many other important nuanced questions to be asked about clinical issues, and interprofessional research needs to be conducted in collaboration with other mental health disciplines, which advances and furthers existing psychotherapy outcome data.

Students are often relieved to learn that the therapeutic alliance accounts for a significant percentage of the therapeutic outcome of psychotherapy. However, the therapeutic alliance is a prerequisite, not a substitute, for empirically supported interventions. Being a good listener, well-intended, and compassionate is not enough to disregard the scientific evidence when making practice decisions, nor is adherence to an evidence-based approach in a rigid, mechanistic manner without a strong therapeutic alliance. The power of the alliance in tandem with research-supported interventions for the particular patient problem illustrates Florence Nightingale's reflection on nursing, that is, putting patients in the best possible condition or environment for healing to occur. Embedding evidence-based interventions in the healing relationship requires clinical expertise and knowledge of the approach and interventions as well as knowledge of your patient's culture, preferences, and characteristics. Practicing without consideration of all these components will result in less potent outcomes.

It is likely that you will gravitate toward one type of approach and feel less comfortable with others, and consequently what you decide to focus on will relegate other dimensions or interventions to the background. If you know only one approach well, that is good news for those who are responsive and receptive to that type of therapy; however, it limits your ability to treat the variety of problems and patients who you will likely encounter in clinical practice. If you do not have the expertise in the approach that has the best evidence, it may be necessary to refer the patient to a colleague who can skillfully provide the evidence-based intervention. Commitment and hard work are necessary to learn new interventions and to integrate various approaches into practice. The ambiguity of psychotherapy can generate a great deal of anxiety and challenge even experienced APPNs. The available research, the relationship-based framework for practice, and the resources presented in this book serve as a compass to guide APPNs toward an ethical, compassionate, empirically based practice. Hopefully, this book is only the beginning of your journey toward expert psychotherapy practice.

Kate Wheeler

Index

acceptance and commitment therapy
   (ACT), 378
accurate empathic understanding, 297
ACE. *See* Adverse Childhood Experiences
acetylcholine, messenger molecule, 73
ACT. *See* acceptance and commitment therapy
"action plans," 798
actualizing tendency, 295
acute stress disorder (ASD), 644–645
adaptive information processing (AIP) model
  EMDR therapy processing, 339–343
  psychotherapy hierarchy framework, 27–28
trauma, 71–72
addicted to crisis, 663
addictions
  case study, 737–740
  cognitive behavioral coping skills and
    relapse prevention, 734
  contingency management, 733–734
  critical goals, 731
  culture, 723
  DSM-5 criteria, 716–717
  etiology, 718–719
  eye movement desensitization and
    reprocessing therapy, 735–736
  integrated family therapy, 734–735
  maintaining therapeutic frame, 731–732
  motivational interviewing (MI), 733
  neurobiology of reward system, 719–721
  older adults, 724–731
    co-occurring disorders, 724–725
    evidence-based psychotherapeutic
      interventions, 730–731
    screening and assessment, 727–730
    12-step peer support groups, 726–727
    trauma-informed care, 725–726
  person-centered care, 721–722
  prevalence, 712–716
  recovery, 718
  relapse, 717
  training and certification requirements,
    740–741
  treatment approaches, 721–722

women, 723–724
adherence, 582–584
adolescent depression, interpersonal
  psychotherapy, 430
adolescents, interpersonal psychotherapy
  with, 791
adult attachment, 125–128
Adverse Childhood Experiences (ACE), 24-27,
  182–183, 447, 571
affective development, 92
  assessment, 121–123
AGPA. *See* American Group Psychotherapy
  Association
Alcohol Use Disorders Identification Test
  (AUDIT), 179–180
alexithymia, 95–96
allostasis, 67
allostatic load, 67
altruism, 475
American Group Psychotherapy Association
  (AGPA), 470
American Nurses Credentialing Center
  (ANCC), 5, 542
American Psychiatric Association (APA), 268
American Psychoanalytic Association, 283
amino acids, 605
amygdala, 60–61
anterior cingulate, 63
anxiety, 17–19
  cognitive model, 380–381
  disorder, in older adults, 831–832
  systemic family therapy, 505
APPN SBAR, 585
arborization, 76
ASD. *See* acute stress disorder
Ashwagandha, 622
assertiveness training, behavioral technique,
  370
assessment
  affective development, 121–123
  belief systems, 129–131
  child psychotherapy, 757–759
  continuum of openness, 111

assessment (*cont.*)
    for dissociation, 654–657
    ego functioning, 116–121
    emotionally focused family therapy, 515
    emotion-focused therapy, 310
    existential psychotherapy, 307
    functional status, 131–134
    genogram, 134–136
    Gestalt psychotherapy, 300
    humanistic–existential psychotherapy, 319–320
    identity diffusion, 120
    interpersonal relationships, 123–128
    mental status examination, 113–114
    person-centered psychotherapy, 296
    present illness history, 110–113
    safety, 189–192
    sample case formulation, 141–143
    screening tools, 136–137
    solution-focused therapy, 314–315
    special populations, 136
    strategic family therapy, 511
    structural family therapy, 507–508
    systemic family therapy, 523
    timeframes, 114–116
    timeline, 658
    for trauma, 654
assessment forms
    Adverse Childhood Experiences Scale, 182–183
    Alcohol Use Disorders Identification Test, 179–180
    CAGE Questionnaire, 178
    case formulation, 159
    Child Attachment Interview Protocol, 181
    clinical assessment, 157–158
    Dissociative Experiences Scale, 160–163
    Generalized Anxiety Disorder Questionnaire, 174
    Geriatric Depression Scale, 168–170
    Hamilton Anxiety Rating Scale, 173
    Impact of Event Scale, 164–165
    Quality-of-Life Scale, 176–177
    SPRINT, 684
    Yale-Brown Obsessive–Compulsive Scale, 175
    Young Mania Rating Scale, 171–172
    Zung Self-Rating Depression Scale, 166–167
assessment phase interpersonal psychotherapy, 432–433
attachment patterns/schemas, 84
AUDIT. *See* Alcohol Use Disorders Identification Test
autobiographical memory, 78
autognosis, 217
automatic thought record, 368, 400

behavioral chain analysis worksheet, 695
behavioral rehearsal, 370–371
belief systems, assessment, 129–131
"betrayal trauma," 574
bibliotherapy, 371
biomedical/allopathic model, 12
biopsychosocial addiction assessment, 729–730
bipolar disorder
    interpersonal psychotherapy, 431–432
    in older adults, 831
body and energy work, 659–660
body awareness, 301
body-based psychotherapy approach, 446–447
"body-based" therapy, 446
borderline personality disorder (BPD), 96, 267, 428, 689, 690, 692, 695, 707
boundaries
    structural family therapy, 506
    therapeutic frame, 215–218, 219
BPD. *See* borderline personality disorder
brain development, 72–77
brain structures
    amygdala, 60–61
    anterior cingulate, 63
    cerebellum, 59
    cerebral cortex, 61–62
    corpus callosum and hemispheres, 63–65
    hippocampus, 59–60
    hypothalamus, 61
    insula, 63
    locus coeruleus, 59
    orbital medial prefrontal cortex, 62
    thalamus, 59
brief psychodynamic psychotherapy, 280–281
burnout, 11

CAGE Questionnaire, 178
Cannabidiol, 622
caring, 14
case formulation
    assessment, 141–143
    assessment forms, 159
    cognitive behavioral therapy, 385–386
    psychodynamic psychotherapy, 262, 272–274
case study
    case formulation and treatment plan, 385–386
    training and certification requirements, 389
    trauma-informed medication management, 589–592
catastrophic thinking, 367
catecholamines, 613
catechol-*O*-methyltransferase (COMT) enzyme, 613

catharsis, 477
CBT. *See* cognitive behavioral therapy
CCC. *See* counseling and coordination of care
Centers for Disease Control and Prevention
    (CDC), 615
cerebellum, 59
cerebral cortex, 61–62
certifications
    addiction nurse, 740–741
    child psychotherapy, 750–751
    cognitive behavioral therapy, 389
    EMDR, 350–351
    family therapy, 530
    group psychotherapy, 489–490
    humanistic–existential psychotherapy,
        322–323
    interpersonal psychotherapy, 435
    psychodynamic psychotherapy, 283–284
    trauma, 677
Certified Group Psychotherapist (CGP), 489
"change talk," 733
child attachment, 128
Child Attachment Interview (CAI) Protocol, 181
child psychotherapy
    assessment, 757–759
    assumptions and principles, 751–755
    case study, 764–768
    common elements approach, 762–763
    evidence-based interventions, 760–762
    evidence-based practice, 755–757
    family-centered care approach, 752
    formulation, 759
    general principles, 759–760
    historical background, 749–750
    principles of
        establishing therapeutic relationship,
            784–786
        initial psychiatric evaluation, 787–789
        involving family in psychotherapy,
            786–787
        setting, 782–783
    self-regulation, 752
    training and certification, 750–751
    treatment planning, 759
children, resources for working with,
    812–814
circle of strength, 359
circular causality, 510–511
classic stress response, 66
clinical assessment
    beginning of, 108
    ending of, 116
    sample form, 157–158
clinical procedural terminology (CPT) codes,
    869–870
    advantages of coding with E/M language,
        870–871

nurse psychotherapists, 871
    timeline and process, 870
clinical rating scales, 133
clonazepam, 672
coalition, 507, 523
cognitive behavioral coping skills, 734
cognitive behavioral therapy (CBT), 793–800
    applications to psychiatric disorders
        anxiety, 380–381
        depression, 378–380
        personality disorders, 381
        substance misuse, 381–383
        termination, 907–909
    behavioral techniques
        assertiveness training, 370
        behavioral rehearsal, 370–371
        bibliotherapy, 371
        contingency management, 371
        guided relaxation and meditation, 372
        homework assignment, 369
        psychoeducation, 369–370
        shame-attacking exercises, 372
        social skills training, 372
    case study, 800–802
        course of therapy, 386
        description, 384
        monitoring and feedback, 387–388
        process and outcome, 388–389
    cognitive techniques for stabilization,
        363–370
    description, 359–360
    evidence-based research, 361–362
    exposure therapy, 373–376
    guiding principles, 360–361
    modifications
        acceptance and commitment therapy, 378
        dialectical behavior therapy, 377–378
        schema therapy, 376–377
    in older adults, 840–844, 842–843
    Socratic dialogue, 363–369
    stabilization
        body and energy work, 659–660
        debriefing, 661
        group therapy, 661
        psychodynamic psychotherapy, 662
    stabilization strategies
        body and energy work, 659–660
        group therapy, 661
    training for, 814–815
cognitive dissonance theory, 401–402
cognitive distortion, 365
cognitive rehearsal, 368
cognitive restructuring, 368
cognitive techniques
    stabilization, 660–661
        advantages and disadvantages, 368
        automatic thought record, 368

cognitive techniques (*cont.*)
    cognitive rehearsal, 368
    cognitive restructuring, 368
    decatastrophizing, 367
    downward arrow, 365
    examining options and alternatives, 367
    idiosyncratic meaning, 365
    labeling of distortions, 365
    paradox/exaggeration, 368
    questioning the evidence, 365
    reattribution, 367
    thought stopping, 368
    turning adversity to advantage, 368
collaborative practice agreement, 542–543
common elements approach, 762–763
    to aggressive outbursts, 764–765
community reinforcement approach (CRA), 381
Community Resiliency Model (CRM), 442, 443
    completion of survival response, 459–460
    gesturing, 451–452
    grounding, 451
    Help Now! strategies, 452
    pendulation, 459
    resourcing and resource intensification, 451
    shift and stay, 452
    for stabilization, 453–457
    titration, 459
    tracking, 451
comorbidity, 578
    older adults, 836
complementary countertransference, 271
complementary identification, 217
complex posttraumatic syndrome, 650
complex reflection, 407
compliant videoconferencing, 197–198
compliments, solution-focused therapy, 316–317
conceptualization, humanistic–existential psychotherapy, 320
concordant identification, 217
conflict split, 311–312
confluence, 300
congruence, 297
Consensus Model, 542
contingency contract, 371
contingency management, 371, 733–734
contract, 237–238
co-occurring disorders, 724–725
coping questions, 316
core negative beliefs, 93
corpus callosum and hemispheres, 63–65
corrective recapitulation, 476
cortisol, messenger molecule, 73
counseling and coordination of care (CCC), 886–894
counter adaptation, 720
countertransference, 216

chronic, 218
complementary, 271
concordant, 217
older adults, 837–838
CPT codes. *See* clinical procedural terminology codes
CRA. *See* community reinforcement approach
creative experimentation, 301–304
cross-cutting assessments, 140
cross-generational coalition, 507
cultural relativity, 21
culture-bound syndromes, 571
cybernetics, 510
cyclical psychodynamics, 251

DBT. *See* dialectical behavior therapy
debriefing, 661
decatastrophizing, 367
declarative memory, 78
defectiveness, negative beliefs of, 93
defense mechanisms, 79–83, 83
deflection, 300
dementia, older adults, 833–834
depression
    cognitive model, 378–380
    interpersonal psychotherapy, 428–429
    in older adults, 828–830, 830–831
depressive symptomatology, 384
devaluing patient, 911
developmental theory, 780–782
developmental trauma disorder, 446
diagnosis, 138–141
Diagnostic and Statistical Manual of Mental Disorders, fifth edition (DSM-5), 13, 21, 643, 716–717
diagnostic assessment tools, 544
dialectical behavior therapy (DBT)
    assumptions, clients and treatment, 690–692
    behavioral chain analysis worksheet, 695
    case study, 702–706
    characteristics of DBT therapists, 691
    cognitive behavioral treatment, 377–378
    individual therapy, 697–699
    principles of practice, 692–694
    skills modules, 696
    skills training, 695–697
    stages of treatment, 694–695
    training, 706
DID. *See* dissociative identity disorder
differentiation of self, 501
dimensional assessments, 140
diseases and disorders of trauma, 651
disengaged family, 522–523
disorders of extreme stress, 650
displacement, 278

dissociation, 68
   assessment/outcome instruments, 654
   client-reported signs, 647
   observable signs, 647
   practice guidelines, 659
dissociative disorders, 646–650
Dissociative Experiences Scale (DES), 160–163
dissociative identity disorder (DID), 643
dopamine, messenger molecule, 73
dreams, 278–280
   condensation, 280
   displacement, 280
   secondary representation, 280
   secondary revision, 280
"drug-facilitated sexual assault," 583
drug selection, 545
dual awareness, 668
dyadic states of consciousness, 85
dysfunctional multigenerational patterns, 504

eating disorders, interpersonal psychotherapy,
   428
EFT. See emotion-focused therapy
ego alien, 271
ego dystonic, 271
ego functioning, 116–121
ego syntonic, 271
e-mails, therapeutic frame, 222–223
E/M codes. See evaluation and management
EMDR therapy. See eye movement
   desensitization and reprocessing
emotion, 91–95
   definition, 309
   instrumental, 310
   primary, 309
   primary adaptive, 309
   primary maladaptive, 309
   secondary, 310
emotional connection, 14
emotionally focused family therapy
   attachment, 513–514
   description, 513–514
   emotions, 513
   goals of, 515
   psychotherapeutic interventions
   assessment, 515
      empathic attunement, 516
      encouraging acceptance, 516
      evocative questions, 516
      images and metaphors, 516
      intimate attachments, 516
      reflective statements, 516
emotional regulation, 91–95, 444–445
emotional safety, 573
emotional-state-dependent memories, 78
emotion-focused therapy (EFT)

definition, 308
emotion schemes, 309
goals of, 310
memory, 309–310
psychotherapeutic interventions,
   assessment, 310
empathic attunement, 516
empathic resonance, 209
empathy, 209–212
empty-chair dialogues, 302–303
enactments, 508
encryption, 198–200
endocrine, messenger molecule, 73
endorphin, messenger molecule, 73
engagement, motivational interviewing
   skills, 407
enmeshed family, 507, 522
Erikson's psychosocial stages, 254, 781
essential vitamins, 605
evaluation and management (E/M) codes
   counseling and coordination of care (CCC),
      886–894
   5-digit, 874
   99212—established patient, 888
   99213—established patient, 889
   99214—established patient, 890–891
   99215—established patient, 891–892
   history, 877–880
   language associated with, 876
   medical decision making, 881–886
   psychiatric single-system exam, 880
evenly hovering attention, 272
evidence-based applications
   adolescent depression, 430
   bipolar disorder, 431–432
   eating disorders, 428
   interpersonal counseling (IPC), 432
   perinatal depression, 429–430
   postpartum depression, 429–430
evidence-based interventions, 760–762
evidence-based practice, 755–757
   child psychotherapy, 755–757
evidence-based research
   addictions, critical goals, 731
   cognitive behavioral therapy, 363
   EMDR therapy, 332
   group therapy, 479–482
   humanistic–existential psychotherapy,
      317–318
   interpersonal psychotherapy, depression,
      428–429
   motivational interviewing, 402–406
   in older adults
      cognitive behavioral therapy, 840–844
      interpersonal psychotherapy, 844–846
      mindfulness-based interventions, 846–847
      reminiscence and life review, 847–850

evidence-based research (*cont.*)
  psychodynamic psychotherapy, 257–261
  stabilization, 658–662
evocation, 401
  questions, 516
evoking, motivational interviewing skills,
    407, 409
exception questions, 315–316
existential factors, group therapy, 477
existentialism, 290
existential psychotherapy
  description, 304–305
  existential themes, 305
  goals of, 306–307
  psychotherapeutic interventions, 307–308
experiential reflection, 307–308
expert nursing practice, 765
  with emotional disorders, 766–767
  with pediatric bipolar disorder, 767–768
explicit memory, 78
exposure and response prevention (ERP),
    374–375
exposure therapy, 373–376
expressive psychotherapy, 268–271
eye movement desensitization, 735–736,
    802–810
eye movement desensitization and
    reprocessing (EMDR) therapy, 573
  case study, 810–812
  circle of strength, 359
  clinical applications, 335–336
  description, 331–332
  evidence-based research, 332
  lightstream exercise, 358
  mechanism of action, 332–337
  meta-analysis, 333–334
  processing
    AIP model, 339–343
    general guidelines, 342–343
    protocols for, 344–346
    therapeutic window, 341
    traumatic memories, 340
  process trauma, 346–350
  randomized clinical trials, 333–334
  stabilization, 337–339
  termination, 909
  training and certification requirements,
    350–351
  training for, 815

false memories, 94
family-centered care approach, 752
family therapy
  assumptions, 499
  case study, 497–498, 528–530
  emotionally focused approach

    attachment injuries, 514–515
    attachment styles, 514
    description, 513–514
    emotions, 513
    goals of, 515
    psychotherapeutic interventions, 515–516
  evidence-based research, 523–525
  evolution of, 499–500
  knowledge importance, 495–497
  practical guidelines
    beginning session, 518–519
    conceptualizing problem, 521
    conducting assessment, 519–521
    diagnosing problem, 522
    facilitating change, 522–523
    forming relationship, 518
  strategic approach
    circular causality, 510–511
    cybernetics, 510
    description, 525–527
    feedback loops, 510
    first-order changes, 511
    goals of, 511
    homeostasis, 510
    second-order changes, 511
  structural approach
    boundaries, 506
    coalition, 507
    disengaged family, 507
    enmeshed family, 507
    family structure, 506
    goals of, 507
    parentification, 507
    psychotherapeutic interventions, 507–508
    subsystems, 506
  systemic approach
    differentiation of self, 501
    emotional cutoff, 502
    family projection process, 502
    goals of, 503
    multigenerational transmission
      process, 502
    nuclear family emotional system, 502
    psychotherapeutic interventions, 503–504
    sibling position, 503
    triangles, 502
  training and certification requirements, 530
feedback loops, 510
feeling-state addiction protocol (FSAP), 736
feeling-state addiction therapy (FSAT), 736
feeling-state therapy (FST), 735
fees, 201–202, 221–222
finances, 577–578
flashbacks, 648, 669, 671
focusing, 302
  motivational interviewing skills, 407, 409
folate (vitamin B9), 605, 613–614

framework
for psychotherapy practice, 30–31
for treatment, 662–665
Fraser table technique, 34, 673–674
Freud's psychosexual stages, 252
frontal lobe, 61
FSAP. *See* feeling-state addiction protocol
FSAT. *See* feeling-state addiction therapy
FST. *See* feeling-state therapy
"functional" medicine, 602
functional status, assessment, 131–134
future-oriented questions, 316

gamma-aminobutyric acid (GABA), 73,
606, 619
Generalized Anxiety Disorder Questionnaire
(GAD-7), 174
genetic assays, ordering and interpreting, 614
"genetic code," 612
genetic testing, 608–613
case example of, 614–615
folate, 613–614
ordering and interpreting genetic
assays, 614
training in, 615
genogram, 134–136, 502
Geriatric Depression Scale (GDS) (Short
Form), 168–170
geropsychiatric nursing (GPN), 851–852
Gestalt psychotherapy
boundary disturbances (interruptions),
299–300
description, 298
figure and ground, 298–299
goals of, 300
layers of personality, 299
organismic self-regulation, 299
psychotherapeutic interventions
assessment, 300
creative experimentation, 301–304
I–Thou relationship, 301
Ginkgo biloba, 622
Global Assessment of Functioning (GAF), 132
glutamate, messenger molecule, 73
goals of treatment
assessment, 654–657
timeline construction, 658
GPN. *See* geropsychiatric nursing
group cohesiveness, 477
group psychotherapy
benefits of, 478–479
case study, 487–489
development of, 482–484
evidence-based research, 479–482
history, 469–471
stabilization, 661

theoretical approaches and focus, 472–474
therapeutic factors, 471, 475–477
training and certification requirements,
489–490
treatment and practice, 484–487
types of groups, 477–478
group therapy, 661

Hamilton Anxiety Rating Scale (HAM-A), 173
healing, holistic paradigm of, 12–14
hippocampus, 59–60
holding environment, 254
holistic model, 12–13, 918
holistic outcomes, 918–919
holistic paradigm of healing, 12–14
homeostasis, 510
homework assignments
behavioral technique, 369
solution-focused therapy, 317
humanistic–existential psychotherapy
beliefs about clients, 293–294
case study, 319–322
characteristics
belief in holism, 292
emphasis on themes, 292–293
experiential techniques, 293
focus, 292
phenomenological perspective, 291
prominence of process, 293
therapist–client relationship, 291–292
evidence-based research, 317–318
historical roots, 290
nursing and, 289–290
training and certification requirements,
322–323
humility, 569
hypothalamus, 61

identity diffusion, 120
imitative behavior, 476
immature defenses, 79, 80
immediacy, 214, 277
immune messenger molecules, 73
Impact of Event Scale (IES), 164–165
imparting information, 475
implicit memory, 78
individual therapy, 697–699
ineffective communication, 523
initial psychiatric evaluation, 787–789
insomnia, 672
instillation of hope, group psychotherapy, 475
"institutional trauma," 574
instrumental emotion, 310
insula, 63
integrated family therapy, addictions, 734–735

"integrative functional medicine," 602
integrative medicine, 601–603
   case study, 627–630
   complementary modalities in psychiatric
      nursing practice, 616–617, 618–626
   genetic testing, 608–613
     case example of, 614–615
     folate, 613–614
     ordering and interpreting genetic
       assays, 614
   gut, 603–604
   integrative psychiatric healthcare, 603
   laboratory testing in integrative psychiatry,
      607–608
   mind-body practices, 626–627
   nutrition, 604–607
   off-label drug use and cam, 616
   post-masters training in, 630–631
integrative psychiatric healthcare, 603
integrative psychiatry, laboratory testing in,
   607–608
interactive dialogue, 425
International Board for Certification of Group
   Psychotherapists (IBCG), 489
International Society of Study for Dissociative
   Disorders (ISSD), 191
interpersonal and social rhythm therapy,
   431–432
interpersonal counseling (IPC), 432
interpersonal learning, 476
interpersonal psychotherapy (IPT)
   with adolescents, 791
   case study, 432–435
   evidence-based applications
     adolescent depression, 430
     bipolar disorder, 431–432
     depression, 428–429
     eating disorders, 428
     interpersonal counseling (IPC), 432
     perinatal depression, 429–430
     postpartum depression, 429–430
   foundational concepts, 419–420
   goals and phases of, 426–427
   nursing theory, 420–421
   in older adults, 844–846
   principles and guidelines, 423–426
   role of therapist, 424
   strategies, 426–427
   termination, 909
   therapeutic alliance, 424–426
   training and certification requirements, 435
   underlying assumptions, 421–422
   vs. psychodynamic psychotherapy,
     422–423
interpersonal relationships, 123–125
   adult attachment, 125–128
   child attachment, 128

interpersonal styles, 126
interruptions, 299–300
intersubjectivity, 256
introjection, 299
invariant prescription, strategic family
   therapy, 512
Inventory of Psychosocial Functioning
   (IPF), 134
IPC. *See* interpersonal counseling
IPT. *See* interpersonal psychotherapy
I–Thou relationship, 301

joining questions, 315

Kava, 622
kindling, 68
Kohut, Heinz, 255

laboratory testing in integrative psychiatry,
   607–608
language of responsibility, 303–304
life review, in older adults, 847–850
lightstream exercise, 358
limbic resonance, 91
listening, therapeutic communication, 206–209
locus coeruleus, 59
long-term potentiation, 76
$_L$-Theanine, 619

Mahler's stages of separation–individuation,
   253
maladaptive schemas, 378
"malicious use of pharmaceuticals," 583
manualized approach, 761–762
manualized therapy, 19, 257
Maslow's hierarchy of needs, 20
mature defenses, 80, 81
medical decision making (MDM), 881–886
medication, 672–673
   safety, assessing for, 588
melatonin, 619
memory
   attachment, 83–86, 85
   consolidation, 309, 720
   defense mechanisms, 79–83
   motor, 78
   reconsolidation, 309, 720
mental health, and culture, 19–22
mental health assessment, 552
mental illness, 22–24
   adverse life experiences, 24–27
mental status examination, 113–114
messenger molecules, 73

meta-analysis
EMDR therapy, 333–334
motivational interviewing, 402
methylcobalamin, 605
MI. *See* motivational interviewing
middle phase, interpersonal psychotherapy, 433–434
mind-body practices, 626–627
mindfulness
definition, 274
meditation techniques, 448
psychotherapy, 9
in stabilization, 666–668
miracle questions, 315
mirror neurons, 85, 209
Model Act, 542
motivational interviewing (MI), 791–792
addictions, 733
case studies, 410–414
complex reflection, 407
evidence-based research, 402–406
guiding principles, 401–402
history, 402
meta-analysis, 402
modifications, 410
phases of change process
engagement, 407
evoking, 407, 409
focusing, 407
planning, 409
simple reflection, 407
training, 414
motor memories, 78
multigenerational transmission process, 502
multiple selves, 255

N-Acetylcysteine (NAC), *619*
narcissistic transference, 255
narrative, 264
National Council of State Boards of Nursing (NCSBN), 542
NE. *See* norepinephrine
negative reinforcers, 371
negative therapeutic reaction, 277
neural networks, restructuring, 86–90
neuroactive molecules, 626
neuroception, 69, 83, 185
neuroleptics, 545
neuropeptides, 92
neurophysiology
polyvagal theory, 69–71
responses to trauma, 65–69
trauma and psychotherapy
AIP theory, 71–72
brain development, 72–77
brain structures, 58–65

memory, 77–86
restructuring neural networks, 86–90
neuroplasticity, 75
neurotic defenses, 81
nocebo, 579–581
nondirective–facilitative counseling, 296–297
norepinephrine (NE), 73
Notice of Privacy Practices, 233–236
nuclear family emotional system, 502
nurse–patient relationship, 10
nurse psychotherapists
history, 8
holistic paradigm of healing, 12–14
learning stages, 6–7
psychiatry codes, 871
qualities of, 7–9
requisites for, 9–12
nursing
geropsychiatric, 851–852
humanistic–existential psychotherapy, 289–290
pediatric bipolar disorder, 759
theory, 420–421
nutraceuticals, 618–626
nutrigenomics, 613
nutrition, 604–607

object constancy, 271
observer-rated ego function assessment tool, 118–119
obsessive-compulsive symptoms, 578
occipital lobe, 62
"off-label use" (OLU), 616
older adults
assumptions and principles, 824–828
case study, 850–851
cohort issues and changes, 826
co-occurring disorders, 724–725
evidence-based psychotherapeutic interventions, 730–731
evidence-based research
cognitive behavioral therapy, 840–844
interpersonal psychotherapy, 844–846
mindfulness-based interventions, 846–847
reminiscence and life review, 847–850
functional status, 825–826
general guidelines
collaboration, 837
comorbidity, 836–837
complementary and alternative medicine therapies and older adults, 838–839
practical issues, 838
termination, 838
transference and countertransference, 837–838

older adults (*cont.*)
  in geropsychiatric nursing, 851–852
  late adulthood development, 824–825
  life context and care considerations, 828
  person-centered care, 721–722
  psychiatric disorders
    anxiety disorders, 831–832
    bipolar disorder, 831
    dementia, 833–834
    depression, 830–831
    gambling, 834–835
    posttraumatic stress disorder, 832
    schizophrenia, 832–833
    substance abuse and gambling, 834
    suicide risk, assessment, and
      intervention, 835
    treatment option, 841–842
  screening and assessment, 727–730
  social support and family issues, 826–827
  societal issues, 827–828
  12-step peer support groups, 726–727
  trauma-informed care, 725–726
Omega-3 fatty acids, 626
OMPFC. *See* orbital medial prefrontal cortex
orbital medial prefrontal cortex (OMPFC), 62
ordeals, strategic family therapy, 512
organismic self-regulation, 299
outcome evaluation, 917–919
overconsolidation of traumatic memories, 68
overdeterminism, 10
oxytocin, messenger molecule, 74

paradoxical interventions, 226–228
paradoxical technique, strategic family
    therapy, 512
parentification, 507
parent management training, 792
patient-identified problem, 108
pediatric bipolar disorder, 759
"peptide bonds," 612
perinatal depression, interpersonal
    psychotherapy, 429–430
personality disorders, cognitive model, 381
person-centered care, addictions, 721–722
person-centered psychotherapy
  actualizing tendency, 295
  belief of human nature, 295
  description, 294–295
  fully functioning person, 295
  goals of, 296
  psychotherapeutic interventions
    assessment, 296
    nondirective–facilitative counseling,
      296–297
    personality growth, 297
  self-concept, 295

physiological arousal, 669–671
Piaget's stages of cognitive development,
    781, 782
placebo, 579–581
"placebo talk," 542
planning, motivational interviewing skills,
    407, 409
plant-based medicines, 619–626
polyvagal theory (PVT), 15, 57, 69–71, 83, 644,
    659, 660, 662, 670
  unmyelinated dorsal vagal, 70
  myelinated ventral vagus, 70, 71
postmodernism, 313
posttraumatic stress disorder (PTSD), 571,
    645–646
practice guidelines, 659, 915–917
prefrontal cortex, 62
preliminary psychoeducation, 442
presence, existential psychotherapy, 307
pre-session change question, 315
pretend techniques, strategic family therapy,
    512
primary adaptive emotions, 309
primary emotion, 309
primary maladaptive emotion, 309
primary maternal preoccupation, 252
primitive defenses, 79
probiotics, 626
problematic reactions, emotion-focused
    therapy marker, 311
problem-solving skills training, 792–793
processing technique
  EMDR therapy
    AIP model, 339–343
    general guidelines, 342–343
    therapeutic window, 341
    traumatic memories, 340
  treatment hierarchy framework, 31–33
process note, 203, 239
process recording
  criteria for evaluation, 241–243
  directions, 241–242
  purpose, 241
progressive muscle relaxation, 686
progress note, 240
projection, 299–300
projective identification, 271
psychiatric database, comprehensive outlines,
    151–157
psychiatric disorders, 644, 649
  CBT applications
    anxiety, 380–381
    depression, 378–380
    personality disorders, 381
    substance misuse, 381–383
  older adults, 841–842
    anxiety disorders, 831–832

psychiatric disorders (*cont.*)
 bipolar disorder, 831
 dementia, 833–834
 depression, 830–831
 gambling, 834–835
 posttraumatic stress disorder, 832
 schizophrenia, 832–833
 substance abuse and gambling, 834
 suicide risk, assessment, and
  intervention, 189, 835
 practice guidelines, 260, 915–917, 921
psychiatric nursing practice, complementary
  modalities in, 616–617, 618–626
psychiatry codes
 add-on codes, 872–873
 CPT codes, 869–870
 eliminated, added, and did not change
  codes, 871–872
 revised, 873–874
 timelines and process, 870
psychic determinism, 275
psychoanalytic psychotherapy, 271–272
psychodynamic continuum, 261–264
 expressive psychotherapy, 268–271
 psychoanalytic psychotherapy, 271–272
 supportive psychotherapy, 265–268
psychodynamic psychotherapy, 790–791
 alliance ruptures repairing, 276–277
 assumptions, 250–251
 brief, 280–281
 brief psychodynamic psychotherapy,
  280–281
 and case formulation, 272–274
 Erikson's psychosocial stages, 254
 evidence-based research, 257–261
 expressive psychotherapy, 268–271
 Freud's psychosexual stages, 252
 Mahler's stages of separation–
  individuation, 253
 meta-analytic studies of, 258
 psychoanalytic psychotherapy, 271–272
 stabilization, 662
 supportive psychotherapy, 265–268
 termination, 908
 training and certification requirements,
  283–284
 vs. interpersonal psychotherapy, 422–423
 vs. relational psychodynamic therapy,
  255, 256
 working-through process, 274–276
 working with dreams, 278–280
psychoeducation, 674–676
 behavioral technique, 369–370
 group therapy, 477
 stabilization, 674–676
psychopharmacology, concepts and, 572–574
psychosomatic disorders, 651

psychotherapeutics
 application to practice, 550–552
 barriers to full scope of practice, 548–549
 case study, 552–555
 practice models, 542–543
 prescribing process, 543–547
 reuniting psychotherapy and
  pharmacotherapy, 547–548
 psychotherapy and medication, 90–91
psychotherapy approaches, 789
 cognitive behavioral therapy, 793–800
 eye movement desensitization and
  reprocessing, 802–810
 humanistic-existential and solution-focused,
  289–323
 interpersonal psychotherapy with
  adolescents, 791
 motivational interviewing, 791–792
 parent management training, 792
 problem-solving skills training, 792–793
 psychodynamic psychotherapy, 790–791
 trauma resilience model therapy, 441–464
psychotherapy practice, framework for, 27–30
PTSD. *See* posttraumatic stress disorder

QOL. *See* Quality-of-Life
Quality-of-Life Scale (QOL), 176–177

randomized controlled trials (RCTs), 257,
  258, 330, 402, 405, 431, 443, 579, 626,
  790, 849
rational emotive therapy (RET), 372
RCTs. *See* randomized controlled trials
reactance theory, 402
reattribution, 367
records, 203
 management, 203
reflection, empathic validation, 211
reflective statements, 516
relapse prevention, addictions, 734
relational psychodynamic therapy, 255, 256
relationship, 14–15, 185–190, 193, 197, 204, 206,
  209, 210, 212–221, 223–226, 228
reminiscence, 847–850
repairing alliance ruptures, 276–277
reprocessing therapy, 735–736, 802–810
resilience, 15–17, 89, 96, 129, 204, 442, 446, 450,
  451, 657, 659, 661, 678, 718, 754, 780,
  790, 815, 825
resistance, psychotherapeutic process, 223–228
resources, 670
restructuring neural networks, 86–90
RET. *See* rational emotive therapy
retroflection, 300
rituals, strategic family therapy, 512

S-Adenosylmethionine (SAMe), 619
safety
    assessment, in therapeutic alliance, 189–192
    therapeutic relationship, 664–665
    safety issues, 662–665
SAMe. *See* S-Adenosylmethionine
sample case formulation, 141–143
sample termination letter, 245
scaffolding, 458
scaling questions, 316
schema therapy, 376–377
schism coalition, 507
scope of practice, 542, 601, 631
screening tools, assessment, 136–137
SD. *See* socratic dialogue
secondary emotion, 310
secondary gain, 227
secondary revision, 278
second-generation antipsychotics (SGAs), 545
selective serotonin reuptake inhibitor
        (SSRI), 580
self-actualization, qualities of, 20
self-awareness, 10, 11
self-care, 11
self-care modality, 443
self-concept, 295
self-disclosure, 220–221
self-help groups, 478
self-interruptive split, 312
self-regulation, child psychotherapy, 752
semantic memory, 78
sensitization, 720
sequential acquisition, 75
serotonin, messenger molecule, 74
SFT. *See* solution-focused therapy
SGAs. *See* second-generation antipsychotics
shame-attacking exercises, 372
shared attunement, 85
Short PTSD Rating Interview (SPRINT), 684
simple reflection, 407
situational briefing model, 584–585
SJS. *See* Stevens-Johnson syndrome
skewed coalition, 507
skills modules, 696
skills training, 695–697
sleep hygiene, 672–673
social constructionism, 313
socializing techniques, group psychotherapy,
        476
social skills training, 372
socratic dialogue (SD), 363–369
solution-focused therapy (SFT)
    goals of, 314
    postmodernism, 313
    psychotherapeutic interventions
        assessment, 314–315
        compliments, 316–317

coping questions, 316
        exception questions, 315–316
        future-oriented questions, 316
        homework assignments, 317
        joining questions, 315
        miracle questions, 315
        pre-session change questions, 315
        scaling questions, 316
        subsequent sessions, 317
    social constructionism, 313
    solution talk, 314
somatic symptoms and related disorders,
        650–651
SSRI. *See* selective serotonin reuptake inhibitor
stabilization
    case study, 676–677
    cognitive behavioral strategies
        advantages and disadvantages, 368
        automatic thought record, 368
        body and energy work, 659–660
        cognitive rehearsal, 368
        cognitive restructuring, 368
        debriefing, 661
        decatastrophizing, 367
        downward arrow, 365
        EMDR therapy, 337–339
        evidence-based interventions, 658–662
        examining options and alternatives, 367
        group therapy, 661
        homework, 369
        idiosyncratic meaning, 365
        labeling of distortions, 365
        mindfulness, 666–668
        paradox/exaggeration, 368
        psychodynamic psychotherapy, 662
        psychoeducation, 369–370
        questioning the evidence, 365
        reattribution, 367
        thought stopping, 368
        turning adversity to advantage, 368
    stages of learning 6-7
state-dependent learning, 77, 273
12-step peer support groups, 726–727
Stevens-Johnson syndrome (SJS), 580
St. John's Wort, 622
strategic family therapy
    circular causality, 510–511
    cybernetics, 510
    description, 510
    feedback loops, 510
    first-order changes, 511
    goals of, 511
    homeostasis, 510
    psychotherapeutic interventions, 511–512
        invariant prescription, 512
        ordeals, 512
        paradoxical technique, 512

strategic family therapy (*cont.*)
  pretend techniques, 512
  rituals, 512
 second-order changes, 511
stress diathesis model, 23
stress response, 67
structural dissociation theory, 652–653
structural family therapy
  boundaries, 506
  coalition, 507
  disengaged family, 507
  enmeshed family, 507
  family structure, 506
  goals of, 507
  parentification, 507
  psychotherapeutic interventions
    assessment, 507–508
    enactments, 508
    problematic interactions, 509
    structural mapping, 508
  subsystems, 506
structural mapping, 508
substance misuse, cognitive model, 381–383
suicide plans, 588
support groups, group therapy, 477
supportive psychotherapy, 265–268
symbolic representation, 278
systemic family therapy
  differentiation of self, 501
  emotional cutoff, 502
  family projection process, 502
  goals of, 503
  multigenerational transmission process, 502
  nuclear family emotional system, 502
  psychotherapeutic interventions
    anxiety and interrupt conflict, 505
    assessment, 503–504
    detriangulate, 505
    dysfunctional multigenerational patterns, 504
    nuclear family emotional process, 505
    repair cutoffs, 505
    self-statements, 504
    sibling position, 503
    triangles, 502

telephone calls, therapeutic frame, 222–223
telepsychiatry, 196
temporal lobe, 61
termination
  case study, 920–924
  cognitive behavioral therapy, 907–909
  EMDR therapy, 909
  intermittent psychotherapy, 910
  interpersonal psychotherapy (IPT), 909
  older adults, 838

practice guidelines, 915–917
  psychodynamic, 907
  reasons for, 908
  sample letter, 245
  therapist initiation, 917
termination phase, interpersonal
    psychotherapy, 434–435
thalamus, 59
therapeutic alliance, 91, 92
  elements of, 186
  first contact, 192–203
    compliant videoconferencing, 197–198
    encryption, 198–200
    ending session, 202–203
    fees, 201–202
    goal establishment, 202–203
    practical arrangements, 195–200
    records management, 203
  interpersonal psychotherapy, 424–426
  ongoing process, 186–187
  relationship-building skills, 188
  safety assessment, 189–192
  strategies, 187
therapeutic communication
  attending, 206–209
  description, 203–206
  empathy, 209–212
  exploration, 212–215
  listening, 206–209
  techniques, 205
  treatment hierarchy and continuum, 205
    focusing, 214
    immediacy, 214
    interpretation, 214–215
    observation, 214
    reflection, 211
therapeutic frame
  addictions, 731–732
  boundaries, 215–218
  cancellations, 221–222
  countertransference, 216
  e-mails, 222–223
  fees, 221–222
  lateness, 221–222
  self-disclosure, 220–221
  telephone calls, 222–223
therapeutic relationship
  existential psychotherapy, 307
  safety issues, 664–665
therapeutic strategies, alliance repair, 226
therapeutic use of self, 217
therapist website resources, 383
thought stopping, 368
TIC. *See* trauma-informed care
training
  addictions, 740–741
  for CBT, 814–815

training (*cont.*)
  child psychotherapy, 750–751
  cognitive behavioral therapy, 389
  dialectical behavior therapy (DBT), 706
  EMDR, 350–351
  for EMDR, 815
  family therapy, 530
  in genetic testing, 615
  group psychotherapy, 489–490
  humanistic–existential psychotherapy, 322–323
  integrative medicine, 630–631
  interpersonal psychotherapy, 435
  motivational interviewing, 414
  psychodynamic psychotherapy, 283–284
  trauma, 677
transference, 579–581
  cure, 276
  definition, 206
  narcissistic, 255
  neurosis, 272
  older adults, 837–838
trauma
  brain development, 72–77
  brain structures
    amygdala, 60–61
    anterior cingulate, 63
    cerebellum, 59
    cerebral cortex, 61–62
    corpus callosum and hemispheres, 63–65
    hippocampus, 59–60
    hypothalamus, 61
    insula, 63
    locus coeruleus, 59
    orbital medial prefrontal cortex, 62
    thalamus, 59
  dialectical behavior therapy (DBT)
    assumptions, clients and treatment, 690–692
    behavioral chain analysis worksheet, 695
    case study, 702–706
    individual therapy, 697–699
    principles of practice, 692–694
    skills modules, 696
    skills training, 695–697
    stages of treatment, 694–695
    training, 706
  focused therapy
    conducting exposure, 701–702
    preparing for exposure, 700–701
    emotions, 91–95
  traumatic stress responses
    acute stress disorder, 644–645
    disorders of extreme stress, 650
    dissociative disorders, 646–650
    posttraumatic stress disorder, 645–646
    practice guidelines, 659
    psychosomatic disorders, 651

somatic symptoms and related disorders, 650–651
  spectrum of, 644
trauma-informed care (TIC), 569, 570, 725–726
trauma-informed medication management, 569–571
  adherence, 582–584
  application of, 584–585
  APPN SBAR, 585
  assessing for medication safety, suicide plans, 588
  case study, 589–592
  clarifying communication, 587
  collaboration and mutuality, 588
  concepts and psychopharmacology
    power and control, 574
    safety and stabilization, 572–574
  deprescribing, 581–582
  discussing side effects, 586
  educational opportunities, 593
  empowerment, voice, and choice, 588–589
  identity, stigma and self-stigma, 575–576
  medication, 579–581
  reorienting to goals of treatment, 587
  starting new medications, 586
  symptoms and wellness, 576–578
  treatment-interfering behavior, 587–588
trauma narrative, 312
trauma resiliency model (TRM), 441
  case study, 453–457, 460–463
  evidence base, 443
  origins of, 442–443
  skills, 448–452
  training for CRM and, 463
  trauma processing in, 457–460
  underlying assumptions of, 443–448
trauma response, 678
traumatic experiences, 569
traumatic memories, 64
traumatic transference, 665
treatment-interfering behavior, 587–588
treatment planning, 759
triangulation, 523
TRM. *See* trauma resiliency model
two-person psychology, 256

unclear felt sense, 311
unconditional positive regard, 297
undifferentiated ego mass, 501
unfinished business, emotion-focused therapy marker, 312
universality, 475

valerian root, 622
vasopressin, messenger molecule, 74

vicarious or secondary traumatization, 11
vulnerability, 312

window of arousal, 70, 71
window of tolerance, 669
working-through process, 274–276

Yale-Brown Obsessive–Compulsive Scale
    (Y-BOCS), 175
Young Mania Rating Scale (YMRS), 171–172

Zung Self-Rating Depression Scale (ZSRDS),
    166–167